HEINEMANN GNVQ

ADVANCED

HEALTH AND SOCIAL CARE

SECOND EDITION

GENERAL EDITOR: NEIL MOONIE

RICHARD CHALONER
KIP CHAN PENSLEY
MARGARET HILTON
KAREN HUCKER
KATE MAKEPEACE
JILL PATEL
BERYL STRETCH
including contributions from
MARTIN SADLER

Heinemann

Heinemann Educational Publishers,
Halley Court, Jordan Hill, Oxford OX2 8EJ
a division of Reed Educational & Professional Publishing Ltd

MELBOURNE AUCKLAND FLORENCE
PRAGUE MADRID ATHENS SINGAPORE
TOKYO SAO PAULO CHICAGO PORTSMOUTH (NH)
MEXICO IBADAN GABORONE JOHANNESBURG
KAMPALA NAIROBI

First published 1996
99 98 97
10 9 8 7 6 5

A catalogue record for this book is available from the
British Library on request

ISBN 0 435 45253 3

Typeset by TechType, Abingdon
Printed in Great Britain by The Bath Press

Front cover
Designed by: Tad Kasa
Photograph by Format Partners

Contents

Preface to the second edition v

Acknowledgements vi

Introduction to GNVQ 1

Equal opportunities and individuals' rights
1 Legal rights and responsibilities in relation to equality of opportunity 26
2 How individuals can be affected by discrimination 42
3 Ethical issues in health and social care practice 54
Self-assessment test 69
Fast Facts 73

Interpersonal interaction in health and social care
4 Interpersonal interaction 76
5 Skills of interpersonal interaction 102
6 Analysing methods of interacting with clients in health and social care 119
Self-assessment test 140
Fast Facts 141

Physical aspects of health and social well-being
7 The organisation of structures within human body systems 146
8 The functions of the main organ systems 160
9 Methods for monitoring and maintaining the healthy functioning of the human body 183
Self-assessment test 192
Fast Facts 197

Health and social well-being: psycho-social aspects
10 Human growth and development 201
11 How individuals function in and are influenced by society 249
12 The effect of socio-economic factors on health and social well-being 265
Self-assessment test 291
Fast Facts 297

The structure and development of health and social care services
13 The provision of health and social care services and facilities 305
14 The development of health and social care provision 319
15 The organisation of health and social care planning and provision 336
Self-assessment test 349
Fast Facts 355

Health and social care practice
16 The planning of care and interventions for individual clients 358
17 Methods for promoting and protecting health and social well-being 385
18 Clients' perception of health and social care services 405
Self-assessment test
Fast Facts

Educating for health and social well-being
19 Health education campaigns 428
20 The reasons for, sources of, and methods used, in health education campaigns 455
21 Evaluating the effectiveness of a health education campaign 461
Self-assessment test 466
Fast Facts 471

Research perspectives in health and social care
22 The research process 474
23 Planning research and gathering data 491
24 Producing and presenting research findings 518
Self-assessment test 528
Fast Facts 533

Core skills
25 Communication 536
Fast Facts 576
26 Application of number 578
Fast Facts 601
27 Information technology 603
Fast Facts 628

Self-assessment test answers 630

Icons for photocopying 636

Index 638

Preface to the second edition

This book has been compiled to support students who are working to the 1995 national standards for Advanced GNVQ in Health and Social Care.

The book is very different from the first edition. Chapters are now organised in terms of elements, rather than by units and the volume of material covered is more extensive than in the first edition.

The second edition aims to help students to gain Merit or Distinction grades by providing:

- An introduction to GNVQs including:
  - levels of awards
  - GNVQ standards and structure
  - grading criteria
  - portfolios
  - tests
- The knowledge, skills and values associated with each of the eight mandatory units:
  Unit 1 Equal opportunities and individuals' rights
  Unit 2 Interpersonal interaction in health and social care
  Unit 3 Physical aspects of health and social well-being
  Unit 4 Psycho-social aspects of health and social well-being
  Unit 5 Structure and development of health and social care services
  Unit 6 Health and social care practice
  Unit 7 Educating for health and social well-being
  Unit 8 Research perspectives in health and social care
- The knowledge and skill associated with the core skills of Communication, Application of Number and Information Technology at level 3. Additional core skills are briefly integrated with theory in Chapters 5 and 6
- Sufficient depth of coverage to support students' development of grading criteria skills – particularly with reference to evaluation, synthesis and command of language.

Special features of the book

- Icons are used to link theory with practice. Icons are provided to suggest areas for:

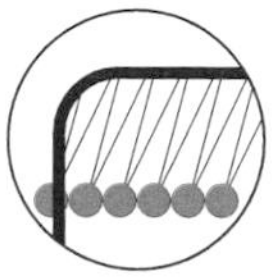
Reflection (*Think it over*)

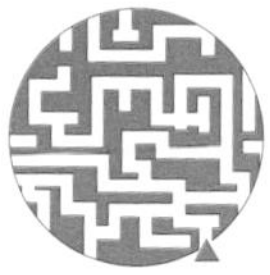
Practical experience (*Try it*)

Meeting evidence requirements (*Evidence collection point*)

Icons are also suggested as a way of labelling work.

- Multiple-choice questions will help preparation for tests and check personal understanding
- Fast Facts will also help preparation for tests and provide a quick reference section for key concepts
- Case studies show how theory links to practice
- Diagrams, drawings and cartoons are used to make sections easier to refer to and remember.

How to use this book

This book is designed to be used as a source of knowledge and ideas. It can be read from beginning to end, but it is also designed so that you can go directly to a section on a particular element. Fast Facts are listed alphabetically at the end of each unit so that concepts can be checked quickly. You may wish to use the book in a very different order from the way it is set out.

In particular, you may want to study the core skills chapters on Communication and interviewing, Application of Number and Information Technology before studying all the mandatory units.

Core skills interlink with the mandatory units, and evidence for them should be gathered with evidence for the units. You will probably wish to dip in and out of these chapters as you study each of the units.

Each reader will have his or her own needs and purposes for this book. For this reason it has been designed with easy reference headings and icons, so that it can be used flexibly - in keeping with the ideas behind GNVQs.

Acknowledgements

The authors and publishers would like to thank the following individuals and organisations for permission to reproduce tables, photographs and other material.

The Controller of HMSO – Crown copyright material reproduced with permission
CameraPress
The Confederation for the Registration of Gas Installers
The Coronary Prevention Group
Family Planning Association
Format Partners
Health Education Authority
The Hulton-Deutsch Collection
Kraft General Foods Ltd
Milk Marketing Board
Oxford University Press
The Portman Group
Quit, The National Society for Non-Smokers
Routledge Publishers
School for Advanced Urban Studies, University of Bristol
Science Photo Library
Science and Community Planning Research
John Walmsley
The Winged Fellowship Trust

Introduction to GNVQ

This section covers:

- What are GNVQs?
- Levels and pathways to qualifications
- What does a GNVQ Health and Social Care qualification lead to?
- The structure of Advanced GNVQ in Health and Social Care
- GNVQ standards – an explanation
- GNVQ assessment
- Meeting evidence indicators – things that count as evidence
- Collecting evidence
- Reflection
- Using concepts and theory
- Assignments
- The grading criteria
- Ideas for evidence for the grading criteria
- The portfolio
- Tests
- Self-assessment of knowledge about GNVQs
- The Health and Social Care Advanced GNVQ Game
- Answers to self-assessment quiz
- Fast Facts

What are GNVQs?

GNVQs are a new system of qualifications designed to fit into a national pattern of 'levels'. GNVQs are also designed to allow students to have some choice in the work that they do. This introduction explains how the national system works and how *you* can manage your own learning while working on a GNVQ programme. GNVQs are not intended to be simple, but this section will help you to manage your own study of GNVQ at an Advanced Level in Caring.

This introduction contains both *theory* and *advice*. Before starting, it may be worth checking what you need to know. Use the list above as a guide to what is on offer. If you know very little about GNVQs then start at the beginning.

Getting a GNVQ qualification may be a bit like learning to drive a car or ride a bicycle. It takes time and, most importantly, it takes *practice*. What is said here will make more sense when you are actually working to get the GNVQ award. Like learning to drive, there is a limit to how much *theory* you might want to learn in one go. It may be best just to read parts of this section as you need them.

When you have finished the introduction you might like to test your understanding with the questions at the end. Another idea is that you look at the questions to begin with and decide whether you need to know about these things. If you just need to understand a technical word, look up Fast Facts.

You are in charge of your own learning, so please see this section as something to explore. Different people might want to use this introduction in different ways and at different stages in their GNVQ programme.

A note on change and development in GNVQs

Learners develop their skills by constantly building on their experience. Good learners are open to change – they drop things that don't work well in practice, and fine-tune behaviours that do seem to work, in order to get the best outcomes.

GNVQs are still new. The detail of how to achieve a GNVQ will almost certainly continue to build on experience and develop over the next few years. The advice and guidance in this introduction is based on the GNVQ system as it was in the early summer of 1995. Fine detail on issues like grading, revising for test questions and portfolio design may continue to develop. You are therefore recommended to check whether new details or new regulations have come about. It is worth checking the latest information with a tutor or teacher if you are enrolled on a GNVQ programme.

GNVQs involve exploring ideas and developing skills in using information and knowledge. You should use your skills to check that the information has not become dated!

The meaning of GNVQ

GNVQ stands for General National Vocational Qualification:

- **General** means that the qualification is not just for a particular job. General qualifications are broad; they are designed to enable people to move on to higher qualifications or to get jobs in a wide range of employment.
- **National** means that the qualification is valuable nationally. The qualification has the same value everywhere in the 'nation'.
- **Vocational** means that the qualification focuses on areas of employment. A vocational qualification in Health and Social Care provides the knowledge and understanding that a person needs to go on to work in many different caring jobs. People with an Advanced GNVQ may go on to take up careers in caring or progress to degree level study.
- **Qualification** means that an individual has passed at a definite standard. Advanced GNVQs are also known as Vocational A-levels. They are A-level qualifications. So 12 units (eight mandatory and four optionals) of GNVQ are 'worth' two academic A-levels; 18 units (eight mandatory, four optional and six additional units) of GNVQ are 'worth' three academic A-levels.

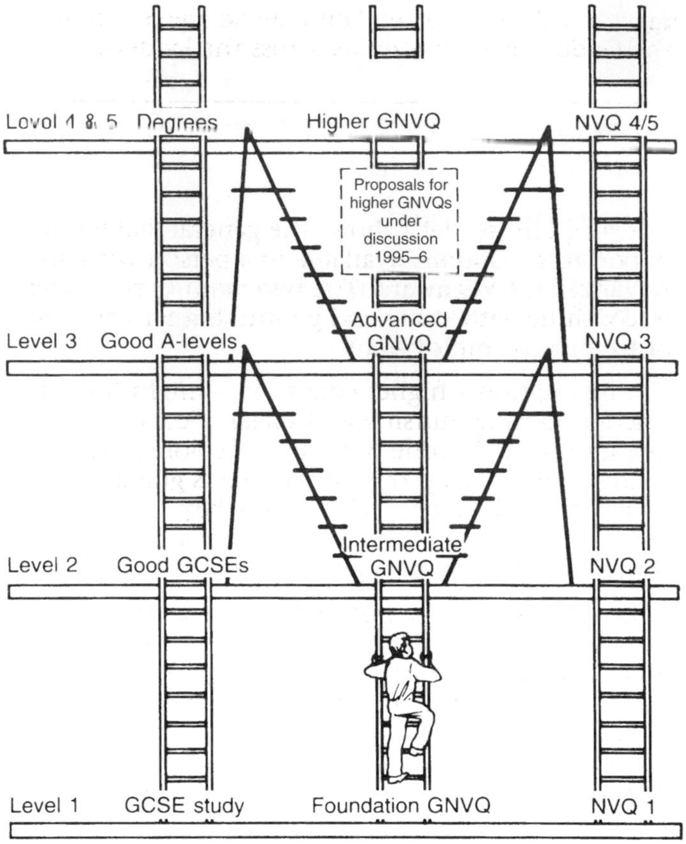

Figure 1 How the ladders work

Levels and pathways to qualifications

There is now a national system of qualifications at five levels, as shown in Figure 1. *Level 1* is the starting point for foundation qualifications. *Level 2* (Intermediate) covers jobs that are more complex, and academically it is worth GCSE at good grades. *Level 3* covers jobs that involve high responsibility and complexity, perhaps including supervising others. This level is designed to provide vocational A-levels. *Levels 4* and *5* cover professional and management jobs and are designed to be degree and post-graduate equivalents.

As well as the five levels, there are three *pathways* to qualifications. The first pathway – the 'academic' one – has been around for many years and has worked well for some people. But in 1986 the government decided to set up the National Council for Vocational Qualifications (NCVQ) so that there would be new ways to obtain qualifications. To begin with, the NCVQ designed qualifications called National Vocational Qualifications (NVQs).

NVQs are designed to provide qualifications for particular jobs or professions. Sometimes NVQs can be studied at college, but many of these qualifications are easier for people to get if they already have a job. For many individuals, NVQs opened up the possibility of getting a recognised qualification for the skills and 'know-how' they had already learned at work. NVQs meant that people could become qualified at work without necessarily having to start at the beginning with their studies again.

The third pathway or ladder is a GNVQ. GNVQs first began in 1992 and their original purpose was to provide a 'middle way' between academic and work-based qualifications.

GNVQs are based on standards in a similar way to NVQs. GNVQs cover a much broader range of knowledge and understanding than NVQs.

There is increasing interest in new types of qualification that will allow students to combine units of GNVQ with units of other qualifications. In the future, the three ladders may become merged. It may even be possible for you to take a mixture of GNVQ units and A-levels, or BTEC, or Open College units at Advanced level. You may be able to climb the ladders using footholds across the ladders.

What does a GNVQ Health and Social Care qualification lead to?

The diagram (see left) shows the general 'ladder of opportunity' options available to a person with an Advanced GNVQ award. The two main options are: to continue with study and go into higher education; or to go into employment.

The first option – higher education – might include teacher training, nursing and social science qualifications. Anyone wishing to explore these routes should seek professional careers guidance, which might include advice on the best combinations of additional units or academic A-level combinations with GNVQ.

Candidates going straight into employment might subsequently be offered the chance to collect an NVQ at Level 3. An Advanced GNVQ qualification will provide much of the 'knowledge base' requirements for NVQ at Level 3. GNVQs may also provide much of the 'know-how' when it comes to coping with NVQ assessment arrangements.

Many people may undertake an Advanced GNVQ out of personal interest. Some people may take GNVQ while they are in employment. Like other academic or vocational A-levels, Advanced GNVQ Health and Social Care should open up a wide range of learning and career opportunities.

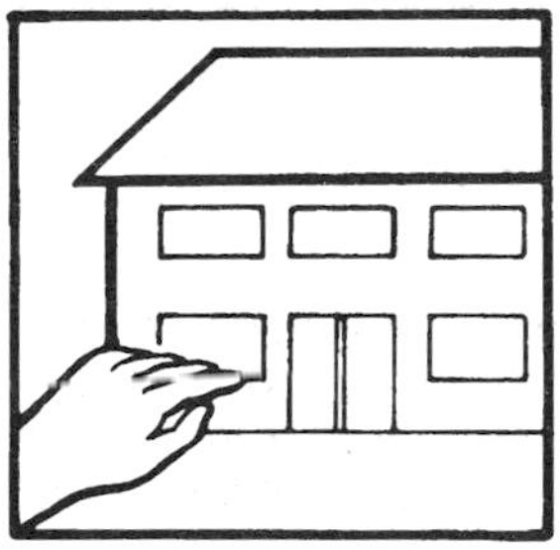

Mandatory Units

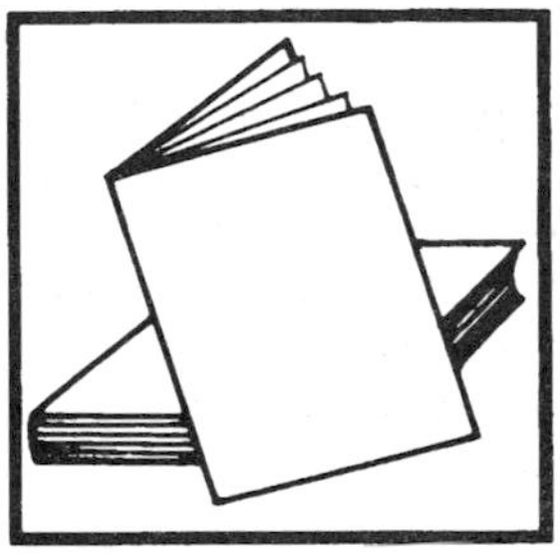

Optional Units

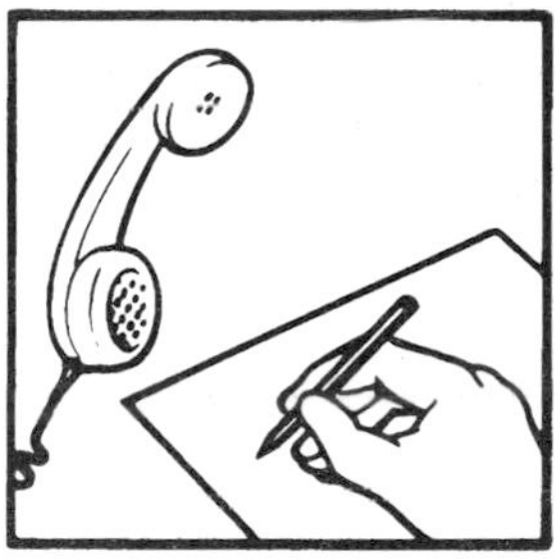

Core Skills Units

The structure of Advanced GNVQ in Health and Social Care

All GNVQs are made up of **units.** Each unit can be 'passed' and then awarded to the person who has achieved it. So GNVQs can be 'passed' bit by bit, unit by unit. If a person doesn't complete a GNVQ programme, they still keep the units they have passed. This means that they could start again without having to go right back to the beginning.

Advanced GNVQs can be taken as a two A-level programme or as a three A-level programme. The standard two A-level programme consists of eight mandatory units, four optional units and three core skills units. The three core skill units may be integrated into the evidence collection work for the other 12 units. Because of this, the standard programme is often referred to as a 12 vocational unit route. This standard GNVQ programme can be linked with the study of academic A-levels. The standard programme can also be extended to include an extra six additional units. This programme is worth three A-levels, and is sometimes referred to as an 18 vocational unit route.

The mandatory units provide a study area which covers a range of knowledge, skills and values central to health and social care work. Most mandatory units are tested. Unit 2 (Interpersonal Interaction) is not expected to be tested.

Core skills units are different from mandatory units or optional units. This is because they are meant to be studied *with* the other units. The evidence needed to 'pass' core skills is meant to be collected with the evidence to pass the mandatory and optional units.

The idea of core skills is that communication, number and information technology skills are needed in *all* work situations. GNVQs will probably cover many areas of work in the future. Core skills *standards* will be the same across all the areas, but the *evidence presented* will be different because it will be linked to practical assignment work for each qualification. In Health and Social Care, evidence opportunities for core skills like information technology will link with assignment work in Caring.

Only core skill units in communication, number and information technology have to be assessed and awarded for the award of a GNVQ qualification. However, there are three other areas of core skills: problem-solving, working with others and improving own learning and performance. These core skills are worth including in a portfolio of evidence because they help towards the achievement of Merit and Distinction grades.

GNVQ standards – an explanation

To collect GNVQ units and qualifications, candidates have to demonstrate that they have achieved a defined **standard of work.** GNVQ standards are definitions of what is required in order to 'pass' and be awarded the qualification. Because standards are definitions, they are not always easy to understand. This part explains the technical criteria, range statements and evidence indicators.

The whole set of standards for a qualification runs to many pages. Most people who sit down and read standards will say that they are boring. Many people will say they cannot really understand them!

Why are standards so complicated?

Standards are difficult for three reasons:

1 *Standards are a system for defining outcomes.*

Because standards define things to be understood or done, they become a bit like legal statements. Standards try to give exact details of what is required rather than discuss ideas about what would be useful. Standards end up being technical rather than interesting simply because they are definitions. Definitions are necessary because they have to be applied in the same way across the country. Standards are a guide to assessment; they explain what has to be done in order to pass the GNVQ. Standards don't really explain what has to be studied; rather, they define what has to be achieved in order to get the qualification. So standards are like goal-posts in football – they define the goal that has to be reached. Standards do not explain how to get there!

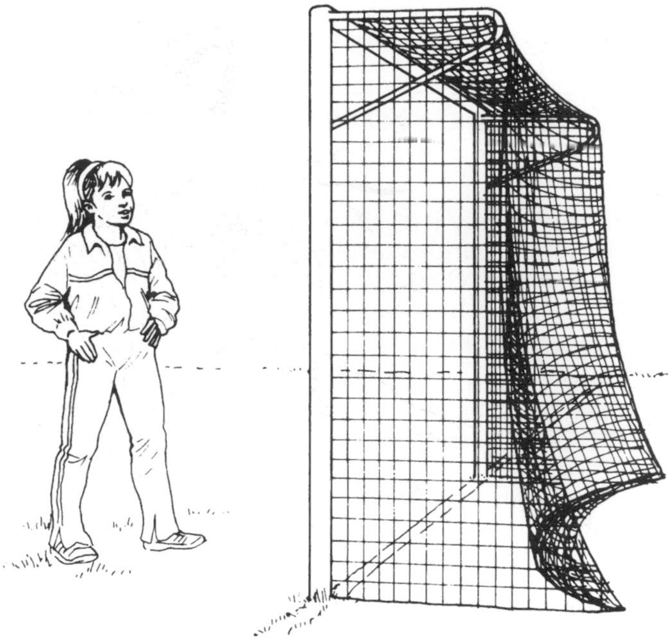

Figure 2 It is boring just standing looking at the goal … it is much more fun if you are doing something with it!

2 *The value of a qualification will depend on the definition of standards.*

There are two kinds of qualifications. One kind is based on what people can do or understand, and the other kind is based on who comes first in a competition. Many qualifications have exams, which are like a competition or a race. The people who run the fastest get to the end first – these people pass. In a running race, the people who come in last are not so good; in the exam, the people with the lowest marks fail. Not all exams are marked in terms of top and bottom, but they all have some degree of competition about them. Standards allow a different way of qualifying – instead of doing better than others in an exam, the candidate has to show what he or she can do or prove that he or she knows the details needed for the qualification.

Exams give people qualifications because they have come in the top group. Standards give people qualifications because those individuals have proved they can do what is needed. The problem with standards qualifications is that the qualification is only as good as the standards. If standards are not well defined, or if they don't cover much, then the qualification is not worth a lot. Standards need to define complicated details carefully if the qualification is going to be worthwhile in the end.

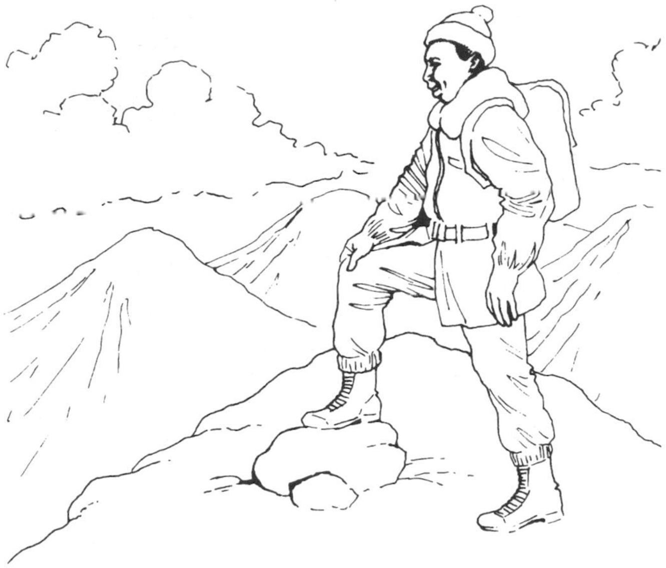

Figure 3 Climbing to the top is like achieving a standard – you can do it in your own way at your own pace. Running a race is different – you have to beat the others!

3 *Standards are impossible to understand without the knowledge of the area they are about.*

Because standards define areas of skill, values and knowledge, they are impossible to understand without the necessary knowledge. At the beginning of a course of study, the standards will be difficult because people will not know all the terms and detail involved. As a person learns about the issues, so the standards should become easier to understand. When a candidate's work is ready for assessment, the standards should be clear.

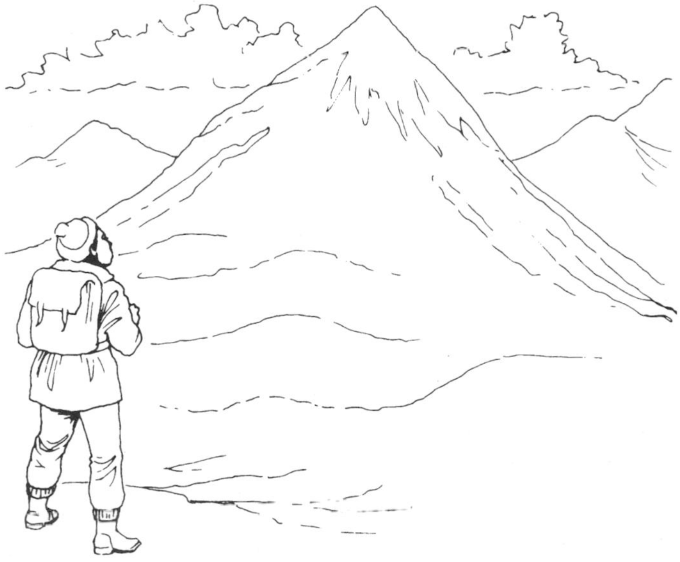

Figure 4 It looks a long way up from the bottom!

The way standards are written

Standards are written for guiding the assessment of GNVQs. They start with units.

- **Units.** GNVQ qualifications are split into units. Units cover particular areas of knowledge, values and skill. For example, Unit 2 covers knowledge, values and skills needed to engage in caring work – interpersonal interaction with other people. A person who achieves Unit 2 will have demonstrated that he or she has the skills and knowledge and can work within the values defined in the standards for that unit. Unit 2 isn't a whole qualification, but it is the first part of an Advanced GNVQ in Health and Social Care.
- **Elements.** Each GNVQ unit is split into elements. Unit 2: Interpersonal interaction is split into three elements. Each element defines an area of values, skill or knowledge. Elements are the smallest areas to be assessed, and evidence has to be presented for each element. When there is enough evidence, an element can be 'passed', but a person has to provide evidence for all the elements in a unit before the unit is awarded. Elements are not awarded. Elements cannot be accumulated as credit or recorded as an award in a National Record of Achievement.

  Elements have titles such as, '2.1 Explore interpersonal interaction'. This may be an appropriate task, but it is not easy to see exactly what it means or how it should be assessed. To explain the element title, elements are described in terms of performance criteria.
- **Performance criteria.** Performance criteria define what is required to pass the element. They help to explain what the element title is all about. When evidence is gathered to 'pass' an element, that evidence will meet the requirements of the performance criteria.

  The element title gives the focus of what has to be done, and the performance criteria help to explain this focus. However, range is also needed to explain what the evidence might cover.
- **Range.** Range explains the area that performance criteria cover. The word *range* comes from archery or perhaps from shooting ranges. If something is in range, then it is within your area of study. If an issue

is not in range, then you would not be expected to know about it when you come to take tests or present assignments.

Each element also has evidence indicators.

- **Evidence indicators.** Evidence indicators explain exactly what your assignment or final portfolio of evidence needs to cover. You will need to check that any written reports or assignments have covered everything that was asked for in the evidence indicator section of the standards. You may want to check that you understand these requirements when you design your action plans. You may need to check that your work has covered the evidence indicators before handing it in for assessment.

  Reports or assignments can cover more than just one element's evidence indicators. You do not have to cover evidence indicators in the order in which they are written. There are often a number of possible ways of choosing to cover evidence indicators. You might choose to write a report on a video you have seen, or you might go out and interview people in order to collect evidence. The way in which you cover the demands of the evidence indicators may be up to you.

  Standards also contain amplification and guidance sections.

- **Amplification.** Amplification increases the amount of detail about the performance criteria. Amplification is intended to make the meaning of performance criteria clearer and to prevent misinterpretations.
- **Guidance.** Guidance provides ideas to help teachers and tutors to cover the issues identified in the performance criteria and range.

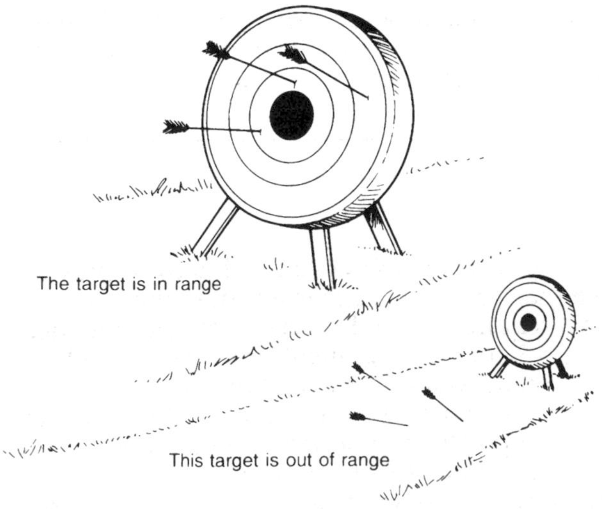
The target is in range
This target is out of range

An example: How to interpret one element

Element 1 of Unit 2 is 'Explore interpersonal interaction'. You will see it referred to as Element 2.1.

The element has six performance criteria which explain how the exploration of interpersonal interaction should be performed. Different forms of interpersonal interaction have to be explained. The influence of interpersonal interaction on health and social well-being has to be described. The effects of gender, age and culture have to be explained. Ways of optimising interaction have to be described. The detailed ideas which are implied in the performance criteria are then explained in the range statements.

The evidence indicators explain what you really have to do. If you turn to Chapter 4 of this book you will be able to review the knowledge needed for Element 2.1 and a summary of ideas which may help you produce a report. Your report needs to explain the different forms of interpersonal interaction and how interaction can be optimised, enhanced and inhibited. Your report needs to provide two examples of positive and negative influences on health and well-being. The report also needs to describe sources of data used for an evaluation of interaction. Finally, you also have to provide a brief summary explaining the effects that gender, age and culture may have on interpersonal interaction.

Each element of each unit has to be assessed before the unit is awarded. Assessment takes place when there is enough evidence to be assessed. In order to know what counts as enough evidence, candidates need to have their own assessment skills. Self-assessment of evidence is necessary in order to achieve good grades on GNVQ.

The individual working for a GNVQ qualification will go through a process of action planning, assignment work, checking and submitting the work for assessment. This is not the whole story, however. When work is submitted or 'given in' for assessment, a whole system comes into operation.

GNVQ assessment

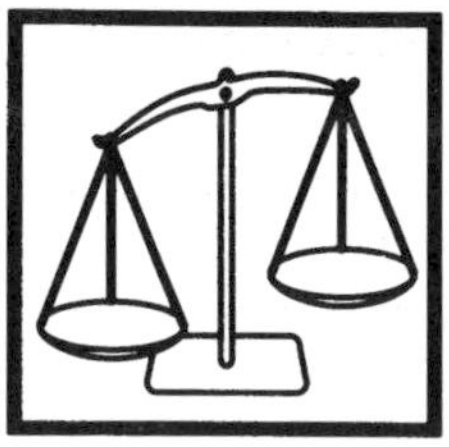

In the past, work was given to teachers or tutors, who marked it. This approach was often much simpler than in GNVQ. Now when work is given in, it is more than just 'work'. Assignments are now designed to provide evidence. Evidence has to be

PERFORMANCE CRITERIA

A student must:

1 explain the different **forms** which interpersonal interaction may take
2 describe how interpersonal interaction **influences** individuals' health and social well-being
3 explain the **effects** of gender, age and culture on interpersonal interaction
4 explain the **factors** which affect the interpersonal interaction
5 describe how effective interaction may be **optimised**
6 describe **sources of data** and **criteria used in evaluating** the effectiveness of interaction

RANGE

Forms: through language, through sensory contact (touch, presence, eye contact, listening, body position), through activity

Influences: positive, negative

Effects due to: use of sensory contact, distance between individuals, body language, accepted forms of respect, items of interest, preferred form of interaction, personal strengths

Factors: enhancers, inhibitors

Optimised through: respect for others' beliefs and views, establishing boundaries, showing interest in the individual, using body language, seeking information (from the individual, from others), taking positive action, seeking feedback, reflective listening, interpretation, self-reflection

Sources of data: feedback, observation, self-reflection, knowledge and understanding of participants

Criteria used in evaluating: participation, quality of contribution, improvements from previous occasions

EVIDENCE INDICATORS

A report which:

- explains the different forms of interpersonal interaction
- explains how interaction can be enhanced and inhibited
- provides two examples of positive and negative influences of interaction on individuals' health and social well-being
- describes the sources of data used for an evaluation of interaction.

A brief summary explaining the effects that gender, age and culture may have on interpersonal interaction.

Figure 5 An example: Element 2.1 Explore interpersonal interaction

judged to decide if there is enough, and if it is the right quality to show that a standard has been reached. The person who decides whether there is enough quality evidence is called an **assessor.** Often the people who act as assessors will be teachers or tutors, but when they collect in the work, they become assessors.

Assessors have to have qualifications and knowledge in the field in which they work. They also have to understand the standards for which they are checking evidence. Assessors will have gained an NVQ award which shows that they understand the GNVQ assessment process. All these checks are required to try to ensure that the quality of GNVQ assessment is fair and works properly. But it is more complicated still. The assessments themselves have to be checked.

Assessments have to be checked by an **internal verifier.** 'Internal' means internal to, or inside, the centre (inside the college or school, etc). 'Verifier' means that the person checks the correctness of assessment. Internal verifiers will look at samples of assessment work and check that evidence is being correctly and fairly measured in relation to standards. If candidates don't think their work is being fairly assessed, they can appeal to the internal verifier to look at their work, and re-check it.

There is also an **external verifier.** 'External' means outside, from outside the centre (a school or college, etc.). External verifiers are appointed by the awarding body. An awarding body is BTEC, City & Guilds or RSA. The awarding body checks the overall quality of the centre's assessment. The external verifier checks the quality of both the assessor's and the internal verifier's decisions. The idea of all this checking is to ensure that standards *really work* – what is accepted as evidence must not become too simple or too complicated. A qualification gained at one college or school should require the same amount and quality of evidence as elsewhere.

Meeting evidence indicators – things that count as evidence

In order to pass your GNVQ you will need to provide evidence that you have done everything that the indicators require you to do. Very often the evidence indicators ask for an assignment or a report which explains certain issues. At the end of your GNVQ programme (or course) you may have collected other evidence in a portfolio (a portable folder). Both assignments and portfolios might include the following examples of evidence:

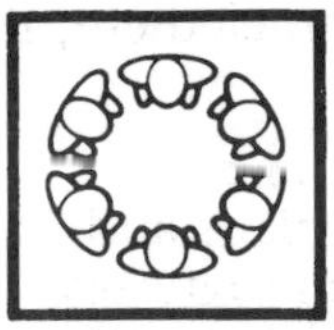

Practical demonstration of skills can be watched by an assessor or they can be videoed or tape-recorded (with everyone's permission).

Reports can provide evidence of knowledge, records of practical work and projects. Many units will require some report writing.

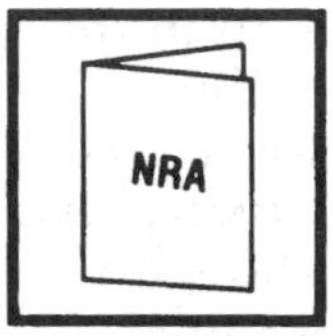

Past records of achievement and qualifications can count as evidence towards GNVQ units. For instance, GCSE work might count towards core skills assessment.

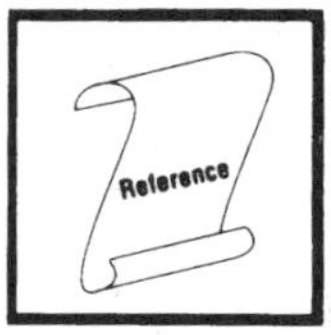

References from other people such as placement supervisors or employers can provide evidence of practical caring skills, and core skills.

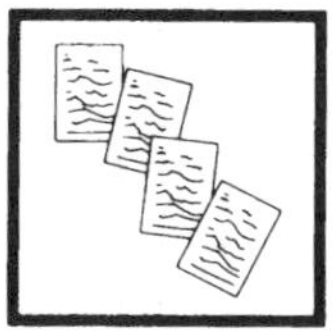

Notes: not all written work needs to be put together into assignments – notes will often be enough to provide evidence for knowledge, or perhaps evidence of planning skills.

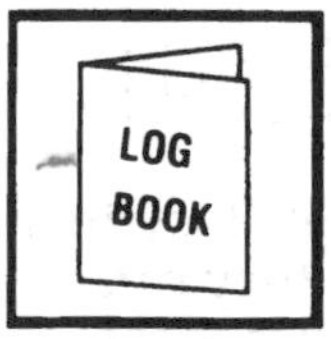

Log books or record books are a way of providing evidence to meet grading criteria standards. Log books may be easier to use than loose notes.

Photographs of placement work, perhaps of events organised by a candidate, can sometimes count as evidence towards achieving standards. Photos can often make assignments more interesting.

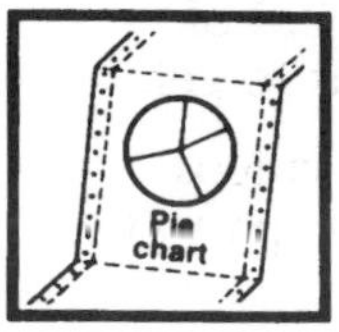

Other work, such as computer printouts, can provide evidence of skills and knowledge. Computer printouts will sometimes need to be 'certified' by an appropriate person to prove that they were done by the candidate.

Collecting evidence

Each element suggests a way of getting the necessary evidence in the 'evidence indicators' section. Usually, tutors will provide more information and ideas on practical ways in which evidence can be gathered. Here are some points to remember:

- **Permission.** It is *always* necessary to have other people's permission before written details about them can be used. For instance, written details of a conversation can give evidence of conversation skills, but things other people have said must not be written down without their permission and knowledge of what is written. Where someone is unable to understand, perhaps because he or she is too young, then the parents or guardians have to give permission.
- **Confidentiality.** If you use written or taped evidence that involves other people, it is important that their confidentiality is respected. One of the most effective ways of keeping material confidential is to keep details anonymous. This means that you should not write the names or any identifying personal details of people you have worked with on your finished work. If you interview people for evidence, you should *not* explain who they were in your assignment, logbook or portfolio of evidence. Instead, you might say that you worked with a friend, a relative, or a tutor or supervisor. Any personal details such as age, place of work, or detailed description of appearance should not be recorded.

So, as well as asking for permission to use interviews or group work, you should also keep your reports confidential. If this is not possible, for example, if you have video evidence where it is obvious who the people are, you should show the video to all the people involved in it and ask for written permission before you can use it as evidence. This might be agreed simply if you are all students. If you video clients on placement, you might need to get written permission from them and from parents or managers – after they have checked your material – that the material may be used as your evidence. This kind of agreement may sometimes be difficult to get.

Of course all written details, tapes or videos should be kept safely and used only as part of your GNVQ work.

- **Group work.** Working with other people is often the best way to plan to collect evidence. Sometimes a group project can meet the evidence requirements for an element. The only problem is that each individual's work has to be separately recorded or noted, so that each has individual evidence of planning and achievement for their portfolio. Naturally, the general outcome can be recorded as well.
- **Evidence from others.** Evidence of skills used on placements is really valuable, but it will need to be confirmed by a manager or supervisor in the work setting. Usually the supervisor will also have to explain that he or she has watched practical work, and give reasons for agreeing with claims for evidence. Sometimes a report or reference will be needed.

Quality of evidence

Being assessed involves convincing an assessor that your evidence is good enough. Usually, candidates will get a lot of help and guidance to make sure the evidence is all right.

The process of assessment will probably start something like this:

1. Teachers or tutors suggest a project, assignment or demonstration to provide evidence for particular evidence indicators. Written guidelines are given out.
2. Candidates discuss the guidelines, probably with a tutor, and think of ways of planning practical work.
3. Each individual designs an **action plan** for the assignment or project (see page 11).
4. Each individual discusses the action plan with a tutor.
5. The individual **monitors** the implementation of the action plan, i.e. he or she checks and revises ideas as the assignment gets going.
6. Candidates do the practical work and write about it.
7. The written work is checked by an assessor. If it is all right, then it counts as evidence. If not, then further work can be done until the evidence is right.
8. When there is enough evidence for an element, it is credited as complete.

At the start of a GNVQ programme, tutors and teachers will probably help with action plans and other practical work. As the programme progresses, candidates will have to do this work without help in order to gain Merit and Distinction grades.

Reflection

Planning to collect evidence can be interesting. It involves a special skill called **reflection.** Think of a mirror. When a person looks in a mirror, his or her image is being bounced back – reflected – from the mirror. Reflection is the bouncing back of the original image. In social care, reflection means the same sort of thing; except here we are thinking about thoughts and ideas rather than images. Thoughts and ideas get bounced backwards and forwards between people.

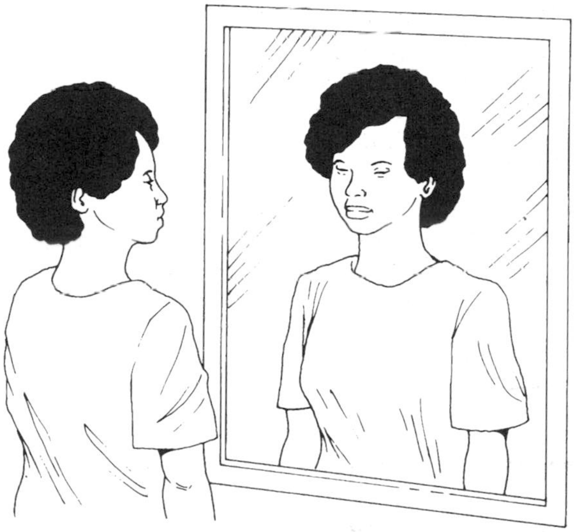

Reflection can be very useful. When people look in a mirror, they can see what they look like; they can change their hairstyle or appearance until it looks right. The same idea goes for thoughts. If an individual can have his or her thoughts mirrored or reflected by another person, then the individual has a chance to change or alter his or her own thoughts. Like changing hairstyle, reflection allows individuals to experiment until their ideas are good.

Reflective listening is a special skill that is explained in Chapters 4 and 5. People who can help others to reflect have a very useful skill. When people get very good at reflecting with others, they can sometimes reflect in their own mind – alone. This becomes a

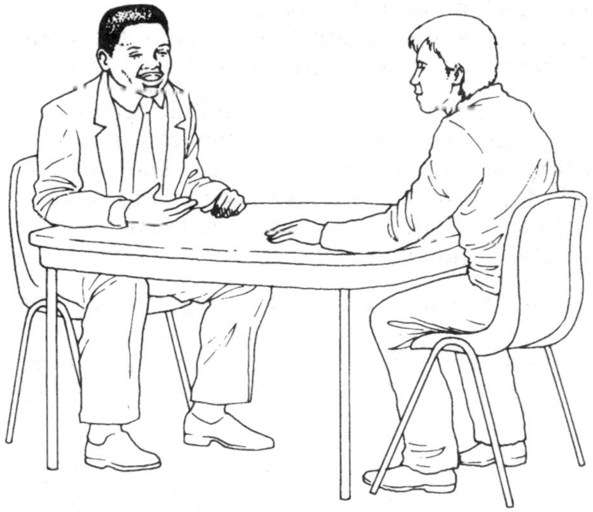

powerful learning skill as people can adapt their own thoughts using an internal mirror, rather than using another person. Reflection is also needed in order to plan the collection of evidence.

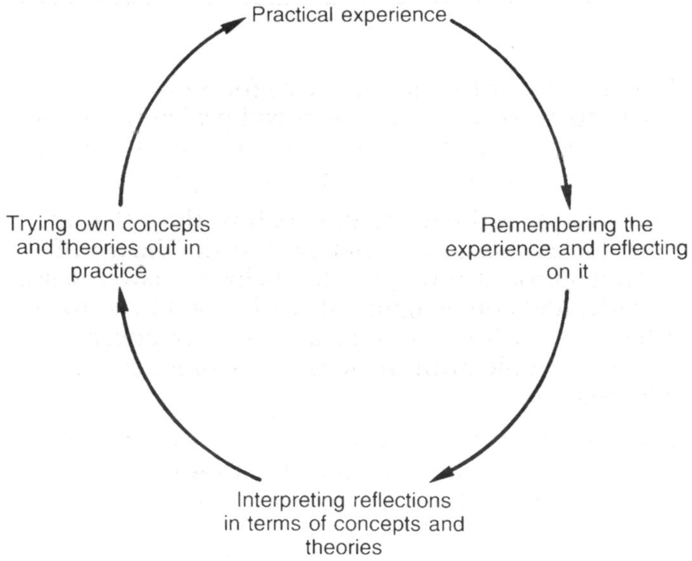

Figure 6 A learning sequence or learning cycle (adapted from Kolb *et al.*, 1979)

Using concepts and theory

As well as using reflective thinking, advanced candidates will need to be able to use care concepts and theory. *Using* concepts or ideas is very different from just being able to state what they are. A famous psychologist, Kurt Lewin, is reported to have once said, 'There is nothing as practical as a good theory.' Our concepts and theories about care help us to recognise situations. Concepts help us to make sense of what we hear and see. We organise our lives around our own personal theories of people and social behaviour. Most importantly, concepts – and theories which are made up of concepts – help us to guess what will happen next. Understanding and using the knowledge involved in the advanced mandatory units is about being able to recognise, understand and predict what clients and colleagues are doing. Advanced skill in caring requires advanced understanding.

One theory of learning – the Kolb learning cycle (Figure 6) – suggests that learning needs to involve practical experience. This experience is not enough on its own. For experience to be remembered and used it may need to be recalled in imagination. Experience may need to be reflected on. But reflection alone may not be enough to enable individuals to understand and predict what best to do. A stage of conceptualising or theorising may be needed. Concepts and theories don't always have to come from books. People can develop their own personal ideas without formal study. The idea of using book knowledge is to improve on personal concepts and ideas. Knowledge of other people's theories may give us a starting point for the development of our own ideas. Other people's ideas may help us to question false assumptions we have made. We may be able to build a better interpretation of other people, and their lives, if we link new theory to our own personal view-points.

The point of theory is that it should be useful in helping us to understand and work in health and social care. Kolb saw this as the fourth stage in learning. We have to use theories if we are really learning, as opposed to just remembering! Using theory might mean checking whether we can explain something, or guessing what we think is the right thing to do, and checking this with tutors or supervisors. Using theory is about checking it out for its practical value. This stage is sometimes called 'experimenting', but here this might best be interpreted as 'trying out in practice'.

The concepts contained in this book may become part of a practical tool kit for work in health and social care. Concepts and theories can become 'tools of analysis' – practical ideas which help us interpret our life experience.

Assignments

Evidence for units will mostly be found in assignment work. Assignments will probably contain most of the evidence for the core skill units, spread across the mandatory and optional units.

Most people will need to discuss how they plan to write assignments or do practical work. The act of talking a project through often helps to clarify ideas. Usually, ideas on assignment writing will need to be reflected on with a tutor. Ideas can be 'bounced' between people until the ideas grow more practical and useful.

Before starting any practical or written work it will be important to construct an **action plan** to help find the necessary information and evidence opportunities. Action plans can be monitored for progress. Keeping notes on progress may help to organise a project. Monitoring may also boost confidence when it comes to sitting down and writing an assignment. Planning involves self-assessment. Monitoring progress with evidence collection involves being in control of personal work. Self-assessment and control of work should provide a very useful starting point for getting a GNVQ qualification.

Action plans

Action plans are records of the ideas that go into getting ready for assignments and evidence collection. They record ideas for the following:

1 *Finding information*

- looking up books for information and ideas
- asking people for their opinions
- asking tutors, learning advisers, librarians for advice on how to find information.

2 *Reflecting on ideas*

- discussing with tutors, with other candidates
- discussing with placement supervisors
- working out what information is needed in order to do assignments, etc.

3 *Preparing to gather evidence – plans*

- for practical activities
- to get evidence during placement
- for doing assignments
- for what to include in notes and written work.

4 *Self-assessment and monitoring*

- self-assessment of evidence before it is formally assessed
- self-checking of own progress
- checking of ideas against assignment guidelines
- checking own study patterns and use of time.

Many people like to use a form to help record their ideas. Forms are useful because they can focus attention on what needs to be done. They also keep a record of planning activities which can fit neatly into a portfolio. Records of planning are needed in order to get Merit and Distinction grades.

Forms are just one way of organising and recording a 'plan for action'. Some people prefer to write everything down in notes or to use notes to go with their forms. Others like to make 'pattern notes' to help display things visually.

Suppose you want to collect information to help with your work on Element 2.1, 'Explore interpersonal interaction'. Pattern notes might help you to decide on the information that you need. By looking at the evidence indicators, you could produce a pattern like the one shown in Figure 7.

Pattern notes can be used for both action planning and for identifying information needs. You may find pattern notes particularly useful for identifying information needs.

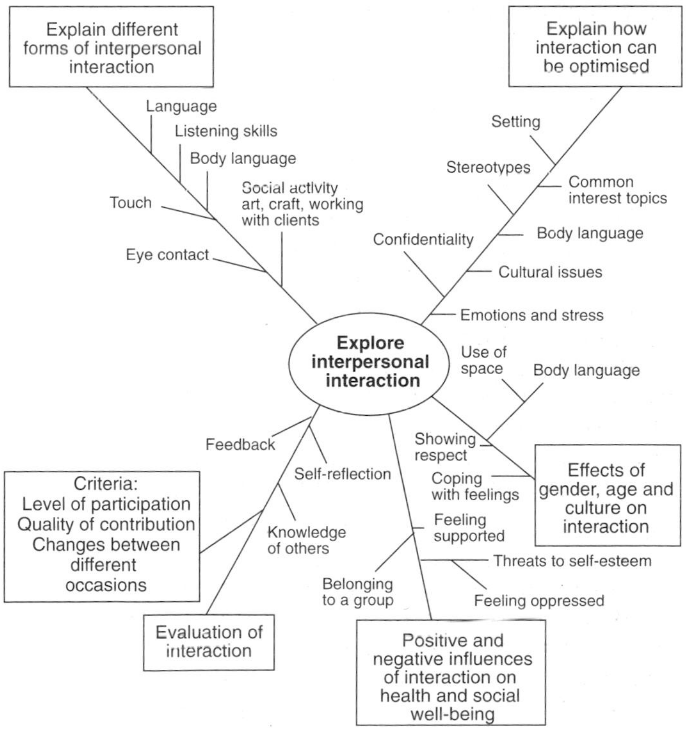

Figure 7 Information needs for Element 2.1

Planning and information seeking are usually required before you will be able to write assignments or produce work to meet the evidence indicators. Planning and information seeking are also part of the grading criteria for the full GNVQ award.

Advanced GNVQ qualifications can be awarded at a Pass, Merit or Distinction grade. At present, these grades are awarded when a student's final portfolio or work is assessed at the end of the programme.

To achieve a Merit or Distinction grade, advanced students have to be able to demonstrate that they have followed a process of planning, information handling and evaluation in at least one-third of their work. This process should lead to a 'quality outcome' in at least one-third of a student's work. The *quality of outcomes* theme requires that students demonstrate command of language and synthesis of ideas in their projects or assignment work.

The process of evidence collection

The process of preparing to meet evidence indicators should always start with planning. Sometimes this planning stage might involve identifying information needs and sources where this information can be obtained. It is important to monitor your plans and your collection of information. You should reflect on whether your plans are working – are you collecting the information that you need? Finally, you should self-assess or check your work before handing it in. Did your work meet the evidence indicators? This is **evaluation.** You should always evaluate your work before handing it in.

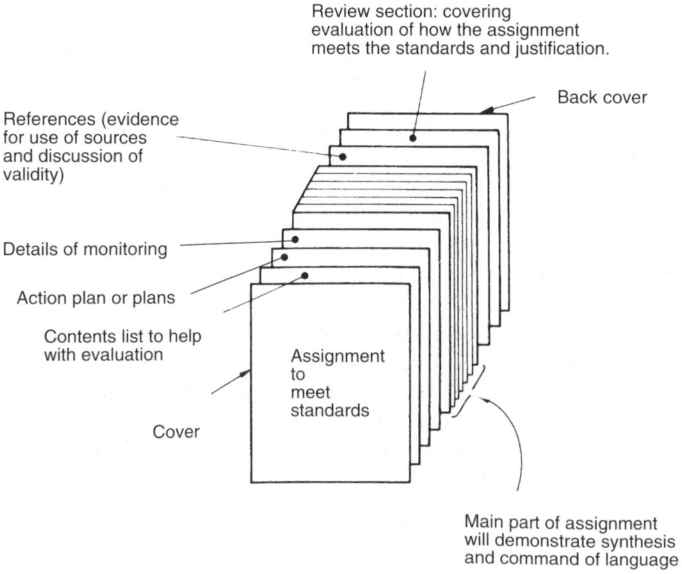

When you design assignments they may be laid out something like the diagram below left.

Outcome of your work

When your assignment work is received, it will be judged to see whether it shows a synthesis (combination) of skills, knowledge and understanding, and whether it demonstrates the right command of language.

If your work demonstrates the right process and outcomes you can be awarded a Merit or Distinction.

The grading criteria

The National Council for Vocational Qualifications has published a guide to grading, and your GNVQ Centre may provide you with up-to-date detailed guidance on the criteria by which your work will be judged.

These notes are intended to explain more about the process and outcomes you are aiming for. You might need to refer to the formal definitions of the grading criteria in order finally to judge your work.

In outline, to get Merit and Distinction grades you must provide evidence for three process grading themes of:

- planning
- information handling
- evaluation.

You must also provide evidence for the 'outcome' grading theme of quality.

Each of these themes is defined in terms of two criteria as set out below:

The planning theme

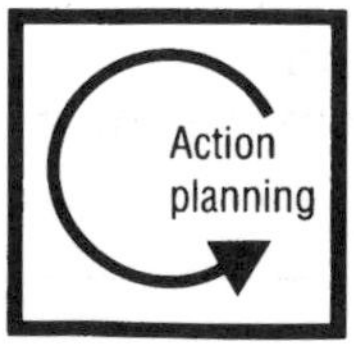

Action plan: Independently draw up action plans for tasks that 'prioritise' or explain the order of activities to meet deadlines. At Distinction grade, this has to cover complex activities rather than just individual tasks.

Monitor: Independently work out where monitoring skills need to be used. This might involve monitoring action planning, revising and changing action plans where necessary. Revision may be made with guidance from a tutor. At Distinction grade, students have to demonstrate that they can make revisions independently.

The information handling theme

Use of sources: Independently identify, access and collect information for tasks. The candidate will identify sources such as libraries and newspapers, but some help with finding material may be given by tutors. At Distinction grade, this skill has to cover complex activities rather than just discrete tasks. Candidates have to use a range of sources and justify why they were used.

Validity: Independently work out what information needs checking for validity. Validity may be checked using methods supplied or given by tutors. At Distinction grade, the selection of appropriate methods must be done independently by candidates.

The evaluation theme

Evaluation: Judge outcomes against plans or perhaps against evidence indicators or other criteria. Identify alternative criteria that could be used to judge the success of activities. At Distinction grade, candidates have to apply a range of alternative criteria in order to judge the success of activities.

Justification: Justify approaches used; indicate that alternatives were (identified and) considered. At Distinction grade, justification must be based on a detailed consideration of relevant advantages and disadvantages. Alternatives and improvements must be identified.

The quality theme

Synthesis: The work has to show an effective linking of skills, knowledge, concepts and understanding in relation to pieces of work. At Distinction grade this understanding and synthesis has to cover complex work such as whole assignments.

Command of language: The work has to show an effective use of terms, ideas and concepts used in health and social care language. At Distinction grade, the work has to demonstrate a fluent use of concepts and terminology.

Your work needs to demonstrate the process of planning, action and reviewing. It then needs to demonstrate quality in terms of knowledge and command of language

Ideas for evidence for the grading criteria

Any practical research or activities with clients might be planned and evaluated using the grading criteria process. Assignments might be designed from the start to meet the grading criteria.

The grading criteria for action, monitoring and use of sources might be fairly easy to build into assignment work.

Before starting any written work you need a plan. An action plan can cover a whole range of issues: what books you should use, what people you could talk to, where and how you can collect evidence, when it should be done by. As well as drawing up plans, you may have to prioritise what you do. Which books are the most important to read first? Which chapters or sections of books will give you the theory you need? Who must you work with in order to collect the evidence needed for the unit standards? Who should you speak to first?

As well as designing an action plan, you will need to monitor how well it is working and you can do this by including dates in your action plan records to review progress. Using dates for review should go some way toward meeting the grading criteria requirement to 'independently identify points at which monitoring is necessary'. Revising action and assignment plans following a review will be important. Never destroy an action plan that needs revision – simply produce a revised plan with dates. This provides evidence for your planning skills.

Writing a quality assignment will require an initial plan for the content, layout and the concepts and theory to be included. Few people can write effectively without planning and monitoring. The only new thing that the grading criteria for planning and monitoring requires is records of the process.

Quality projects and assignments will require concepts, theory and information to be related to practical issues. Candidates will need to identify and use sources of information to plan and to develop assignment work. The action plan could record the identification of key texts, people to interview, places to phone for information, and so on. A carefully laid out reference section (a list of sources used or bibliography) at the end of the assignment will also provide evidence towards this.

Look at the style of reference layout used in this book to help design the bibliography, or follow your centre guidelines if different. Identifying sources involves finding useful details and showing how these help you to meet the standards. Just copying a list of book titles at the end of an assignment is not evidence of using them for tasks or complex activities. As well as identifying sources of information in an action plan, and listing them later, you would need to include references to them in the assignment work. The usual way of doing this is to quote the author's name, put the date of the work in brackets and then put full details in your reference section. When writing or recording details of information gained on visits, you may record details of how you identified appropriate information in a sources section at the end of your assignment.

Naturally you will be given lists of references and guidelines on using information technology, libraries and so on. You job as an independent researcher is to work out how to get the necessary information out of books, libraries, databases or interviews. You have to work out exactly what information is needed: which quotations to use, which questions to ask people, which issues to write about. Using sources is a skill, and like all skills it will develop with practice and with reflective feedback from others.

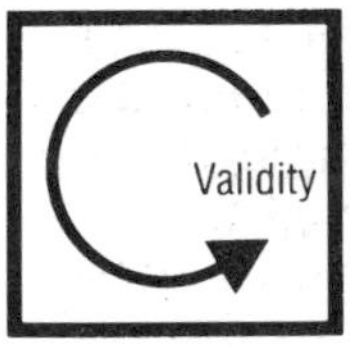

Establishing the validity of information involves a depth of thinking about what is being written or recorded. How do you know you have got the ideas right? If you are using another author's theory, are you sure what you have put down is valid, or a true representation of their ideas? If you are drawing conclusions from an interview, are you sure that they are reasonable? If you are writing your own views about a topic, how can you back up your views so that they are valid?

Identifying information which requires to be checked or supported involves self-assessment skills. It also involves being critical of what you write or record. The validity skill involves frequently asking yourself: 'How do I know that this is correct? What evidence could I use to support this point?'

Creativity is important at advanced level, and each candidate may develop a range of methods for demonstrating and checking validity. Methods may vary between units. Checking validity in Application of Number may involve double-checking calculations; checking validity in Unit 8, 'Research', may involve checking a conclusion by using more than one research technique. Below are a few general ideas which you might like to develop into your own style of writing or recording.

- Review the quality of books, journals or newspapers that you are using. How credible or reputable are these sources? Write short notes about your sources listed in your reference section. Evaluate your references.
- When writing about an author's views, quote the page numbers of your source and select some quotes on those pages which establish the validity of your interpretation. Use the author's own words to support your case.
- When interpreting views from interviewees, check what you have written with the people you interview. Ask them if your interpretation is correct – check the validity of your views.
- Suppose you were writing about placement, work or visit experiences, and you were quoting details like the number of clients or the size of the building. You might ask a workplace supervisor to check your statements and validate them for accuracy.
- Always quote the reference for any theories you write about. Quote more than one author or more than one set of statistics to support complex arguments you wish to make. This demonstrates a weight of evidence for your argument. It doesn't prove that you are right, but it does show that what you are saying is reasonable and appropriate.
- Cross-check any tables or statistics you quote. Explain that you have double-checked your reasoning.

Demonstrating that you have built validity into your assignment is another **self-evaluation** or self-assessment task. One way of doing this is to write a short set of notes at the end of each assignment. These notes might explain how you have checked your work. The notes might also point out page numbers in your assignment where you have checked the validity of what you are arguing or saying. As a self-check, you could put a small pencil 'V' in the margin to note your performance. Whatever methods you use to demonstrate the validity of information, you might need to discuss this concept with your teacher or tutor. Sometimes it may be necessary to use a reflective learning process like the Kolb cycle (Figure 6) in order to develop your style of work.

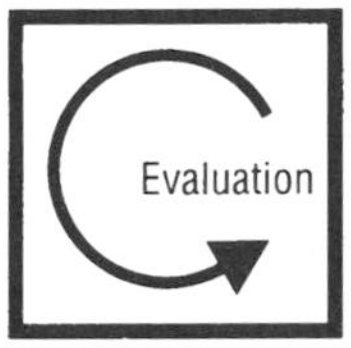

Evaluation is another self-assessment skill. As a higher education skill, evaluation involves being able to make comparisons and see similarities and differences between ideas, theories or situations. It may involve contrasts between viewpoints. At advanced level, evaluation implies the ability to review your own work.

Evaluation means that when working on Advanced GNVQ assignments, it is not good enough simply to produce a good assignment – you have to know that you've done a good assignment, and know why it's a good assignment! Then you have to explain what you know – evaluate and 'own' your achievement. Evaluation skills involve taking control of your own assessment, at least in the first instance.

Providing evidence for evaluation might involve producing a set of notes at the end of each task or assignment that you complete. This set of notes would cover your own judgement as to how your work met the national standards – the element or unit standards that you were working towards. If, for example, you had written an assignment to cover Element 2.1, you might provide a contents page which would list how you had met the evidence indicators. The evaluation or review section at the end of an assignment could explain that particular communication techniques had been recorded on video or audio tape, and that evidence for the element could be found there.

As well as evaluating how an assignment meets assessment criteria, you need to evaluate how aspects of your performance worked. This will involve judging the outcomes of behaviour in terms of theory. You will need to analyse your own ideas and performance in relation to alternative concepts and theories. A thorough knowledge of a range of concepts and how they can be used in practice will usually be needed for Distinction grades.

When you evaluate your knowledge and performance, you are beginning to argue a case for your work; this will also call on the skill of 'justifying approaches'.

Justifying the approaches used and their alternatives, advantages and disadvantages, is the final self-assessment skill. Like evaluation, this skill will involve analysing approaches and techniques used in assignment and evidence-collection work. Like evaluation, it will involve a wide range and depth of knowledge if you are to be able to make an effective case for yourself. Justification involves the questions: Why did I do this work the way I have done it? What advantages were there in doing it this way? What were the alternatives? Why didn't I choose them?

Justification involves producing an argument to support your design work.

You will often need to use theory and value statements in order to be able to justify your approach. Again, concepts and theory will often provide a basis for considering alternatives and relevant advantages and disadvantages.

Providing evidence for justification might involve producing a set of notes at the end of each assignment. These notes might be written together with the notes on evaluation. Alternatively, they might be written under a separate subheading or written on a form supplied by the centre.

When you pass a driving test, you have to demonstrate that you can drive effectively and answer a few questions at the end of the test. To pass an advanced driving test you have to be able to explain or evaluate your driving as you go along. Advanced GNVQs may be like advanced driving – both evaluation and justification skills are needed to demonstrate that you really know what you are doing. To achieve Merit and Distinction grades you have to review and evaluate your work. Even more importantly, you have to be able to explain and justify the way your work has been done.

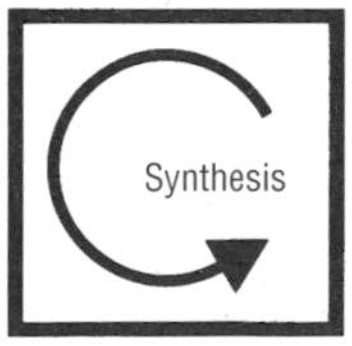

The outcomes criteria depend on your ability to analyse and interpret knowledge, skill and understanding. The verb *synthesise* means to build up ideas into a connected whole, or into a theory or system of thought. Demonstrating an effective synthesis could mean being able to explain how theories and practice relate to each other. The ability to explain events during a work placement in terms of theoretical concepts might be evidence of synthesis in a limited area. If you can understand how a range of concepts and theories link, if assignments explain how theories may link and how they relate to practical issues, then this may provide evidence for synthesis in relation to complex tasks.

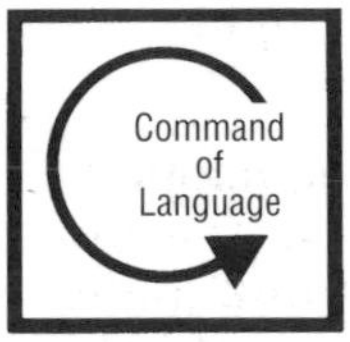

Command of language may be evidenced in work which demonstrates that you are confident in using the ideas, concepts and technical vocabulary involved in sciences, such as biology, and social sciences, such as psychology and sociology. You will also need to demonstrate confidence in the use of health and social care concepts and terminology.

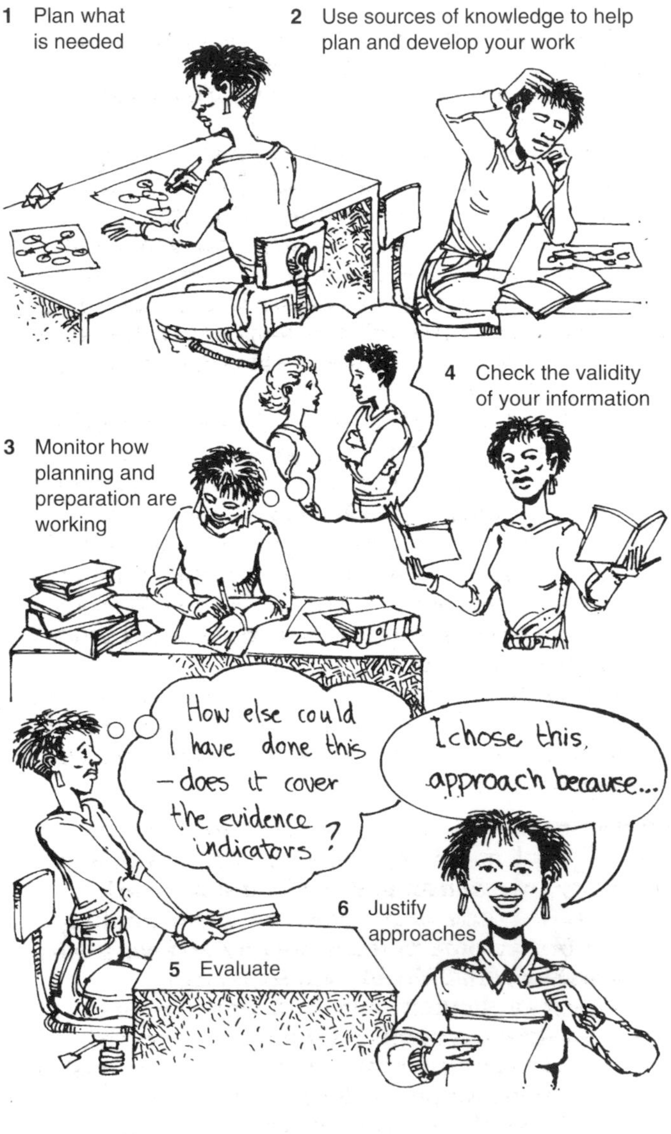

Figure 8 Grading criteria – the process

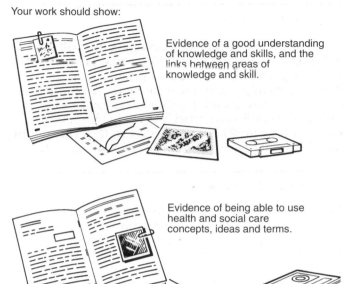

Figure 9 Grading criteria – the outcome

The development of synthesis and command of language is likely to be a gradual process which will require regular reflective feedback and discussion with your tutors or teachers.

Collecting evidence for the grading criteria might begin with each piece of written work, each report or assignment that you design. As you begin to pass a number of units, you will need to think about the presentation of your work in a final portfolio. The overall design of your portfolio might also be something which could be evaluated and reviewed to provide extra evidence of your skills.

The portfolio

A GNVQ portfolio is your collection of evidence for the award of the qualification. Evidence for the qualification will probably be contained in:

- assignments
- a record or log book
- extra notes and forms.

Evidence has to cover:

- mandatory and optional units
- core skills units
- grading criteria.

Assignment work

Evidence for mandatory and optional units will mostly be found in assignment work. There may be one or more assignment per element or sometimes assignments might run across elements. Assignments may be straightforward to present at the end of the course. They will also probably contain most of the evidence for core skills units. However, the evidence for core skills will probably be spread *across* assignments.

Record or log book

Another way of collecting evidence for the unit standards, core skills and the grading criteria, is to use a log book. By keeping a diary of study activities, it may be possible to provide evidence for the process grading criteria. A log book used on placement might provide evidence of communication, information technology and even use of number core skills. Placement activities might often provide opportunities for demonstrating skills. Records of performance might need to be signed by a supervisor or manager before they can count as evidence.

Notes

Sometimes candidates might prefer to use action plan forms for planning. Core skills in information technology might be demonstrated by designing action plan forms, or other record sheets. These sheets might be separate from the assignments or from other log books or notes.

What the portfolio might look like

By the end of the GNVQ programme, there could be a great deal of evidence to be reviewed for the award of the qualification.

All this evidence could be collected together, dumped in a bag and given to the assessors and verifiers. But no-one would be able to understand it. A disorganised portfolio will not communicate quality, nor will it suggest good planning, monitoring or evaluation. So a portfolio is more than a bag of bits!

Think it over

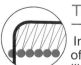

Imagine your assessor checking the quality of assignment evidence. What sort of things will he or she be looking for?

If you can use you imagination to reflect on and visualise this situation, then you have the planning skills to organise a good portfolio of your work.

Your portfolio needs to be carefully planned and organised. The planning of the portfolio might provide evidence for the grading criteria.

The portfolio might be a ring binder, an envelope folder or a file of some sort. The portfolio at the end of the programme might need more than one folder. What matters is that there is an explanation of how the evidence in the portfolio meets the standards for GNVQ and the standards for a Merit or Distinction grade if this is claimed.

So, looking inside the folder there might be:

1. *A title sheet* stating your name, the centre's name (school or college) and the name of the qualification (Advanced GNVQ in Health and Social Care).
2. *An index of assignments, evidence and assessments* which have already been made.
3. *A statement* or *claim* explaining that the assignment work meets the unit standards and has been assessed as meeting the standards (dates of assessment and forms might be included here).
4. Photocopies of the *unit standards* which the work claims to demonstrate (or workbook containing the standards).
5. An *index of core skills evidence*. This index would explain where evidence could be found for information technology, application of number and communication skills. Page numbers in assignment work might be quoted. Notes would be placed in order in the portfolio and numbered. Core skills demonstrated by other records (floppy disk, video, etc.) would also be noted, and disks and boxes labelled.
6. An *index of evidence for the grading criteria*. Most of the evidence would probably be in project reports, assignments or on forms. Page numbers should be quoted.

You do not have to supply evidence for the core skills of problem-solving, working with others and improving own learning. It could still be worth putting in for these units, however, as the grading criteria often require problem-solving and improving own learning skills. Health and social care assignment work often links with working with others. To design a really good portfolio you will need to self-assess your own learning. A high-quality portfolio might supply evidence to claim the additional core skills linked to achieving Merit or Distinction grades.

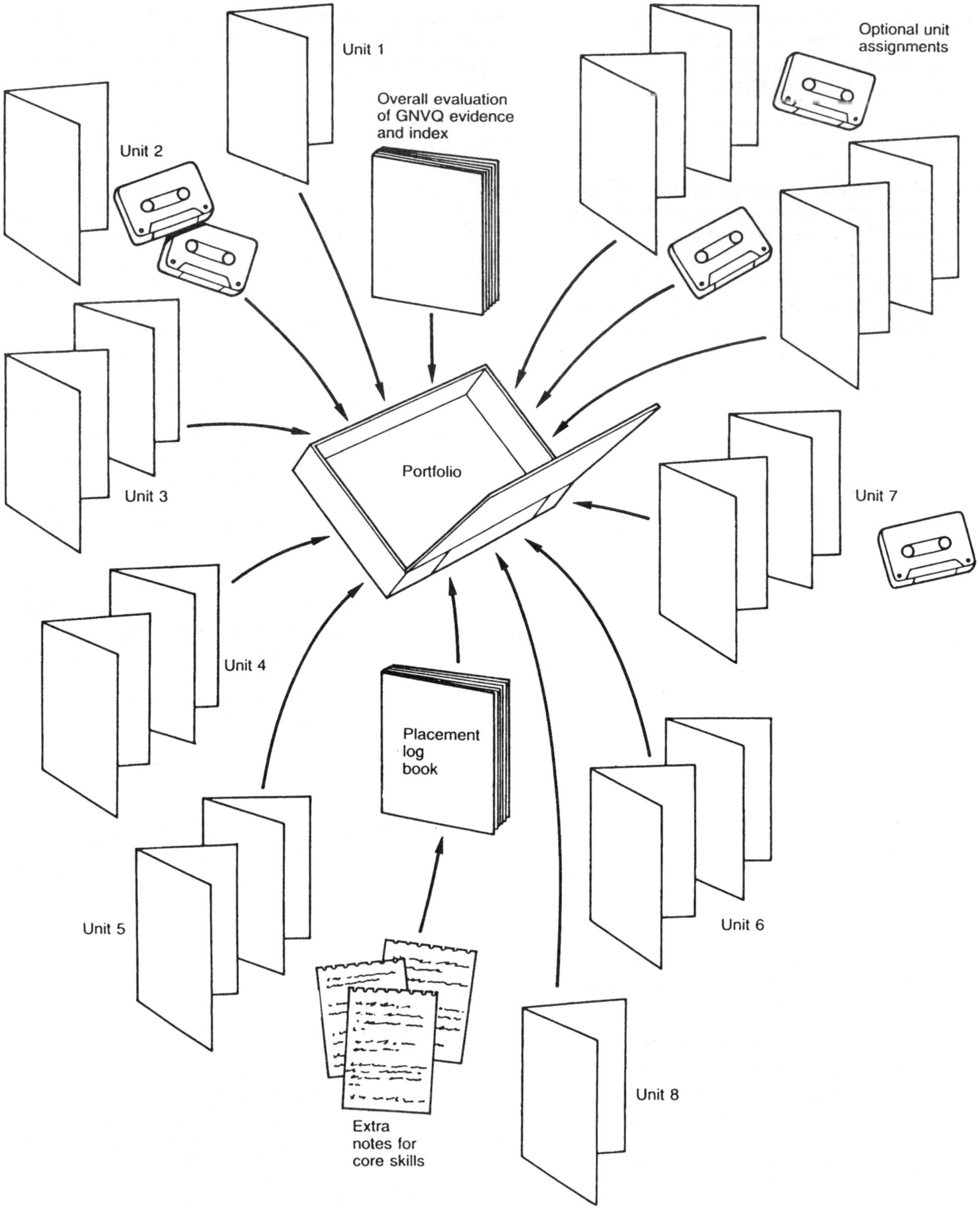

Figure 10 A visual map of portfolio evidence

So, in summary, the portfolio will include indexing, the standards and the evidence. The portfolio can also contain explanations and arguments which support the claim for a Merit or Distinction grade.

Using icons to organise the portfolio

One idea to make indexing easier is to use symbols or 'icons' to label your evidence. A range of icons appears at the back of this book – these can be photocopied for use with GNVQ evidence, free of copyright restrictions. After photocopying, they can be cut out and stuck to notes or pages of assignment or log-book work. When an icon is stuck next to a piece of writing, or on a tape box, etc. it means that evidence is being claimed. An icon states, 'Look, this is evidence'.

Portfolio design

Designing a portfolio to achieve a Distinction grade will involve a good deal of self-assessment work. Usually, this work will have to be started *early* in the programme and developed as the programme goes on. Good grades may be difficult to achieve if portfolio design is left until the end of the programme.

Designing a portfolio of evidence will eventually require you to self-assess your own evidence. You will have to be able to show that:

1 The work is your own.
2 There is enough work to cover the evidence indicators.
3 There is enough evidence to meet the grading criteria.
4 There is enough evidence to meet core skills standards.

Doing all this involves using imagination and checking ideas with tutors or assessors. Designing a good portfolio is a major learning task.

As you gradually put together your design for your portfolio, you will have opportunities to include new evidence to meet unit standards, to cover core skills or to meet the grading criteria. You are putting your own book together! The portfolio is the final record of your achievements. It can be more than just a box of assignment work. The portfolio can be the final review of all your learning. The indexing and the claim statements can make an argument for the grade of qualification that you are seeking.

Designing a portfolio is the final check that all the necessary evidence has been collected. The grade of the GNVQ qualification will be awarded in relation to the quality of the portfolio and its contents.

Getting started

Imagine trying to learn to drive a car by reading a book. Very few people could do it. To drive a car you have to *practise* doing it. Collecting evidence and designing projects, assignments and portfolios, will be the same kind of learning – try it, imagine how to do it better, listen to advice … or listen to advice, imagine it and then try it. The order is not important. What can't be done is to learn the whole idea in one go and then do it.

Evidence collection will look very complicated at first – there is so much that can go into a portfolio. It is important to get some ideas, think about them, try them out in practice and then get advice. If this is done over time, it should become much easier. Like driving a car, it gets easier once you have tried it for real.

Some of the ideas here might make more sense after evidence for the first assignment has been collected. So, if you are reading this before starting your GNVQ why not plan to read it again in a month's time or in two months' time? Some of the ideas about assignment and portfolio design will make more sense when they are tried in practice.

Tests

Mandatory units are expected to have tests, except in Unit 2. Tests provide evidence that all detail involved in the units has been covered. Some people think that test evidence will mean that GNVQ

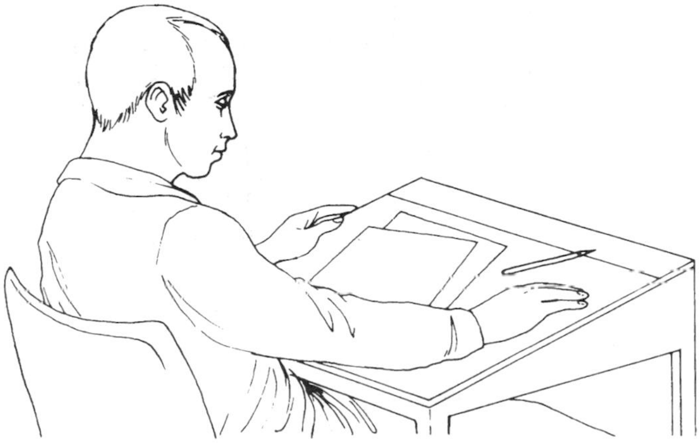

qualifications will be more valued and respected by the public and by future employers.

GNVQ tests should usually be taken after all the other evidence collection work for a unit has been done.

Tests will ask a number of short questions about the unit and will probably last about one hour. Tests have to be passed in order for a unit to be awarded. If a test is not passed first time, it can be taken again. Indeed, it should be possible to take the test several times if necessary. Fear of failing often worries people when they have to take tests. GNVQ tests *shouldn't* cause fear because the tests can be retaken.

You will probably have achieved lots of practical learning for the unit before you take a test. You will have planned evidence collection, reviewed your own knowledge, reflected on knowledge with others in discussion and written assignments or notes. All this work will have been assessed. It should mean that there is not a lot of extra work and revision to do for the test.

Before doing the test, it might be worth organising discussion sessions with others so that practical work and information can be shared. *Talking* about knowledge can be one of the best ways of learning to remember it for a test.

The knowledge contained in this book should help cover the needs of the test. Fast Facts won't always cover every question possible for a unit, but they should cover many. Use Fast Facts for revision.

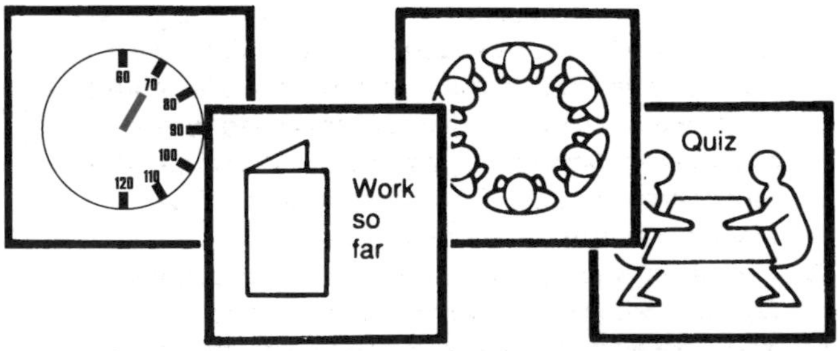

Another idea is to combine group discussion and Fast Facts to make up your own quiz game, along the lines of 'Trivial Pursuit'. Making revision fun can provide a good way of checking learning. Turning revision into a game may also remove anxiety.

Preparing for tests

You will need a lot of knowledge in your head to pass the test. Sometimes people imagine that getting this knowledge is like filling up a mug with water. The idea is to keep learning until the mug is full. Big mugs hold lots of water, little mugs can't hold so much. Sometimes people try to stretch their memory to hold lots of information – they try to become big mugs.

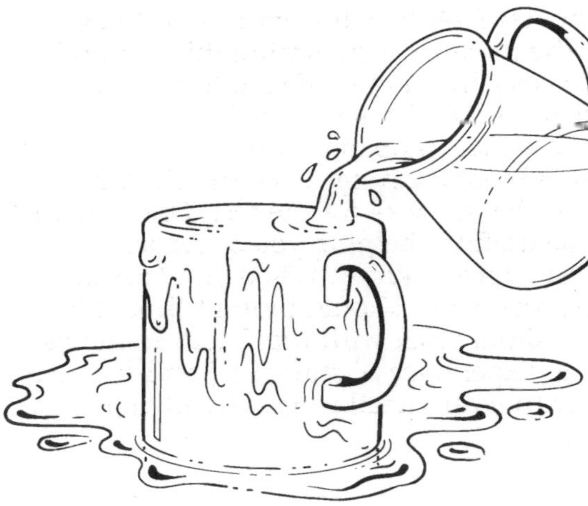

This idea of stretching memory is usually unnecessary and it makes taking a test a very unpleasant experience. In caring, it should not be necessary to 'strain' your memory.

For example, a student starting a placement may have lots of clients' and colleagues' names to remember. One idea could be to stretch the memory and go around trying to list all the names over and over again until they stick. Usually, carers do not do this. An alternative idea is to talk to each person and to get to know them one by one. After a while it becomes easy to remember all sorts of details about people. Their names become easy – and sometimes automatic – to remember, because names link to all the other details about the people. This kind of automatic knowledge feels natural; sometimes people feel that it just happens to them. It may be that this kind of learning is 'deeper' than the kind where a memory gets 'full up'.

GNVQ tests won't be as natural as remembering people on placement, but the ideas about learning may still work. If you have done project work, written assignments, shared ideas with other people, taken notes from other people's explanations and so on, then learning may feel more real and natural. This deeper learning may be interesting. It could even make the tests feel like a fun challenge, rather than an unpleasant pressure.

Whatever the test feels like, it is important to avoid 'overfilling' the memory – cramming things into it for a test. It is usually a better idea to learn from practical experience and then to use Fast Facts to help revise. Fast Facts probably won't work very well as starting points for learning. They should not be crammed into the memory for the test. One way that they might be useful is helping you to recognise things that you already know. When you look at a Fast Facts list, the words should prompt thoughts. The thoughts should link with the details under each 'fact' heading. Experience of studying Fast Facts may make it easier to recall detail when actually taking a test for a unit.

Self-assessment of knowledge about GNVQs

1. What are 'standards'? Why are standards used in assessment?
2. Why are standards sometimes difficult to understand at the beginning of a GNVQ programme?
3. Why is it necessary to produce evidence in order to be awarded GNVQ units?
4. What are action plans? Why is it important to keep records of action plans?
5. Can a person plan to get a Distinction or Merit grade and be confident of getting it?
6. What is needed in order to get a Merit or Distinction grade?
7. What is a portfolio? When should work on a portfolio start?
8. How might students prepare to take a GNVQ test?
9. Why is it important for GNVQ candidates to assess their own learning?
10. Why is 'reflection' useful when learning in health and social care?

Answers to these questions can be found below and on page 23.

Answers to self-assessment quiz

1. Standards are definitions of what has to be demonstrated and assessed in order to get GNVQ awards and qualifications. Standards don't explain what has to be studied – only what gets assessed. Standards provide an alternative to exam-based qualifications. Exam-based qualifications are like a competition; only the people who come top do

Getting there: the Health and Social Care Advanced GNVQ Game

Goal

The object of the game is to get to Distinction grade as quickly as possible and in as few moves as possible. If you feel competitive you can try and get there before other players. If you want a short game you can aim for just a Merit grade or even just a Pass grade!

Rules

1. Place your marker on the Start square at the start of the game.
2. Use only one six-sided dice.
3. Throw the dice and move up or sideways to the exact number thrown. You may choose to move in any up or sideways line, provided you stay on the board and you finish on the exact square that your dice throw indicates.
4. Skills squares give you an extra free go, and you can move diagonally to any square that is counted by your dice number. You may only move diagonally from a skills square.
5. You must keep a list of the 'evidence' you collect, and which squares don't provide evidence – try not to land on them.
6. Empty squares don't provide evidence – try not to land on them.
7. Hazard squares cause you to miss a turn – try not to land on them.
8. You have to collect evidence for each element on every unit that you will need for a 12-unit GNVQ. So you will need to land on three squares (marked M) for each numbered mandatory unit, and three squares (marked O) for your four options. You will also need to land on four element squares for Information Technology (IT), four element squares for Communication (C), and three element squares for Number (No.).
9. Only when you have recorded landing on all these squares can you get through the 'pass' barrier.
10. You must land on the eight different grading criteria squares marked Merit in order to get a Merit.
11. You must land on the eight different grading criteria squares marked Merit, and the eight different grading criteria squares marked Distinction to get a Distinction.
12. As soon as you have all the evidence for Merit or Distinction grade, and all the evidence for the necessary units, you have to throw a number that will take you across the 'pass' barrier. You have then won.

In real life the game is a little more complicated and usually takes two years to play.

GETTING THERE: THE HEALTH AND SOCIAL CARE ADVANCED GNVQ GAME

DISTINCTION ESTABLISH VALIDITY				M 7.3	DISTINCTION USE INFORMATION SOURCES		✹ SELF CONFI-DENCE			⚠ NO CAREER PLANS	PASS	MERIT	DISTINC-TION
	M 6.1		M 7.2			02.1	IT ELEMENT 3	03.1		M 6.3	PASS	MERIT	MERIT
		✹ USE OF THEORY					DISTINCTION SYNTHESIS			⚠ MISS A TUTORIAL	PASS	PASS	PASS
	DISTINCTION EVALUATION			02.3		DISTINCTION COMMAND OF LANGUAGE		✹ **APL** SYSTEMS		✹ LOG BOOK	⚠ NO INDEX IN PORTFOLIO	⚠ NO CLEAR CLAIM FOR GRADE	⚠ NO CLEAR CORE SKILLS INDEX
M 7.1			03.2		IT ELEMENT 2		M 6.2		03.3		04.1		⚠ NO LOG BOOK RECORDS
				✹ USE OF PLACEMENT EVIDENCE	M 8.1		No. ELEMENT 1	No. ELEMENT 2		DISTINCTION ACTION PLANS		04.2	
	M 5.2				M 8.2		MERIT SYNTHESIS	No. ELEMENT 3			MERIT JUSTIFICATION		04.3
		M 4.3				02.2		C ELEMENT 4				✹ REFLECTIVE THINKING	
⚠ CAN'T FIND STANDARDS	IT ELEMENT 1		M 4.2	C ELEMENT 3	M 4.1			DISTINCTION JUSTIFICATION			MERIT EVALUATION		IT ELEMENT 4
⚠ MISS A TUTORIAL				✹ PORTFOLIO DESIGN		⚠ CAN'T FIND REFERENCES				MERIT ESTABLISH VALIDITY			
	01.2	C ELEMENT 2	M 3.3		M 2.3				MERIT USE INFORMATION SOURCES				
C ELEMENT 1	M 3.1	M 3.2		M 2.2		M 5.1		MERIT MONITOR ACTION				MERIT COMMAND OF LANGUAGE	
M 1.1	M 1.2	01.1	01.3				✹ SELF ASSESS-MENT			⚠ NO GUIDANCE ON PLACEMENT			
START	M 1.3	M 2.1		⚠ MISS A TUTORIAL	⚠ NO NOTE TAKING SKILLS			M 5.3					M 8.3

Key:
M = Mandatory unit
0 = Optional unit
C = Communication (core skill)
IT = Information Technology (core skill)
NO. = Application of Number (core skill)
⚠ = Hazard square
✹ = Skills square
APL = Accreditation of Prior Learning

well. With standards, it only matters if people can demonstrate what's needed.

2 Standards often contain technical words and descriptions. People will need to know a great deal about an area before standards for that area can be easily understood. At the beginning of a programme, people often do not have the knowledge to understand what is meant by particular element and performance criteria statements. Understanding standards are part of the learning goals for GNVQ.

3 Assessment of standards requires evidence. The standards define what is needed for an award; evidence is the information that shows that individuals have done what was needed. They have reached 'the standard'. When all the appropriate standards have been reached, individuals have qualified.

4 Action plans enable individuals to work out how they will collect evidence to meet 'evidence indicators'. Action plans can also be used to plan assignments, practical demonstrations and placement and project work. Action plans might be useful in helping candidates to meet standards requirements. Action plans are necessary for Merit and Distinction grades, as candidates have to show skills in planning and in monitoring courses of action. Records of planning will be needed to provide evidence of planning and monitoring skills.

5 Yes! Candidates can work out what is needed and, provided they do the work and submit the necessary evidence, they should be able to guarantee the grade they want. GNVQs are not a competition – grades do not depend on some final assessment of group results. Candidates can get advice and guidance as they go through the programme, to ensure that they have the necessary evidence for Merits or Distinctions.

6 Evidence of independent action planning monitoring, use of sources, validity, justification, evaluation, synthesis and command of language.

7 A portfolio is a portable collection of evidence, including assignment work, which aims to demonstrate that national standards have been met. The portfolio will, therefore, include an index of assignment evidence, core skills and grading evidence. This will be used by assessors and verifiers who will check the quality of a candidate's work.

The portfolio will be complicated and work on it should start early in the programme. Leaving the design of the portfolio to the end of the programme may make it difficult to achieve Merit or Distinction grades. If the collection of evidence is regularly 'self-assessed' or checked, then candidates can change their work to ensure that it meets the requirements for these grades.

If the records are not kept, or not checked, then it may become too late to do the right kind of work at the end of the programme.

8 They should revise their own portfolio of evidence and assignments for the unit, discuss unit content with other people and make notes of their work! Discussion might help memory. Use the Fast Facts sections of this book as an aid to recognising concepts and ideas.

9 Good grades on GNVQ depend on reflection and self-assessment. Students have to provide enough evidence to meet the grading criteria. A good way to make sense of all this work is to self-assess the evidence before presenting it. The development of self-assessment skills would cover much of what is needed to meet the grading criteria.

10 Reflection is a skill which enables people to experiment with their ideas until the ideas work in a useful way. Reflection is a skill that will enable self-assessment and evidence collection.

Fast Facts

Action planning. Evidence has to be collected in order to pass a GNVQ. The collection of evidence needs to be *planned.* What action will produce enough evidence to demonstrate (pass) the standard? Action plans are the same as plans to get evidence. Evidence of good action planning helps towards Merit and Distinction grades.

Assessors These are the people who assess evidence to decide whether it meets the requirements of national standards. In other words, they assess work to see if it should pass. Assessors will also assess the grade of a GNVQ qualification when the portfolio is presented for assessment. Assessors will often be tutors or teachers.

Assignments Assignments are one way of collecting evidence to demonstrate (pass) an element or unit of GNVQ. Assignments should be planned and negotiated with an assessor or tutor.

Awarding body City & Guilds, BTEC or RSA will check the quality of courses and candidates' work. They award the GNVQ qualification (the National Council for Vocational Qualifications does not award qualifications – it designs and checks the national system).

Candidates People who collect evidence to get GNVQs are called candidates – they are candidates for assessment. Colleges call all people who study 'students', and 'students' and 'candidates' are the same.

Command of language To achieve Merit or Distinction grades, students must demonstrate an effective or fluent use of the terminology, ideas and concepts used within health and social care.

Concepts Concepts are ways of thinking which enable people to understand and make more sense of the world.

Core skills The skills of communication, application of number and information technology are needed to get the GNVQ qualification. They are assessed using evidence gathered to pass mandatory and optional units. Core skills of problem-solving, improving own learning and working with others can also be assessed.

Criteria Criteria are standards by which things are judged, i.e. measured.

Elements The smallest parts of standards to be assessed. *Units* are usually made up of three or four elements. Once an element is 'passed', it has to be collected with other elements to pass a unit.

Evaluation An advanced grading criterion. Evaluation will require the ability to judge or self-assess work in relation to criteria. Evidence should be *evaluated* by candidates in order to check that it meets the standards.

Evidence This is the key to passing a GNVQ and getting good grades. Evidence is information which confirms that a standard has been reached. Evidence can be gathered in assignments. There are many ways in which evidence can be presented, such as by video or tape recordings. Demonstration of skill can be observed and recorded to provide evidence. Tests also provide evidence of knowledge.

Evidence indicators Part of GNVQ standards. Each elements concludes with evidence indicators, for which evidence must be produced, but different assignments or projects may be designed to cover the indicators in different ways.

Grading GNVQs are graded Pass, Merit or Distinction. GNVQs cannot be failed, but they are not awarded or 'passed' until all the necessary units are passed. Merit or Distinction grades depend on extra evidence of performance with regard to grading criteria standards.

Grading criteria At Advanced level, candidates have to demonstrate the processes of action planning, monitoring, use of sources, validity, evaluation and justification. Students' work has to demonstrate an outcome of synthesis and command of language

Justification Advanced level grading criteria. Justification requires the ability to design an argument which supports the approach taken in practical and assignment work. Justification might be written alongside the evaluation of a piece work.

Knowledge The work covers information, facts, concepts, theories and also the way people use their ideas to guide their work. GNVQs in Health and Social Care will involve using knowledge in practical situations. Just remembering things won't be enough for most units.

Levels Both GNVQ and NVQ qualifications are structured in five levels: Level 1 is Foundation; Level 2 is Intermediate and equal to good GCSE qualifications; Level 3 is Advanced Vocational A-level; Levels 4 and 5 are graduate and post-graduate equivalents.

Mandatory unit Mandatory units are a fixed part of the GNVQ qualification. They have to be achieved or passed to get the GNVQ.

Methodology The approach taken, or methods used, to organise or design outcomes.

Monitoring Monitoring means checking what's happening. In GNVQs plans have to be monitored, or checked, and developed, in order to achieve Merit and Distinction grades. Monitoring links with self-assessment, where individuals check their evidence before having it assessed. A log book or notes will often be needed to provide evidence of monitoring.

NRA A National Record of Achievement.

NVQ National Vocational Qualifications are more narrowly focused than GNVQs. They are structured in different units, but designed with the same qualification levels as GNVQs.

Optional unit Advanced GNVQs have four optional units. These are not formally tested.

Performance criteria These define the performance necessary to reach the standard (or criteria) necessary to achieve an element. Performance criteria explain what is to be covered.

Planning A necessary part of all practical and assignment work. Independent planning forms part of the grading criteria for Merit and Distinction grades.

Portfolio A portable folder (or collection) of evidence. Action plans lead to the collection of evidence to meet unit requirements. All the evidence should be put together into a folder – or perhaps a file box if photos, tapes and videos are included. The portfolio can then be assessed and verified.

Programmes GNVQs are usually called programmes because units can be taken in any order, and passed in any order. Individuals could – at least in theory – take different pathways to achieving a GNVQ.

Qualification The whole Advanced GNVQ in Health and Social Care. GNVQ units are *not* qualifications.

Range Range provides details of what should be covered when providing evidence for an element.

Reflection A skill which helps in the process of evidence collection, self-assessment and planning. It is also a skill necessary in health and social care work.

Self-assessment Achieving Merit or Distinction grades will require candidates to monitor and evaluate their work. These skills require candidates to assess their own work before formal assessment takes place.

Skills Abilities which people have and can demonstrate. GNVQ standards cover instances of knowledge, skills, understanding and values.

Sources Use of sources is one of the advanced level grading criteria. Candidates have to show evidence that they have identified books, articles, databases, people to interview, places to visit, materials to use, etc. Evidence will often require a references or bibliography section at the end of an assignment. Further discussion of sources may also be required in review and action planning sections.

Standards The basis for assessment – national standards are all the unit, element, performance criteria, range and evidence indicator descriptions for GNVQ areas. Standards don't explain what must be studied, but they do explain what is to be assessed.

Synthesis Means putting things together to make a whole. In GNVQs, knowledge, understanding and skills have to be synthesised, or put together in order to achieve Merit or Distinction grades.

Tests Seven mandatory units are tested at present. Tests last about one hour, and involve multiple-choice questions.

Theory Theories are systems of ideas which interpret and explain things. Theory will involve the use of concepts. In health and social care work, it will often be necessary to use theory to interpret events. Theoretical knowledge will be needed to evidence the evaluation and justification grading criteria.

Tutorials A term for the discussions with a tutor or teacher which will guide action planning, evidence gathering and project work.

Understanding Deep or thorough knowledge and skill that can be used in many different circumstances and settings; also, practical knowledge that can be used to solve problems. GNVQ evidence will often show that concepts can be used in practice, or in practical situations.

Units The building bricks of qualifications. Units are the smallest part of a GNVQ to be awarded. They can be recorded in the NRA. Units are made up of elements.

Validity Advanced level grading criteria requiring candidates to check and self-assess their work. Validity requires evidence that details are checked and that arguments are supported. Evidence for validity might often be found within a candidate's assignment work.

Values Viewpoints which are the foundation of professional practice. Values are part knowledge and part skill. They are partly a skill because they have practical applications in decision-making. In health and social care, values are emphasised because other caring skills cannot work without them.

Verifier A person who checks assessments. When assessments are made of people's evidence, these assessments themselves have to be checked. The *internal verifier* checks a sample of tutors' assessment work within a GNVQ centre. The *external verifier* checks the operation of systems in GNVQ centres on behalf of the awarding body.

Reference

Kolb, D., Rubin, I., and McIntyre, J., 1979 (Third edition), *Organizational Psychology: an Experimental Approach*, New Jersey, Prentice Hall

Chapter 1

Legal rights and responsibilities in relation to equality of opportunity

Equality of opportunity, and the rights and responsibilities people have under equality of opportunity, as well as the ethical base underlying equal opportunities are important facets of all work in health and social care. This chapter gives you the opportunity to learn about the underlying principles. As well as studying this chapter you should draw on media coverage of these issues to develop your own understanding of the topics.

Principles which underpin equality of opportunity

All human societies, and large-scale social groupings, need to have rules or principles which establish how people are expected to behave in relation to other people. One of the oldest and most well known set of principles for regulating society is the 'Law of Moses', known as the Ten Commandments in the Old Testament of the Bible. These principles have established a foundation for Jewish, Christian and Islamic societies. They include rules about the importance of human life, 'Thou shalt not kill', laws about property, 'Thou shalt not steal', and laws about family life, 'Thou shalt honour thy father and mother' and 'Thou shalt not commit adultery'.

Foundational principles such as these provide a structure for the organisation of a society. However, whilst all effective societies must have principles, not all societies share the same principles. Even the importance of human life has not been accepted or seen in the same way by all human societies. There have been societies which have made a virtue of male aggression and where the social status of a man, including his right to marry and have children, has depended on the number of people he has killed. The philosophy behind this was that a high level of aggression would increase the military power of the society and enable it to conquer and exploit other societies. However, the lesson of history appears to be that a society which develops this way tends to become completely disorganised as individuals compete with each other. Far from achieving military dominance, such societies may collapse and be taken over by more socially cohesive and organised cultures.

Some societies have avoided the idea of property rights. Tools, clothes and equipment are 'owned' communally, i.e. people use things as they wish and as they need them – they do not belong to any individual. Such a principle might work, and it is possible to find examples of successful communities which share everything. The problem lies in organising very large-scale societies, with millions of people, so that everyone is fed, housed and has their basic needs met. Without the 'institution' or social belief in property rights there may be difficulties in organising a society.

The principles of equality and individual rights and choice are not merely simple ideas about being nice to others or about being 'good'. Like principles about the importance of life, or rules about property, equality and individuality are foundational values which will influence how a society functions.

Modern Western societies describe themselves as *democracies*. The democratic theory is that political power and economic control depend on the wishes of a majority of the population. The majority voice their wishes by electing a 'party' to power. The party then makes day-to-day decisions about the operation and regulation of society.

As a generalisation, a democracy depends on the principle of individuals having the freedom to voice differing political opinions. Democracy balances a wide range of individual freedoms with the general wishes of a *majority* (or 'greater number of people'). Respect for individual rights, and having individual rights to make choices, are an essential part of the principles which underlie a society organised as a 'democracy'.

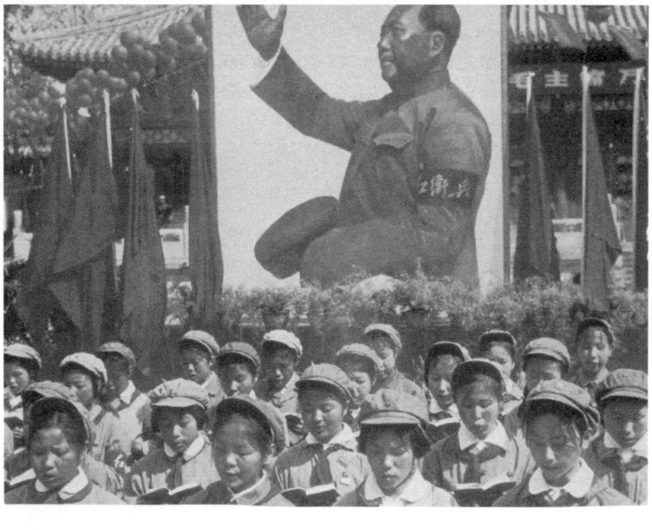

By contrast, centralised Communist societies do not organise themselves around principles of individual rights. In some recent Communist societies it was essential that people understood themselves not as individuals but solely as members of a large group. Conformity to group belief systems and behaviour patterns was seen as a foundational principle of some Communist societies. Sometimes the Communist system has been confused with personality cults.

Western democracies adopt the notion of competition as an organisational principle of society. Individuals must compete with one another to make money and achieve economic success. Part of this competitive ethic, or principle, is that no group should be discriminated against or prevented from the opportunity to compete. Equality of opportunity legislation is aimed at ensuring that factors like gender, race and disability do not exclude certain groups of people from the chance to compete. This principle of equality does not necessarily mean that every person has the same chance in the 'competition'. It is a principle of not excluding people because of their group membership or origins.

Another reason for equal opportunity principles relates to the multicultural nature of Western societies. Britain has been a society with a variety of religions, including people of different racial origins and different customs and practices, for many centuries. There is an argument that Britain has a long history of being multicultural (meaning, many customs, cultures and beliefs). For a multicultural society to function smoothly it may be important that the equality between different cultures, as well as individual rights, are respected.

These principles of democracy, individual rights and choice, and equality have resulted in laws aimed at promoting equality of opportunity. These principles and laws will influence how our society functions. From a care perspective, a person's rights to equality of care and individual rights are defined in the value base unit for National Vocational Qualifications (NVQ).

The value base for health and social care

Most professions have ethical codes or **value bases** which guide the behaviour of members of that profession. Care work is an area where values are particularly important. People often receive health or social care services because they are vulnerable. Clients may often be afraid, in pain, unhappy or just simply young and easy to influence. The value base is considered to be at the heart of NVQ qualifications in Care. Care workers are required to use 'caring values' in all of their work with clients. In the NVQ awards the value base is referred to as the 'O' Unit of Competence.

Elements of the NVQ value base 'O' Unit

- 'O' a Promote anti-discriminatory practice.
- 'O' b Maintain the confidentiality of information.
- 'O' c Promote and support individual rights and choice.
- 'O' d Acknowledge an individual's personal beliefs and identity.
- 'O' e Support individuals through effective communications.

Values need to be defined because they establish the expectations for all people who use the caring services. The 'O' Unit value base specifies how quality might be understood in care. A high quality of interpersonal care will mean that clients are not discriminated against. Information is treated as confidential; clients are empowered to make personal choices. Clients' personal beliefs and identity are respected and clients are supported through effective communication. Poor quality care may not maintain these principles.

Carers will be able to check and monitor their own work in relation to these care values. Most importantly, carers will be able to decide how they should behave towards clients using the value base to guide their actions. Clients and their relatives might be able to refer to the value base to establish whether an appropriate level of care is offered or not. The value base provides a set of principles that allows everyone to understand what they need to do and what is expected. The 'O' Unit provides a framework for the social care profession.

The 'O' Unit value base reflects the basic principles of equality, individual rights and choice. The 'O' Unit values go further in that they define what quality caring needs to involve. The values also offer principles to guide interpersonal interaction. (See Chapter 3.)

Without such basic principles and values as a framework, carers may be confused about what they are trying to achieve. Without principles and values it might be difficult to find constructive guidance as to the quality of care services. Without any principles at all, it is likely that society would be confused and disorganised. Social expectations, laws and trading arrangements would probably break down. Such a society might be very unpleasant indeed.

Individual and organisational responsibility under equal opportunity legislation

Equal opportunity is a concept which arises from legislation to address issues around direct and indirect discrimination. Originally the legislation was seen in terms of equal pay, gender, race and disability issues in employment. Equal opportunity has now been widened to include discrimination of *all* types, wherever it is found; for example, discrimination against those who are HIV-positive or who have AIDS, or on the grounds of sexuality or age. It is important to note that only discrimination in terms of gender, race and disability in the workplace have legislation to outlaw them.

In health and social care terms it could be argued that equal opportunities can be defined as 'the right of an individual to have access to provisions and services. All people should have equal access to services and opportunities, *irrespective of ability, age, ethnicity, gender, religion or sexuality.* All staff working within the health and social care setting need to take full responsibility for implementing the principles which underpin the concept of equal opportunity.

Each health and social care organisation has a responsibility to provide high quality care for every client. All organisations should have an equal opportunity policy or, at least, a statement of intent agreed by members of the organisation. This policy will outline the commitment of the organisation to honour the principles of equal opportunities.

However, having a policy which has been agreed and adopted by an organisation is one thing – implementing that policy may well be another! In order to be effective, a policy must be well known and understood by all members of staff within the organisation at all levels. This has implications for the recruitment and selection of staff, induction to the organisation when appointed and ongoing staff development for all staff to raise awareness of the issues.

It is important to remember that each individual has had a unique experience of life, i.e. two people who have been through the same life events will interpret their experiences differently. A person's interpretation will rely on past experience in order to make sense of new experiences. Interpretation of life events will also depend on the attitudes and values which have been learnt through the process of socialisation.

An individual's awareness of equal opportunities will also vary. Some people may have had a wide experience and have seen, or sadly experienced, discrimination and therefore will know the damaging effects this has on the individual. But others may have had very limited experience of religious intolerance, racism, sexism and abilism. (These are all terms used to describe discrimination against a particular group.) People who have experienced discrimination may have a clearer understanding and may be able to empathise with individuals, whereas people who have not experienced discrimination may have to work harder to try and understand the issues.

Managers in health and social care work have responsibilities to support staff individually and as a group, to help everyone to work in harmony to implement an equal opportunity policy – thereby upholding the core values of health and social care. Management must also have an effective monitoring system to ensure the policy is implemented consistently. There should also be clear guidelines stating what steps will be taken should the policy be infringed, i.e. a disciplinary procedure.

Individuals themselves have the responsibility to attend any staff development sessions and to reflect on their own attitudes and values in the light of that training. This can be a difficult and lengthy process. As awareness levels rise, individuals may be faced with the realisation that they have unwittingly been placing certain groups of people at a disadvantage. This can be painful for carers who might perceive themselves as 'caring' people which implies being understanding and supportive of others. This realisation may well be a threat to such a person's self concept or identity.

Colleagues must accept the responsibility to support others as they work to raise their awareness of the complex issues of equal opportunities. It is also important to take responsibility to challenge appropriately any incident of discrimination, should the situation arise. This may be particularly difficult if a colleague has negative attitudes to certain groups of people or individuals. For example, leaving a client until last 'because they are always complaining', refusing to take someone on a trip 'because they might become incontinent', avoiding giving an individual physical care 'because they are gay'. A colleague could be subtle in their discrimination yet the effect on the individual is still damaging.

Think it over

What would you do if a colleague makes discriminatory remarks about a client when working with you? You may wish to discuss this in a group and see what solutions you can propose. The difficulty is an ethical one as you are trying to balance your loyalty to a colleague, yet uphold the basic principles of care! It involves balancing the importance of friendship and a harmonious working relationship against supporting a possibly vulnerable client. The implications of any decision may have far-reaching effects for you, your colleague and the clients; but can you ignore the situation and hope that things will improve on their own?

Government charters, such as the Patient's Charter, outline the standards of service which should be a right for all service users. In this instance the responsibility lies with the hospital or trust to interpret the Patient's Charter, by stating what patients may expect from that particular hospital.

Think it over

Next time you visit your local hospital collect a copy of their Patient's Charter; note such things as the published waiting times in the out-patients department etc. Collect a copy of the government Further Education Charter and also the one from your college, or a copy of the Parents' Charter and the one published by your school. Note how each has interpreted the standards as set by the government; each will have used the government Charter as a basis for designing the service provided in their organisation. This will include recommendations on the ways in which a complaint may be lodged and how that concern will be dealt with.

As citizens in Britain today we are bound by the laws of the land. This means that we each have individual responsibility to uphold the law or face the legal consequences, which could include an appearance in court and a charge and sentence under a particular Act of Parliament. In terms of the laws relating to equal opportunities it will be useful to place each in an historical context, to gain a broader understanding of the many issues involved.

The historical background of equal opportunities legislation

A good starting point is 1942, when the **Beveridge Report** looked at the state of the nation. The Second World War continued until 1945 and the role of women had changed dramatically in order to take over work in the factories and on the land while the men (and some women) were in the forces. A radically new concept emerged from the Beveridge Report, which aimed to rid the country of what was termed the 'five giants' of *want, disease, ignorance, squalor* and *idleness*. The idea of the Welfare State had been conceived.

The Welfare State was set up to provide for the welfare of every citizen 'from the cradle to the grave'. The Education Act 1944 provided education for all from the age of 5 to 15 years. The National Health Service was created in 1948 to provide medical care and advice for all ages. This system included Social Services, dentists, general practitioners and pharmacists: no longer would poorer people suffer because of their inability to pay for medical help. Mothers would receive care and advice before, during and after the birth of their children. Children would be monitored by health visitors, and seen by doctors and dentists, to ensure their appropriate physical and mental development. Housing and social security benefits meant that those who were on low incomes, or were unemployed, had somewhere to go for advice and assistance. In all, the aim was to rebuild a nation following two devastating world wars: a nation where provisions and services were more widely available to all.

Many changes have taken place in the fifty years since the introduction of the Welfare State, not least in the rise in population and the change in the population in terms of the ethnic mix. Britain in the 1990s is a multicultural society; industry has become more complex and competition from around the world is greater. The demands on the Welfare State are very great compared to those of the 1940s; social values and roles have changed as society evolves to keep pace with events.

There is not space here to go into the detail of the many changes, but it may be helpful to have a basic awareness of the background to the current changes. You may find it useful to read about the development of the Welfare State to gain a better understanding of the issues.

In order to ensure that all members of society have equal opportunities in the workplace, several pieces of legislation have been implemented over the last thirty years in particular.

Equal Pay Acts

The rising number of women in the workforce, in the late 1960s and early 1970s, saw the introduction of

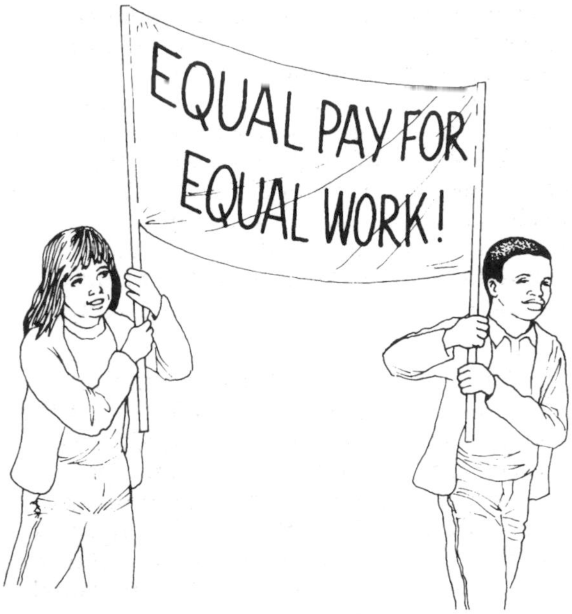

the **Equal Pay Act 1970.** This made it unlawful for firms to discriminate between men and women in terms of their pay and conditions in the workplace. This Act came about as a direct result of the Treaty of Rome (1957), Article 119, which stated that,

> *Each Member State shall during the first stage ensure and subsequently maintain the application of principle that men and women should receive equal pay for equal work.*

Later, the Equal Pay Act 1975 and the Equal Pay (Amendment) Regulations (1983) made it possible to claim equal pay for work which was considered to be of 'equal value' to that done by a member of the opposite sex. This, too, came about following proceedings by the European Commission against the British Government. This amendment to the original Act brought Britain further into line with mainland Europe.

Sex Discrimination Acts

The **Sex Discrimination Act 1975** built on the Equal Pay Act of 1970 by further ensuring that women were not discriminated against in education or employment on the grounds of their gender or marital status. It is interesting to note that the provisions of this Act apply equally to discrimination against both sexes. Women are the major beneficiaries, however, as they are more likely to face inequality on the grounds of their gender in the workplace.

The Sex Discrimination Act is concerned with the recruitment, training and promotion of employees, as well as other aspects of employment. In all these aspects it is essential that an employer does not discriminate against a person on the grounds of gender.

The Act established two forms of discrimination – direct and indirect – both of which are unlawful. *Direct discrimination* arises when a person of one sex is treated less favourably than another purely on the grounds of their gender. So it is unlawful to refuse to employ a woman because a position is a 'man's job'; for example, the position of school caretaker has in the past been seen as a man's job. If a woman applied for such a post and fulfilled all the relevant criteria, then she should be given equal consideration for the job; failure to do so could lead to a case being brought before a tribunal if the evidence is clear that the woman was not appointed solely because she was a woman.

Discrimination is illegal on the grounds of marital status for either sex. In the past, women who have childcare responsibilities were often seen as a potential liability to a firm or business. Under the Act it is illegal to take this into consideration to the detriment of the individual; for example, no questions should be asked at an interview regarding domestic or childcare arrangements. It has to be assumed that the person would not have applied for the job without considering the implications for their personal and family life. If an employer considers such a question to be important then they must ask all applicants and not just women; this is, however, most unlikely. Equally it is good practice to try and gain a gender balance on an interview panel where possible.

Indirect discrimination arises when conditions are applied which favour a person on one sex rather than another. If these conditions cannot be justified, then the employer is deemed to be acting illegally. For example, in 'Hurley v. Mustoe', the applicant for a waiter/waitress job was a woman with four young children. The manager decided to give her a trial but on the first night the proprietor of the restaurant asked her to leave. He said that it was against his policy to employ women with young children as he thought they were unreliable. The woman took her case to a tribunal, who ruled that she had been directly discriminated against on the grounds of sex contrary to Section 1(1)(a) and indirectly discriminated against on grounds of marital status contrary to Section 3(1) (b).

Equal Opportunities Commission (EOC)

At the same time as the Sex Discrimination Act was passed, the Equal Opportunities Commission (EOC) was set up to monitor, advise and provide information regarding the Sex Discrimination Act and its implementation. Individuals have the right to bring proceedings before an industrial tribunal should they face discrimination under this legislation. Help and advice is obtainable from the EOC should an individual feel that they have a case.

The EOC has issued a document, 'Guidance on Employment Advertising Practice'. This document helps employers to consider appropriate wording for advertising jobs. Appropriate wording is essential to remain within the law. It is unlawful to advertise a post in such a way as to discriminate against one sex in favour of another. The use of terms such as waitress, barman, steward and postmistress imply that applicants should be either male or female.

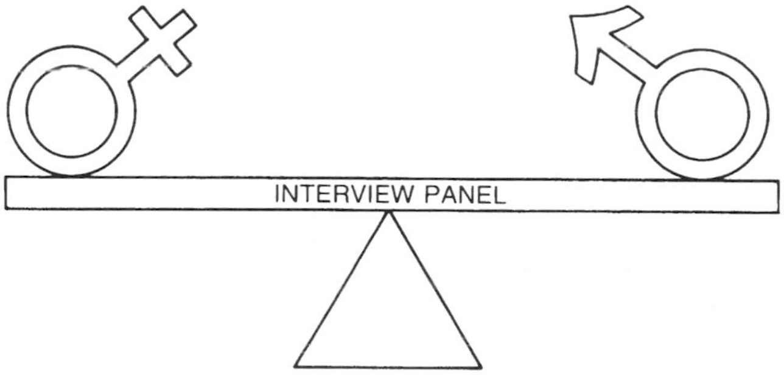

Figure 1.1 Achieving a gender balance on the interview panel is one of the principles of good recruitment practice

Following the EEC Equal Treatment Directive (76/207/EEC), major amendments were made to the Sex Discrimination Act 1975. These amendments affected discrimination in collective agreements, employment for the purpose of private households, employment in firms with five or fewer employees and retirement age. All were brought together to widen the scope of the original Act and to bring Britain in line with mainland Europe through the **Sex Discrimination Act 1986.** The EEC Directive also means that decisions made by the British courts and tribunals are subject to the overriding views of the European Court of Justice applying Article 119 of the Treaty, and the Equal Pay Directive. In the event of any disputed interpretation of these issues, it is European Law which will apply.

In 'Worringham v. Lloyd's Bank', female clerical officers under the age of 25 were not required to contribute to a pension scheme. However, male clerical officers under the age of 25 were required to contribute 5 per cent of their salary to the scheme. To compensate for this, male staff were paid 5 per cent more than female staff. The Equal Pay Act (Section 6) (1A) (b) excluded terms relating to death or retirement, or any provision made in relation to death or retirement. Contributions to a pension scheme are therefore outside the scope of the Equal Pay Act.

The female clerical officers took their case to the European Court of Justice as they considered that they were not being afforded equal pay and conditions. The European Court of Justice ruled that, under Article 119, there was an enforceable Community right on all individuals within the EEC. The right to equality of pay meant that the Bank was in violation of Article 119 which took precedence over the Equal Pay Act: the female staff won their case!

Race Relations Acts

In the same way that Europe influenced British social policy in terms of discrimination on the grounds of sex, so it did with race. The treaty of Rome 1957 made it unlawful to discriminate against EEC workers on grounds of nationality and citizenship.

The British government introduced the **Race Relations Act 1965** which made it unlawful to discriminate on the grounds of colour, race, ethnic or national origins in places of public resort. The Act also made it an offence to incite racial hatred. The Race Relations Board was set up to enforce the law, acting as a 'watch-dog'. A Local Government Act 1966 made money available to local authorities for work with 'immigrants' from the New Commonwealth. Some of this money was used to create 'section eleven' posts to meet specific need, for example to pay for staff to support learning in schools and colleges.

The 1965 Act was replaced by the **Race Relations Act 1968.** The provisions under the Act were widened to include areas of employment, education, and the provision of housing and services.

This law was repealed by the introduction of the **Race Relations Act 1976.** This law, currently in force, seeks to close several loopholes left by previous legislation. Modelled closely on the Sex Discrimination Act, the Race Relations Act 1976 identifies direct and indirect discrimination in the area of race.

Direct discrimination occurs when a person treats another person less favourably because of their 'group membership'. In the case of racial discrimination, the actual race of the person discriminated against is immaterial. It is possible, for example, for Jonathan to discriminate against Stuart on the grounds of Jamal's colour: i.e. Jonathan may dismiss Stuart in order to give Jamal a job because Jamal is black. Stuart would win his case for unfair dismissal at a tribunal under Section 1 (1)(a) of this Act.

Equally, it is unlawful to segregate a person on racial grounds, as this constitutes less favourable treatment. Providing separate facilities for black and white staff is unlawful. However, if a group of black care staff negotiate to work together on a particular shift that is acceptable – unless the manager states that all black staff should work a specific shift. The former is negotiated by choice, the latter imposed by reason of race.

Indirect discrimination occurs when a condition(s) is applied which places people from one race in a more advantageous position than people of another race. Any criteria for a job which an applicant 'must' have is deemed discriminatory if it disadvantages a person of one race in favour of another. If a firm can demonstrate that the requirements or conditions are justified, then the complaint will not succeed. For example, in 'Panesaar v. Nestle & Co Ltd.' a factory rule prohibited beards and long hair. This was seen as indirect discrimination against the applicant who was a Sikh. However, the Court of Appeal held that the condition was justified on the grounds of hygiene and safety.

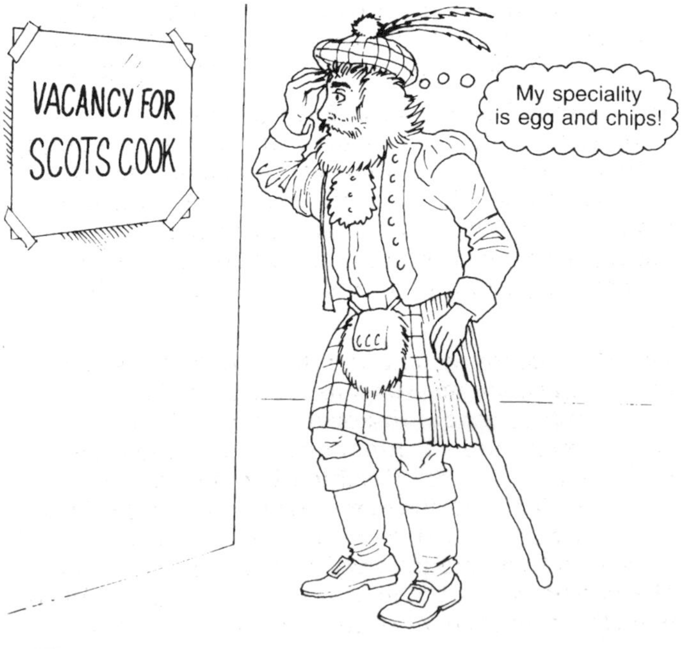
VACANCY FOR SCOTS COOK
My speciality is egg and chips!

The Race Relations Act makes it unlawful to discriminate on *racial grounds*. The Act defines racial grounds as being colour, race, nationality or ethnic or national origins. A House of Lords ruling in 'Ealing Borough Council v. Race Relations Board', held that the term 'national origins' meant race rather than citizenship. This is now overruled, being replaced by the term 'nationality' to cover both meanings.

This is a complex issue, as was demonstrated by a much publicised debate about an advert for a 'Scots cook'! It was ruled that it was unlawful to advertise in this way and it was suggested that the advert should read, 'a person skilled in Scottish cooking'!

The debate centred on whether Scotland is a separate nation, or an ethnic or racial group. This is a matter of concern for several groups. The Act does not appear to cover religion as such, which can cause confusion. Are all Muslims deemed to be of the same racial, ethnic or national origins? What about Hindus, Christians or Jews? The law as it stands is not very clear.

In 'Mandla v. Dowell Lee', the House of Lords held that the term 'ethnic' was appreciably wider than 'race'. What constitutes an ethnic group? Under the Act, such a group must be able to demonstrate particular characteristics:

a they must have a long history shared and kept alive by all its members
b a cultural tradition with shared social traditions and customs.

Other factors which may be relevant include:

- a common geographical origin or common ancestors
- common language (this may not necessarily be peculiar to the group)
- common literature
- common religion different from their neighbouring groups
- being either a minority or a dominant group within a large community.

An example of a racial group using these criteria would be Sikhs. They share common religious beliefs, have social customs and traditions which are shared by all.

The 1976 Act denotes important exemptions, such as 'positive action'; for example, a Social Service

Department wishing to recruit a social worker to have responsibility for meeting the needs of a particular ethnic group. It is perfectly acceptable within the law for positive action to be taken to advertise the post by stating that the post is for someone from that particular ethnic group. The rationale for this is that a person from the same ethnic group will have a better understanding of the needs of the group. The person will therefore be in a more favourable position to identify and meet those needs. This is covered by Section 5 ,'genuine occupational qualifications'.

Commission for Racial Equality (CRE)

The Race Relations Act 1976 abolished the Race Relations Board and set up the Commission for Racial Equality (CRE). This body monitors the Act, acts as an adviser and has extensive powers to investigate discrimination. Individuals have new rights to bring proceedings before an industrial tribunal should they be the victims of discrimination. The CRE may be asked to give information to an individual who wishes to take a case to a tribunal.

Disabled Persons Acts

Legislation is also available for people with disability. **The Disabled Persons (Employment) Act 1944** and **1958** lay down the main provisions for the legal obligations placed on employers towards people with disabilities. The Acts were initially passed to support the many men who returned from the Second World War with disabilities.

The Disabled Persons Act produced a requirement that all companies employing twenty people or more should ensure that 3 per cent of the workforce were registered as disabled. A register of disabled people was set up, as were records to demonstrate that the Act was being complied with. Designated employment by the Secretary of State included car park attendants and lift attendants.

Certain exemptions were made to the Act. This included special industries where the employment of people with disabilities might be hazardous, for example the steel and mining industries, steeplejacks etc. It is also possible for a special permit to be obtained if a firm can show that the work is unsuitable for people with disabilities, or that the firm has not reached its quota because few people with disability had applied. Few cases have ever been brought under this Act. A special Advisory Committee hears the case from the employer before deciding whether to prosecute. Persuasion is considered to be a better policy than compulsion!

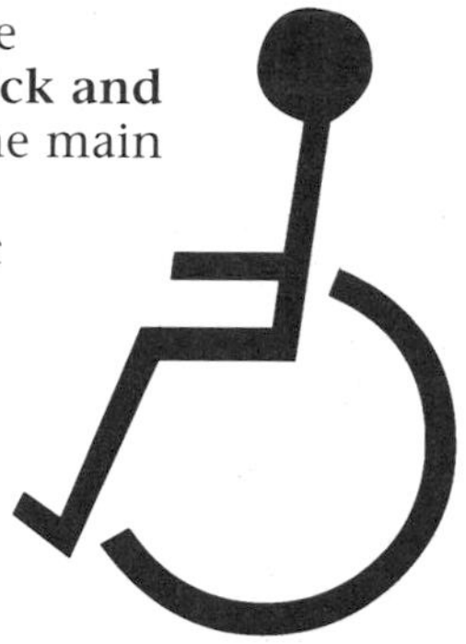

The Acts of 1944 and 1955 were followed by the **Chronically Sick and Disabled Persons Act 1970.** The main focus of this legislation was to ensure physical access to public buildings and educational establishments, to maintain parking spaces, provide toilets for people with physical disabilities and to provide appropriate signs.

This Act was amended by the Chronically Sick and Disabled Persons (Amendment) Act 1976 to ensure that the provisions outlined above were extended to places of employment.

The Companies (Directors' Report) (Employment of Disabled Persons) Regulations 1980, states that companies which employ more than 250 people (on average over a year) must include a statement in the Directors' Report regarding company policy on recruitment, training, career development and progression of people with disability within the company.

What was then called the Manpower Commission produced a Code of Good Practice on the Employment of Disabled people in the 1980s. This document had no legal status but it did foster good practice for the employment and training of people with disability. It set out clear aims and objectives which could be incorporated into company policy.

The **Disabled Persons Act 1981** places a responsibility on the providers of premises to comply with standards set by the Code of Practice, for access for disabled people in buildings (British Standards Institute). This legislation also covers highways, placing an obligation on highway authorities to '... have regard to the needs of disabled and blind persons'.

The EEC Recommendation (OJL 86/225/43) states that appropriate measures to '... provide fair opportunities for the disabled in the field of employment and vocational training', should be made. This led to the **Disabled Persons (Services, Consultation and Representation) Act 1986.** This Act requires that people with disability, or their representatives, are involved in planning their care. The person with disability or the carer has a right to request an assessment of their need for services.

It gives the person with disability the right to representation by another person, for example to have an advocate. It places the responsibility on the local authority to provide the necessary resources to meet the needs of people with disability within their area.

Think it over

Heather, a black woman in her mid-twenties, has multiple sclerosis which is a degenerative disease affecting the covering (sclera) of the nerves supplying muscle. The condition means that Heather experiences weakening of some muscle resulting in loss of movement. Heather does go into remission from time to time, when all symptoms disappear. Currently the condition has worsened, resulting in Heather having difficulty in speaking and moving as the muscles in her larynx and legs are affected.

Under the current legislation Heather has the right to request an assessment of her physical needs by a social worker, who will liaise with an occupational therapist to identify her need for a wheelchair and any adaptations in her home to allow for her independence.

The social worker will liaise with the district nurse to ensure that Heather's physical requirements are met in terms of hygiene and medical care. A bath attendant may be called to assist with personal hygiene, and a home carer to offer support with getting up and going to bed if there are no family members able to assist Heather. 'Meals on Wheels' may be organised or a stay in respite care facilities, to relieve relatives for a week or two during the year.

A plan of action to meet Heather's physical and social needs will be drawn up to include the above network of support. Her cultural, intellectual and emotional needs will need to be addressed by any such care plan.

As Heather has difficulty in speaking because of her condition, she may nominate a relative or friend, or request a social worker, to act on her behalf as an advocate. This person works with Heather to gain help and advice, attending hospital or meetings with her to speak on her behalf. Any decisions are made by Heather in conjunction with her advocate; she does not give up any of her legal rights.

The **NHS and Community Care Act 1990** builds on the legislation outlined above for people with disability. It is widened to take into account all people in need of care in the community. The Act ensures that all individuals in need of care have the right to be assessed for services to meet their need. A care manager works to meet individual need by providing a 'care package' for each individual. The Act also ensures that all individuals have a right to complain about services. Greater detail regarding this far-reaching legislation is given in Chapter 15.

Children Act 1989

Children have rights within the law. The Children Act 1989 followed several well-publicised cases of child abuse and seeks to simplify the great complexity of child care law. The law applies to all statutory and voluntary organisations providing care for children and their families. It is essentially a balancing act between the rights of the child and the parents and the duty of the state to protect children deemed to be in need or at risk.

Children in need are defined as, '.... children whose health and welfare may suffer significantly without support from social services.' Any child with a disability is automatically deemed to be in need. The local authority must provide services to meet identified need, for example nurseries and family centres.

Race and culture are, for the first time, recognised as essential factors to be given consideration. Local authorities must carefully consider a child's race, religion, language and culture when deciding on fostering, day or residential care services. Department of Health guidelines state that day care services should promote the self-esteem and racial identity of the child. Any provider of child care services must be able to satisfy the local authority that they are able to meet the racial and cultural needs of the children in the area, in order to gain registration.

The Act requires local authorities to 'take preventive steps', to ensure that children may live as normal a life as possible. Care must be taken to ensure that children are safe from suffering and that disabilities are minimised. Care must also be taken to ensure that children do not commit offences, so avoiding the need for placing them in secure provision.

Other key features of the Act lie in a principle termed **paramountcy.** This term means that the child's welfare is paramount (the most important issue). Any decision made about the child has to be made in the child's best interest. Where a child is either mature enough or old enough, they have a right to be consulted about their wishes. These wishes must be given priority.

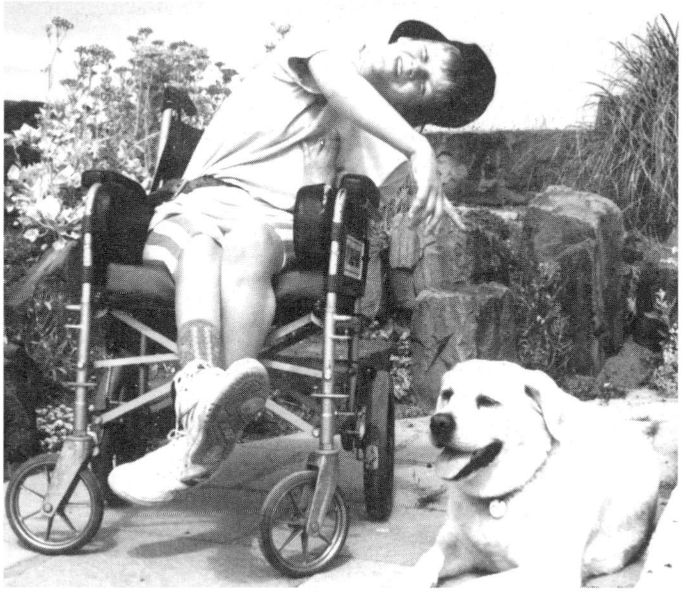

Figure 1.2 A child's own wishes must be given priority (*Photo courtesy of Winged Fellowship Trust*)

The Act requires caring agencies and parents to work in partnership. Both work to plan and organise to meet the needs of the child at all stages. Parents are also still responsible for their child, even when that child is living in a local authority establishment. Any person may apply to be deemed responsible for the child, such as a friend or relative if it is appropriate; for example, the grandmother of a boy orphaned whilst his parents were on holiday in Eastern Europe.

Collaboration between parents, child care agencies and the child is essential to meet the needs of the individual child at all stages.

The Department of Health produces a useful series of booklets about the Children Act.

The Children Act and Local Authorities – A Guide for Parents (CAG1)
The Children Act and You – A Guide for Young People (CAG3)
The Children Act and Getting Help from Social Services (CAG5)
The Children Act and the Courts – A Guide for Children and Young People (CAG6)
Living Away from Home, Your Rights – A Guide for Children and Young People (CAG7)

The UN Convention on the Rights of the Child was formalised by international agreement to protect the rights of children. This was in response to concerns raised across the world about the rights of children being ignored or forgotten.

The articles (statements) identify the rights of all children in the world, whether rich or poor, up to the age of 18. Three main rights were stated:

1. All rights apply to all children whatever their race, sex, religion, language, disability, opinion or family background. In other words, there will be no discrimination. (*article 2*)
2. Adults must always consider the best interests of the child when making decisions for them. (*article 3*)
3. Children must be listened to carefully and their opinions heard. Courts must take note of a child's wants and feelings. (*article 12*)

Other rights include civil and political rights, economic, social, cultural and protective rights. All are important issues which should be part of good child care practice. For example, Article 24 states that children have the right to live in a safe, healthy and unpolluted environment. Article 18 notes that children should have proper care from day to day with the family, but with government support if necessary. Article 20 looks at the day-to-day care with other families, or in a children's home if there is no family. Due respect must be taken of a child's race, religion, culture and language when a new home is sought.

Think it over

Does this sound familiar? You can clearly see how important this UN Convention was when looking again at the Children Act 1989!

You may wish to obtain a booklet, *The Rights of a Child – A Guide to the UN Convention* (CAG9), from the Department of Health, to further your understanding.

The implications of the Children Act for those working in health and social care are great. Children must be provided with a safe environment where they may grow and develop to their full potential. That environment must acknowledge the child's race and culture, religion and language. This is essential for the child to develop a positive self-esteem, which will enable the child to grow into a confident adult, able to take his or her place in society.

Charters

The British government has produced a series of charters which aim to improve a wide range of services. A **Parents' Charter** looks at education, denoting performance indicators which a school must make public; for example, exam results and truancy rates. It looks at the rights of parents when they consider the education they require for their child.

The **Patient's Charter** looks at the Health Service, again noting performance criteria; for example, the waiting time in an out-patient department. It sets targets in order to improve the quality of care available. The Charter outlines complaints procedures throughout the hospital. An ombudsman for health can be contacted if there is concern about administration, but would not deal with complaints about professional malpractice. In such a case there will be an independent review, with reports sent to the Regional Health Authority.

Concerns about doctors (GPs), dentists, opticians and pharmacists go through the Family Health Services Authority. The Community Health Council is available for advice on matters concerning community health. If required they will attend a tribunal to support a complainant.

There is a **Citizen's Charter** which aims to work for better quality in public services: to offer more choice and to ensure that all know the kind of service that they have a right to expect. Each charter also states what can be done if the service provided does not meet the expected standard.

Other Charters cover **further education** and **higher education.** They outline the criteria to ensure high quality services are provided. They look at the way each service identifies and works to meet the needs of its service users, and review the complaints procedures.

Consistencies and inconsistencies in the rights of individuals under equality of opportunity legislation

As stated earlier, the law clearly provides for people on the grounds of race, gender and disability. There is an organisation to deal with race and gender issues with a specific brief to provide information about rights under the respective Acts and to offer support for any individual who may wish to take a case to an industrial tribunal.

Organisations are increasingly aware of the areas of race and gender and work to promote equality of opportunity, with varying degrees of success (as has been highlighted earlier). Test cases under these Acts are well reported in the press, which keeps the issues in high profile.

Yet, despite this, women often have difficulty obtaining senior posts – even when they comprise the majority of the work force in a particular field of employment. There are many more women than men currently employed in the caring professions but, if you review the senior posts in health and social care organisations, it is often men who are in the most senior positions! In the same way, people with non-English sounding last names may find they are not invited for job interviews. All of which shows inconsistency in what the law might be seen as intending to happen and what is in reality happening at present.

To gain further understanding of inconsistencies in the opportunities available to individuals, we will look at two aspects in particular in this chapter: disability and sexuality. The first one has given rise to legislation to promote equality; the latter has little.

Disability

Public attitudes and opinions play a significant part in government decision making. Much pressure has been applied over the years to ensure equal pay and equal rights for individuals on the grounds of race and gender. But the public attitude to those with any kind of disability has been (and continues to be) ambiguous. Many of the general public see people with disabilities either as objects to be pitied or as a drain on national resources, as they may require help from the State rather than being a productive member of society contributing to the economy.

A brief historical perspective on disability issues will help to place the current situation in context.

Historical perspective

During the nineteenth century the response to people with disability began to alter and with it came a change in public attitude.

The Poor Law Amendment Act of 1834 created the Poor Law Commission, which decreed that all aged and infirm people ('the deserving poor') should be separated from the able bodied. Medical science had improved in leaps and bounds. Institutions were created offering specialist treatment. Education for children with disability included residential care, and the 'medical model' of disability was born.

This model viewed people with disability as patients who needed treatment and nursing care. Patients were seen as having limited potential and therefore had limited opportunities. They were also seen as in need of 'protection' from the general public.

The enormous number of young disabled soldiers returning from the First World War became a turning point once more. Society valued people with active productive lives, so what was to become of these returning 'damaged' young men? The government response was to create special workshops, have 'reserved' occupations such as lift and car park attendants, and to ensure reserved places on public transport.

The Second World War saw yet another change. This time there were relatively few men returning with disabilities. The key factor was the economic situation, which promised a prolonged boom yet was coupled with a chronic shortage of labour. This created a market-driven force to find ways to employ those with disabilities. There were, however, problems as the new improved machinery, the enforced discipline and time keeping, were not always suitable for those with disability.

It was also during this time that the Welfare State was created, as great strains were placed on families trying to support someone with disability.

Various attempts to redress the balance for people with disability have been made to date. But it is interesting to note that a post for Minister for Disability was not created until 1974! There are two important events to note. In 1977, Alf Morris MP, as Minister for the Disabled, set up a Committee to review the impact of the Chronically Sick and Disabled Persons Act 1970. The findings, published in 1979, reported that there was little awareness of the Act and little improvement in access. Consequently, recommendations were made to have mandatory building codes to improve access.

The second issue was the creation of the Committee on Restrictions against Disabled People (CONRAD) in 1979. The remit was to examine the exclusion of people with disability and to propose ways to combat it. The Committee presented its report in 1982, recommending that broad anti-discriminatory legislation should be adopted. Successive Conservative governments since then have opposed this, despite a series of attempts from MPs like Jack Ashley.

In 1985 the Voluntary Organisation for Anti-discrimination Legislation (VOADL), comprising representation from voluntary organisations for the disabled, was established to co-ordinate lobbying activities. They have been instrumental in bringing about the Civil Rights (Disabled People) Bill which was introduced as a Private Members Bill at the end of 1991, reaching its second reading in February 1992. The Bill was reintroduced in 1993 as a Private Members' Bill by Dr Roger Berry MP (Labour).

An intensive campaign to gain public support included wide use of the media and the distribution of over 250,000 postcards in support of the Bill, in addition to lobbying in Parliament. The Minister for Disabled People was forced to offer a series of further consultations on measures to fight discrimination and to provide:

- possible legislation for employment
- a Code of Practice for the insurance industry
- the extension of building regulations
- the establishment of a new advisory body on disability.

Time will tell what the outcome of these consultations will be!

There is no real 'watch-dog' for people with disabilities in the way that the EOC and CRE oversee gender and race issues; although there are many charities for specific conditions which work tirelessly to raise public awareness. The main issue is that, to date, there has been no monitoring of legislation for people with disability – so any legislation lacks 'teeth'. Public attitude to people with disability will have to change to support pressure groups like VOADL if the current Bill is to be made law and enforced.

Sexuality

It has been said that the last great taboo in society today is sexuality. *Homophobia* (an irrational fear of anyone who is gay) is still rife in Britain. It is a fear based on ignorance, viewing others who conduct their lives in different ways as socially deviant and therefore social outcasts.

In recent years there has been increased pressure from members of the gay community to raise public awareness of the discrimination faced by gay and lesbian people. Legal action has been taken by men and women against the armed forces for their dismissal on the grounds of homosexuality. This is seen by the leaders of the armed forces as being incompatible with service life.

Pressure groups have also lobbied Parliament, resulting earlier in 1994 in a law that reduced the age

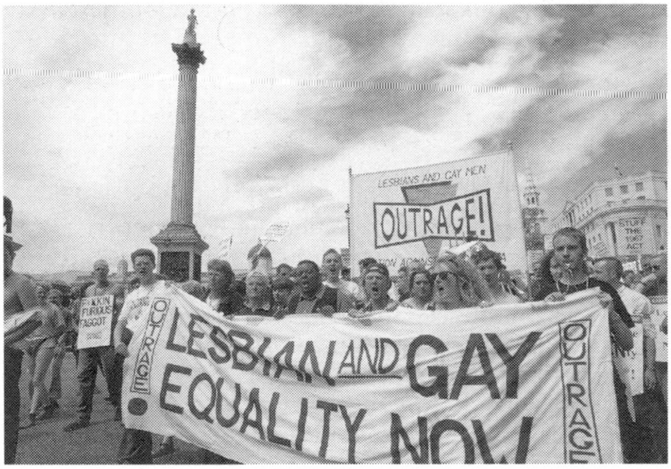

of consent for homosexual acts between consenting males in private from 21 to 18 years. It had been hoped to reduce the age of consent to 16 years, which would be in line with heterosexual relationships. There is no law covering an age of consent for homosexual females.

Other inconsistencies in equal rights

In the same way that people with disabilities may be denied equality of opportunity, older people may also be viewed as a drain on resources rather than as contributors to the economy. In some cultures older people are revered for their wisdom, but this is not necessarily the case in Britain. Here, the elderly are frequently stereotyped as being physically and often mentally incapable of caring for themselves or of making clear decisions about their lives.

On retiring from paid employment at the designated age of 60 or 65 years, a person is perceived as being different. In periods of recession organisations often bypass more experienced older applicants in favour of younger, less experienced, and therefore cheaper applicants for the job. This may leave an older applicant feeling devalued and robs the organisation of that person's experience and expertise.

Recently publicised cases of patients who require expensive long term treatment being denied the right to register with a particular general practitioner, or gaining access to hospital treatment, may further highlight the potential inconsistency between what care principles require and what the market forces in the current economy are willing to provide.

Other examples of inconsistencies in equal rights for all include the many people with learning difficulties or mental health problems now living in the community. Many of these people have lived some considerable time in institutions, being completely 'cared' for. The transition from institution to independence in the community with, at times, little active support, has resulted in several tragedies in recent years and raised public concern about safety under community care. It begs the question of the rights of these individuals to dignity and support if economics appear to be the main concern!

In terms of religion, history very clearly shows the effects of religious intolerance with, for example, the rise of anti-semitism leading to the Holocaust in Germany during the Second World War. It is therefore vitally important to combat discrimination on the basis of religion. Education may play its part here by making provision for pupils from different religions, for example in colleges providing a quiet room for prayer for Muslim students and staff. Schools can ensure that books, pictures, music, celebrations, customs and food encourage awareness and the value of all religions. The idea is to raise awareness and understanding rather than to convert children to any particular religion. In the home each family will raise their children in a particular culture or religion until such time as the children are able to make their own informed decisions about their faith and customs.

Routes by which individuals may seek redress under equality of opportunity legislation

In terms of employment, workers who consider that they have been discriminated against have several avenues which they may explore. Information regarding the individual's rights may be obtained from the Commission for Racial Equality, if the issue is regarding race, or the Equal Opportunity Commission if the discrimination was on the grounds of gender – for either male or female employees.

A questionnaire has to be completed and returned within three months of the alleged incident. The next stage is then to go before an industrial tribunal or county court. In the event of the discrimination being direct and intentional the industrial tribunal or county court can award damages and make recommendations and a declaration of the law.

An incidence of discrimination on the grounds of race or gender which is outside employment may also be addressed by an industrial tribunal or county court. If the discrimination was direct and intentional then, again, the industrial tribunal or county court can award damages and make recommendations and a declaration of the law.

In either case, if the direct or indirect discrimination is proven to be unintentional, then the industrial tribunal or county court can only make a declaration and/or recommendations; but no damages can be awarded.

Other routes to gain information regarding individual rights may be gained by visiting the local Law Centre or the Citizens' Advice Bureau. Trade unions will also be able to offer advice to their members.

It is possible to appeal against a decision made by an industrial tribunal or county court. An appeal can only be made on a point of law to the Employment Appeal Tribunal. Any such appeal must be made within six weeks of the decision being given. In certain circumstances the case may be passed to the House of Lords and, finally, to the European Court in Luxembourg.

There is an Ombudsman for health and social care. The role is to consider any complaint about the service provision in this area. If an individual considers that his or her legal rights have been infringed, or that there has been unfair treatment or maladministration, then the Ombudsman may consider the case – unless it has already been to a court of law or industrial tribunal.

The Ombudsman will require full details of the situation and will try to settle the dispute between the two parties. Failure to achieve this means that the Ombudsman will make a decision on the information received. Any decision made may be accepted or rejected; in the latter case the decision will lapse and the individual may take legal action against the organisation.

As stated earlier, organisations will have an equal opportunity statement or policy. Government Charters will have been interpreted by the organisation to form the basis for their own Charter or standards. These will include the method for making a complaint and the time element involved.

Most professional bodies have a code of practice for their staff; perhaps one of the best known is the Hippocratic Oath taken by doctors. The British Association of Social Workers, the United Kingdom Central Council and the British Psychological Society all provide such guidelines for staff, to name just a few.

Residential care, too, has seen a series of reports and codes of practice to ensure clients' rights and the quality of service are maintained. The **Wagner Report** stated that people moving into residential care should have real choices. These rights and choices include: the continued right as a citizen, for example, to vote in local and government elections etc; having access to community services and the right to complain if need be; the right to manage their own affairs, including their pensions; the right to make decisions and, where this is not possible, the right to a six-monthly review; and the right to have their cultural needs met.

In 1986 **Home Life: A Code of Practice for Residential Care** was introduced. This stated that clients have the right to: individuality, dignity, esteem, fulfilment, autonomy, be able to take risks, have a quality of experience and have emotional needs met through personal/intimate relationships, if they wish.

Community Life 1990 went a step further by saying that all care packages should reflect the informed choice of the client. Individuals should know their rights and responsibilities. They have the right to an advocate, and to make complaints if required. This placed responsibility on the providers

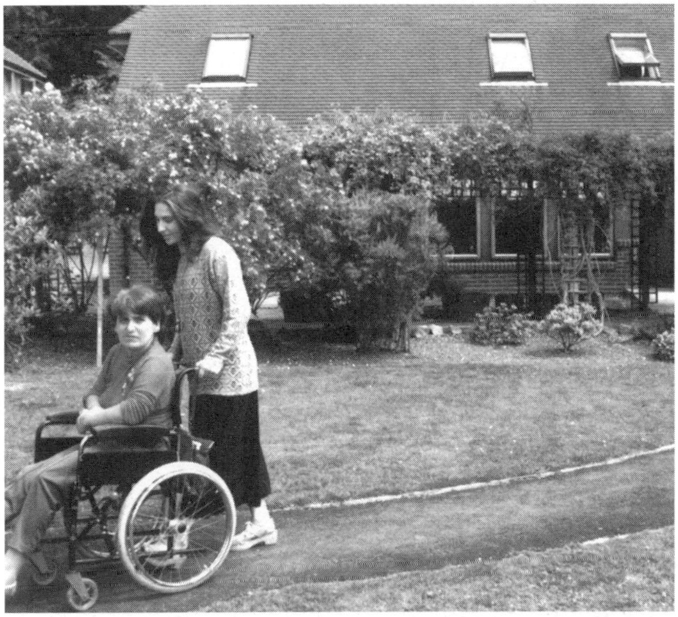

Figure 1.3 People in residential care have rights and choices
(*Photo courtesy of Winged Fellowship Trust*)

of services to ensure that a complaints procedure was implemented and that provision for advocates was made. Providers have to ensure that all the service users are aware of possible choices and the potential outcomes of those choices. This also meant that clients could decide to take a calculated risk: for example, to make their own cup of tea despite some physical difficulty. The provider should take all necessary steps to minimise the risk but not prevent it.

Complaints procedures are made available to all service users; for example, a complaint regarding the service in a residential home would be made to the manager. Should the service user remain unsatisfied, the next step is to refer to the Social Services Department or to the Registrar of Residential Establishments (the person who registers such establishments).

If it is a member of staff who has a complaint, this would be addressed to the immediate line manager. The staff member may wish to take the matter to the union for advice and guidance before taking the matter up with the employers. Should the case be one of discrimination on grounds of race or gender, then the matter may be referred to a tribunal as described earlier.

Evidence collection point

Produce a report, choosing one issue from the range covering the principles of equal opportunity legislation, describing its importance to workers in health and social care. Outline the responsibility of the organisation and the individual worker to uphold these principles. Review any consistencies or inconsistencies which may be found. Give details of any system of redress available to individuals under each area of the range. Explain three of the factors which influence the formation of equality of opportunity legislation, giving one example of each.

Factors which influence the formation of equality of opportunity legislation

As has been stated earlier in this chapter, there are many factors which may influence the formation of equal opportunity legislation. One of the most significant factors is the state of the economy.

Many changes have been seen in Britain this century. The role of women has gradually changed, with the rise of the Suffragette movement which was a key factor in obtaining the right of women to vote. Women's role in society and their perception of themselves as individuals began to change with the increased awareness of contraception. Contraception became more socially acceptable unless there were strong objections on religious grounds. This gave women the choice as to when they started a family and how many children they wanted. This afforded some women a choice – to follow a career and/or be a mother and home-maker (although in many jobs a career and marriage were still mutually exclusive until much later this century).

During the two World Wars women became an essential part of the work force, both on the land and in the factories. The economic boom following the Wars also gave rise to job opportunities, although there was also pressure to increase the population.

The advent of the Welfare State was as a direct result of the need of the country to ensure that all citizens had adequate medical care. In addition, good housing and social security support when ill was seen as essential to rebuild Britain after the Second World War.

Education was also regarded as a significant factor, to ensure that children gained the appropriate knowledge and skills to enable them to become active and productive members of society. The many Education Acts, in the last twenty years in particular, have been a way for the respective governments to try and influence the education sector to develop those skills so essential for the growth of the economy.

Think it over

Consider the kind of subjects you studied at school. Was there any difference between those subjects taken by girls and those by boys? Arrange to talk to someone of 70 years and over, concerning the subjects boys and girls were taught then. Consider, too, the age people started and left school then and today. Why do you think this is?

The economic boom after the war also saw an increase in immigration of people from Commonwealth countries in particular. It was in the concern to ensure equality in terms of pay, gender, and race, that the Equal Pay Act, Sex Discrimination Act and the Race Relations Acts were introduced. At the same time, the rise of feminism gave further voice to women's issues and, particularly, women's rights to equal pay and opportunities.

The government set up two specific organisations to monitor gender issues and race issues, the EOC and the CRE, as described earlier.

It has been shown that the power of pressure groups plays a significant role in determining policy. The current debate regarding the legal age of consent for homosexual men, and the activists promoting the rights of people with disabilities, are the result of two such pressure groups. They are concerned to lobby MPs of all parties and often look to the action being taken in the USA and other parts of Europe as encouragement of what can be achieved by concerted effort.

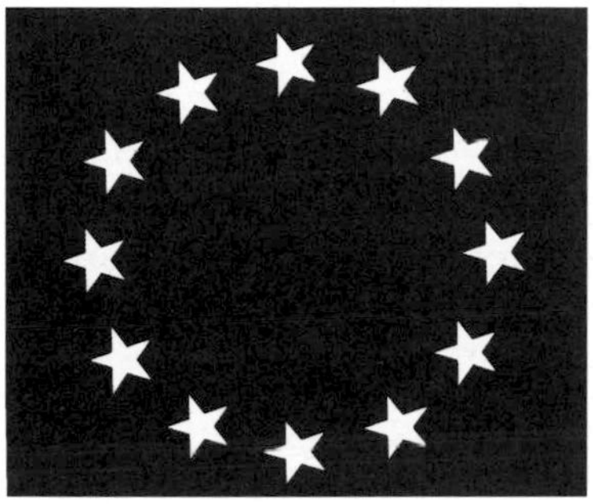

Once Britain became a member of the European Community (now the European Union – EU) then directives began to have a significant impact on matters here. As was seen earlier, it is possible to appeal to the European Court of Justice on human rights issues. Any ruling there must be accepted by Britain. However, different political parties have different views about Europe; indeed, many MPs in the same party may have differing opinions regarding the sovereignty of Westminster and may feel concerned that Britain is 'losing out' to Europe.

Think it over

Collect articles from the quality press on European issues which affect Britain. You might collect information about the different manifestos from each political party to note how each perceives the EU. Discuss your findings.

It is not difficult to see how the different political parties think about the economy. Very simplistically, each party has an underpinning philosophy regarding the role of the government. One idea is that the government should always create ways to support those in society who need additional help. Business is there to create wealth for the community and so should be regulated by the state.

An opposing view is that wealth is created by encouraging competition – private ownership rather than public ownership. The idea here is that motivation is higher if individuals own and are therefore responsible for their own business. This has led in recent years to the selling off of public organisations, for example the water and gas utilities. It has also led to incentives to encourage individuals to buy their own homes rather than to live in council-owned property.

Other political parties may well share some views of the two major parties, yet have some significant differences which include some state ownership and some encouragement of private ownership to boost the economy.

The creation of Charters for different aspects of public services, like the Patient's Charter and Parents' Charter, are a way for the government to outline clearly the standards the public should expect from these services. It also places responsibility on the individual organisations to interpret the standards for themselves.

Organisations like the Further Education Funding Council, set up by the government, employ inspectors to make regular checks on colleges of further education to ensure that high quality is achieved, mapped against very specific criteria. The results of inspection are then made public through a report.

There are similar bodies for the Higher Education sector and schools; in fact, league tables showing success rates and attendance records are now published which again increase competition and public knowledge and aim to raise standards everywhere.

In terms of the National Health Service, the Family Health Service Authority monitors the service provided by the community health service, e.g. GPs, dentists, chemists. The Community Health Council is a body with local councillors who also monitor the health service provision in its area and can offer advice to service users. Registration Officers of Social Service departments act as Inspectors in homes for elders to monitor the provision there.

So it may be seen that, where possible, there are systems in place to outline the standards expected of a service, then to monitor the service and provide a means whereby individuals may complain should their rights to that service be infringed.

It has also been seen that having a system which may be supported by legislation does not always mean that every individual in society has an equal chance in the 'competition'. The next chapter reviews ways in which some people are disadvantaged in society.

Chapter 2

How individuals can be affected by discrimination

This chapter explores the ways in which individuals can be affected by discrimination. Society places value on individuals based on such perceptions as gender or race, or other social constructs, such as occupational status.

Try it

Arrange to interview two people who have had very different experiences of life. This may be because of a difference in their age, ability, gender, ethnicity, social class or religion. Try to determine the factors which have led to the formation of their current view of themselves and the world. Who were key people in their lives and why?

Bases of discrimination

Individuals valued by society for their knowledge, experience, or authority gain high status and power. Those who are deemed to be of low status have little power and are disadvantaged by society. This is a difficult issue as the value placed on a particular social role varies between cultures; for example, males are valued by many in Third World countries as they are the providers of food for the village. Sons also care for their elders in their later years, whereas daughters marry and go to a new family or village.

In Eurocentric cultures, value has been awarded to those who contribute to the economy. Those who are not able to contribute are deemed to be of little apparent value. Such people include those over retirement age (i.e. 65 years), those who are physically or mentally unable to contribute for whatever reason and those who are unable to find employment (in the recession in the 1990s). In Britain, society demonstrates the value placed on individuals by the monetary rewards made available, e.g. high salaries. Unemployed people rely on benefits set by the State, on the one hand, and on strategies devised to enable them to contribute in some way or the other, e.g. retraining schemes.

There is a problem when those in work become frustrated by rising taxes, necessary in order to support financially those who are not in work. The stage is set for one group in society to marginalise another. Those in work may construct a mental picture of those who are unemployed. The mental picture could include a range of characteristics (*stereotype*) which are applied to all unemployed people; for example, lazy, work-shy, inadequate, unskilled etc. This description is unfairly attributed to all unemployed people. A stereotype is an irrational and unfair label. Some unemployed people may be unskilled but many are highly skilled; some may be content not to work, others write endless job applications. It should be clear that it is *discriminatory* to assume that such a range of characteristics may be applied to all in the same predicament.

Stereotyping is a way of making a collective sense of the world by grouping objects together into a fixed pattern or image; it makes life easier to organise. The word comes from the printing industry; but people are not words, people are unique individuals and cannot be grouped in such a way.

Discrimination is the ability to notice differences between things. In an equal opportunities context, discrimination means to notice differences between groups of people and then go on to deny one group the same quality of opportunity or service that a different group receives. Discrimination may mean favouring one group more than another when it comes to maintaining rights or access to services.

Positive action may be taken to redress an imbalance to ensure that equality of opportunity is afforded to disadvantaged groups. For example, special equipment may be provided in a college to enable a student with a hearing impairment to participate fully in all sessions; or special arrangements might be made for testing candidates who have dyslexia, so they are not disadvantaged.

Discrimination may involve basing decisions on attitudes acquired during socialisation. These attitudes are based on beliefs about people or prejudices. *Prejudice* involves the use of stereotypes to try to explain or categorise particular groups in society. Secord and Backman (1974) describe discrimination as: 'The inequitable treatment of individuals considered to belong to a particular social group.'

Attitudes, values and beliefs are formed in early life through primary socialisation. During secondary socialisation, the individual begins to reaffirm or change existing values in the light of wider experience and learning.

Discrimination in a health and social care context is seen as a negative practice. Discrimination involves the power of one group to place people in other groups at a disadvantage. Disadvantaged groups in current society include the young and the aged, and people with physical disability or learning difficulties. Others face discrimination because of religious beliefs, their gender, race, social status (class) or sexual orientation.

Contexts in which discrimination may occur

Discrimination may be direct or indirect. **Direct discrimination** is obvious, for example: a child bullied at school because of an unsightly skin disorder, such as psoriasis; an Asian youth beaten up by a gang of white youths, as he waits for a bus, just because he is Asian; a black family suffering hate mail to get them to move from a mainly white district; an elderly resident handed clothes to wear, without being allowed the opportunity to choose for him/herself.

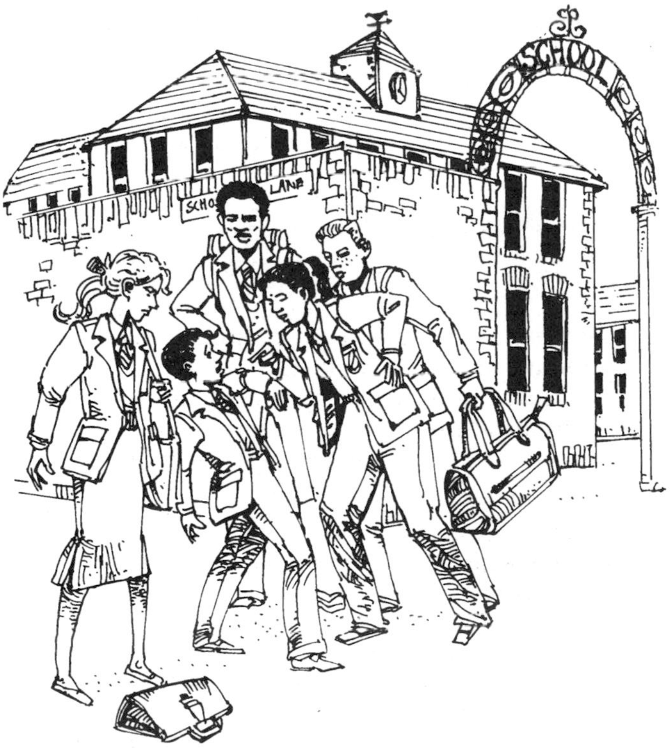

Disability

Think it over

When I was in a clothes shop with a disabled friend in a wheelchair, the assistant politely asked me about a range of outfits I might wish to see. The assistant assumed that I was buying for my friend as she was unable to make decisions for herself just because she was in a wheelchair! She was openly discriminating against my friend, by making assumptions about her abilities. This assumption led the assistant to ignore my friend – denying her the dignity of making her own choice. When people are regularly exposed to discrimination like this it may threaten their self-esteem.

Such an example shows how discrimination can occur unwittingly. The shop assistant was young and relatively inexperienced; she had never been in close contact with someone in a wheelchair before. The stereotype she had in her mind was that people in wheelchairs were cognititively disabled as well as physically! A gentle word in the assistant's ear helped her to understand the situation, and afterward she could not have been more helpful.

It would have been easy to get cross with the assistant and to have marched out of the shop in anger; but what would the assistant have learnt? That people pushing wheelchairs should be avoided at all costs because they were as difficult as the occupant of the wheelchair!

Individuals should not be blamed for making errors because of their lack of awareness. It may be a different story if the person does not change their behaviour, once their awareness of discrimination has been raised.

Race

Think it over

A black woman, employed in a busy bank, was made to feel very welcome by her white colleagues who included her in all the social activities. It was a different story when opportunities for staff development and training came along. The woman was not included in such training, which meant no opportunity for promotion despite her undoubted capabilities. The woman successfully took her employers to an Industrial Tribunal and won her case under the Race Relations Act 1976.

Discrimination may be individual, as has been explained above, or institutional. Institutional discrimination includes any systems which disadvantage others; for example, – shops with baby – changing rooms in inaccessible places when the baby is in a pram or pushchair.

An example of institutional discrimination might include a firm employing many people with young children but not providing creche facilities; museums and galleries providing lifts and ramps for people in wheelchairs, but giving no thought to those with sight or hearing impairment – just assuming that such people would not want to visit!

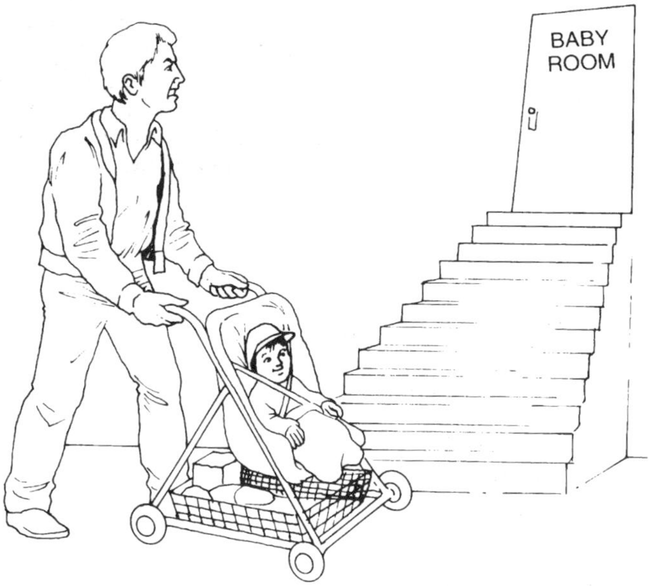

Health status

Indirect (or covert) **discrimination** is far more subtle and hidden. For example: not inviting someone with a disability to a party because you feel embarrassed by their disability; avoiding a friend who has been diagnosed as HIV positive; a restaurant set out so that people in wheelchairs will be unable to gain access; providing information in English only, when it is known that people using other languages might also benefit from the same information.

Psychologists are interested in why individuals discriminate against others. Minard (1952), looked at the co-operative interaction of black and white miners when relying on each other underground. This co-operation ceased for many of the miners as soon as they returned to the surface. The norms above ground meant separation not co-operation! Underground, co-operation could mean the difference between life and death; above ground there were no such concerns, only the need to be accepted in terms of the dominant white group.

Studies have been undertaken to see if there is a personality type more likely to be prejudiced, for example Adorno *et al.* (1950); whilst others looked to see if competition for resources was a factor, for example Sherif *et al* (1961), Typerman and Spenser (1983), Brown (1988).

Discrimination in education

Psychologists studying the behaviour which contributes to prejudicial attitudes and discriminatory behaviour sometimes study what might be a fragment of a much wider picture. Factors to be considered include individual, social, cultural, political and social policy issues.

Sociologists have undertaken research in a range of areas to gain insight into the way some groups are marginalised by others. Education is one such area where discrimination has been clearly demonstrated. The Swann Report (1985) highlighted a range of factors that led to the death of an Asian boy in a school in northern England. The factors ranged from systems and practices within the school to social factors within the locality.

Other studies look at the way different groups are perceived by teachers and the effect of low teacher expectation. Jackson and Marsden (1962), and Keddie (1975), noted that black children, in particular, were not expected to do well. These children were not stimulated to achieve their potential in the way that their white peers were.

Discrimination in education is about race but also about gender and social class. Bernstein (1959) and Gould (1965) noted that children from working-class families were disadvantaged because they used a different 'language' code. Bernstein alleged that children from working-class families adopted a restricted language code from their carers. These children would use simpler language and were not encouraged to think in an abstract way. For example, in answer to a question, 'What is this?' (holding up a drinking glass), a reply would name the object (glass) and that would be the end of the conversation. Bernstein considered that children from middle-class homes used an elaborated 'language' code. A child from a middle-class group, asked the same question, was likely to give the name of an object and also describe the object's function 'it's a wine glass – for drinking wine'.

Such a difference between two groups means that whereas one is encouraged to think things through and explore, the other is not. This has implications for children in school as some teachers use an elaborated code. The elaborated code might disadvantage those who have only experienced a restricted code.

The introduction of the comprehensive school system, following the Education Act 1976, was intended to offer wider opportunities for all. Prior to that, children sat an 'eleven-plus' exam which determined whether they moved to a grammar school, and so to university and a profession with corresponding pay and social status; or, if they did not pass the eleven-plus, a secondary modern school, where the emphasis was on more practical trades for the future in business and industry, which meant lower status and lower pay in many instances. Some children did progress to higher education from secondary modern schools but they were the exception rather than the rule!

The emphasis in education since 1979 has been to meet the needs of industry and business in a very competitive world market. The introduction of training schemes, the National Curriculum in schools and the emphasis on core skills in GNVQ is part of that movement.

The Warnock Report (1978) reviewed the educational provision for children deemed in the terminology of that time to be mentally or physically handicapped. The recommendations of that report helped to change the focus of provision for people with disabilities and indeed the terminology used. Children considered to have *special needs* were to be offered a range of options and, where possible, the segregation in special schools was to cease.

Think it over

Integrating children with special needs into mainstream schools has been slow; perhaps you have noticed this development during your own time at school?

Language

Language is a uniquely human skill. Birds, fish and animals communicate by body language; some even make vocal sounds, for example the songs of a whale, or the clicks of a dolphin. But only humans have a complex language by which information is transferred.

Discrimination can take place in language through the choice of words and even the tone adopted during conversation. Calling people names that are aimed to make them feel bad or different is an example of the way language may be used in a discriminatory fashion. For example, to call someone an imbecile implies that they are mentally less able; the term 'imbecile' was at one time used as a label to denote people who we would today say have learning disabilities.

Consider why people may take offence at certain words; for example, most black people today prefer to be called 'black' and not 'coloured'. However, many older people were taught to say coloured, as it was then more polite than to say black. Look at this poem, whose author is unknown; it gives an insight into why black is a more appropriate term.

When I was born
  I was black
As I grow up
  I am black
When I go in the sun
  I am black
When I am cold
  I am black
When I am ill
  I am black
When I die
  I will be black

When you were born
  You were pink
As you grow up
  You are white
When you go in the sun
  You are red
When you are cold
  You are blue
When you are ill
  You are green
When you die
  You are purple.

And you have the audacity to call me coloured!

Anon

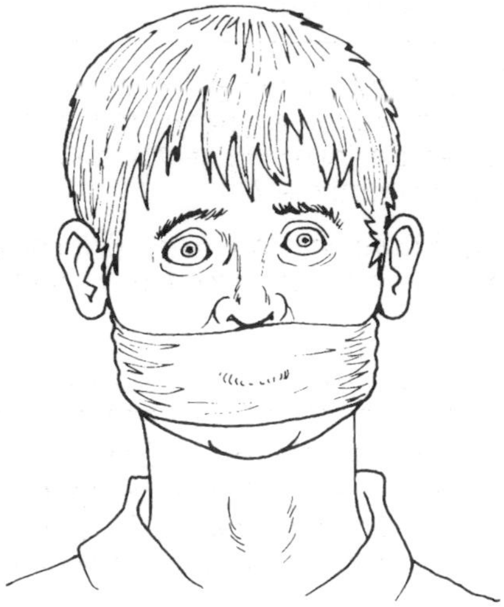

Figure 2.1 An awareness of language does not mean that one has to feel trapped by it

However, there is a problem in that black has sometimes been seen as the colour to symbolise bad things in Western culture. When did you see a good fairy in a children's book dressed in black or the wicked witch dressed in white? This association has been so much part of Western culture that some people may accept it as the way things are. But this can cause offence to many of the population, so maybe the situation needs to be reviewed. Perhaps now is the time to be more aware of the power of language, in that it can be used to discriminate against others.

English is the most widely spoken language in the world. It is used in British schools and is taught as a second language in nearly every country worldwide. The result is that many British people have never seen the value of learning a second language themselves. The root of this view may lie in an imperial past, when Britain ruled many foreign countries – imposing her language and culture on others.

It is easy to be trapped by language and to feel that one has to watch everything that is said, to be 'politically correct' in speech. A more sensible view is that it is important to be aware of the possible implications and roots of language; to check with people what they would prefer, so that offence is not unwittingly given.

Today, those for whom English is a second language may well feel that in Britain their own language is unimportant. Being taught in English at school, spoken to in English at the doctor's surgery or at Social Services offices, means learning the language quickly to survive. Some young people can cope well with learning a new language, but other people may well find this difficult.

Think it over

Imagine falling ill on holiday in a foreign country. You are far from home, feeling unwell and unable to make people understand what you need. You are also unable to understand what they say to you and can only watch as they start any treatment. What emotions would you have? What would help to reassure you?

Children in school who need to learn English may well speak several languages. Those same children may be seen as slow learners by the teachers until their English improves. Imagine then what a teacher would think of an English-speaking child of the same age who could also speak fluent French, German or Spanish. That child would be seen as clever; but the Asian child of the same age who can speak Hindi and Gujerati but who has a poor command of English, may be viewed less favourably!

If little value is placed on original languages, children may begin to value original languages less favourably and so lose part of their culture. It is an undeniable fact that children do need to learn English. It will enable them to cope with life in Britain. But this does not need to be at the cost of losing their mother tongue.

Body language

We live in a hearing world, so what happens to those who are hearing-impaired? Since the Education Reform Act 1988, children with hearing impairment may be learning in a mainstream school with support. Some theatres have special performances with a person at the side of the stage signing. Efforts have been made to sign for musicals and opera, so that people who are hearing-impaired can enjoy this form of art. BBC2 has news programmes with a signer but in the main little is done for those with hearing impairment. Try watching your favourite TV soap with the sound off. Is it not frustrating to miss half of what is going on? Especially if several people speak at once – who do you watch if you have to read their lips?

People who are hearing-impaired are perhaps more keenly aware of the signals people give with their

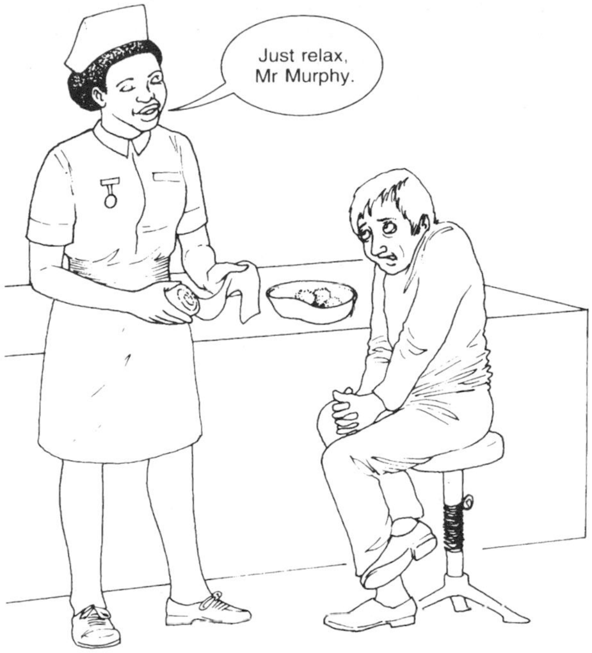

Figure 2.2 Body language sends messages

bodies. Think again about feeling ill in a foreign country: you will be sensitive to people's facial expressions, tone of voice and body posture (body language).

We use body language to assist the verbal messages, to act as a reinforcer to help get the point across. Imagine a person angry with another: words will be used to express feeling but body language will also send a message. The body will perhaps lean towards the other person, possibly pointing a finger at the other's face, or shaking a fist; the face will be contorted into a twist, the corners of the mouth down and the eyes staring directly at the other person. Even if you could not hear the words you would know exactly how the other person felt!

We also use body language to discriminate against others. It may be by turning your back on another, blocking them out of your sight. It may be by making a sign which shows your feelings; indeed body language may result in abusive gestures such as two fingers put up to show anger and contempt. Putting your finger to the side of your head and rapidly twisting it denotes that you think the other person is mad, or mentally affected in some way.

Think it over

Imagine that you are learning a new skill and the person demonstrating the skill makes the following gestures while you are practising, how will you feel?

Raising the eyebrows, looking to the sky, showing anger or impatience, giving at the same time a loud sigh.

Think it over

Think of a time when you said 'no' to someone. A soft 'no', accompanied by a smile, will be seen as playful, perhaps really a 'yes'! A sharp 'no', accompanied by a frown is clearly understood.

'You cannot do that, you are only a girl', said with disdain is a way of implying girls to be less able than boys. 'Real men do not do such things', said with a look of horror, or a sarcastic smile, implies that you are less than the accepted norm of a man! In both instances you may feel a whole range of emotions, one of which will be hurt, as you have been discriminated against. If an individual is constantly put down by others, because they are seen as different, they may lose confidence. A child repeatedly told that they are 'stupid' or 'bad' may begin to believe it and stop trying; in addition, they may incorporate the idea of being poorly valued into their identity. A self-fulfilling prophecy may be established as the labelled person comes to believe that they really are 'bad'.

> *Labelling a person may begin to create a self-fulfilling prophecy.*

A young person facing name-calling, because of their skin colour, may begin to feel awkward and different. Such a person may become stressed if they do not get positive support for their identity. A person with physical disabilities, or with learning disabilities, may be told so often that they cannot do things for themselves that they begin to believe it. The individual takes on board the opinions and actions of others, incorporating those opinions into their perception of themselves.

Think it over

A young girl, badly scarred by a fire at the age of six years, is shy and withdrawn as a teenager. She is unwilling to go out to meet new people, because people show their horror at her scars even though most try not to stare. She feels ugly in a world that only values beauty and perfection. She knows that the world values such things because she has never seen anyone like herself on the TV or as a model in a magazine.

Perhaps part of the appeal of such plays as *Beauty and the Beast,* the *Phantom of the Opera* and the *Elephant Man,* is that at last someone has seen below the surface to the real person: seen the ability not the disability!

Think it over

Think again of the times as a child when you waited to be chosen by someone in your group to join their team. Remember the feelings?

People who have faced perhaps a lifetime of discrimination will feel devalued which can lead to a feeling of powerlessness, feeling that it is not possible to change their situation. This leads to low self-esteem, i.e. 'I must be less valuable because that is what others think'. So it is vital to recognise the importance of other people in the formation of our pictures of ourselves as individuals. Other people matter: we all have a basic need to understand ourselves in relation to others.

How can individuals who feel less valued than others claim their rights in society? Such people may well feel that they are not entitled to any services and they probably will not have the confidence to assert their rights to such services. For example, it may be difficult to ask a doctor why a certain treatment has been prescribed, when the doctor is perceived as being of a higher status than you. Assumptions about social value lead to discriminatory attitudes. For example:

1 'What right has someone with a disability to ask for alterations to their home, when they do not work and therefore do not pay taxes'?
2 'What right has a woman to a job when many men are out of work, when the woman believes that men have a higher social status than women'?

Other assumptions about social status might include the mixture of apprehension and anger when a group of travellers settle in a field near a town or village. People draw on their stereotype of travellers rather than looking at the individuals. The power of the stereotype results in prejudicial attitudes and may result in discrimination. A further example might be a single parent putting up with unsuitable bed and breakfast accommodation because society currently sees single parents as a drain on resources. All these people may well feel unable to make full use of all services, particularly if – in their experience – they are put down when they do try.

Prejudice

Preconceived opinions (usually negative) or prejudice may result in discrimination. For example: a home carer who wears a mask and thick rubber gloves when working in the home of a person with AIDS; a nurse who is brusque with the person being treated for a drug overdose, considering it to be self-inflicted; the social worker who shows disdain for someone suspected of abusing others; the teacher who expects little from a black child but much from a white child in the same class. Such prejudicial attitudes from these people reinforce a feeling of inferiority in the individual, compounding the discrimination given by others.

Health and social care staff have a responsibility to ensure that they remain impartial and non-judgemental at all times in their working lives.

Think it over

Consider the following case study: Mrs Ahmed, an Asian woman in her late seventies, was admitted to a residential home for the elderly. Mrs Ahmed had arrived in England from Calcutta twelve years previously. She lived with her son and family, rarely went out and had not learned very much English. The family had fallen on difficult times after the recent death of her daughter-in-law. Mrs Ahmed had been given a place in the residential home for three weeks to enable her son to come to terms with his new situation. The staff in the residential home had no experience of Asian elders.

Imagine what must have been going through Mrs Ahmed's mind: a strange land, language and customs and no family to turn to whilst in the home. The staff, though concerned and caring, had asked about diet but not about customs such as different hygiene, dress etc. Mrs Ahmed was expected to conform to 'the way we do things here'. Unable to communicate, Mrs Ahmed became withdrawn, stopped eating, refused to get out of bed and was quickly labelled as 'awkward' by the overworked staff. Frustrated care workers showed their annoyance by the body language and tone used when working with her. Being unable to understand the language, but interpreting the frowns and sighs of staff, did little to reassure a bewildered and frightened woman.

Imagine the horror of the son on finding his mother in such a state. The guilt of giving up his duty of caring for her, by agreeing to respite care, would be reinforced by seeing her so unhappy and confused. However, the situation could have been avoided if the staff had ensured that as much as possible was learnt about Mrs Ahmed's culture before she arrived. The ideal would have been to have Asian staff but this may not be possible. An interpreter should be found and the staff could learn a few words of greeting to break the isolation. Learning about dress and hygiene codes would avoid offence. Checking about diet and any religious practice would also help. Ensuring that Mrs Ahmed had access to others who spoke her language, and people who could provide books or music for her, would be useful.

Staff would also need to watch for any possible discrimination from other residents – whether intentional or not. Pulling faces or exchanging glances at the dining table when Mrs Ahmed ate her food using her hands rather than the strange knives and forks; making comments about the smell of unfamiliar Asian food in a tone that would leave Mrs Ahmed in no doubt as to their disapproval; refusing to sit next to her, or turning away from her; all these things would show discrimination. Mrs Ahmed would feel very vulnerable and devalued, no wonder she did not wish to face such discrimination – apparently giving up the will to live.

Think it over

Consider also the case of Robert, a young man aged 23, attending a Social Education Centre for adults with learning difficulties. Robert is the only child of an elderly couple who were in their forties when he was born. The joy of having a child, after nearly twenty years of marriage, turned to grief on discovering that he had Down's syndrome.

Robert's parents over-protected him as a child. They felt guilty for producing a child whom they saw as being less than perfect. In their guilt they showered him with love and affection. The result, however, was to treat him as a young irresponsible child rather than as a growing

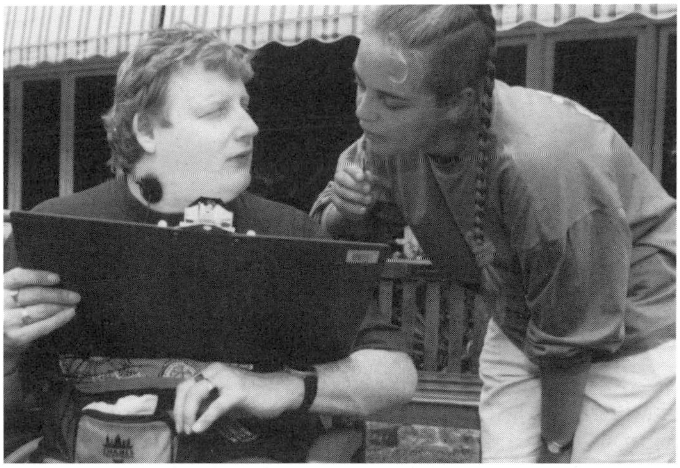

(Photo courtesy of the Winged Fellowship Trust)

adult. Robert was dressed in short trousers, led around by the hand and spoken to as if he was a young child despite being in his twenties. Never allowed to go out alone, even to the shop next door, he was unable to develop the skills required for independence. Robert was encouraged by his parents to 'play with his cars' and to read books more suited to a nine-year old child. But Robert's parents genuinely felt that they were giving him the best care possible.

Imagine the difficulties facing Robert at the Centre he now attends. The staff there will work with him to build his social and life skills required for independence. He will mix with a range of people and learn many new things which could bring him into conflict with his parents. The staff have a sensitive task to work with Robert and his parents to meet his needs as a man in his twenties.

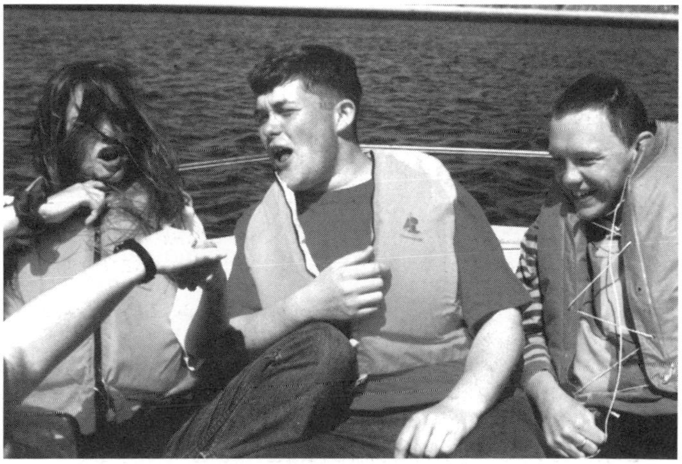

Figure 2.3 Mixing with people brings social skills
(Photo courtesy of the Winged Fellowship Trust)

It is important for Robert to gain some independence, to encourage him to make the most of his abilities. It is also important that he has the support of his parents as his world begins to expand. The importance lies in his rights as an individual to reach his own potential within society.

Primary socialisation is very powerful. Robert had limited secondary socialisation from his school. His experiences at the Social Education Centre will build on the socialisation process so that Robert can be accepted more readily in a wider society.

People often show sympathy to children with any form of disability. Generally, people feel protective of these children and tolerate behaviour from them which would be deemed unacceptable if they were perceived as being 'normal'. However, once the child grows to a physical adult, attitudes change. People may often think of other people like Robert as overgrown children – to be patronised – or as a threat – because their behaviour is considered unpredictable. Think of the confusion for individuals who have been allowed to do what they like as children, because they were perceived as being less capable. But anti-social behaviour tolerated as a child is frowned upon in an adult world.

One of the results of the National Health Service and Community Care Act, 1990 is that large hospitals and institutions for people with learning difficulties are closing. The residents of these institutions are being prepared for integration into the community. Unfortunately, the community is not necessarily prepared to welcome them and discrimination may and indeed does take place. Comments from potential neighbours may show irrational fear for the safety of residents and the value of property. Only education and time, with support from professionals for all concerned, will see true integration.

Try it

Choose a client group, perhaps the client group you are currently working with on placement. Identify any stereotypes associated with this group. Stereotypes may enable people to try to predict likely behaviour of anyone in this group. Many in the group may have some of the characteristics, but rarely all!

Identify any areas of overt discrimination which are common in society against this client group. What effect does this have on the individual? Think of any more subtle ways in which people discriminate against this group. What action would you consider necessary to improve the situation?

Think about the different social contexts where discrimination takes place and note the possible effect this has on the individual. (Think about when someone is applying for work, housing, education or health care.)

What do you consider to be your personal responsibility to ensure that you do not discriminate against others? What, in your opinion, should be done in the health and social care field to prevent discrimination?

To summarise: it has been argued that attitudes and values are formed through the socialisation process. Stereotyping people, by attributing a range of characteristics to the members of that group, is a way of trying to predict behaviour. The dangers of generalisation may lead to discrimination and the formation of prejudicial attitudes. This means that members of other groups can be treated less favourably. Discrimination has been described as either being openly displayed or more subtle. All forms of discrimination may lead to individuals perceiving themselves as less valuable than others. Once individuals believe themselves to be devalued they are less able to claim their rights assertively in society.

The effects of discrimination on Individuals

Think it over

It could be that you have faced discrimination in one form or another during your lifetime. If this has happened you will be aware of the emotions and feeling of powerlessness. Most people are resilient enough to cope with these feelings for short periods of time. But constant daily discrimination has a profound effect on the individual, requiring skilled support to combat the low self-esteem.

Have you ever experienced the situation when two members of your class at school were told to choose a team? Can you recall the feeling of unease as members of your group were gradually called to join one team or another? Do you remember the feeling of relief when you were chosen? Perhaps even a sense of smugness as you looked at the discomfort of the few remaining children left until last? Were they last because they were considered to be no good at the game to be played and therefore a liability? What effect do you think it had on the child who was *always* the one to be left until last? Why did you feel

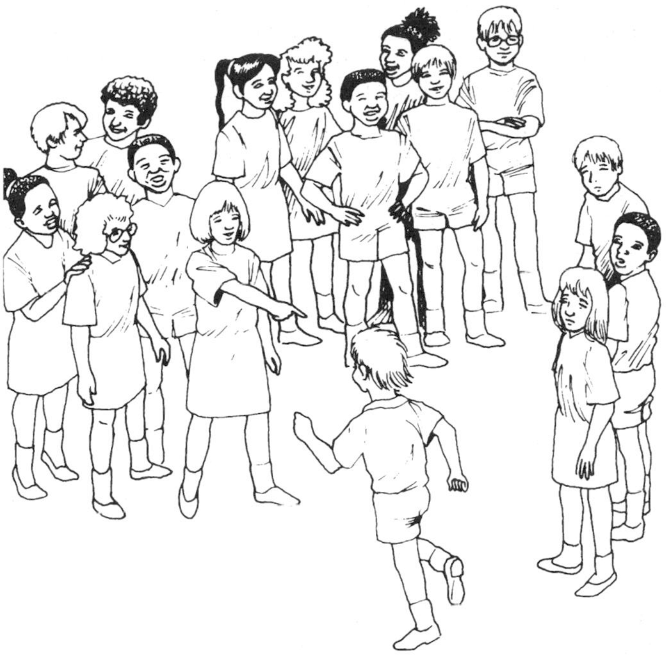

Figure 2.4 It can be hard if you're the last one chosen

smug when chosen early on? People can be fickle and self-centred, even cruel, particularly, (but not exclusively) in childhood.

You might have never had the experience of waiting to be picked for a team. Think then of a time when you had been 'put down' by an adult; remember how it felt, particularly if you believed their actions were unjust in some way. Can you remember the anger and frustration, the feeling of powerlessness? As a child you were expected to do what the adult said. Adults had power to control situations, whereas you as a child did not.

Think it over

Imagine now some adult experiences: the worker made redundant, the individual made homeless, the couple going through a divorce process, the ending of a relationship you felt would last forever. All these would have a profound effect on the way the individuals perceive themselves and the value they place on themselves. It takes time and support from others to rebuild a bruised and battered self-esteem.

Imagine that all your life people have put you down by the way they have spoken to you or behaved towards you. Perhaps at school there was a subject you found particularly difficult. However hard you tried you could not get it right. If the teacher at school – and also perhaps your family at home – were less than sympathetic to your efforts, and kept making comments about your low marks, you might begin to believe that you would never be any good at that subject. So in the end you stop trying – and then you never do succeed at that subject! Motivation to succeed when things are difficult comes from determination on the part of the individual – but also from the understanding and support of others.

Think it over

A young child struggling to dress herself may put clothes on back to front, or button things wrongly. It the carer is impatient, ignoring the child's attempts and dressing the child properly and quickly, the child is likely to lose confidence and not feel good about trying to do things for herself. On the other hand, if the carer smiles and rewards the child with praise for her efforts, the child will be eager to try again – to learn independence and to gain further adult approval.

Read the poem (below) by Dorothy Law Nolte.

Children Learn What They Live

If children live with criticism
They learn to condemn.
If children live with hostility
They learn to fight.
If children live with ridicule
They learn to be shy.
If children live with shame
They learn to feel guilty.

If children live with tolerance
They learn to be patient.
If children live with encouragement
They learn to be confident.
If children live with praise
They learn to appreciate.
If children live with fairness
They learn justice.
If children live with security
They learn to have faith.
If children live with approval
They learn to like themselves.
If children live with acceptance and friendship
They learn to find love in the World.

This poem looks at children's needs but it could equally be applied to people of any age; although the early years are particularly important for a child's developing self-confidence and self-esteem.

Anyone, who has experienced a life event such as the loss of a job, an accident or illness which leaves them less physically or mentally able than before, or any form of discrimination, will experience a loss of self-esteem. They are likely to feel less valuable in society – that their social role is now less important, i.e. that they have lost social status.

Social status

Members of society hold different positions within that society. These positions are known as social status; for example, they proclaim the status in the family – such as son, daughter, mother, father etc. Other social status is associated with work, e.g. lecturer, nurse, social worker, cleaner etc. In some cultures status comes with age or knowledge, or by being the first-born son.

Status can be related to biology, as in gender (male or female), or race (nationality, black or white). Status can also be culturally defined in other ways, such as the leader of a group, or a pop star or artist.

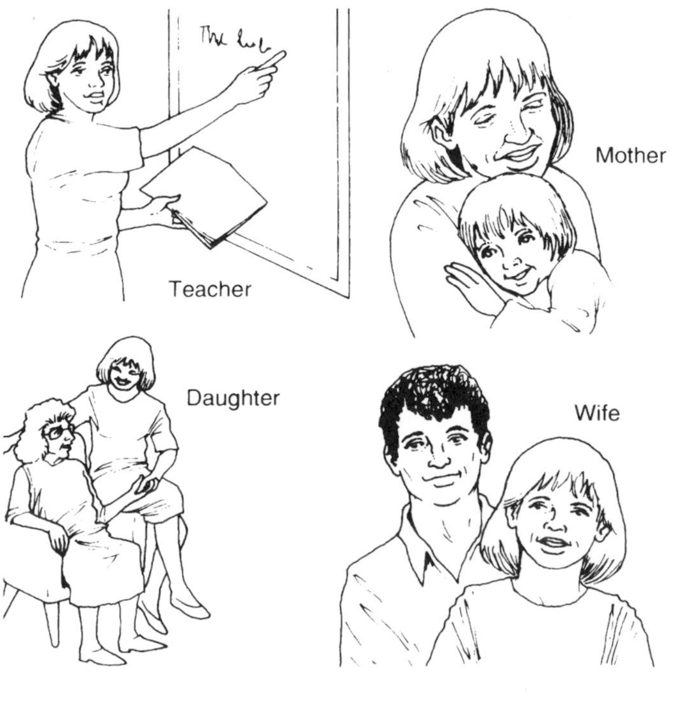

Figure 2.5 Social status is associated with different roles

Social roles

Along with positions of social status come norms. Norms provide a kind of blueprint as to the expected behaviour associated with the position or social role. The social status of a nurse is defined and associated with the role of the nurse who wears a uniform as a symbol of the role. Patients expect the nurse to have specific knowledge to meet their needs when ill. They also expect the nurse to have certain qualities, for example to be calm, efficient, patient, understanding, etc. In turn, the nurse will look to the person who is unwell to fulfil the social role of patient. In this way each is clear about the accepted norms for their role and the two are able to work together to aid recovery.

Social roles assist in the organisation of behaviour by regulating that behaviour in a way that is acceptable to society. They help individuals to be able to predict the probable behaviour of others, so that they can adopt the corresponding role themselves.

Try it

Make a list of the many roles that you have played today; these may include son or daughter, parent, brother/sister, student, friend, customer. Write down against each role the possible behaviour that others would expect of you in that role; check your ideas out with others.

Then make a list of the behaviour you expect from a lecturer. Check your ideas out with one of the lecturers – any surprises? You might ask the lecturer to list the behaviour they expect from a student and compare your ideas!

When people experience discrimination, it has a profound effect on them as individuals. Each person will find a different way of coping. For example, a black comedian may make jokes about the colour of his or her skin as a self-defence mechanism – before others can put them down for being black.

We all have coping mechanisms or strategies which we adopt to protect us from the hurt others can cause. Some people withdraw into themselves, others become angry and aggressive. People can be deeply affected by discrimination and prejudice – whether they are willing to acknowledge it or not.

If people feel themselves to be of little value, then they do not always have the confidence or motivation to stand up for their rights in society.

They may appear passive, accepting whatever service is offered without comment or complaint.

Such people are 'handicapped' by this lack of self-esteem and motivation; they are therefore at a disadvantage in a competitive society. The result, in health and social care terms, is a poorer service for those individuals – unless they can be empowered by others to rebuild their feelings of self worth. This will motivate individuals to aim higher, to be more assertive and to speak up for themselves; i.e. to claim their rights to enter the 'competition' and to gain the services which are due to them.

Evidence collection point

Identify a health or social care setting with which you are familiar. Write a report to outline the way the service users could be discriminated against in terms of the bases for discrimination. Outline the many ways society may discriminate against the service users as individuals and also on an organisational basis. Give details of the differing effects discrimination may have on an individual, giving one example from each area of motivation, self-esteem, rights and opportunities.

Chapter 3

Ethical issues in health and social care practice

This chapter examines a variety of ethical issues in health and social care practice. The responsibilities of care workers are outlined and explained, and case studies are used to highlight a range of ethical issues which could arise in care work.

In recent years there has been an increasing interest in the field of professional ethics. Some authors, for example Don MacNiven (1990), argue that this is due to the Western world being in a period of moral decline. He argues that greed has become the norm in business and industry, as well as in the professions such as the law and medicine, resulting in declining standards.

It is doubtful whether the authors of the Welfare State in Britain in 1948 could have accurately envisaged the huge increase in demand for services to be seen today. It is unlikely that they could have envisaged the great leaps forward made by medical science which have directly contributed to the increasing population – so that more people now live for longer than ever before. Yet it is these factors which underlie the ethical problems faced by workers in the health and social care field, as well as for those in other professions such as the law and for religious leaders.

In the 1990s professionals are faced with trying to provide the best service possible for clients during a period of limited finances. The National Health Service tries to cope with treating as many people as possible whilst balancing the budget. Elderly people requiring residential care need financial support from the State when their own resources are exhausted. The high level of unemployment necessitates an increased budget to support those unable to find work to support themselves and their families. Many people have become accustomed to the concept of the State providing for those in need. Many in Britain today have never known anything other than a Welfare State and, after a lifetime of making contributions through the National Insurance system, expect to have their needs met.

The cost of meeting the diverse and often complex needs of individuals in the 1990s may mean increased taxation or reduced services. Most people want better services, but few people welcome the idea of increased taxes: perhaps this is one of the issues behind the argument of greed mentioned earlier? In the context of increased demand for a wide range of services within a limited or restricted budget, there is a need to explore ways in which professionals may make difficult decisions.

Responsibilities of health and social care workers

Professionals in the health and social care field are required to balance the needs of one individual against the needs of others within a fixed budget for a given year. This can cause tension for both the professional and those for whom they care.

To gain a deeper understanding it is important to look at the underpinning principles or **values** which form the bedrock of the health and social care professions. Simplistically, a value is a learned principle or thought system which enables individuals to choose between alternatives and make decisions. Values guide behaviour in relation to what is judged to be 'valuable'. Values are learnt in a cultural context and will develop in relation to the beliefs and norms which exist within a cultural group.

NVQ value base 'O' unit

In the context of health and social care, the value base is the framework which informs and supports all systems and processes in practice. In other words, it becomes the guide to the way professionals work with clients. It is outlined very clearly in the 'O' unit for NVQs in health and care.

There are five elements of the 'O' unit, which clarify responsibilities, as outlined below.

Promote anti-discriminatory practice

To discriminate means to be able to tell things apart from one another. We discriminate when we distinguish between things and put them in different categories. It is necessary to categorise things in order to make sense of the world. But in care work, discrimination has a more specialised meaning than simply to notice and categorise things. In care, discriminating against people means to disadvantage them, to provide a different quality of service for people from different social categories. People may receive a poorer quality of service because of their age, disability, gender, health status, ethnic status, religion or sexuality.

Anti-discriminatory practice involves being able to identify prejudices, assumptions and stereotypes which are used to devalue people. It involves trying to meet the varied needs of different people, rather than giving everyone the same service. If everyone is spoken to in the same way, given the same diet, given the same level of physical assistance and so on, then some clients will have their needs met and others will not. The people who do not have their needs met will be discriminated against.

Anti-discrimination involves being able to identify differing individual needs and meet them with different types of service. Anti-discriminatory practice also aims to identify organisational systems which might result in some people being treated less favourably than others.

Maintain the confidentiality of information

Confidentiality is an important value in nearly all professional services for people. Medicine, law and financial services all impose a strict duty of confidentiality on workers. The key issues that make confidentiality so important are the issues of trust and client safety. Personal information about health, about finance or about feelings, needs to be restricted to people who have a 'need to know'. Individuals must be sure that they can talk freely and openly to their carers. Clients will want to feel that they can control what is repeated to others.

The value base states that the confidentiality of records and information should be discussed with clients wherever possible. Some clients may not wish their relatives and friends to know about their finances or their medical details, or even to know about some day-to-day details of life. Knowing that conversations and personal details will be kept private may help to create a feeling of emotional safety and trust between clients and carers.

Confidentiality is an important responsibility in order to provide clients with security. If details of an older person's money and possessions are openly talked about, an individual may be at greater risk of exploitation or perhaps even burglary. Individuals may have personal secrets which they might wish to confide. Sometimes these secrets might make the individual vulnerable to the prejudices or assumptions of others if they were made public.

Confidentiality also preserves privacy. It may be hard for individuals to maintain a sense of dignity or self-esteem if all their actions and personal habits or behaviour are on public display. A client's emotional security may depend on the maintenance of confidentiality.

Promote individual rights and choice

Clients' rights include freedom from discrimination. Clients also have a right to dignity. This means that they are treated as being worthy of respect, and that their feelings are considered in the care they receive.

Some clients are vulnerable to a loss of dignity because of the level of help they need from others. Infirm elders or disabled people may need assistance with many personal aspects of their care. It is important that the dignity of the client is respected when providing this care. Clients who feel that they are being treated as though their feelings do not matter may find that their self-esteem is affected by their experience of care. Maintaining the dignity of clients in situations where they are dependent on others is a skill; it is a right of clients to have their dignity respected.

Being able to choose what we wear, how we look, what we eat, where we go, who our friends are – these are the ways in which we express our self-concept or identity. When we were very young our parents may have made all the choices for us. As we grow up, freedom to make our own choices becomes more and more important.

Children learn to become independent through learning how to make decisions. Adults need to be able to make choices about their lifestyle in order to preserve dignity and independence. Therefore carers need to empower clients to make their own choices and to control their own lives as far as possible. Not to have choices is to be controlled by others; being controlled by others is to be disempowered. Empowering care tries to help clients to make decisions and choices about their lifestyle.

Empowerment is about giving choices and encouraging clients to make their own decisions. In

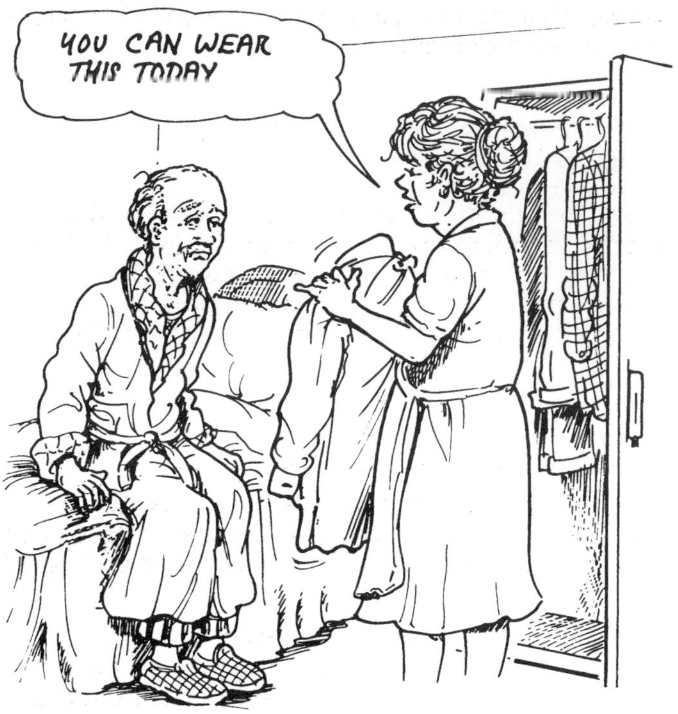

this way individuals are able to make informed decisions about their lives.

However, clients may not – for example – always be given the chance to choose what to wear. Yet clothes are a way for people to make a statement about themselves as individuals.

Think it over

Think about the clothes you wear and what they say about you as an individual. Think about how you would feel if you were told what to wear each day. Think too about the power a worker has. A client may not be able to speak up for themselves or fear that, if they do, they may be seen as a nuisance by staff.

Acknowledge an individual's personal beliefs and identity

This responsibility requires that carers try to learn about and to understand the individuals that they work with. Each child has a social background and context that will influence how they come to understand themselves. Each adult and older person may have developed a self-concept or sense of personal identity (see Chapter 10). When clients are ill or frail, or when they are young, they are emotionally vulnerable to the way carers treat them. It is a responsibility to help to build clients' self-esteem and to acknowledge and maintain clients' sense of themselves – their personal identity. This responsibility is also contained in the Patient's Charter.

The First National Standard in the Patient's Charter is:

> *Respect for privacy, dignity and religious and cultural beliefs. The Charter Standard is that all health services should make provision so that proper personal consideration is shown to you, for example by ensuring that your privacy, dignity and religious and cultural beliefs are respected. Practical arrangements should include meals to suit all dietary requirements, and private rooms for confidential discussions with relatives.*

It is important to recognise that gender, ethnicity, culture, religion, social status and sexuality all contribute to the way clients perceive themselves. To deny clients any aspect of their identity is to deny their personal uniqueness. Care workers need to review their own value systems to ensure that they do not impose their own values on the client and so disempower or belittle the client by making that person feel less worthy.

Support individuals through effective communication

If carers are to understand clients, work in an anti-discriminatory way and meet the self-esteem and emotional security needs of clients, then carers must have effective communication skills. These skills are discussed in detail in Chapters 4 and 5. Communication has to be adapted to the needs of individuals; it is important that carers can convey respect in all their conversations and in all the body language that they use when working with clients.

Empowerment

These five responsibilities contribute to acting in the best interests of clients; they imply the need to provide access to necessary information and they may result in giving power to the client. The five principles in the value base are intended to show how important the client is and to guide carers to put the needs of clients first. Carers should not take power over their clients and try to control them. Rather, carers should try to make clients feel

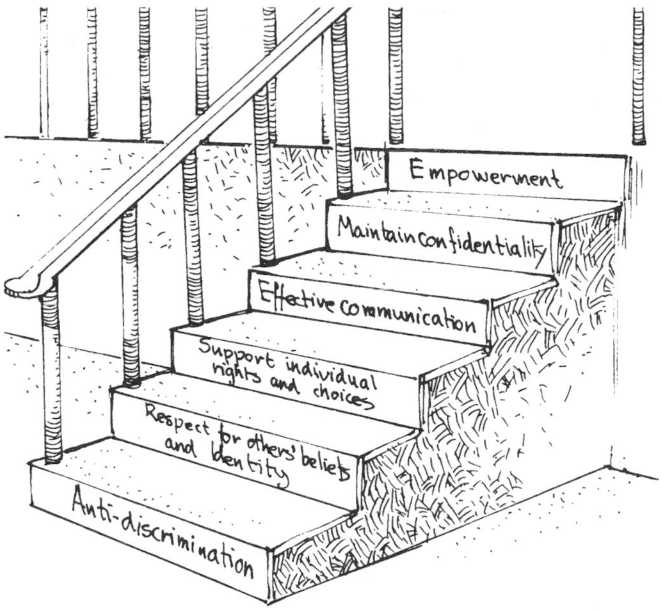

Figure 3.1 Five steps towards empowering clients

important and valued. Clients should be empowered to control conversation and information as much as possible. **Empowerment** means that clients should be in control of their daily lives and activities as far as possible, rather than being dependent on a carer who controls them.

As well as being the principles of care, the five care values might be seen as steps which enable clients to become empowered during interactions with their carers (see Figure 3.1).

Care workers have a responsibility to ensure that the client is fully informed about the service provided and their rights within it. The worker should encourage the client to express their own needs and wishes and should offer choices where possible. Ensuring that clients have all the relevant information available is the beginning of empowerment. If knowledge is power then to withhold information is to disempower an individual. If a client feels devalued, and is not aware of all the facts, how can they make a realistic judgement about their life?

As well as having a responsibility to empower and act in the best interests of clients, carers must be mindful of the risks to clients' health and safety. This may often involve the need to assess the likelihood of risks that exist in relation to the client's lifestyle or the care environment.

Ethics

Ethics (or morals) are the principles an individual adopts, in order to make decisions in life and when applying the values of a given profession. The value base informs the decision-making process for the individual, but ethical principles also have to be used.

Think it over

Imagine professional ethics as a bunch of specially made keys. These keys have been carefully prepared to uphold the value base of health and social care staff.

When faced with a problem a decision has to be reached. The keys enable the worker to open the appropriate door, thereby making a sound professional judgement. Ethics are the essential tools of the trade to uphold professional standards of care.

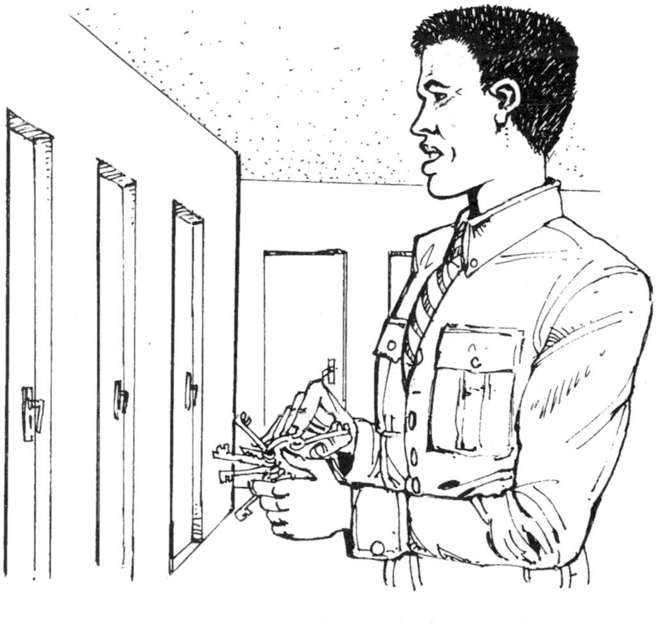

Ethical dilemmas

There are different schools of thought regarding the function of professional ethics. Each school of thought will tackle situations in different ways.

Utilitarianism, or **consequentialism,** was developed by Jeremy Bentham (1748–1832) and John Stuart Mill (1806–1873). A utilitarian will believe that a morally right act has to bring about the greatest happiness for the greatest number of people. Utilitarians equate happiness with good, so a morally right act (from this viewpoint) is one which creates the greatest good for the greatest number of people.

Utilitarian philosophy holds that all knowledge comes from experience (*empiricism*). The situation or social context is a major factor, as is the effect or consequences of any action; i.e. whether a doctor tells a patient that they are terminally ill will depend on the doctor's knowledge and experience of that individual and on the effect the news is expected to have on the person. It can be seen that utilitarian philosophy, like most ethics, involves making personal judgements, rather than following strict rules in a given situation.

Ethical systems of thought always encounter problems. It is difficult sometimes to define what is good. How can you guarantee that all possible consequences have been considered prior to action being taken? The concept of the greatest good for the greatest number of people is not straightforward. At face value this idea seems an admirable concept but does it always work in practice? For example, keeping an ailing business going to prevent redundancy may in time bring down the whole business. If some staff had been made redundant in the beginning then the jobs of the majority might have survived.

Think it over

If every decision was made simply on the basis of the greatest happiness of the greatest number of people then all sorts of injustice and abuses could be justified. If the people in a particular neighbourhood wanted to prevent a care home being built, they could argue that there were more of them and that more happiness would result from their ability to exercise their prejudice than would result from providing care for people with learning disability. Tax payers could argue that more happiness for more people would result from not paying tax rather than meeting the needs of people with disability and so on. It was for this reason that John Stuart Mill argued that utilitarianism had to be just a principle of decision-making: a principle that could only be used after the more important principle of justice had been checked through.

The idea of creating the greatest happiness for the greatest number of people has to be used as a principle to *guide* the construction of codes of

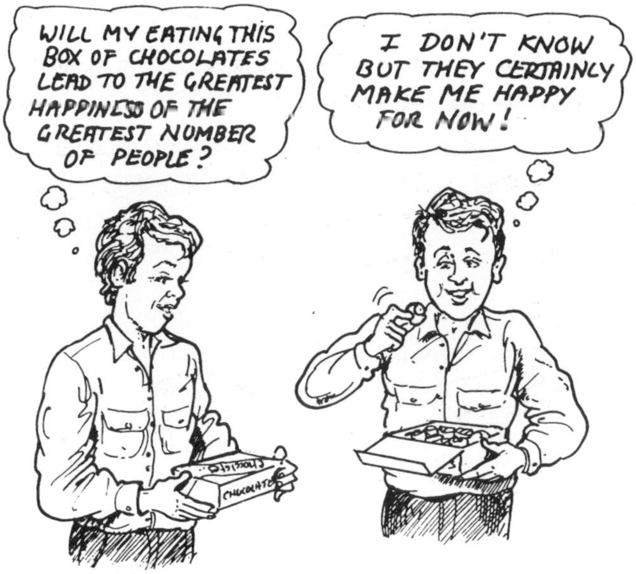
WILL MY EATING THIS BOX OF CHOCOLATES LEAD TO THE GREATEST HAPPINESS OF THE GREATEST NUMBER OF PEOPLE?
I DON'T KNOW BUT THEY CERTAINLY MAKE ME HAPPY FOR NOW!

professional conduct, or for designing laws and systems of social regulation. Utilitarianism does not work very well when it is applied to day-to-day decisions, or day-to-day actions. The first reason for this is that very few people can predict the future and manage to work out what will create future happiness.

The second reason that utilitarian principles don't work well when applied to acts of behaviour is that most people are very biased in their judgement of happiness.

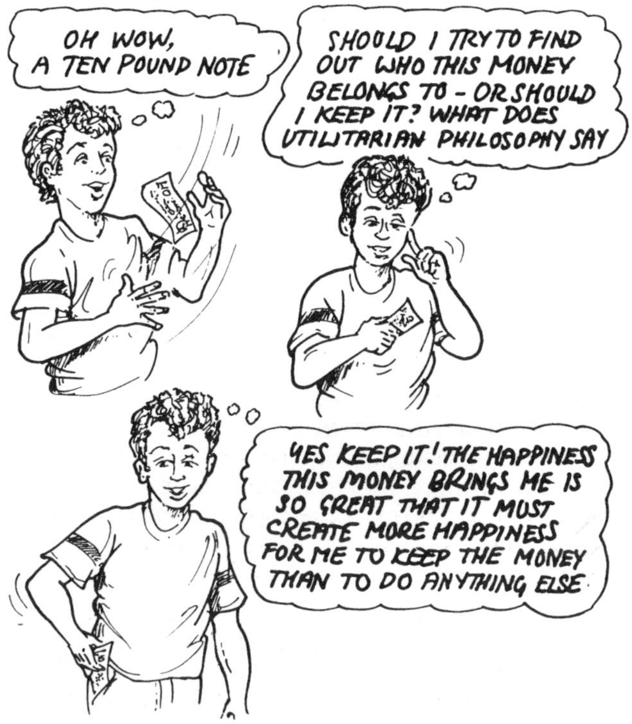
OH WOW, A TEN POUND NOTE
SHOULD I TRY TO FIND OUT WHO THIS MONEY BELONGS TO - OR SHOULD I KEEP IT? WHAT DOES UTILITARIAN PHILOSOPHY SAY
YES KEEP IT! THE HAPPINESS THIS MONEY BRINGS ME IS SO GREAT THAT IT MUST CREATE MORE HAPPINESS FOR ME TO KEEP THE MONEY THAN TO DO ANYTHING ELSE

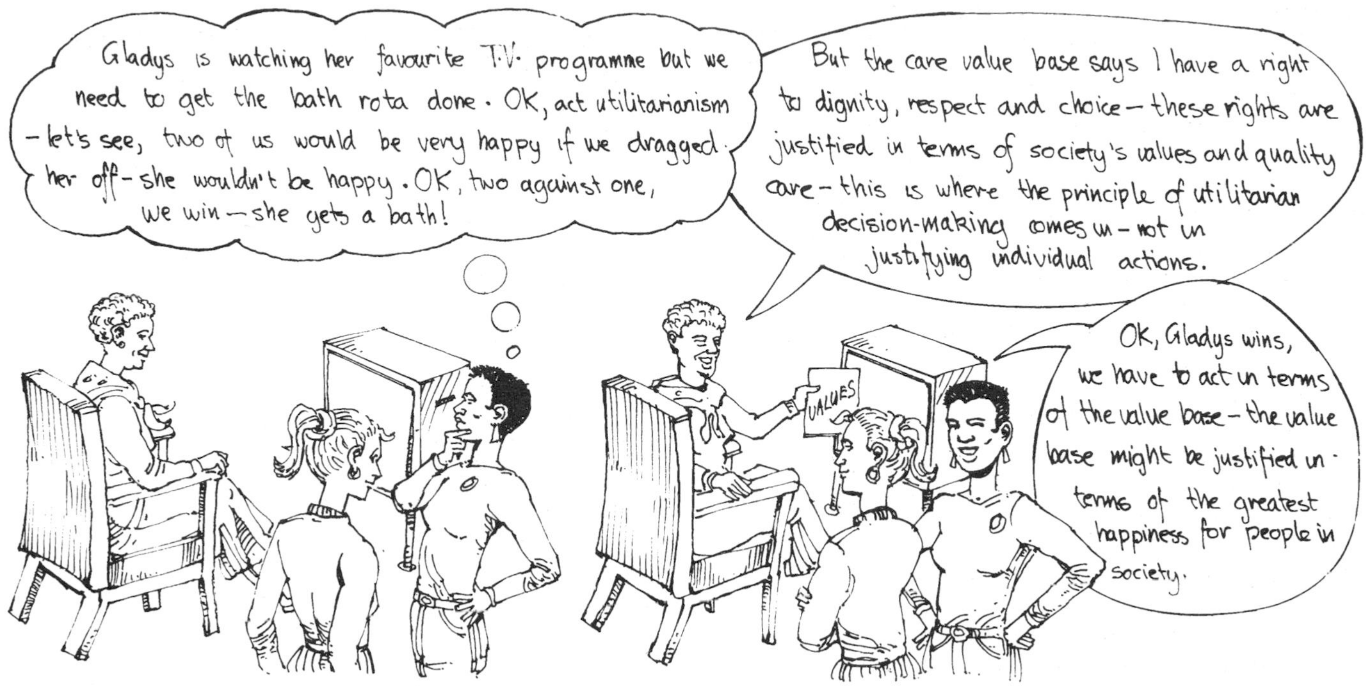
Gladys is watching her favourite T.V. programme but we need to get the bath rota done. OK, act utilitarianism – let's see, two of us would be very happy if we dragged her off – she wouldn't be happy. OK, two against one, we win – she gets a bath!
But the care value base says I have a right to dignity, respect and choice – these rights are justified in terms of society's values and quality care – this is where the principle of utilitarian decision-making comes in – not in justifying individual actions.
VALUES
OK, Gladys wins, we have to act in terms of the value base – the value base might be justified in terms of the greatest happiness for people in society.

Figure 3.2 An alternative logical theory of ethics

So the idea of greatest happiness may be a helpful principle of social justice, but not a useful way to make moment-by-moment decisions in care work.

Immanuel **Kant** (1742–1804) argued that the same rules should apply to all people and that knowledge comes from a process of reasoning. Whether an action is right or wrong will therefore depend on the motives for the action.

Kant's theory is universal, i.e. everyone has to follow the same moral rules whatever the situation, and is therefore objective, i.e. there are set rules which all should follow. According to this viewpoint a doctor would always tell a terminally-ill patient the truth. It is deemed an essential duty always to tell the truth because Kant believed that in this way respect for the individual is demonstrated.

Kantians argue that it is impossible to have a meaningful relationship unless it is based on truth. In this example, the patient has free will and, if he asks for a diagnosis, the truth must be told. In this way the doctor has done the right thing by telling the truth to the patient and has therefore demonstrated respect for that individual.

Critics of Kantianism state that the definition of duty can be interpreted in different ways by different people. The essential dictate (rule) always to tell the truth may place an individual in an impossible situation; for example, being told something in confidence by one person then instructed to tell the truth about the confidence by another. Kant would expect both!

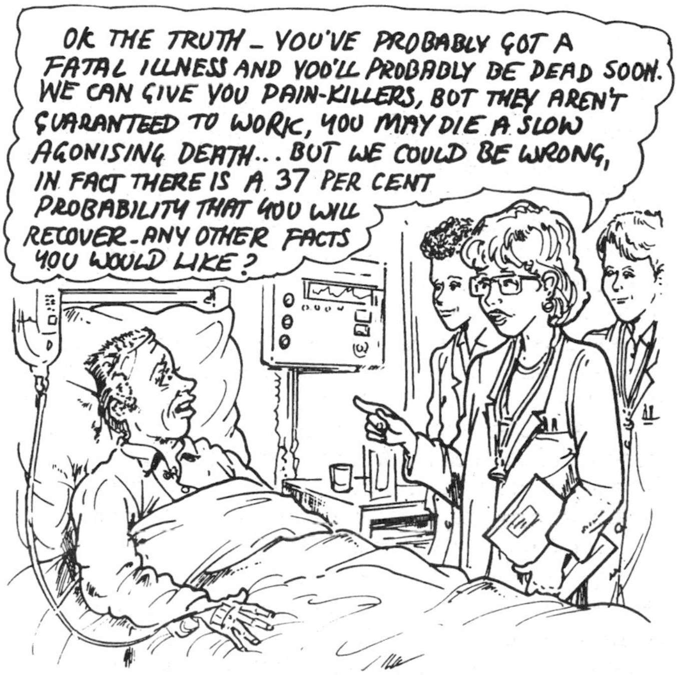
OK THE TRUTH – YOU'VE PROBABLY GOT A FATAL ILLNESS AND YOU'LL PROBABLY BE DEAD SOON. WE CAN GIVE YOU PAIN-KILLERS, BUT THEY AREN'T GUARANTEED TO WORK, YOU MAY DIE A SLOW AGONISING DEATH... BUT WE COULD BE WRONG, IN FACT THERE IS A 37 PER CENT PROBABILITY THAT YOU WILL RECOVER – ANY OTHER FACTS YOU WOULD LIKE?

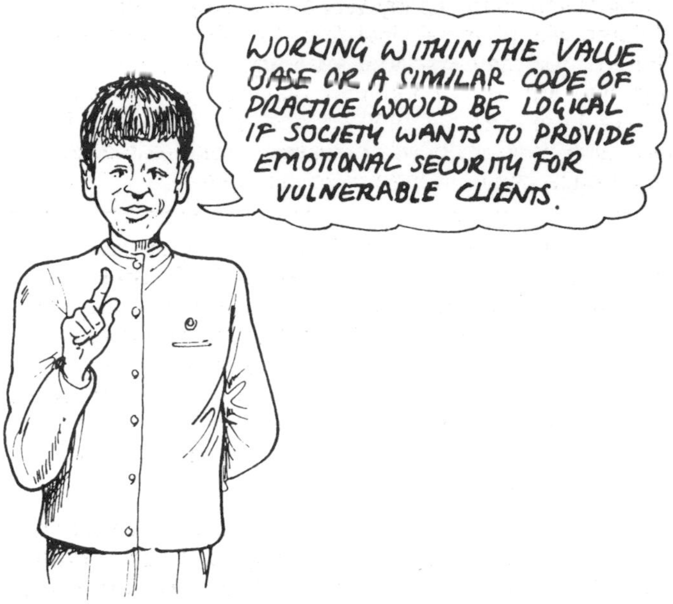
WORKING WITHIN THE VALUE BASE OR A SIMILAR CODE OF PRACTICE WOULD BE LOGICAL IF SOCIETY WANTS TO PROVIDE EMOTIONAL SECURITY FOR VULNERABLE CLIENTS.

Pure logic and absolute truth seem a good idea at first, but when used as a basis for day-to-day decision-making the idea does not lead to acceptable practice on its own. It is not enough simply to be logical or truthful. Communication has to show respect for individual beliefs and identity. The care value base does not suggest that it might be acceptable to lie or mislead clients, but it does suggest that truth and logic are not the sole issues in care work.

Decision-making in health and social care cannot depend on simple principles like utilitarianism or logic: but nor can decision-making be left to the beliefs that individuals have been brought up with, or socialised into. Professional value bases or codes of practice are needed to help workers make decisions. The problem is that decision-making is still a difficult task, even when staff understand value bases and codes of practice. Many situations require professional levels of judgement.

Think it over

What makes a person a skilled and valued professional? In the past many people may have answered that it is knowledge that is important; it's what a person knows that makes a professional lawyer, doctor, engineer and so on. But nowadays a vast amount of factual knowledge is available from a CD-ROM and anyone can obtain detailed information if they try. Professionals deal in more than information – they have skills in making important decisions, skills of judgement. Ethical decisions and judgements are part of the skill base of professional workers.

There is a debate about duty and morals. **Morals** are the rules whereby society defines what is right and what is wrong. They are general rules which should be kept, but there could be circumstances whereby they are broken for the good of the many.

Think it over

Imagine that you have a friend who has a drink problem which she has so far hidden from her employer. She operates machinery and could endanger herself and others. The dilemma is the risk to the friendship by telling the employer, or the risk of harm to people through an accident. Kantians would argue that duty states the friend should be told of your concerns, thereby demonstrating respect for her as an individual. Your individual perception of right and wrong could conflict with the values of society at large, as society might see it as your duty to tell the employer of the possible dangers. A utilitarian might have no such qualms: the good of the many may outweigh the good of the one. So different ethical beliefs can lead to different conclusions.

In the past there has been a great divide between the academic study of ethics and the practical application of ethics in a given organisation or profession. But in recent years the appreciation of the diversity of moral dilemmas which now face professionals has prompted the wider study of ethics, both in education and the professions, hence the inclusion of them in the standards for GNVQ.

A growing school of thought advocates a combination of the best elements from utilitarianism and Kantianism. Rowson (1990) and Tschudin (1992) both see value in using a combination of the two schools of thought to help professionals solve difficult ethical problems. The flexibility of being able to review the consequences of general actions, combined with the logical use of a set rules, such as codes of professional conduct, gives great potential for developing decision-making skills.

Ways in which organisations handle ethical issues

Daryl Kohen (1994) and Geoffrey Hunt (1994) both see the introduction of codes of ethics for a range of professionals as a response to the decline outlined by MacNiven at the beginning of this section. Codes of practice may provide a way of focusing ethical decision making.

Think it over

Review the Code of Professional Conduct produced by the United Kingdom Central Council (UKCC) responsible for Nurses, Midwives and Health Visitors or the Code produced by the British Association of Social Workers (BASW). See pages 62–3. Note any similarities and differences and the value base inherent in each.

You may also wish to look at codes of practice from other professions; for example, the Hippocratic Oath taken by doctors, those from the Law Society, dentists, psychologists, pharmacists and the code of ethics regarding research.

It is important to review the ethics involved in drafting care plans for individuals. Having made an assessment with a client to determine their needs, the professional may then have to perform a balancing act to meet these needs – possibly in the light of a restricted budget. Knowing what is considered to be the best for an individual unfortunately does not always mean that the best is possible, and a compromise must often be reached.

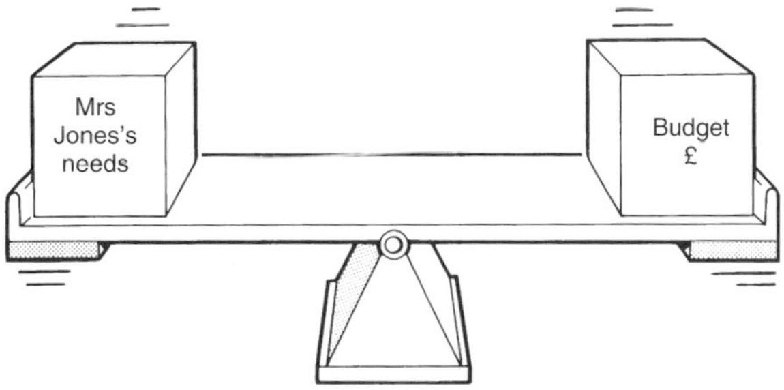

Chapters 22 to 24 provide another application of ethics, with a review of the ethical issues involved in undertaking research.

Dealing with ethical issues

Think it over

How would you decide if you had the choice: *either* of taking two children with terminal illness to Disney World *or* taking several children with physical disabilities to a theme park in Britain? You may wish to make a list of for's and against's for each option, then discuss your ideas with others. Look carefully at the factors you choose; how is the value base used? It's not easy! Look again at the value base given on the previous pages.

A utilitarian view could involve looking at the consequences of any action taken. All children would benefit from a trip: the excitement of new things to see and do, the magic of the rides etc. All children have a right to fun, to play, to experience new sensations, tastes, sounds, smells, ideas. In each case the children involved would gain from the experience. If the choice was to take the two then the many would be denied the experience.

Kantians, on the other hand, would consider that the duty was to take the two terminally-ill children rather than the many on this occasion. A justification would be that the two children only have limited time to gain such an experience, whilst the many will have other opportunities. The problem presents a difficult scenario and one which has no right or wrong answer!

The role of a carer in the health and social care field is to provide care which is in the best interest of the client. However, as we have seen, the best interest of the client may not always be possible. More importantly, who decides what the best interests of the client are?

The value base provides a guide which may help to answer the question. Respecting individuals, and empowering those individuals to make informed choices about their lives, means that where possible it is the client who should determine their own best interest.

Empowerment places a great deal of responsibility on the care staff. It is the staff who must ensure that clients are kept informed of their rights. There are several guides which may help here: these include the Patient's Charter, Community Care Charter, professional codes of practice, Equal Opportunities Policy and the complaints procedures held by organisations/institutions. Legislation such as the Children Act 1989, NHS and Community Care Act 1990, Criminal Justice Bill 1994, Mental Health Act 1983, the Data Protection Act 1984, the Access to Personal Files Act 1987, the Access to Medical Records Act 1988 and the Access to Health Records 1990, all outline client rights.

A working knowledge of the relevant information, or knowing how and where to obtain that information

12 Principles of Social Work Practice

1. Knowledge, skills, and experience used positively for the benefit of all sections of the community and individuals.
2. Respect for clients as individuals and safeguarding their dignity and rights.
3. No prejudice in self, nor tolerance of prejudice in others, on grounds of origin, race, status, sex, sexual orientation, age, disability, beliefs, or contribution to society.
4. Empowerment of clients and their participation in decisions and defining services.
5. Sustained concern for clients even when unable to help them or where self-protection is necessary.
6. Professional responsibility takes precedence over personal interest.
7. Responsibility for standards of service and for continuing education and training.
8. Collaboration with others in the interests of clients.
9. Clarity in public as to whether acting in a personal or organisational capacity.
10. Promotion of appropriate ethnic and cultural diversity of services.
11. Confidentiality of information and divulgence only by consent or exceptionally in evidence of serious danger.
12. Pursuit of conditions of employment which enable these obligations to be respected.

UKCC CODE OF PROFESSIONAL CONDUCT

FOR THE NURSE, MIDWIFE AND HEALTH VISITOR

Each registered nurse, midwife and health visitor shall act, at all times, in such a manner as to:

- safeguard and promote the interests of individual patients and clients;
- serve the interests of society;
- justify public trust and confidence and
- uphold and enhance the good standing and reputation of the professions.

As a registered nurse, midwife or health visitor, you are personally accountable for your practice and, in the exercise of your professional accountability, must:

1. act always in such a manner as to promote and safeguard the interests and well-being of patients and clients;
2. ensure that no action or omission on your part, or within your sphere of responsibility, is detrimental to the interests, condition or safety of patients and clients;
3. maintain and improve your professional knowledge and competence;

4 acknowledge any limitations in your knowledge and competence and decline any duties or responsibilities unless able to perform them in a safe and skilled manner;

5 work in an open and co-operative manner with patients, clients and their families, foster their independence and recognise and respect their involvement in the planning and delivery of care;

6 work in a collaborative and co-operative manner with health care professionals and others involved in providing care, and recognise and respect their particular contributions within the care team;

7 recognise and respect the uniqueness and dignity of each patient and client, and respond to their need for care, irrespective of their ethnic origin, religious beliefs, personal attributes, the nature of their health problems or any other factor;

8 report to an appropriate person or authority, at the earliest possible time, any conscientious objection which may be relevant to your professional practice;

9 avoid any abuse of your privileged relationship with patients and clients and of the privileged access allowed to their person, property, residence or workplace;

10 protect all confidential information concerning patients and clients obtained in the course of professional practice and make disclosures only with consent, where required by the order of a court or where you can justify disclosure in the wider public interest;

11 report to an appropriate person or authority, having regard to the physical, psychological and social effects on patients and clients, any circumstances in the environment of care which could jeopardise standards of practice;

12 report to an appropriate person or authority any circumstances in which safe and appropriate care for patients and clients cannot be provided;

13 report to an appropriate person where it appears that the health or safety of colleagues is at risk, as such circumstances may compromise standards of practice and care;

14 assist professional colleagues, in the context of your own knowledge, experience and sphere of responsibility, to develop their professional competence, and assist others in the care team, including informal carers, to contribute safely and to a degree appropriate to their roles;

15 refuse any gift, favour or hospitality from patients or clients currently in your care which might be interpreted as seeking to exert influence to obtain preferential consideration, and

16 ensure that your registration status is not used in the promotion of commercial products or services, declare any financial or other interest in relevant organisations providing such goods or services and ensure that your professional judgement is not influenced by any commercial considerations.

This Code of Professional Conduct for the Nurse, Midwife and Health Visitor is issued to all registered nurses, midwives and health visitors by the United Kingdom Central Council for Nursing, Midwifery and Health Visiting.

The Council is the regulatory body responsible for the standards of these professions and it requires members of the professions to practise and conduct themselves within the standards and framework provided by the Code.

to help clients, is important. Copies of the relevant Charters or Codes of Practice should be available in each establishment.

Try it

Analyse the following problem:

An elderly person is having increasing difficulty coping independently at home. She agrees to a visit from a social worker to review the situation. The woman lives in a large old house, requiring considerable repairs, which she cannot afford. Well-meaning neighbours are vocal in their opinions that it would be in her best interest to 'go into a home to be looked after'.

Under the NHS and Community Care Act 1990 the woman is entitled to an assessment of her needs. The social worker must work with her not only to assess her needs but to explain all the options available, including residential or day care or support services within her own home.

In this case empowerment is therefore the encouragement to review all the options. By ensuring that the woman actively participates in the decision-making process, the social worker is demonstrating respect for her as an individual. The danger would be to fall into the trap of stereotyping the woman as elderly and therefore incapable of making her own decisions.

However, remember that it was said earlier that cost has implications for the care which is available. The social worker will need to have an *holistic overview* (i.e. insight into all the factors involved), in order to work with this client.

It will be important for the social worker to liaise with a range of other professionals, and any family the woman may have, in order to meet her needs. It is important therefore that the social worker reaches an agreement with the client that the situation may be discussed with these people.

Confidentiality

One of the values inherent in health and social care work is confidentiality. What do you do when a client confides information to you as a health or social care worker that you feel should be shared? Is it ethical to break a confidence? You have a moral duty to your client to maintain confidentiality, yet you may decide that the situation is outside your abilities to cope.

Clear boundaries for a given role should be defined when a worker takes up a post. This ensures that the worker is aware of the expectations of others and the limits of the duties required. Equally, it is important to set boundaries with clients so that they are aware of the role and responsibilities you each have in your relationship.

If the worker considers that the information received should be shared with a senior member of staff for the benefit of the client, then that should usually be stated to the client. It is important to explain why it is necessary to share the information and to reassure the client that boundaries of confidentiality will still be maintained. It is better still if the client can be persuaded to give the information directly to the senior member of staff.

Cultural needs

Britain today has a multicultural society. Therefore in health and social care it is important to have some understanding of different cultures in order to meet the needs of all those who require care. It may often be necessary to provide a care worker from a particular ethnic group to meet the needs of particular people; for example, a Bengali-speaking social worker employed to work with that particular ethnic group in the community.

The charity Age Concern reviewed the needs of many elders from different ethnic groups in a video produced in the late 1980s, *According to need.* You may wish to review this to gain a clearer insight into what can be achieved to meet the needs of particular groups.

The key points raised by the video include the requirement to recognise the needs of elders growing old in an alien culture. Many may have little or no English, and little contact with people who understand their culture and religion. The video also reviews the setting up of day centres and the special provision necessary in the community and residential settings. The training needs of home care and residential staff, and the responsibilities of Social Services, are reviewed.

Think it over

Meeting the cultural needs of a particular individual may include issues about diet and the preparation of food. What do you do if a new client has particular dietary requirements which may mean that food has to be prepared separately? The establishment has a limited budget and one cook who has been there for sometime. How do you balance the needs of the majority and the needs of the one within that budget?

There are many issues that arise from the concept of equal opportunities. Do you challenge an elder who makes a sexist or racist comment? Or do you ignore it, 'because they don't know any better'? Many white elders hold stereotyped views of people from different ethnic groups. They may well have no understanding of different cultural needs, for example, eating with fingers instead of with cutlery. Some might complain about the smell of food, the accents, dress, etc.

It is the responsibility of all staff in health and social care to ensure that the rights of all clients are upheld – including their dignity and respect as individuals. This may well mean challenging inappropriate comments in a straightforward but supportive way to enable all to learn. Staff should also be positive role models for clients – a great responsibility! But in order to support clients, and to ensure that they maintain a positive view of themselves, a respect for the clients' culture is essential.

Think it over

Respecting culture is about the environment in which the client lives. Look at the pictures on the walls, the books, videos, music, papers and magazines; do they reflect the ethnic and cultural mix of residents and staff?

If the only provision is for white people, what is the hidden message being given to those from different ethnic and cultural backgrounds? Food is often an issue that staff consider, but it is also important to recognise different eating habits, such as eating with fingers.

Body language can give offence in a powerful way: people pulling faces, moving away or refusing to sit next to an Asian person for instance, because of their eating customs.

Care workers need to be aware of the situation and to deal with it when it arises. One way of doing this might be to take the person who makes the remark to one side in private, explaining that such comments are hurtful and not appropriate. Another way might be to point out to the client that the staff work to respect *all* their clients, that this is the way this person has been taught to eat their food and that there are strict rules about eating in that culture as well as in a white culture.

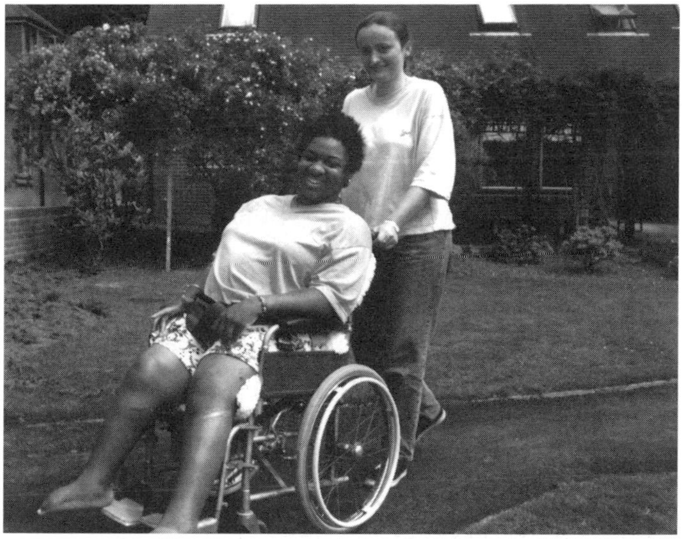

(Photo courtesy of Winged Fellowship Trust)

Continuing with this example, it would also be important to support the Asian person and to acknowledge that they may be hurt by the reaction of white clients. It might be helpful to work together to resolve the situation for the benefit of all.

Staff have a great responsibility as they must ensure that an equal quality service is given to all. Individual needs are assessed with clients and an agreed way of working has to be reached to meet those needs.

Personal needs

Other ethical issues which may arise include dealing with clients who may become disturbed or aggressive. As a carer, do you keep these clients restrained for their own safety and for the safety of others? You are responsible for the well-being of all in your care. In certain circumstances training programmes are provided for staff, to help them to cope effectively with violence in as safe a way as possible for all concerned.

A difficult situation arises when the client has limited understanding. This places particular responsibility on staff to ensure that, as far as possible, the client is made aware of their rights and given opportunities to choose options. The danger is that staff could stereotype the client and make decisions on their behalf based on the stereotype After all, it is quicker to say, 'You do like tea – here it is' than to offer a choice which may take time!

An important issue arising out of the movement of clients from large institutions into independent living is the inability to make choices. If a person's total experience of life is to be told when to get up, what to wear, when to eat etc., then it becomes the norm; and the norm is safe because it is the daily pattern. It is difficult – and possibly frightening – to have to make even simple everyday decisions.

Staff in the health services and in social care have been working hard with many clients who have been institutionalised. Working to give the individual the confidence to make decisions for themselves is very demanding, requiring a great deal of patience and diplomacy. But the time and effort is well spent when looking again at the value base of health and social care: working to provide the best quality of life for each individual by meeting needs; empowering the individual to make informed choices and encouraging independence displays ethical professional practice.

Sexuality

One of the dilemmas facing those working with adults with learning difficulties is the question of sexuality. The stereotypical view of someone with learning difficulties is as an overgrown child who is asexual (has no sexual feelings). This stereotype discriminates against people with learning difficulties. All humans need the company and respect of others to a greater or lesser extent. Puberty brings with it an awakening of the physical body, a need to be seen and accepted as a man or a woman, and it happens to all of us – regardless of our intellectual capabilities.

Much debate has gone on in the education sector to try to determine when children should be taught sex education. In the past it was thought that this was unnecessary for those with physical disabilities or those with learning difficulties. This denied the rights of those individuals to express themselves and to gain the satisfaction of a sexual relationship should they so choose. There has also been debate regarding the sterilisation of some people with learning difficulties – denying them children and a family life. Organisations such as the Association of Spina Bifida and Hydrocephalus (ASBAH) have set up an advisory service to help those with physical disabilities. For those with learning difficulties it may well be the key worker or advocate of a client who needs to work to help the client gain understanding.

Sexuality has been a taboo subject and still may be so for many people. It is an area where care workers may unwittingly impose their own views and values on a client. However, to do so can be argued to be unethical as it denies the rights of individuals to make their own decisions. It may be desirable to stop a client from masturbating (i.e. stimulating their own genitals for sexual pleasure) in a public or open lounge because masturbation is seen as unsociable behaviour. It may be preferable to suggest that they go to their room for privacy. However, making that client feel dirty or guilty by the oppressive behaviour of staff may be argued to conflict with the value base and to be unethical. Staff may therefore need to be in touch with their own feelings about sexuality before they are able to work effectively with others.

Sex education should be dealt with when the individual is ready. It needs to include the importance of relationships as well as the mechanics of sexuality and safety issues regarding unwanted pregnancy, HIV and sexually transmitted diseases. This should be achieved in a way that is easily understood by the individual and at their own pace.

Think it over

The officer in charge of a residential establishment for people with physical disabilities had agreed that partners could stay for weekends if they so wished.

Over a period of time it was noticed that one resident was withdrawn and quiet; he had many visitors but no-one was asked to stay. Eventually his key worker managed to get him to talk about his concerns and was taken aback to learn the reason for his depression.

The man confided that he was gay and had had a stable partner for many years. He very much wanted his partner to stay but felt unable to ask. He felt that the culture of the establishment was towards heterosexual relationships and that he would be discriminated against.

Here was a staff team who were trying hard to meet the needs of all the clients but they had made certain assumptions about the clients. Those assumptions that all clients were heterosexual had indeed discriminated against this man, making him feel vulnerable and isolated. Effectively, his rights to express his sexuality as he chose had been denied, leading to discrimination and disempowerment by the staff.

The resident agreed to his worries being shared with the officer in charge and the staff team. A staff development programme helped staff to work through the issues, and the man had his partner to stay.

During the course of a day's work, staff in the health and social care field are faced with many ethical issues. These may include: the sharing or withholding of information; balancing the rights of one client against the rights of others; and client safety balanced against their wish to take risks, for example, a client wishing to discontinue medication.

In each case it is the responsibility of the care worker to ensure that the clients are able to make an informed decision where possible. Staff may have the policy of the establishment as guidance and, if necessary, must tell the client if they cannot deal with the situation themselves, but must inform a senior member of staff.

Think it over

An elderly man has been admitted to a care home as a short-stay client, to give his family a much-needed break. He is a pipe smoker and makes it clear that he enjoys his pipe and wishes to continue smoking. But several clients object to tobacco smoke in the lounge and come to you to complain. What do you do?

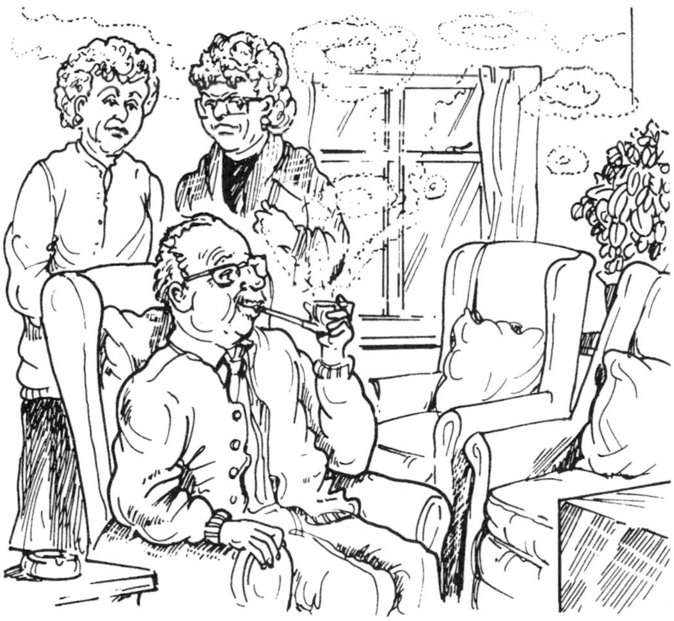

Carers have a responsibility to meet the needs of all clients. At first sight it might appear that in order to uphold the rights of those who are making a complaint, the carer must deny the right of the one. But the right to choice is part of the value base!

One way to approach the problem might be to acknowledge the concerns of those who are complaining but also to acknowledge the right of the individual. It might be useful to check to see if the home has a policy on smoking; if it has a policy then it might be important to see if the man was aware of it. If there is no policy then a compromise might be reached, perhaps about smoking in a designated room, for example.

Some establishments have a residents' committee which meets to review the needs of all the residents. Such a committee might be run for and by residents, perhaps with a staff representative. If such a committee exists then the issue of smoking could be raised there. It is important that the value base of care should be involved in all decisions about what is good practice.

Medical ethics

The health service faces many similar dilemmas to social care but there are also some significant differences. Care of those who are terminally ill may raise special issues. It would not be appropriate here to discuss euthanasia (ending someone's life) and in Britain it is against the law. But the issues surrounding euthanasia are often debated at many levels in the health field.

It may be appropriate, however, to look briefly at the issues facing medical staff working with seriously ill people. There is a distinct difference between giving a lethal injection (an injection which will kill) to end a person's life and withholding treatment in certain circumstances.

It has been argued that to hasten a person's death is a moral and not a medical decision; the decision does not solely concern the medical profession. To stop or withhold treatment *is,* however, a medical decision and can legitimately be made by doctors.

A doctor may seek the permission of relations to end treatment; for example, to turn off a life support machine if there are no signs of recovery. For a person close to the end of a terminal illness the doctor may ensure that all nursing care is given to the patient but no further treatment, for example for lung infections etc., will be given. The patient is therefore allowed to die with as much dignity as the situations allows. So a doctor may stop treatment, but a doctor may not take direct action to end a patient's life.

Think it over

A doctor in a casualty department is faced with the decision whether to save a life by performing a minor operation to enable a paralysed patient to breathe. The decision has to be made in a hurry or the patient will suffer from damage to the brain due to lack of oxygen. One of the thoughts going through the doctor's head might be that the patient will have a restricted life, as he is likely to be paralysed from the neck down with only a slim chance of recovery. The care implications and cost of such paralysis are enormous. To do nothing would mean death from lack of oxygen to the brain.

A Kantian view might be to say that the doctor's duty is to perform the operation because of the principle of preservation of life. A utilitarian might try to review the consequences. What general approach would you choose and why?

The emphasis in the health service rests on the preservation of life. Individuals also undergo operations and extensive treatments in the hope of gaining a better quality of life. Much has been learnt from such operations as bone marrow, kidney, heart and liver transplants. Many patients have benefited from such treatment; sadly, some have not.

The ethical dilemma facing the surgeons treating such cases is to decide whether the operation is in the best interest of the patient. Some sections of the media are quick to criticise the medical profession for undertaking such treatment when the chances of success are slim. The families and friends of very ill patients, however, may often prefer to risk the slim chance rather than to acknowledge no chance of survival. The surgeon therefore has all these factors to consider when coming to a decision.

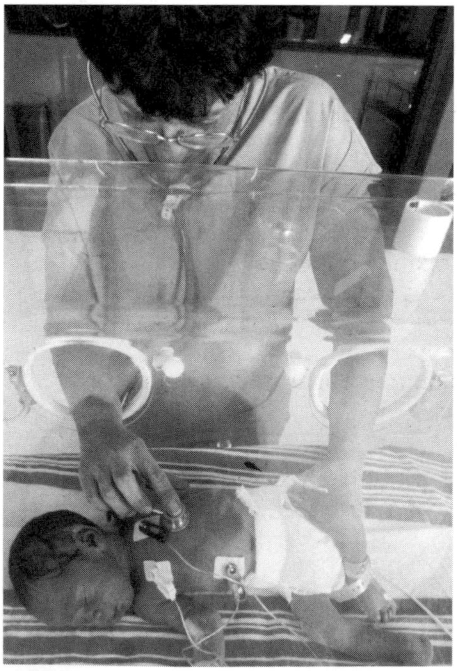

Nurses may well be faced with a patient who refuses medication or refuses to eat. Failure to take medication or refusing food could lead to the death of the patient. The role of the nurse is to preserve life, so can he or she stand back and watch someone die?

This is a very complex issue and needs to be reviewed on an individual basis with each patient concerned. If the patient is conscious, and is knowingly refusing food, then an exploration of the reasons behind this may be essential. It could be the only way in which the person feels able to assert themselves in an alien environment. The change of environment, meal-times, diet and concern about the patient's condition and future may all be issues which have to be addressed by the nurse or other professional.

If the person is unconscious, or mentally unable to make rational decisions, then again the issues vary. The decision whether to feed through a naso-gastric tube or intravenously will have to be made by the medical staff.

Nursing staff may be asked to try to coax a reluctant but conscious person to eat. The danger in this case is the nurse being aware that a certain amount of food is deemed to be essential during a given time period, which might lead to the nurse pressurising the patient to eat. This could result in a loss of trust between the patient and the nurse and a further refusal to eat. (Chapter 4 of Hunt, 1994, gives an excellent account of these complex issues.)

The key issue is the need to be very clear about the role of all staff involved in patient/client care. Knowing one's own boundaries is as essential as the awareness of the value base expressed through an ethical and professional code of practice.

Overview

Workers in health and social care provide a range of skilled personal services to clients. Many problems can arise about individual and community rights and how to provide a high quality service. Because ethical problems are often very difficult to resolve, many professions and occupations are defining the principles of good practice in value bases and codes of practice.

In health and social care the 'O' unit value base for NVQ qualifications may be argued to provide a framework for outlining the responsibilities of care workers. This framework includes the principles of working in the client's best interests and empowering clients.

Many care workers and care professionals may also have to assess the risks which their policies and actions may create. Health and safety at work legislation requires managers to assess the risks associated with practice and to minimise risks to personal safety and health.

The complexity of services to meet individual needs can create an almost infinite range of ethical problems and decision-making tasks in practice. Workers need to develop their own skills of personal judgement and ethical decision-making. Codes of practice and value bases may assist with decision-making. The principles of logical decision-making and utilitarianism may also provide a starting point for the development of decision-making skills.

Organisations may tackle complex ethical issues by holding discussions with clients, relatives and workers; by defining organisational policies and by referring to value bases and codes of practice; by maintaining staff development and training policies; by ensuring that practice complies with the law and by taking advice from professional bodies.

Evidence collection point

Prepare a report which will explain a variety of different ethical issues faced by health and care workers. Explain the responsibilities of health and social care workers. Describe ways in which organisations and individuals might handle ethical issues, and analyse the handling of two ethical issues.

Self-assessment test

1 All societies share the same underpinning principles.
True or false?

2 Competition is central to the principles of Western societies.
True or false?

3 The purpose of equality of opportunity legislation is to ensure all groups of people have an equal chance to compete.
True or false?

4 Legislation ensures that everyone has the same chances in the 'competition' for wealth and social status.
True or false?

5 Ethical codes are based on the values which guide professional conduct.
True or false?

6 Health and social care staff have important social roles in relation to equal opportunities because:
- **a** They are able to ensure equal access to service
- **b** They have a range of knowledge and skills
- **c** They have control within the care setting
- **d** They are able to provide a safe environment

7 Respecting the culture of a client is most important because it will:
- **a** Demonstrate tolerance
- **b** Demonstrate flexibility
- **c** Reinforce self-esteem
- **d** Reinforce individual learning

8 Institutionalised racism is:
- **a** Racism through violence on the streets
- **b** Racism through the culture of an organisation
- **c** Racism through verbal attacks
- **d** Racism through failure to employ black people

9 The Sex Discrimination Act is principally designed to:
- **a** Protect women in employment
- **b** Protect men in employment
- **c** Ensure equality in the workplace
- **d** Ensure fair play

10 Professional Codes of Practice aim to:
- **a** Outline the expected behaviour of workers
- **b** Outline working conditions
- **c** Outline hours of employment
- **d** Outline the expected behaviour of clients

11 There is legislation to cover discrimination on sexuality.
True or false?

12 The legal age of consent for homosexual relations is:
- **a** 16 years
- **b** 19 years
- **c** 21 years
- **d** 23 years

13 It is illegal to discriminate against a person due to age.
True or false?

14 If you think you have been refused a job because of your gender, you should complain to:
- **a** The Commission for Racial Equality
- **b** The Advisory, Conciliation and Arbitration Service
- **c** The Crown Court
- **d** The Equal Opportunities Commission

15 If you think you have been denied promotion because of your ethnic origins, you may first gain information and support from:
- **a** Your local council
- **b** Your local MP
- **c** The Equal Opportunities Commission
- **d** The Commission for Racial Equality

16 An example of inconsistency in enforcing the law is:
- **a** The monitoring of race issues
- **b** The monitoring of gender issues
- **c** The lack of monitoring for disability issues
- **d** The lack of monitoring of sexuality issues

17 An appeal may be taken further following an industrial tribunal.
True or false?

18 An example of a pressure group trying to influence equal opportunity legislation is:
- **a** Age Concern
- **b** Save the Children Fund
- **c** Voluntary Organisation for Anti-discrimination Legislation
- **d** Shelter

19 The legislation intended to help people with disability get a job is:
- **a** The Equal Pay Act
- **b** The Mental Health Act
- **c** The NHS and Community Care Act
- **d** The Disabled Persons Employment Act

20 Equal Opportunities legislation in Britain is influenced by which European body?
- **a** The European Court of Justice
- **b** The European Parliament
- **c** The European Council of Ministers
- **d** The Euro MPs

21 Direct discrimination means:
- **a** Subtle ways of showing disrespect
- **b** Failing to monitor an equal opportunity policy
- **c** Hiding true feelings about a given group
- **d** Blatant ways of showing disrespect

22 Indirect discrimination takes place when:
- **a** You move your seat when a person with a learning disability joins your table
- **b** You avoid any potential insult to your black friend by not inviting him or her to a party where all the other guests are white
- **c** You give a look of disgust and comment about a person who has disfiguring facial scars
- **d** You speak to the person pushing the wheelchair about the occupant, but ignore the person in the chair

23 State which of the following is an example of direct discrimination:
- **a** You refuse to work with a client that you can't get on with
- **b** You cross the road to avoid speaking to a person you know to be gay before he or she sees you
- **c** You deliberately tell racist jokes at a party where there are black and white guests
- **d** You choose not to join a club as you consider the members are 'old fogies'

24 Discrimination can take place on different bases. Some of these are:
- **a** Gender
- **b** Physical ability
- **c** Age
- **d** Race

A selection of statements from job advertisements include the following. Indicate the discriminatory base for each statement:
- **i** Child models required, must be fair skinned
- **ii** Sales representatives required, only active car drivers need apply
- **iii** Housemaid required for hotel

25 Language may be used to discriminate by:
- **i** tone of voice
- **ii** choice of words
- **iii** body language
- **iv** assumptions

Which of the following applies?
- **a** Putting milk and sugar in the tea of an elder who has been labelled 'confused'
- **b** Saying 'you are *only* a girl'
- **c** Pulling a face and laughing at a person with learning difficulties when he or she becomes confused with money

26 Which of these statements demonstrates discriminatory language?

- **a** New theatres should have access for wheelchair users
- **b** Retired people should be banned from this health club
- **c** Society should be more tolerant of gay people
- **d** Pubs should make provision for families

27 An important aspect of discrimination is the way in which language is used. Decide which of these statements is true and which is false:

- **i** The meaning of a sentence can be changed by the tone of voice adopted
- **ii** Words can be used as a powerful tool to put other people down

Which option best describes the two statements?

- **a** **i** (T) **ii** (T)
- **b** **i** (T) **ii** (F)
- **c** **i** (F) **ii** (T)
- **d** **i** (F) **ii** (F)

28 Failing to promote women in the company is an example of:

- **a** Sexual harassment
- **b** Racial harassment
- **c** Indirect discrimination
- **d** Institutional discrimination

29 Refusing to employ workers who are Muslim as they will want time to pray contravenes which legislation to promote equality of opportunity?

- **a** Equal Pay Act
- **b** Sex Discrimination Act
- **c** Race Relations Act
- **d** Health and Safety at Work Act

30 Positive action means:

- **a** Actively recruiting certain people to redress an imbalance of staff in an organisation
- **b** Actively recruiting only women in an organisation
- **c** Actively recruiting only men in an organisation
- **d** Actively recruiting people of a certain age in the organisation

31 Which is an example of using body language to reinforce discrimination?

- **a** A black teacher smiling and nodding as a child tries to answer a question
- **b** A female member of an interview panel leaning forward to listen to a male candidate's responses
- **c** A careworker gently touching the arm of an elderly client during conversation
- **d** A group leader who keeps his or her back to a person with disability during group discussions

32 Direct and indirect discrimination take different forms. Which of the following is true (T) or false (F)?

- **i** Direct discrimination involves open belittling of female staff
- **ii** Indirect discrimination involves quietly avoiding tea breaks with someone with severe facial scars

Which option best describes the two statements?

- **a** **i** (T) **ii** (T)
- **b** **i** (T) **ii** (F)
- **c** **i** (F) **ii** (T)
- **d** **i** (F) **ii** (F)

Questions 33 to 35 share answers a to d

Individuals may be discriminated against because of their:

- **a** Gender
- **b** Race
- **c** Level of cognitive ability
- **d** Level of physical ability

Which form of discrimination is occurring in each example?

33 Denying choice to a man 45 years of age with Down's Syndrome

34 Refusing to admit a black applicant to a youth club

35 Refusing an application from a female for an electrician's post

36 Discrimination in the context of health and social care results from people:

- **a** Treating all people equally
- **b** Recognising individual differences
- **c** Respecting individual differences
- **d** Recognising inequalities in society

Questions 37 to 39 share answers a to d

Jim, a young married man with two children, has recently returned home from hospital following an accident at work which has left him blind. The family feel very protective of him but Jim needs to:

- **a** Rebuild his self-confidence
- **b** Adjust his self-image
- **c** Gain new skills for employment and daily living
- **d** Learn about the choices and services available to him

Which of these will be affected most if his family:

37 Encourage him to join his friends at their weekly social events?

38 Encourage him to join a retraining programme?

39 Encourage him to take an active role with the children?

40 A carer can *best* avoid discriminatory practice by:
- **a** Sticking to a strict routine
- **b** Avoiding stereotyping clients
- **c** Speaking slowly to all elderly clients
- **d** Treating everyone the same

41 Health and social care professionals work within a defined value base.
True or false?

42 A well-defined value base will reassure clients about the quality of service they may expect.
True or false?

43 Confidentiality of information is a core value in health and social care. This is important because:
- **a** Carers need to know everything about the client
- **b** Carers need to gain the trust of the client to work effectively
- **c** Carers need to know what to tell relatives
- **d** Carers need to keep records on all clients

44 A client confides information which you consider must be shared with senior staff. What is your *first* course of action?
- **a** Keep the information to yourself to maintain confidentiality
- **b** Discuss the issue with a colleague but do not identify the client
- **c** Discuss the issue with a close friend outside work, but do not identify the client
- **d** Discuss the issue with the client, explaining why the matter needs to be taken further

45 State which of the following is true (T) or false (F).
- **a** Clients have a right to see their personal file
- **b** Under certain circumstances some information in a personal file is withheld from the individual

Which option best describes the two statements?

i	**a**	(T)	**b**	(T)
ii	**a**	(T)	**b**	(F)
iii	**a**	(F)	**b**	(T)
iv	**a**	(F)	**b**	(F)

46 A central care value is to promote anti-discriminatory practice. Decide which statement is true (T) and which false (F).
- **a** Health and social care staff have a duty to recognise and appropriately challenge any discriminatory behaviour
- **b** It is acceptable for older people to have negative attitudes to people they perceive as different.

Which option best describes the two statements?

i	**a**	(T)	**b**	(T)
ii	**a**	(T)	**b**	(F)
iii	**a**	(F)	**b**	(T)
iv	**a**	(F)	**b**	(F)

47 It is the responsibility of a carer to ensure a client is aware of his or her rights to a given service. This may best be done by:
- **a** Reading them to the client when first meeting
- **b** Providing written policies and charters
- **c** Continually reinforcing a client's rights whilst working
- **d** Checking the client understand his or her rights

Questions 48 to 50 share answers a to d

Bwahema, a young West African, has been admitted into care. The staff are anxious to give her time to adjust to her new situation. She needs:
- **a** Her culture and values to be respected
- **b** Information to remain confidential
- **c** To be encouraged to make choices about her life
- **d** To have clear and effective communication with staff

Which of these will best be addressed when staff encourage her to:

48 Make informed decisions?

49 Attend classes to learn English?

50 Keep in contact with members of her community?

Questions 51 to 53 share answers a to d

Care staff may demonstrate respect for different cultures by ensuring that:
- **a** A broad range of decorative pictures reflects the ethnic diversity in the care environment.
- **b** Appropriate dietary needs are met.
- **c** Clients have access to an appropriate religious leader should they wish.
- **d** All staff are aware of personal/religious customs.

Which of these will be demonstrated when staff:

51 Check to see whether a client prefers a bath or shower.

52 Check to see if a client wishes to observe religious ceremonies

53 Check the care environment to ensure it reflects the ethnic diversity of clients.

54 An elderly client wishes to sit up late to watch the football in his own room. He has the volume turned up as he is hard of hearing. Several of his neighbours complain that they cannot sleep. What might be the best action for the night carer to take?
- **a** Negotiate with the man to turn the volume down and just watch the pictures.
- **b** Negotiate with the man to watch the TV in the lounge away from the other residents.
- **c** Negotiate with the other clients to wear ear plugs for the night.
- **d** Negotiate with the man to turn the TV off, promising to record the match for him.

55 Fund-holding GPs have to gain the best possible treatment for all patients within a set annual budget. A new treatment may greatly improve the quality of life for a young child. The treatment is lengthy and expensive which will limit the treatment available to many other patients. The GP will reach a decision using either the view of ethics held by Kantians or that by the Utilitarians. Decide which is true (T) and which is false (F).
- **a** Following the Kantian view, the GP is likely to elect to give the child the new treatment.
- **b** Following the Utilitarian view, the GP is likely to elect to treat as many patients as possible.

Which option best describes the two statements?

i	**a**	(T)	**b**	(T)
ii	**a**	(T)	**b**	(F)
iii	**a**	(F)	**b**	(T)
iv	**a**	(F)	**b**	(F)

Questions 56 to 58 share answers a to d

Organisations have a responsibility to ensure that staff and clients have equal opportunities. This is achieved through:
- **a** Equal Opportunity legislation
- **b** Access to Personal Files Act
- **c** Patient's Charter
- **d** Professional Code of Conduct

Which applies to the following?

56 Ensuring that waiting times in hospital clinics are kept to a specified time limit.

57 Ensuring that selection and interview procedures do not disadvantage people on the grounds of race, gender or marital status.

58 Ensuring that all staff actively uphold the core values of the profession.

59 Ethics are a way of health and social care staff to agree what is in the best interest of their clients. This is best done by:
- **a** Negotiating with the line manager
- **b** Negotiating with relatives
- **c** Negotiating with the client
- **d** Negotiating with colleagues

60 A wheelchair user, in a residential setting, wishes to go to the shops unescorted. The carer is concerned because he must cross a busy main road. The young man is an experienced wheelchair user, but has not been out unattended to date. Which action will best demonstrate the carer's understanding of professional ethics?
- **a** Refusing permission because it is too dangerous
- **b** Discussing the dangers and agreeing a compromise
- **c** Insisting he or she accompanies the client as it is dangerous
- **d** Insisting he wait until a relative or friend can accompany him

Fast Facts

Attitude Socially-learned reactions to and likes and dislikes of people, objects or situations.

Belief Ideas which we draw upon to make sense of our own particular view of the world.

Black A term used to describe physical characteristics, e.g. skin colour and racial features. The term is also used in a political context to include all people who are oppressed by racism and discrimination because of skin colour or ethnic and cultural background. Much work has been undertaken in the last two decades to redefine the term to highlight positive issues.

Confidentiality The right of clients to have private information about themselves restricted to people who have an accepted need to know.

Consequentialism See Utilitarianism

Culture A collection of ideas and habits shared by a given group, i.e. the norms and value base for the group. These help to reinforce the identity of the group, making it different from other groups. Individuals learn the roles acceptable to others within their culture.

Discrimination To be able to distinguish between things. In health and social care, it refers to a decision to deny one group the same rights as another.

Discrimination, direct Very open and obvious methods of disadvantaging a person or group of people, e.g. name calling, refusing to employ someone because of their age or religion etc.

Discrimination, indirect Subtle ways of disadvantaging an individual or group, e.g. not providing access for people in wheelchairs, or selecting people only from certain housing areas, in order to discriminate.

Disempower To deny clients the opportunity to take control of their life. To deny choice, to withhold information so the client is unable to make an informed choice. The opposite of empowerment.

Empathy A conscious effort to try to see the world as another person sees it. Empathy is an attempt to gain a closer understanding of another's feelings.

Empiricism Knowledge gained through experience.

Empowerment Encouraging an individual to take control of own life. This is achieved by sharing information with the client, so that they may make informed choices, and by working within the care value base.

Equal opportunity Aims to ensure that all people are afforded equal access to services and have equal rights in law and society. Ensuring that all have an equal right to develop to their full potential.

Ethics The moral codes which form the basis for decision making and, therefore, the behaviour of workers in a given profession.

Ethnic group A group who share the same cultural tradition, perhaps a common ancestry or geographical place of origin. The group may share a common language, literature, music etc.

Ethnic minority A commonly used term in Britain to describe groups from the black community. The term also covers such groups as Chinese, Greek, Turkish people, etc. This broad term covers a range of factors e.g. race, religion, culture and language.

Eurocentric Viewing the world solely from a white European value base. This does not address issues raised within other cultures and may assume the superiority of European culture.

Hypothesis A projection or idea which is proposed and then tested out to see if the idea is valid or not.

Identity Put simply, a person's identity is how they see themselves and make sense of their life in relation to other people and society.

Kantianism The philosophy of Immanuel Kant whereby duty means that the same rules apply to all people. It is an essential duty always to tell the truth.

Marginalise In health and social care terms it is to push a group to the outer edge of society and social concern, and so disadvantage them. Such groups may be oppressed due to age, ability, gender, race religion or social class.

Norms The accepted attitudes and values which underpin the behaviour of a particular social group, i.e. the 'rules' by which the group functions.

Peer group A group who share a common purpose or who are in a similar situation. For example, a youth club or a study group may have members of different ages but all have come together for a specific purpose.

Positive action A positive step which aims to benefit individuals or groups who face discrimination, e.g. employing an interpreter to assist a student with hearing impairment in the classroom. In this way the student is not disadvantaged by the hearing loss.

Prejudice An attitude which is based on pre-judgements made about others, leading to discrimination. Prejudice is often based on ignorance and stereotyped views of an individual or group.

Primary socialisation The socialisation that takes place during early childhood when the rules and norms of the society into which an individual is born are acquired. Through the family a child learns the patterns of acceptable behaviour expected by their social group. The attitudes and values of the culture of that society are also formed.

Race The idea of a group based on perceived biological differences between people. In practice, a person is assigned to a particular race on the basis of the subjective impressions of others, not on the basis of measurable biological differences.

Racial discrimination Unequal treatment on the grounds of being a member of a particular racial group.

Racial prejudice An unfavourable attitude towards another because they belong to a particular race. This attitude may be based on negative stereotypes of that particular race.

Racism Attitudes and procedures (economic, political, social and cultural) which advocate and seek to maintain the superiority of one racial group or groups over others.

Secondary socialisation Wider experience of the world outside the home exposes the child to different attitudes and values in society. The main agents of secondary socialisation are the media, education and peer groups.

Sexism Attitudes and procedures (including economic, political, social and cultural factors) which seek to maintain the superiority of one gender over the other.

Social context A particular social setting in which individuals have a preconceived notion about acceptable behaviour. There is clear definition of the roles and the behaviour associated with those roles in this setting. For example, in a hospital ward, the nurse is expected to behave in a caring and professional manner.

Social role The 'part' that an individual plays in a given situation. The accepted behaviour expected by others of that role, e.g. a college student being ready to learn, asking questions etc.

Social status The value a group places on a particular social role, giving credibility and respect. For example: the leader of a teenage group, because they can organise others or perhaps control the group through fear; a judge, because of the knowledge they hold and the power to uphold the laws of society. Status may be due to money or possessions and will vary depending on the culture of groups within society.

Stereotype A way of grouping people, objects or events together, attributing individuals with the same qualities and characteristics. Stereotyping can help the individual to make sense of the world by making predictions easier. Stereotyping may have positive or negative consequences.

Utilitarianism A philosophy originally developed by Jeremy Bentham and John Stuart Mill. It holds that a morally right act is one which benefits the greatest number of people.

Values Learned principles or thought systems which enable individuals to choose between alternatives and make decisions. Values guide behaviour in relation to what is judged to be 'valuable'. Values are learned in a cultural context and will develop in relation to the beliefs and norms which exist within a cultural group.

References and further reading

Adormo, T.W., *et al*, 1950, *The Authoritarian Personality,* Harper

Bernstein, B., 1959, A Public Language: Some Sociological Determinants of Linguistic Form. In *British Journal of Sociology* 10

Brown, R., 1988, *Group Processes,* Blackwell

Ellis, P., 1993, 'Role of Ethics in Modern Health Care: 2' in *British Journal of Nursing,* Vol 2 No. 3

Gould, J. (ed.), 1965, *A Socio-linguistic Approach to Social Learning,* Social Science Survey, London

Hunt, G., 1994 (ed.) *Ethical Issues in Nursing,* Routledge

Jackson, B., and Marsden, D., 1962, *Education and the Working Class,* Routledge Kegan-Paul

Keddie, N., 1975, *Knowledge and Control,* M. Young ed.

Kohen, D., 1994, *The Ground of Professional Ethics,* Routledge

MacNiven, D., 1990, *Moral Expertise, Studies in Practical and Professional Ethics,* Routledge

Minard, R., 1952, 'Race Relations in the Pocationtas Coal Field' in *Journal of Social Issues,* 8, 9, 29–44

Rowson, R., 1990, *An Introduction to Ethics for Nurses,* Scutari Press

Secord, P.T. and Backman, C.W., 1974, *Social Psychology,* McGraw-Hill

Sherif, M., *et al*, 1961, *Intergroup Conflict and Cooperation: The Robbers' Cave Experiment,* University of Oklahoma Book Exchange

Swann, Lord, 1985, *Education for All: A Brief Guide,* HMSO

Tschudin, V., 1992, *Ethics for Nursing: The Caring Relationship,* 2nd ed.

Typerman and Spenser 1983 as cited in: Gross, R., 1991, *Psychology: The Science of Mind and Behaviour,* Hodder and Stoughton, pages 289–90

Warnock, M., 1978, Warnock Report, HMSO

Chapter 4

Interpersonal interaction

This chapter explores the nature of interpersonal interaction: what it is, how it might influence health and well-being, some issues that influence human interaction within Western culture, and how interaction might be optimised and evaluated.

The word inter means 'between', so interpersonal interaction means 'action between people'. Health and social care work depends on skilled interpersonal communication. Interpersonal interaction is essential for:

- **making and maintaining social relationships**
- **enabling the existence of social groups and society**
- **effective social, emotional and intellectual development**
- **understanding social roles and self-awareness**
- **happiness – few people are happy without worthwhile relationships**
- **coping with work – most jobs involve a degree of interpersonal interaction.**

The skills of interpersonal interaction are likely to influence how happy people's relationships with others are (including loving relationships), how popular people are and how people succeed or fail at work. The study of interpersonal skills is a vital area of interest for most individuals and many professions.

Interpersonal interaction involves a wide range of abilities and covers a vast range of behaviours. The most obvious form that interpersonal human interaction may take is through language.

Language

There are perhaps about 4000 different spoken languages in the world, and these are complemented by sign languages. Language naturally enables people to communicate with each other and send messages. It may be possible for some creatures to use limited language systems but, in the main, language ability seems to be one of the main characteristics that set humans apart from other species on earth.

The tremendous potential of language is not simply that it enables people to communicate – because people could communicate anyway by using 'body language' and actions.

Think it over

Suppose you wanted to teach a child to brush his or her teeth, how would you do it? Would you really go into great long descriptions of how to open your mouth, how to hold a toothbrush and so on? Surely, instead of giving a lecture, you would show the child what to do! All you really need to do is to get the child to copy your actions, and guide him if he seems to be getting the actions wrong. You can say things like, 'Do it like this': but you don't always need spoken or signed language systems to interact with others.

The real value of language is that language guides human thinking. You think in a language! Humans use language *concepts* to clarify and make sense of everyday experience. Concepts help people to understand their lives and to know what to expect in the future. Language therefore gives humans a special ability to understand and control their environment (see Chapter 10).

The most valuable aspect of language lies in its value for influencing thought; but spoken language or verbal communication is still an important part of interpersonal interaction.

Verbal and non-verbal communication

Communication can be divided broadly into two parts: what we say and what we don't. Initially it may be thought that the words we use are of the greatest significance, and we often take great trouble to 'say the right things'; but is this enough? Have you ever been in a situation where someone says 'the right thing' but you don't believe a word they are saying?

For example, imagine a middle-aged woman meeting a man for the first time. He gazes into her eyes and

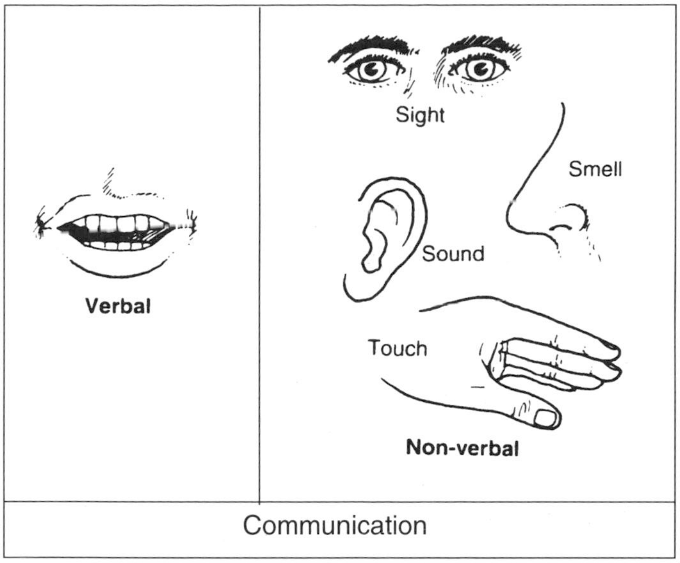

Figure 4.1 All communication involves sensory contact. The main distinction which is drawn is between verbal and non-verbal communication

swears that he thought her daughter was her sister. She would have to be very gullible to believe what he was saying (and he would have to be a very accomplished liar for his non-verbal communication to support his words).

Barriers to communication

We use more than words to 'say' what we mean. We use non-verbal messages either to support our spoken words or to undermine them. Using non-verbal signals involves using our eyes and our bodies to send messages. We can think of them as signs associated with sight, sound, touch and smell.

People with certain disabilities will therefore not be able to use the full range of communication.

Think it over

What type of disabilities will limit communication? If we consider verbal and non-verbal communication we can understand the difficulties of someone unable to hear or to see, or unable to move certain parts of their bodies or to speak.

Different communication systems have been developed to help people. So people unable to speak can have an electronic board made for them, called a Bliss system. The board shows different words or phrases which the person is likely to want to use and the user touches the areas they want to indicate what they wish to 'say'. Blind or partially-sighted people may use Braille. This is a touch system where words are converted into raised dots on the paper, so that the 'words' can be felt rather than seen. Many people with some sight can use computers with facilities to enlarge the print. Computers which 'speak' the print being typed in or scanned are also available. In these ways people with visual problems can access print and produce things for themselves in a written format.

Think it over

James is partially sighted and about to leave home to go to university. He has been in touch with the support staff at university and they have provided him with the technical equipment he will need. What other difficulties might he expect in his new life?

James has been provided with access to verbal communication but he is unable to 'read' some non-verbal communication. He cannot see the expressions on people's faces unless they are very near and he may not recognise other students as they pass by. He may be thought anti-social if he does not speak to someone he has recently met; and going to large 'fresher' events in dimly-lit bars will be difficult for James because it will make it even harder for him to recognise new people. James has no glasses, white stick or guide dog, so his is a hidden disability which people may be unaware of. New people and new environments will be more stressful for him than for others. He will have to rely on his auditory skills to pick up meanings from people's voices, rather than relying heavily on non-verbal communication. Hopefully, his intellectual progress will not be impaired but he will need support and understanding from his peers if he is to settle emotionally and socially.

People who are deaf or have partial hearing have the opposite difficulties to James. They will rely much more heavily on non-verbal communication. Some hearing-impaired people will lip-read, which means they need to face speakers who should take care not to put their hands on their faces. Most hearing-impaired people will use a combination of careful observation of others' body language and signing.

British and American Sign Languages have been developed to a high level of sophistication. Makaton is another system of sign language. It is a fairly simple way of signing basic needs and is sometimes used to help people with learning difficulties.

Body language

Understanding people involves understanding their non-verbal communication as well as what they say. People use their bodies to send non-verbal messages, so non-verbal communication is sometimes called **body language.**

Body language is always present, even though people are not always conscious of the messages given out. Most people are usually careful about what they say and usually explain why they have said what they did. Body language or non-verbal communication is different – most people do not think about it, they just experience it.

Some of the most important body areas to use, and to watch others use, are:

- the eyes
- the face
- voice tone
- body movement
- posture (how people sit or stand) and head angles when looking at others
- gestures (use of arms and hands).

Important special messages are sometimes sent by:

- touch
- how close people get to each other
- mirroring of body postures and movements (i.e. copying the postures and movements of others).

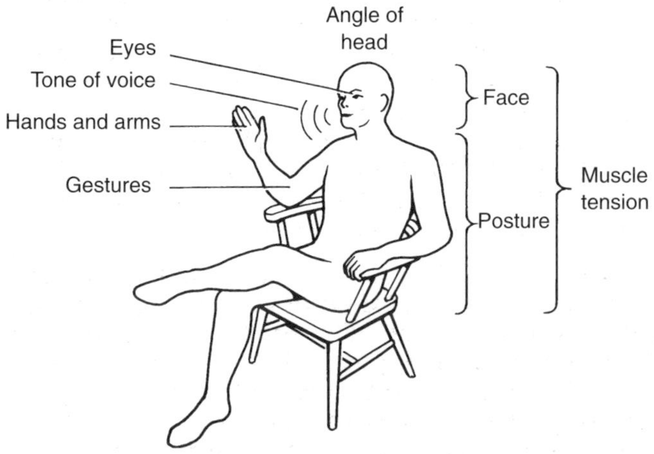

Figure 4.2 Body language sends messages

Non-verbal interaction: visual communication

How we *perceive* someone is influenced greatly by how we *see* them. Think of someone you have met recently, perhaps a member of your course group, and try to think of how what you first saw of them influenced the way you first thought of them.

You were probably influenced first of all by the clothes they wore and their hairstyle. We make conscious decisions about these things because we are very much aware that they portray us in a certain way – how we wish people to perceive us. This may be one reason why there can be friction between adolescents and parents. Adolescents are trying to assert their own views and project an independent image of themselves to the rest of the world. They often adopt images exactly opposite to those of their parents to accentuate their difference. This may cause much family unease in the process!

We are sometimes constrained by circumstances to project a 'suitable' image, often in terms of a more formal one than we would wish. Does the way we present ourselves influence the way we behave?

Think it over

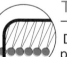

Do you behave differently when you are presenting yourself in a formal or non-casual way?

There has been much discussion about whether, for example, pupils at school should be required to wear uniforms, because it is thought that wearing specific clothes influences the way people behave. Even reminders of authority can influence people; for example, cardboard figures of policemen in supermarkets are known to reduce petty theft. Certainly, appearing in court in front of a judge wearing robes and a wig is likely to give the occasion, and the judge, much more authority than if the meeting took place in an ordinary room with the judge wearing casual clothes. Clothes certainly give messages; for example, the victim of an accident might feel comforted by, and confident in the ability of, someone approaching who is wearing a nurse's uniform.

Think it over

Perhaps you know staff who wear a uniform at work. If so you could speak with the people you work with, both colleagues and clients, and ask them whether they think the uniform inhibits or helps personal interaction.

Facial expressions

People often make judgements about others based on their physical appearance. Included in this is their facial expression. Because the face is such a sensitive guide to a person's feelings we often try hard not to let ourselves reveal too much by our expressions. Only when we are overcome by our feeling do we allow our faces to 'say' what we feel.

Can you remember an occasion when you felt very strongly about something but managed not to let your feelings show? Perhaps you were furious with a customer but had to remain polite, or felt amused by a child with whom you were trying to be stern.

Our facial expressions reveal our emotions in several ways; for example, by the pupils of the eyes expanding and contracting, or by blushing or sweating. Our eyebrows will rise or fall and the mouth smiles, raising upwards, or tightens with anger, turning down to show displeasure. A nervous person's mouth may twitch and they may feel a need to lick their lips. Even the muscles in our face and neck tighten if we feel angry or tense.

Different cultures may have different ways of behaving in terms of displaying feelings. Japanese people, for example, often do not display – or expect others to display – facial expressions showing anger or displeasure.

Gaze

An important part of the facial expression is how we use our eyes to gaze at others. The very act of making or having eye contact implies recognition of some sort.

The eyes can send a vast range of messages and may often be the most important part of the body when sending non-verbal messages. One poet called the eyes 'the window of the soul', meaning that sometimes people can see the feelings and thoughts of another person by looking at their eyes. Looking at the eyes might be like looking through a window into the other person's feelings.

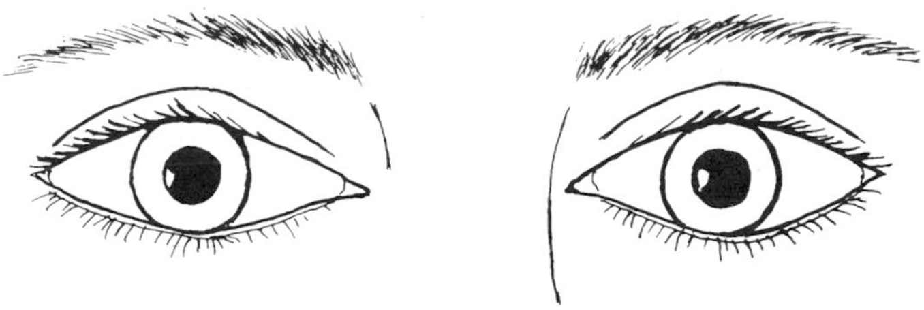

This may sound romantic, but the eyes will usually send messages about how a person feels emotionally. Skilled actors learn to control their eyes by remembering an emotional feeling and then trying to send that feeling with their eye movements. Most people do not learn to act to that level of skill, but their eyes still send messages.

The eyes tend to widen when people are excited or interested in something. If we feel attracted to a person we will probably send him or her this message just with the look in our eyes. Equally, if we are angry, the eyes also quickly send this message.

The way the eyes widen and narrow may not be as important as the way people use their eyes to make contact with others. People who think you are interesting, or attractive, will want to look at you. If your eyes meet someone else's there is often a momentary widening (excitement) in the other person's eyes, this is followed by quickly looking away, followed by looking back (perhaps to see if you are still looking). A person who is not interested and just happened to be looking your way may move his or her eyes more slowly – there will be less jumpiness in the way the eyes move.

Have you ever used gaze to tell someone how you were feeling? It may have been to tell people you were annoyed with them. For Europeans, refusal to meet someone's glance at you is a very powerful means of rejecting them. Long gazes of more than six seconds indicate high degrees of intimacy or liking. However, long gazes can also be used to intimidate and show aggression, 'to stare someone out'. Ellsworth (1975) found that staring motorcyclists at traffic lights caused motorists to move off much more quickly than usual.

Glances are used in conversations to indicate a wish to enter into the discussion or to signal agreement. People look more when they are listening than when they are talking. So if you look at someone while they talk it is an important way of supporting someone's views and letting them know you are interested in what they are saying. Amongst Europeans, if someone is attempting to lie, or find what they are saying difficult, they are likely to look away from the people they are talking to: they will break or avoid eye contact. However, different

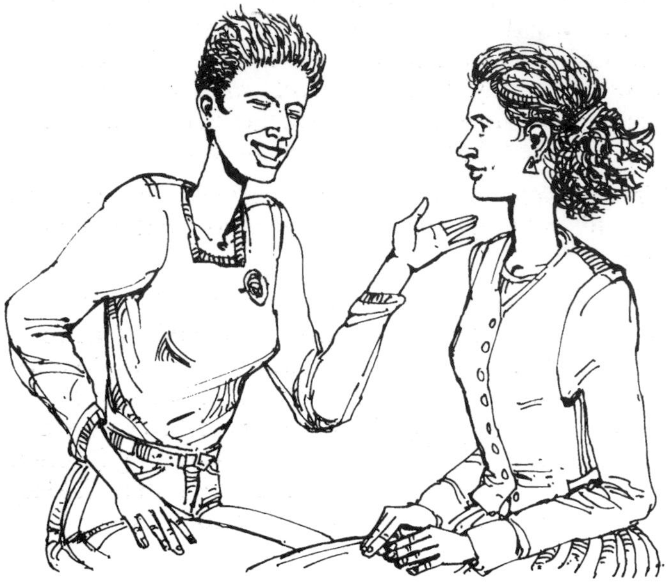

Figure 4.3 Looking at someone whilst talking is an important way of showing support

cultures use gaze differently and it is important to check the cultural norms of an individual before interpreting their non-verbal behaviour.

When communicating with clients it is important to take their individual needs into account. If someone cannot see well, the use of *gaze* will be impaired. Parents of blind children may sometimes find it difficult to establish a bond with their child because much early communication between babies and adults is in eye contact. It is important to use other communication skills when gaze is not available.

A number of studies of people with schizophrenia note that they look at psychologists on average only about 65 per cent as much as non-schizophrenics. However, a study by Rutter (1976) showed that when talking to another person about impersonal problems their gaze was of normal level. They, and people suffering depression, may avoid eye contact when talking about personal matters.

Think it over

Have you ever been instructed on 'correct' gazing or found yourself instructing others?

Again, gaze is also subject to cultural interpretations. Most people in Northern European and Asian cultures will have been told that it is rude to stare at strangers. Parents tend to demand that their children look at them at certain times, notably when they are being told off for a wrongdoing! ('Look at me when I'm talking to you!') Too much gaze, however, is seen as insulting, disrespectful and threatening (Watson, 1972). By way of contrast, in Southern European, Arab and Latin American cultures, too little gaze is seen as being insincere, dishonest or impolite. There may also be rules about who to look at or not, as well as how to look. Some Kenyans may not look directly at their mother-in-law or Nigerians at a person of high status. Some South American Indians must look at outside objects during a conversation and Japanese people prefer to have the gaze directed at the neck rather that the face (Argyle, 1983). It is important to remember that a client is an individual and individuals have different experiences. Carers need to learn to 'read' people and understand their different responses.

Gestures

Gestures vary from society to society and between groups within society. In Britain there are about twenty commonly used gestures while in Southern Italy there are about 200!

Can you think of cultures where gesture is extensively used to communicate? Specialist gesture languages have been developed in certain working environments; for example, in broadcasting where speech would interfere with the work being staged, or at race tracks to send messages over a distance. Noisy mills and mines are also places where workers will use signs to supplement mouthed words. Gestures in general usage are often involuntary, and of no particular use, for example, pointing to give directions when on the telephone! However gestures can sometimes betray emotions, such as clenched fists indicating aggression or anxiety.

As mentioned above, hearing-impaired people may use signs to communicate. As with spoken languages, sign languages are constantly evolving. For example, the signs to indicate full breasts for women and a moustache for men have been changed to a tap on the forehead for men and on the cheek for women. These changes reinforce the status of sign languages as evolutionary and responsive to the societies in which they are used.

Other visual elements of non-verbal communication include **proximity, orientation** and **posture.** The

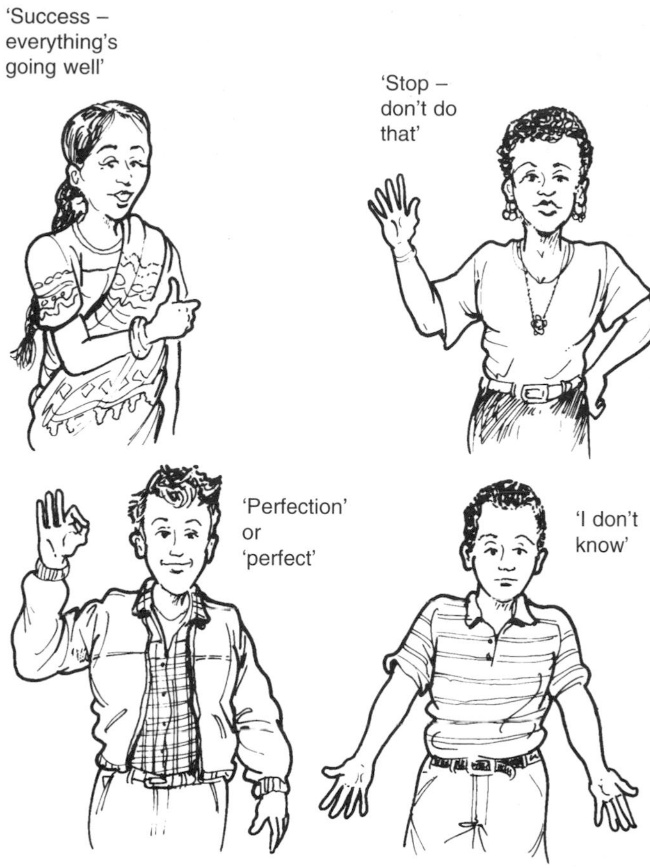
'Success – everything's going well'
'Stop – don't do that'
'Perfection' or 'perfect'
'I don't know'

Figure 4.4 Some gestures common in Britain

nearness or distance, **proximity,** between people, may be a good indication of how they feel towards one another. The ritual of shaking hands may have evolved as a measure of a polite distance between two people meeting formally (to keep someone at arm's length). It is interesting to note that within some cultures, such as the Southern European, Arab and Latin American cultures, greeting may often involve a hug and kiss rather than just a handshake. You may have experienced the person who needed less personal space than you did – and had the feeling of being edged into a corner as you moved away from their closeness. In northern European culture this may be a way of intimidating people; standing too close can make others very uncomfortable!

Body movements in interpersonal interaction

Very few people keep still when they communicate with others. They move their arms, their hands, their feet, their eyes, head, facial expressions and so on. The speed and type of movement can send many messages. People can signal how interested they are by the way they move. They send messages of affection and attraction by the way they tense and relax their body. The way people walk, turn their head, sit down, etc. sends messages about whether they are tired, happy, sad, bored and so on.

Many people use 'head-nods' to signal 'I am listening to you' and 'I agree', or 'I understand what you are saying'.

Posture is the way a person sits or stands, and it gives messages about how they are feeling. Tension in the back and shoulders indicates stress, as do arms clasped around the body. Someone with an 'open' body posture, leaning slightly forward towards the speaker, indicates a relaxed, non-threatening listener. But someone sitting with hunched shoulders, folded arms and crossed legs might not be so relaxed!

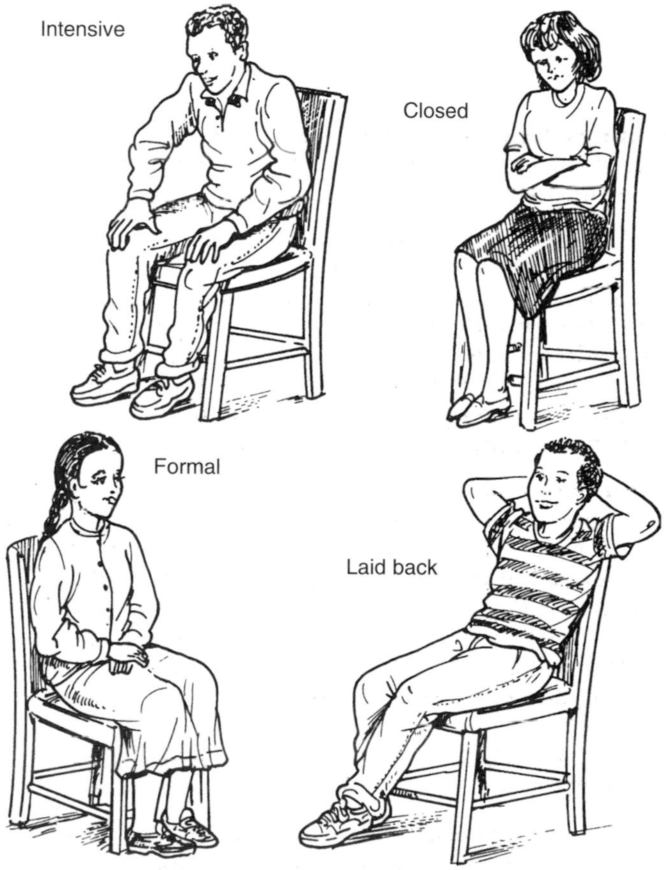

Figure 4.5 Body postures that send messages

Face-to-face interaction

The way people face each other can send many different meanings. Many of these meanings can involve strong emotions. Is it always a good idea to face another person 'eye-to-eye'? 'Eye-to-eye' or 'square-on' postures might mean: intimacy, attachment or love, confrontation, hostility or aggression, honesty or openness in commercial dealing.

Sitting face-to-face can indicate formality or a confrontational conversation. However, in *informal* settings it can imply the opposite – closeness, intimacy or love. A face-to-face position is nearly always an intensive one.

Standing at a slight angle, on the other hand, can indicate informality and being relaxed. It can send non-verbal messages of: 'I'm calm' or even 'I'm cool!' Sitting at angles can also send messages of 'This is informal', and 'We can be relaxed'. As well as keeping a body angle to the other person, if you want to communicate a relaxed, calm message it may be important to adopt a very slight angle to your head. Some people feel that this communicates interest and involvement.

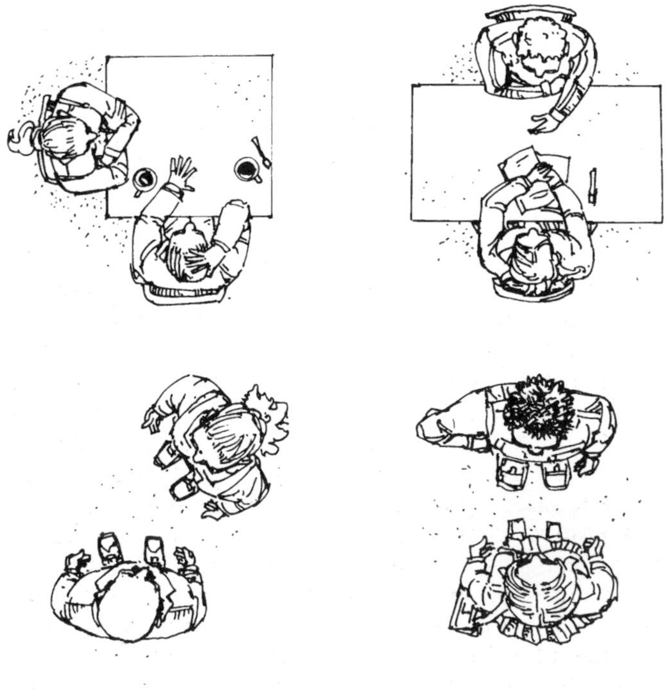

Figure 4.6 Face-to-face interaction

Muscle tension during interaction

Feet, hands and fingers can give signs of being relaxed or tense. When people are tense they sometimes clench their hands or press their fingers together. Continuous moving of feet or changes of body posture can indicate tension.

When someone gets very tense, their shoulders stiffen, their face muscles tighten and they sit or stand more rigidly. When the face becomes tense, the mouth will be closed and the lips and jaw tightened. With a lot of stress, people develop wrinkled lines where the face is always tensed – this may show in the person's forehead.

Tense people always breathe more quickly, and their heart will work faster. It is important to be able to recognise these signs of tension in others. If a person becomes tense during conversation, maybe something is wrong. Perhaps the person is becoming tense because of emotional feelings like grief. The best thing here might be to stay with the person while he or she cries. There may be nothing to say, but emotional support might be provided through body language. The **presence** of a person, interacting with appropriate body language, may be enough to provide clients with support at such times.

Orientation is an important element of non-verbal communication. Orientation means organising your own or others' positions in the space available. Consider the court-room again. It is no accident that the judge is placed physically on a higher level and apart from the rest of the court. Judges are automatically perceived as 'higher' and in control. All variations of positioning make statements about the participants' roles. An interview with the bank manager or head teacher will often take place with a desk between the participants, which forms a barrier; while a counselling session is more likely to be between people seated on the same level, with no barriers between them. The way you organise your environment will support or obstruct your communication.

Olfactory communication

Newborn babies are known to recognise their mothers by her smell and people with visual disabilities may distinguish landmarks in buildings and towns by their particular odours. Whilst the smell of fish and chips may be enticing or otherwise to sighted individuals, to a visually disabled person it might be an essential part of the geography! Smell is also very powerful in evoking memories of past events. The mind will respond to a certain smell by conjuring up vivid images and events associated with that particular odour – perhaps the smell of a dentist's surgery is one of the most unpopular!

To some extent, smell may be a much weaker influence in communication than it was to our prehistoric ancestors. Without the benefit of deodorant it would have been all too easy to tell when people were frightened or anxious by the smell of their perspiration. Psychologists believe still that humans are attracted to each other by the presence of *pheremones,* barely detectable smells which either attract or repel. However, generally these days it is not socially acceptable to have 'natural' smells and there is a large market in covering them and projecting different images of ourselves by the way we smell. Manufacturers of washing powders compete to produce the 'cleanest smelling wash', so, commercially at least, a person's status can be defined by their smell – provided it is unnatural!

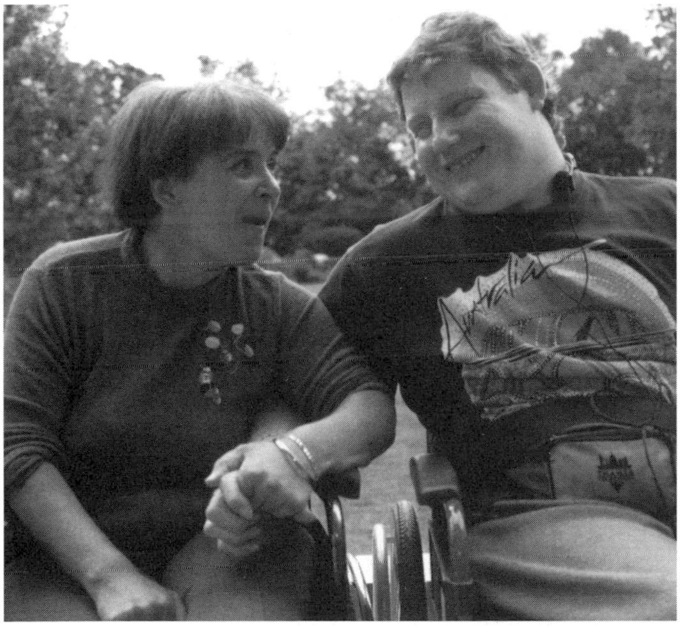

Figure 4.7 Tactile communication can be important (*Photo courtesy of Winged Fellowship Trust*)

Tactile communication

The use of the sense of touch is one which is surrounded by cultural taboos. Many northern Europeans are not inclined towards body contact, except formally when shaking hands or within a close relationship. In the British culture tactile messages are most often concerned with aggression, greeting, guiding or caressing. Depending on how comfortable a client feels about touch, tactile contacts can be very important.

Think it over

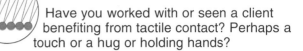

Have you worked with or seen a client benefiting from tactile contact? Perhaps a touch or a hug or holding hands?

Many disturbed or severely disabled people may find massage comforting or soothing. Elders who no longer have close friends or relatives may lack the comfort of touch. However, remember that it is essential to gauge the client's reaction to a tentative touch, say on the arm, and caution must be exercised when working alone with clients.

It is also important that your touch is appropriate to the client's culture and age. It would obviously be abusive to pat a middle-aged person with learning difficulties as one might a very small child.

Auditory communication

Auditory communication covers what we hear. This includes not only the language and words that are used, but also the tone of voice and the speed with which words are spoken.

Certain clients may give the answers they think they should give, either because they don't want to be thought a nuisance, or because they fear what will happen if they complain. It is the carer's job to listen to the tone, timing, accent, speed of delivery and rhythm to judge whether the words mean what they say. If, for example, you were to say, 'YOU LOVELY LITTLE THING' to a baby in a loud and threatening voice it would probably cry. The baby makes a judgement about your attitude based on how the words are said, because it doesn't understand their meaning. The opposite is often true with adults: they will use the right words but their meaning can be obscured by the way they say them. Can you remember saying, 'Sorry' because you were made to – not because you were sorry? It is likely that you didn't sound it!

Listening

It is useful to separate the idea of listening to what people say from the idea of hearing the noise that people make when they talk!

Here, **listening** means hearing another person's words, thinking about what they mean and planning what to say back to the other person. **Hearing** the other person means picking up the sounds they make.

Listening is a skill. It is far more than just being around when something is said. Listening involves **hearing** and then **remembering** what has been said. If we are going to remember what someone else has said, we have to **understand** it first.

Some psychologists believe that people usually only remember about one out of every 2000 things that are heard in a day! Most of the sounds that come to our ears are not important enough to bother about remembering.

Think it over

Last night you may have watched TV or talked to family and friends. Just how much can you recall of what you heard?

If you cannot remember much about what you watched on TV, perhaps it does not matter; the important thing may be that you enjoyed it. But listening is a vital skill in health care and social care work. Listening skills enable carers to develop an understanding of clients and their needs.

To understand another person it is necessary to know something of his or her background, lifestyle and personal situation. As well as knowing about these, it is important to be able to make sense of them, to feel that you understand and have some idea of what to expect. This understanding develops from experience of listening to people. Perhaps we gradually get better at it.

Sometimes, getting ready to listen involves switching into a store of knowledge and understanding. For some people this is a conscious 'switching-on' process. We switch on by remembering another person's name or face; perhaps we can recall when we last talked to them and what they said. Listening skills depend on being able to remember important details about other people.

Listening can be hard mental work. Instead of just living in our own private worlds, planning to say whatever we think, we have to think about other people. So, if someone is saying that he or she is sad about something we *first* have to hear their words and *then* imagine how the other person feels. We have to make sense of what is said, perhaps imagining how we would feel if it happened to us. Having thought through what we have been told, we have to think again before we speak.

Listening takes time. Because real listening takes thinking time, sometimes people do not bother to listen. Listening can often be difficult. If you are going to listen, then the other person has to keep talking.

Reflective listening

Think it over

Imagine that you are caring for an older man and start talking to him. He is very miserable and perhaps angry about things that have not gone right. Suddenly he turns and says: 'Nobody cares about me. Do you know what my son said to me last time he came to see me? He said: "Well, you won't live much longer, you'll be dead soon and then I won't have to bother visiting you".' He then goes quiet and looks at the floor.

You're the carer – what do you do now?

This is a difficult situation. First, you cannot just walk away because that would look as if you did not care either. It might be possible to ask a question, but what would be a sensible one? You can't say: 'Ah, so do you think you son does not like you then?' The man has made the situation clear – it would be insulting to get the question wrong.

It would be possible to go silent too. Silence can be a good technique (see below) – but not here. Going silent might look like not knowing what to do.

If your own response is one of shock; if you feel 'that's awful', and if you are lost for words, what is left to say? You could just repeat the words, 'He said you'll be dead soon and I won't have to visit you'. If the client's words are repeated with the right tone of voice – a tone that gives the message 'that's awful' – then you have proved that you were listening to the client, and that you have taken him seriously. The simple act of repeating the statement also invites him to keep on talking: having proved that you were listening, and that you are concerned, is there anything he can add to what he has said?

Simply repeating the client's message can keep the conversation going, but it is not a good idea to do this too often. If you keep repeating what the client says, you will sound like a parrot. The client could think he is being made fun of. However, repeating the client's words once can keep the conversation going a bit longer. It is now the client's turn to speak again. Perhaps he will give some details about his life; perhaps you will learn more about his needs and understand more.

Repeating the client's words in this way is the simplest kind of reflection. But a better way is to put what the client said into your own words. For example, something like: 'Your son does not want to visit you and does not care whether you are alive or dead.' When you use you own words, it almost becomes a new question – you are testing your understanding of the client's message. This type of reflection is also called **paraphrasing.**

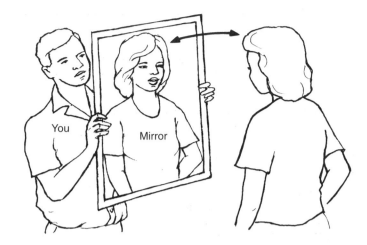

Figure 4.8 Helping another person to 'see' her thoughts and feelings

Paraphrasing

Summing up what another person has said, is called **summarising.** Both paraphrasing and summarising are types of reflective listening.

Putting the client's statement into your own words is usually better than just repeating what has been said.

1. It shows that you thought about what he said.
2. Your statement is not mechanical – you speak in your own usual way.
3. The other person has to do more thinking to check that what you said is what he meant. He is more likely to keep talking, after this extra thinking.
4. Because using your own words often sounds more caring and sociable, you can use this reflective technique more often.

So, repeating what another person said is a useful way of keeping a conversation going. However, it can be more than that. If the right non-verbal messages are used and the words do make sense to the other person, then repeating the other person's statement is like holding a mirror for them. He can see his thoughts and feelings in the 'mirror' that the words have created.

A person may say, 'no one likes me, nobody talks to me here'. The technique of reflective listening can mirror this: 'No one cares at all?'. The person may then want to say more: 'Well, you do, you listen – but nobody else does.'

Because of this 'mirror' (reflective listening), the person has now thought things through a little further. It is not that 'no one cares' – you are providing emotional support, so 'you care'. This can be very important. Learning the technique of reflective listening can help people to sort out their thoughts.

Reflecting back what someone has just said is a very powerful caring technique. In order to make it work properly, it should not be done too often in a conversation and it is vital to be careful not to twist and change what other people might mean when they speak.

If a person said, 'No one likes me, nobody talks to me here', and the carer said, 'Perhaps no one likes you because you are always sitting here'; would this be a reflection? It can only be reflection if it acts as a mirror – if it bounces back just what the person says. This example twists things. The carer talks about where the client sits, and that's not reflection.

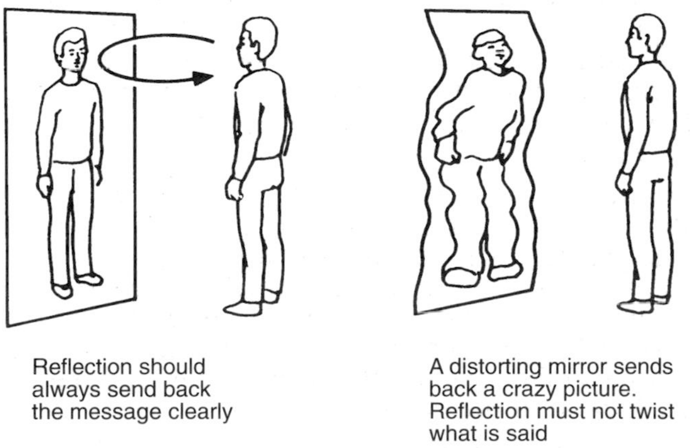

Reflection should always send back the message clearly
A distorting mirror sends back a crazy picture. Reflection must not twist what is said

Figure 4.9 Ensure accurate reflection!

Reflective listening can lead to reflective learning. When the carer bounces the client's message back like a mirror, clients can hear their own message and think about it: is it exactly what they were thinking, can they improve on it, make the meaning clearer, add more detail? The idea behind reflective listening is that it makes both the speaker and the listener think more. This thinking sometimes becomes a kind of reflecting inside the head – i.e. reflective learning.

Try it

Try reflective listening in practice. Find someone who is studying this unit and get a tape recorder. Sit down with him or her and explain everything you know about reflective listening. Describe what it is, how you do it, when it could be useful, what would help make it work, what would stop it from working. Ask your colleague to listen and to use some reflective listening, if possible, with just an odd question, probe or prompt. Tape record what you say.

There is a Chinese saying: 'I know what I think when I hear what I say'. Listen to what you said!

Trying reflective listening in practice, and thinking the idea through, probably means learning more than if you read this chapter many times! You will be doing thinking work. If your colleague reflects what you say effectively, you will be able to sort your ideas out by talking them through. Reflective listening may lead to reflective learning.

Summary

- Reflective listening may help people to think things out.
- Thinking things out helps people to learn.
- Thinking things out may help some people to feel better.

Silence

When a person is having a conversation with someone and cannot think what to say, it may feel embarrassing. A long silence seems to mean, 'I can't think properly', or, 'I do not understand' or, 'I wasn't listening.' A pause puts pressure on the conversation; some people may feel that they have to invent something to say to avoid a silence.

One definition of friends can be people who can sit together and feel comfortable in silence. Silence can mean different things depending on the situation. If a person has only just met someone and is trying to get to know them, a silence may look like incompetent questioning. If the person is not a stranger, however, then silence might be all right. Silence might mean, 'take your time', 'think about things,' 'reflect in your own mind'.

When people need time to collect their thoughts, they might signal non-verbally that they are thinking. Respect can be shown by simply communicating non-verbally, and not speaking.

Imagine, for example, that a doctor or nurse has to tell a patient some bad news. If the person breaks the bad news then immediately continues with details of the next thing to do – what hospital the patient will have to go to and so on – the patient may not be able to take it all in, and is likely to be shocked and unable to think of questions to ask.

A more caring way might be to tell the patient the bad news and wait. The doctor or nurse could ask if the person had any questions, and could communicate a caring attitude non-verbally. Leaving a silence would give the patient time to think. The silence would be caring.

Sometimes, too, it can be better to stay silent when a person has told you something. It is possible to communicate your feelings non-verbally, to communicate, 'I'd like you to say more about it' using head-nods, eye-contact and facial expressions. This use of silence can encourage the other person to reflect and to keep talking. Silence is sometimes a good alternative to repeating the verbal message. Silence can be another reflective technique.

Summary

- Silence can link with reflective listening.
- Silence can give people a space to think.
- Silence can be a skill in caring communication.

Social context

Human interaction is strongly influenced by the social context, i.e. where people are when a conversation takes place. As long ago as 1930, two researchers called Hartshorne and May asked children questions about

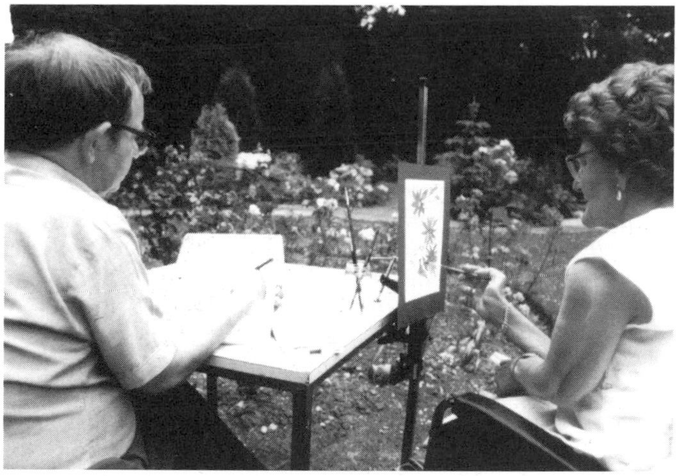

(*Photo courtesy of Winged Fellowship Trust*)

what was right and wrong. The researchers found that the children questioned were not consistent in what they said and did. Children might say that an action is wrong in one context – perhaps when they are with adults, and yet they might give a different opinion when with friends.

People are likely to say and do different things in different ways, depending on where they are. A conversation between colleagues at work might be rather formal. There might be strict rules for turn-taking. Colleagues might have to choose their words very carefully and prepare what they are going to say; something that a person says at work might be quoted back later. However, a conversation with friends at a party could be very different – people don't need to bother with turn-taking! Friends will not worry if you say something silly, you can relax and just say whatever you like. If a person says whatever comes into their head in a formal work meeting they may find that they break the unwritten rules or values of the work group.

In care work, activities are often used to create a context for social interaction. Craft activities, exercise sessions, exercise to music, learning to play music, listening to stories and so on, all provide a social setting. Within this setting clients and workers will interact and attempt to maintain clients' sense of self-esteem. Activities provide a valuable social context for building and maintaining social relationships. With some client groups, such as children and people with learning disability, such activities can provide a context for learning the social skills involved in interpersonal interaction.

How interpersonal interaction influences individual health and social well-being

Social relationships

During almost all of our lives we are interacting with others and forming relationships. As very small children our contacts are limited, often to our immediate families or care givers. As we grow older and begin school we gradually extend our circle of friends. By the time people have reached their teenage years the importance of friends begins to draw level with, and sometimes overtake, the importance of families.

Contacts with other people are vitally important to us emotionally. Prisoners who have been kept in solitary confinement may report the feeling of being out of touch with reality or of feeling they are going insane. It is of great importance that we gain skills at making social contacts and, as carers, help our clients to communicate effectively.

Sometimes, when personal lives get difficult, it is tempting to wonder why we bother making friends. However, research shows that people with good strong relationships are usually happier and healthier than those without. Argyle (1987) shows that people who are married or living with a partner and have a close relationship have the best support. People who are widowed or divorced are more likely to take time off work, and to see the doctor more often, than married or single people. Death rates for divorced or widowed people are higher, and this is likely to be because of their lifestyle. Lonely people may drink and smoke more, or not bother to make themselves nutritious meals. They are more likely to become mentally ill or commit suicide than married people.

After a partner or spouse, family and children are the next most important form of social support. Research shows that even when the children have left home the parents' health is better if they see their grown-up children often.

Contact with friends is also important. Interestingly, it is the *quality* of interaction that is important, not the number of times they meet. Steve Duck (1992) found that people who were good friends often had the same ways of thinking and similar views. People with a good quality relationship will discuss problems, and give and receive support. A good friend makes the other person feel accepted. This does not mean they think they are perfect, but that they are prepared to accept them along with their faults.

Think it over

Make a list of all your social contacts and try to put them in order of importance. Your list might look something like this: partner or spouse, parents or children; close friends; college or work-place friends; neighbours and local organisations; people you see during your daily life, shop-keepers etc.

Interaction with friends, family and colleagues may help to protect us from the risks and stresses that we might otherwise face in life. Parents may provide a safe social context during early life, whilst adult relationships with partners and friends may help us to cope with transitions and changes in life (see Chapter 10).

Michael Argyle (1987) describes the social value of relationships as **buffering.** A buffer is a kind of shock-absorbing barrier which gives protection. (Buffers are used to protect trains at stations.) Arglye's idea is that partners, family and friends act as the shock-absorbers which protect us from the knocks that we take in life. When we change jobs, move home, get married or have children, become ill, become unemployed and so on, our partners, friends or relatives can help us. Relationships with friends help us because they can take the shock out of these events.

Relationships depend on people's interactive skills. Steve Duck (1992) states: 'Talking is fundamental to relationships – whether they are starting, getting better, getting worse, or just carrying on. Also, such talk is one obvious vehicle for creating change in relationships, for expressing emotion, for handling conflict and for indicating love and affection.' (*Page 1.*)

Michael Argyle (1987) points out that some people say they have friends, but really they still feel lonely. Simply being with people isn't always what is needed. Just being able to talk with others about sport, cars or magazines can be boring. Good relationships are ones where people can talk about their feelings. Being able to talk about worries, share interests and talk confidentially about personal things may be the basis of real friendship. Argyle suggests that lonely people may feel lonely because they cannot talk about interesting and important personal issues. Good relationships may depend on people being good at conversation. The best friends may be people who are good listeners – people who are honest, concerned and understanding.

Argyle (*page 29*) states:

> *It has recently been discovered that lonely people do not have sufficiently intimate conversations with their friends, do not make enough self-disclosure (telling others about themselves and their feelings). Talking for hours about sport is not enough ... Conversations with females do more to relieve loneliness, for members of both sexes, because these conversations are found to be pleasanter, more intimate, to involve more self-disclosure, and to be in general more 'meaningful' than those with men ... lonely people lack social skills in other ways too; they take less interest in other people, for example asking fewer questions, are less rewarding and like and trust others less, and fail to send positive non-verbal signals via facial expression or tone of voice.*

So effective interpersonal interaction may have the positive influence of helping people to make happy and lasting relationships in work and in private life. Poor interpersonal interaction may have a negative influence on life, resulting in people being lonely and isolated. For many individuals, loneliness and isolation may result in poorer health and even a shorter life expectancy. (See Chapter 10.)

Relationships are also about the membership of social groups. Groups develop a feeling of belonging together because people interact or communicate with each other. Good interactive or communication skills are necessary for groups to form and develop. Interaction will influence whether a person feels they belong to a group or not. (See Chapter 5.)

Development

Interaction influences personal, social, emotional and intellectual development. Individuals build an idea of who they are as they develop through childhood, adolescence and adulthood. The messages that other people communicate to us influence our ideas. The way people react to us, what they say and the way we compare ourselves with others, all affect our concept of self. Our communication with others affects our self-confidence and self-esteem. Therefore, interaction influences how we develop emotionally and socially.

To sum up: we communicate by using language. The concepts we learn help us to build our intellectual ability. Concepts help us to understand our experiences and to know how to act; they help us to understand our lives. Even practical concepts about movement can help us to swim more effectively. (See Chapter 10.)

In the same way, using concepts about listening, body language, verbal and non-verbal communication might help individuals to develop insights into the way social relationships work. Because interaction with others is central to relationships, the positive or negative impact of interaction will have a strong influence on happiness and success in life in general. Career success is likely to be influenced by our skills of interacting with others.

Individuality, self-esteem and the effects of gender, age and culture on interpersonal interaction

When people begin to grow up, they gradually start to become aware of a sense of who they are – a thinking and feeling of self. Everyone needs to be 'someone' and to have a feeling of being something to call 'I' or 'myself'. This sense of being someone motivates people to the things they do, choosing the clothes to wear, making friends with particular people and so on.

Being able to study depends on choosing to be a person who is keen to study. Going to school, college or work depends on a person's sense of who they are – it is often nicer to stay in bed, but people make themselves do other things because of this sense of being a special individual, or having an idea of what they would wish to be like.

Think it over

What are your earliest memories of choosing things to buy? How did the things you bought influence your sense of independence and 'self'? What are your earliest memories of being told you were good at something? How did this influence how you understood yourself – your sense of individuality?

A person's sense of their own 'individuality' or 'self' develops and changes during a lifetime. The sense of self is influenced by the physical body and feelings, and a person's family or care relationships. As a person grows, their individuality is influenced by the community, culture, friendships and group situations that they experience. Many adults believe that their sense of self is something that is consciously chosen to develop. Words like 'self-development' and 'personal growth' are used to describe this process.

Three things which many people include in their sense of self are:

1 **A need to feel special.** We are different from everyone else. There is no one else exactly like us.
2 **A need to feel that we have 'roots'.** We have a personal history. While we do change, we never stop being the person we were born to be.
3 **A need for self-esteem.** People need to value or 'esteem' their sense of who they are.

Think it over

Think about these three ingredients of the sense of self. Do you choose clothes or jewellery that make you feel special? Do you ever think about your past and how your life has changed? Does this give you a sense of having 'roots'? Are you glad to be alive? Do you enjoy life in general? How is your sense of self-esteem?

If a person has problems with feeling special, or with feeling a sense of life-long development, or with self-esteem, then this may lead to personal unhappiness. Sometimes people become depressed if they lose their sense of self, or are unclear about personal identity.

Understanding other people

All people have their own special view of themselves. For many people this might involve thoughts and feelings which could be listed under headings like 'culture', 'religion', 'gender', 'age', 'physical appearance', 'physical and mental abilities', 'sexuality'.

To care about individuals, is to want to make them feel special. To do this means finding out about them and making it clear that their individuality is respected and valued. Learning about other people's sense of self involves looking at how they present themselves – what clothes they choose, what jewellery they wear, what non-verbal messages they send. People will often display something of their individual sense of culture, religion, gender and age just in their clothes and non-verbal behaviour. By talking to people it is possible to learn so much more.

Communicating **respect** involves learning about other people, remembering what has been learned and reflecting it back. For instance, learning the names of people you are working with – the name that the client prefers to be called by. Then it is important to remember things you have been told and use them later, 'Hello Mrs Andrews, how did your son get on at that job interview you told me about?'

Communicating respect involves getting into conversations with others and showing that you listen to them. It is important to show that you value what they have told you enough to remember it. You 'switch on' your memory when you next meet. Naturally, the way you make people feel special will involve sending non-verbal messages of interest and respect as well. So you could greet Mrs Andrews with a smile and make eye-contact (both are messages which say, 'I'm interested in talking to you'). If Mrs Andrews wishes, use hand movements to signal interest and then say, 'How did your son get on at that job interview you told me about?' You are sending the message 'I'm interested in you and I remember what you told me. I respect and value you as an individual.'

Not everyone does this. Sometimes people don't even bother to learn the clients' names: 'There are too many of them so I call all the male old people "pop" and all the women "dear"!' This kind of behaviour sends the message, 'You are not special. I don't care about you as an individual.'

Also words like 'dear' can convey the message, 'I am more important than you', 'I have power over you', 'I have more status than you'. These messages can be dangerous. They can mean that the client will dislike the carer, and the carer may come to dislike the client.

Another important point is to be sure not to label people. Because each person is an individual, it is important not to make **wrong assumptions.**

Imagine two people are having a conversation. One is a Muslim and the other person is not, but the second person has tried to learn about the Islamic faith. Perhaps the non-Muslim has heard of Ramadan, a time of fasting during daytime. The non-Muslim might say, 'Oh, it's Ramadan so I did not get you a drink.' What this person has done shows that he or she was trying to learn about religion – but forgot about individuality. Each individual will keep his or her own religious observances, so the speaker should have checked what the other person thought, before jumping to conclusions. Many Muslims do not drink during the days of Ramadan, but is that the code this individual actually follows? It is essential to understand culture and religion on an individual level when working with individuals. Failure to do this may lead to stereotyping others.

When trying to communicate with others it is also important to show respect for **individual self-esteem needs.** People should always be offered choices so that they can express their individuality, i.e. asking their opinion, rather than guessing what is needed. The idea is this: if people make their own choices and are asked for their views and opinions, then they are *in control.* People express their sense of self by making choices and having opinions. Carers should be sensitive to this and thus increase a sense of self-worth in others.

Body language and culture

Body language is just that –it's a language. There are many languages in the world and they do not all have the same concepts and sounds. Body language is not the same everywhere.

For example, in Britain the hand gesture with palm up and facing forward, means 'Stop, don't do that.' In Greece it can mean, 'You are dirt' and is a very rude gesture.

Why do the same physical movements have different meanings? The answer lies in culture. One explanation for the hand signs is that the British version of the palm-and-fingers gesture means, 'I arrest you, you must not do it'; whereas the Greek interpretation goes back to medieval times when criminals had dirt rubbed in their faces to show how much people despised then.

Without looking at history and culture, it is confusing to consider why gestures mean what they do. No one knows all the history and all the cultural possibilities of body language and non-verbal communication. But it is vitally important that carers should always remember that people have different cultural backgrounds. The carer's system of non-verbal communication may not carry the same meanings to everyone. We can easily misinterpret another person's non-verbal messages.

Sometimes cultural differences are very marked. White British people are often seen as 'unusual' or odd when they go outside Europe, because they keep a large personal space around them. Other people are not allowed to come too near when they speak, or to touch them. In many other cultures, standing close is normal and good manners – touching an arm or shoulder is just usual behaviour. Some British people feel threatened by such non-verbal behaviour because it is not what they have grown up with. For some British people, strangers who come too close or who touch are trying to dominate or have power over them. They become afraid or defensive. However, things work out when this need for space and distance is understood and allowed for by people from other cultures.

From a caring viewpoint, respect for other people's culture is the right attitude. People learn different ways of behaving, and good carers will try to understand the different ways in which people use non-verbal messages. For instance, past research in the USA suggests that white and black Americans may have used different non-verbal signals when they listened. It suggests that black Americans may tend not to look much at the speaker. This can be interpreted as a mark of respect – by looking away it demonstrates that you are really thinking hard about the message. Unfortunately, not all white people understood this cultural difference in non-verbal communication. Some individuals misunderstood and assumed that this non-verbal behaviour meant exactly what it would mean if they had done it. That is, it would mean they were not listening.

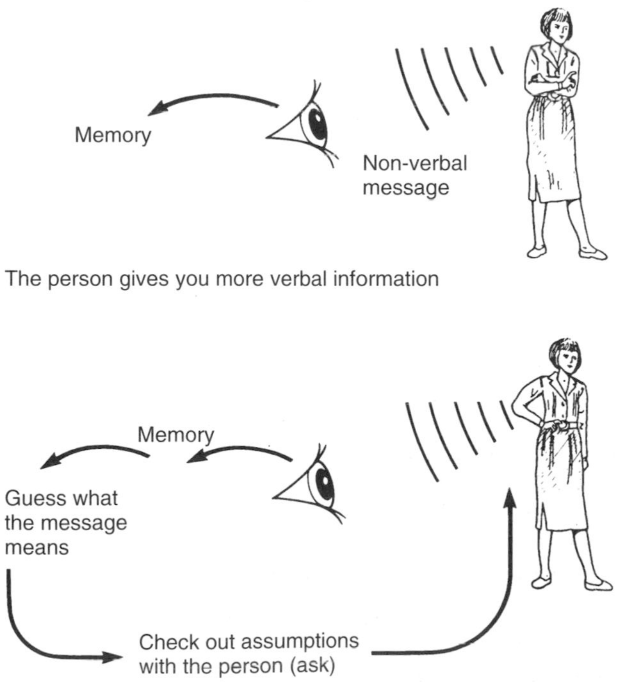

Figure 4.10 The process of understanding another person's body language

Learning the cultural differences

There is an almost infinite variety of meanings that can be given to any type of eye contact, facial expression, posture or gesture. Every culture develops its own special system of meanings. Carers have to understand and show respect and value for all these different systems of sending messages. But how can you ever learn them all?

In fact, no one can learn every possible system of non-verbal message – but it is possible to learn about the ones people you are with are using! It is possible to do this by first noticing and remembering what others do – what non-verbal messages they are sending. The next step is to make an intelligent guess as to what messages the person is trying to give you. Finally, check your understanding (your guesses) with the person: ask polite questions as well as watching the kind of reactions you get. So, at the heart of skilled interpersonal interaction is the ability to watch other people, remember what they do, guess what actions might mean and then check out your guesses with the person.

Summary

- Never rely on your own guesses, because often these turn into assumptions.
- If you don't check out assumptions with people, you may end up misunderstanding them.
- Misunderstandings can lead to discrimination.

Think it over

You are working with an older person. Whenever you start to speak to her she always looks at the floor and never makes eye-contact. Why is this?

Your first thought is that she might be sad or that you make her sad. Having made such an assumption, you might not want to work with this person – she is too depressing and you do not seem to get on. You might even decide that you do not like her. But you could ask: 'How do you feel today; would you like me to get you anything?' By checking out what she feels, you could test your own understanding. She might say she feels well and is quite happy, and then suggests something you could do for her. This means that she cannot be depressed.

Why else would someone look at the floor rather than at you?

1 It could be a cultural value. She may feel it is not proper to look at you.
2 She may not be able to see you clearly, so she prefers not to try to look at you.
3 She may just choose not to conform to your expectations. Looking at the floor may be important to some other emotional feeling that she has.

So it would be unfair to assume that she was difficult or depressed just because she did not look at you when you talked to her.

Good caring is the art of getting to understand people – not acting on unchecked assumptions. So non-verbal messages, should never be relied on; they should always be checked. Non-verbal messages can mean different things depending on the circumstances of the people sending them. But all messages are like this. Words can be looked up in a dictionary, and yet words do not always carry exactly the same meaning.

As well as looking at the whole picture of people's words, their non-verbal messages and where they are, it is also necessary to understand their culture, their individuality and how they see their social situation. This is why caring is such a skilled area of work. People can improve their skills constantly through experience, and through linking new ideas to their experience. The main thing is always to check out assumptions. It is important to remember that it is easy to misunderstand others. By checking out ideas it is possible to reduce the risks of being uncaring or discriminatory.

Culture, age and gender

A person's understanding of him or herself will be strongly influenced by past personal history and current social context. Socialisation into the rules of a culture has a major part to play in the way individuals form a self-concept or identity. (See the sections on self-concept and socialisation in Chapters 10 and 11.)

Perceptions of age-appropriate behaviour and gender-appropriate behaviour are strongly influenced by culture. Culture is the term used to describe the norms and values which belong to an identifiable social group. People are socialised into the norms and values of a culture; they learn the socially accepted rules of their group. Group norms and values – the 'rules' for behaviour – vary between different religious, ethnic, class, gender and age groups.

Norms and values which influence interpersonal interaction vary a great deal between different class groups and different regions of Britain. Not only do norms of interaction vary, but they also constantly evolve and change. It might be possible to invent a dictionary of rules for understanding the meanings of verbal and non-verbal behaviours; but such a dictionary would need constant revision for it to be accurate.

People of different age groups have usually been socialised into different norms with respect to interpersonal behaviour.

Think it over

Florence Tucknell was born in 1912. When she was young there was a cultural norm that only close friends and family would call her by her first name. She was Miss Tucknell to everyone else. For a stranger to call her 'Florence' would be a sign of disrespect, a sign that they thought they were socially superior or more powerful than her. When Florence went into a respite care home for a week she was upset that everyone used first names. She knows that this is what goes on nowadays, but this was not how she was brought up to behave.

Miss Tucknell was very pleased to be greeted by her key worker who introduced herself as, 'I'm Anthea Shakespeare, may I ask your name?'. Miss Tucknell replied, 'I'm Miss Tucknell, please.' 'Shall I call you Miss Tucknell then?' 'Yes please.' Miss Tucknell was annoyed with one of the other staff who said 'Hello Flo, I've come to take you into lunch'. Miss Tucknell avoids this care worker whenever she can.

Age norms and gender norms may interact.

Think it over

Martin Howarth was born in the north of England in 1949. He recently moved to the south-east of England and took a job as a care worker. Martin was shocked to find that many of his younger female colleagues were complaining about his behaviour. Martin has been socialised into the norm of calling women 'Flower' or even 'Petal.' When Martin used these terms he was expecting to communicate approval, comradeship and warmth. Martin believed that these were universal terms of endearment, i.e. 'You are likeable, we're all working together, we get on – don't we?' His new colleagues in the south had never been referred to as 'Flower' before and saw it as sexist and degrading: 'You are saying that I am weak, short-lived and that all that matters about my existence is my degree of sexual attractiveness!' Martin soon learned that age, gender and region affect how words are understood. Words change their value with time.

Think it over

When Jason was 13 years old he used to call really interesting clothes or bicycles 'wicked'. He is now 19 and recently started helping at a local youth centre. When he said, 'Cor, that's a wicked set of trainers', the younger adolescents all laughed at him for being out of touch. 'Wicked' no longer meant you belong to the 'in-group' of 13-year-olds: not at this centre anyway!

The way verbal interaction is understood depends on the influence of norms within group culture. The same is true for body language.

Enhancing and inhibiting interpersonal interaction

Enhancing interaction for people with sensory disabilities

Think it over

If someone has a hearing impairment but can sign and lip read does this mean they have no difficulties?

Signing and lip reading work well on a person-to-person basis, providing both can sign, but public information systems, for example, over a loud speaker or in a lecture hall mean the speaker cannot be seen. A system has therefore been devised for large public halls called a *loop system* which relays the sound to a person's hearing aid.

Watching films and television can be difficult for hearing-impaired people because sometimes the words heard are from people not facing the camera. You may like to experiment with this by turning off the sound on a television programme and trying to understand what is happening. Sometimes vital information is verbal and anyone not hearing it would miss the point of the programme. Some programmes carry subtitles but these are relatively infrequent.

Hearing impairment may also cause problems socially. If someone is in a large gathering of hearing people it can be difficult to follow the conversation which may jump rapidly from person to person.

Think it over

Ibrahim has recently begun a catering course at college. He is a quick worker and remembers what he has been shown. However, he has a hearing impairment. The result of this is that he tends to work in isolation, concentrating on his task. Some of the other students are less able than Ibrahim and need help. The staff ask Ibrahim if he will lend them a hand but he signs to say, 'No, I have done my work, I want to have a break now.' If the other students are talking and laughing Ibrahim sometimes reacts angrily, banging his equipment around. What effect is Ibrahim's disability having on his learning experience?

Ibrahim is isolated socially from his group because of his hearing impairment. He is unused to co-operating as part of a group and his refusal to help others is not gaining him friends. Because he can't join in the incidental chatting and joking he sometimes thinks that the laughter is directed at him. This is emotionally upsetting and further erodes Ibrahim's confidence to become part of the group. The college are trying to provide a communicator to work alongside Ibrahim. This would make it easier for him to understand what is happening informally and, if he understands others better, he may be more prepared to work as part of a team.

The environment and social context

We choose different situations and ways of communicating depending on what we want to 'say' and to whom we want to express it.

Think it over

The columns below list different types of communication and situations. Select which you would choose for each communication:

- telling someone they are terminally ill
- helping someone sort out their bills
- celebrating a birthday
- deciding on clothes for a holiday

- disco
- department store
- quiet room
- at a desk

The situations above may not have been hard to sort out. But as the old saying goes, 'There is a time and place for everything'. Places which are entirely appropriate for some types of communication are not suitable for others. It would not be easy to have an in-depth conversation on a serious issue in a disco. Aronson (1994) quotes Baum and Valins (1979) in a study which showed that students who lived in crowded dormitories were more withdrawn socially and less likely to solve their own problems than ones who lived in less crowded conditions. People who are unhappy and stressed need privacy and peace in which to discuss their problems. Loud music and bright lights would add to their pressure and mean quiet conversation would be impossible.

Care workers must provide clients with the appropriate time and space to communicate. Think carefully about the surroundings. A mother who has her very small children with her is unlikely to feel at ease in a room full of ornaments and plain light-coloured carpets! It is important that the type of words used are right for the person and circumstances. Anyone who has found themselves in a situation where the slang or formal language used is different from what they are used to will know how difficult communication can be. Even people speaking the same language can have difficulties with local dialect. For example, consider a student from the north of England who moved to Newcastle to go to university. The distance away from his home is only about 100 miles and not too many difficulties were expected. However, his request for, 'A Newcastle Brown, please' in the local pub was met with a blank stare until the barmaid responded with, 'Why aye, pet, a Brun'. Even getting a drink speaking the same 'language' can be confusing if you are unfamiliar with the slang.

Think it over

Lindsay, a trainee teacher, was instructed to join her multicultural studies group at the local Sikh temple one Sunday.

When she arrived she could not find her group but she decided to go into the service anyway. She was directed to the women's entrance where the females left their shoes. At this point she realised she had no head covering and had to borrow a scarf to put on her head. She followed the rest of the women into the temple and sat with them on the floor, feeling very conspicuous. She could not speak the language or understand the service and was wearing inappropriate clothes.

Everyone Lindsay met had been friendly and helpful. The barriers to communication were that she did not understand the language, dress codes or religious procedures. If she had joined her group she would have had the benefit of a guide who would have interpreted the service. She should have remembered to take a suitable head covering, but if she had been sitting with others wearing Western dress she would have felt less conspicuous.

A client arriving in a new care situation may feel like Lindsay. They will not know the layout of the establishment, what is expected of them or how to behave. It is very helpful for anyone in this situation to be 'attached' for a short time to someone else who is familiar with the place and routine and who will help them to understand what happens when. Such a person is called a 'mentor' and a mentor system is useful in many situations where there are newcomers, for example, at work or college.

To sum up: it is likely that carers will find their clients' experiences different to their own. The best way to deal with uncertainties is to ask questions. Carers should not make guesses but should read the non-verbal signs carefully. They should then check to see if they are right with their interpretations.

Factors which inhibit communication

There is a range of problems that may prevent people from communicating with each other.

Some of these may be physical factors and are quite obvious. If people cannot hear one another because of background noise, or if they cannot see one another properly because of poor lighting, then they will not be able to understand non-verbal messages. Furniture can act as a block. For example, if desks or tables are arranged badly, then people may not be able to see or hear one another easily.

Less obvious problems include those that arise when people do not attempt to respect one another or to respect the self-esteem needs of the people they are talking to. Both conversations and relationships break down when people do not attempt to communicate respect. Respect involves trying to understand the language and terminology that other people use. Sometimes people talk in their own 'slang' language or in jargon (technical talk that is hard to understand). If people really wish to communicate, they will alter their way of speaking to meet the needs of others. There are several other reasons why people do not listen to one another.

1 Listening takes up too much mental energy – a person might be too tired to listen properly.

2 People say they have too little time and too much work to do. Sometimes this might be true, but sometimes it might be an excuse.
3 It seems like someone has heard it all before and there is nothing to be done to help – it feels easier to switch off.
4 Some clients in care are seen as unimportant and their worries are not considered worth listening to – so they are not treated with the respect they deserve.
5 Sometimes people do not understand the backgrounds and lifestyles of others. It becomes easier not to have to learn about people who are different – not listening means not having to adjust our views and beliefs.
6 Sometimes clients can make carers worry. They might talk about pain, suffering and grief. People can be afraid to talk about such things, so not listening means that they do not have to.
7 Some people like to control clients. It is quicker and easier just to get on with practical day-to-day tasks – asking the client's opinion gets in the way of serving the meal quickly.
8 Most important of all, some people imagine that they should always be able to offer simple advice to anyone with a worry or a problem. They feel that they have to have an answer for everything. This belief stops them from listening to what the problem is.

Optimising effective interaction

Do good relationships just 'happen?' It might be comforting to think that fate has our life in hand and we just have to wait for things to happen, but in reality we have to work at it!

A good basis for starting friendships is to be interested in the same things. This provides opportunities for conversations and outings, perhaps to a football match or to the theatre. Clients who have difficulty in expressing themselves can find safe self-expression through activities like drama. It can be easier to confront behavioural problems in the context of art or drama than on a personal level. For example, watching a TV soap opera with someone may bring an opportunity to talk with them about a situation which may also be happening to them. So a teenager could say to a parent, 'What would you do, mum, if I were pregnant?' in the context of watching a TV programme. The teenager might not be pregnant but the context of the TV programme provides an opportunity to explore reactions and gauge feelings, or even just open a discussion.

A good way to learn to share is to play a team game where everyone has a part and is working towards the same end. It helps people to begin to co-operate and work with each other rather than just for themselves.

Optimising a conversation may involve close attention to both verbal and non-verbal behaviour. Before starting a conversation with another person you will both probably:

- make eye-contact
- smile
- nod
- have the appropriate facial expression
- change position (e.g. stand up, sit down)
- use a gesture.

All these things are likely to happen before any words are spoken and will give indications of what type of conversation is likely to take place. If the exchange is not a friendly one, the facial expression, position and gestures will easily be seen as being threatening.

Depending on how well the people know each other, some form of greeting will be used, for example, 'Hi', probably followed by a remark such as 'How are things?' In a friendly and warm encounter, general remarks might continue with topics such as the weather, etc. In contrast, if the encounter is an interview with a boss who is not pleased about something, it is likely that the subject of the meeting will be introduced straight away.

If a conversation is to be satisfactory to both or all the people taking part in it, it is necessary to take turns to speak and for one person not to dominate the conversation. Consider how a young baby 'talks' with an adult.

Humans learn turn-taking rules even before they can speak. The young baby will babble then stop and wait for the other person to speak. When the person stops, the baby will babble again. The baby will babble for a similar length of time to the person he or she is 'talking' with. If the person 'talking' were to speak angrily or scowl and look fierce, the baby would become upset and probably cry.

All this takes place without the baby understanding the words used. It says a lot about the power of non-verbal communication. Remember, you are giving and receiving messages all the time without saying anything at all.

There are a number of ways by which people judge when it is their turn to speak. It is possible to try this out by closing your eyes during a conversation and

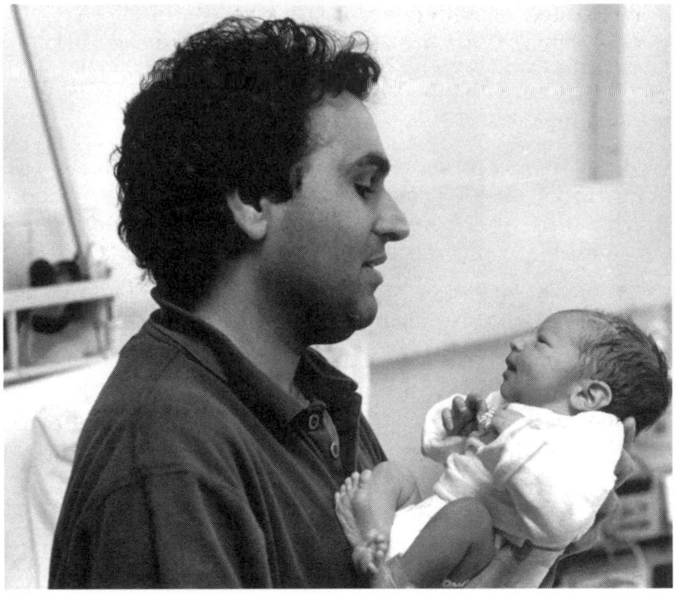

trying to judge when it is your turn to come in. Think carefully about what clues you are receiving.

Think it over

You should notice:

- There is a tendency for the last part of the speech to be drawled or slower.
- There is a drop in pitch (a change in voice tone).
- The statement is completed.

But having your eyes closed means missing some of the clues that are available – those of non-verbal or body language. When a person has finished his part of the conversation, he may use a hand gesture or relax his body position.

Seeking information – questioning skills

Many people may enjoy talking about themselves, so someone who is a skilful questioner can easily become a good conversationalist. Care workers may also need to get information from clients to understand how to respond to their needs effectively, so good questioning skills are important here.

Think it over

Sometimes the answers that are given to questions do not tell us what the person really thinks. Think about some reasons why someone might not say what he or she really thinks.

A client may be worried about upsetting staff, being thought of as a trouble-maker, if he or she complains. The client may, therefore, say what he or she thinks you want to hear rather than what he or she really wants to say. Many people have done this at some point. It may have been when a teacher or parent asked them why they were acting in a certain way. Often, when we do not know how to start telling someone how we really feel, we say 'Nothing' when asked what is bothering us.

In other circumstances a person may want to look good, so will agree with the person speaking even when he or she really disagrees. A person may also make up an answer to a question, rather than admit ignorance of the the true answer, to avoid looking silly.

Obviously, then, while asking questions can be a useful way of getting a conversation going, it can also seem threatening to the person being questioned. Most of the reasons above for not giving true answers were based on the fact that the people being questioned did not feel confident, or needed to protect themselves in some way. It is important not to make others feel they are on trial or being harassed! It means watching carefully to see how the person you are talking with is responding and knowing how far to go and when to stop.

Closed and open questions

Some types of questions are known as **closed** questions. This is because it is possible to answer them simply without widening the conversation.

For example a person might ask children if they have been to school that day. Many children would simply say 'yes' or 'no', which does not extend the conversation very much. If, however, an open question was used – such as 'What did you do at school today?' – there is a better chance of them giving an answer that can be used to carry on the conversation. Of course, the answer may be just 'nothing'; but at least there is a possibility of getting more information!

Open questions therefore can keep the conversation going. But sometimes it is useful to structure the conversation to focus on a specific subject. For example, a carer may want to plan some leisure activities for an older client group. If asked directly what they wanted to do, they might all say they do not know. If the carer were to use a questioning technique called **funnelling,** more information might be forthcoming.

Funnelling means starting with an open question and then narrowing down to concentrate on something definite. For example:

Care worker: What sort of things did you do in the evenings before television came along?
Client: Oh, all sorts really. We used to have some fun though.
Care worker: I suppose you had to make your own entertainment?

Think it over

Try to think of some more questions and answers following on the above conversation.

It might be possible to develop the above conversation to see whether the client group would enjoy having some recordings of old singers or inviting someone in to play the piano/accordion for a sing-song, or perhaps getting some crafts going, such as rug-making, or comparing old photographs. This technique is based on the idea of knowing where you want to steer the conversation, while allowing the other people time to collect their thoughts and develop them in their own way.

Another technique that may be useful with all client groups, but particularly with older people, is to use recall questions such as, 'Where did you live when you were a child?' However, it is necessary to think carefully about the questions you are asking, because some areas of their lives may have been painful.

Think it over

Try to remember a time when you were talking with someone about an experience that was painful to him or her. Make a note of what you needed to do when listening.

It is important to be very aware of non-verbal signals, such as:

- facial expression
- whether the person leaned forward or pulled back
- how near he or she was positioned to you
- how much eye-contact was used
- the tone of voice
- the speed at which he or she spoke
- the rhythm of the speech (smooth or jerky).

The person is always 'saying' more than the content of their verbal communication.

Conversational skills

Being sensitive to others involves listening and memory. An understanding is built up which helps you to say the right things, and to send the right non-verbal messages.

It is also necessary to express **warmth.** Warmth involves not being critical about other people, but being accepting of differences between yourself and others.

Think it over

Think of a person you have met who is totally different from you – someone with different interests, habits, lifestyle, culture, etc. Do you think first about what is 'wrong' with the other person – for example, the things you would disagree with, what you would argue against? Or do you think first about what is exciting and interesting in this other person?

'Warmth' can describe the feelings of excitement and interest when we meet different people. Judging others in a critical way is uncaring and unsupportive.

When thinking about other people and their life situations, we are bound to notice the difference between their ways of thinking and ours. Where differences exist, one response is to argue about them, to challenge the other view as 'wrong'. In other words, when people lead different lives or have different problems from our own, there can be a tendency to assume that we have a better way of thinking, a better lifestyle, etc., and that we do not really need to know about theirs!

To show 'warmth' is to have the ability not to sit in judgement on someone. It is the ability to listen, understand and not criticise other people's individuality. Carers must accept that other people have the right to be the way they are.

Finding the right behaviours to communicate 'warmth' will help carers to work in an anti-discriminatory way with clients.

Finally, showing respect for others requires carers to be sincere. Respect needs to be real or genuine. It needs to be an expression of a person's own self.

When trying to listen, understand and be warm, as a carer you still have to 'be yourself'. Attempts to use stock phrases, or to copy a performance, can destroy the safety and trust that develop if people are to believe they are understood and accepted. Clients must also understand a little about their carers in order to trust them. So there must be an **openness** in the way a carer communicates understanding and acceptance for it to mean anything.

It is important that carers help their clients to feel emotionally secure. This security comes from having a high level of self-esteem. Carers need to be able to observe people carefully to see what messages they are sending out, and to be able to respond to these messages. The messages will often be unspoken, so the skill is in understanding non-verbal signs as well as verbal or spoken ones.

The best way to get an understanding of what other people are feeling is to attempt to see things from their point of view, to 'step into their shoes'. Before this, however, it is helpful to get a picture of how you feel you communicate at present, so you can begin to work on the areas that need improving.

Evaluate your conversational skill

Think it over

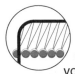

Ask yourself the following questions. (Cover up the scores – there is no point in fooling yourself!)

When someone tells you something, do you:

1 **a** note the content of what they say?
   b watch their face, gestures, posture etc.?
   c think of the context in which they are saying it?

Score: a=1; a and b=2; a, b and c=3

2 **a** pick up on something that interests you, and reply straight away?
   b listen to all of what is said, then reply?
   c think of what the speaker is wearing?

Score: a=0; b=2; c=0

3 **a** start thinking of a reply before the speaker has finished?
   b allow the speaker to finish before beginning to think of a reply?
   c interrupt with your own view?

Score: a=0; b=2; c=0

4 **a** look around you?
   b nod and give eye-contact?
   c position yourself appropriately to the speaker?

Score: a=0; b=2; c=2

Interpreting your score

If you have scored between 7 and 9 in total you have a high level of conversational skill. The questions covered some of the most common listening problems.

In question 1 it is important to take account of all the clues the speaker has provided. This means taking notice of the *context* in which the conversation takes place and the non-verbal clues available, as well as what is actually said. (You will realise from this that communicating by telephone means it is much more difficult to get a full 'picture' of what the speaker is saying.)

Question 2 deals with the way we can allow ourselves to be side-tracked into picking up mainly on what interests us, by hearing only what we want to hear. This is sometimes called 'selective hearing'.

Question 3 identifies a tendency to start thinking of a reply before the speaker has actually finished saying everything. This is a very common fault and we can all remember the frustration of talking with someone who finishes our sentences for us! Sometimes we do this because we want to avoid silences or gaps in the conversation. Sometimes we are more interested in what we ourselves want to say than in what the speaker is saying. Sometimes we are bored and want the speaker to get to the point. However, we must give the speaker space to make their point and say what they mean, not assume we know what they mean.

Question 4 deals with the importance of letting someone know you are listening to them, by looking at them and being in an appropriate position. If you are gazing around and not giving eye-contact, it is difficult for them to judge what your reactions are.

Evaluating effective interaction

Not all the relationships we form will be deep ones. We do not have the emotional 'space' to have a large number of very deep relationships and this would not always be appropriate or desirable; so the levels of intensity in relationships will vary. We know that, as professionals caring for other people, it is necessary to monitor interaction and not just 'hope' to get on well with others. Hopson and Scally (1988) have suggested the following criteria to monitor behaviour, in order to convey the intentions of respect, sincerity and empathy to other people:

- *Respect*
  - giving positive attention
  - active listening: show you are giving the other person your full attention by your body language and noting the feelings behind the words
  - giving your time: try to make the person you are listening to feel that what they are saying is the most important thing, not that you are anxious to stop the conversation so you can get on with something else
  - remembering the person's name: this means paying proper attention when you are introduced and not letting your mind wander on to other matters
  - introducing yourself
  - asking questions
  - checking assumptions: make sure you are understanding correctly by asking for clarification and not making assumptions
  - not stereotyping or making critical evaluations: listen to what the person is really trying to say, rather than agreeing or disagreeing
  - giving the other person 'air space' and not interrupting.
- *Sincerity*
  - talking appropriately about yourself: it helps people to know you if you tell them bits about yourself but be careful not to be so busy talking about yourself that you don't listen to them!
  - responding naturally: don't be afraid to show your feelings. Of course you shouldn't become so upset you are no longer any use to the client, but there is nothing wrong in showing you share a client's distress
  - sharing feelings appropriately
  - being spontaneous: a spontaneous hand on the shoulder or a hug can speak volumes, but make sure this is appropriate behaviour, i.e. you know your client well enough to judge how they would receive spontaneous words or gestures
  - your verbal behaviour is consistent with your non-verbal behaviour
  - not being defensive: if someone makes a justified criticism, accept it; no-one is expected to be perfect
  - not pretending to be someone or something you are not.
- *Empathy*
  - deflecting back the other person's feelings: 'you must feel very angry'
  - sharing related experiences of your own
  - mirroring: smiling when the other person smiles, frowning when the other person frowns.

Evaluation

All effective interpersonal interaction involves moment-by-moment monitoring of your own and others' behaviour. Monitoring involves being able to reflect or think about what is happening while a person is actually holding a conversation.

Experienced health and social care workers may be able to ask themselves questions whilst a conversation is in progress. They might think about:

- eye-contact
- body posture
- facial expression
- body movements
- muscle tension
- gestures

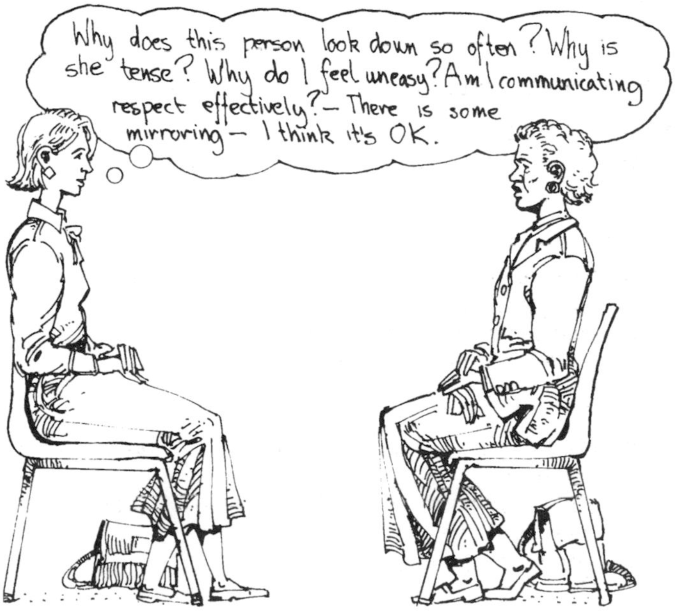
Why does this person look down so often? Why is she tense? Why do I feel uneasy? Am I communicating respect effectively? – There is some mirroring – I think it's OK.

Figure 4.11 Monitoring

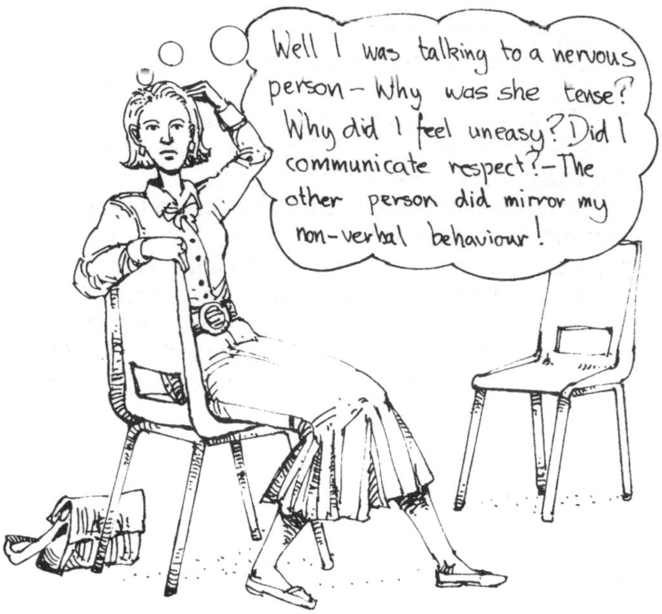
Well I was talking to a nervous person – Why was she tense? Why did I feel uneasy? Did I communicate respect? – The other person did mirror my non-verbal behaviour!

Figure 4.12 Reflecting

- tone and speed of verbal communication
- touch
- verbal messages.

At first this kind of monitoring is very difficult. Sometimes it may take all of an individual's mental energy just to understand what is being said and what to say next. The best way to build optimal monitoring skills may be to practise monitoring in the imagination first.

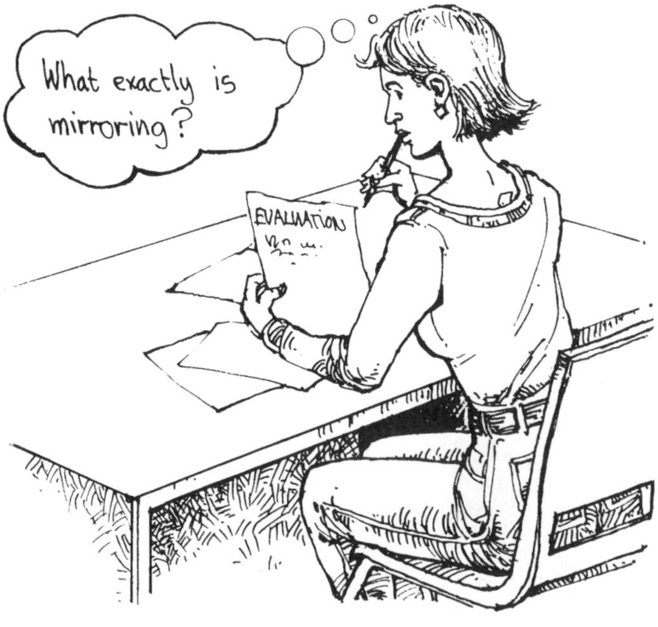
What exactly is mirroring?
EVALUATION

Figure 4.13 Using concepts

When using imagination in this way a carer is using evaluative skills, to review the value of an action or a piece of behaviour. Imagination or reflection is a good way of linking theory to practice. Concepts of 'eye contact,' 'mirroring' (copying each other's non-verbal behaviour) and so on, can be used to review what may have happened. However, just thinking about things is rarely enough to develop advanced skills; usually people need feedback from others as well.

If you have to put ideas into words, you may have to think them through more carefully than usual. It can be valuable to produce written evaluations, because the act of writing develops an ability to concentrate on ideas.

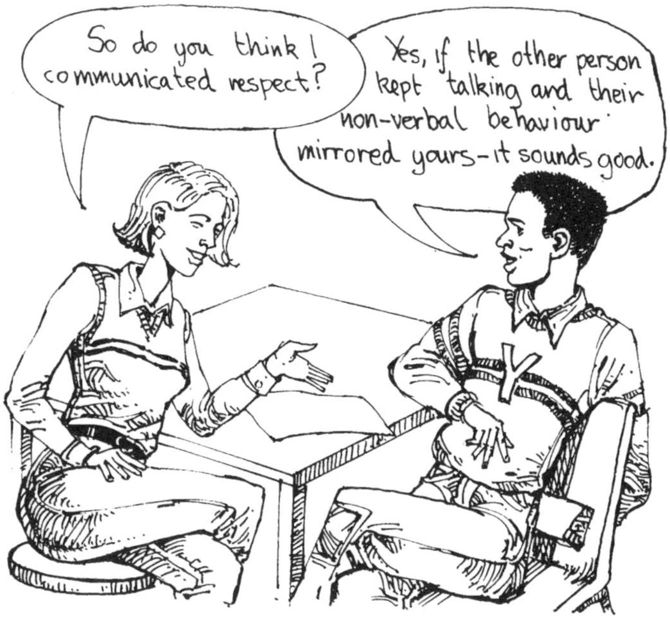
So do you think I communicated respect?
Yes, if the other person kept talking and their non-verbal behaviour mirrored yours – it sounds good.

Figure 4.14 Feedback

Talking your thoughts through with someone else may give you an opportunity to gain feedback on your ideas. Other people can ask you questions and you can ask them for their interpretation of your observations. Friends can provide a vital source of feedback on your use of concepts and ideas. Teachers and tutors can give more formal guidance. Group discussion can provide an excellent source of feedback if the group is supportive and caring.

Data for evaluating an interaction will be your records of conversations or other interactions. These could include tape-recorded or video-recorded records in addition to your memory or written notes. As well as the interaction itself, you will have your knowledge of verbal and non-verbal behaviour, your knowledge of other people and your own skills of observation, imagination and reflection.

The skill of monitoring one's own and others' behaviour might grow out of the practice of evaluation, imagination and using feedback from others. So very expert, experienced carers may not always be able to explain how they monitor their clients' reactions. After years of experience these skills may become automatic – people forget how they developed them or even that they have them!

Evidence collection point

For Element 2.1 it may be best to undertake practical work based on one-to-one interaction, work that can also be used as evidence for Element 2.2. This practical work could be the basis for a report which: explains different forms of interpersonal interaction, explains how interaction can be enhanced, inhibited and optimised, provides two examples of positive and negative influences of interaction on health and social well-being and describes the sources of data which might be used to evaluate interaction. Notes on the effects that gender, age and culture may have on interpersonal interaction are also required.

Chapter 5

Skills of interpersonal interaction

This chapter builds on the theory outlined in Chapter 4 and explores the theory of interpersonal interaction as applied to group interaction. Evidence indicators for Element 2.2 require a practical demonstration of interactive skills. Theory to support the organisation and evaluation of skilled interpersonal interaction is provided.

Interpersonal interaction in groups

In everyday language 'group' can mean a collection or set of things, so any collection of people could be counted as a group. For example, a group of people might be waiting to cross the road. These people have not spoken to each other, they may not even have communicated non-verbally – they are simply together in the same place at the same time. They are a group in the everyday sense of the word, but not in the special sense of 'group' that is often used in health and social care work.

In caring, working with a group implies that the people belong together and would identify themselves as belonging to a group. Groups have a sense of belonging which gives the members a 'group feeling'. This could be described as group identity.

A group will usually have some task or some common purpose or social role which acts as a focus for meeting. A group of people studying for a GNVQ might meet to try out practical ideas together. They would be a group in the care sense if they feel that they belong together. The learning tasks might contribute towards making the group feel that they belong together.

How groups get started

Usually, a collection of people will come together because they have a **common goal**. In order to get a group started, its members will need to have good communication skills and may need a 'leader'. The individual skills associated with providing emotional support will be a good foundation for assisting in group development, or in becoming a leader in the group.

People need a group identity in effect to get a group going; people have to feel that they will belong to the group. Initially, the group will need a clear task or purpose, in which all the members feel they want to join. For example, a playgroup for young children will need to be organised around particular activities. A reminiscence group for older people will involve photos or objects from the past. The organisation for these groups would have to be planned in advance. A discussion group (perhaps to discuss GNVQ skills) would require such planning considerations as: who would introduce the topic, what material would be needed, and whether the discussion would be recorded on video.

Use of space

An important aspect of a discussion group is how the group sits. When working with a discussion group it is very important that everyone can see and hear one another. Non-verbal communication will be important, and if people cannot see everybody's faces, this will not be possible. Usually, chairs are placed in a circle when planning a discussion group. In a circle everyone can get non-verbal messages from everyone else.

Organising a group to sit in a circle may suggest that everyone is equal, that everyone is expected to communicate with everyone else. This freedom to communicate is also linked with creating a feeling of belonging: 'We can all share together – this is our group!' (Figure 5.1a).

Other patterns of seating will send different messages. Teachers might sit in the middle of a half-circle. This sends the message 'We are all equal and we can all communicate with each other, but the teacher is going to do most of the communicating!' (Figure 5.1b).

At a formal lecture, people sit in rows. This sends the message 'The lecturer will talk to you. You can ask questions but you should not talk to one another!' (Figure 5.1c).

Some less formal seating arrangements can be chosen to create blocks. Sometimes a desk or table acts as a block. For example, in Figure 5.1d, the two people on

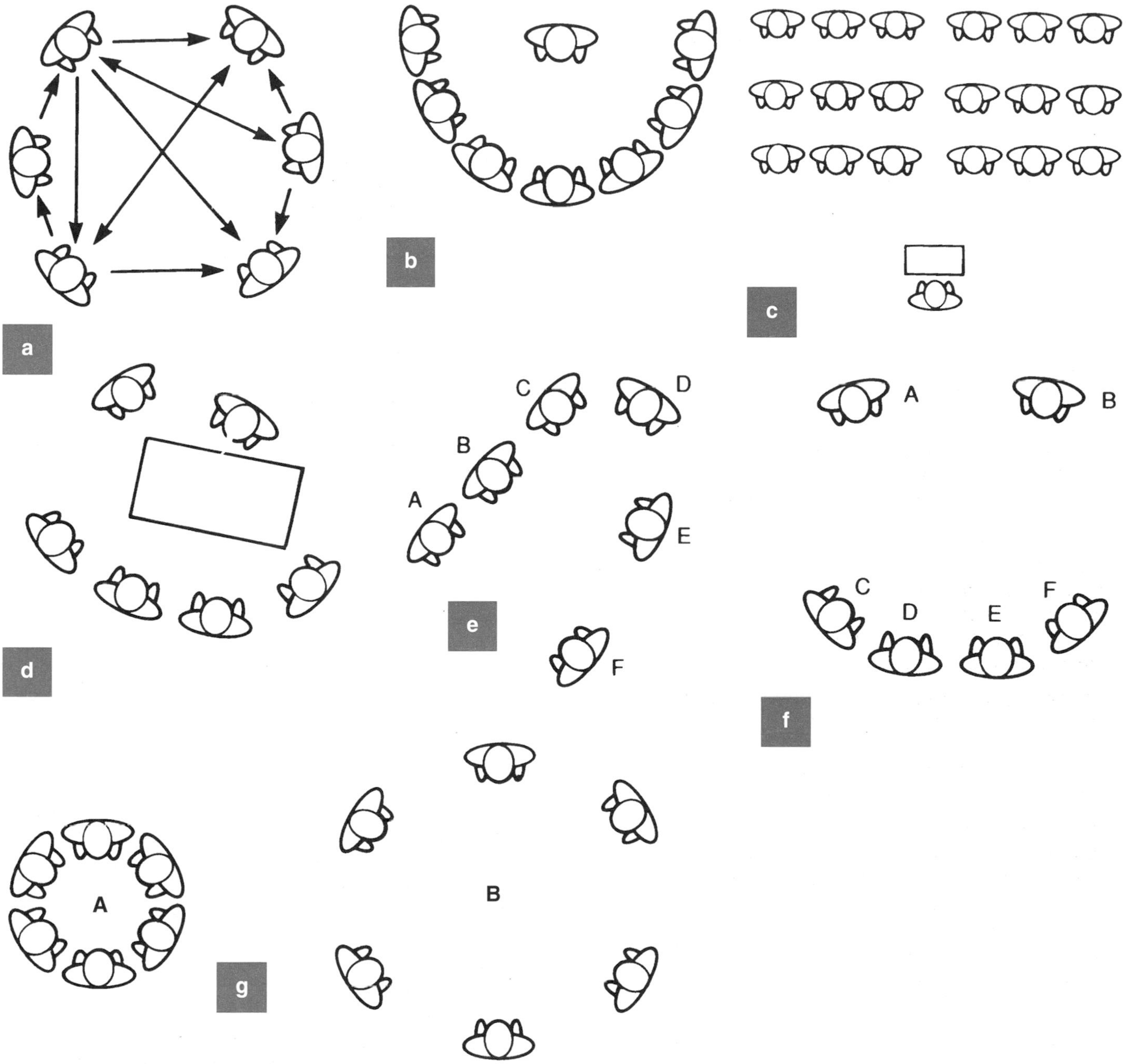

Figure 5.1 a–g 7 seating patterns

their own might be sending the message, 'We are not sure we want to be with this group'. The table can make them feel separate, 'We'll join in only if we feel like it'.

Sometimes space can be used to create a gulf. In Figure 5.1e, person A cannot see person C properly – so the two of them are unable to exchange non-verbal messages. Person A sits 'square on' to person F. Perhaps A does not want to talk to C. Perhaps F and A do not trust each other. The layout of seats makes it look as though there could be tension or reluctance in this group.

Space can also signal social distance – see Figure 5.1f. A and B are keeping their distance from the rest of the group. There could be many reasons, but perhaps they are sending the message 'We do not really belong with you four!'

How close together or spaced out a group of people is sitting should also be considered. In Figure 5.1g, group A are huddled together, whereas group B are more spaced apart. There might be a number of reasons why people get closer or further apart in groups. For example: being close can signal that it's noisy – the group has to get close to hear. It can suggest that the members like each other and are very interested in the discussion topic.Alternatively, it might be that group members feel unsafe – that being together gives more confidence that everyone will be supportive.

Whenever a discussion group is encountered, it is worth studying how people sit and where they sit. It may be possible to work out just by watching how people choose to arrange the seats.

Advantages and disadvantages of groups

If you are taking a course or working in a social care environment it is likely that you will often be asked to work as a part of a group.

Try it

Make a list of the advantages of working in a group during a course for: (a) the individual; (b) the group as a whole.

Below is a list of advantages of working in groups. Compare it with your own list and decide which apply to the individual and which to the group as a whole.

Advantages:

- broader base of knowledge/skills (shared between people)
- motivated by others (having company and support)
- shared responsibility (having others around you)
- security (safety with others)
- confidence (in the group, and in their view of you)
- role models (people whose behaviour can be copied)
- power (the group may have more power collectively than a single person has)
- division of tasks (between people; people can do what they are best at)
- able to work to own strengths (people do the things they are best at)
- improve weaknesses (people to help you)
- question assumptions (people to check your ideas)
- give feedback (people can give advice and help with learning)
- fun (groups can be!)
- synergy (the whole is greater than the parts, interacting parts fitting together)
- richer decisions (better analysis and evaluation).

Think it over

As can be seen there are many advantages to working within a group but, in an imperfect world, there can also be disadvantages. From your own experience of working with others, now make two lists of disadvantages you have experienced: one for individuals and one for groups.

For a group to work well together and gain the advantages identified earlier, its members will have had to go through a process of learning to work with each other. If this does not happen problems may arise:

Individuals' difficulties which may occur in group work:

- one person may dominate the group
- the leader may 'lean' towards one or more person's views
- there may be confused aims
- insecurity if individuals feel they don't 'fit'
- loss of own identity
- specialist jargon might be used
- excess risk-taking
- co-leaders may create a power point, making it difficult to challenge their assumptions
- peer pressure (others might put pressure on you to agree with them)
- difficult to challenge group values
- individuals might shelve personal responsibility
- group pace may differ from own pace
- lack of personal satisfaction
- roles could be forced upon individual
- individual may be tired or overworked.

General problems which may exist for groups:

- groups might be inclined to greater risks
- badly used space, crowded or 'split', inappropriate seating

- factions/disagreements may occur
- inertia (not getting things done)
- conflict of aims
- time-wasting discussion
- power struggles
- unequal commitment
- the group may refuse to take responsibility for actions or decisions.

You may have worked in groups which have been very successful – but why was this so? Success does not always happen automatically; so to ensure it does, it is necessary to consider what conditions are ideal or optimal.

For a group to work it is often necessary for it to have a common aim. After all, groups come together because of a sense of common purpose. So what do groups need in order to be successful?

Groups need to co-operate, be supportive, and be open with members. it usually becomes important to adopt a group identity, become cohesive, stable and, in order to plan, dynamic (or full of energy). Within social care, groups such as support groups are often formed to help those in need.

Creating a successful group

When a group is formed its purpose or objective might need to be defined. Organisations define their objectives in **mission statements.**

Think it over

Some of the organisations you have worked for on placement will probably have mission statements. Do you know what they are?

Within a mission statement the objectives have to be realistic, clear and understood by all. Unfortunately, establishments often have very admirable mission statements, for example about client dignity, but workers do not always abide by them. There is no point in having mission statements about respect and dignity and then barging into people's rooms without knocking! Conversely, while objectives should not be unattainable, they should be ambitious – otherwise no progress would be made.

Groups need to be of an appropriate size and to contain people with the right skills and training. They also need members who are likely to remain with the group. It is demoralising to have to restart a group because people leave. It is important, therefore, when you are working as a team member, to realise that others are depending on you and not to let them down. (For example, do not be away when you have some important material for the group's presentation!) The members of a group need to know what is expected of them in order to carry out their part of the task. Many groups also need a leader who is experienced, skilled and committed to the group's aims.

Finally, resources are important. It is difficult to achieve much without such basic resources as a place and time to meet, support, materials and finance. Power is an important factor, but sometimes, as in the case of support groups, their very function is to *create* power to achieve unmet ends.

Once the objectives have been defined and values identified, the members of a group might analyse their strengths and weaknesses and decide on roles to work together. Tasks have to be allocated to decide who will do what and, eventually, review progress.

It is important that there is a balance of personalities within a group, although all members should take an active role. A certain amount of flexibility is needed in the sharing of tasks. If the group is mutually supportive members should feel able to make mistakes and fail without blame. If this is not so, the dynamism (or energy) of the group is curtailed with everyone 'playing safe' so as not to take risks. The

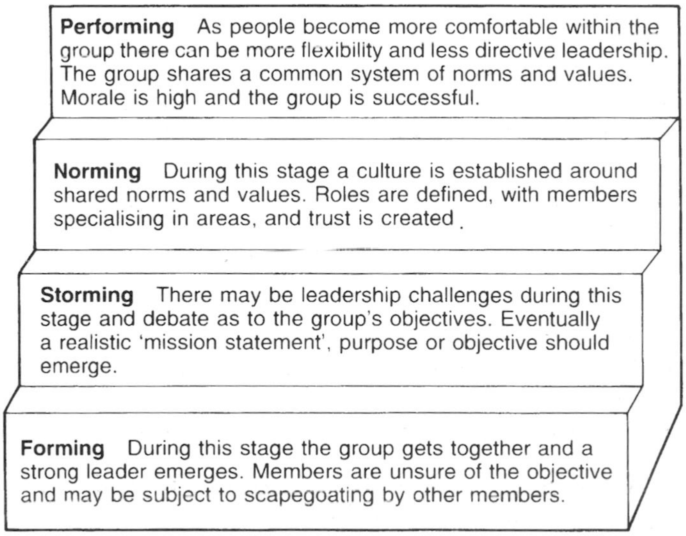

Performing As people become more comfortable within the group there can be more flexibility and less directive leadership. The group shares a common system of norms and values. Morale is high and the group is successful.
Norming During this stage a culture is established around shared norms and values. Roles are defined, with members specialising in areas, and trust is created.
Storming There may be leadership challenges during this stage and debate as to the group's objectives. Eventually a realistic 'mission statement', purpose or objective should emerge.
Forming During this stage the group gets together and a strong leader emerges. Members are unsure of the objective and may be subject to scapegoating by other members.

Figure 5.2 Tuckman has suggested that groups go through a process of maturing before they function efficiently

group will then be less proactive (able to plan) and will achieve less in the long run. Finally, members must be committed to attend meetings and show good timekeeping.

If a group consists of people working towards common goals, and if a group which works well together can accomplish much more than one person alone, why don't all groups work? Much research has taken place on this subject and many people feel that groups have to go through a process of maturing before they function efficiently. Tuckman (1965, pp. 384–99), divided the process into four stages, as shown in Figure 5.2.

In an ideal world, all groups would progress through these stages to successful outcomes, but not all do. Woodcock (1979) says that some groups get stuck in the *forming* stage and need to be pushed through the next two stages before becoming mature and reaching a *performing* stage.

Think it over

Within an educational situation the aim of a group might be to help people learn. How can you, as a group member, help yourself and others?

You may decide that groups can help the learning process by:

- offering information and advice
- listening to problems
- careful questioning
- summary and reflection
- encouragement
- providing opportunities.

Group interaction

In any form of group interaction individual people will adopt different ways of behaving. The same person will probably behave differently within different groups. As a group goes through its maturation process. individuals will adapt their behaviour. Bales (1970) observed groups in action and defined the following types of behaviour:

1 Proposing – a behaviour which puts forward a new concept, suggestion or course of action.
2 Building – a behaviour which extends or develops a proposal which has been made by another person.
3 Supporting – a behaviour which involves a declaration of support or agreement with another person or their ideas.
4 Disagreeing – involves a declaration of difference of opinion, or criticism of another's ideas.
5 Defending/attacking – a behaviour which attacks another person or defensively strengthens a person's own position. Defending/attacking behaviours tend to involve open value judgements and often contain emotional overtones.
6 Blocking/difficulty stating – a behaviour which places a difficulty or blockage in the path of a proposal without offering an alternative proposal, or which states a difficulty without full reason.
7 Open – a behaviour which exposes an individual showing it to the risk of loss of status or to ridicule. Admissions of mistakes or inadequacies made in a non-defensive manner.
8 Summarising – a behaviour which summarises, or otherwise restates in a compact form, the ideas of previous discussions.
9 Seeking information – a behaviour which seeks facts, ideas or clarification from another member.
10 Testing understanding – a behaviour which seeks to establish whether or not contributions have been understood.
11 Giving information – a behaviour which seeks facts, ideas or clarification from another member.
12 Bringing in – a behaviour which offers facts, ideas and opinions to others.
13 Shutting out – a behaviour seeking to exclude another.

Try it

In order to begin to analyse how you and others function in groups you will need to identify the types of behaviour used. A method known as the 'goldfish bowl' technique enables an observer to record on a chart each person's behaviour within a group discussion. A possible discussion might be based on the 'plane crash' exercise. Imagine a group of people in a plane that crashed as it crossed a desert. Fifteen people survived the crash, as did a motorcycle which was in the hold of the plane. The temperature in the desert was very high and the survivors were not likely to last more than a few hours without water. Only two people can be selected to board the motorcycle and head for an oasis twenty miles to the south. There is a working compass on board.

Form into two groups. The discussion which follows should last for fifteen minutes. One group will discuss which of the fifteen passengers described below should go for help. The other group will select one member each of the first group and monitor their part in the discussion by marking the boxes on the chart. Do not say who is monitoring whom.

Chart to profile individual's interaction

Group member: ------------------------------

Time intervals — Minute by minute: 10 to 15 minutes

Proposing															
Building															
Supporting															
Disagreeing															
Defending/attacking															
Blocking/difficulty stating															
Being open															
Summarising															
Seeking information															
Testing understanding															
Giving information															
Bringing in															
Shutting out															
Total															

List of survivors

1. Pilot, appears to be in shock
2. Doctor
3. Army sergeant (female)
4. Mother of ten children
5. Priest
6. Man in remission from cancer
7. Orienteering expert, wanted by police for murder
8. World-renowned plastic surgeon
9. Taxi driver
10. Old-age pensioner on way to see newborn grandchild
11. Manual labourer, native of desert
12. RAF (engineer), male, accompanied by person number 13
13. Eleven-month-old son (of RAF engineer)
14. Air hostess
15. Long-distance runner.

When you have completed the exercise, the monitor and the person being monitored should discuss the pattern of communication shown on the chart. It is sometimes surprising to see your behaviour recorded in this way!

Group polarisation

Much research has taken place as to whether decisions reached by groups of people differ radically from those made by individuals. Bem, Wollach and Kogan in a number of studies between 1962 and 1965 believed that groups were more inclined to take greater risks than individuals and this became known as the 'risky shift' effect.

However, subsequent studies found that groups may not necessarily be less cautious but that they tend to be more extreme either in caution or risk than the individual. If the individuals were initially cautious,

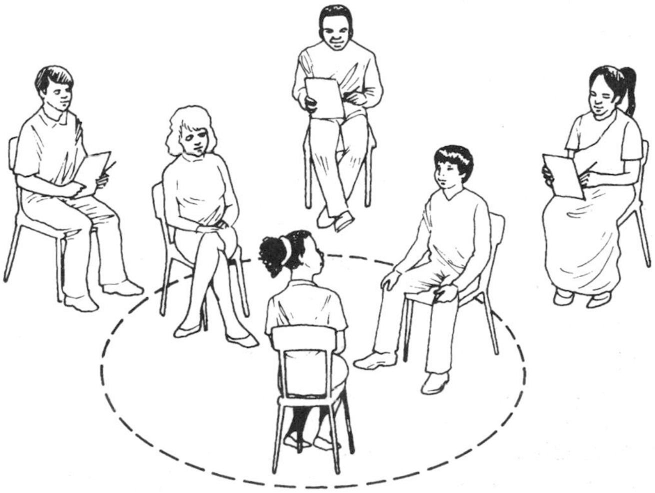

Figure 5.3 The 'goldfish bowl' technique

the group would become more cautious. If the individuals were inclined to take risks, the group would take greater ones. It is the norms or values which become adopted by the group which cause 'polarisation'. The group becomes more extreme or polarised when people focus on shared beliefs.

Think it over

When formulating a group response why might individuals take a more or less cautious view than their own original one ?

You probably realised that there are two basic reasons:

- people tend to be influenced by others
- they gain more information on a topic after discussion.

These two effects have been classified as:

- the *normative* influence and
- the *informational* influence.

The group provides a forum in which the person can get extended information and can re-evaluate their position. Studies have shown that either the informational influence or the normative influence can work independently, but that the informational effect is greater.

Sometimes norms become so ingrained that people really believe this is the 'correct' way to behave. These are accepted ways of behaving and people don't have to think; they are comfortable that they are behaving appropriately. Sometimes, however, norms can be prejudices or restrictive to a particular group and may reflect prejudiced attitudes.

When carers are dealing with clients, it is important to keep the clients' culture in mind and try to understand as much as possible about the norms of their culture. For example, many organisations now follow the American habit of addressing everyone by their first names. Some elders may find this disrespectful. In order not to give offence it is best to ask clients if they would like to be called by their title and last name or by first name.

Try it

You could test out these ideas of norms and influences by having a group discussion.

First, read the scenario below and on a scale of 1 to 10 write down a score each for Peter and the assistant on the justification of stealing drugs. (10 is high and 1 is low.) Do not tell the rest of the group what your scores are. When you have read the scenario discuss your views and reach a group score each for Peter and the assistant. You can then compare your individual scores and see if they have been influenced by the group.

Peter's fiancée Thelma has lung cancer. She is twenty-eight and they have a six-month-old son. Thelma has seen a hospital consultant who tells her the pharmacy at the hospital has a new, very expensive drug which could treat her. The drug could, at best, hold the disease in remission for around ten years.

However, the consultant refuses to treat Thelma unless she agrees to give up smoking. The hospital cannot afford to treat everyone and there are other people who do not smoke needing the drug. Thelma has smoked since she was a child and feels, with the pressure she is under, she would not be able to do this.

Peter knows the assistant at the hospital pharmacy. The assistant has a disabled mother who needs extra support, more than he can afford to give her on his wages. Peter persuades the assistant to steal a week's supply at a time for payment and to continue doing so until the consultant confirms the disease is in remission. This is likely to take at least a year and the cost to the hospital of the stolen drugs will be many thousands of pounds.

Is Peter justified in asking the assistant to steal for him and Thelma?

Is the assistant justified in stealing the drug?

When you have written down your scores and without saying what they are, have a group discussion. Eventually you should arrive at two group scores. Compare them to your own original ones.

Try it

From what you have learned about yourself and seen of groups operating make a list of what *you* feel makes groups succeed or fail. You can do this alone or in a group.

Some of the reasons for groups succeeding are listed below. You may have thought of others, there are many reasons, which will vary depending on the circumstances of the group.

Success in groups

- composition of group – right people
- agreement on objectives
- outcomes agreed, even if it is not what the individual might want
- openness about agendas etc.
- agreement on way of operating
- good quality information
- experience of respect for others, active listening, feeling valued
- not feeling pressurised
- ability of individuals to pick up signals and respond
- role of leader (see below).

Failure in groups

- no clear agenda or objectives
- participants not feeling equally valued, balance of contribution
- lack of trust, suspicion, hidden agendas – for individual or organisation
- avoidance tactics, avoiding work
- different power levels within group
- too much time or not enough time.

Chairing a group

One of the key people in a group is the person who chairs it. The chair (or chairman or chairwoman) is responsible for making sure that the meeting covers the agenda and progresses as it should.

Think it over

Make a list of what you think a chairperson needs to do within a meeting.

A chairperson can have a long list of duties – no wonder many people avoid chairing meetings! Some key points are listed in Figure 5.4.

It is important to remember that both the chairperson and group members can positively or negatively influence people's feeling of inclusion. All members of groups positively and negatively influence the feeling of openness, and thus trust, experienced by their colleagues, as well as people's feelings of control and ownership.

- define objectives, set a time-scale and keep to it unless it is renegotiated
- pay attention to the process and people as much as to the task/content
- keep the session moving
- involve people in the discussion, control any 'dominators'
- clarify points of discussion
- bring people back to the point if things start to drift
- summarise progress
- check out the views of non-contributors
- ensure an outcome to any discussion
- summarise points, identify key issues, check for agreement, action

Figure 5.4 Key duties that a chairperson may have

Difficult behaviour in groups

Despite being aware of the roles you and others play when working in groups, almost everyone will experience difficult behaviour from group members at some time. It is impossible to predict what form this might take, or the reasons for it, but the grid that follows offers one strategy that could be adopted to try to work through the difficult behaviour. Enter your ideas for handling the difficulty in the boxes.

Actions to prevent difficult behaviour			
	Before (meeting)	During (meeting)	After (meeting)
Self			
With other person			
With the whole group			

Types of difficult behaviour may include: (1) people who are unmotivated or reluctant to join in; (2) those who put others down; (3) aggressive people; (4) those who are dominant or just talk too much.

Think it over

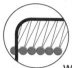

Taking each of the four types of difficult behaviour, brainstorm how you might deal with the problems they present.

People who are reluctant to join in can be encouraged in by the chairperson the following ways:

- encourage contributions and reinforce their offerings
- try to find why they are resistant or reluctant to join in
- allow them to choose their task
- offer alternative work
- give time
- give responsibility
- encourage others in the group to respond to the reluctant person's suggestions
- get them to work with a supportive group member
- attend to what they offer
- be patient
- work on relationships within the group
- challenge if appropriate
- if appropriate, invite to leave the group.

People who put others (or the task) down can be helped towards less difficult behaviour. It might be possible to:

- set ground rules
- give the group responsibility – use others to rebuff criticism
- build a contract for membership
- support/reinforce/model other behaviours
- give feedback
- confront behaviour
- allow 'time out' for the group.

To help deal with aggressive people in the group the chairperson could:

- confront behaviour
- give feedback
- focus on difficulties and feelings produced by behaviour
- reinforce more appropriate behaviour
- discuss effect on group
- set ground rules
- seek causes for behaviour
- discuss with person outside group.

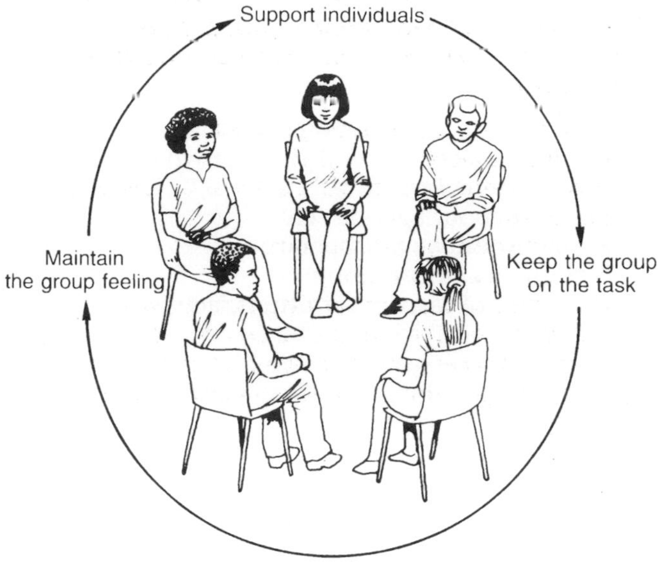

Figure 5.5 The dynamics of a care group

Dominant or talkative people can be encouraged to work better with others. You might decide to:

- agree to share time for discussion
- divide into small groups – to give less opportunity for dominance
- discuss the effect on the group
- give a specific task, e.g. taking notes for group!
- encourage others to contribute more
- seek others' views about confronting the culprit in the group
- speak with the person outside the group situation.

Group values

Groups can form around all sorts of purposes and values. Some people just want to belong to something and will go along with anything. Some groups create a sense of belonging by breaking social rules (taking drugs and so on). Other groups unite around values, like opposing fox hunting – they share a common value in being opposed to something.

In care work it is important that groups respect and value individual group members. Valuing individual people is one of the unwritten rules for working together. Group work in social care should also reflect the NVQ value base. (See box below.)

Demonstrating respect and value for others and demonstrating supportive behaviour are not just skills;

> **All individual conversations, group work and professional care work have to demonstrate these values:**
>
> - Support individuals through effective communication.
> - Acknowledge individuals' personal beliefs and identities.
> - Promote individual rights and choices.
> - Maintain confidentiality.
> - Promote anti-discriminatory practice (which includes identifying and challenging discrimination based on race, gender, culture, religion, age, physical appearance, physical ability and mental ability).

they also provide the value base for creating the sense of 'belonging' among individuals in a discussion group.

Getting care groups to work

Most care groups have a purpose or task to work on. Children get together to play games, adults may get together in recreational groups. Groups often need a focus – a game to play, an activity to join in or a topic to discuss.

1. If individuals are going to join in a supportive group meeting, then someone will need to introduce the activity – start the conversation. From time to time when the conversation wanders, someone will need to steer it back to the right topic.
2. Occasionally group members will need to clarify, or make sense of, what is being said.
3. Throughout the group meeting people will need to exchange ideas on the activity or topic being discussed.
4. Towards the end of a meeting, group members will need to agree on what has happened or what the group has decided. The group will come to some kind of conclusions.

As well as performing their tasks, groups have to be 'maintained'. Group maintenance consists of encouraging a sense of belonging and keeping the whole meeting enjoyable. The following are some behaviours to maintain group discussion in a caring setting:

a A bit of laughter can help to relieve tension and create a warm, friendly feeling that everyone can join in.

b Show interest in the people in the group – learn about the 'identity' of group members.

c Be 'warm' and show respect and value when listening to people who are different from yourself or who have had different life experiences. This behaviour makes it safe to be in the group.

d Express feelings honestly and with sincerity. This will help others to understand *your* identity. Help others to understand you as well as trying to understand others.

e Take responsibility for everyone having a chance to speak and contribute. Some people may need to be encouraged or invited to speak, some people may need organising, so that turn-taking works!

f If necessary get people to explain what they have said, and to talk through disagreements. Group members need to feel that their shared values will make it possible to arrive at solutions when people disagree.

A group leader must keep reflecting on what is happening in the group. Does the group need to come back to the task? Is this the right time for a funny story? Should I make it clear that I am listening and that I value what is being said by this person? Every other group member who really wants the group to work will also monitor how the group is getting on with its task.

To summarise: care groups need to provide a task, keep a sense of belonging going and make sure each individual is supported and valued.

Undertaking practical work

Demonstration of the skills of interpersonal interaction will also require the core skills of 'working with others' and the ability to evaluate personal work involved in the core skills of 'improving own learning and performance'. The background to these skills is described in the following sections.

Improving own learning and performance

Think it over

What is learning?

Many people think of learning in terms of memorising facts. Taking notes from lecturers or books is seen as the main way in which people learn. Yet most of the life skills that enable people to work with others, make relationships with others, bring up children,

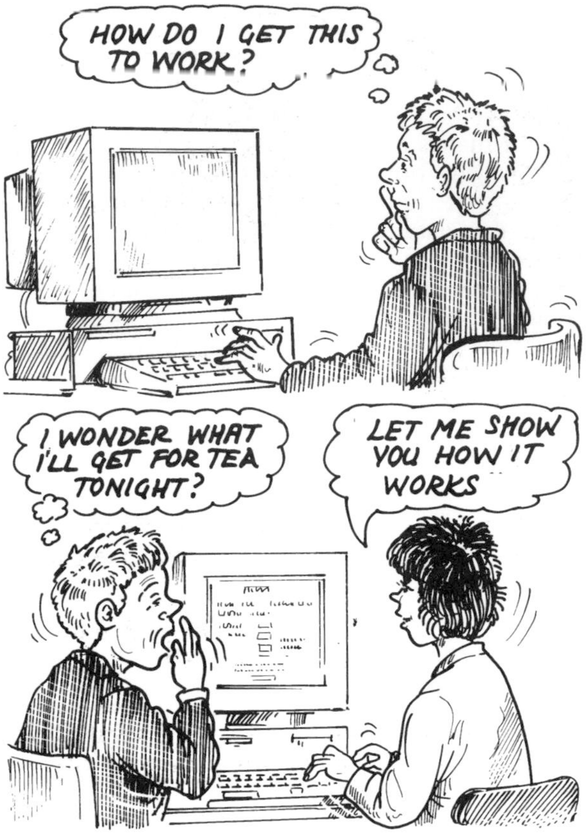

Figure 5.6 People learn from active involvement – not just 'being around'

shop, find their way round cities, drive cars and so on, are not learned by memorising facts, not are they learned from lectures or reading books.

Much of the skill and knowledge that enables people to lead happy successful lives is learned practically – through practical experience. Practical experience means being actively involved in trying to learn something through practice. People rarely learn from experiences which 'just happen to them.'

If you are actively motivated to learn from experience you may be able to do so. Just being around is not always good enough! Both learners in Figure 5.6 might have done a six-week computer course – they have had experience, but only the person who is actively involved will necessarily learn.

So the first principle of practical learning is wanting to learn or being motivated to learn.

Think it over

What motivates people to learn? One answer may include social approval – people want to be seen as clever, skilled or useful. Learning may be one way in which both children and adults achieve social status.

Skills and ability may lead to respect. Status and respect lead to high self-esteem, self-confidence and a positive self-concept or identity.

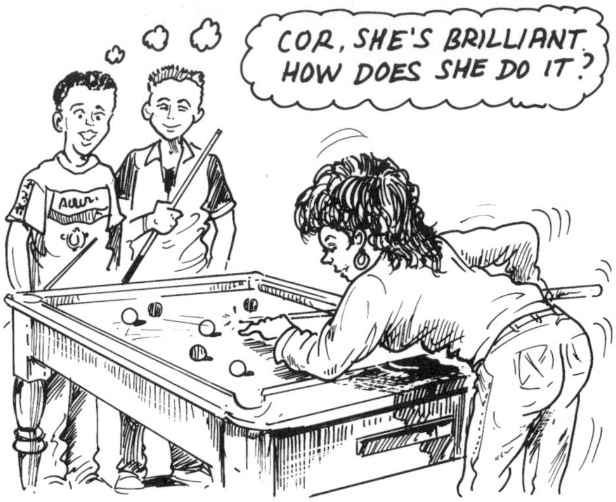

As well as self-esteem goals, many people learn knowledge and skill in order to establish a career and make money. Careers and money are important for a person's status in Western society.

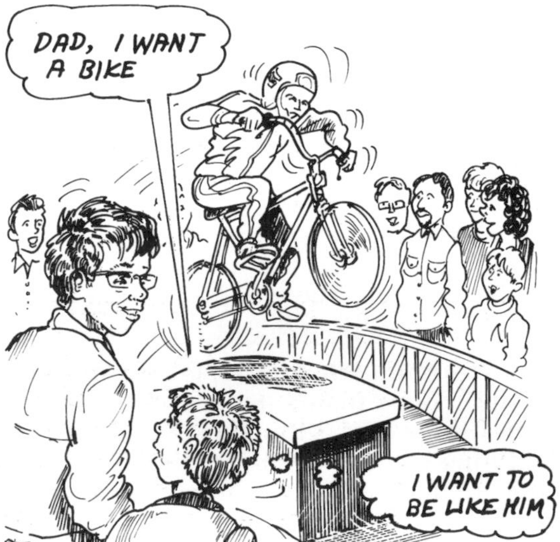

Figure 5.7 People may want to learn in order to copy others

The key issue is that the desire to learn something needs to have a social goal or at least a social context. People are often motivated to learn skills because of the social context they are in.

There are individuals who gain pleasure from memorising bus timetables or football results, but most people will only behave in this way if there is a social value for their effort – such as being able to use the information for a game of Trivial Pursuit.

Learning through practical experience often involves getting feedback from other people. It is possible to learn things from trial and error – but people often fail to learn in this way.

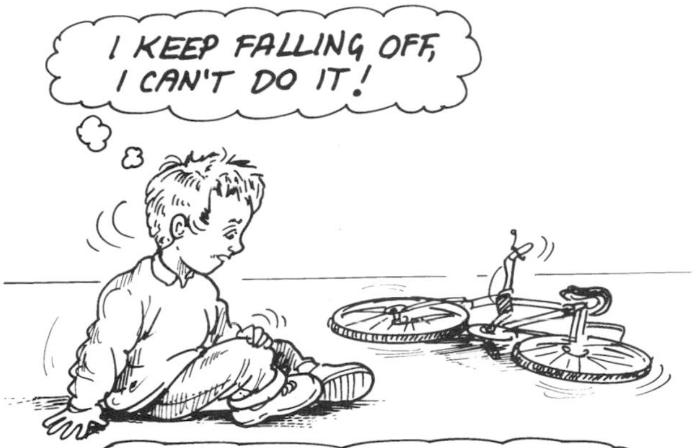
I KEEP FALLING OFF, I CAN'T DO IT!

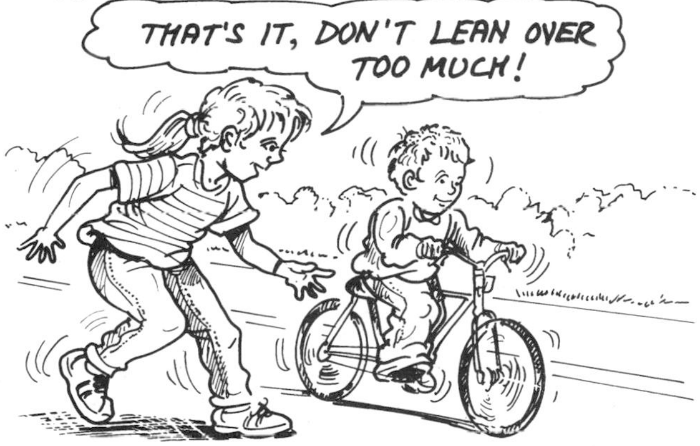
THAT'S IT, DON'T LEAN OVER TOO MUCH!

So a young child can experiment with riding a bicycle and may learn how to do it – it may come naturally, but many people need feedback from others. An older sister might show her brother how to ride his bike by watching what he does wrong and then guiding him to get it right. A driving instructor will guide a novice driver in the same way. Many people need feedback on their performance before they can learn.

The other thing that most people need for learning is imagination. It is not enough simply to watch what

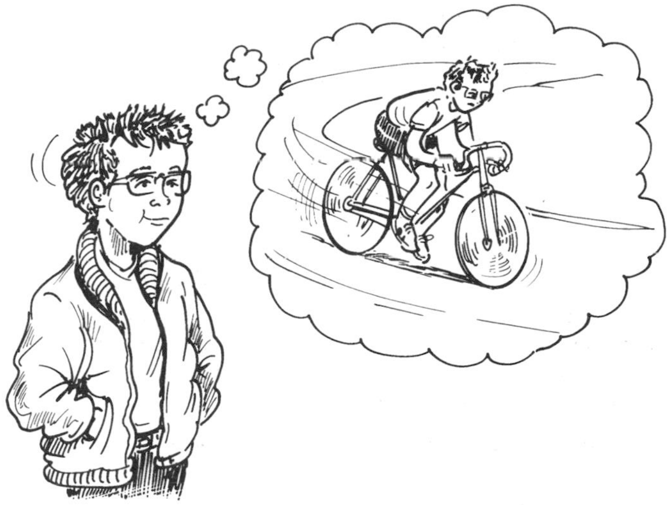

other people do; usually we have to be able to imagine ourselves doing something before we can copy or imitate others.

Imagination becomes a key skill in being able to learn from experience and improve own performance.

So **motivation, social context**, use of **feedback** and **imagination** may be the key principles that help with practical learning.

Practical learning

Nearly 50 years ago Kurt Lewin suggested that practical problem-solving and 'real life' learning might be developed using a four-stage sequence of **planning, acting, observing** and **reflecting**. Planning involved imagination, identifying what needs to be done, what the problem is. Acting means 'doing' – trying something out. Observing means

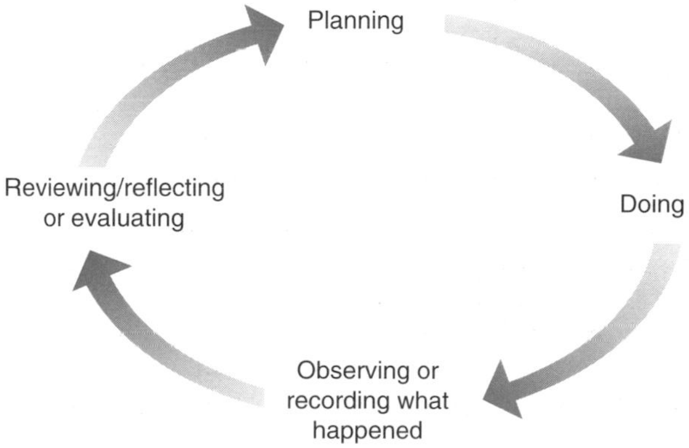

Figure 5.8 Four stages of practical learning

taking note of what happened, perhaps getting feedback from others. Reflecting means using imagination to think something through, perhaps evaluating the outcome of a piece of work. Practical learning could be seen as a four-stage process, as in Figure 5.8.

For example: Alesha wants to involve a small group of adults who have learning disabilities in a cookery class. Alesha's idea is not to train the group to make cakes, but to provide an enjoyable social experience which the group could join in with and maintain their social skills. Before she could start, Alesha would need to plan. She would need to plan what ingredients to buy, and her own preparation of the ingredients, before the session began. She would also need to organise the use of an oven for baking cakes, etc.

As well as this, Alesha would need to plan how to support the group. Who does or doesn't get on with others? Who might be able to help with tasks? How could she interest and motivate the individuals? How would she keep the atmosphere enjoyable? All this planning would depend on Alesha's ability to use her imagination, perhaps to picture the group and work out how to organise the session.

Alesha would need to ensure that the tasks were enjoyable and appropriate to each individual. Before moving on to do the activity, she could also get feedback on the plans from a senior member of staff – just to check that the activities were appropriate.

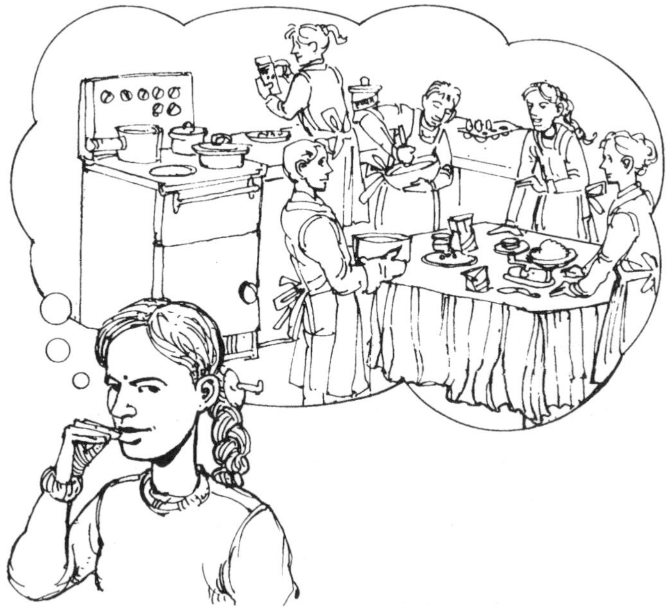

Doing the session would not necessarily be straightforward. Alesha would need to monitor how the session was going: did the verbal and non-verbal messages from her group suggest that they were enjoying themselves? Did the session promote interpersonal interaction and social skills? Alesha would need feedback, so she could ask the group members what they thought. Another member of staff might help her by joining in and providing feedback. Whilst leading the cookery session Alesha is also observing or taking in what is happening.

After the session is over Alesha would need to evaluate what had happened. Evaluation would depend on imagination. The evaluation would enable Alesha to make recommendations to improve her work in the future by thinking her work over before, during and after the cookery session. Alesha is thus able to develop her own self-awareness and sense of skill.

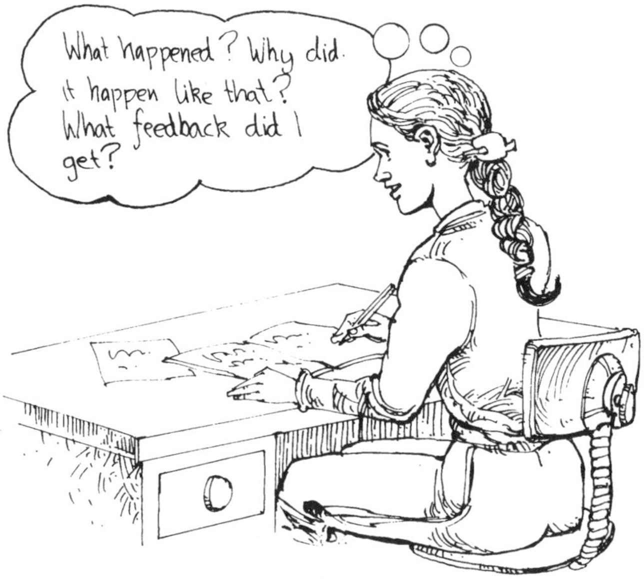
What happened? Why did it happen like that? What feedback did I get?

A process of planning, doing and reviewing may enable individuals to understand how their own skills influence others. The ability to imagine and understand how an individual's behaviour will influence outcomes lies at the heart of improving one's own learning skills and the skills involved in working with others.

Think it over

If practical learning focuses on 'doing' and using imagination to plan and review, what is the point of listening to lectures, classroom learning or reading about theory?

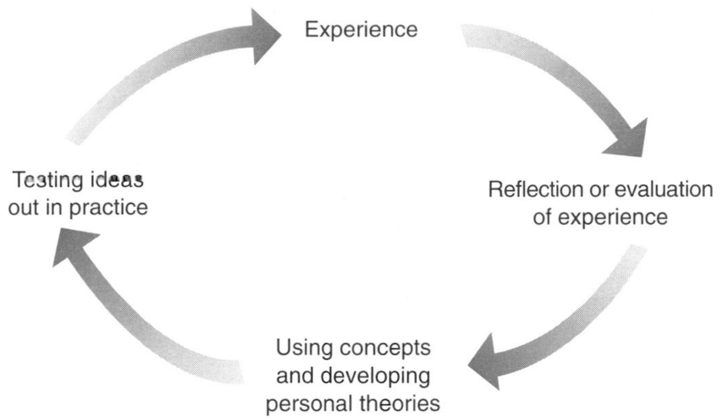
Experience
Reflection or evaluation of experience
Using concepts and developing personal theories
Testing ideas out in practice

Figure 5.9 Diagram based on the 'Kolb learning cycle'

The whole point of theory is that it can influence imagination: it influences what people can imagine and, therefore, how he or she can manage to plan or evaluate. A non-medical person might look at an X-ray film for a few minutes. The person will know that the film shows bones, but will not be able to interpret it – he or she would need theory to guide that evaluation, in order to be able to diagnose illness in the same way as a doctor.

David Kolb saw the importance of theory in his version of the practical learning process. An interpretation of Kolb's theory is that learning starts from practical experience. If practical experience is really to lead to learning then an individual will need to reflect on, or evaluate, that experience. Concepts and theories can guide individuals' understanding of their experience, and new experiences can help individuals to develop their own personal theories. Finally, learning really takes place when people try out their ideas in practice.

In real life, many practitioners do not find the idea of four-stage processes to be useful. Not everyone has 'an experience,' sits down to reflect on it, links it to their concepts and then goes on to try ideas out in practice. Real-life learning is much more 'messy.' People have to imagine or reflect at the same time as they are monitoring, experiencing and testing their ideas out. People use concepts all the time. Learning may not depend on a nice, neat four-stage process. Even so, it is important to think about the importance of concepts and theory in guiding personal understanding of experience. (See the section on Piaget in Chapter 10.)

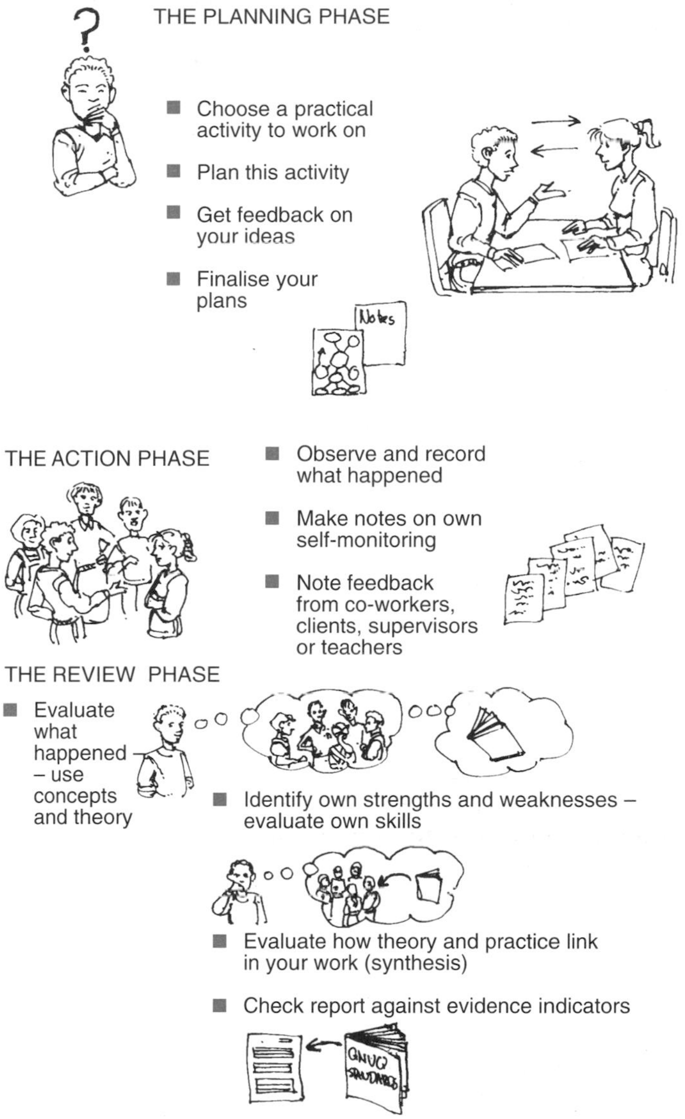
THE PLANNING PHASE
Choose a practical activity to work on
Plan this activity
Get feedback on your ideas
Finalise your plans
Notes
THE ACTION PHASE
Observe and record what happened
Make notes on own self-monitoring
Note feedback from co-workers, clients, supervisors or teachers
THE REVIEW PHASE
Evaluate what happened – use concepts and theory
Identify own strengths and weaknesses – evaluate own skills
Evaluate how theory and practice link in your work (synthesis)
Check report against evidence indicators

Figure 5.10 Three phases in the 'improve own learning' skills process

Demonstrating skills of interpersonal interaction

A demonstration of interpersonal skills may run through the stages involved in developing own learning and performance. There will need to be a planning phase, which focuses on the use of appropriate forms of interaction. There will need to be monitoring of interaction in order to optimise it.

An evaluation of the practical session will be

required. This evaluation may include an evaluation of a person's own strengths and weaknesses and conceptualisation of his or her own skills. This may be one way of evaluating 'the contribution of self' to the interaction.

Recommendations for the future may follow from this evaluation. Practical work of this nature may go some way to meeting the additional core skills standards for 'improve own learning and performance' and 'working with others'.

In order to plan, monitor and evaluate a practical demonstration of skill, it will be necessary to use theory. Concepts or interpersonal interaction will guide imagination during the planning stage. Concepts and theory are necessary to optimise interaction. Concepts will inform the interpretation of feedback. Concepts and theory will be necessary to guide evaluation (Figure 5.11).

Returning to the earlier example of Alesha: she plans to describe her practical group work to a group of colleagues. By describing her work with people with learning disability, Alesha hopes to meet the performance criteria for 'Demonstrate skills of interpersonal interaction'.

Before Alesha can demonstrate her skills she will need to plan the talk. This planning stage involves

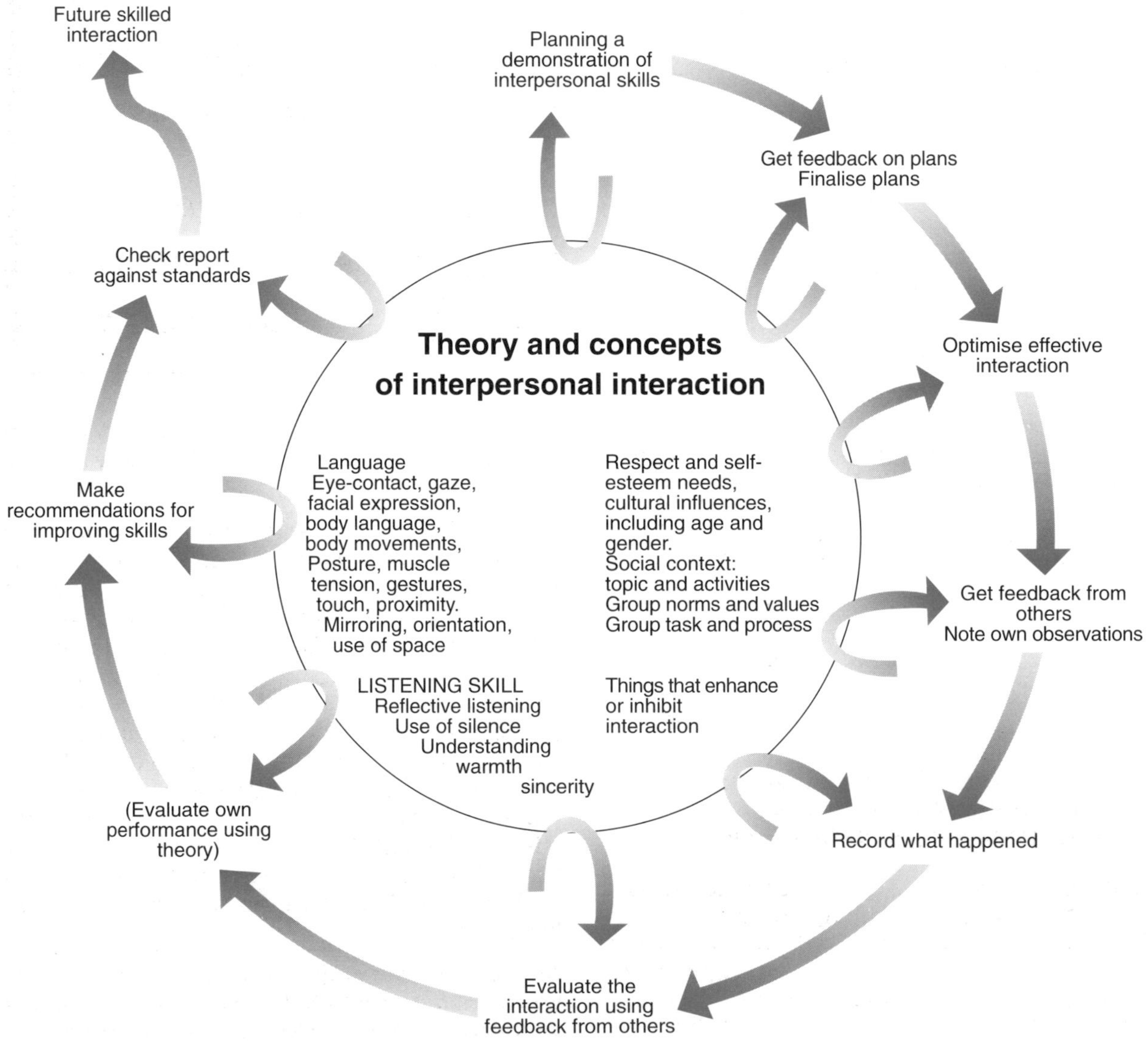

Figure 5.11 Theory will guide practical skills

imagining the group she will be talking to. If the talk is going to be interesting, she will need to support her colleagues by involving them. This might mean that Alesha needs to plan some questions to ask. Appropriate support might cover ideas to make the talk clear, interesting and easy to follow. Alesha will need to plan how much to say, and what objects, images or diagrams she might use to keep the talk interesting. Alesha will need to think about the environment – for example how the seats are arranged. Will everyone be able to see everyone else? Should the seats be arranged in a circle? Will the discussion be uninterrupted? Can she enhance the talk by inviting others to discuss issues which would involve them with their own practical projects?

As well as the content of the talk, Alesha needs to think about the process of group discussion and the self-esteem needs of individuals. This is hard to plan for, but Alesha can imagine jokes or diversions that some individuals may come up with. Because Alesha can imagine what to expect, she is able to feel confident that she will have the right replies.

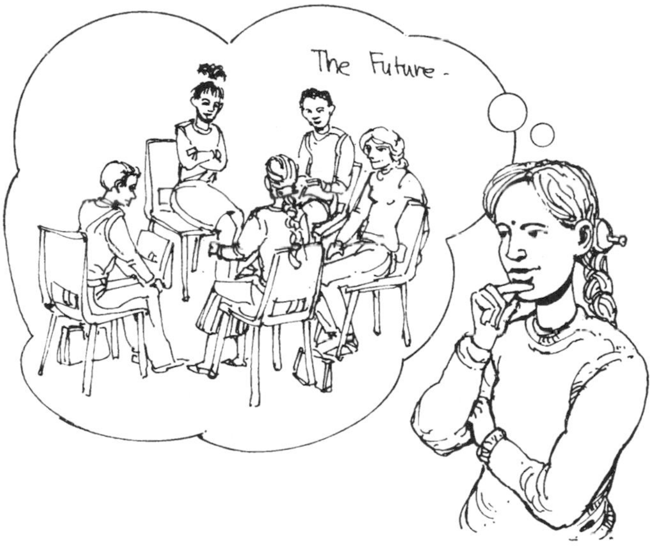

As well as planning the talk, Alesha also has to plan how to collect feedback. Alesha decides to design a short questionnaire to ask people their views.

Before finalising the details, Alesha checks her ideas with a tutor who will join the group and give feedback. She also thinks of an activity that everyone is likely to enjoy. If she can get everyone's agreement she could bring some of the cakes in and get her colleagues to try them – that would support the group's need for activity and create a fun atmosphere. So the planning list includes:

bring in cakes

bring in evaluation form (photocopied)

bring in recipe for cooking

write out three quotes that the cookery group said

have four questions written out on a note pad ready for the discussion

In order to use this activity for the GNVQ grading criteria, Alesha also makes detailed notes of the planning work.

When the discussion starts Alesha is a bit nervous. She is concerned about optimising the interaction. She starts her talk by explaining her work and the needs of the adults that she has worked with. As the talk gets under way Alesha realises that she knows the group well enough to switch on to signs of interest or boredom. At first the group are very polite, but as the time goes by several members begin to fidget. Because Alesha knows them, and is monitoring their behaviour, she decides to ask them a question about their own practical work with clients. The use of questions comes just at the right time. People start to answer and to have discussions with one another. The interest level in the group has been raised.

As Alesha's talk continues she is able to optimise the interaction by appropriate eye contact, using body language to convey interest, asking questions, leading the group and monitoring when people need a change from listening to her. Towards the end of the

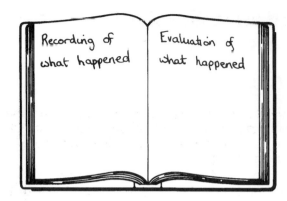

talk Alesha produces the cake tin and asks people to try the cakes. This creates a very happy and positive atmosphere in the group. Because the group is sharing food together there is a feeling of 'belonging' to the group, a feeling that the group is united and shares the same values. Everyone compliments Alesha on her talk and the way she has been able to optimise interaction, through careful planning and sensitive monitoring of the group atmosphere.

Although the practical work is over, and Alesha has written feedback on her questionnaire, she is concerned to make notes about the interaction as soon as possible. Alesha knows that if she doesn't make notes soon after the practical work, she will forget all the fine detail of the group's verbal and non-verbal behaviour.

Alesha uses a notebook to record her memory of the discussion. Later she will use these recordings, on the left-hand page, together with the tutor's comments and the questionnaire results, to write an evaluation on the right-hand page. Her final piece of writing is to evaluate her own skills and how a discussion like the one she led might be improved in future. Alesha decides that she could have 'broken the ice' with the group by asking a question right at the start. She remembers that she felt nervous at the beginning of the session. By getting the group to join in earlier she could have reduced this stress. Finally Alesha has to check that her report covers the evidence indicator requirements and the grading criteria requirements.

Evidence collection point

A record or practical demonstration is required covering one-to-one interaction, interaction with a small group, and interaction with a large group. At least one of the group interactions should be with people of a different status. At least one of the interactions should be through an activity.

Notes are also required which show how 'support needed' was established and how effective interaction was optimised.

Chapter 6

Analysing methods of interacting with clients in health and social care

This chapter provides an overview of the possible effects which care settings may have on clients and explores the possible effects of caring relationships. The theory of optimising interaction in care settings is developed with reference to the care sector value base and the theme of empowerment. Ideas which may contribute to improving interaction in the caring relationship are discussed. The possibility of researching interactions, as a basis for making recommendations for improvements, is briefly explored.

The effects of care settings

As we grow from dependent babies to children to independent adults we gradually take on more responsibility for our own lives. At eighteen years of age we are considered 'adult'. In some cultures adulthood is conferred earlier. Adult status offers choice and independence as well as responsibilities, and an eighteenth birthday is generally something most people regard as an important milestone.

Provided that we enjoy good health, and do not meet with any accidents, we expect to have our independence until old age. However, fate can sometimes intervene and make us reassess out lives – our independence– in a way we had not imagined. 'Independence' is defined as 'opportunities to think and act without reference to another person, including a willingness to take a degree of calculated risk'.

Think it over

Read the following descriptions of life events and decide how being affected by one of them might change your life.

- A motorbike accident leaves you paralysed from the waist downwards.
- A rare genetic condition causes you to lose your sight.
- An arthritic condition means you can hardly use your hands.

You could join with a partner to simulate one or more of these conditions. You could get someone to blindfold you, push you in a wheelchair or bind your fingers together with tape.

All the conditions described above would mean that you had to adapt your life and become more dependent on others. Being put in a wheelchair, blindfolded or unable to use your hands may not seem so dramatic while you are being escorted round, say, a college or school building for a while, but most people would not stay 'in character' when the time came to eat a meal or visit the toilet!

Care can be given in many settings. Sometimes this may be within the client's own home, a day centre, clinic, residential establishment or in hospital. As you probably discovered, if you tried the exercise above, receiving care may create an intrusion into privacy.

Think it over

If you were paralysed in a road accident, and being cared for at home, what would you have to allow your carer to do for you?

You might have to allow someone you had never met before into your home. He or she would probably have to go into your cupboards and drawers, use your kitchen and bathroom. Some people have cupboards and drawers the state of which they wouldn't want their best friends to see – but this is a stranger!

In addition to having someone in your home you would have to allow this person to help with intimate parts of your life such as going to the toilet, bathing and dressing.

Receiving care can involve a loss of independence or control over individual lifestyle. This may be a particular risk for adults and older people who receive day or residential care, or adults who are admitted to hospital.

All people who receive care are likely to be vulnerable in some way or another. Young children going into a nursery will be vulnerable because they do not know what to expect or how to behave. The nursery setting may have a strong influence on how they learn to understand themselves and how they value themselves.

People going into hospital may be vulnerable because they are afraid of pain; they may also fear a loss of dignity. They may fear a loss of function, i.e. they may not be able to walk or move as they used to be able to do. A person visiting a doctor can be vulnerable – a patient may be fearful of the diagnosis that the doctor will make. People can be afraid that they may have a serious illness or that their lifestyle will be disrupted. Some illnesses are so serious they create a fear of dying or a fear of the treatment and its side-effects.

Many adults hold negative views on disability and ageing. When these people perceive themselves as disabled or old, they are likely to stereotype and label themselves. The experiences that a person has in care may tend to confirm or challenge these stereotypes. Where people do stereotype themselves they are likely to experience a loss of self-esteem. They may feel they are no longer 'the person they used to be'. Being in a position of receiving care may lead to individuals feeling that their concept of themselves – or their personal identity – is now threatened. The way self-perception may affect people in care is explained in more detail in the section on humanistic theories of personality in Chapter 10.

When a person faces any new situation some degree of fear or stress is likely to be created. Just having to live in a new setting can create a sense of insecurity, uncertainty or disorientation (for example, in students leaving home to go to college). Not knowing what to expect can create feelings of inadequacy.

For many clients, receiving care involves a stressful life transition. The child starting at a nursery is changing from being a person who could depend on his or her mother to a person who has to cope without a mother; it is a transition in children's lives and in their sense of who they are. An adult going into hospital is changing his or her social role to that of a patient. It is now necessary to be 'treated' by other people. Older people who have regular home-carers may go through a transition which involves re-thinking their roles in life. They may begin to regard themselves as dependent. A person going into residential or day care may see himself or herself as facing the last stage of life. Some people will find this an exceptionally stressful transition. (The theory of life-stage transitions is explained in detail in Chapter 10.)

Because clients of health and social care services are likely to be vulnerable, and because some clients will feel afraid or inadequate and tend to become dependent or withdrawn, care settings have to create an atmosphere which supports the individual. Both the care setting and the interaction with staff need to be organised to value clients and to provide a sense of physical, emotional and social well-being.

Kornfield (1972), quoted in Broome and Llewelyn (1995), described the impact a residential care situation could have on someone. Being in care can cause:

- *Geographical confusion*
  Where should I go?
  Where can I go?
  What is 'patient' territory?
- *Subcultural confusion*
  Who is who?
  Who does what?
  When are things done?
  What is good or bad conduct on the part of the staff?
- *Role confusion*
  How should I relate and behave?
  What is appropriate communication with staff?

From his research in total institutions, Erving Goffman (1959), also quoted in Broome and Llewelyn, found that many people adapt to new situations by going through stages. At first people tend to watch what is happening and not join in. They are trying to make sense of their situation. Gradually they become part of the life around them and sometimes even work out ways of making it work to their own advantage! You may remember from being in new situations how helpful it is to have someone to show you around and tell you what is likely to happen.

The physical care setting

Think it over

Imagine you entered a home where you had to share your room with a stranger. There are only hard floor coverings (no carpet) and all the chairs and furniture are old and look the same. You are given food and told when and what you can eat. You have to eat with plastic cutlery and drink out of plastic mugs.

How reassured would you feel? How valued and important would you feel if you had to live in such a setting?

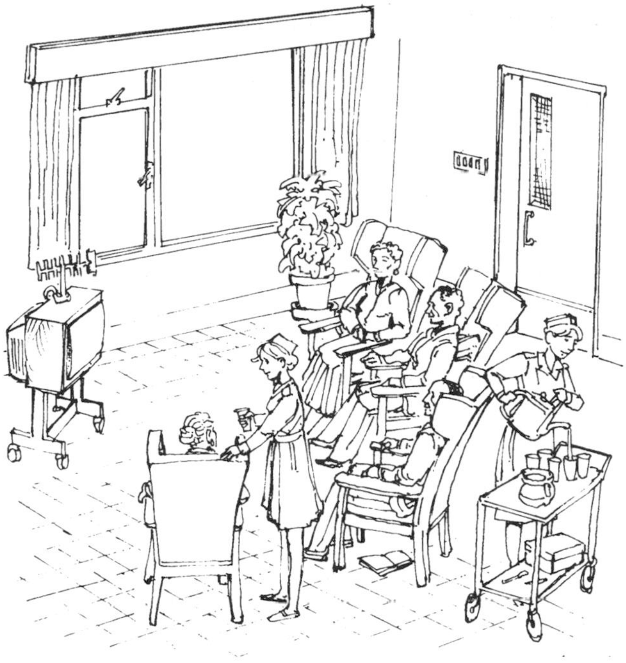

Poor, 'institutional' surroundings may send the message: you don't matter any more. You are expected to be incontinent – that's why the home doesn't bother with carpets. You are expected to drop your drink – that's why you get a plastic cup. You are expected to be disorientated – that's why we give you your food and drink without asking you about it! A setting like this is likely to threaten many clients' sense of well-being straight away.

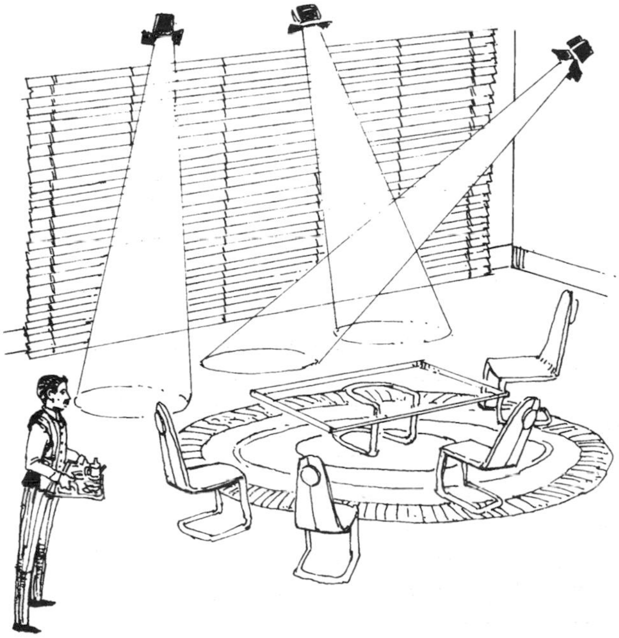

It is possible to go to the other extreme and design a super-modern setting for older people. Such a setting sends the message, 'This is a striking setting – you have to be special to be here.'

The problem is that such a setting may still not value older people. The environment might not fit their cultural expectations. Bright lights and dim areas may not suit some clients' visual needs. The chairs might look good but prove very uncomfortable. Fine bone china may have small handles and some clients may find this type of cup very difficult to use. The effect might be to intimidate rather than to relax clients.

So what principles guide the design of care settings? Naturally, buildings and facilities have to be fit for their purpose and function efficiently. There have to be adequate washing, toilet, catering facilities; adequate heating, insulation, lighting, etc. The design of rooms and facilities has to accommodate disabled access and prove functional for the staff and residents.

As well as the functional aspects of the physical care environment, the physical setting needs to convey a sense of value for clients. This sense of value might come across in the quality of furniture, carpets, curtains and general fixtures and fittings. Quality is a subjective concept, however, and different individuals will have different ideas about the details they would like to see. The key issue is that a residential or day care setting should convey the idea that the clients matter – they are valued and valuable people.

Because people always have individual needs, and individual perceptions of what creates quality will vary, it will usually be important that individuals can make choices. In a residential rest home for older people it may be important to have different types and styles of chair. Different people will prefer different types of seating. Residents may require types of furniture in their bedroom, different types of assistive equipment – to meet the varying physical, social and emotional needs of different individuals. The key principle here is *choice*. Can residents choose chairs, furniture (or choose to bring their own furniture and equipment), assistive equipment, eating utensils, etc. to suit their own needs? Or is it a setting where everyone is treated the same and staff insist that clients use what they are given?

The physical environment can involve more than just equipment and facilities, it can also include cultural messages. For instance, in the 1970s it was possible to walk into clean, bright, warm nurseries for children

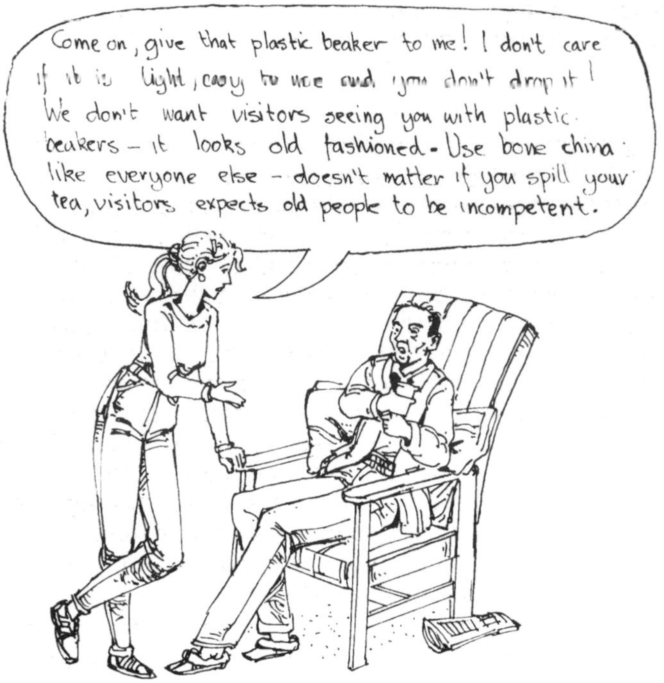
Come on, give that plastic beaker to me! I don't care
if it is light, easy to use and you don't drop it!
We don't want visitors seeing you with plastic
beakers – it looks old fashioned. Use bone china
like everyone else – doesn't matter if you spill your
tea, visitors expects old people to be incompetent.

Figure 6.1 The key issue about facilities is client choice – not just what things 'look like'

which were well equipped yet not welcoming to black children. Pictures, toys and artwork all showed white children and white parents. Although a young child would be unlikely to be able to explain cultural issues in language, this does not mean that the child would not be influenced and made to feel as if he or she did not belong. The images, artwork and pictures in a care setting need to reflect the cultural identity of the clients that the care setting serves.

The caring relationship

The relationship between care staff and clients will often be more important than the physical surroundings. In a care setting, however, physical surroundings can influence the assumptions that staff and relatives make.

Positive relationships will reduce the vulnerability and the potential fear and insecurity that some clients might feel. Relationships will do this by making the client feel safe. Clients will need to feel 'safe,' both physically and emotionally.

Professional staff can assist clients to feel physically safe by performing in a competent and skilled way. If staff are competent with administrative and physical care tasks it may contribute to the clients' sense of safety. Emotional security, however, is likely to depend on the client feeling valued, respected and in control of their own lives.

In order to achieve emotional security, staff will need to perform within the value base requirements for social care. This will mean that staff will need to understand the stereotypes and assumptions which surround various groups of people. If staff can recognise and avoid false assumptions about gender, race, disability, age, sexuality and so on, then this will contribute to working in an anti-discriminatory way. If staff can understand and convey value for others' beliefs and identity, then this will also contribute to anti-discriminatory practice. To understand others, and convey a sense of value, staff will need skilled listening and interpersonal skills. If clients are to feel safe, then confidentiality must be maintained. If clients are to feel in control, then they must be able to make choices and their dignity must be respected.

The care value base provides a set of principles which guide the delivery of interpersonal care. If staff work within the principles of the value base, clients should feel some degree of confidence in the staff. Clients

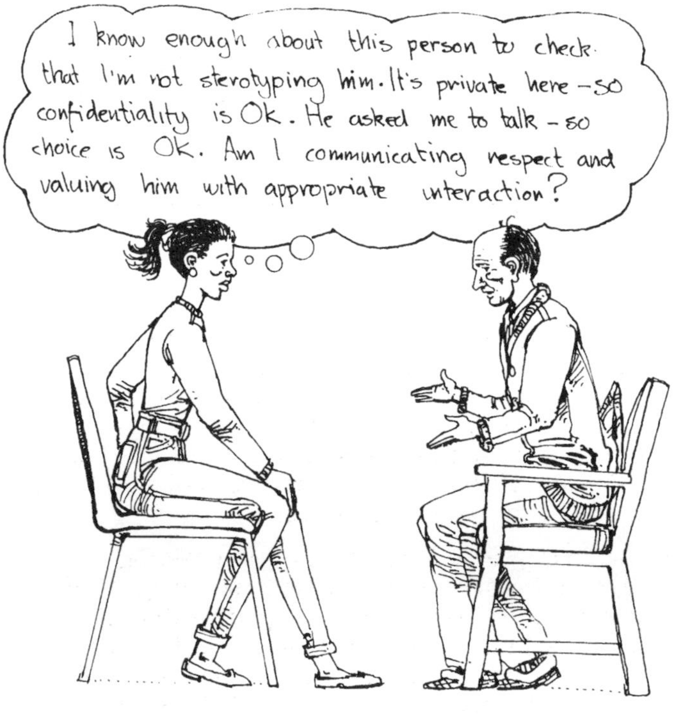
I know enough about this person to check that I'm not stereotyping him. It's private here – so confidentiality is OK. He asked me to talk – so choice is OK. Am I communicating respect and valuing him with appropriate interaction?

Figure 6.2 Working within the value base needs reflective thinking and time!

may still feel anxious about the future, fearful of pain or angry with relatives and so on. The staff may be able to create a degree of emotional security with the quality of their relationship skills.

Reducing clients' vulnerability may depend on competent caring skills and working within the principles set out in the care value base.

To be able to work within the value base, staff will need training, supervision and time. Without adequate time to spend with clients, and especially in care settings that are short staffed, the positive effects of the caring relationship may be reduced.

Working within the value base may also be assisted if the quality of a client's care is monitored as part of the client's 'micro' care plan. (See Chapter 16.) A care plan which accurately meets a client's physical, social or emotional needs is likely to result in an increase in health or social well-being. The nursery which provides a welcoming environment for the young child is likely to enable that child to develop his or her intellectual and social skills. The child will become more confident in interaction with other children and adults; the child may also become more confident in his or her own learning skills. A lonely housebound person who receives home care may feel safer when she has someone she can trust to shop for her and someone she can confide in.

As people feel safer or more confident, so their levels of anxiety or stress should be reduced. A reduction in stress or anxiety should result in improved health and well-being.

Problems within the care setting: abuse

Not all care is delivered within the principles of the value base, however; and not all care is monitored in terms of a client's care plan or 'micro' care plan. Some care settings may experience a shortage of resources resulting in a lack of staff time. The social, emotional, cultural and identity needs of clients can be overlooked under this pressure.

People being cared for in a clinic, day centre, residential home or hospital are likely to spend their time surrounded by many more people than they may be used to. When they first arrive they will be unfamiliar with the routine of the place and uncertain of what to do or expect. This lack of control over their environment can cause people to feel inadequate, as if their adult status has been taken away. Some people may react with uncertainty or fear whilst other adults may become dependent.

Think it over

Nicola, a new mother in a maternity hospital, was 'told off' in front of others in the ward for taking a bath without asking. As an adult she had been used to taking a bath when she felt she would like one and, although there may have been good safety reasons for asking or informing staff of her intention, she felt humiliated by the way in which she was reprimanded. Many of the events of childbirth had been outside her control, and being confronted in this way contributed to her feelings of lack of control and inadequacy. Imagine how much more difficult this situation would have been for someone functioning in a second language, or for someone with a hearing impairment, or for a person from a culture which has very strict personal privacy rules.

In extreme cases the term 'abuse' can be applied to care that seriously ignores the needs of clients. Every year there are instances of care facilities where clients have experienced neglect, or physical or emotional abuse. Clients in the community are occasionally at risk of financial or sexual abuse. Abuse can include the following issues:

- **physical abuse:** hitting, pulling, pushing or causing physical pain to another person
- **emotional abuse:** sometimes called psychological abuse, this might involve humiliation and intimidation or undermining another person's identity
- **financial abuse:** exploiting or using another person's financial resources
- **sexual abuse:** exploiting another person for sexual gratification (sexual pleasure)
- **neglect:** sometimes called passive abuse, neglect involves ignoring a person's needs to the point where health or emotional well-being are affected.

Abuse does not always happen because of a straightforward desires to exploit or dominate other people. Li McDerment (1988) raises the issue of abuse that 'just happens' in care settings. This abuse is not caused because of hatred or anger, or because of a desire to 'use' people. This abuse comes about because of the way some 'care' settings work. The *system* causes abuse, not the individual staff. McDerment identifies three factors which may lead to abuse in care settings. These are: (1) dependent clients; (2) stressed staff; and (3) power belonging to the staff alone.

Dependency is where children, people with learning disability or elders rely on staff for general support in daily living. Elders, in particular, may be vulnerable to threatened identities.

Stress occurs when staff are short of time; when they feel that they can't deliver care effectively because of the demands made on them.

Power involves the staff making all the decisions, feeling that they have to control the routine of the home or day centre; staff feeling that they know best. Power being centred on the staff means that they will not bother to ask clients for their thoughts or wishes.

McDerment believes that when these three things occur together then abuse is likely to result. The staff of a home may feel responsible for the residents, yet they have no time to listen to them. They have no time to show respect and value for residents' past lives and beliefs. There is no time to offer choice, and no time to find out about the residents' social or 'personal' identity so that discrimination can be prevented. A lack of time could even lead to breaches of confidentiality if records and notes are not maintained and requests are not respected.

McDerment calls this situation 'the abuse triangle' (see Figure 6.3, below).

All of the care values can be violated and not used. Residents' basic rights and needs may not be met. As staff become more stressed they may seek more power to control the residents. As residents become more controlled, so they become more dependent. As residents become more dependent, their sense of self-esteem and self-concept becomes threatened. Residents will, in extreme cases, be driven into withdrawal or into isolating themselves from others. Personal identity and dignity may be denied if the residents end up conforming to a strict routine aimed at reducing the stress for staff.

Both physical and emotional abuse are likely to result from the kind of situation described above. A lack of care values will result in unintentional stress and deprivation for residents. It may become important always to hurry residents. Physical abuse can result if staff have to struggle with 'difficult' people. When staff are exhausted, neglect becomes an ever-more tempting possibility; yet the staff may not intend any of this abuse. Indeed, accusing the staff of abuse may threaten their sense of self-esteem and self-concept. The system creates the abuse, not the personalities of the people involved .

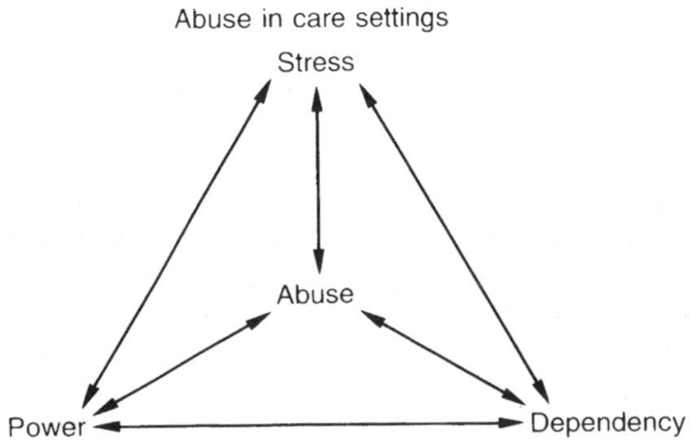

Figure 6.3 The abuse triangle (adapted from Li McDerment, 1988)

Effects of abuse

The effects of abuse on clients may include fear, initial aggressive behaviour, withdrawal, depression, loss of self-confidence, loss of self-esteem, loss of control and doubt about their own abilities (loss of a sense of self-efficacy). Abuse may also cause loss of identity, attention seeking, imitation of abusive behaviour, increased dependency, stress and possibly mental illness, or even death from a combination of helplessness, frailty and despair.

Emotional abuse is often likely to result where caring values (as defined in the NVQ standards) are not used in health and social care practice. Part of the function of the value base is to reduce the vulnerability experienced by clients.

Answers to the abuse triangle should centre on: (1) providing care which is *empowering* – this is where residents are encouraged to keep their own routines and make their own choices; (2) working within a care value base which promotes anti-discrimination and respect for individual identity; (3) reducing pressures and stresses on staff.

Optimising interaction with clients

Key principles which might guide interaction are defined within the NVQ value base. The key values are:

1 To promote anti-discriminatory practice.
2 To maintain confidentiality.
3 To promote individual rights and choice: many people would include the right to independence and dignity as of central importance.
4 To acknowledge individuals' personal beliefs and

identity; and to show respect for others' individuality or identity.

5 To support clients through effective communication.

These principles might help to optimise interaction in the following ways.

Freedom from discrimination

Discrimination on the basis of race or gender is against the law. Nevertheless. people are sometimes discriminated against on these or other grounds within our society. (No doubt many of you are aware of the 'does he take sugar?' syndrome.) It is essential that all care-workers look at their own attitudes and behaviour in order to ensure that no individual or group of people are treated less well than others.

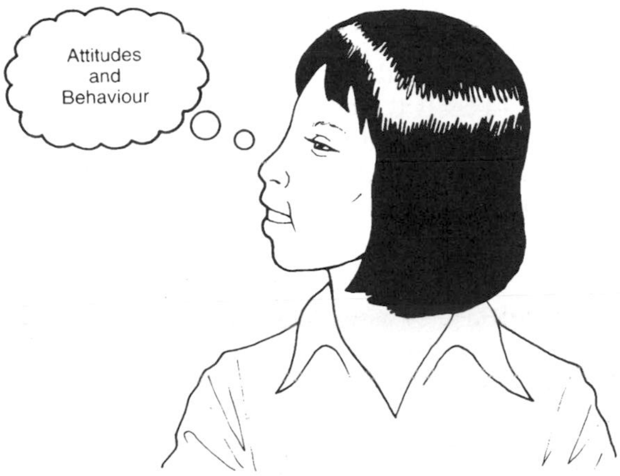

Care-workers should be aware of what is happening if they make assumptions about a person based on preconceived stereotypes; for example, making an assumption about a person because of his or her appearance.

Discrimination may also occur within systems. For example: residential, day care and meals-on-wheels services may not cater for preferred or special diets; or buildings may be inaccessible to people with a physical disability, thus preventing the individual from using the services offered within. Provision of service delivery should take account of the needs of potential clients in all aspects of planning. Failure to do so is a form of discrimination against those who are excluded.

Each agency and workplace should have its own local policy on how to deal with acts of discrimination. The policy should assist care-workers to promote anti-discriminatory practice. Challenging discrimination can sometimes be very difficult; however, if left unchallenged, discrimination is likely to continue. A knowledge of the local policies may indicate what actions may be appropriate.

Confidentiality

Health and caring agencies need to keep detailed information about clients in respect of their needs and to ensure their care and well-being. However, only certain people should have access to this information and workers should only have access on a 'need to know' basis. Systems through which information about a client is handled should allow appropriate access, but must also maintain confidentiality.

Care-workers will be given information about a client which will help the worker to provide the care that is required; however, this information should not be passed on to others unless it is necessary to do so in order to maintain that care. A client may choose to give the care-worker additional information, but in these cases it is also important that the worker keeps this confidential. Breaches in confidentiality could result in a care-worker being disciplined.

Situations may arise when the care-worker feels the need to pass on confidential information given to by the client (for example, if a client is depressed and has indicated that he or she is contemplating suicide). When a client starts to tell a care-worker something that might need to be passed on, it is important that the worker stop the client and says that he or she may need to pass the information on, if more is said. However, if the client does not want comments to go further, then his or her wishes should be respected wherever possible. The care-worker may need to discuss the particular situation with a line manager when in doubt as to what action, if any, should be taken.

Choice

In many cases the needs of clients will dictate the type of care that they receive, and so the amount of choice that the individual has may be limited. However, if clients are made aware of this, and are informed about the alternatives that are available, they will be able to contribute to the decision-making process.

Working practices should promote as much client choice as possible. For example, in a residential unit, there should be a certain amount of flexibility in mealtimes; there should be a choice of menu and residents should be able to retire to bed at a time that is suitable to them. Residents should also be encouraged to personalise their rooms and be offered some choice in the arrangement of the environment.

Some clients may have difficulty in expressing their wishes, either because of a disability or because their past experience of care has discouraged them from doing so. Care-workers can help by assisting people to speak for themselves: this is called *self-advocacy*. Helping people to understand their rights, and helping them to develop skills to express their wishes, are the principles on which self-advocacy is based.

Programmes aiming to promote self-advocacy may be built into a care plan. Increasing a person's ability to express their feelings and wishes will result in increasing his or her participation in decision-making.

In some instances, the client may not be able to develop skills in self-advocacy, for example where the client has advanced dementia. It will then be necessary for another person to take on the role of advocate, such as the carer, care-worker or some other independent person. Advocacy for others requires sensitivity and care, in order to ensure that the feelings and wishes of the client are being accurately relayed.

Dignity

People must be treated with a great deal of respect in order for their dignity to be maintained, especially in situations where the person's needs include high levels of personal care. It is easy to destroy people's dignity if they consider that their feelings are not being taken into account when personal care tasks are being carried out. Systems and care-workers must operate in a way that helps to preserve the dignity of clients. For example, when a client is being assisted to a bath he or she should be helped to undress in the bathroom, not undressed in another room and then transferred to the bathroom. Only one care-worker should be in the bathroom. If need be, appropriate equipment, such as a hoist, should be used. People can feel at their most vulnerable when they are undressed and so they should always be given as much privacy as possible.

Other ways in which a person may feel that dignity has been disregarded may include: a care-worker conveying feelings of disapproval when carrying out unpleasant tasks, such as dealing with the effects of incontinence; impatience or lack of interest when a client has difficulty in expressing himself or herself and carrying on a conversation with a third party as if the client were not there.

Clients should feel comfortable with the care that they receive and must never be made to feel that they are causing problems because of their needs.

Independence

Promoting independence can be achieved by involving clients in their own care as much as possible; i.e. doing things *with* clients where possible, not *for* them. Clients and their carers should be involved in the decision-making processes regarding the care to be provided. People need to be *empowered* to take control of their lives – and encouraged to do so.

It is important to find out what people can do for themselves. Even if it could be quicker for the carer or worker to do it for them, clients should be encouraged to do things for themselves. Clients should be allowed time to find out how to help

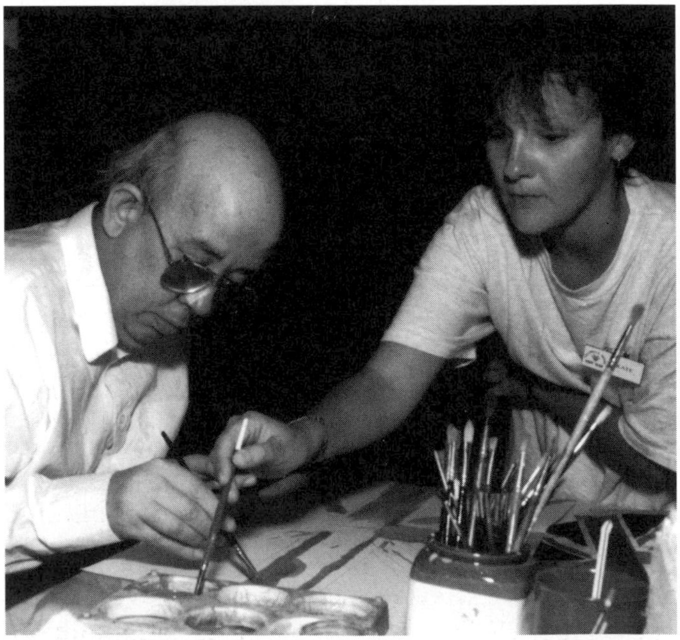

Figure 6.4 By being encouraged to do things for themselves, clients are empowered to take control of their lives
(*Photo courtesy of Winged Fellowship Trust*)

with their own care. It may be that the only contribution they can make is in discussing the issue of how their care is to be carried out, but this may also increase their feelings of independence and self-esteem.

Clients can be further empowered by ensuring that they have the necessary equipment to help them. They should be helped to make the best use of the equipment that is available to them so that their independence is improved (Figure 6.4).

Acknowledging beliefs and supporting clients

Acknowledging a client's personal beliefs and identity entails first understanding what clients' self-concept of their beliefs and identity involve.

Information about basic beliefs, like a person's broad category of religion, can sometimes be found in a client's records. This basic information is usually not enough to enable a carer to understand a client's beliefs about personal issues. For instance, it would be quite wrong to assume that all Christians fast during Lent or go to church on Sundays. It would be quite wrong to assume that all Jewish people celebrate every Jewish festival or that individual Muslims always pray at specific times during the day. Guessing at a person's beliefs from an outlined knowledge of his or her social group classification can be offensive. People develop their own personal beliefs. Your individual right to personal beliefs can be denied when someone else tells you what you are supposed to believe in, or think.

Being able to understand a client's personal beliefs usually involves learning about the client using skilled or optimal communication. Carers use listening skills and adapt their verbal and non-verbal behaviour to help them learn about their beliefs and identity of their clients. When adult clients can communicate in the same language as their carers it is possible to develop communication skills which promote a supportive relationship.
A supportive relationship is where the carer tries to understand the way a client thinks. If a carer can understand or empathise with clients, then he or she is likely to be able to provide emotional support and convey respect and value to clients.

Developing supportive skills may be one method for optimising conversational skills in the caring relationship. Like all worthwhile skills, it is likely to take time to learn to be supportive. Practice-based supervision and self-monitoring skills will be important to guide the development of personal conversation skills.

Supportive relationship skills

Carl Rogers (1902–1987) identified three necessary conditions for creating a *safe* conversational atmosphere which *valued* a client. Originally these were seen as a basis for counselling relationships, but they have since become adopted as a basis for any befriending or supportive relationship. The three conditions for a caring supportive conversation are that the carer must show (or convey) a sense of warmth, understanding and sincerity to the client. The *conditions* for valuing others sometimes have other names:

- warmth (sometimes called acceptance)
- understanding (originally called empathy)
- sincerity (originally called gentleness).

Conveying warmth

Conveying warmth means being seen by the client as a warm, accepting person. In order to influence another person to view you this way you will need to demonstrate that you do not stereotype and label others. You will need to demonstrate that you do not judge other people as good or bad, right or wrong. This is sometimes referred to as a *non-judgmental attitude*. Warmth means not even comparing people to see who is best!

Conveying warmth means being willing to listen to others. It means being able to prove that you are listening to a client because you can remember what he or she has said to you. Warmth involves using reflective listening. That is, you give your attention

Client 'I hate it here, you don't know what it's like, there's no one to talk to, they're all too busy, no one cares about me.'
Carer 'I suppose they are busy and you feel that no one cares.'
Client 'That's right, they don't – you aren't so bad, but you won't be here tomorrow.'
Carer 'Well that's right, I can't come in tomorrow but we could talk for a while now if you would like that.'

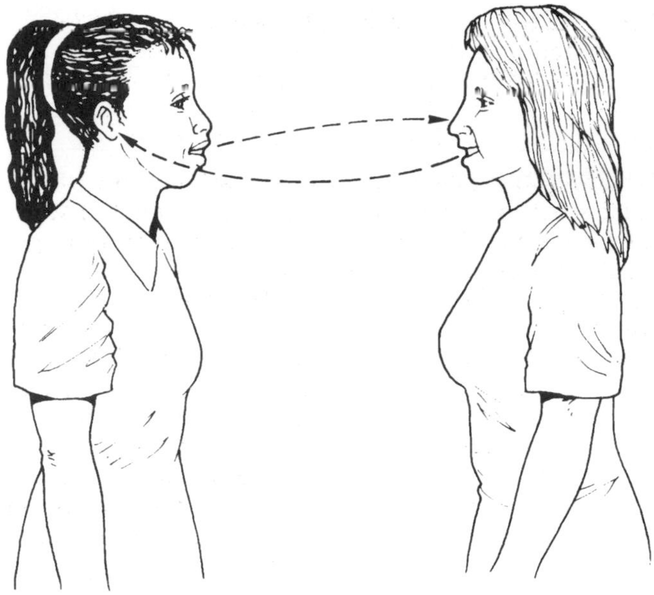

Figure 6.5 Warmth involves using reflective listening

to clients when they talk, and remember what they say. You can then *reflect* the words back again.

The carer is able to show the client that he or she is listening by repeating some of the things that the client has said. The repetition is not 'parrot fashion' – the carer has used his or her own way of speaking. The carer has also avoided being judgmental. When the client said that no one cared, the carer did not argue. The carer might have felt like saying, 'How can you say that – don't you know how hard we work for you? You want to think yourself lucky, there's plenty of people who would be pleased to be here, and other people don't complain'. This advice to think yourself lucky and the comparison with other people is judgmental, it does not value the client, it is not warm. If the carer had said these things it would have blocked the conversation. *Warmth* makes it safe for clients to express their feelings. Warmth means that the carer could disagree with what a client has said, but the client should feel safe that he or she will not he discriminated against or put down.

As a care-worker you will come across a wide range of clients, many of whom will have ways of thinking and life experiences completely different from your own. You will usually choose as friends people who have views similar to your own, but you will not be able to choose your clients.

Think it over

Even within a group of friends or a family, there are likely to be areas of disagreement. Write down three areas in which you disagree with your friends or your family.

You have probably found that you have differences of opinion in areas such as:

- choice of clothing and hairstyles
- choice of foods – vegetarian, non-vegetarian, etc.
- choice of leisure activities
- responsibility for household chores.

So, even our family or people we choose as friends do not always think or feel as we do ourselves.

In developing the skill of showing warmth, it is important not to judge, not to compare yourself with others. Carers accept that clients have the right to be the way they are, and to make their own choices. While you may disapprove of a client's behaviour, you must show that you do not dislike him or her as an individual person. This is particularly important when working with clients with difficult behaviour. It is essential that clients know it is the behaviour which is disliked, not them as individuals.

Conveying understanding

Understanding means learning about the individual identity and beliefs that a client has. Carl Rogers saw the idea of understanding or empathy as 'the ability to experience another person's world as if it was your own world'; the key part being the 'as if'. We always keep an idea of our own world and we know that the clients have different experiences from our own. It is

Client	'So anyway, I said to the doctor, look these pills are only making me worse, I don't want them.'
Carer	'So you told him to stop them.'
Client	'That's right, I don't believe in pills – you end up rattling round with all that lot inside you – if you're meant to get better you will, that's what I say.'
Carer	'Have you always believed that pills don't help?'
Client	'Yes, well ever since I was young, I put my faith in God.'

important to try to really understand clients' thoughts and feelings.

Reflective listening provides a useful tool to help carers gradually to learn about their clients. By keeping a conversation going, the carer may help clients to feel that they are understood; the carer is warm and non-judgemental, so it becomes safe to tell the carer something about their lives. If the carer checks that he or she understands the client, the client may feel valued. As the client gets value from the conversation so they may talk more. The more the client talks, the more the carer has a chance to learn about his or her views.

By listening and conveying warmth the carer is being given the privilege of learning about the client's religious views and perhaps even needs. Understanding can grow from a conversation which conveys value for the client.

If you can get to understand your clients a sense of trust may develop. If clients are understood and not judged they may consider it safe to share thoughts and worries with their carers.

Conveying sincerity

Being *sincere* means being open about what you say and the way that you speak. It means not acting, not using set phrases or professional styles which are not really you. In some ways, being sincere means being yourself – being honest and real! Being real has to involve being non-judgemental, however, and trying to understand people rather than trying to give people advice. If being honest should involve giving other people your advice – don't do it! However, when you listen and learn about other people, do use your own normal language. Think about ways you might describe yourself and occasionally share details of your own life with clients. Sometimes it is necessary to share your thoughts to keep a conversation going.

Sharing information from your own life might help to convey sincerity or genuineness in some situations.

Client	'But what's the point in talking to you? I mean you don't really care, it's just your job.'
Carer	'It is my job, but I do care about you, and I would be pleased to talk with you. I chose this work because I care and because I can make the time to listen if you want to talk about it.'

Understanding, warmth and sincerity have to be combined in order to provide a safe, supportive setting. Ideally, carers might combine these approaches with the broader caring value base to develop a *personal style* of working with clients.

Learning to create a supportive relationship with clients will involve practice and a great deal of self-monitoring and reflection. It will be necessary to get feedback from colleagues, supervisors and most importantly clients, if you practise conveying warmth, understanding and sincerity. Carers may be able to tell if their communication is effective because the client may reflect their behaviour. That is, if carers are warm and understanding and the client comes to trust them, then carers may find that the client is warm and friendly back towards them. When carers are honest and sincere, their clients may be honest and sincere with them. The quality of a supportive relationship can become a two-way process. Working with clients may become more enjoyable when carers become skilled at warmth, understanding and sincerity.

Although supportive relationship skills cannot be used in every care relationship, the basic idea of trying to build an understanding of the client's beliefs and identity is still central to care work. When carers work with people with dementia, for example, they may not be able to befriend or build a supportive relationship with clients. But it will still be possible to learn some details of a client's past and to observe how the client responds to different care situations. People with dementia will still have their own personal history, their own customs, culture and beliefs. Carers can still use imagination to try to understand client need, and they can still change their own behaviour in response to things that the client does. Carers can try to communicate an acknowledgement of others' beliefs and identity to all clients.

The care value base

An outline checklist of the value base as applied in care settings might include the following headings.

Freedom from discrimination, confidentiality and respect for identity

A 'good' care setting will seek to:

1 ensure that clients are not subject to abuse including degrading treatment, or compelled to undertake domestic or other tasks against their will.

2 encourage freedom of conscience, thought and religion, and facilitate participation in political process and in chosen activities, religious or otherwise
3 encourage freedom of expression – meaning the right to complain, to hold opinions, and to receive and impart information and ideas, particularly regarding personal care and treatment
4 maintain the right to liberty, including from participation in care and treatment
5 respect private and family life, confidentiality of personal affairs and personal space
6 permit and facilitate close personal relationships, sexual or otherwise and including marriage, between residents and between residents and other acquaintances
7 permit and facilitate opportunities for social and other gatherings for whatever purpose, inside and outside the home, and place no restrictions on participation
8 supply information to residents and apply appropriate types and levels of support to encourage and enable them to exercise their rights
9 safeguard individual rights without discriminating on any grounds, including gender, age, race, colour, language, religion or other status, or political or other opinion
10 ensure that where it is deemed necessary to interfere with or restrict an individual's rights, for the protection of that person or the rights and freedoms of others, or for any reason, such actions are recorded, explained to the individual and other interested parties, and reviewed regularly according to an agreed procedure
11 have mechanisms for monitoring the care setting's performance in safeguarding residents' rights.

Choice

A 'good' care setting will seek to:

1 recognise the inherent value to clients' well-being of their being able to exercise some choice about the content of their daily lives
2 have a clear picture of clients' physical and mental capacities and knowledge of the extent to which each person wishes – and is able – to make choices
3 ensure that clients have adequate information on which to base decisions
4 promote a care regime which facilitates and encourages clients to exercise choice regarding personal affairs, care and lifestyle in the context of an agreed notion of acceptable risk and the constraints of communal life
5 create a physical environment in which clients can choose to use a variety of spaces and facilities, and one which is safe from hazards and has aids for people with physical disabilities; so that inaccessibility or fear of accidents should not limit scope for exercising choice
6 monitor each client's condition and behaviour so as to ensure that a reasonable balance is achieved between self-determination, degree of risk involved and impact on other people
7 create safeguards to ensure that any limitations placed on residents' right to exercise choice are explained, justified and reviewed regularly.

Independence

A 'good' care setting will seek to:

1 have some knowledge of clients' previous lifestyles and consult with them and their relatives/advisers so as to understand their expectations and wishes regarding independence
2 help and encourage clients to think and act independently as far as this is compatible with their own abilities, their impact on other people, the constraints of communal life and the risks involved
3 encourage and enable clients to participate in making decisions about home-life in general, insofar as they wish and are able to do so
4 provide a physical environment which enables clients to do as much as possible for themselves without having to rely on staff assistance or having things done for them
5 monitor each client's condition and behaviour so as to ensure that a reasonable balance is achieved between independence and risk taking
6 create safeguards to ensure that any limitations placed on clients' scope to act independently are explained, justified and reviewed regularly.

Privacy and dignity

This is defined as, 'the right of individuals to be left alone or undisturbed and free from intrusion or public attention into their affairs'. A 'good' care setting should:

1 have some knowledge of clients' previous lifestyles so as to understand their expectations regarding personal privacy
2 identify clients' preferences regarding the extent to which they wish to associate with other clients and in what circumstances
3 ensure that clients can meet people, have conversations, make or receive telephone calls, correspond and receive visitors, without being overlooked or overheard, and without having to account to anyone for their actions
4 ensure that clients can bathe, wash and use the toilet without being overlooked or overheard, and that they are protected from intrusion whether accidental, deliberate or routine
5 ensure that where staff assistance is required to enable clients to dress, bathe, wash or use the toilet this is kept to the minimum commensurate with the residents' abilities and is performed with due regard to the need to safeguard the privacy of the individual
6 make suitable arrangements for clients to discuss personal matters with staff and visitors in private
7 ensure that staff deal discreetly with the affairs of clients and safeguard the confidentiality of information held about them
8 ensure that essential housekeeping and administrative procedures intrude as little as possible on the privacy of individuals or groups.
9 create safeguards to ensure that any erosion of privacy that is considered by 'management' to be necessary in order to provide essential care for individuals is explained, justified and reviewed regularly
10 create a physical environment which protects people from the public gaze, which allows the choice of whether to be alone or in company, which provides personal and private spaces for every individual, which provides for security of information and personal possessions, and in which shared facilities such as bathrooms and toilets are designed to ensure that personal activities can be conducted in complete privacy.

Try it

Below is a charity's own interpretation of the value base which is used with young people with learning difficulties. Against the policy they match the evidence they have to show how it is put into practice. This matching practice takes place on a daily, weekly, termly and annual basis. From your own experience of social care placements, try to complete the second half of the chart with examples you know take place.

Value base	**Practice**
continuity and consistency	
choice	
dignity	
confidentiality	
Respect – empowerment	
communication	
access to relationships	
open access to records	
challenging disadvantage	
independence	
fulfilment	
Potential development	
hope	
creating opportunity	
partnership	
working together	
Membership sharing and caring	
responsibility	
the environment	
privacy	
Rights – empowerment	
involvement in decisions (participation)	
health and safety (protection, welfare, care)	
access to education	

You may see from the value base examples that attempts are made to give individuals control over their lives in as many ways as possible. The examples are broken down into daily, weekly, termly and annual examples to remind staff that this is an ongoing process and not something which is documented at an annual review and then not practised .

If, for example, a pupil arrived at the school he or she would immediately be encouraged to make choices and be independent within the daily structure. Pupils are offered choices about food, going to bed and getting up. In order to foster community responsibility there are negotiations for certain chores to be done by individuals. They will be offered opportunities for privacy by having their own personal space in their bedrooms and the use of bathrooms. Leisure activities will be individually planned with the opportunity to participate in a group or not. They will see people valued as individuals through the presentation of certificates. All pupils will be shown the records kept about them and know that they have

Value base – examples of practice

Daily
- individual interactions between young people and staff
- access to: daily planning and decisions, documentations e.g. daily diaries, incident reports
- access through complaints procedure
- participation in academic and social skills programmes
- food, mealtimes
- waking up
- going to bed
- work activities
- personal space, use of bedrooms, bathrooms etc.
- sharing, participation, certificate presentation
- weekend activities

Weekly
- in-house meetings/team meetings
- shares
- access to agenda, planning, decisions
- contact with range of people
- money management – pocket money/ allowances etc

Termly
- participation in planning regarding:
- activities
- holidays
- celebrations and special events
- leisure
- cultural events
- home visits
- places of worship
- medical issues
- money, clothing grants
- transitions: new young people joining, new staff joining, moving base house
- decision-making through school council planning discussions

Annually
- annual reviews
- annual reports

access to the planning and decision-making process. They will be aware of how to complain if they feel they are being unfairly treated. By itemising examples in this way every opportunity to use this value base is maximised.

Empowerment

Another general principle which might guide interactions in care settings is the principle of 'empowerment.' Smale *et al* (1993) contrast a historical way of working with the idea of empowerment. In the past, carers, social workers or nurses would often regard themselves as experts on people. Professionals would assess a client's needs and then present the client with a possible range of service to meet the carer's view of the client's needs. The power in this situation all lies with the carer. The carer learns about the client, the carer decides what his or her needs are and then the carer might set about 'helping' the client. The client becomes a passive 'patient', someone who shows patience whilst undergoing treatment.

Smale *et al.* (1993) propose that carers should always work from the principle that 'people are, and always will be, the expert on themselves' (page 13). Whilst people may not be expert on their own biochemistry and may need treatment for biological illness, people themselves *will* be the experts on their own social, emotional and cognitive needs. The idea is that power should be given to the clients, that clients should be *empowered* to make their own decisions about their own life. In principle this sounds fine, but many clients receive social care because they are not able to make or not confident in making their own decisions.

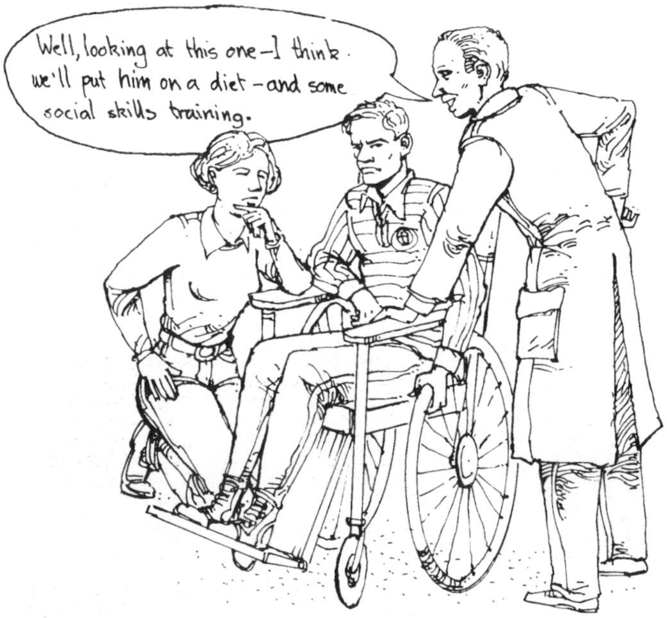

Figure 6.6 Disempowering problem-solving: the expert professionals decide the client's care needs

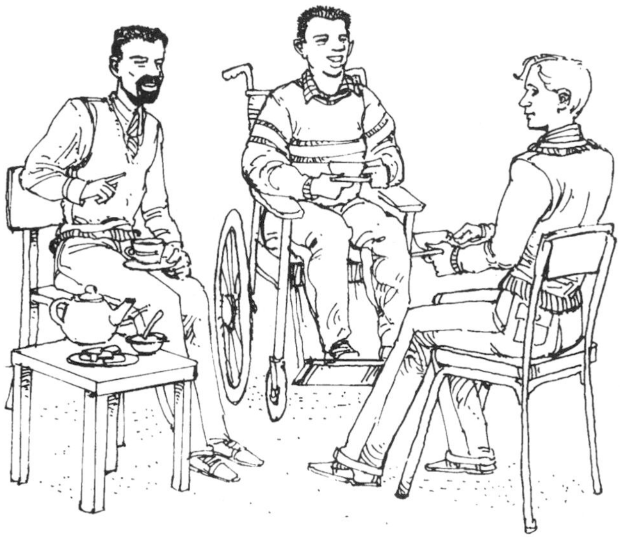

Figure 6.7 Empowering problem-solving: care-worker, client and relatives share their interpretation of the issues

If the carer can build an understanding with a client, if the carer can empathise with a client, then the carer and client can work together to solve problems. This approach links with the idea of self-advocacy, where the worker enables a client to speak for himself or herself.

Very often, meeting clients' needs may depend not only on interacting with clients but also interacting with relatives or friends in the clients' social 'network'. Where clients are not able to express their own beliefs, or communicate about their personal and cultural identity, it may be important for the care-worker to discuss problems with relatives to get information about the client. Rather, the care-worker is trying to understand the relatives and the client's viewpoint. A relative may understand the client's personal or cultural identity in a way that the care-worker does not. A relative may be in a position to speak for the client or act as an advocate for the client. For example, a wife may be able to explain the needs of her husband who has dementia. The wife may also be able to provide information about her husband's beliefs and previous lifestyle. If the care-worker can talk to the wife, then he or she may be able to learn ideas for communicating effectively with her husband. Learning about the husband's life might enable the care-worker to ensure that routine, diet, social activities and so on fit with the husband's past identity and lifestyle.

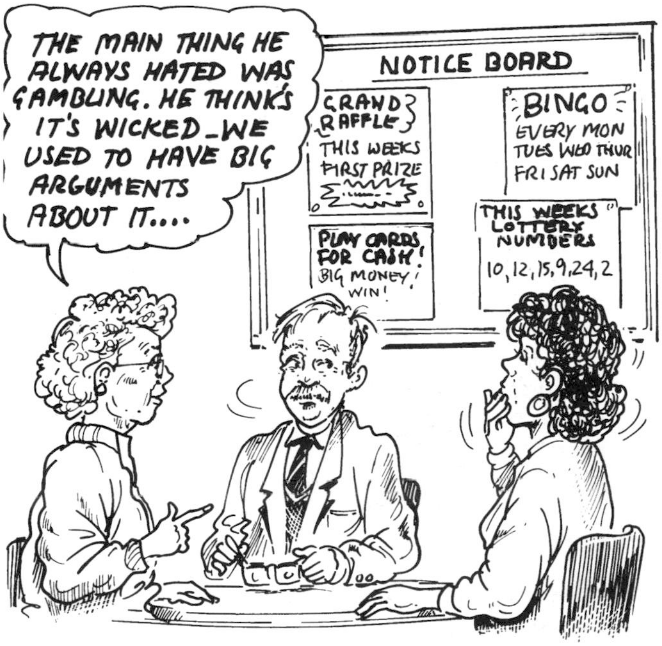
THE MAIN THING HE ALWAYS HATED WAS GAMBLING. HE THINK'S IT'S WICKED – WE USED TO HAVE BIG ARGUMENTS ABOUT IT....
NOTICE BOARD
GRAND RAFFLE
THIS WEEKS FIRST PRIZE
BINGO
EVERY MON TUES WED THUR FRI SAT SUN
PLAY CARDS FOR CASH!
BIG MONEY! WIN!
THIS WEEKS LOTTERY NUMBERS
10, 12, 15, 9, 24, 2

The principle of empowerment implies that the client's problems are solved through building an understanding between the client and the care-workers. The client's problems are not solved by professionals or care staff on their own. The principle of not keeping power solely with the staff, but empowering clients to control their lives, will follow from the principles involved in the NVQ value base.

Try it

Consider this as an example of disempowering interaction. How many of the five care values are ignored in the following interaction? It takes place at lunch-time in the lounge of a rest home with other residents listening.

Carer	Come on Bill, it's time for lunch. What's the matter, don't you want any?
Resident	What's the time?
Carer	12 o'clock, come on now, look lively.
Resident	But I'm not hungry.
Carer	You're not? Well, you don't have to eat, you know. But why don't you just come along with me, your appetite will come back, I'm sure it will!
Resident	What's for dinner?
Carer	Can't you remember? You had a menu yesterday.
Resident	I never did – I don't remember it.

Carer	Well, don't worry yourself, we'll give you something, you're not fussy are you?
Resident	I'll not eat pork and I'll not eat all that sweetcorn rubbish – chicken food, that's what that is. I want decent food.
Carer	Well, just leave anything you don't like. Look – here we are – just sit here.
Resident	But this isn't where I usually sit.
Carer	Well, it's all change today. Have a change, Bill, do you good. Now don't start on me, will you?

1 **Discrimination**: Did the resident want to be called Bill? It may be that he would have preferred 'William' or 'Mr Sidewell.' The resident's past culture may have been ignored here. The carer took no interest in the resident's reasons for not wanting pork or sweetcorn. The resident may have had lifelong customs, religious or moral beliefs which are not being supported here. Attitudes towards food are dismissed with 'You're not fussy are you?'

2 **Confidentiality**: It's one thing to inform the client that it's lunch-time, another to ask questions like, 'Don't you want any food?' 'Can't you remember?' and 'You're not fussy are you?' These questions could undermine the client's privacy. Why should the other residents learn all about this resident's memory failings?

3 **Rights and choice:** The resident seems to have no choices – he is told to 'look lively', told that he'll 'get something to eat', told 'to leave it if he doesn't like it' and told where to sit. The lack of choice is likely to undermine the resident's sense of self-esteem and personal dignity. His life is controlled by the wishes of the care-worker.

4 **Respect for others' beliefs and identity:** There is little evidence of respect here. The carer makes no attempt to learn about the client's past life, his culture, beliefs or sense of self or identity. The carer seems to be in a hurry, just wanting to sort out the client's physical needs. The client's opinions and wishes seem to be largely ignored. The client has to follow the carer's routine rather than being treated as an individual.

5 **Effective communication:** Most of the communication from the carer seems to be about getting on with the current task. The carer seems very pushy. There is no attempt to understand the resident's viewpoint, no warmth, no listening. The carer may have come across as patronising and concerned only to avoid the possibility that Bill will express his anger.

An empowering interaction

A verbal interaction in this care setting which fulfilled the value base requirements might have gone something like:

Carer	It's lunch-time, Mr Sidewell, do you want me to help you to the dining room?
Resident	What's the time, then?
Carer	It's 12 o'clock. Do you want lunch yet?
Resident	I'm not really hungry. What's for dinner anyway?
Carer	Well, I'll just check with the menu. Ah yes, you could have an egg salad, ham salad or the cooked choice.
Resident	Egg salad would be all right – there's none of that rubbish in it – that sweetcorn, is there?
Carer	I'll make sure you get one without. Would you like to come now, or later?
Resident	Oh I'll come now, I want to watch the news later.
Carer	I'll make sure there's no sweetcorn – but why do you dislike it so much?
Resident	It's rubbish, we used to feed it to pigs and chickens in the war – I'm not being treated like that now. I don't see why I should put up with it.
Carer	Oh, I didn't know it used to be fed to animals. We don't do that nowadays.
Resident	Well, there's some strange things nowadays; help me over there will you, that's where I want to sit.
Carer	Yes, of course – then I'll get your lunch for you.

In this interaction there is evidence that the carer wants to empower the client. The client has the power to choose whether he wants to go in for lunch or not and whether he wants help or not. The client's questions are answered with respect and there is no suggestion of the carer having a right to control or take power over the client. As well as providing a choice for the client, the carer is careful to listen to the client. The carer reflects the statement about sweetcorn: 'I'll make sure there's no sweetcorn – but why do you dislike it so much?' The carer is actively interested in the client and is trying to build an understanding of his needs. The carer is rewarded by finding out the answer – sweetcorn is only fit for animals, according to the client. The client's dignity would be offended if it was offered to him.

By carefully asking the right questions the carer is working in an anti-discriminatory way – and avoids making inappropriate assumptions. The carer is also able to demonstrate respect for the client's beliefs and to support and value the client with effective communication. The client's right to confidentiality and privacy is not infringed.

The key issue which makes this an optimised interaction is the fact that the carer seems to empower, or give power to the client rather than disempowering or taking power from the client.

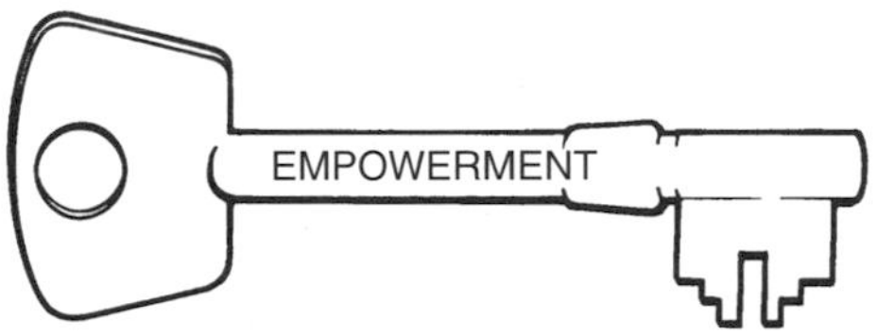

The principle of empowerment follows from working within the NVQ value base. Empowerment is an important goal of all caring interaction.

Solving problems in the care context

The principles which might optimise interaction in care can be described, but the full range of circumstances and possible interactions which can take place in care is potentially infinite. Individual care-workers cannot learn a simple set of behaviours which will enable them to work effectively. If care work was just a matter of fixed actions or routines, then it might be performed by robots. Humans are still better at work that requires a complex sense of judgement or decision-making.

Care work involves constant problem-solving; but not solving other people's problems – only they can do that. Care work is a constant struggle to optimise the *quality* of relationships and service.

Kahney (1986) explains that problem-solving is needed wherever a person has a goal which is blocked or which cannot be achieved directly.

Every care setting involves day-to-day problems. Three children want the care-worker's attention at the same time: who should the care-worker go to? An older person keeps complaining that he has no food, yet he has had a great deal to eat and suffers from dementia – how should the carer respond? A new manager says a room looks institutional, yet there is no money for re-decoration – how can the setting be improved?

These types of problems do not have simple, straightforward answers that can be listed in a book. Care-workers solve these problems using the experience and knowledge they have gained through practice, reflection and feedback from others (see Chapter 5). Hopefully, values and concepts will also guide day-to-day problem solving. The complexity of the caring task is often overlooked; care work is sometimes stereotyped as being simple or 'common sense'.

It is important to see practical problem-solving as a key part of the carer's role. It may be important to emphasise the skill of problem solving in order to enhance the status of health and social care work. Most of all, it will be important to take a problem-solving approach to practical care work, in order to avoid thinking which makes too many assumptions! Care work can be very tiring; it is too easy to slip into a way of thinking which stops enquiring and stops trying to solve problems.

Going back to the problems above, it's easy to see the situations as fixed. The children always want attention at the same time – just ignore them. The older person always complains – it's dementia, nothing we can do! The room has always looked bad – but we don't have any money. A problem-solving attitude involves checking assumptions. Some problems don't have answers – but at least as carers we can check out assumptions and try to see if there might be any new possibilities.

Think it over

There is a story of King Robert the First of Scotland. He had lost all of his battles, was depressed, lonely and hiding in a cave. His only company was a spider who entertained him by continually trying and failing to build a proper spider's web. Eventually the spider succeeded and the web was built. King Robert decided never to give up but to keep trying – a problem-solving attitude. King Robert went on to achieve great success and fame.

There are several interesting points to this short story:

1 You need time to reflect in order to solve problems. King Robert had time to sit around and think in his cave.

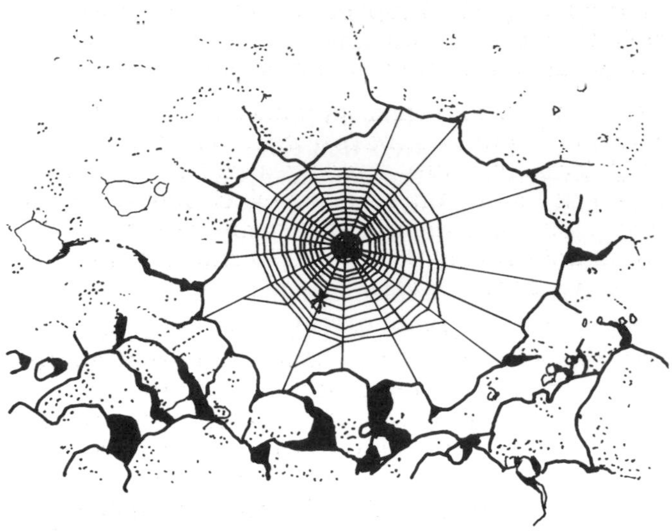

Figure 6.8 There are all sorts of learning experiences in life – but only if you have an open mind

2 There is usually more than one way to do things – the spider was good at experimenting and learning from feedback.
3 A spider can make a good tutor – anything can; changing attitudes and challenging assumptions depends on the frame of mind of the learner more than the teacher.
4 Never give up – unless you know why!

A **problem-solving attitude** involves:

1 Being able to identify difficulties as a challenge, as a problem to be overcome – rather than as situations where nothing can be done.
2 Being able to talk to others to share ideas and make sense of the situation. A problem shared is a problem halved. In care work it is vitally important to involve clients and service users in making sense of problem areas.
3 Being able to think of a range of ideas to try out. Plan to try out the best ideas.
4 Being able to reflect on practical work and evaluate ideas.

Think it over

For instance, a room looks institutional – but there is no money!

1 Just because there is no money it doesn't mean nothing can be done.
2 What do clients and others who use the room think? What makes something look institutional? What ideas do other people have? Reflect on their views.
3 Could the room layout be changed? Could new activities take place in the room – perhaps the problem is the way the room is used? Could furniture be swapped with other rooms? Would it be possible to get second-hand furniture from outside sources, such as voluntary groups? Could anyone bring in cheap extras, for example, plants, posters, anything to alter the way the room looks?
4 Try the ideas out on the client group and on the manager who thinks the room looks institutional. Surely one idea could be tried? Evaluate the success or failure of the idea.

The key issue is not to become stuck with assumptions – and to take a problem-solving attitude to work.

Evidence collection point

You will need to produce a summary of your knowledge of one domestic and one 'institutional' (residential, day care or centre-based) care service. This summary must explain and contrast the possible effects of care on clients; explain two positive and two negative effects of the caring relationship for one client group; and explain four ways of optimising interpersonal interaction.

It may be important to use practical experience of care services related to theory in order to present evidence for positive and negative effects and to explain the use of care values and associated skills for optimising interaction.

Methods for improving interaction in the caring relationship

Information

People need information in order to understand care services. People will become anxious if they do not know what to expect. (This is true of any situation, but particularly when people require health or social care services.)

People who are ill, worried or unhappy find it more difficult to deal with life and its problems than people who are unstressed. This means that professionals explaining matters must take great care to go through things carefully, often more than once. This does not mean they should be patronising, but just take time and care in the way they explain things. Broome and Llewelyn (1995, page 79) found that the greater the clients' understanding of their condition and treatment, the more at ease they felt. The problem is that often medical jargon is used and information given involves complicated medical explanation. Clients may need several opportunities to discuss matters with staff. People can be overwhelmed with large amounts of information all at one time and will benefit from having opportunities to talk frequently with carers who use short sentences and simple words.

Giving clients information in a written form has been found to help. Broome and Llewelyn (1995) quote studies by Young and Humphrey, (1985) and Wallace (1986) which show that distress can be reduced by giving people written information. It is important, however, that the written information is carefully matched to the skills of the reader so as not to be too complex to be understood.

Schain (1980) writes, 'In any given anxiety-provoking situation, especially in the face of major illness or radical surgery, people need to feel that they have some control over their lives . . . the absence of power is strongly correlated with feelings of helplessness and is a precipitant to depression.'

Clients who become passive and dependent often fail to take charge of some aspects of their condition which only they can control. For example, if diabetics do not take charge of their condition, and carefully monitor food and insulin intake, their condition may deteriorate causing severe degeneration of their eyes and kidneys.

Nichols (1993) reports on a team at Exeter hospital which has tried to establish a partnership between patients with kidney disease and the medical staff. Their aim is:

(1) Not to have passive patients but clients who are 'associates' to the health care team and are included wherever and whenever possible.

(2) To ask clients to honour the following responsibilities in terms of education and self-care: (a) to use the informational care facility in order to keep informed, thus reducing the stress of 'not knowing' and allowing participation in medical objectives and decisions; (b) to use the educational facility in order to achieve self sufficiency in dialysis, diet, exercise and physical self-care; (c) to use the emotional care and support facility in order to prevent isolation with stress and to promote a self-care awareness in stress and problem management.

Many care establishments produce a booklet which gives the client information about how the establishment is run. It is helpful to have charts showing where things are and which staff do which jobs. Again, it is important to pitch written communication at the right level and print in different languages and/or Braille.

Types of help will vary according to client group. Some establishments find clients prefer staff not to wear uniforms. However, people who associate uniforms with professional competence may prefer staff to wear them and so be easily identifiable . Others, perhaps, feel a badge will be sufficient; however, this may not help if clients are unable to read the badge, perhaps because of language or sight problems.

Try it

If you work or have a placement in a residential care situation, note how new clients are introduced and how they behave over the first few days and weeks. Note what techniques are used to help them settle in. Explain the possible effects of the care setting on the client.

Giving clients information, in order to help them understand the service they are receiving or services they may receive, is a contribution toward the broader principle of improving interaction in the caring services.

Methods for improving interaction might be grouped under three broad headings: these groupings interact with each other.

1 Service delivery

From the client's viewpoint, clients have a right to expect interaction that:

- **(a)** is consistent with the care sector value base, including rights to dignity and independence
- **(b)** is aimed at involving and empowering clients to remain or become in control of their own lives
- **(c)** where appropriate, involves communication skills which provide emotional support and, in all circumstances, conveys value and respect for clients
- **(d)** is competent.

2 Care-workers' self-development

From the careworker's point of view, care-workers may need to develop personal skills and knowledge in order to be able to provide optimal interaction. Personal skill and knowledge will include:

(a) a problem-solving attitude to day-to-day care situations
(b) the ability to improve one's own learning and performance by using reflective thinking and feedback from others and self-monitoring skills
(c) the ability to work with others using interactive skills that convey value and respect for others, and possibly more advanced skills to create emotional support
(d) the development of day-to-day problem-solving skills into more formal research skills (although this may only be appropriate for workers engaged in advanced or higher education).

3 Organisational systems

To support quality service delivery and care-workers' self-development, care services will need to provide:

(a) induction training – to familiarise new staff with the care setting
(b) regular supervision to assist staff to practise and develop problem-solving skills and use reflective thinking and feedback
(c) training sessions to explore new ideas, knowledge and skills relevant to self-development and service delivery
(d) opportunities for obtaining further qualifications or to take part in further educational programmes. These programmes may enhance workers' knowledge and self-development skills, and the more multi-skilled a worker is, the more effective their work with clients may be
(e) access to counselling or support services. People who feel cared for and supported may tend to treat others in a caring and supportive way. People who feel devalued or stressed may tend to devalue and stress others. Whilst this idea is a little superficial – human behaviour is more complex than this – there is some truth in the idea that enabling staff to experience skilled emotional support may help many to copy the skill and provide emotional support to others
(f) care plans. Organisations will need to review and monitor client well-being. A system for monitoring client need whilst clients receive caring services may be necessary to ensure effective service delivery for clients.

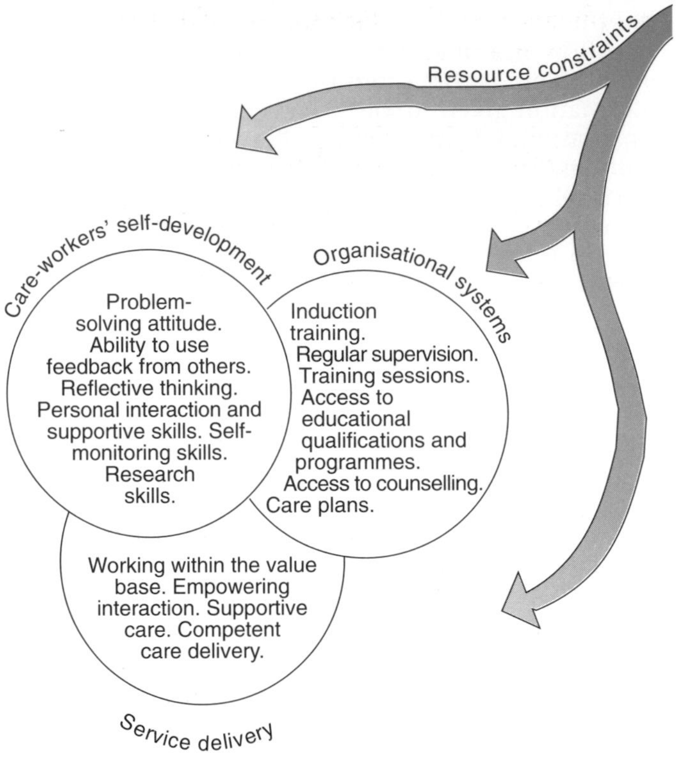

Resource constraints

The fourteen broad 'methods' outlined above might be combined to improve and optimise interaction in the delivery of care services.

Think it over

In your own experience of care, how many of the 14 points above (1a–3f) are really in operation in the services you know?

The methods outlined above will be influenced by resources, however. The development of personal skills requires time. Supervision and training costs money. The quality of emotional support may be influenced by resource constraints on time and money. If recommendations for improving care are to be realistic and valid then the issue of resource constraints may need to be evaluated in relation to any proposals put forward.

Some areas of self-development may not depend on the time and money available to an organisation; yet it is easy for staff to become de-motivated if self-development and service delivery do not support the goals of a care-worker's own self-development. The effectiveness of methods to improve interaction will be influenced by the resources available to care organisations.

The care environment

The environment can influence clients' well-being. The 1993 Community Care Act emphasised the importance of treating people in their own surroundings wherever possible and, if not, in small groups in the community.

Case study

People who have been involved in the closing down of large institutions and seeing clients move to the community have sometimes been amazed at the changes in people they have known for years.

Jim had been a patient in a large mental hospital since he was in his teens. He never spoke but made a series of grunts which the staff responded to by supplying him with a cigarette or whatever they guessed he wanted. Many staff had never heard him speak. However, when Jim's hospital ward was closed he was moved to a small unit in the community where he had a room of his own for the first time. Staff who had known him for years were amazed to hear him speak in short phrases and to see his interest in the plants around the home. He had a key worker who has been able to spend time with him and help him discover his choice of food and clothes. Jim is now able to make trips to town with his key worker and choose food and goods for himself.

'Advocacy' is the term used to describe encouraging people to speak for themselves, to make up their own minds, be assertive and not just accept what happens to them. It is particularly important for clients who have communication difficulties, or who have a different first language, to be provided with a means of communication either through an interpreter or some other system.

Jim's next challenge is to be taught how to travel independently so he can join a part-time horticulture course at the local college. Through effective interaction with a key person, Jim is gradually being empowered to take control of his life. He has taken control of his daily routines, when to get up, have a bath, eat etc. He no longer smokes through boredom, although he likes to go to the local pub and have a drink and a cigarette sometimes. At present he does not control his own finances, but he is becoming aware, through his outings to buy food, that if certain items are not bought they will not be available to eat later. He no longer lives in a hospital environment surrounded by people in uniforms. He has a worker dedicated to spending time with him talking things through and encouraging him to take control of his life where possible.

Staff working in the community – as opposed to institutions – are expected to carry out a greater range of tasks than before and they often have no one on a day-to-day basis to whom they can refer. Previously, in a large institution, it was likely that other staff would be around to discuss problems with. Now, working in the community in small units, staff are less likely to have ready support. This can increase their stress.

As a response to this isolation and stress, carers are setting up support groups. Gray-Toft and Anderson, described in Broome and Llewelyn (1995), discovered that such groups showed that measured stress diminished for nurses and satisfaction with co-workers increased. Techniques such as role play and communication exercises were used to increase group support and individual skills. Besides supporting their members, groups such as these can be a focus for sharing information and debating practice methods.

Making recommendations for improvements in interaction

Each individual care situation and setting will have its own special circumstances. The general theory outlined in this chapter will need to be related to real situations and real constraints. One way of doing this might be to research views and beliefs within a care setting to which you have access. It may be possible to use in-depth interviewing techniques with care staff to try and get their ideas on the quality of care and the constraints that influence it. Work for this section might be combined with work for Unit 8 Research.

There are important ethical considerations involved in interviewing clients. It may be inappropriate to attempt to research clients' views in any formal way. If you have day-to-day contact with clients it may be that you will have experience which will inform your recommendations (clients will tell you what they think anyway). It will be vital to preserve confidentiality in your work (see Introduction, page 8) but it may be possible to use your own experience as a basis for problem-solving to produce evidence.

Evidence collection point

You need to provide a report which explains four methods used to improve interaction in a caring relationship and which recommends how interaction in a caring relationship familiar to you might be improved.

Self-assessment test

1 Which statement is closest to the truth?
- **a** People with partners and close family have a high quality of emotional support.
- **b** People who are rich have a high quality of emotional support because people want to please them.
- **c** Young people have a high quality of emotional support because of their friends.
- **d** Poor people have a high quality of emotional support because they have to stick together.

2 Non-verbal messages are messages:
- **a** Delivered in writing.
- **b** That do not use words.
- **c** That depend on electronics.
- **d** That do not involve sound.

3 Empowerment means:
- **a** Agreeing with whatever clients say because they have the power.
- **b** Involving clients or their advocates in decisions and working within the value base.
- **c** The staff taking power over clients because they are the trained experts.
- **d** Giving more money to clients so that they are more economically powerful.

4 Effective interaction with clients will involve:
- **a** Reflective or active listening and conveying respect and value.
- **b** Always agreeing with the clients to keep them happy.
- **c** Always being available for clients when they want to talk.
- **d** Never being silent when with a client.

5 It is likely that carers will find:
- **a** Clients' experiences the same as theirs.
- **b** Clients' views the same as theirs.
- **c** People have different perspectives.
- **d** It is best to treat everyone the same.

6 Co-operating in a group involves:
- **a** Always being at meetings.
- **b** Talking a lot in meetings.
- **c** Supporting and encouraging others.
- **d** Making sure the meeting ends on time.

7 The value base for care requires carers to respect the clients' dignity, privacy and independence. This means:
- **a** Listening to the clients' wants and not intruding on their space.
- **b** Making the clients dress themselves.
- **c** Never getting involved with the clients' financial affairs.
- **d** Only talking when necessary.

8 Methods which improve interaction include:
- **a** Helping clients understand by writing information down and explaining carefully.
- **b** Wearing a uniform.
- **c** Making jokes with clients.
- **d** Saying 'Don't worry, everything will be all right.'

9 How can the environment influence the clients' well-being?
- **a** They can get more fresh air in the community.
- **b** Clients can be empowered to control their own lives.
- **c** They can be provided with friends.
- **d** They can choose their own television channel.

10 Activity-based interaction means:
- **a** Playing ball games.
- **b** Using an activity to interact with others.
- **c** Going to bingo.
- **d** Learning to swim.

11 Support can be offered through:
- **a** Sensory contact
- **b** Leaving the room when someone is upset.
- **c** Buying someone a drink.
- **d** Meeting a lot of people.

12 Communication will be effective if:
- **a** We say the right thing.
- **b** We monitor others' behaviour and respond appropriately.
- **c** We don't have silences in the conversation.
- **d** We always speak quietly.

13 If a care-worker looks steadily at a client who is speaking about his or her problems, the care-worker's gaze could not be interpreted as:
- **a** Attraction.
- **b** Anger.
- **c** Rejection.
- **d** Feeling too busy to listen.

14 Which of the following would indicate that a listener is not paying attention?
- **a** Assuming an open body posture.
- **b** Smiling, nodding.
- **c** Reorganising his or her file.
- **d** Tolerating silences.

15 Which of the following is an essential component that a group could not function without?
- **a** A room to meet.
- **b** Someone to take minutes.
- **c** A common aim.
- **d** Money.

16 Which of the following would be least effective if a chairperson was experiencing difficulties with a group member?
- **a** Build a contract within the group to support each other.
- **b** Tell the person the chairperson is the boss and he or she must obey instructions.
- **c** Discuss the matter with the person outside the group.
- **d** Reinforce or support acceptable behaviours.

17 Which of the following reasons is least likely to cause a group to fail?
- **a** Lack of trust, suspicion.
- **b** Members avoiding work.
- **c** Meeting in a poorly decorated room.
- **d** Not having enough time.

18 Non-judgemental behaviour means:
- **a** Not making decisions.
- **b** Always going along with the client.
- **c** Not helping a client.
- **d** Not judging someone by his or her appearance or views.

19 Being independent means:
- **a** Clients should do everything for themselves.
- **b** We should not ask or expect others to help us.
- **c** We should have the opportunity to make our own choices and decisions.
- **d** Teenagers should be allowed to go anywhere they want.

20 Which of the following does clients' entitlement to privacy not include?
- **a** Having regard for the extent to which they wish to associate with other residents.
- **b** Having somewhere for visitors and telephone calls which is private.
- **c** Ensuring that clients can use the toilet and bathe without being seen or heard.
- **d** Having an en-suite bathroom.

Fast Facts

Anti-discrimination Practical work which aims to stop members of particular age, class, cultural or other groups from receiving a lower standard of service than others.

Appearance How we look. People use different clothes, hairstyles, cosmetics and adornments to express their membership of particular age groups, class groups, cultural and friendship groups.

Assumptions These are ideas which we assume to be correct but which we haven't checked. In care work it is very important that we do check our ideas about other people and their needs. Wrong assumptions can lead to the breakdown of conversations and to the breaking up of groups. They can also be discriminatory.

Auditory The form of communication taken in through the ears (hearing).

Body language This is the language of non-verbal communication, messages we send with the body. It consists of signs that other people can read in the way our body looks, or the way it moves. Non-verbal communication has a slightly wider meaning than body language. 'Non-verbal' covers everything which is not actual words (for example, tone of voice). Body language focuses on the way the body, face, eyes, hands etc. look and move.

Body movements The speed and type of people's movements can send a vast range of messages. We can interpret tension, anger, attraction, happiness and many other emotions by watching how people move their hands, eyes, head and body.

Boundaries A boundary may represent a line that you may go up to, but must not cross. Boundaries divide areas into different sections. In practical care work, boundaries define the limits of a carer's role.

Buffering Partners, friends and family may help to protect a person from the full stress of life changes and conflicts. Michael Argyle called this protection 'buffering'.

Confidentiality A care value and part of the NVQ value

base. Confidentiality means keeping information that you have about others to yourself; only sharing it with individuals who have a 'need to know'.

Culture The customs and ways of thinking that people learn define their culture. It is the social learning that influences how people understand themselves, and so has a very important influence on how people explain their own individuality. Differences in culture lead to non-verbal messages being interpreted in different ways.

Dependence Having to rely on others in order to maintain physical, social or emotional well-being. People can also become dependent on drugs and aids to daily living.

Devaluing Stereotyping the views and beliefs of others as worthless or ridiculous. Devaluing a person's culture and beliefs can undermine his or her personal development.

Discrimination Treating a person or group in a different way from how others are treated. Discrimination can be either negative or positive; but when used on its own, the word usually refers to negative discrimination, which is to treat certain people less well than others.

Distance Distance is one of the things to look for when trying to interpret other people's non-verbal messages. Distance has no fixed meaning, but in some cultures, standing or sitting close can mean: affection or love, anger or aggression, fear, or difficulty in hearing one another. Standing or sitting back might mean feeling comfortable or feeling separate. The cultural setting and other communications help us to work out the best interpretation.

Emotional support A general term, used to include listening and conversational work, to support other people's individuality and self-esteem.

Empowerment Giving power to others. Using your situation to enable other people to make their own decisions and to control their own lives.

Eye contact This happens when people's eyes 'contact' each other and send non-verbal messages. Eye contact is important in both individual and group communication. Turn-taking in conversation often relies on eye contact. Messages of interest, attraction, affection, hostility and many other emotions can be sent by eye contact alone.

Facial expression The face is an important area of the body for sending non-verbal messages. Even line diagrams can convey instant meaning to people. Facial expression is often easier to control than our eyes. Much non-verbal communication using the face is conscious if not always deliberate. People think about their faces and control them.

Feedback Getting information from others which is 'fed' to you to help you learn, adjust and develop your skills.

Gaze Allowing the eyes to meet with other people's eyes and exchange looks. Gaze is part of the non-verbal system of eye contact which is a central component of non-verbal communication.

Gestures These are non-verbal messages sent (mainly) with the arms, hands and fingers. Gestures are especially sensitive to cultural interpretation. A hand-signal can mean 'everything is fine' in one culture, and can be a serious insult in another.

Groups In social care a 'group of people' means people who feel that they belong together. They will share some common purpose, common culture, or common values.

Group formation Groups take time to build a sense of belonging. A collection of people will probably be very cautious at first. There is often tension until people feel that they belong – that they share common values. Once people feel that they all belong together, the group may work well.

Group values These are shared beliefs which everyone agrees with or supports. Respect and value for other people's individuality, using supportive communication, preventing discrimination and encouraging choice and control in others are caring values.

Independence Freedom from dependence on others. The right to choose and control one's own lifestyle.

Individuality This is a general term covering the sense of self that people develop from culture, religion, gender, age, race, social circumstances and their own physical and intellectual nature. Individuality is everything that makes the individual special. Recognising individuality is a necessary starting point for creating equality or a feeling of being equal. Recognising individuality involves not making assumptions about people.

Interest Communicating interest is a step on the way to building an understanding of other people during conversation.

Interpersonal interaction Interpersonal interaction includes every type of communication between people.

Labelling Identifying individuals as members of a particular group, whether or not they see themselves as members. Labelling is linked to stereotyping, and people are expected to conform to the behaviour associated with the stereotype with which they have been labelled.

Learning Any change in what you are capable of doing which is not due to impairment, growth or some other purely physical process.

Listening skills The ability to build an understanding of another person's views when expressed verbally. Listening skills may include reflective listening, questioning skills, ability to understand non-verbal behaviour, ability to show respect for others, use of silence and self-monitoring skills.

Meshing When the contributions to a conversation link in a smooth and effective way, they are said to mesh. They fit together like links in a 'wire mesh' fence.

Mirroring Not to be confused with reflecting. Mirroring is when a person copies another person's non-verbal messages. A person who is attracted to someone may copy his or her way of sitting or standing when talking. For example, a person may cross his or her legs if the other person has crossed legs. Successful mirroring sends the message: 'I like you'.

Mission statement A group's or establishment's statement about its aims, objectives and methods of operating.

Monitoring own behaviour This is a really important skill for developing caring abilities. Monitoring involves reflecting on your own behaviour and on the reactions of other people. It involves thinking about what is happening within group or individual communication.

Muscle tension This is one type of non-verbal message. Tension can communicate messages about the other person's emotions, especially when linked with body posture. It is something else to look for when trying to understand other people.

Non-verbal signals Using our eyes, faces and bodies to send signals. Messages which do not involve words. Tone of voice is often regarded as non-verbal, because verbal relates only to the words used in a message.

Observational skills Observation of others will involve trying to understand their appearance, verbal and non-verbal communication. Observational skills may imply the ability to monitor own and others' behaviour.

Olfactory Our olfactory sense is the ability to smell.

Optimised interaction Optimised means 'made as good as possible in the circumstances'. Optimised interaction in care might need to conform to the value base, aim to empower clients and employ a wide range of skills.

Orientation Organising your own or others' positions in the space available. The way people face or look when communicating. (Orientation relates to direction.)

Pace of communication The speed of a person's conversation. Speech that is too fast or too slow can be hard to understand. Some people may require you to speak more slowly than normal so that they can understand your everyday speech.

Personal space This is an area of space which an individual tries to keep other people out of. It can be seen as the distance between people when they communicate with one another. Like many non-verbal messages, distance is used in different ways by different cultures. How closely people stand will depend on their culture, their feelings for one another and the physical and social situation.

Pheremones Barely detectable scents which may attract or repel.

Pitch The degree of high or low tone in someone's voice. A high-pitched voice is used in baby talk.

Posture This is the way a person positions his or her body. Posture usually sends messages about the individual's degree of tension or relaxation. It can also send all sorts of social messages, such as 'I'm really interested', 'I don't want to be here', and so on.

Questioning This is an important skill for keeping a conversation going. Questions can be open or closed. A closed question is where the kind of answer required is simple and fixed. 'How old are you?' is a closed question because the answer has to be a number – once you've said it there is little else to say. 'How do you feel about your age?' is open because the other person could say almost anything – how long they speak for is 'open'. Giving a short quick number is a 'closed' reply. Closed questions are of limited use in working with people. Open questions are often much more valuable for building an understanding.

Reflective listening This is a care skill which involves either using your own words to repeat what another person said, or repeating the words exactly, or using non-verbal messages with silence. The idea of reflection is to use conversation like a mirror, so that the other person can see his or her own thoughts reflected. They can then be altered more easily.

Responding skills Use of verbal and non-verbal communication to respond to others. Responses may use reflective listening, questioning and skills focused on understanding the other person.

Role boundaries Boundaries to the commitment or duties involved in a 'caring relationship'.

Self-confidence An individual's confidence in his or her own ability to achieve something or to cope with a situation. Self-confidence may influence and be influenced by self-esteem.

Self-disclosure This happens when we tell other people about our own experiences, thoughts and feelings. Some self-disclosure can be useful when trying to understand others. It can create a sense of trust.

Self-esteem How well or badly a person feels about himself or herself. High self-esteem may help a person to feel happy and confident. Low self-esteem may lead to depression and unhappiness.

Self-image The kind of person we think we are. If there is a big gap between our ideal self and our self-image we are likely to have a low self-esteem.

Sensory contact Touch, smell, vision, hearing or other sensations which give us information about other people.

Silence Silence is a useful part of some conversations. Sometimes silence is better than just talking to fill a gap. It can provide an opportunity for feelings to be expressed non-verbally.

Sincerity This involves being real and honest in what we say to others. Without sincerity, warmth and understanding, relationships usually break down or 'go wrong'. Honesty with clients is an important part of relationship and supportive work.

Social context A setting where social influences affect an individual's learning and development.

Social role The behaviour adopted by individuals when they are in social situations. Group norms and individual status help to define a role such as mother, sister, engineer etc.

Status A measure of the power or prestige of a person. Status helps to define how people are treated by others and how they see themselves.

Stereotyping Judging an individual to be a certain type of person by his or her appearance or behaviour. A stereotype is not a description of a real person. It is a collection of characteristics which members of a particular group are expected to possess. People who have been stereotyped are expected to behave as 'typical' members of the group to which they have been assigned.

Stress A physical condition. Symptoms may include tiredness, irritability, lack of clear thinking, difficulties in sleeping and physical illness.

Submissiveness Feeling that others' needs are more important than your own, giving in to them so as to avoid trouble.

Supportive skills Warmth, understanding and sincerity can be used together to create a safe, caring conversation.

Tactile Something which can be touched.

Tone of voice Voice tone is the sound of the voice, rather than the words that are spoken. The tone of someone's voice can send messages about attraction, anger, sympathy and other emotions. Because voice tone is separate from spoken words, it is classed as 'non-verbal'. The sound of our voice is separate from the word messages we send.

Touch This is another way of sending non-verbal messages. Touch can be a very important way of saying 'I care', or 'I am with you'. Touch can be interpreted in various ways. It can send messages of power and dominance, and can be sexual as well as caring. The important thing is how a person understands touch, not what you intend.

Understanding An important goal of caring is to learn about other people's individuality. It is necessary to build some understanding so that you correctly communicate respect and value.

Value base A system of values to guide the care profession. The NVQ value base is defined in the NVQ '0' Unit. This covers the promotion of anti-discriminatory practice, the maintenance of confidentiality, the promotion of individual rights and choice, the acknowledgement of individuals' personal beliefs and identity, and the support of individuals through effective communication.

Values Values are learned through systems which enable individuals to make choices and decisions. Values may guide communication skills.

Valuing others Promoting a sense of self-esteem in other people.

Verbal communication Spoken messages – messages which use words – are 'verbal'. The opposite is non-verbal communication, which means messages sent without words. Non-verbal language is often harder to understand than verbal language.

Warmth A supportive skill which displays the ability to be non-judgemental and to listen to clients. Warmth can help to create a safe conversational atmosphere which may lead to a sense of trust.

References and further reading

Adler, T., 1993, *Looking Out/Looking In*

Argyle, M., 1983, *The Psychology of Interpersonal Behaviour*, Pelican

Argyle, M., 1987, *The Psychology of Happiness*, Methuen

Argyle, M., 1994, *The Psychology of Social Class*, Routledge

Argyle, M., and Henderson, M., 1985, *The Anatomy of Relationships*, Penguin

Aronson, E., *et al.*, 1994, *Social Psychology: The Heart and Mind,* HarperCollins

Atkinson, R., 1993, *Introduction of Psychology,* Ted Buchholz

Bales, R., 1970, *Personality and Interpersonal Behaviour,* Holt, Rinehart and Winston

Bem, Wollach & Kogan, 1965, *Journal of Personality and Social Psychology*

Broome, A. and Llewelyn, S. (ed.), 1995, *Health Psychology – Processes and Applications,* Chapman and Hall

Dion, K.K., 1972, What is good is beautiful. In *Journal of Personality and Social Psychology*

Duck, S., 1992, *Human Relationships,* second edition, Sage

Ellsworth, P., 1975, *Direct Gaze as a Social Stimulus,* Plenum

Hartshorne, H., and May, M., 1930 *Studies in the Nature of Character,* Macmillan

Hopson, B., and Scally, M., 1988, *Lifeskills Teaching Programmes,* Southgate Publishing

Kahney, H., 1986, *Problem Solving,* Open University Press

McDerment, L., 1988, *Stress Care,* Social Care Association

Meichenbaum, D.H., 1983, *Stress Reduction and Prevention,* Plenum

Nichols, K. A., 1993, *Psychological Care in Critical Illness,* Chapman & Hall

Rogers, C.R., 1951, *Client Centred Therapy, Its Current Practices, Implications and Theory,* Houston

Rutter, D., 1976, Visual interaction in recently admitted and chronic long-stay schizophrenic patients. In *British Journal of Social and Clinical Psychology* volume 5

Schain W. S., 1980, Patients' Rights in Decision Making, In *Cancer*, 46

Smale, G., *et al.*, 1993, *Empowerment, Assessment, Care Management and the Skilled Worker,* NISW: HMSO

Tuckman, B., 1965, Development sequence in small groups. In *Psychological Bulletin,* LXIII(6)

Walsh, F., 1993, *Normal Family Processes,* Guildford Publications

Watson, J.B., 1972, Conditioned emotional reactions. In *Journal of Experimental Psychology*

Chapter 7

The organisation of structures within human body systems

This chapter focuses on:

- **human body cells, their structure and functions – endoplasmic reticulum, ribosomes, mitochondria and nucleus**
- **tissues and their functions – epithelial, connective, muscle and nervous tissues**
- **cellular respiration – aerobic and anaerobic respiration, including glycolysis and the Krebs cycle.**

It also provides micrographs of the main tissue types for interpretation.

Human body cells

Cells are considered to be the basic structural and functional units of the living body. The word 'cell' was originally used by Robert Hooke in 1665 when he viewed slices of cork bark under one of the first simple microscopes. He did not realise at the time that he was looking at dead cell walls, but they looked like little rooms – hence the term cell, which was the name given to the small rooms used by monks. As microscopes became more and more sophisticated and capable of higher magnifications, more cellular structure was revealed. However, a limit was reached using light microscopes due to the problems of blurring with greater and greater magnification. (See Figure 7.1.)

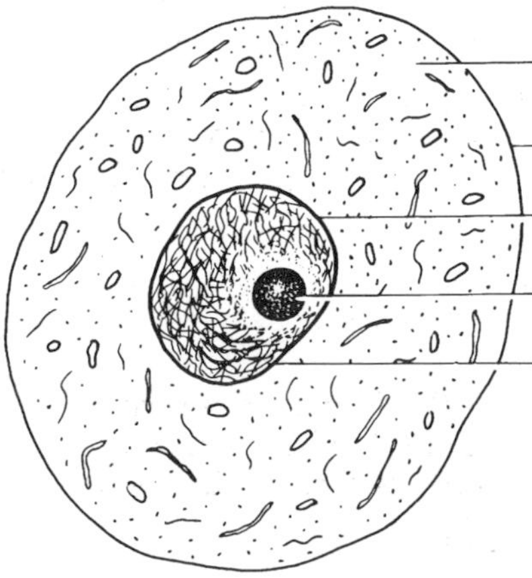

Figure 7.1 A cell viewed under a light microscope (magnified × 300)

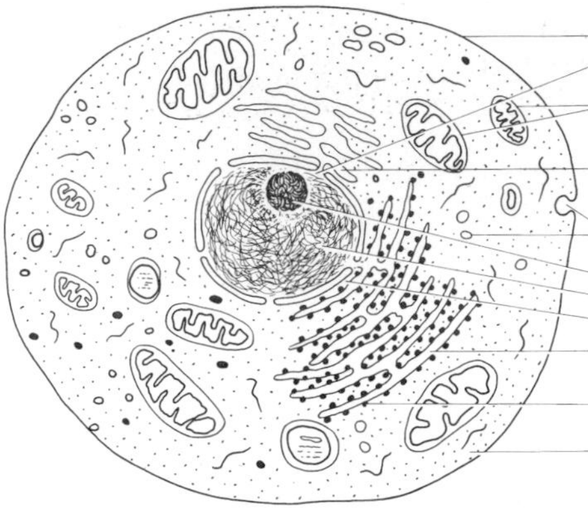

Figure 7.2 A cell magnified under an electron microscope (magnified × 1000)

A giant leap forward was made in the 1940s when a commercial electron microscope was developed. An electron microscope can magnify cells over 5000 times. A whole new science was born called *cytology*, the study of cells. The interior of a cell was found to be more organised than was previously thought. (See Figure 7.2.)

Cell structure

The outer limit of a cell is known as the *plasma* (or *cell*) *membrane*. Visualised simply as a line under the light microscope, it takes the appearance of a protein sandwich with the electron microscope. The function of the plasma membrane is to regulate substances passing into and out of cells. The plasma membrane is approximately 50 per cent lipids (fatty substances) and 50 per cent proteins by weight. However, proteins are much larger than lipids, so there are many more lipid molecules than proteins. The current theory of cell membrane structure is called the *fluid mosaic model* (see Figure 7.3).

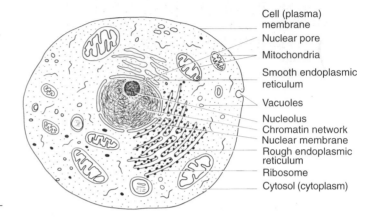

Most of the lipids are *phospholipids*, which consist of a 'head' of phosphate and two 'tails' of fatty acids (see Figure 7.4). The significance of these lies in the fact that the head is *hydrophilic* (water liking) and the tails are *hydrophobic* (water hating). Two layers (a *bilayer*) of phospholipids line up together

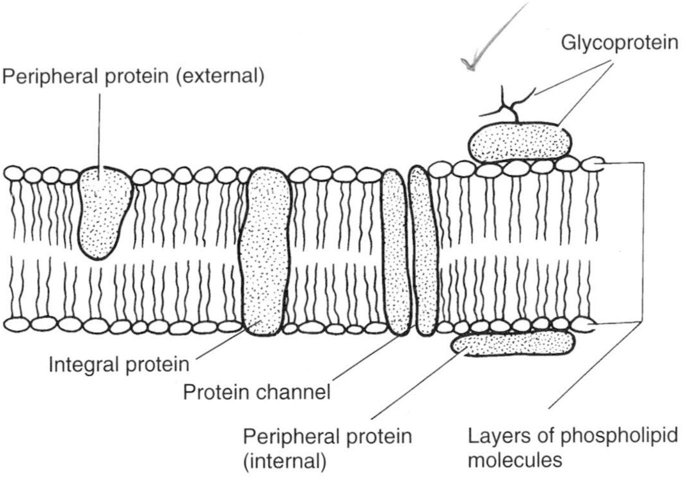

Figure 7.3 A schematic diagram of the fluid mosaic model

in the plasma membrane. The heads face outwards to the fluid surrounding cells (*extracellular fluid*), while the tails face inwards towards each other, away from the extracellular fluid. The phospholipids can move sideways in their position, hence the fluidity of the membrane. One advantage of this is that the layer is self-healing. Proteins may protrude all the way through the phospholipid bilayer, or be inserted only into the inner or outer surfaces (*membrane proteins*). Proteins which pass all the way through tend to have sugar chains attached which face the extracellular fluid, these are known as *glycoproteins*.

Glycoproteins often have channels or pores which act as gates through which substances may or may

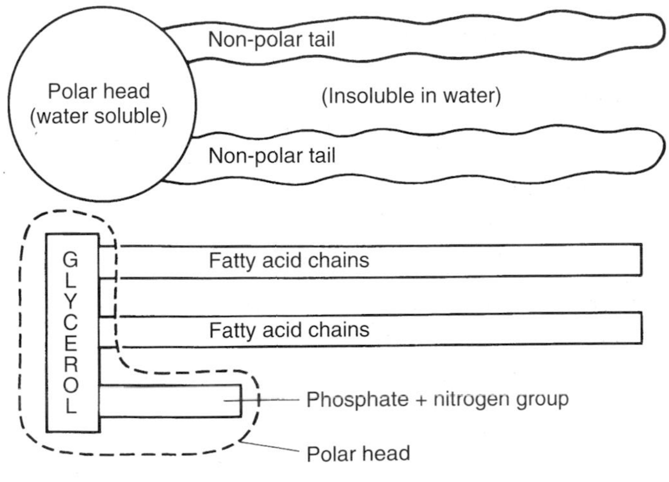

Figure 7.4 The structure of phospholipids

not pass to the cell interior. Others are carriers which transport some molecules in a similar way.

Membrane proteins either serve as cell identity markers or as receptor sites for molecules of importance to the cell. Plasma membranes exert selectivity over some substances which pass into and out of the cell (*selective permeability*). Those substances which dissolve easily in lipids have no problems gaining access to the cell (*freely permeable*), neither does water. However, substances carrying an electric charge known as *ions* can have great difficulty getting through. Ions largely depend on suitable protein channels for their passage. Generally, ions bearing positive charges (*cations*) are more favoured than negatively charged ions (*anions*).

Think it over

Make a list of the main cations and anions you know. If you are not familiar with any at all, look up hydrogen, oxygen, hydroxide (OH), phosphate (PO_4), sodium, potassium, chloride (see Figure 9.7, page 189).

The contents of a cell can be referred to as *protoplasm*, but this is more usually divided into the central darker staining *nucleus* and the remainder which is the *cytoplasm* (plasm means stuff or material, hence this name is cell material). See Figure 7.1.

Cytoplasm is a semi-fluid base (the *cytosol*) in which other components are suspended. Cytosol has a large fluid part (*intracellular fluid*) in which chemicals are dissolved. Many chemical reactions are carried out here. The sum total of chemical reactions occurring can generally be referred to as *metabolism*.

Also present in the cytoplasm are the *inclusions* which are chemicals, such as glycogen (a storage form of sugar) and melanin (a pigment responsible for hair or skin colour).

Cell organelles and their functions

Components of cells with distinct structures and functions have been likened to little organs and received the name *organelles*. Organelles include:

- endoplasmic reticulum
- ribosomes
- mitochondria
- nucleus.

Endoplasmic reticulum

'Endo' means within, and 'reticulum' a network. Hence, the *endoplasmic reticulum* (ER) is a network of channels enclosed in membranes which fills the cell interior and is continuous with the membrane surrounding the nucleus. (Only a small part is shown in a cell diagram for clarity.) There are two distinct types:

- *rough* (or granular) *endoplasmic reticulum* (ER)
- *smooth* (or agranular) *endoplasmic reticulum* (ER).

The difference between them is that the rough ER is studded with *ribosomes,* whereas the smooth ER has none. Rough ER together with its ribosomes makes the cell proteins and acts as a temporary storage area. It can also add on sugar chains to make glycoproteins. Smooth ER makes fatty materials such as steroids, phospholipids and fatty acids.

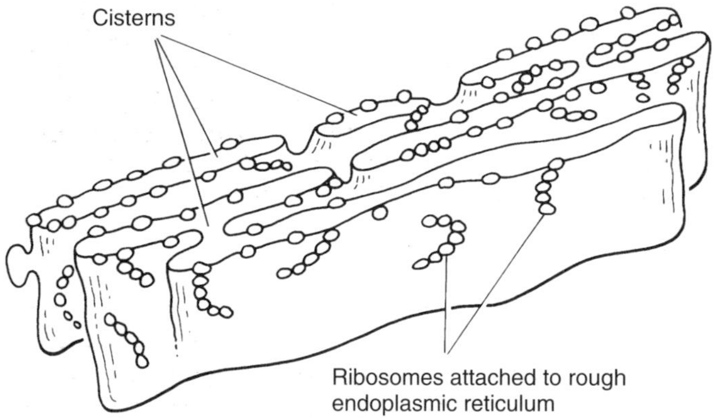

Figure 7.5 The structure of endoplasmic reticulum

Ribosomes

Ribosomes appear as small spheres floating freely in the cytoplasm (*free ribosomes*) or attached to the rough endoplasmic reticulum. They have been identified as possessing two sub-units, one half the size of the other, and containing the nucleic acid, ribonucleic acid, more commonly referred to as RNA. See Figure 7.6. We shall return to nucleic acids in the section on the nucleus (see opposite). Ribosomes are named after the RNA found inside them. RNA is found elsewhere in a cell, so this type of RNA is often known as rRNA where the r refers to ribosomal RNA.

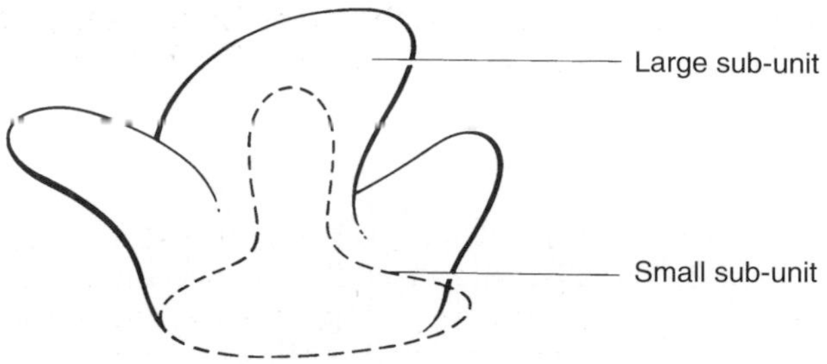

Figure 7.6 The structure of a ribosome

Free ribosomes make the proteins used inside the cell, whereas endoplasmic ribosomes make proteins used in the cell membrane or transported outside the cell for use elsewhere.

Mitochondria

Usually around a thousand in a cell, mitochondria replicate themselves as a cell divides or if there is a need for increased energy storage in the cell. Cells which are very active, like muscle and liver, have larger numbers of mitochondria than other cells.

Mitochondria are capable of generating a compound rich in energy, known as *adenosine triphosphate* (ATP) from the oxidation of glucose. This will be referred to again under aerobic respiration (page 157). Each mitochondrion (singular) has a double membrane, similar in structure to the plasma membrane. The outer layer is smooth, but the inner layer is folded to form shelf-like ridges. The enclosed central part is the matrix. The folds are called *cristae* and house the enzymes responsible for the last stages in the

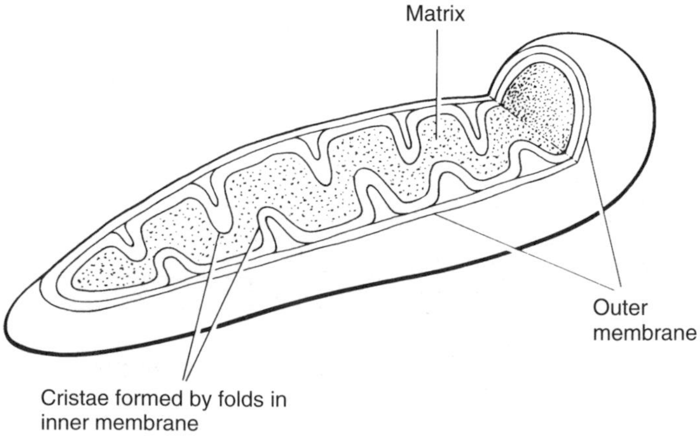

Figure 7.7 The structure of a mitochrondrion (part removed)

oxidation of glucose. Mitochondria have often been called the 'powerhouses' of the cell. See Figure 7.7.

Nucleus

The largest structure in the cell usually stains very darkly and is easily picked out – this is the *nucleus*. There may be no nucleus, as in mature red blood cells, or several of them, such as in a skeletal muscle fibre. A cell separated from its nucleus usually dies, and red blood cells do not survive for very long (average 120 days).

The nucleus is separated from the cytoplasm by a double layered nuclear membrane similar in structure to the plasma membrane. The nucleus is usually spherical or oval in shape, but some cells have unusually shaped nuclei (plural), the most common being the lobed nucleus of white blood cells known as *phagocytes*. (See the next chapter and Figure 8.33.)

Nuclear membranes contain relatively large pores through which substances like RNA and proteins move into the cytoplasm.

There may be other smaller spherical bodies visible in a nucleus, and these stain even more darkly than the whole nucleus. These are called *nucleoli* and represent the part of the cell where ribosomes are formed.

When a cell is not undergoing cell division (*mitosis*), the interior of the nucleus looks like a tangled mass of material – the *chromatin network*. During cell division, the chromatin network shrinks and thickens to form rod-shaped bodies called *chromosomes*. Chromosomes are made of another nucleic acid, deoxyribonucleic acid (DNA) and various protein molecules. The DNA is folded and coiled around a protein core and this represents the genes or units of heredity. The nucleus of a cell controls all the activities going on inside the cell.

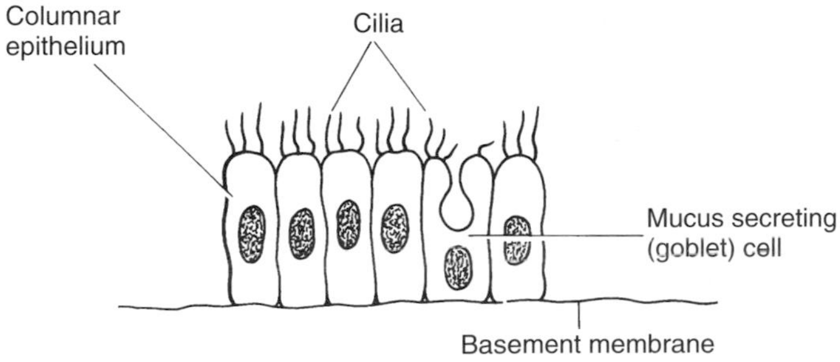

Figure 7.8 Ciliated cells

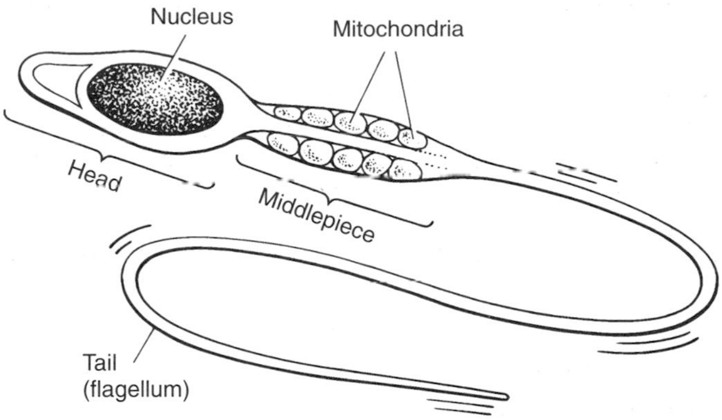

Figure 7.9 A spermatozoon

Throughout the body there are numerous variations of a typical body cell such as the one described. Some cells contain extra projections from the surface. If there are many such projections which appear hair-like, they are called *cilia* (Figure 7.8). Cilia move materials on surfaces and are mainly associated with mucus secretions, such as the lining of tubes between the ovary and the uterus and cells lining the trachea. *Flagellae* occur singly or in pairs, they are longer than cilia and usually cause movement of the cell, for example a sperm cell (Figure 7.9).

Evidence collection point

Write an illustrated report on the main parts of a cell and their functions. You may choose a specific cell, such as a liver, muscle or skin cell, or provide a more general account of cell parts.

Tissues and their functions

Cells carry out functions, but in practice they do not work in isolation. They usually form groups and work together carrying out their particular function. A group of similar cells carrying out a particular set of functions is called a *tissue*. The cells of a tissue can be fastened together in several ways, called *cell junctions,* but there is always fluid between these fastenings. The fluid is known as *interstitial* or *tissue fluid*. It transports materials to cells and carries out chemical reactions. This fluid is where bacteria are found in bacterial infections. Viruses, on the other hand, can reproduce only when inside living cells. This is why chemicals such as antibiotics are effective against bacteria, but not against viruses as the cell would be damaged as well.

The study of tissues is called *histology* and, for simplicity, tissues can be classified into four major groups:

- epithelial tissues
- connective tissues
- muscle tissues
- nervous tissue.

Epithelia

These tissues cover internal and external body surfaces, including the lining of ducts, body cavities, hollow organs and gland formation. Epithelia consist of closely packed cells either in single layers (*simple epithelia*) or in several layers (*compound epithelia*).

The lowest layer of epithelia always sits on a basement membrane. This is a thin membranous layer secreted by the epithelial cells themselves, which provides support and attachment. Epithelia have nerve supplies, but are nourished by diffusion from blood vessels in neighbouring connective tissue.

As epithelia line surfaces and organs, it follows that they are subject to considerable wear and tear, so their capacity for repair is greater than most other cells.

Simple epithelia

The simplest type is *squamous epithelium* which consists of cells so flat that the nucleus forms a lump in the centre, giving an appearance something similar to the yolk of a fried egg when viewed from above. They fit together rather like crazy paving with very little tissue fluid between them (see Figure 7.10).

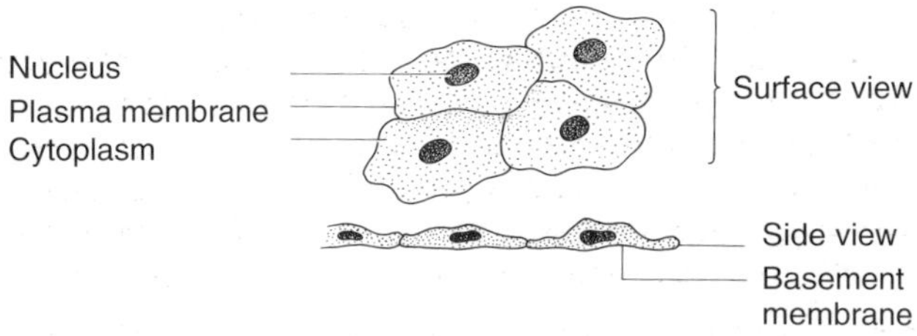

Figure 7.10 Simple squamous epithelium

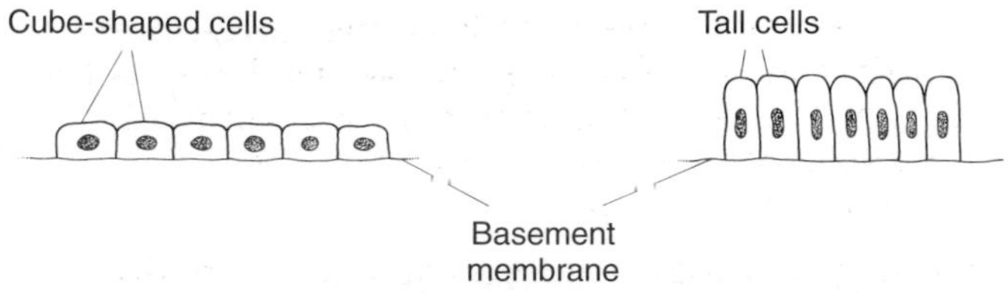

Figure 7.11 Cuboidal and columnar epithelium

Squamous epithelium cells are found in the wall of blood capillaries (in this location called *endothelium*), Bowman's capsule in kidney nephrons and lung alveoli. They are located in areas where diffusion and osmosis take place, or where filtration and secretion occur.

Other types of simple epithelia are *cuboidal* and *columnar epithelia* which have shapes like cubes and columns respectively (see Figure 7.11). Columnar cells are often associated with the presence of cilia and mucus-secreting cells (see Figure 7.8).

Compound epithelia

These consist of several cell layers which can be cuboidal, columnar or mixed with squamous cells forming the upper layer. This last type is called *stratified squamous epithelium* (see Figure 7.12) and it lines the vagina, oesophagus, mouth and tongue. The skin is similar, but with the added protection of a layer of dead cells forming a barrier to the outside world (*cornified stratified squamous epithelium*).

The lower layers of stratified squamous epithelium are formed of cuboidal or even columnar shapes which gradually become flattened (squamous) as

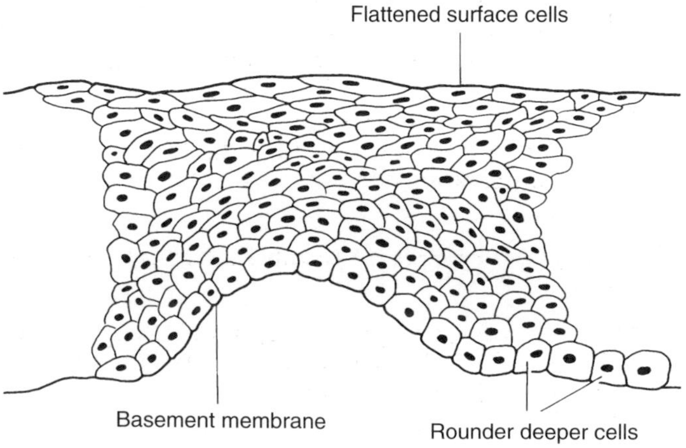

Figure 7.12 Stratified squamous epithelium

they near the surface. This is due to the multiplication of cells in the lowest layer as they divide. The newly-formed cells are gradually pushed upwards. The lowest layer sits on a basement membrane.

Clearly, by forming several layers, the main function of this type of epithelium is the protection of deeper structures.

Connective tissue

This is the tissue found most widely in the human body. Some connective tissues are liquid like blood, flexible like cartilage or rigid like bone. Connective tissues lie deeper than epithelial tissues. They support, connect and strengthen other tissues while some protect and insulate body structures.

Connective tissues consist of cells located in a matrix (background substance). The matrix surrounds cells, which are therefore not attached to each other, and is often called *intercellular matrix*, because it is between the cells. The matrix is usually secreted by the cells themselves and gives the tissue most of its characteristics. Matrix can be fluid as in blood, semi-fluid as in the general white, sticky connective tissue around muscle fibres, nerves, etc. (*areolar connective tissue*), flexible and firm as in cartilage, or calcified and rigid as in bone. Many types of matrix also contain fibres such as collagen, which give added strength, or elastic fibres, which give elasticity. Some contain both.

Blood

This connective tissue consists of a fluid matrix called *plasma* in which cells or fragments of cells are suspended. Plasma is a straw-coloured liquid consisting of water in which nutrients (like glucose and amino acids), ions (sodium, chloride, etc.), enzymes, hormones and gases are dissolved. Plasma proteins found in plasma have important functions in the body.

Blood cells have diverse functions and comprise the following:

- red blood cells, or *erythrocytes*, which carry oxygen to body cells and have a role in transporting carbon dioxide away from them
- white blood cells, or *leucocytes*, which come in different forms:
  - *phagocytes* which engulf foreign materials and microbes
  - *lymphocytes* which play an important role in immunity
  - *monocytes* which behave in a similar way to phagocytes
  - *basophils* which produce an anti-clotting agent
  - *eosinophils* which are involved in allergic reactions.

Cell fragments are the platelets (or *thrombocytes*) concerned with blood clotting mechanisms.

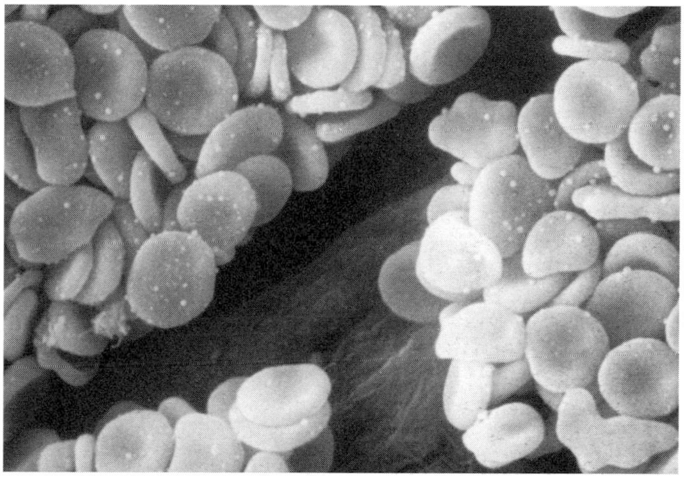

Figure 7.13 Scanning electron micrograph of normal red blood cells in a vessel lumen

Compact bone

This is the dense bone found on the outside of all bones and in the shafts of long bones of the skeleton.

The other type of bone is *spongy bone* (Figure 7.14) which forms the bulk of the heads of long bones and irregular bones. Spongy bone contains spaces filled with bone marrow and is less rigidly organised than compact bone.

Compact bone is constructed to withstand the weight of the body carried by the long bones and to protect and support other tissues. Under the microscope, this tissue is seen to be made of series of concentric circles called *Haversian systems* (or *osteones*) each with a central canal containing blood vessels and nerves (see Figure 7.14). These connect with larger blood vessels and nerves which penetrate the bone from its outer covering, the *periosteum*.

Each Haversian system has rings of hard calcified material visible and these are called *lamellae*. At

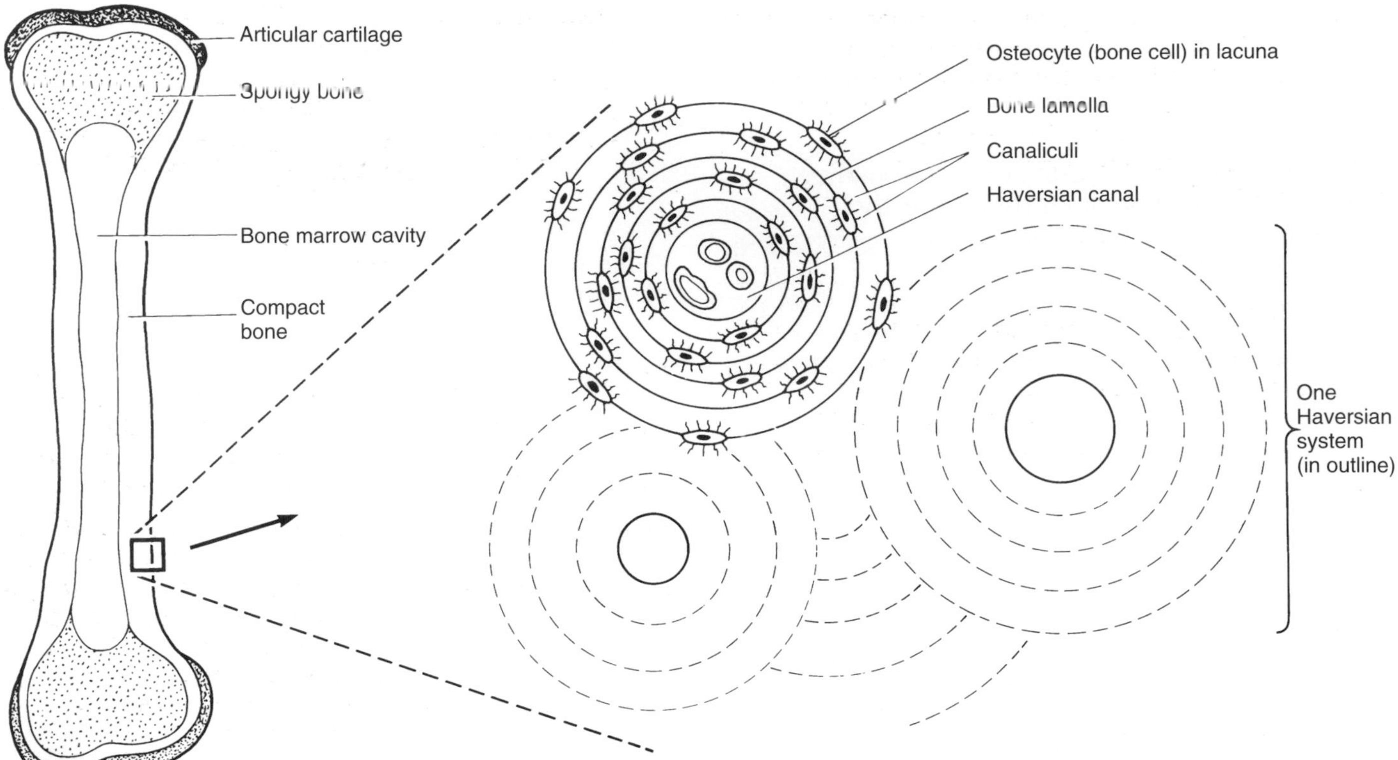

Figure 7.14 A long bone and the microscopic structure of compact bone

intervals close to the lamellae are small spaces, or *lacunae*, which house mature bone cells, or *osteocytes*. In the immature state, these cells are *osteoblasts* which secrete the matrix and become imprisoned in it. Running outwards in all directions from the lacunae are tiny channels (*canaliculi*) which are filled with fluid and contain long, finger-like processes from the osteocytes. These channels connect with other osteocyte canaliculi and eventually the Haversian canal, and in this way the cells are nourished and able to get rid of their waste products.

The matrix of bone has two major components:

- *mineral salts*, mainly salts of calcium, like calcium carbonate and a form of calcium phosphate, which form around collagen fibres and give the bone its hardness
- *collagen fibres*, which give bone its ability to bend under strain and prevent it from being too brittle like an eggshell.

Try it

Obtain two chicken (or similar) leg or wing bones. The bones should not be too large or the experiment will take too long. Clamp one bone and place in a bunsen burner flame until grey. You have burned away the collagen fibres and left the mineral salts. When the bone is cold, unclamp it – it will probably fall apart as you do this, demonstrating its brittleness.

Now take the other bone and leave it in a bath of dilute hydrochloric acid for a few hours. This dissolves out the mineral salts and leaves behind the collagen. Wash the bone in water before handling and then bend it. You will probably be quite surprised at the ease with which this can be done. Remember to observe safety rules when you carry out this experiment – you are dealing with heat and acid.

Muscle tissues

There are three types of muscle tissue in the human body:

- skeletal muscle (also called voluntary, striated or striped muscle)
- smooth muscle (also called involuntary, unstriated or unstriped muscle)
- cardiac muscle.

Each type consists of special cells known as *muscle fibres* which are capable of contraction, or shortening. In this way they cause movement or help to maintain posture. All muscles generate heat as a side effect and this contributes to maintaining body temperature. All muscles have blood and nerve supplies.

Skeletal muscle

As its name suggests, this is always attached to bones of the skeleton – it is the familiar meat we see in butchers' shops. It can be made to contract or relax by an individual's conscious control via nerve impulses, hence the alternative name of *voluntary muscle*. The individual muscle fibres show alternate bands of light and dark, thus appearing striped or striated (see Figure 7.15). Fibres in a muscle lie parallel to each other and are cylindrical in shape. There are hundreds or thousands of fibres in each individual muscle, depending on its size. The thickness and length of individual muscle fibres is variable – the largest fibres can be up to one third of a metre long and one hundredth of a millimetre thick.

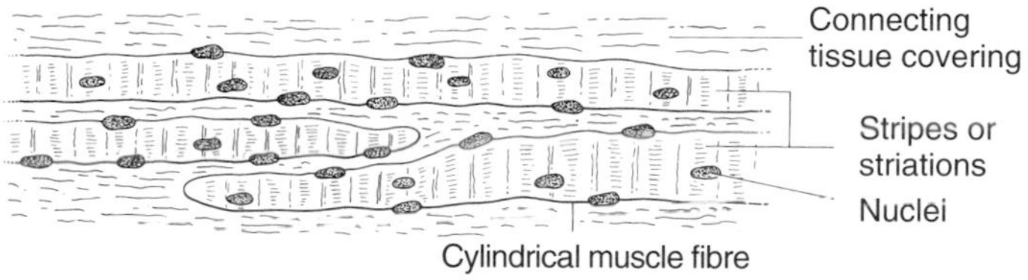

Figure 7.15 The microscopic structure of skeletal muscle

Each fibre is composed of many *myofibrils* and these are made up of tiny protein filaments. The cell membrane of a muscle fibre is called the *sarcolemma*. It encases the myofibrils and many nuclei located close to the sarcolemma. The fibre is said to be *multi-nucleate*. Large numbers of mitochondria lie close to the myofibrils in parallel rows, able to supply ATP to the fibre for the contraction process.

Smooth muscle

This type is found in the walls of arteries and veins and in sheets running in different directions around hollow organs such as the stomach, intestines, bladder and uterus. It is not attached to

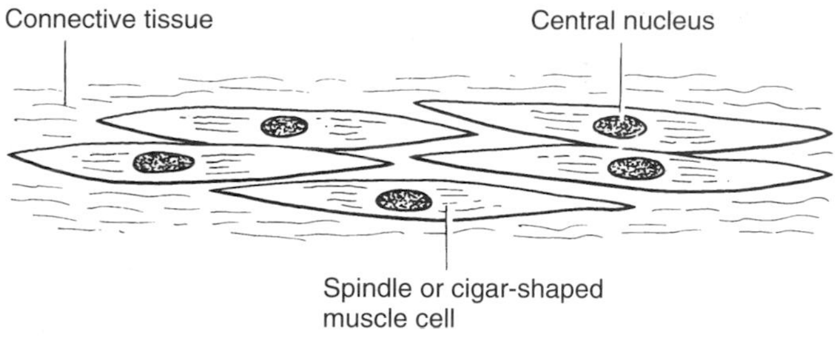

Figure 7.16 The microscopic structure of smooth muscle

bones. If you think about it, you cannot control the contraction of these muscles, hence the alternative name – *involuntary*. There are also no bands visible so it is unstriped or unstriated.

Each fibre is spindle-shaped, with a central nucleus, surrounded by a sarcolemma (see Figure 7.16). They lie dove-tailed with one another in sheets. Although these fibres still contain protein filaments they do not lie in an orderly fashion so this is why there is no light and dark banding. Recent evidence suggests that shortening or contraction occurs because the fibre twists and coils up.

Cardiac muscle

As its name suggests, this is found only in the walls of the heart. The fibres interconnect and branch with each other forming a network. Each cell is roughly rectangular with a central nucleus and packed with mitochondria. Like skeletal muscle, it shows banding but, like smooth muscle, it cannot be controlled at will. When isolated from a nerve supply, it is still able to contract and relax – a property known a *myogenicity*. The sarcolemma between adjacent cells is thickened to produce a disc-like appearance known as *intercalated discs*. This enables nerve impulses to pass very swiftly from one cell to another. When one fibre is

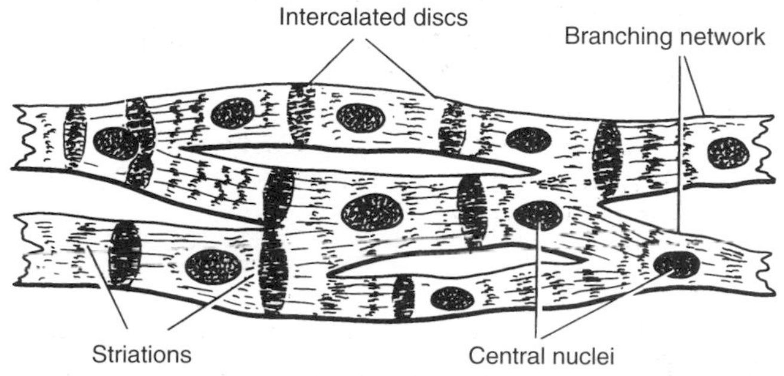

Figure 7.17 The microscopic structure of cardiac muscle

stimulated, the impulse rapidly spreads through the network of cells. See Figure 7.17.

Nervous tissue

Surprisingly, this consists of only two types of cell – nerve cells (*neurones*) and supporting cells called neuroglia. The latter are not important at this level of study.

Neurones are highly specialised cells which are either sensitive to stimuli, converting them to nerve impulses, or capable of transmitting nerve impulses to effectors or other neurones. Effectors are structures which do (or effect) things in response. In practice, these are muscles which respond by contracting or glands which respond by secretion. So basically, there are three types of functional neurones – sensory, relay and motor neurones.

All types of neurone have similar structural components:

- cell bodies, which contain nuclei and other organelles
- axons, which are single, long processes which conduct nerve impulses away from the cell body
- dendrones, usually multiple processes which carry nerve impulses towards the cell body.

Sensory neurones are mainly located intimately with sensory receptors or have their terminal portions adapted to receive stimuli themselves.

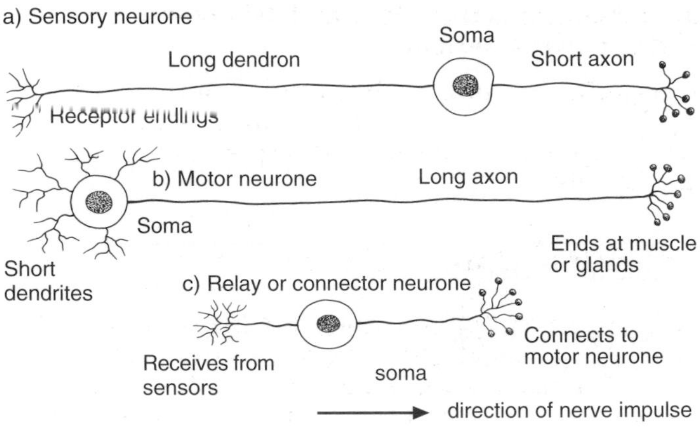

Figure 7.19 Schematic diagrams of sensory, motor and relay neurones

They usually have quite long dendrons which carry the impulses close to the brain and spinal cord where their cell bodies are located. Axons, on the other hand, have only a small distance to cover inside the central nervous system, and are therefore short.

Motor neurones are intimately associated with effectors. Their axons are long, with specially adapted endings called *neuromuscular junctions*. The dendrons travel only a short distance within the central nervous system and are short.

Relay neurones, also called *connector* and *internuncial neurones*, have relatively short axons

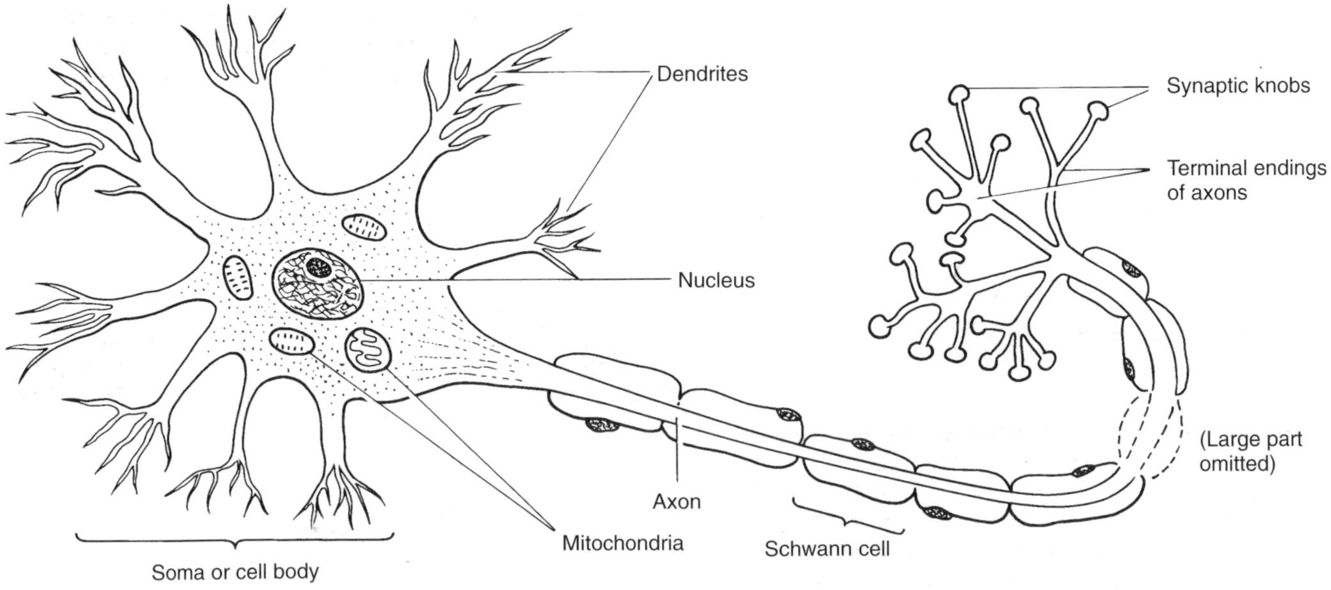

Figure 7.18 The general features of a nerve cell (neurone)

and dendrons as they lie completely within the central nervous system.

Nerve cells, like muscle fibres, are excitable cells capable of responding to stimuli by producing nerve impulses or contraction responses respectively.

Evidence collection point

Study micrographs 1–4 (page 156) carefully. (A micrograph is a photograph of a microscope image.) Identify the type of tissue shown in each micrograph and describe, using your own words, the main features of the four main types of tissue. Relate these features to their functions.

Cellular respiration

Many people confuse respiration with breathing, so it is necessary to have a clear picture of what is meant by cellular respiration. Obviously, this is a process carried out *within cells*, which carry out a number of different activities. Muscle cells contract, nerve cells transmit impulses, epithelia have a lining function so need constantly to be replaced, connective tissues support and bear strain, etc. All these activities require an energy supply. The energy has to be obtained from food. All food can be traced back eventually to green plants which carry out a process called *photosynthesis*, the chemical process by which green plants make food from carbon dioxide in the air around us, water from the soil and energy from sunlight. The energy becomes temporarily fixed in the chemical bonds which link the carbon, hydrogen and oxygen together in the molecules which make up our food. The chemical equation for photosynthesis is:

$$6CO_2 + 6H_2O + \text{sunlight energy} = C_6H_{12}O_6 + 6O_2$$

carbon dioxide + water + sunlight energy = glucose + oxygen

Digestion occurs when humans take in the long complex, often insoluble, molecules which make up our food and break them down into small units of soluble material which are capable of passing through the epithelial linings of our digestive system into the blood. However, these units, although much smaller, still lock up most of the energy in their chemical bonds. It is only inside cells that the 'equipment' exists for releasing that energy so necessary for cells, tissues, organs and organ systems to carry out their functions. Cellular respiration, then, is the release of energy inside cells. Breathing and gaseous exchange between air and lungs are part of the respiratory system, which gets the vital oxygen necessary for cellular respiration to the cells. Cellular respiration is also known in biology textbooks as *tissue* or *internal respiration*.

The overall equation for cellular respiration can be represented as:

$$C_6H_{12}O_6 + 6O_2 = 6CO_2 + 6H_2O + \text{energy}$$

glucose + oxygen = carbon dioxide + water + energy

However, it must be emphasised strongly that this is only a summary of the enormous number of chemical reactions taking place in a cell to effect respiration.

ATP (adenosine triphosphate) has already been referred to in the section on mitochondria inside cells (page 148). A base called adenine is combined with ribose sugar to form adenosine and this can attach to one or more phosphate groupings. In ATP there are three phosphates. Another compound involved in energy release is ADP (adenosine diphosphate) which has two phosphates attached. The last phosphate ATP is special – it attaches to the rest with what is termed a high energy bond. This means that the bond requires more energy to build it up, and that when it is broken it releases more energy than other bonds. When the bond breaks the

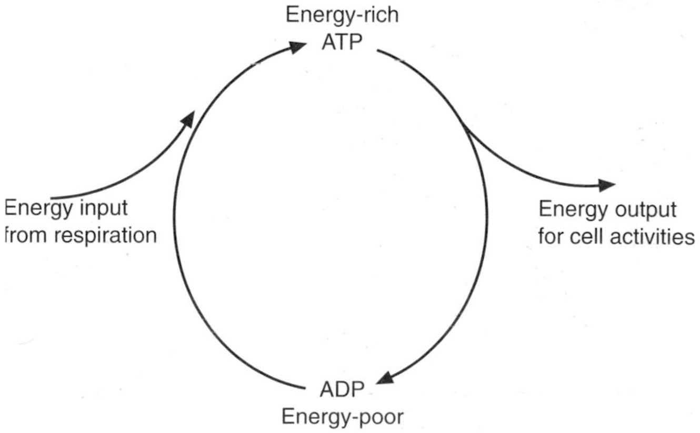

Figure 7.20 The interconversion of ADP and ATP

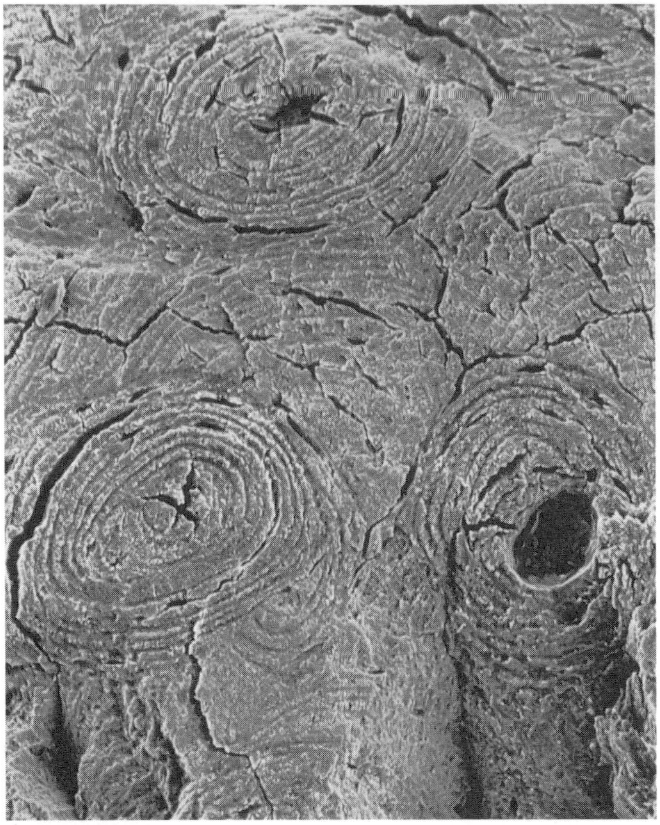

Micrograph 1

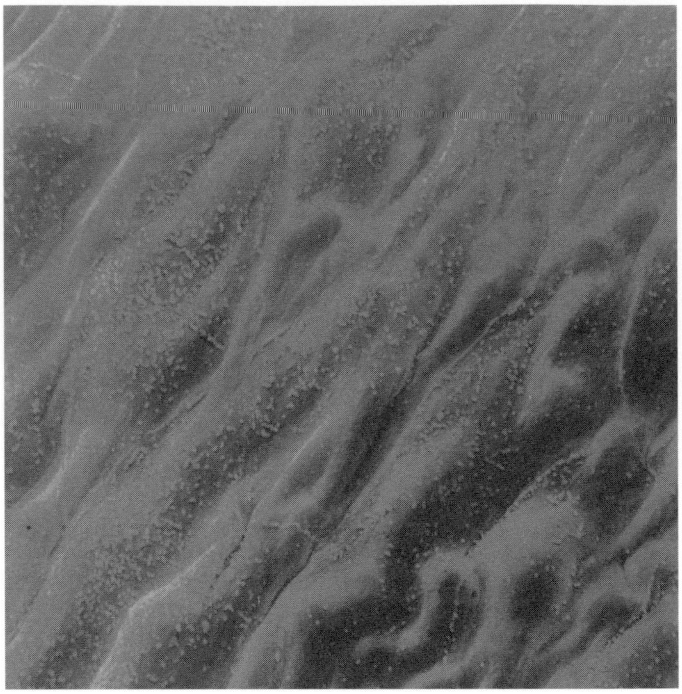

Micrograph 2

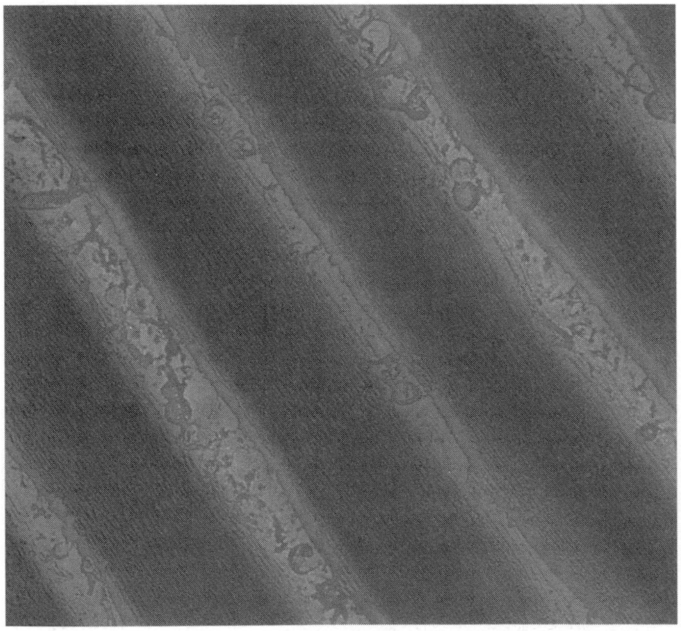

Micrograph 3

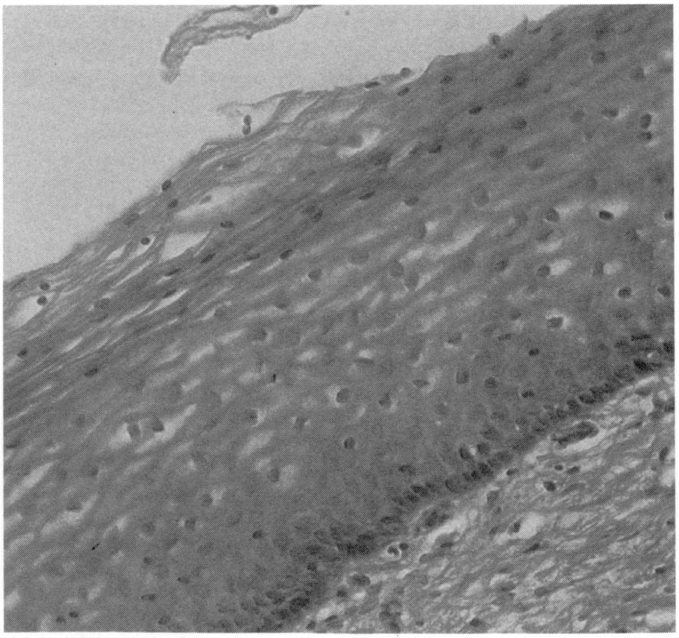

Micrograph 4

phosphate is freed and ATP becomes ADP and vice versa. The situation can be represented as shown in Figure 7.20.

ATP can hold energy and release it as required, breaking down to ADP in the process. ADP can acquire another phosphate group to become ATP providing that there is sufficient energy available to form the bond. The action is rather like a rechargeable battery.

Think it over

You wish to use your personal stereo on a caravan holiday. There is mains electricity on site but no shops. Think about the way you would do this.

To 'recharge' ATP, the cell releases energy chiefly from glucose in food. This is a relatively slow process, so ATP is used as the 'middleman' to store the energy until it is required, often in large amounts, to carry out activities. When energyless, ATP has become ADP ready to take up more energy from the oxidation of glucose. All of this takes place inside the cell's mitochondria.

Aerobic respiration

Respiration taking place when there is adequate or normal oxygen supplies available to the cell is *aerobic respiration* – it is the norm. The equation on page 155 represents aerobic respiration. The process is in two stages:

- glycolysis
- Krebs cycle.

Glycolysis

When glucose passes through the plasma membrane and into the cytoplasm, it is immediately converted to a substance called glucose-6-phosphate by the addition of phosphate from a molecule of ATP. This *phosphorylation* has the effect of trapping glucose inside the cell so that it cannot move back out again. Another ATP molecule is used as glucose-6-phosphate further breaks down to form 3-carbon fragments, each of which goes through the processes described. Altogether, there are around ten enzyme-controlled reactions which take place in glycolysis,

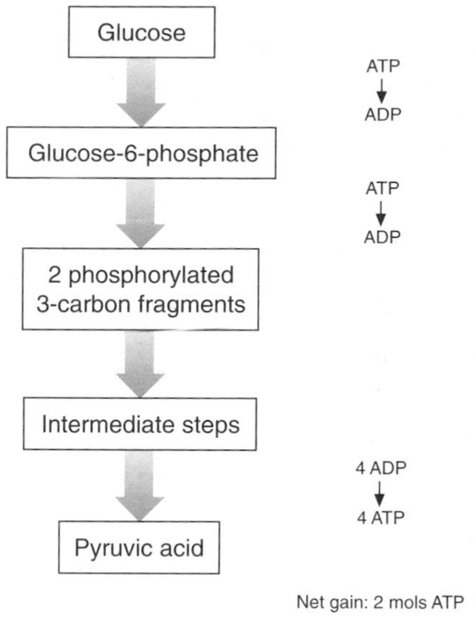

Figure 7.21 The stages of glycolysis

resulting in an intermediate product being produced known as *pyruvic acid*. See Figure 7.21.

It is not necessary to know the chemistry taking place in these ten reactions. Four molecules of ATP are generated from every molecule of glucose used during glycolysis, but remember two were used up in 'pump-priming' the process in the beginning, so there is a net gain of two molecules of ATP. This has all taken place in the cell cytoplasm.

One other interesting feature has importance here and must be mentioned. At the end of the glycolysis stage, no oxygen has yet been used. This is often known as the *anaerobic stage* of aerobic respiration but it must not be confused with anaerobic respiration although it is part of it, as we shall see.

Krebs cycle

Pyruvic acid now has to enter the mitochondria to combine with a substance called Co-enzyme A to form Acetyl Co-A, which undergoes reaction with an organic 4-carbon acid to become citric acid, a 6-carbon organic acid. An alternative name for this complex chemical cycle is the *citric acid cycle*.

Gradually the 6-carbon acids are broken down to 4-carbon acids with the redundant carbon being oxidised into carbon dioxide, a waste product. Hydrogen ions are also liberated at various points and they become converted to water molecules.

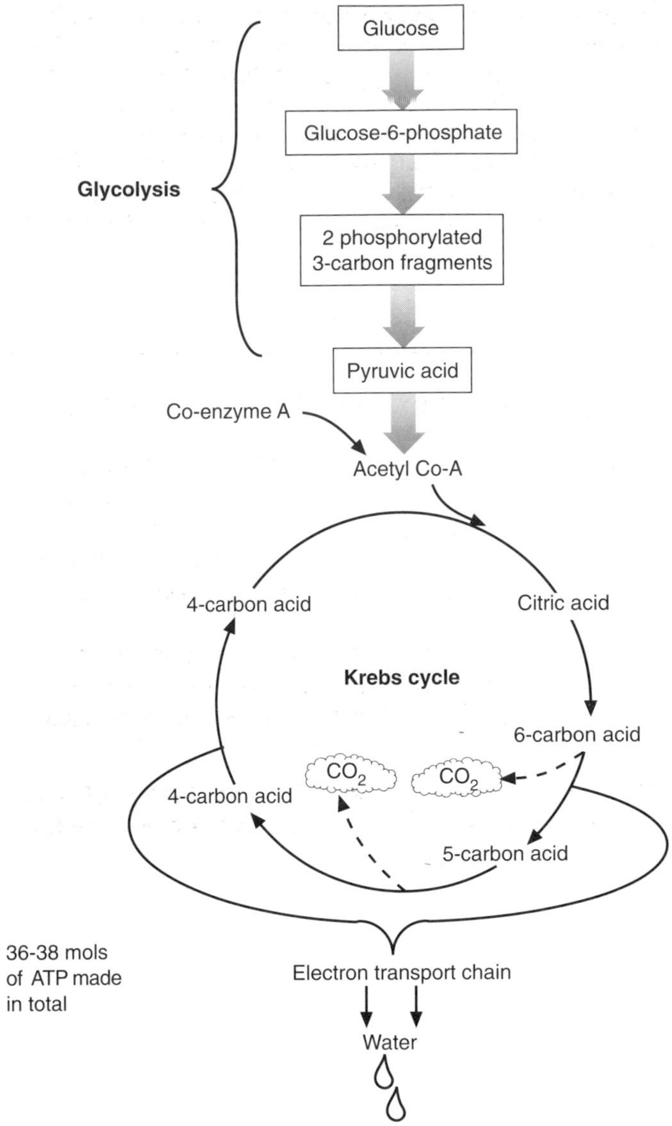

Figure 7.22 The stages of aerobic respiration

At the end of the Krebs cycle a net 36 (or 38 in some cases) molecules of ATP have been formed, including those made during glycolysis, from each molecule of glucose. The process depends on electron carriers functioning as a chain, passing ions along like buckets in a water chain. These are present on the inner folds of the mitochondrial membrane.

Krebs cycle does involve using oxygen to form carbon dioxide and water, so this is the *aerobic stage*. See Figure 7.22.

The process began with glucose molecules, but other molecules (fats and proteins) can also provide energy for the human body. Acetyl Co-A is an entry gate for intermediate products from both fat and protein breakdown to access Krebs cycle.

Anaerobic respiration

This type of respiration occurs when oxygen is in short supply and it cannot be delivered by the heart, lungs and circulation in the quantities required to meet the energy demands. It is helpful to visualise this in terms of an athlete taking strenuous exercise, where the muscle cells are not getting the oxygen in the amounts required, therefore resulting in being short of breath – anaerobic respiration.

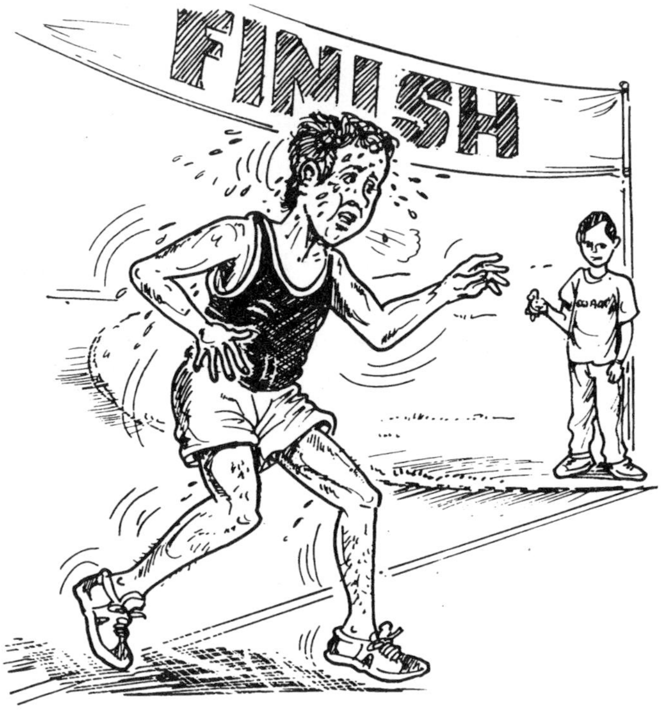

You will recall that the first stage of aerobic respiration, glycolysis, did not use oxygen at all. The process can proceed to the formation of pyruvic acid, but not into Krebs cycle. Pyruvic acid acquires extra hydrogen ions from the electron carriers and becomes lactic acid. This is the product of anaerobic respiration. Only two molecules of ATP have been formed, so the process is not efficient in the production of energy and is time-limited. A further disadvantage lies in the fact that an acid is produced, and enzymes essential to the respiratory process become

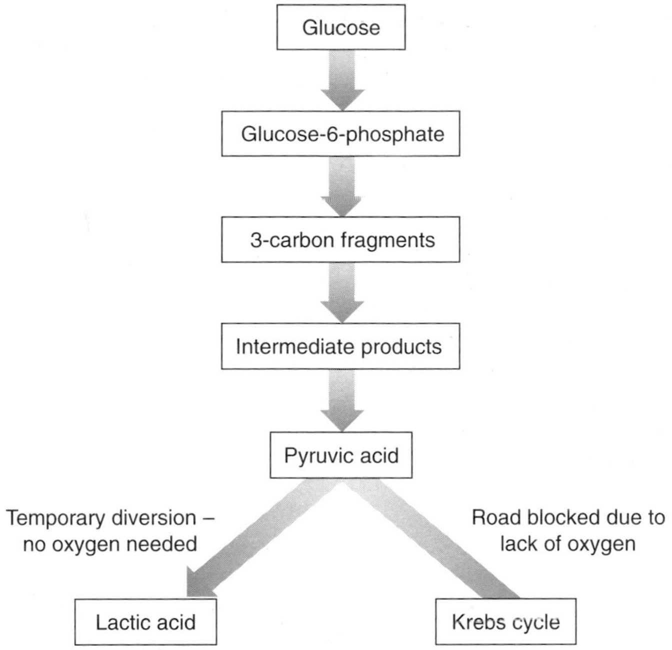

Figure 7.23 The stages of anaerobic respiration

denatured, or inactivated, in the presence of too much acid.

Lactic acid diffuses from the muscle cells into the blood and eventually reaches the liver where it is oxidised, when oxygen becomes available again, to form carbon dioxide and water. An oxygen debt is built up when the oxygen available for the work or exercise does not match the oxygen taken in through the respiratory and cardiovascular systems. As we all know, debts have to be paid back after borrowing so this is why we carry on breathing fast for some time after the exercise has finished.

Evidence collection point

Write a report explaining the following:

a what is meant by the term cellular respiration
b the role of ATP in energy storage and release
c what happens to a glucose molecule when it enters a cell in the presence of oxygen until the final production of carbon dioxide, water and energy release (aerobic respiration)
d the sequence of events taking place in muscle cells during strenuous exercise, when oxygen intake does not match oxygen needs (anaerobic respiration).

When you have completed all the evidence collection points in this chapter you will have the evidence for your portfolio for Element 3.1.

Chapter 8

The functions of the main organ systems

This chapter focuses on:

- how body systems perform functions – communication, support and locomotion, reproduction, energy supply, excretion, defence
- homeostatic mechanisms – body temperature, blood sugar, water, respiratory rate
- the effect of ageing on body systems – support and locomotion, reproduction, homeostasis.

How body systems perform functions

Communication

The human body consists of millions of *cells,* each with its own complicated internal structure which carries out a large number of different functions. Some cells are newly-formed, others undergoing reproduction; some are functioning at the peak of their performance and others are in decline or even dying. Yet all these cells must be able to function together as a whole for healthy performance of the human body. New examples of the way in which cells act together are constantly being discovered by medical researchers. For the purposes of organisation of study, cells are grouped together to form *tissues* (see Chapter 7), tissues are grouped together to form *organs* and organs carrying out special functions are classified as *organ systems.* Although all organ (body) systems must have methods of communicating, some have a more well-defined communication role. Those described in this section will be:

- circulatory system
- nervous system
- endocrine system
- sense organs.

Circulatory system

To understand the principles of communication, it is necessary to have a basic understanding of how the circulatory (or cardiovascular) system is organised and how it functions.

The circulatory system comprises the heart and its associated blood vessels, i.e., arteries, veins and capillaries.

The heart

The heart is about the size of a clenched fist, situated in the chest (or thoracic cavity). It lies behind the sternum and in front of the oesophagus, protected on either side by the ribs and their cartilages (see Figure 8.1). The heart is surrounded by a tough double-layered fibrous sac called the *pericardium.* There is a thin fluid film between the two layers of the pericardium which reduces the friction of the heart's movement.

At first sight, the heart appears to be a single organ but, in reality, it consists of two muscular pumps working side by side. It will help us to understand the way the heart works if we consider these pumps to be separate to begin with.

Imagine that the heart is sliced vertically through its central partition, which is known as the *septum.* Each pump now has an input tube (or vessel) and an output vessel. *Note:* an important point to remember with any textbook diagram is that the heart drawn on a page is opposite to the way it is sited in the body. To place the diagram as it is in the body you could lift the book or page and place it in front of your chest, facing outwards – the sides now correspond to your left and right sides.

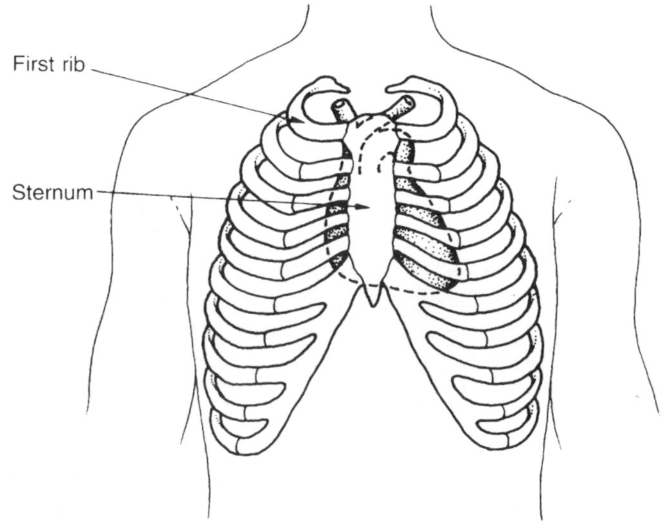

Figure 8.1 The position of the heart

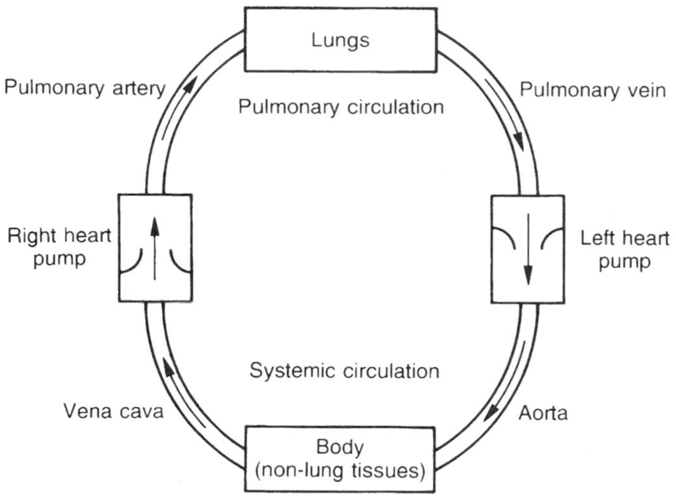

Figure 8.2 Blood flows around the body in a circle

Each pump consists of two chambers: an upper chamber called the *atrium* (plural, atria) and a lower, the *ventricle*. Atria have *veins* supplying them with blood and ventricles have *arteries* taking blood away from them. The right pump receives blood from the body (or non-lung) tissues and sends it to the lungs. The left pump receives blood from the lungs and sends it to the body. In this way (as you can see from Figure 8.2), blood flows around the body in a circle.

Blood vessels taking and receiving blood from the lungs are said to form the *pulmonary circulation,* while those concerned with the non-lung tissues form the *systemic circulation.* Arteries carry blood away from the heart, so there is the *pulmonary artery* serving the lungs and the aorta delivering blood to the rest of the body. Veins bring blood back to the heart, so again we have pulmonary veins from the lungs, but *vena cava* from the body. In fact, there are two venae cavae: the *superior* from the head and neck, and the *inferior* from the trunk and lower limbs.

The term *double circulation* is often used in human physiology because there are two circulations and the blood passes through the heart *twice* (through each half pump). The function of the pulmonary circulation is to allow the blood to release carbon dioxide and take up oxygen to supply the tissues. The systemic circulation acts in the opposite way: to release oxygen to the tissues and take up carbon dioxide to carry to the lungs. Following this through, the right side of the heart carries blood poor in oxygen, called *deoxygenated* blood, while the left side distributes oxygen-rich, or *oxygenated,* blood to the body or *somatic* tissues. The two pumps can now be imagined working side by side (see Figure 8.3).

As blood flows in a circle, it must flow at the same rate through the blood vessels, whether they are large, near to the heart, or very small, supplying a group of cells. If the flow of blood was not at the same rate serious 'traffic jams' of blood could occur – causing a lack in other parts of the body. This might prove fatal if the part of the body concerned was a vital organ such as the heart itself, the brain or the kidneys. There are about five litres of blood in the human body, more in males than females, and resting blood flow is approximately five litres every minute. So, on average, all the blood in a person flows around the body once every minute. There will be more details about blood flow later in the chapter.

You can understand that with such importance attached to these circulations, blood could not be permitted to flow in a reverse direction – particularly through the heart. To ensure this never happens, the heart is fitted with four *one-way valves.* Two are located deep inside the heart, between the atria and the ventricles on each side; and two more are

The *myocardium* is the name for the heart muscle.
The *endocardium* is the name of the smooth endotherlial lining of the cavities.

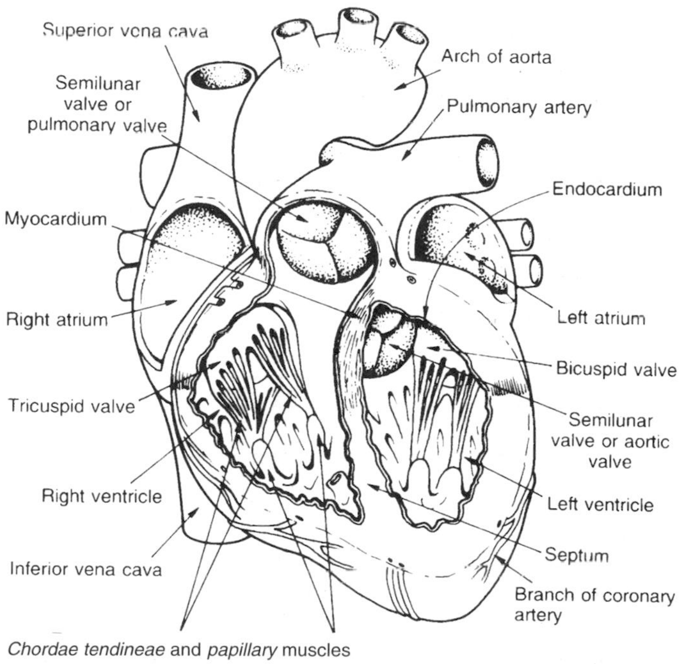

Figure 8.3 A section through the heart

situated just inside the major blood vessels which carry blood away from the heart. The one-way valves cannot operate on their own; they are relatively flimsy and do not contain any muscle. They open and close due to the forces which push them from either side. This force is called *blood pressure* and it is the force which blood exerts on the walls of the heart or the blood vessels. (See Chapter 9, page 184.)

The valves between the atria and the ventricles are often termed *right* and *left atrio-ventricular valves,* but you will find their older names more commonly in text-books. The left-hand valve is known as the *bicuspid valve* and the right-hand one the *tricuspid valve.* (A cusp is the meeting point of two arcs, so 'bi' means two meeting points and 'tri' means three.) The valves lie in a fibrous ring which separates the atrial muscular wall from that of the ventricles. The valves are tethered to the walls of the ventricles by *tendinous cords* and small lumpy *papillary muscles.* These exert tension on the valves and prevent them being turned inside out during periods of extreme pressure; rather as an umbrella can do in a high wind! They function like guy ropes on a tent. The other two valves take their names from the vessels in which they are found, namely the *aortic* and *pulmonary valves.*

Cardiac muscle

The muscle that makes up the heart is of a special type found only in that place and, not surprisingly, is named *cardiac muscle.* Its fibres interconnect to form a network, along which the nerve impulses can pass rapidly to make the heart beat. This muscle, however, is capable of contracting without nerve impulses and this is called being *myogenic.* (See Figure 8.4.)

Cardiac muscle cannot rely upon the blood flowing through for its essential raw materials; it has a special blood supply from the *coronary* arteries and veins. These can be seen running over the external surface of the heart. They bring dissolved oxygen and nutrients to the heart muscle and carry away carbon dioxide, water and other waste products.

The atrial muscle beats at a faster rate than that of the ventricles so, practically, nervous control is important in making the heart contract in a coordinated and purposeful way. Sometimes, if the nervous route is not functioning correctly or is even interrupted, the heart can adopt an irregular pattern; this usually occurs as part of a disease process.

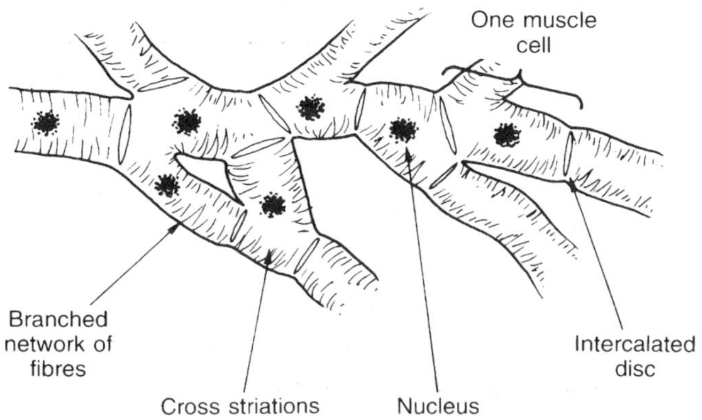
One muscle cell
Branched network of fibres
Cross striations
Nucleus
Intercalated disc

Figure 8.4 Cardiac muscle tissue

Nervous conduction through the heart

A cluster of special cells lie in the upper part of the right atrium and every few moments they become excited, sending nerve impulses across the branching network of the atrial muscle fibres to cause contraction. This cluster is called the *sino-atrial node* (shortened to the S-A node) or more commonly termed the *pacemaker,* because this is indeed what these cells do. These impulses are caught by yet

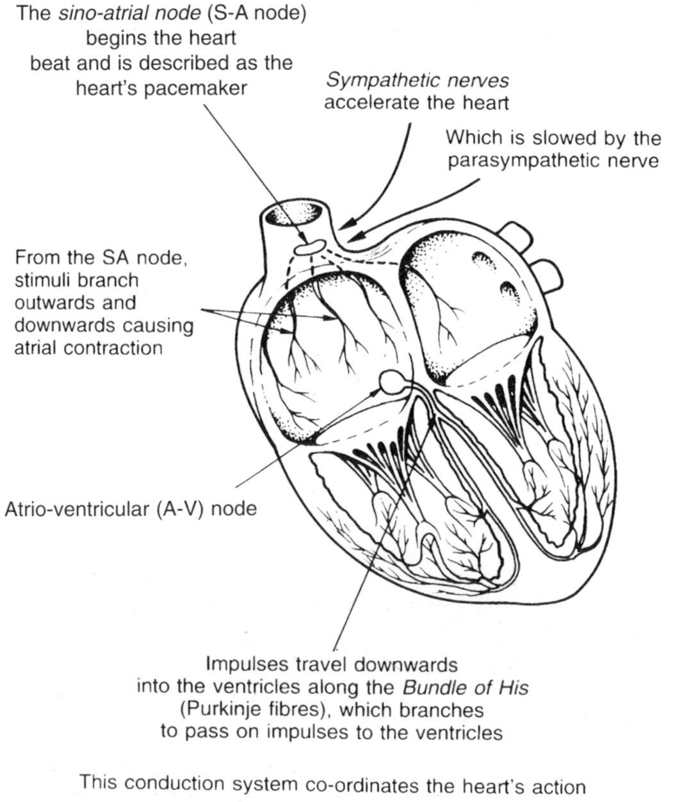
The *sino-atrial node* (S-A node) begins the heart beat and is described as the heart's pacemaker
Sympathetic nerves accelerate the heart
Which is slowed by the parasympathetic nerve
From the SA node, stimuli branch outwards and downwards causing atrial contraction
Atrio-ventricular (A-V) node
Impulses travel downwards into the ventricles along the *Bundle of His* (Purkinje fibres), which branches to pass on impulses to the ventricles
This conduction system co-ordinates the heart's action

Figure 8.5 The heart's conduction system

another group of cells forming the *atrio-ventricular node* (A-V node) and relayed to a special band of tissue made of large *Purkinje fibres,* adapted to conduct impulses efficiently. The A-V node delays the transmission to allow the atria to complete their beat. The Purkinje fibres form the *Bundle of His* (or A-V bundle) which crosses the fibrous ring separating atria and ventricles, and then divides into *left* and *right bundle branches* running either side of the septum before spreading over the ventricles. (See Figure 8.5.)

Impulse conduction is very fast so that the two ventricles beat together to force the blood around the body organs.

If the conduction system fails artificial pacemakers can be fitted which supply electrical stimuli from their batteries to stimulate the cardiac muscle direct.

Nervous control

Despite this elaborate conduction system, the heart also has a nervous control to allow for an almost instant response to the dangers and stresses of everyday life. There are two sets of nerves constantly making a play for control over the heart's rate by influencing the S-A node, which is only rarely allowed to beat at its own pace. Both nervous commands form part of the *autonomic nervous system* which co-ordinates and controls the internal organs (or viscera) of the body. One set continuously tries to calm the heart down, slowing its pace and reducing the strength of the beat. This is the *parasympatheic* branch of the autonomic nervous system, which unceasingly aims for peace and contentment. The other branch is the *sympathetic,* aiming for increased strength of heartbeats and a stirring of pace. It is called into action during muscular work and stress (see Figure 8.5). The sympathetic branch is closely associated with the release of the hormone *adrenaline.*

Cardiac cycle

The events which take place during one heartbeat form the *cardiac cycle.* If the heart-rate, at rest, is counted at around 70 beats each minute, then the time for each beat is 1 ÷ 70 minutes or 60 ÷ 70 seconds. This works out as approximately 0.8 seconds for each beat of the heart.

If this is represented by 8 small squares, each to the value of 0.1 second, then we can produce a diagram as shown in Figure 8.6. If we wish to show events happening in the atria and ventricles during this period, we can have two 'timelines'. The shaded squares represent when the cardiac muscle is contracting and the plain squares, relaxation. Contraction phases are called *systole* or *systolic periods* and relaxation periods *diastole* or *diastolic periods.* (See Figure 8.7.) These names are also used for the two figures in a blood pressure measurement (see Chapter 9, page 184).

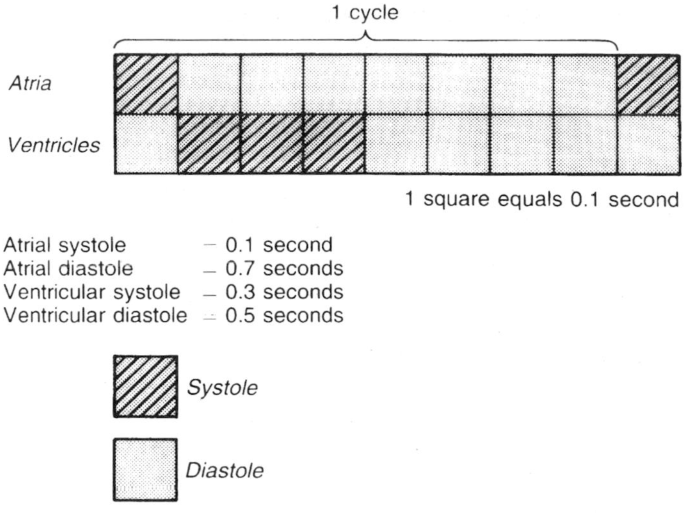

Figure 8.6 Timed events in the cardiac cycle: allocations of systole and diastole

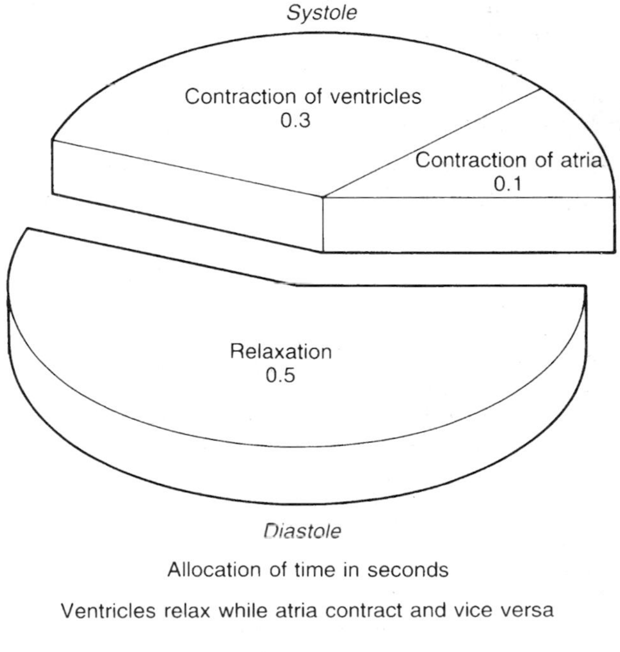

Figure 8.7 Cardiac cycle: resting phase

The events in the cardiac cycle can be described as follows:

1 Atria contract, blood is pushed into ventricles under pressure.
2 Ventricles bulge with blood, pressure forces the tricuspid and bicuspid valves shut. This causes the first heart sound to be heard with a stethoscope; it sounds like 'lub'. Atria relax and begin to fill with blood.
3 Ventricles begin contraction, pressure in blood rises and forces open the aortic and pulmonary valves.
4 Systole in the ventricles pushes blood into the aorta and pulmonary artery. These are elastic walled and begin to expand.
5 Ventricles begin to relax and blood falls back with the effect of gravity for a few moments and catches in the pockets of the semi-lunar valves of the aorta and pulmonary artery, pressing them together and closing off the opening. This causes the second heart sound which, through a stethoscope, sounds like 'dupp'.
6 Tricuspid and bicuspid valves are forced open and blood rushes from the filled atria into the ventricles during their diastolic phase. On being filled to about 70 per cent capacity, atrial systole occurs and the heart has completed the cycle at the point where it started.

Note: in a healthy heart, both the two atria and the two ventricles contract simultaneously.

Blood vessels

These tubes, together with the heart, make up the circulatory system. The main types of blood vessel are:

- arteries
- veins
- capillaries.

Each type has functional and anatomical differences which are summarised in Figure 8.8.

Each organ has an arterial and a venous supply bringing blood to the organ and taking blood away respectively. The link vessels supplying the cells of the tissues of the organ are the *capillaries*. A protein-free plasma filtrate driven out of the leaky (selectively permeable) capillaries becomes the tissue or interstitial fluid which supplies the cells. It is through the blood and tissue fluid that raw materials for respiration, hormones, enzymes, etc. get to the cell organelles (see Chapter 7). This is also the route for communication, as the circulatory system must go to all organs.

Arteries	Veins	Capillaries
Functional differences Carry blood away from heart to organs Carry blood under high pressure	**Functional differences** Carry blood to heart from the organs Carry blood under low pressure	**Functional differences** Connect arteries to veins Arterioles and capillaries cause greatest drop in pressure due to overcoming the friction of blood passing through small vessels.
Usually contain blood high in oxygen, low in carbon dioxide and water *What are the exceptions?* Large arteries close to the heart help the intermittent flow from the ventricles become a continuous flow through the circulation.	Usually contain blood low in oxygen, high in carbon dioxide and water	Delivers protein-free plasma filtrate high in oxygen to cells and collects up respiratory waste products of carbon dioxide and water.
Anatomical differences (see diagram) Large arteries close to the heart are almost entirely made of elastic tissue to expand and recoil with the outpouring of blood from the ventricles during systole. Arteries have thick walls with corrugated lining and round lumens. Walls consist of three layers, endothelial lining, muscle and elastic tissue, and outer tough fibrous layer.	**Anatomical differences** Veins have thinner walls than arteries Veins have oval spaces in centre (lumina) Veins over a certain diameter contain valves which prevent blood flowing backwards under the influence of gravity. Veins usually lie between skeletal muscles which squeeze blood flow onwards during muscular activity. Walls have three coats but far less muscle and elastic tissue and more fibrous tissue.	**Anatomical differences** Capillaries have walls which are only one cell thick. Capillaries have leaky walls (permeable) enabling small molecular nutrients and dissolved gases to exchange with cells. No cell can lie more than a few cells from a capillary. Capillaries often smaller than red blood cells which must distort to pass through.

Figure 8.8 Functional and anatomical differences between arteries, veins and capillaries

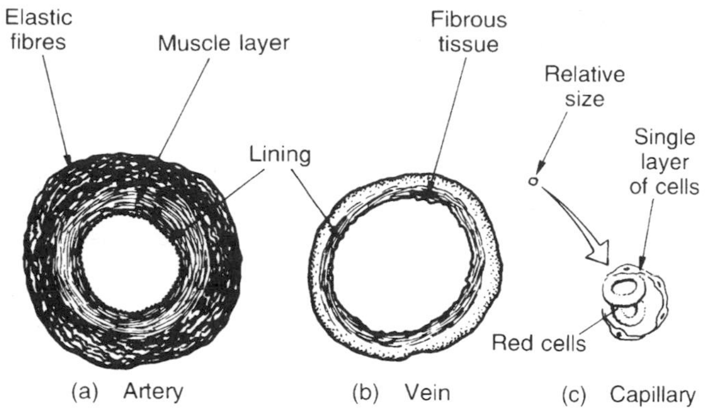

Figure 8.9 Blood vessels, transverse sections

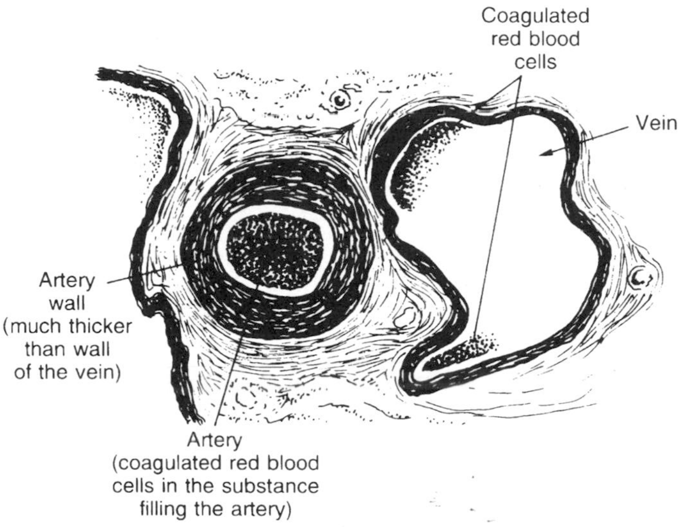

Figure 8.10 Transverse section through a vein and an artery

Nervous system

This system is the fastest means of communication in the human body, used to control, co-ordinate and inform organs of change. The nervous system consists of:

- the central nervous system (brain and spinal cord)
- peripheral nerves (cranial and spinal nerves)
- the autonomic nervous system.

All consist of nerve cells (or neurones), their fibres and supporting cells (neuroglia). Features of neurones have been discussed in Chapter 7, page 154.

Neurones bringing nerve impulses from sensory receptors to the central nervous system (CNS) are

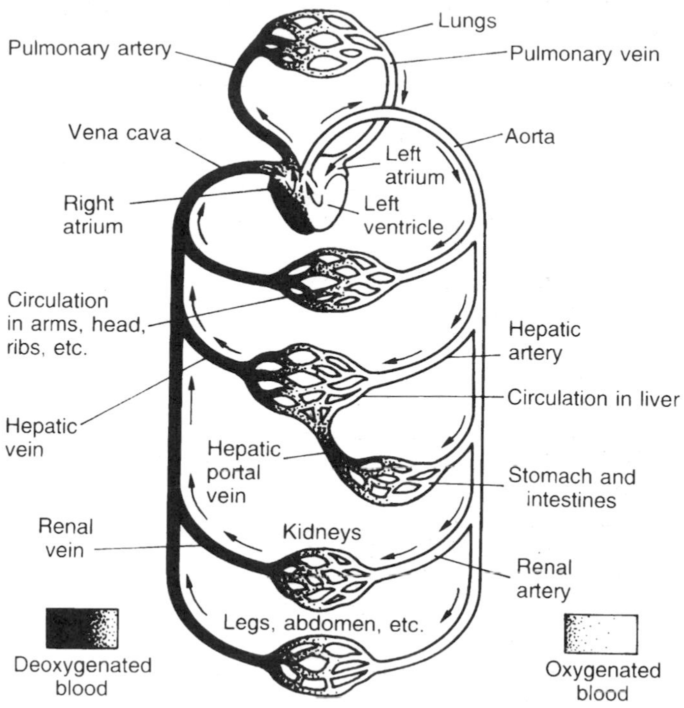

Figure 8.11 The human circulatory system

sensory neurones and those bringing impulses from the CNS to effect change are *motor neurones*. Where neurones link these, they are known as *relay, connector* or *internuncial neurones*. Information from external sources such as the skin receptors responding to environmental temperature change, pain, pressure, touch, light, sound, taste, smell, etc. are said to be under the influence of the *somatic nervous system* (CNS and peripheral nerves). Changes

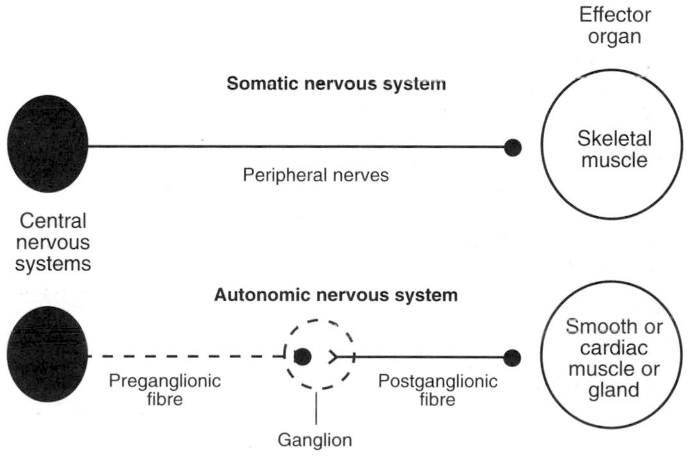

Figure 8.12 The somatic and automatic nervous system

within the body, such as alteration of heart and breathing rate, rhythmic contractile activity of smooth muscle, are under the control of the autonomic nervous system.

There are large numbers of sensory receptors of different types in the human body, each type responding to a particular type of stimulation. Some reach our conscious levels, like pain, change of external temperature, etc., while many others are continually monitoring at a subconscious level, such as changes in blood pressure, flow of digestive juices, etc.

A stimulus may be defined as a change in environment which activates sensory neurones. The role of sensory neurones is to respond to such a stimulus and convert it to nerve impulses. This process is known as *transduction* and sensory receptors function as *transducers*. It must be emphasised at this point that all impulses are similar. In other words, impulses derived from pain receptors are no different from impulses, say, from a change in temperature. How then, are we able to tell the difference? The subsequent pathway and destination of those impulses cause us to interpret them differently. For example, light impulses activated photoreceptors in the light sensitive retina of the eye travel to the hindmost part of the brain, the *occipital cortex,* to be interpreted as pictures – we describe this as seeing or visualising. Impulses from sound receptors in the organ of Corti (the audioreception part of the ear) travel to a completely different part of the brain, the *temporal lobe,* to be interpreted as sound. The actual impulses are identical. It is possible in theory to 'transplant' the nerve carrying the impulses from the organ of Corti to the occipital lobe and have sounds interpreted as vision, and vice versa. So, if you rang a bell in such circumstances, the ringing could be interpreted visually, though it probably would appear as a series of flashing lights rather than an organised scene. This produces another problem – how do we know whether a stimulus is slight or marked if the outcome is the same? Each impulse, once produced, has exactly the same magnitude as the next impulse, i.e. there are no small or large impulses. Differentiation of information comes through in the spacing and frequency of impulses. This can be seen in Figure 8.13.

The nerve impulse, also known as an *action potential,* is a wave of electrical excitation produced by migration of ions (charged particles) across the cell membrane of a neurone. The stimulus results in changes in ionic concentrations. This wave of excitation travels down the neurone until it reaches the branched endings known as *synaptic knobs*. Once there, a minute break in protoplasmic continuity between neurones or neurone/gland or muscle interface must be overcome. The tiny gap between excitable cells like this is called a *synaptic cleft* and is filled with extracellular fluid. At synapses, impulses cause the release of neurotransmitter molecules to flood the cleft, diffuse across and attach to specific receptors on the next (or post-synaptic) neurone's cell membrane. Once the receptors are 'filled' sufficiently, a further wave of excitation is triggered down the post-synaptic neurone.

It can be seen from this description that a wave of electrical excitation becomes transformed into chemical signals across synapses and converted back to electrical phenomena in the next cell.

It is interesting and vital to note that impulses are able to travel in only one direction across a synapse as the facilities for producing neurotransmitters are present only at the expanded endings of the first (or pre-synaptic) neurone.

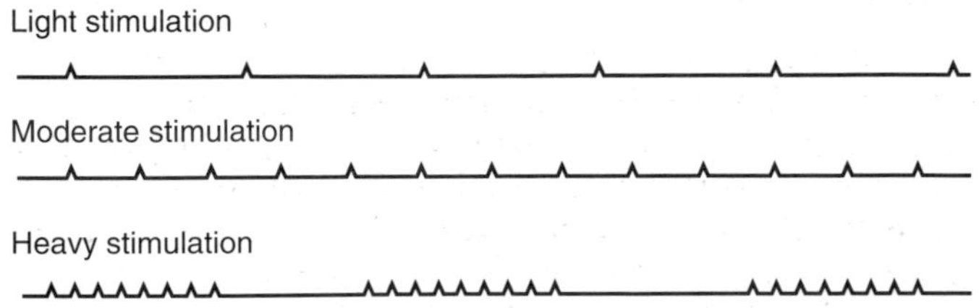

Figure 8.13 Differences in spacing and frequency of impulses

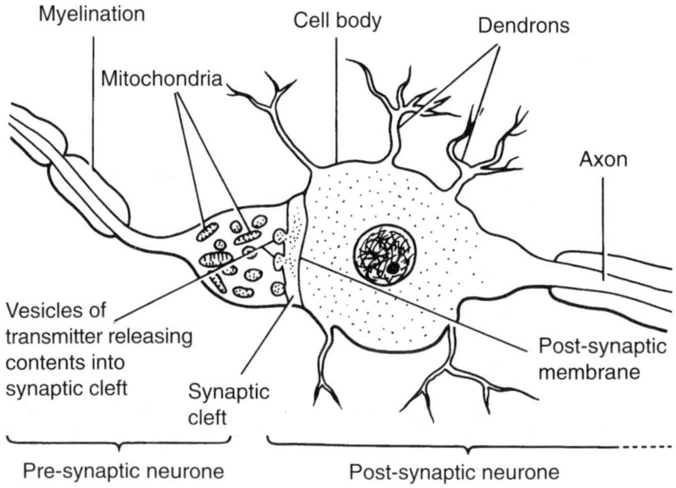

Figure 8.14 A synapse

Neurotransmitter chemicals form the main vehicle for drug action on the nervous system. Any inhibitor of the transmitter must slow down the action of impulses crossing the synapse and vice versa. Once released the transmitter is broken down fairly rapidly (or impulses begin to merge) and the products of the breakdown are recycled into neurotransmitter molecules again using energy from ATP in the neurones' mitochondria. This process takes time and, if there has been continued stimulation over a steady period, neuronal fatigue might occur due to depletion of neurotransmitter molecules. There may be hundreds of synapses impinging on one neurone.

Usually several synaptic endings need to release transmitters at the same time for a nerve impulse to be set up in the post-synaptic cell (*spatial summation*). When one synaptic ending receives impulses several times in rapid succession, these also may be added together to create a post-synaptic impulse and this is known as *temporal summation* (see Figure 8.15). Impulses generated by weak stimuli may not be adequate to summate either in space or time, so the impulse gets no further than the first synapse.

In this way, sensory overload is avoided – we are not constantly aware of the feel of our clothes on our skin, for instance and the feel of chairs, patterns of noise, etc. do not pass into the memory part of the brain. If selection from the constant bombardment of our senses did not occur, human brains would be enormous. Synapses therefore act as 'goalkeepers' of information, passing on only the essential in communication and co-ordination.

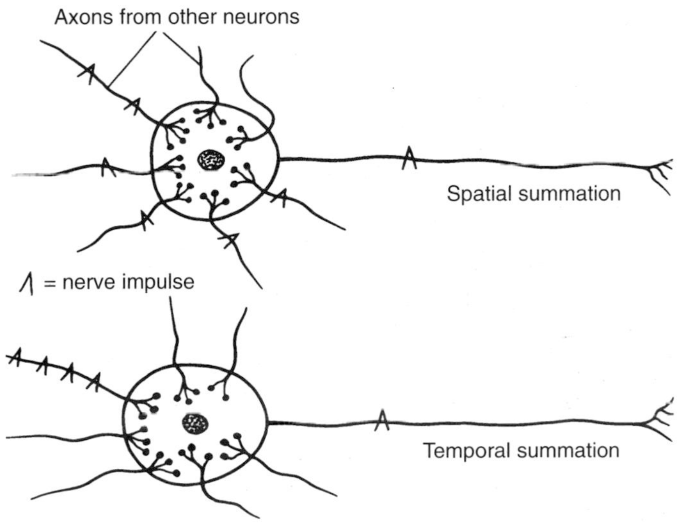

Figure 8.15 Spatial and temporal summation

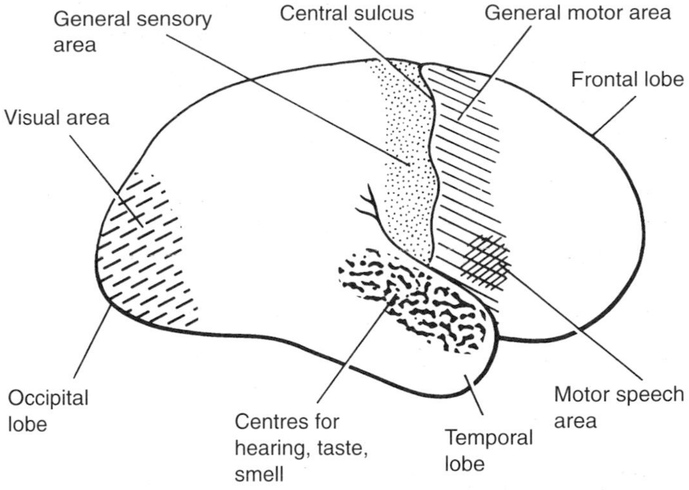

Figure 8.16 The functional areas of the brain

The greatest bulk of neurones used in communication function in the brain. There are two types of matter in the brain, *grey* and *white matter.* Grey matter contains the vital cell bodies of the neurones, while white matter consists of the tracts of fibres, in practice axons and dendrons, on their way to and from other parts of the brain or other organs. The large cerebral hemispheres, which occupy most of the skull, have grey matter on their surface holding billions of neurones. The *cerebrum* is the seat of intelligence, giving us the ability to read, write, speak, remember, plan ahead and, above all, think.

The sensory part of the cerebrum lies mainly behind a large central fissure (or *sulcus* as it is called) in the brain. Information arriving here enables us to locate with precision where the sensation is coming from. Otherwise we would feel pain, for instance, but be unable to locate exactly where the pain was coming from. The intact sensory area of the cortex is essential for this. Centres for speech, hearing, taste and smell lie below the general sensory area in a protruding side lobe – the *temporal lobe.* The visual area lies at the back of the brain. (See Figure 8.16.)

The motor area of the brain lies in front of the central sulcus in the cerebrum. Stimulation in this area leads to muscle contraction in a specific location on the opposite side of the body. Conversion of speech into thoughts and thoughts into speech take place in an area close to the temporal lobe, but within the motor area. Transference of impulses between the CNS and other parts of the body uses the routes provided by the peripheral nerves. These are collections of axons (motor nerves), dendrons

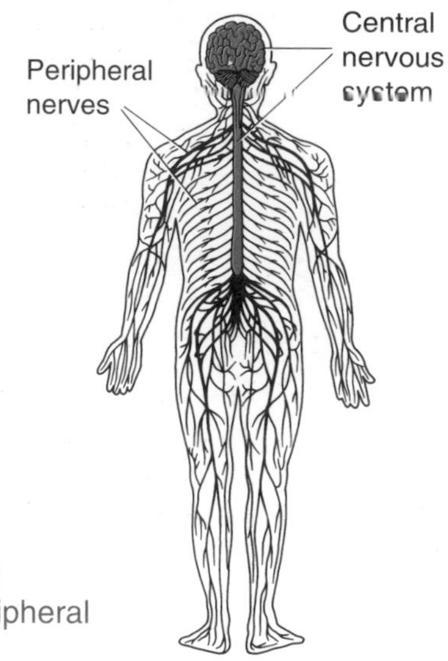

Figure 8.17 The central nervous system and peripheral nerves

(sensory nerves) or, more commonly, a mixture of both (mixed nerves).

Communication from the brain to the internal organs of the body is the role of the autonomic system. This system has two distinct parts known as the *sympathetic* and *parasympathetic branches*. These serve to act rather like a brake, slowing activities down, or as an accelerator, speeding activities up. Unfortunately, it is not possible to say that the sympathetic is the accelerator and so on, because both systems carry out a combination of activities. There is some value, however, in considering the role of each system and this can lead to a satisfactory understanding.

The role of the sympathetic nervous system is to prepare the body for emergencies, commonly known as *fright, flight* and *fight* reactions. This is a response built to enable survival from predators and is not wholly suitable for modern-day living, but unfortunately we have to live with it. The main activities of the sympathetic system are:

- releasing more energy-rich glucose from storage
- providing more oxygen to unlock the glucose energy
- distributing the energy, providing raw materials to muscles and a few other places
- bypassing most organs not useful in an emergency, such as the skin and the alimentary canal
- activating any other activity useful in an emergency, such as sweat secretion, making skin slippery to predators and aiding cooling
- enhancing the activity of the nervous system by harnessing hormonal communication as well.

As you will see from Figure 8.19 these functions involve

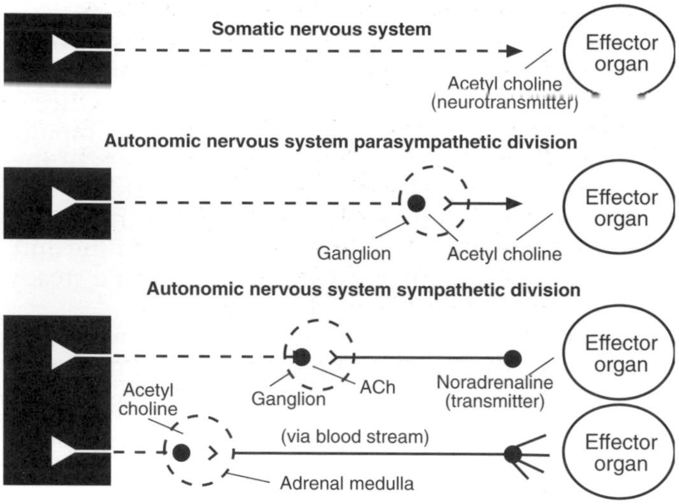

Figure 8.18 The sympathetic and parasympathetic systems of the autonomic nervous system

the cardio-respiratory system to a great extent. The parasympathetic system, by contrast, is activated more during peace and contentment, calming the heart and breathing rates, yet speeding up digestive processes.

Endocrine system

This system interlocks and works with the nervous system to provide communication and co-ordination throughout the human body. Whereas the nervous system is based on waves of excitation passing down specialised neurones, the endocrine system consists

	Sympathetic nervous system	Parasympathetic nervous system
1	Leaves thoracic and lumbar sections of spinal cord	Leaves cranial and sacral regions of the central nervous system
2	Short pre-ganglionic neurones and long post-ganglionic neurones	Long pre-ganglionic neurones and short post-ganglionic neurones
3	Ganglionic chain at the side of the spinal cord	Ganglions in the walls of organs
4	Associated with fight, fright and flight response	Associated with peace and contentment
5	Closely linked with medulla of adrenal gland	Not linked in this way

Figure 8.19 The differences between the sympathetic and parasympathetic nervous systems

of several glands secreting chemicals known as *hormones* to effect change. Hormones, literally meaning to urge on, are secreted directly in to the bloodstream and use the circulatory system as a route for distribution. A common analogy is often made that the nervous system is like a telephone system, fast and efficient but only able to go if the correct wiring is available, whereas the endocrine system is like the postal system, much slower but able to get to every cell. Figure 8.20 summarises the differences between the two systems.

Nervous system	Endocrine system
Electro-chemical phenomena form 'message' – action potentials or nerve impulses	Chemical molecules for 'message' – known as hormones
Travels down nerve fibres	Travels in blood stream
Has rapid transmission	Much slower transmission
Travels to cells supplied only by nerve fibres	Travels to all cells in body

Figure 8.20 The differences between the nervous system and the endocrine system

Hormones can be steroids (derived from cholesterol), proteins or products of proteins (peptides, amines). They affect certain cells which are fitted with cell membrane receptors for that particular hormone, either directly through an enzyme-based system or via the nucleic acids in the nucleus. Most hormones are secreted in short bursts with little or no secretion in between. Under stimulation the bursts become more frequent, so raising the blood concentration of that particular hormone. In the absence of stimulation, the bursts become less frequent and the blood hormone levels decrease. This is part of a feedback process, see page 177.

Hormones are generally used where the effect is long-term or where time is not an important factor, such as growth and control of reproduction.

Figure 8.21 shows the location of major endocrine glands.

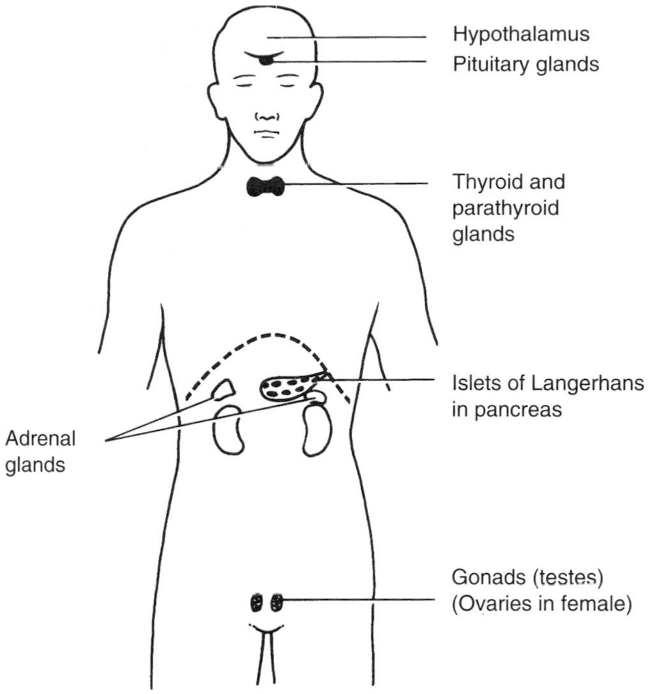

Figure 8.21 The main endocrine glands in the body

The basic functions of hormones are:

- control of most stages of reproduction
- significant role in growth and development
- assistance with smooth and cardiac muscle contraction
- regulation of metabolism, including energy release
- control of extracellular fluid volume and composition
- maintenance of homoeostasis, even in emergency situations.

Specific hormone action is discussed on page 178.

Sense organs

Sense organs are associated with the nervous system, being reliant on it for the interpretation of impulses and subsequent action. Sense organs are collections of sensory receptor cells gathered together to perform a special function.

The special senses comprise seeing, hearing, smelling, tasting and balance (equilibrium). Their reception of stimuli is more intense and more complicated than the general senses like touch, temperature, etc. The sense organs have particular areas of the brain devoted to their interpretations. If these are seriously damaged, the sense is diminished or even absent. The sense organs and associated sensations are:

- vision – eye
- hearing – ear (cochlea)
- smell – nose
- taste – tongue
- balance – ear (semi-circular canals).

Sense organs detect change in the external environment and inform the central nervous system.

Support and locomotion

Skeletal muscle and compact bone have already been described in Chapter 7. An overview is now required to examine the functions of these tissues for the activities of the human body.

The human skeleton provides a bony framework for the support, not only of the whole body but also for individual parts, for example, the skull (cranium) supports and protects the soft brain and the vertebral column supports the spinal cord.

Essential movements such as lifting food to the mouth, breathing and giving birth would be impossible without the support given by the skeleton. Bones may be *long bones* (femur, humerus), *short bones* (wrist, ankle) or *irregular* (bones of the face, vertebrae). They are connected to each other at *joints*. Joints may be fixed, allowing no movement at all, slightly moveable or freely moveable (synovial). It is only at joints that parts of the skeleton change their relative positions. Bones which are attached to the centre or axis of the body form the *axial skeleton,* while the limbs and their girdles make up the *appendicular skeleton.*

Freely moveable joints

The ends of the bones participating in the joint are covered in *articular cartilage,* a glassy slippery surface which reduces friction and protects the bone ends from wearing away. A strong articular capsule surrounds both bone ends, completely enveloping the moving parts. The outer layer of the capsule is tough and fibrous, but the inner lining is of synovial membrane and is more delicate. *Synovial membrane* secretes *synovial fluid* which occupies the capsule and separates bone ends. The outer part of the capsule is usually further reinforced by bands of parallel, slightly elastic fibres. These are the *ligaments* and are there to prevent a joint from over-stretching. External to the ligaments are *tendons* from surrounding muscles. Tendons attach muscle to bone, whereas ligaments attach bone to bone. Tendons are constructed of collagen fibres which interlink and merge with bone collagen. When surrounding muscles contract they pull on tendons and cause the bones to move at the joints.

Different synovial joints cause movement in different planes, but they all have the characteristic features described. Some joints have additional structures, particularly those which are weight-bearing and

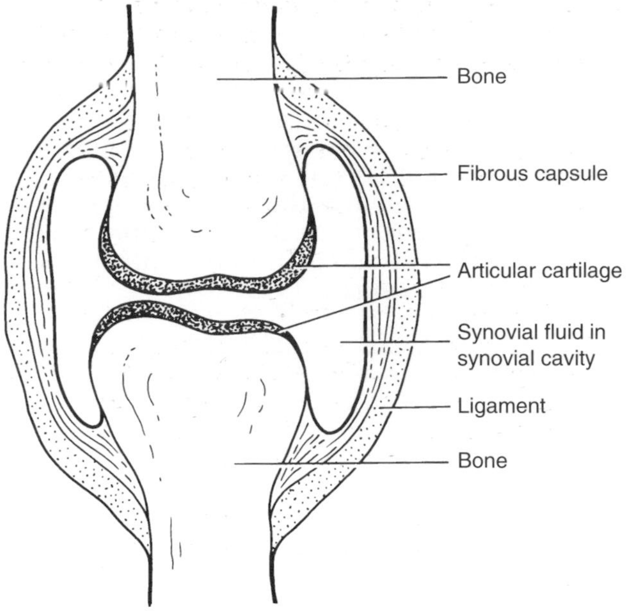

Figure 8.22 A synovial joint

subject to twisting movements, such as the knee joint. This has extra discs of cartilage in the joint and also extra internal ligaments which hold the joint surfaces together. Both of these structures are liable to injury in people who pursue vigorous sports with considerable twisting, for example footballers.

Skeletal muscles are encased in tough connective tissue which extends beyond the muscle fibres to form the tendons. Only when the muscle fibres receive nervous impulses do they undergo contraction or shortening. The nervous impulses flow from motor neurones in the grey matter of the spinal cord. A motor neurone and all its associated

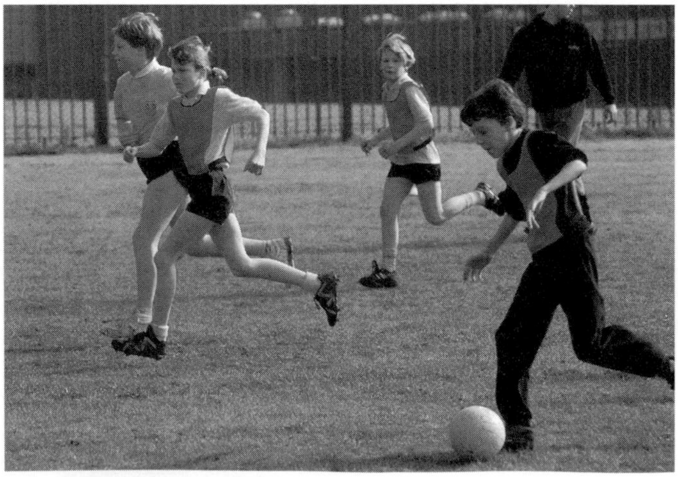

muscle fibres is known as a *motor unit*. Large powerful muscles like the quadriceps in the thigh may have 2000 muscle fibres supplied by one motor neurone, yet small precise muscles, such as those responsible for moving the eyeball in its socket, may have around five muscle fibres in each motor unit. When a motor neurone is stimulated all of its associated muscle fibres contract.

The point at which the motor neurone ending enters the muscle fibre is specially adapted, usually this is around the mid-point of the fibre. Basically having the same structure as a synapse, this is called a *neuromuscular junction*. The post-synaptic membrane is, of course, the membrane of the muscle fibre and it is the *motor end-plate*. Motor end-plates contain neurotransmitter receptors and, when these are filled by neurotransmitter, a muscle action potential spreads outwards in both directions, initiating the contractile process in both directions along the muscle fibre. Contraction of muscle requires energy, which is obtained from a small ready-made supply of ATP inside the muscle fibre and from oxidation of glucose within the fibre. Glycogen, the storage compound of glucose, is found within muscle fibres.

Muscles only pull and never push, which means that muscles must function in pairs at the very least. One muscle to pull the bone into a new position and another situated in an appropriate position to return the bone to its original location. Pairs of muscles acting in this way are acting *antagonistically*. Such action is best illustrated by the action of two muscles in the upper arm, the biceps and the triceps (see Figure 8.23).

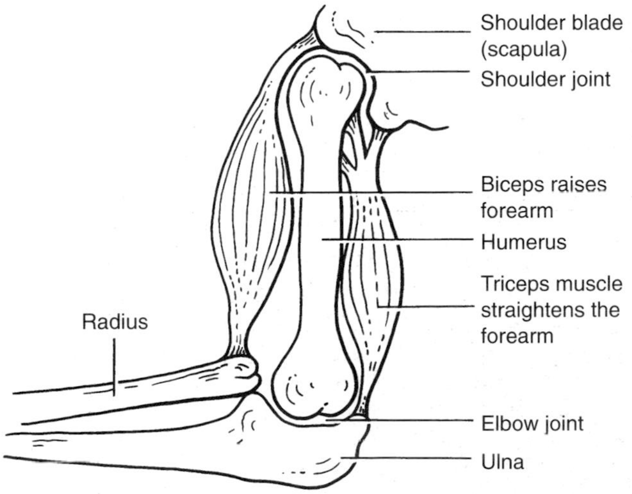

Figure 8.23 The action of the biceps and triceps muscles

The action of biceps is to pull the arm upwards, known as *flexion*, whereas triceps straightens the arm, *extension*. Clearly, if both muscles contract at the same time, the bones will remain stationary, so when one contracts the other relaxes, and vice versa.

For most movements, more than one pair of muscles are in action – whole groups are involved. Some of these will be steadying nearby joints and helping to support the body against the pull of gravity.

Reproduction

In the processes which cause new individuals to be born, reproductive organs, hormones and the circulation are intimately woven together. Primary sex organs, also known as *gonads*, produce *gametes* and *hormones*. Gametes are cells which cannot develop further unless united with another gamete from the opposite gender. Females produce *ova* and males *spermatozoa*, each has only half the chromosome content (*haploid*) found in a normal somatic cell (*diploid*). Gonads are associated with ducts (tubes) which are capable of transporting, storing and receiving gametes. Other organs produce supportive materials and are known as *accessory glands*.

The male reproductive system

Male gonads, or *testes*, hang in skin bags below the abdomen where it is cool enough for sperm to be

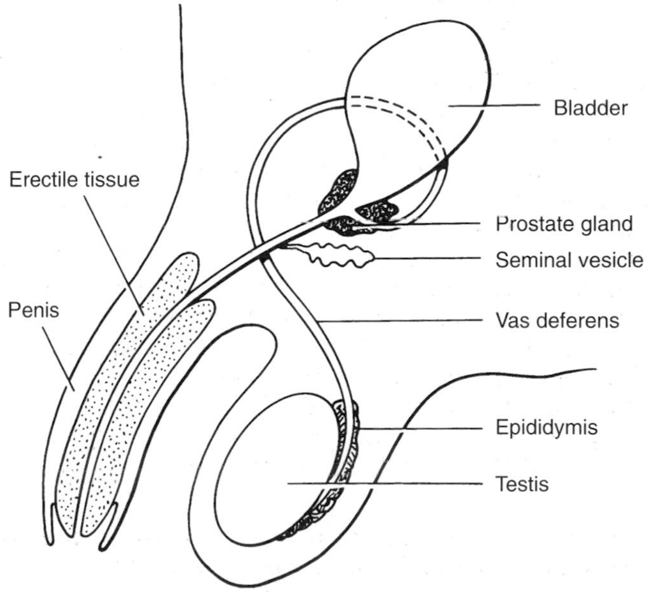

Figure 8.24 The male reproductive organs

manufactured. Testes consist of large number of coiled *tubules,* whose lining cells are constantly dividing, ending in the formation of immature spermatozoa. One of these divisions is the reduction division to halve the number of chromosomes and is known as *meiosis,* the remainder follow the usual pattern of cell division, *mitosis.* The complete process is known as *spermatogenesis* and is under the control of a hormone from the pituitary gland lying at the base of the brain, *follicle stimulating hormone* (FSH). A second pituitary hormone (these two hormones are collectively known as gonadotrophins), *luteinising hormone* (LH) stimulates special cells lying between the seminiferous tubules of the testis where spermatogenesis is occurring, to produce the male hormone, *testosterone.* Testosterone is responsible for:

- the development which occurs at puberty
- sexual behaviour
- sex drive
- the physical changes which differentiate males from females.

All these hormones travel to their target cells via the circulatory system.

The female reproductive system

The system in females is somewhat similar in its hormonal associations, but different in the length of fertility, the number and production of gametes.

The formation of eggs (*ova*) is by a process called *oogenesis* and has similar meiotic and mitotic cell divisions. Generally, one ovum is produced every 28 days, compared to a possible 300 million mature sperm daily from a male. The lining of the uterus is shed and replaced every month from adolescence to middle age. After the menopause is reached, fertility decreases and finally ends. A male may go on producing sperm well into his eighties!

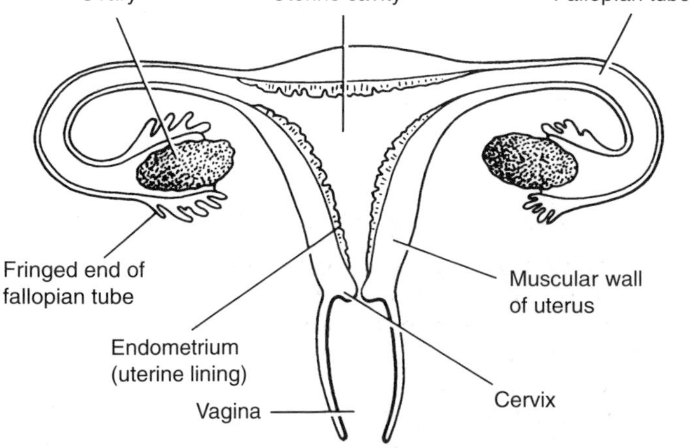

Figure 8.25 The female reproductive organs

A female is born with all the eggs in her ovaries to last her lifetime – no new eggs are made. After puberty has been reached, pituitary FSH starts an ovum ripening at the beginning of the 28-day menstrual cycle and LH causes this ovum to burst out of its fluid-filled sac in the ovary around day 14 (*ovulation*). In the meantime, as the ovum and its surrounding collar of follicle cells has developed, *oestrogen* has been secreted into the bloodstream. Oestrogen is the female equivalent of testosterone and is responsible for promoting:

- growth and development of the female reproductive tract
- development of secondary sexual characteristics such as curvy outline, breast development, etc.
- some fluid and electrolyte control
- some physical characteristics.

The ovum enters the fallopian tube where it may or may not be fertilised by a male sperm.

The rest of the follicle undergoes healing and becomes a minute endocrine gland in its own right. Secreting progesterone, it prepares the lining of the uterus for implantation by the embryo should the ovum be fertilised. If fertilisation does not take place, the lining is shed from the body with a small loss of blood in menstruation, and the whole process begins again. If fertilisation is followed by successful implantation, pregnancy has begun. Oestrogen and progesterone levels must be maintained at a high level to prevent the next menstruation from occurring. All these hormones travel to their destinations via the circulation.

Energy supply

Cell respiration has been discussed in Chapter 7. We will now consider how the digestive system, respiratory system and circulation work together to deliver raw materials to the cells to enable cellular respiration to occur and release energy. Circulation has been mentioned previously and it will suffice to emphasise those parts which serve the lungs.

Blood vessels taking and receiving blood from the lungs form the *pulmonary circulation.* The pulmonary artery leaves the heart with blood low in oxygen and high in water and carbon dioxide. The pulmonary vein returns blood to the heart having received oxygen and delivered carbon dioxide and water. The process between these two states is referred to as *gaseous exchange.*

Gaseous exchange

This involves the exchange of dissolved gases between the alveoli and the blood in the capillaries of the pulmonary vessels. The exchange depends on a process called *diffusion.*

Diffusion is defined as the movement of molecules from a region of high concentration to one of low concentration. (In the respiratory system the important molecules are dissolved gases – oxygen and carbon dioxide.) In reality, this is sound commonsense: if one starts with a lot of anything in one place and a few in another, after a period of time and random movement the numbers should become more even! This is exactly what happens in the lungs. Air, with a high percentage of oxygen molecules, is inside the alveoli; while pulmonary artery blood in the capillaries surrounding the alveoli is low in oxygen molecules. Diffusion occurs because the two single cell layers of the alveolar and capillary walls allow the molecules to 'even up' and oxygen passes into the blood.

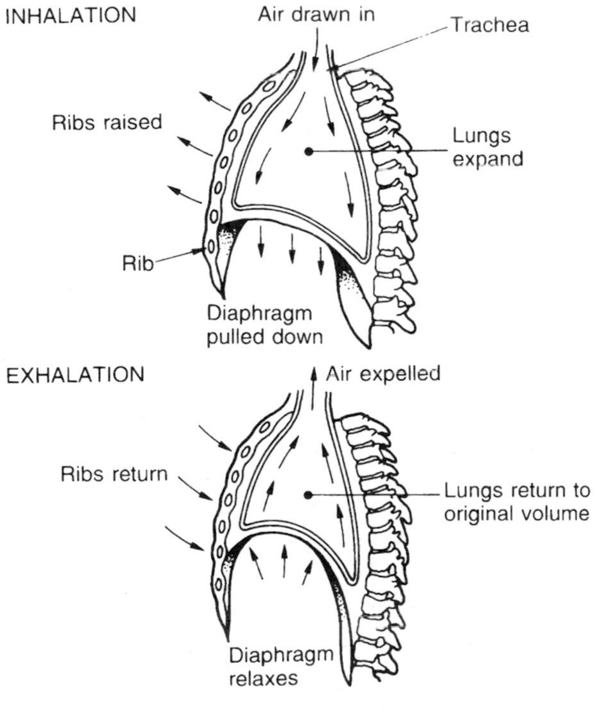

Figure 8.26 Inspiration and expiration

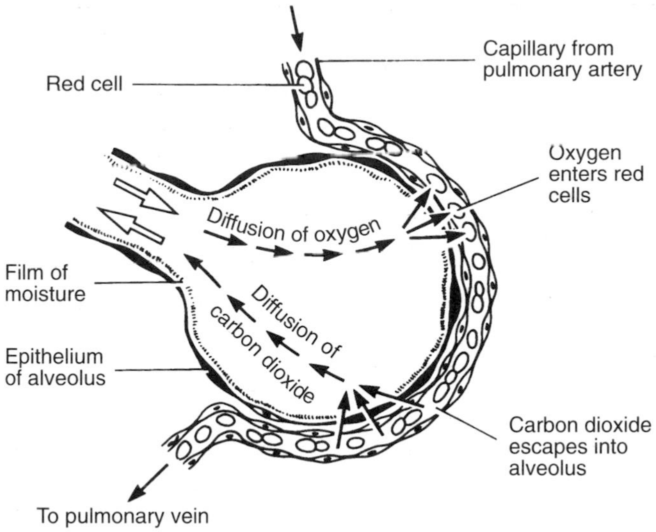

Figure 8.27 Gaseous exchange in the alveolus

Exactly the same process happens with carbon dioxide (and water vapour) but in the reverse direction, because the high concentration is in the capillary blood and the low concentration is in the air in the alveolus. Atmospheric air contains 0.04 per cent carbon dioxide, i.e. virtually none. This exchange means that air breathed out contains less oxygen and more carbon dioxide and water than inspired air (see Figure 8.28).

Content	Inhaled %	Exhaled %
Oxygen	21	16
Carbon dioxide	0.04	4
Water vapour	Variable	Saturated
Nitrogen	79	79

Figure 8.28 The composition of breathed air

The lungs are well adapted to this function because:

- they have a very large surface area due to the millions of alveoli present inside them
- they have an intimate association with the pulmonary capillaries; only two single cell layers separate them
- the constant refreshing and removal of air maintains the concentration gradients between the diffusing molecules

- the capillaries amalgamate to form the pulmonary vein which takes away the diffused oxygen via the blood. You may realise that the pulmonary vessels are opposite in their oxygenation to other arteries and veins – see the table in Figure 8.8

Carriage of dissolved gases

Blood is also well-adapted for this function of gaseous exchange. There are five million tiny red blood cells (*erythrocytes*) in every cubic millimetre of blood. Average blood volume is 5 to 6 litres, depending on the gender and size of an individual.

Erythrocytes contain a very special pigment called *haemoglobin*. This is able to form a compound with oxygen known as *oxyhaemoglobin*. It does this very readily in the conditions of high oxygen concentration which exist in the lungs. Even more remarkable, oxyhaemoglobin breaks down to release its oxygen under the low oxygen conditions which exist in cells. Cells are low in oxygen because oxygen is continually being used up in the process of cell respiration. Thus oxygen is carried to body cells by the red pigment, haemoglobin, found in the erythrocytes.

Carbon dioxide is carried in the watery part of the blood, the plasma, and only has brief contact with red cells. It uses parts of water molecules to form hydrogen carbonate (HCO_3), and on reaching the lungs breaks down to form carbon dioxide and water again.

The digestive system converts the large insoluble molecules which make up our food into simple soluble substances capable of being absorbed through the lining of the small intestine to enter the blood. To accomplish this in the short space of time between swallowing the food and its arrival in the small intestine (at most about three hours) demands the use of some miracle food 'bulldozers' called *enzymes*. Digestive enzymes are secreted in digestive juices from the appropriate parts of the alimentary canal. For example, the mouth secretes *amylase* in saliva and this breaks down starchy food to sugars and the stomach secretes gastric juice which secretes *protease,* capable of breaking down proteins to shorter chain molecules known as *polypeptides*.

Amylases and other enzymes belonging to the carbohydrate group gradually break down complex carbohydrates until sugars, particularly glucose, are produced. This is now a simple enough compound to pass through cell walls to participate in cellular respiration. However, it should be noted that a hormone is essential for glucose to actually pass through cell membranes – insulin (see page 179). Having brought together oxygen and glucose through the cell membrane, internal or cellular respiration can proceed to release energy via glycolysis and Krebs cycle (see Chapter 7, page 157).

Excretion

Excretion is the removal of waste products of metabolism. Metabolism is the sum total of chemical reactions taking place in the body. Many people do not realise that for a substance to be an excretory product it must have entered the flesh of the body. The alimentary canal is considered in this regard to be a hole through the centre of the body and faeces (excreta) are not excretory products as they have never been part of the flesh (except for bile pigments).

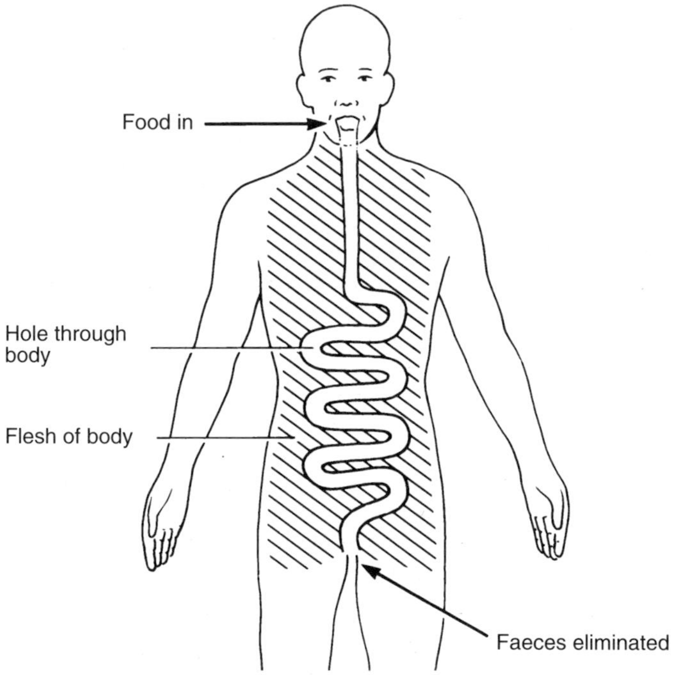

Figure 8.29 The formation of faeces

What the are the true products of excretion? Carbon dioxide and water must be, as they have been formed as a result of cellular respiration. Urea passed out in urine and bile pigments are too, as they were once haemoglobin and part of a red blood cell.

Now the excretory products are known, which are the organs responsible for the elimination? This is explained in Figure 8.30.

Excretory organ	Excretory product	Mode of excretion
Lungs	Water Carbon dioxide	Saturated expired air
Skin	Water Salts	Sweat
Kidneys	Urea Water Salts	Urine
Liver	Bilirubin Biliverdin	Pigments colouring faeces

Figure 8.30 The excretory organs and their products

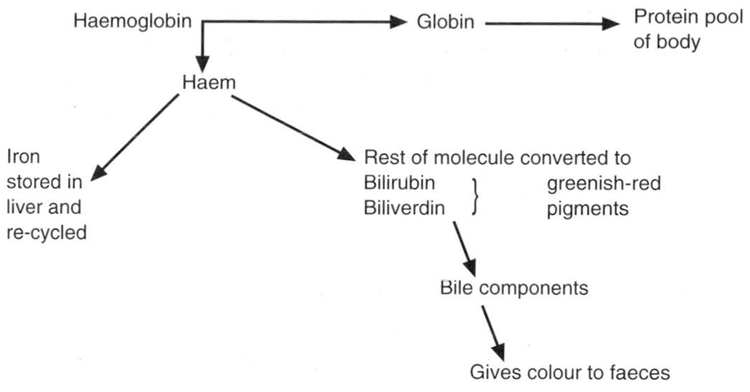

Figure 8.31 The excretion of bile pigments

Water is removed from the body in expiration, urination and through sweat. Expiration and the removal of carbon dioxide have been described previously in this chapter (page 173) and the other methods will be discussed under water homoeostasis (see page 180).

Urea is manufactured as a waste product of metabolism by the liver, but eliminated from the body by the kidneys. Protein in our diet is broken down to simple soluble substances known as *amino acids*. These are the basic building blocks of cells, which can be thought of as fatty bags of protein in their simplest sense. However, most of us take in more dietary protein than we need. The surplus amino acids cannot be stored in the human body. They can be broken down further and used for energy (passing through the Krebs cycle process), but this leaves the nitrogen-containing part of the molecule yet to be eliminated. The breaking-down process occurs in the liver and is known as *deamination* – the nitrogenous group becomes converted into ammonia.

If you have ever put smelling salts (based on ammonium compounds) to your nose, you will understand how toxic ammonia can be to human cells. Clearly, ammonia can only exist for a brief moment as it needs to be converted to a less toxic compound – urea. Toxic at certain concentrations, urea is far less toxic than ammonia and can be removed in a more or less continual cycle in urine formed by the kidneys. It is dissolved in the water of plasma and transported to the kidneys for removal by the circulatory system. Urine is fundamentally a watery solution of urea in which other salts surplus to requirements can also be removed.

The liver is involved in the elimination of bile pigments. Haemoglobin contains precious iron, which must be recycled to form new red blood cells in the bone marrow. The first step is to break the iron-containing haem from the protein *globin*. The latter enters the body reservoir of amino acids/protein and can be used elsewhere. Iron is removed and recycled by bone marrow and the rest of the molecule is converted to two bile pigments *bilirubin* and *biliverdin* which pass in bile through bile ducts into the small intestine. Here they have no specific role in digestion, but are removed as part of the faeces and are, in fact, responsible for their brown colour. The liver also has a role in breaking down excess hormones and the products are removed by the kidneys in urine.

Defence

It is ironic that humanity as a species is by far the most intelligent and the most complex living organism able to survive in extreme conditions, yet it is the most threatened by the smallest group of living creatures – micro-organisms. The body has an elaborate defence mechanism, which occasionally is turned upon human cells with devastating results (auto-immune diseases).

Our skin, when intact, forms a most effective barrier between the internal environment of the body and the external environment which teems with micro-organisms. We even harness some innocent micro-organisms to live on the surface of our skin and act as guardians, preventing more harmful disease-causing microbes (*pathogens*) from 'squatting' there and causing disease. When these harmless microbes are removed by antiseptics or other means, we destroy this natural protective barrier. Skin has on its outer surface layers of dead cells and it is these which form the protection.

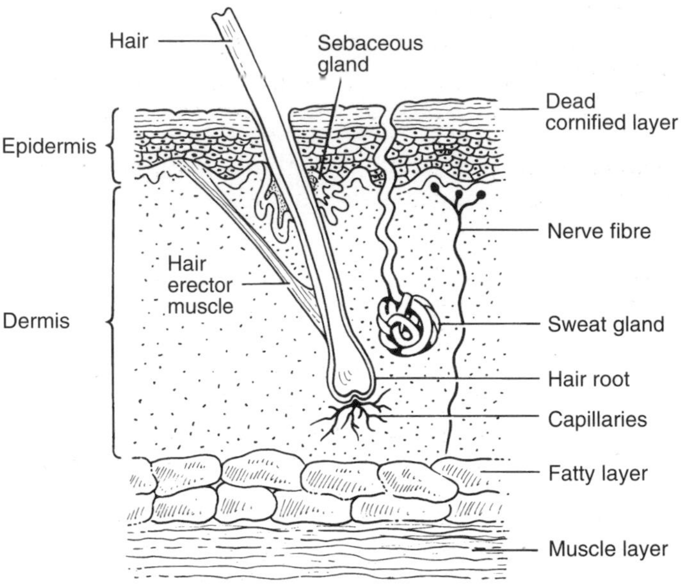

Figure 8.32 A section through the skin

If the skin is breached by accident, injury or disease an infection by microbes can occur. The blood then takes over this defence role. White blood cells (*leucocytes*) play a major part. They can be divided into two main types:

- granulocyctes
- agranulocytes.

Granulocytes

Granulocytes are the most common white blood cells, with numerous darkly-staining granules in the cytoplasm and a 2-6-lobed nucleus. They move like amoebae and carry out *phagocytosis* (digestion of microbes). They are quickly attracted to an area of infection by chemicals released into the tissues (*chemotaxis*). After phagocytosis has occurred, strong antibacterial chemicals are released to effect destruction.

These cells can leave the circulation by squeezing through capillary walls 'a bit at a time' making their shapes as long and thin as possible, a process called *diapedesis*. Once outside the circulation they are able to move through epithelial and connective tissues towards their destination. Granulocytes are the first line of defence, rather like the infantry in war.

Agranulocytes

Much slower to arrive are the *monocytes*, part of the agranular faction, but when they do come they are more effective phagocytosers. They come in larger numbers (rather like artillery or tank brigades) destroying more microbes. Monocytes also leave the circulation and become *macrophages* (literally 'large eaters'), wandering through tissues cleaning up cell debris and microbes.

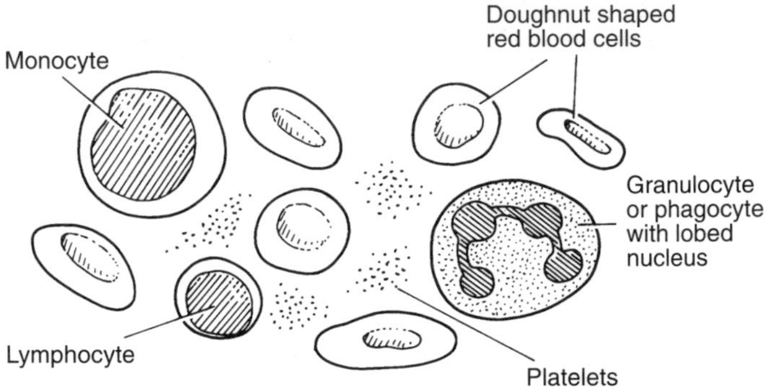

Figure 8.33 White blood cells

The other cells constituting the agranulocytes are the lymphocytes. Much smaller than monocytes, they play a different role in defence, producing immune responses Any substance which stimulates an immune response is called an antigen. In practice, antigens are usually proteins foreign to the human body but part of microbial structures, enzymes or toxins. When lymphocytes are exposed to antigens, they manufacture antibodies, specific proteins capable of binding with and inactivating the antigens. This is known as the *antigen–antibody response*. The response is actually much more complicated than this, but beyond the scope of this

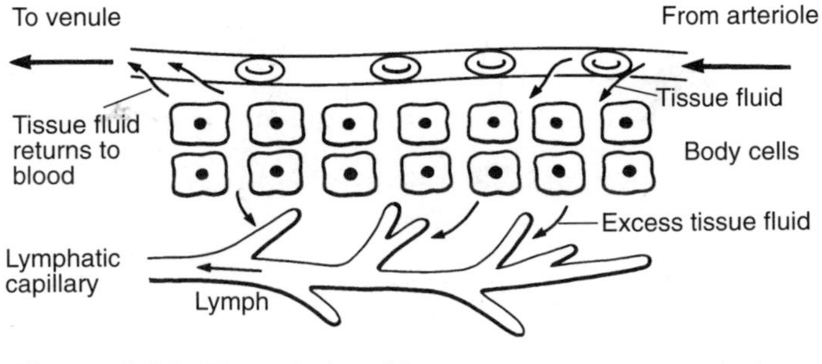

Figure 8.34 The relationship between blood capillaries, cells and lymphatic capillaries (lymph vessels)

chapter. Microbes are then removed by the phagocytosers.

The lymphatic system begins as closed-ended *lymphatic capillaries* which lie in the spaces between cells (see Figure 8.34). They unite to form larger and larger vessels passing upwards eventually to join the great veins in the neck. At several points in this lymphatic circulation, the lymph fluid passes through small nodules known as *lymph nodes,* which are scattered about the body in groups (see Figure 8.35). Lymph nodes contain lymphocytes and macrophages which destroy any microbes which have entered the lymphatic vessels from the tissue spaces. They do this by initiating the antigen – antibody response (sometimes called the *immune response)* and by phagocytosis.

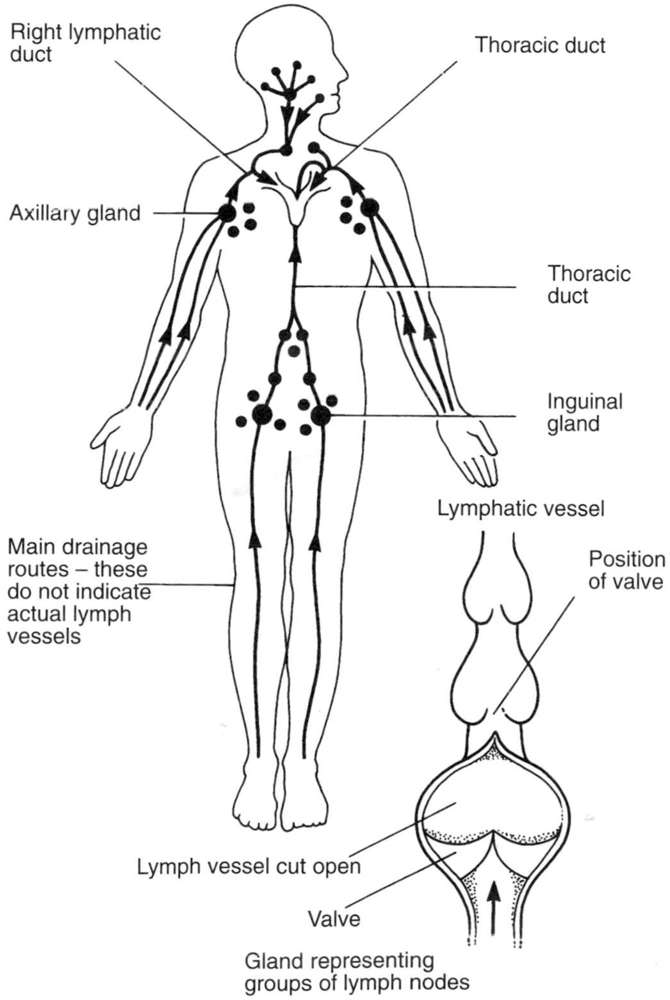

Figure 8.35 The position of the main lymph nodes and vessels

Evidence collection point

Using your own words, write an illustrated report describing how body systems interrelate to carry out the functions of communication, support and locomotion, reproduction, energy supply, excretion and defence.

Homoeostatic mechanisms

In order that body cells function properly, and indeed survive, conditions around their cell membranes must remain stable or within physiological limits. This is often called the *internal environment* and consists of the extracellular fluid which bathes cells. *Homoeostasis* is defined as the maintenance of the constant internal environment. It means that concentrations of ions and nutrients, water, temperature, pH, and more must be kept within a range compatible with correct functioning of cells.

Homoeostatic responses are controlled by the nervous and endocrine systems. The nervous system has receptors which detect when deviations from the normal start to occur, impulses are sent to a control centre, often within the brain, and impulses are then sent to effectors to counteract the change. Endocrine organs work in just the same way, but they use chemicals in the form of hormones instead. Such a system needs constant monitoring to ensure that the mechanism for counteracting the change does not act too far. Such a system incorporates a feedback loop of which there are two types: negative feedback and positive feedback.

- *Negative feedback loops* check the original deviation to ensure that the original state has returned, such loops are very common in the body as we shall see. Examples of negative feedback loops are body temperature regulation and water balance.
- *Positive feedback loops* enhance the original stimulus pushing the change onwards. This does not return the status quo, tends to produce a 'bust' situation and is therefore not in common use in the human body. An example is uterine contractions leading to the birth of a baby.

Homoeostasis of body temperature

Humans are the only animals that can survive in both tropical and arctic conditions and this is largely due to negative feedback homoeostasis mechanisms

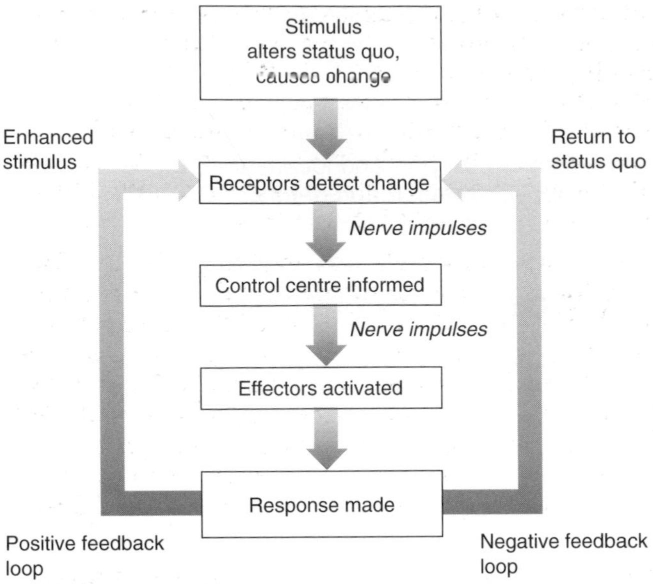

Figure 8.36 Positive and negative feedback loops

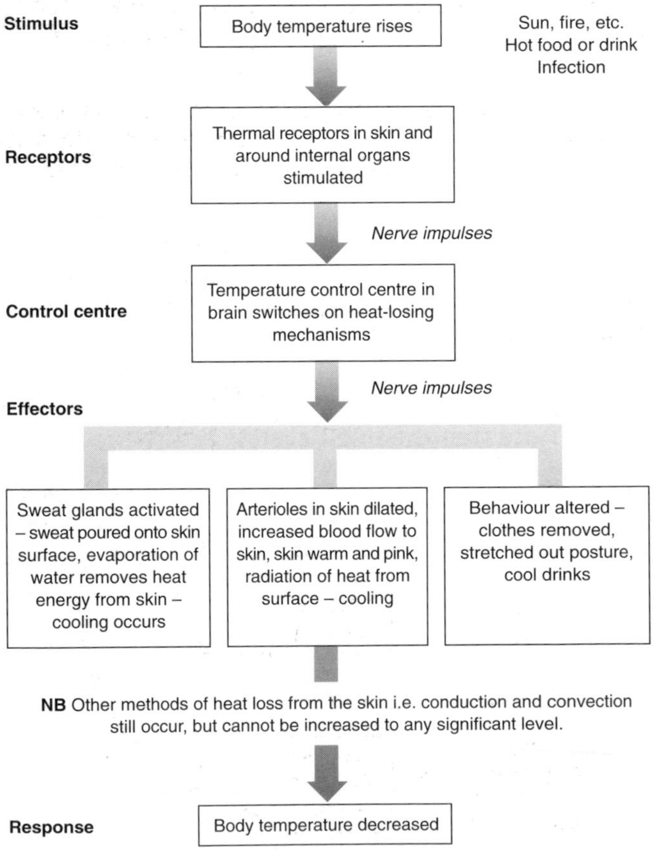

Figure 8.37 The homoeostatic mechanism for regulating rising body temperature

for thermo-regulation, which means that under these conditions body temperature varies very little. The mechanism is shown in Figures 8.37 and 8.38.

At all times, the main aim of the thermo-regulatory systems is to maintain the vital organs of the human body (often referred to as the *core*) at a constant temperature, at the expense of the peripheral areas, chiefly the skin.

Homoeostatic mechanisms regulating blood sugar

The constant requirement for glucose by cells will be apparent from the section dealing with energy supplies in Chapter 7. This sugar is transported to body cells via the blood plasma and tissue fluid. However, given that the supply needs to be constant, but that meals are taken at intervals of about three to

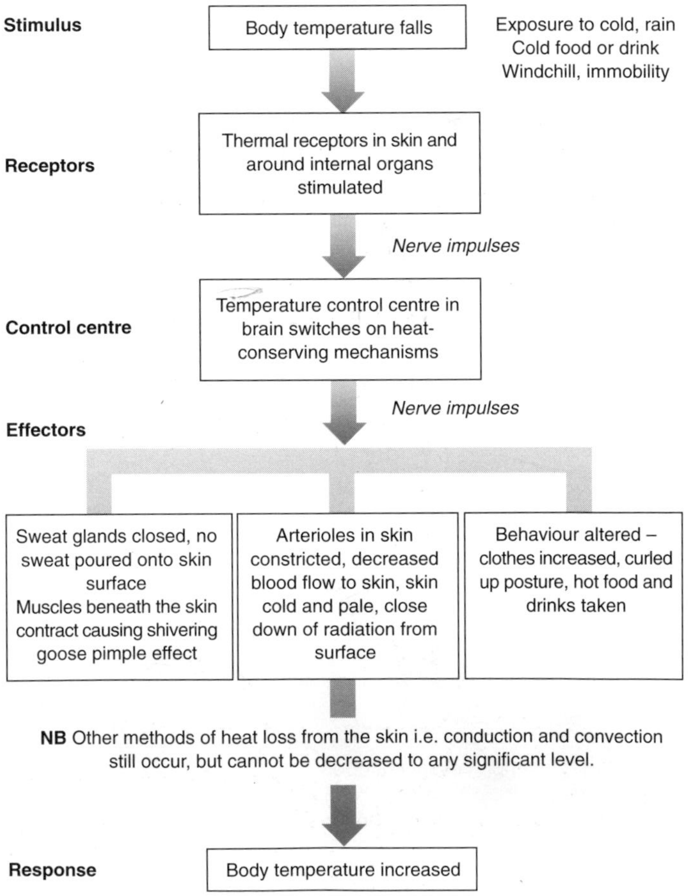

Figure 8.38 The homoeostatic mechanism for regulating falling body temperature

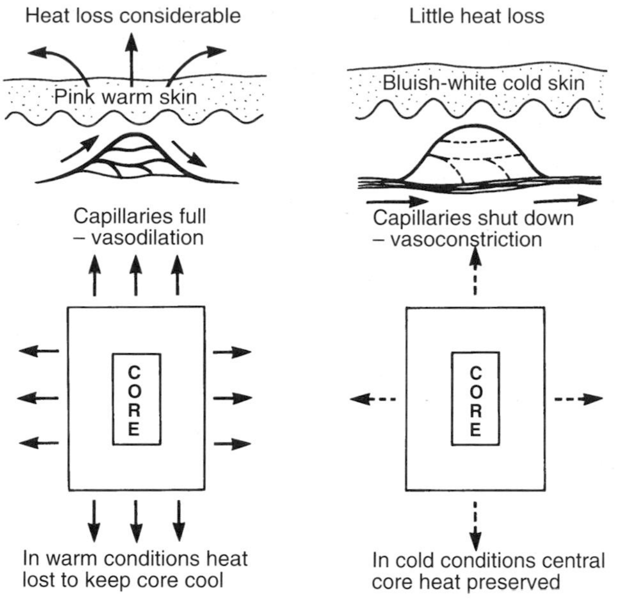

Figure 8.39 Temperature regulation

four hours in Western societies, it is clear some homeostatic mechanisms must be involved.

Glucose does not pass very readily through cell membranes to enter cells. It needs a 'helping push' from a hormone, *insulin*, released from cluster of cells (*the islets of Langerhans*) scattered throughout the pancreas which lies slightly below and behind the stomach (see Figure 8.40).

There are several types of cells in the islets of Langerhans, but the two major types are *alpha* and *beta cells* responsible for insulin secretion. During and after a meal, the digestive system breaks down complex carbohydrates to produce glucose which is absorbed through the gut lining into the bloodstream. As the level of glucose in the blood rises, the islets are stimulated to produce insulin which acts to reduce blood glucose level. As the level falls towards normal, the stimulation is inhibited, a clear example of negative feedback.

Insulin causes blood glucose level to fall by making it easier for the entry of glucose cells through the cell membranes. In addition, it converts glucose into a storage compound, *glycogen*. It is particularly good at doing this with skeletal muscle fibres and liver cells. Minor roles also involve increasing protein and lipid synthesis. Once inside cells, the glucose is either oxidised in respiration and converted to glycogen for storage, or (if glycogen stores are full) converted to fat.

When blood glucose needs to be replenished from the 'store', another islet hormone, *glucagon* (this time from the alpha cells), reverses the actions of insulin and tops up the blood glucose by converting glycogen into glucose. Glucagon is also regulated by negative feedback, controlled by the falling level of blood glucose.

Glucagon is not alone in mobilising stored glucose. A very important hormone called *adrenaline* (released from the *adrenal medulla*, the central part of the

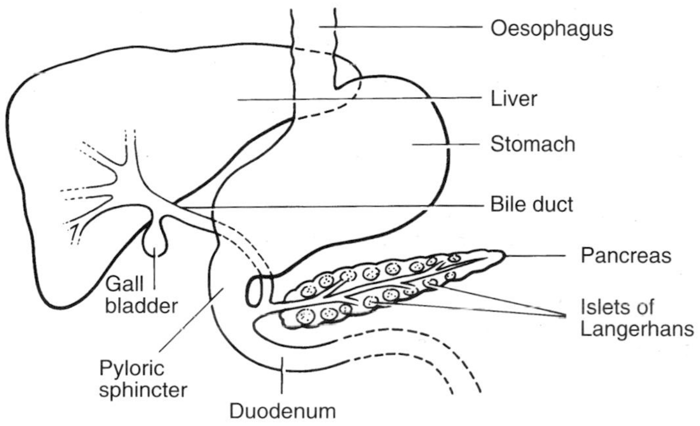

Figure 8.40 The pancreas and islets of Langerhans

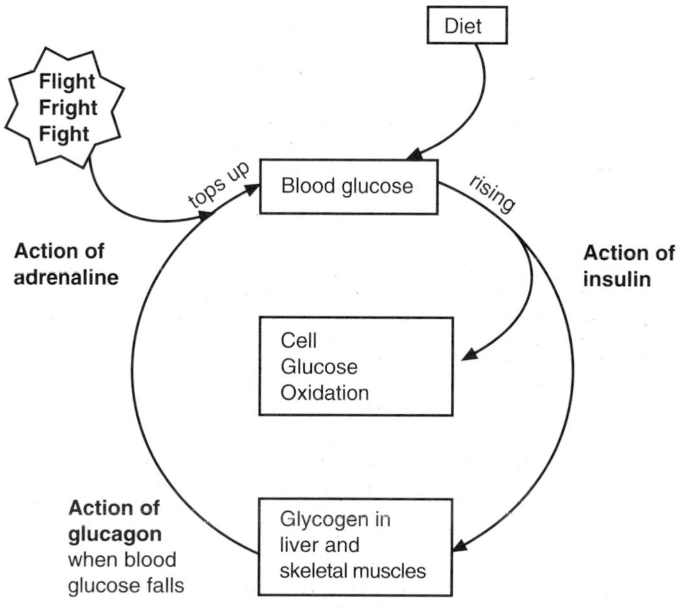

Figure 8.41 A summary of the influences of blood glucose

adrenal glands, when the sympathetic branch of the autonomic system is stimulated) carries out the same function. Previous reference to the sympathetic nervous system emphasised its fight, fright and flight response to stress. One of the facets of this response is the release of large amounts of glucose into the bloodstream for energy. This occurs because adrenaline converts glycogen to glucose as well. A summary of these main actions is shown in Figure 8.41.

Control of blood glucose is a complex interplay of hormone actions, energy demands, state of health and outside influences. Only the major actions have been discussed here.

Homoeostatic mechanisms regulating water levels

Most people are aware that the human body cannot survive for long without a supply of water. It is the most frequently occurring substance in the body, but like most other chemicals, its levels must be kept as constant as possible. Too little water leads to cell *dehydration* and too much to 'waterlogging' or *oedema*. Both conditions result in cell dysfunction and therefore there is a homeostatic mechanism for water regulation.

Water levels themselves are not detected by receptors, but the effect of water concentrations on *osmotic pressure* is. Special sensory receptors, called *osmoreceptors,* lie close to blood vessels in part of the brain called the *hypothalamus*. The hypothalamus is connected to a most important endocrine gland, the pituitary gland, by a short stalk. The gland itself is composed of two major areas – the anterior and posterior lobes of the pituitary gland. The osmoreceptors have long axons which run down the posterior pituitary stalk to end as synaptic knobs among the posterior pituitary cells.

When the osmoreceptors are stimulated by high osmotic pressure of blood (i.e. less water in blood so it is more concentrated) they rather surprisingly synthesise *antidiuretic hormone,* usually referred to as ADH, which is released from the cells of the posterior pituitary gland. Diuretics are substances which increase the flow of urine (many people refer to prescribed diuretics as 'water tablets') so antidiuretic describes a substance which decreases the flow of urine.

The flow of urine from the minute nephrons in the kidneys can be increased by cutting down the volume of water reabsorbed back into the bloodstream in the last part of each nephron. If water is re-entering the blood, it cannot be exiting from the body in urine and vice versa! If the water concentration in blood is greater than normal, i.e. the blood is more dilute, then osmoreceptors are not stimulated, ADH secretion is markedly reduced, little reabsorption of water in the last part of the nephron occurs (they behave more like steel tubes) and the excess water is eliminated in the urine, thus returning osmotic pressure to normal.

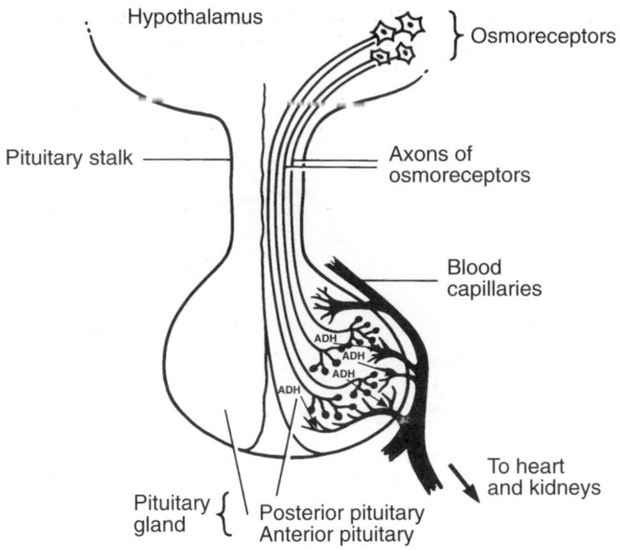

Figure 8.42 ADH secretion

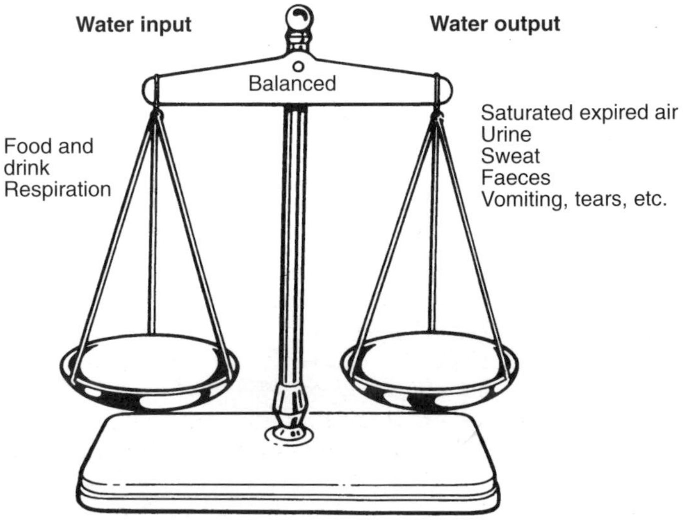

Figure 8.43 The water balance

Most water input is from food and drink, but about half a litre of water is made daily from the respiratory process. Although water can be lost in several ways from the body only two are significant in health – urine volume and sweating in hot weather.

Homoeostatic mechanisms regulating respiration

The skeletal muscles effect an increase in thoracic volume leading to decrease in pressure and inspiration. But they can contract only on receipt of nerve impulses. Breathing, however, is cyclical but skeletal muscle has no built-in automatic rhythmicity like cardiac muscle. It is the respiratory centre in the brain medulla which exhibits rhythmical activity – impulses are generated from the inspiratory centre to pass down nerves leading to the diaphragm and the intercostal muscles initiating muscular contraction and inspiration.

Inspiration normally lasts for about two seconds and expiration three seconds. During quiet breathing, inspiration ends because the muscles become relaxed. There currently exists some controversy over the precise nature of this finish. Elastic or stretch receptors in the walls of the alveoli play some part, sending off impulses when stretched, allowing the lungs to recoil to the resting position. Connections between the inspiratory and expiratory parts of the respiratory centre may also play a part, as may the *pneumotaxic centre* higher up the brain stem in the *pons*.

A wider variation in both rhythm and depth of breathing occurs with many factors influencing the degree of variation. Chemical receptors (*chemoreceptors*) are present both in the brain medulla (where they are called *central chemoreceptors*) and in the small swellings known as the *carotid* and *aortic* bodies (where they are called *peripheral chemoreceptors*). They are sensitive to chemical changes in the blood, particularly carbon dioxide and oxygen levels. When blood levels of CO_2 are increased, the chemoreceptors stimulate the inspiratory centre to increase the rate and depth of breathing. When CO_2 levels fall, the chemoreceptors fail to be stimulated and the inspiratory centre returns to its former level of activity. Thus, the centre sets its own rhythm. Increased rate and depth of breathing is called *hyperventilation* and the decreased shallow breathing, *hypoventilation*. Many other factors affect breathing rates. It is a complex interplay of cardio-respiratory, nervous and hormonal influences.

Normal ranges of factors regulated by homoeostasis

Body temperature

In most people body temperature varies between 36.5°C and 37.2°C. These days most temperatures are measured in the armpits (*axillae*). Temperatures are generally slightly higher in the mouth and in the rectum. Temperature is affected by the time of day (or night), state of health, exercise, sleep, menstrual cycle, eating and drinking. If a single average figure for body temperature is required this is usually taken to be 37°C.

Blood sugar

The normal limits on blood glucose are rather narrow, being 4.5–5.6 mmol per litre of blood or 70–110 mg per 100 cm3 of blood. An increased amount of glucose in the blood is known as *hyperglycaemia* and too low is *hypoglycaemia*.

Respiratory rate

Normal resting respiratory rate is between 13 and 17 breaths per minute for an adult, with a newborn baby breathing at 40 breaths per minute. During exercise, the breathing rate may reach 80 breaths per minute.

Evidence collection point

Make a series of illustrated notes to describe how body temperature, blood sugar, respiratory rate and water levels are kept within normal body ranges by homoeostatic mechanisms. State the normal ranges for body temperature, respiratory rate and blood sugar.

The effects of ageing

The information in Chapter 10 on human growth and development and the information in this section should provide enough underpinning knowledge for the evidence collection point below.

The effects of ageing is one of the most researched subjects in history and there are many theories proposed which are still largely unproven. There is a myth that a fortune can be made if the ageing process could be halted. Some experts believe that the cells of our bodies are pre-programmed with a life span. Some other theories propose that cell replacement cannot keep pace with cell death or that cell replacement processes wear out. Whatever the reason, we know the facts: we do age, metabolism slows, cells do not work as efficiently and that means the functions of organs and organ systems decrease.

Joint mobility decreases with age. Young children can often perform dramatic contortions of their trunk and limbs due to the stretch in ligaments and the mobility of joints. But, sadly, as we get older most of us become much stiffer in the joints and ligaments become far less elastic so that the range of movement at joints becomes more restricted. In the middle to late years, osteoarthritis occurs in many people. In fact, elderly people have come to expect some degree of arthritis. The articular cartilage becomes rough and flaky, leaving bone ends more exposed to friction and its consequent pain. Adhesions form within the joint capsules and limits of movement become closer. People who exercise to maintain mobility of joints will largely prevent these adhesions from forming. Osteoarthritis also brings bone distortion and enlargement. The degeneration affects three times more women than men. Loss of elasticity also affects the focusing power of the lens of the eye, resulting in the long sight of old age (*presbyopia*), and lung function, as inelastic lungs cannot recoil in expiration as they did in younger days.

A decreased ability to reverse falling body temperature is particularly relevant to a discussion on ageing. Both the newborn and the elderly have difficulty in maintaining body temperature once it begins to drop. Both client groups are, therefore, susceptible to the condition known as *hypothermia,* a serious condition which frequently results in death. In the newborn, the brain may be just too immature to make the necessary changes, while in the elderly the cells have become inefficient.

Evidence collection point

Write a short report describing changes occurring with age in the reproductive and support/locomotion systems.

Chapter 9

Methods for monitoring and maintaining the healthy functioning of the human body

This chapter focuses on:

- **monitoring the cardio-respiratory system at different levels of activity, observing safe practice**
- **how to use secondary source data to assess physiological status**
- **the role of imaging techniques.**

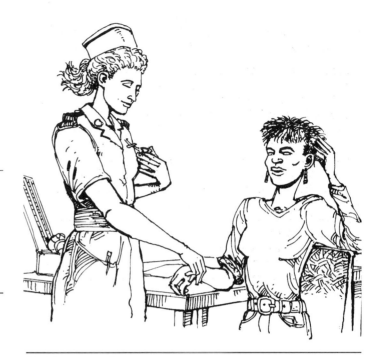

Monitoring the cardio-respiratory system

This section describes the monitoring of pulse rate, blood pressure, breathing rate, lung volumes and peak flow.

Pulse rate

The pulse rate is usually checked during a medical examination as it can give hints about a person's state of health. Other characteristics of the pulse can also be important, such as its strength, rhythm and the feel of the artery concerned.

A pulse can be felt wherever an artery crosses a bone. The most usual place to feel for a pulse is at the wrist, just below the base of the thumb where the radial artery crosses the bones of the wrist. However, in an emergency, if the circulation is shutting down, the *carotid artery* is the main one to feel as this comes straight off the aorta which leads blood away from the heart. This pulse can be felt in the neck on either side of the windpipe. Pulses can also be felt in the groin (*femoral artery*), temple and upper surface of the foot.

A baby's pulse is often difficult to find and the bronchial artery on the inner side of the upper arm is often easier to locate.

The pulse rate corresponds to the contraction of the ventricles of the heart, which forces blood through the arteries causing a shock wave which travels along the arterial system. The shock wave is the pulse that you are feeling. The blood actually travels more slowly.

Taking a pulse

To take a pulse, press lightly against the artery wall with two or three fingers. Do not use the thumb, as this has a pulse of its own and you may find that you have counted your own pulse instead! You will also need a time-piece which is capable of reading seconds. Count the number of beats in a set period and multiply by the correct multiple to make up to

Causes of a faster than normal resting adult pulse rate	Causes of a slower than normal resting adult pulse rate
Being a baby or young child	Being a very fit adult
Exercise or exertion	Fainting
Fright	Compression of the brain
Haemorrhage	Some disorders of the heart
Fever (pyrexia)	
Some illnesses	

Figure 9.1 The causes of variations in pulse rate

60 seconds, i.e. one minute. The minimum you must count for is 20 seconds, and in this case you would multiply by three to get the rate per minute.

The pulse rate is usually between 60 and 80 beats per minute.

Evidence collection point

Take your own pulse or that of a friend:

- at rest (for at least ten minutes)
- after a short spell of minor activity such as waving your arms in the air
- after some strenuous activity like running on the spot for several minutes.

Check that an activity of that sort is all right for that person. Record your readings and convert to pulse rates per minute.

Blood pressure

Blood pressure is the pressure exerted by the blood on the walls of the blood vessels. To measure it, you will need a special piece of equipment called a *sphygmomanometer,* which measures blood pressure, and a stethoscope for listening to the blood flow. Some modern sphygmomanometers have a stethoscope built-in. Sphygmomanometers in the traditional form consist of a cloth cuff which encloses an air bladder connected to tubing and a rubber or plastic bulb used for pumping air into the bladder. The tubing connects to a measuring device or gauge – traditional ones still in use are filled with mercury.

Measuring the blood pressure

You should only measure blood pressure if there is a trained person with you.

The cuff is wound round the upper arm with the bladder (which can be felt) located just above the elbow joint and facing forward. Place the stethoscope over the artery at the elbow, it should be quite flat to the skin surface. The bladder is inflated using the manual pump or bulb until the gauge measures around 200 units, measured in millimetres of mercury. This has the effect of blocking off the supply of blood to the arm, so clearly the inflation must not be left at this level for more than a few seconds.

The cuff is slowly deflated by turning a thumbscrew between the bulb and tubing, while listening carefully through the stethoscope. At the first sounds of blood rushing into the artery, read the gauge. This is known as the *systolic pressure* and it represents the contraction of the ventricles and the recoil of the elastic walls of the aorta as blood passes through. This is the highest level you will record and represents the *numerator* of the fraction depicting blood pressure.

Continuing to deflate the cuff slowly, the beats appear to get gradually louder and then suddenly begin to die away, this is usually described as a muffled sound. Once again, note the reading on the gauge. This is the *diastolic pressure* representing the pressure which exists between heart beats, and the load against which the heart has to work. The diastolic pressure is the more important value of the two, and forms the denominator of the fraction.

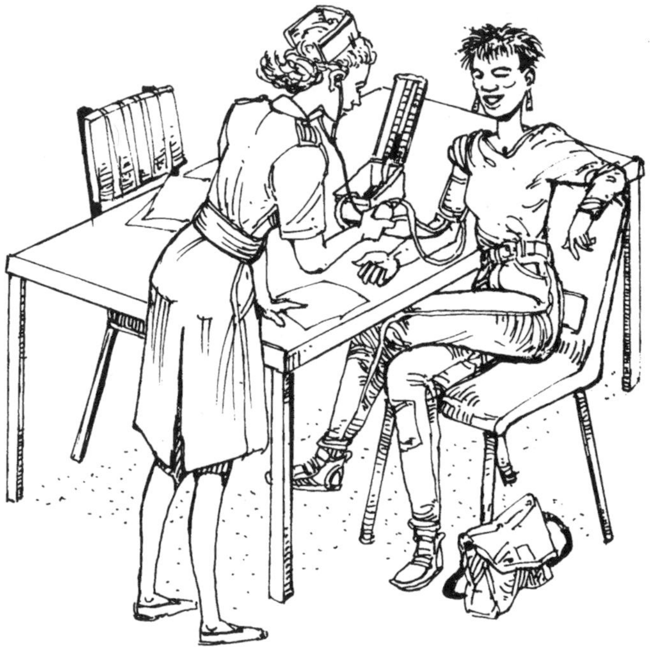

A healthy young adult has a blood pressure reading around 110/75 mm Hg, but an older person has higher blood pressure 130–140/90–100 mm Hg. Hg is the chemical symbol for mercury and is used to shorten the term 'millimetres of mercury'.

Blood pressure varies with activity and circumstance. It rises during pregnancy, exercise, smoking and being anxious about things. Blood pressure falls during sleep and relaxation. Abnormally high blood pressure is known as *hypertension* and low pressure is *hypotension.*

Evidence collection point

In the presence of a trained person, form pairs and take one another's blood pressure:

- at rest
- during exercise
- perhaps immediately after a maths test or some other stressful challenge

Record readings and add them to your pulse rates. If possible, work with the same person as you did when taking a pulse.

Breathing rate

This is the number of breaths in any given time period, usually one minute.

Breathing is the process by which air is drawn into and out of the lungs to allow blood to take up oxygen and expel carbon dioxide. A person can alter the breathing rate by conscious effort, but mainly it occurs unconsciously, controlled by the respiratory centre in the brain.

The normal range of breathing rate is 13 to 17 breaths per minute during rest, but during strenuous exercise this can rise to 70–80 breaths per minute. Like the heart rate (pulse rate), a baby breathes much faster than an adult, around 30–40 breaths each minute. Between 0.4 and 0.5 dm^3 (cubic decimetres – a decimetre is 10 centimetres) of air is taken in at each breath, but only one fifth of this is the desired oxygen.

Evidence collection point

With your partner from the previous exercise, try to count the number of breaths taken each minute:

- at rest
- during mild exercise
- during strenuous exercise.

Record these values and file them with your previous work.

Lung volumes

A deep breath taken in and a forced breath out is familiar to all of us. So, we are aware that lung (or pulmonary) volumes can be altered. In physiology, these volumes are given names and can be calculated. One can never fully empty the lungs, there is always a *residual volume* left behind (1200 cm^3). The volume of an ordinary breath has been mentioned above and is known as the *tidal volume,* because it is air which ebbs and flows, just like the tide. The greatest amount of air which can be taken into the lungs after a forced expiration (breathing out) is called the *vital capacity.* This volume is usually around 4800 cm^3, or just under 5 dm^3. A person with a larger chest, provided that it is healthy, will have greater lung volume than a small person. For this reason, males produce larger figures for lung volumes than females.

Lung volumes are best measured with a *spirometer.* Medical spirometers are slightly different to laboratory spirometers and measure forced expiratory volumes with the client breathing out through a mouth piece. Lung volumes are generally reduced in cases of lung disorders, and this is why such tests are

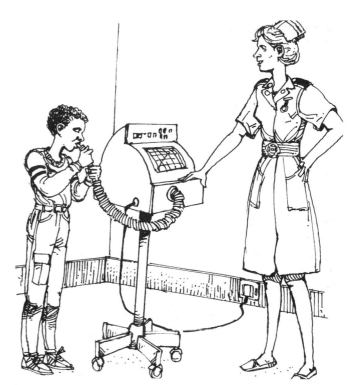

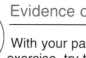

Figure 9.2 Recording rate and total volume of air exhaled from the lungs using a clinical spirometer

carried out. They are often known as *pulmonary function* tests.

Laboratory spirometers are basically calibrated boxes filled with water. Oxygen is pumped in from a cylinder and carbon dioxide is removed by passing the expired air through a container filled with caustic soda, which absorbs this gas. If there was no system for oxygen inflow and carbon dioxide removal, the spirometer box would be filled with carbon dioxide and nitrogen after a few breaths – a very dangerous situation. A large quantity of air is trapped in the box and as the person breathes in and out the pen pointer marks the volumes on a revolving drum or *kymograph*. After recording tidal volume for a few breaths, vital capacity can be demonstrated by breathing in as deeply as possible after a forced expiration.

If such equipment is not available for you to use, a simple apparatus can be substituted. This incorporates a large water trough or bucket, rubber tubing and a calibrated container, at least 5 dm^3 capacity. Calibration means that correct graduations have been placed on the container.

Try it

Turn your calibrated container filled with water upside down in a water-filled trough, being careful either to hold your hand over the opening or put a stopper in the neck of the container. Still holding the container opening under water, remove your hand or the stopper. Some water will flow out, but mainly it will still be filled with water. Read and record the level of the water.

Push a length of rubber tubing through the container opening until it pushes through into the space *above* the water. Take as deep a breath as you can and exhale into the rubber tubing. Take care, water may flow over the trough! Now, read and record the water level in the container again. The difference between these two levels will indicate your *vital capacity.*

Repeat the experiment, but this time breathe in and out quietly. Get your partner to record the readings of inspiration and expiration. This is the *tidal volume.*

Note on analysis:

If you are part of a group performing any of these techniques, you will be able to collect a number of readings and display them in the form of a statistical chart and use graphical techniques to give an instant visual presentation.

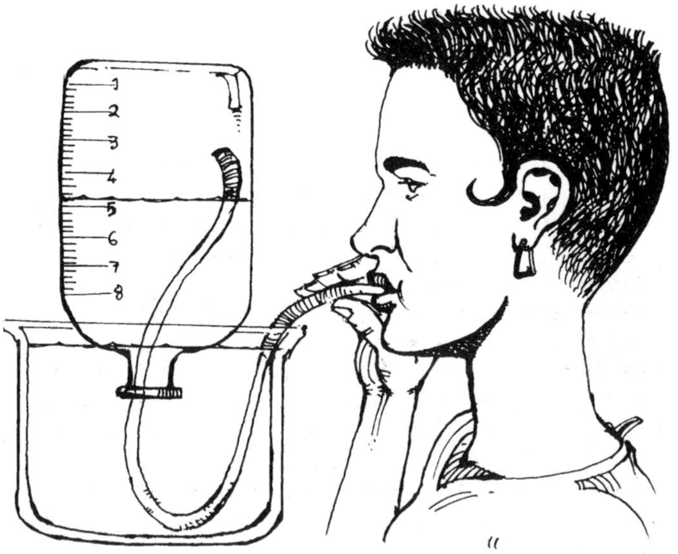

Peak flow

A *peak flow meter,* which records the maximum speed at which air can flow out of the lungs, is simpler and more portable than a spirometer. It is used to assess the width of the 'tubes' (the trachea and bronchi) of the respiratory system. Narrowed tubes make air rush out more slowly so peak flow readings are a useful monitoring device for people with bronchospasm or narrowed bronchi.

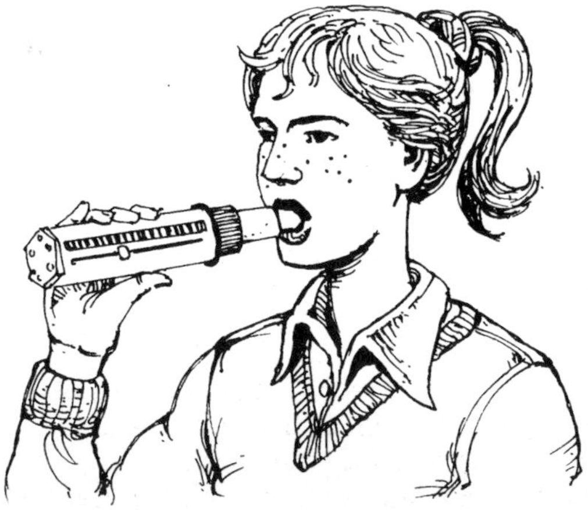

This happens most commonly in people who suffer from asthma, who may be on drugs which widen the tubes. Clients who suffer from asthma are often asked to monitor their peak flow every day, rather like diabetics monitor blood or urine sugar levels. Normal levels for peak flow range from 400–600 dm^3 per minute.

A client takes a deep breath and breathes out as fast as possible into the mouthpiece of the meter. Readings are kept alongside a diary of symptoms. In this way symptoms can be related to circumstances of the time, such as the presence of animals or high pollen counts.

Monitoring and analysing measurements of pulse rate, blood pressure, breathing rate and lung volumes, may enable others to make valid conclusions about the physiological status of an individual. Below is a case study as an example.

Case study – Fred Taylor

Fred Taylor is 72 years old and lives in a flat on the ground floor of a high-rise block of flats. He used to work as a coal miner, and has bronchitis and emphysema as a result of his long-term exposure to coal dust, damp conditions and many respiratory infections. He also has angina and cannot walk far without stopping for a rest. On his last visit to the hospital, he went as usual for the electrocardiogram (ECG), lung function tests, blood cell counts and blood pressure measurement.

His medical notes record the following:

Pulse rate at rest: 83 beats per minute
Pulse rate on minor exertion: 98 beats per minute
Blood pressure (resting): 160/120
Breathing rate: 21 breaths per minute
Tidal volume: 410 cm^3
Vital capacity: 4150 cm^3
Peak flow: 398 dm^3 per minute.

Evidence collection point

Analyse Fred's physiological status from the information above.

Here are some questions to guide you:

a Look at the data collected about Fred's pulse and breathing rates. What do you notice about them? What do you think this could mean?

b Do the figures obtained from the lung volume test support your conclusions in (a)? What reasons would you give to support your answer? Does the peak flow reading further support your conclusions? Why?

c Fred suffers from angina. What do you think about his blood pressure? Are the two related in any way? State how, if you think they are, and why not, if the answer is negative.

d What final conclusions could you come to about the physiological state of Fred Taylor?

You can either use this case study practice as guidance in preparation for your own monitoring of an individual or actually use it as evidence. Your decision might depend on how much assistance you have had from your tutor; if you have had quite a lot, it will be much better if you collect your own data and analyse your results. However, if you accomplished this mainly on your own, then the work you have done will provide sufficient analysis for some of your evidence. You will, of course, need to read some of these sections over again, to check the underpinning knowledge required for the analysis.

Secondary source data

This is data collected by someone else and used by yourself. If you have used the case study provided then you will have been using *secondary source* data. If you have analysed your own readings, then this is *primary source data.*

Element 3.3 requires you to be able to understand some secondary source data which will probably be impossible for you to collect yourself, as you probably will not have the equipment, skills or experience to do so. This secondary source data includes:

- ECG traces
- blood cell counts
- spirometer tracings
- electrolyte concentrations.

ECG traces

Just before heart muscle in the various chambers contracts, there is a succession of electrical impulses to the muscle fibres. The ECG recorder captures this electrical activity and produces either a trace (an inked record on graph paper) or a display on a screen. Sensors to pick up electrical impulses are connected to the client's chest, wrists and ankles and then to the recorder, but this causes no pain to the client. Careful reassurance and explanation is required as the client could be quite frightened by the electrodes, fearing that they might receive electric shocks. The electrical impulses from the heart muscle are very small voltages and cannot be felt.

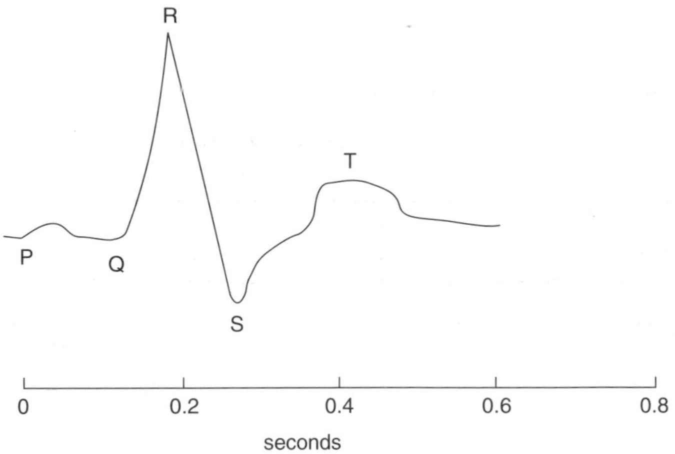

Figure 9.3 The normal pattern of an ECG

Figure 9.3 shows a normal resting ECG. The waves show the spread of excitation over the chambers of the heart, They are lettered for analysis and description purposes:

P wave – just prior to atrial contraction
QRS spike – just prior to ventricular contraction
T wave – represents recovery of the ventricles.

NB Atrial recovery is masked by QRS spike.

In many heart disorders, the ECG is altered so it is a useful aid to diagnosis of heart conditions. In angina, for example, an ECG taken at rest is usually normal, unless previous damage has occurred, so a *cardiac stress* test is used. In this, the client is asked to undertake exercise while the ECG is recording. The exercise is usually performed in the clinical department, which is equipped with a treadmill for this purpose. It continues until the client experiences chest pain. Some alteration of the ECG trace may then be noticed.

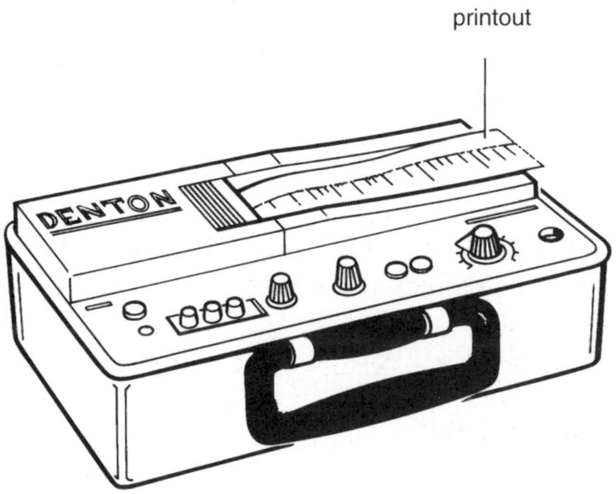

Figure 9.4 A portable ECG recorder

Other conditions which may be diagnosed from an ECG are cardiac muscle disorders, coronary thromboses, myocarditis (inflammation of the cardiac muscle) and pericarditis (inflammation of the membranous sac surrounding the heart).

Blood cell counts

A small volume of blood is obtained from a vein by syringe and needle and sent for analysis in a haematology department. This is the most common blood test used for diagnosing anaemias, leukaemias, genetically-inherited blood disorders and the presence of infections.

A blood count will reveal:

- numbers of red blood cells
- numbers of white blood cells
- numbers of platelets
- the size and shape of red and white blood cells
- numbers of different types of white blood cells.

} in 1 mm^3 of blood

All of these have normal ranges for different individuals, and provide important diagnostic information when at the limits of range or outside the normal range.

Figure 9.5 summarises the types of blood cells and their normal values. Use the chart for information, but do not attempt to memorise it.

Electrolyte concentrations in body fluids

Electrolytes are substances which, when dissolved in body fluids, break up (known as *dissociate*) into their individually-charged ions. For example, sodium chloride dissociates into sodium ions (cations) and chloride ions (anions). The most common ions are those of sodium and chloride, but other cations are potassium, calcium and magnesium, while anions are hydrogen carbonates (formerly bicarbonate), sulphates and phosphates. (See Figure 9.7.)

High sodium concentration leads to dehydration, thirst and restlessness. Low sodium levels cause low blood pressure, rapid heart rate and shock. High calcium values result in weakness, nausea and mental

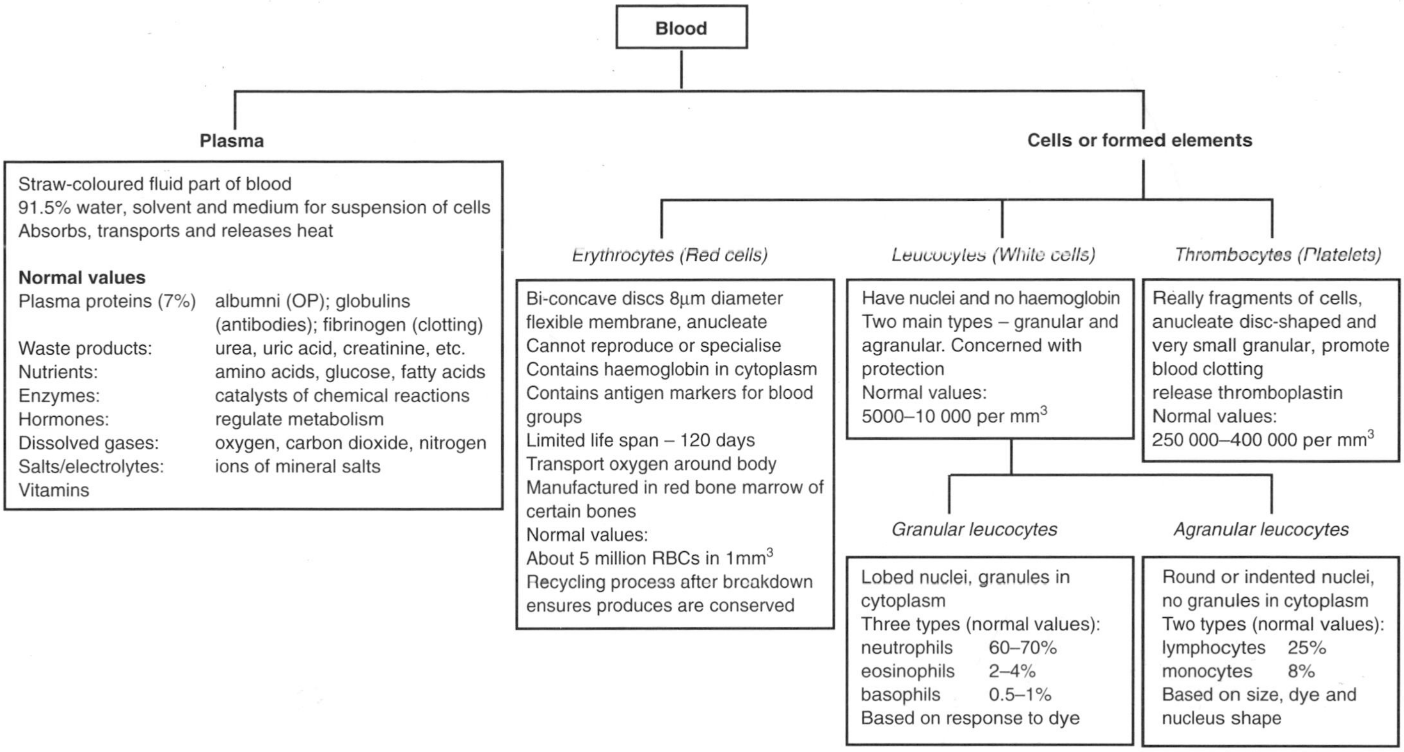

Figure 9.5 Types of blood cells and their normal values

Abnormal feature of blood	Implication
Red blood cells	
Too few	Form of anaemia
Too many	Polycythaemia
Sickle shape	Sickle cell anaemia – inherited form
Immatured	Another form of anaemia
Less haemoglobin	Form of anaemia
White blood cells	
abnormal	Form of leukaemia
too many granulocytes	Infection present
too few	Possible side effect of medication
too many eosinophils	Allergic reactions, parasitic infections
too many basophils	Allergic reations and inflammation
too many monocytes	Infection
too many lymphocytes	Form of leukaemia
Platelets	
abnormal	Bleeding disorder
too few	Bleeding disorder

Figure 9.6 The implications for blood components outside the normal range

Cations positive charge	Anions negative charge
H (hydrogen)	Cl (chloride)
Na (sodium)	OH (hydroxyl)
K (potassium)	HCO_3 (hydrogen carbonate)
Ca (calcium)	PO_4 (phosphate)
Mg (magnesium)	SO_4 (sulphate)
	NO_3 (nitrate)

Figure 9.7 Anions and cations

confusion, while lowered values result in numbness, cramps and convulsions. Potassium is particularly important for its effect on the functioning of the heart, nervous system and muscle.

You will need to research particular effects of abnormal values of electrolytes as you come across them in secondary source data. Many abnormal values cause mental incapacity, coma and even death.

Spirometer tracings have already been covered on page 185.

Evidence collection point

Returning to the case study of Fred Taylor, he also had a blood cell count like this:

RBCs: 3 800 000 per mm^3
WBCs: 9000 per mm^3
Differential WBCs: normal
Haemoglobin: 12.8g/100 cm^3 blood
Blood electrolytes within normal range.

What additional information does this secondary source data provide to add to the original statements about Fred Taylor's physiological status?

You will need to consult the information provided earlier in this section to draw conclusions of this nature. You will also need to investigate the normal range for haemoglobin content as this has not been provided for you.

Write it into your report.

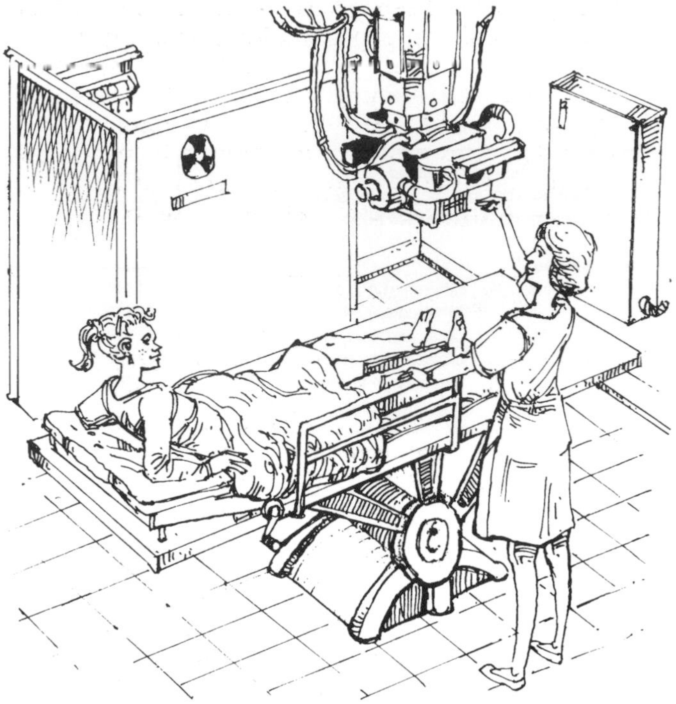

Imaging techniques

The last part of this chapter will investigate plain and contrast X-rays, body scans, ultrasound techniques and magnetic resonance imaging (MRI) and their roles in displaying anatomical features.

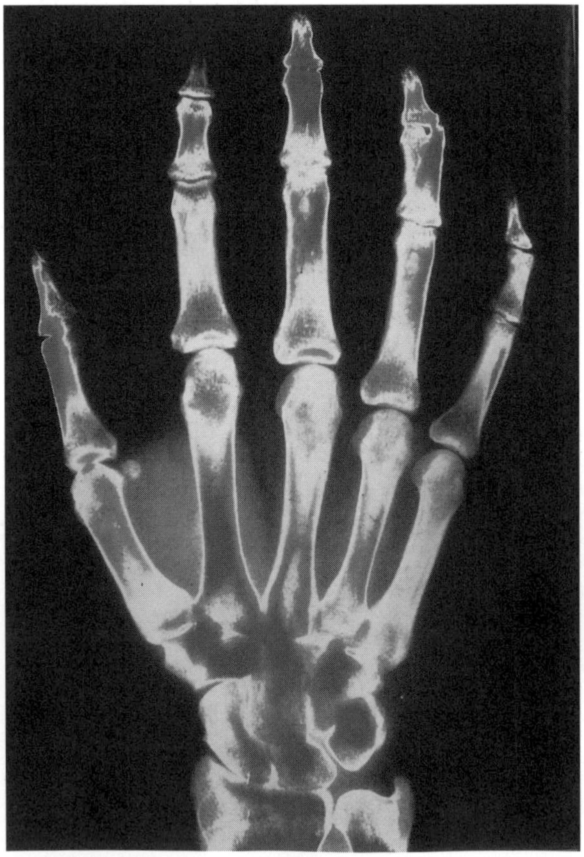

X-rays

Plain X-rays

When electrons, which are travelling very fast, collide with a heavy metal (tungsten), short-wave electromagnetic energy is produced – these are X-rays. Medically, they are used for both diagnosis and treatment, but in this section only the diagnostic imaging will be discussed.

Body tissues absorb X-rays at different levels. Bones, for example, absorb a lot of X-rays, while less hard tissues, like muscle, absorb much less. These different absorption patterns cast different shadows on to photographic film (or fluorescent screens), so that bones appear white and muscle appears grey.

X-rays are, therefore, particularly useful for imaging bones, and most people will have had a chest or bone X-ray at some time in their lives. Modern X-ray machines are capable of producing very good pictures while exposing the client to as little radiation as possible.

Once an X-ray has been taken and developed, rather like a photograph, an expert radiologist interprets the image produced. All doctors and radiographers have the ability to interpret X-rays, but they are all subsequently passed to the expert, the radiologist (who is a doctor as well), for a report to be produced. Plain X-rays are used to detect fractures, arthritic changes, swellings, skeletal features, erosion, etc.

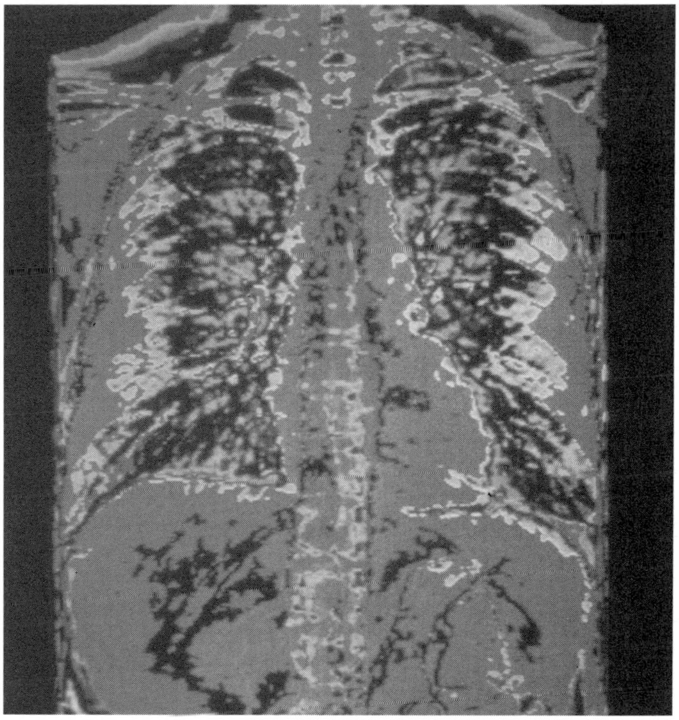

Use of contrast media

As softer tissue does not show up so well on X-ray pictures, various special techniques have been devised to produce more details. One of these techniques is the use of radio-opaque materials, known as *contrast media,* which can be introduced into hollow organs. In this way, the alimentary canal, renal system, blood vessels, joints and many other organs can be successfully imaged. The most useful contrast medium is a barium compound, which can be swallowed (*barium swallow* or *barium meal*), introduced by rubber tubing into the intestine (*barium follow through*) or given as an enema (*barium enema*). In many cases, these have been replaced by *endoscopy,* which uses a rigid or flexible fibre optic instrument through which the medical examiner may directly view the lining of the hollow organ.

Body scans

A scan results when special X-ray equipment is used to produce 'slices' either through the body or a particular organ. This technique is known as *tomography.* If tomography is combined with a computer, the result is called a *CT scan.* Scans of this type use many X-rays passing at different angles, and may also involve the use of contrast media to highlight certain parts. The different rates of X-ray absorption are interpreted by the computer to produce the image.

CT scanners are relatively new and very expensive. As a result, they are usually available only in large hospitals serving a district or region. Scans of this type are particularly useful for investigating the brain, the trunk, locating tumours and aiding the taking of needle biopsies (small samples of tissues by needle) from certain more dangerous locations.

Some three-dimensional computers attached to scanners can produce body images that appear as if the examiner could look inside the body.

Ultrasound scanning

This is not unlike X-ray scanning, but uses high frequency sound waves instead of electromagnetic waves. The waves are not audible to human ears, but do produce echoes as they 'bounce' off structures so producing a 'sound image'. Ultrasound waves pass through fluid and soft tissue easily, but not through gases or bone. They would be of no value in detecting musculo-skeletal abnormalities, or

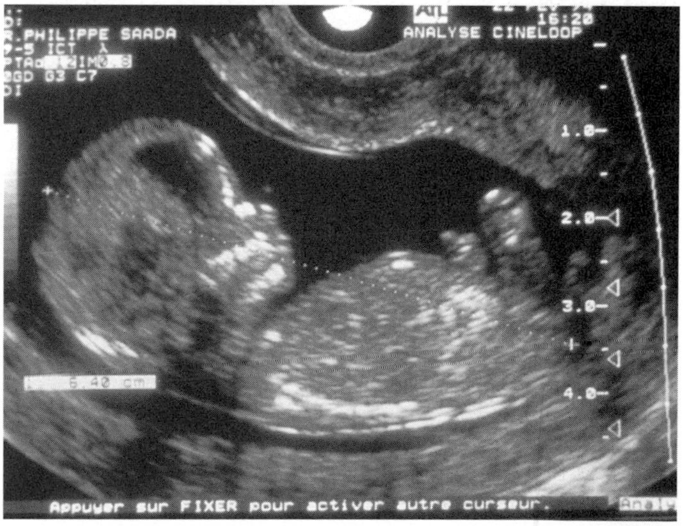

anything encased in bone like the brain, or filled with gas like the lungs (air-filled) or the intestines.

Ultrasound scanning is considered to be extremely safe and its main use is in ante-natal care. Many centres caring for pregnant women offer two ultrasound scans, one early in the pregnancy (around 17–20 weeks) and one later. Scans are also done if a problem is suspected during the pregnancy. *Amniocentesis* and *chorionic villus sampling* is done in conjunction with an ultrasound scan, which is used to locate the placenta and foetus. The needle can then be placed in a site well away from both, ensuring the safety of both mother and child.

The liver is an organ which scans well, showing up cysts, tumours and other abnormalities. Other organs suitable for ultrasound scanning are:

- gallbladder and associated tubes
- pancreas and spleen
- kidneys, bladder and associated tubes
- thyroid gland
- ovaries, testes and breasts
- eyes.

Magnetic resonance imaging (MRI)

MRI produces similar slices, or 3-D images, of body parts like CT scanning, but without the use of potentially harmful radiation. The equipment uses a hollow magnet, in which the client lies, and short

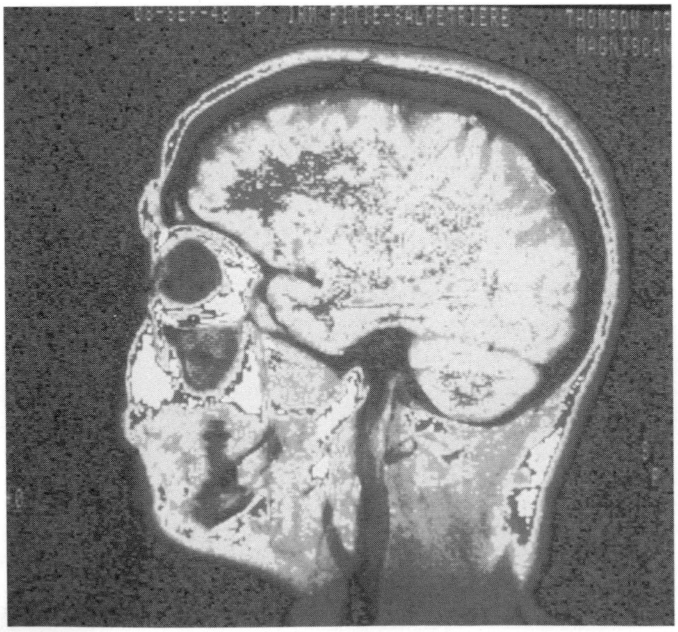

bursts of radio waves which temporarily make parts of a chemical (hydrogen) atom shift their position. As they return to their original position, a radio signal is produced which is interpreted by the scanner. MRI produces better images of some tissues and organs than CT scans. For example, the difference between white and grey matter in the brain and spinal cord is more easily detected, hence accurate positioning of tumours can be done.

MRI is used mainly for examination of:

- the central nervous system
- eyes and ears
- heart and main blood vessels
- joints, particularly the knee.

Like CT scans, the availability of MRI is limited to large medical centres and it is expensive.

Try it

If you live close to a large medical centre, it may be possible for a group to visit and view scanning techniques. Make sure that you have investigated the techniques before the visit, so that you can ask relevant questions and understand the answers.

Make a record of your learning and use it for supplementary evidence.

Most people will live within travelling distance of an X-ray or ultrasound department and may be able to arrange visits to one or both of these also.

Evidence collection point

Write a report, using your own words, on the role of imaging techniques in showing anatomical organs and parts of the body.

Self-assessment test

1 The function of a ribosome is to:
- a Release energy.
- b Manufacture proteins.
- c Control substances entering and leaving cells.
- d Control the cells' activities.

2 The units of inheritance or genes are found in the:
- a Nucleus.
- b Ribsomes.
- c Mitochondria.
- d Endoplasmic reticulum.

3 ATP is mainly found in the:
- a Nucleus.
- b Cell membrane.
- c Endoplasmic reticulum.
- d Mitochondria.

4 A cell viewed under the electron microscope could be drawn as shown below. What are the correct labels for A, B, C and D?

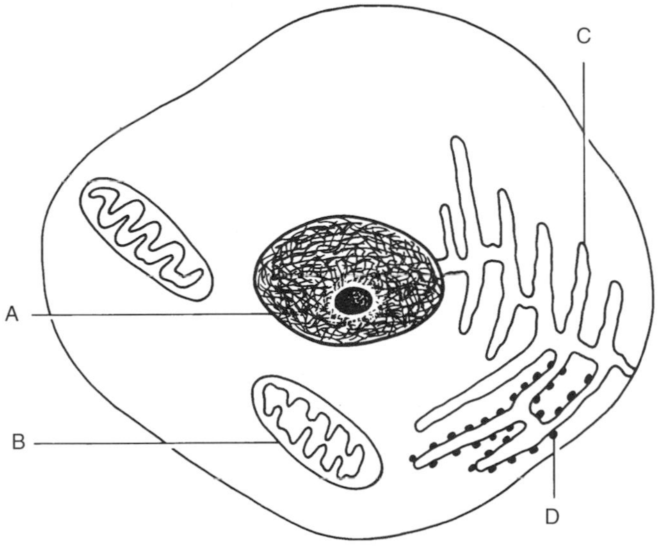

- a Nucleus, mitochondrion, ribosome, or endoplasmic reticulum.
- b Nucleus, ribosome, mitochondrion, or endoplasmic reticulum.
- c Mitochondrion, nucleus, ribosome, or endoplasmic reticulum.
- d Nucleus, mitochondrion, endoplasmic reticulum, or ribosome.

5 Which cell organelle enables materials to move through the cell cytoplasm?
- a Ribosome.
- b Mitochondria.
- c Cell membrane.
- d Endoplasmic reticulum.

6 Which type of tissue consists of cells, fibres and matrix?
- a Connective tissue.
- b Muscle.
- c Epithelia.
- d Nervous tissue.

7 Axons of nerve cells:
- a Detect stimuli.
- b Are supporting structures.
- c Transmit impulses away from the cell body.
- d Transmit impulses towards the cell body.

8 Skeletal muscle has:
- a One nucleus and striped banding.
- b One nucleus and no striped banding.
- c Many nuclei and striped banding.
- d Many nuclei and no striped banding.

9 The tissue drawn below is:

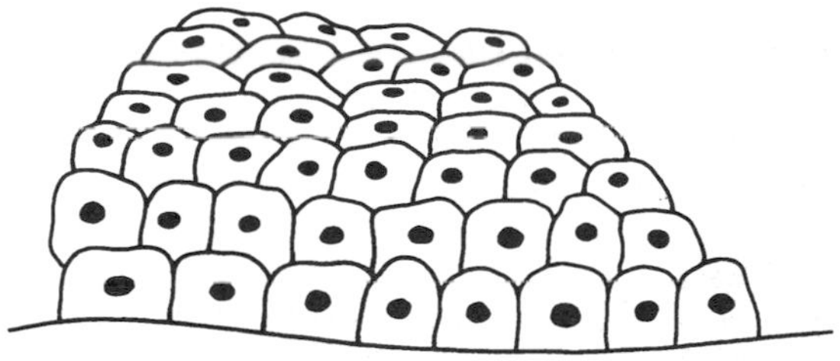

- a Skeletal muscle.
- b Nervous tissue.
- c Compact bone.
- d Compound epithelium.

10 The type of tissue which lines surfaces is called:
- a Connective tissue.
- b Epithelia.
- c Muscle.
- d Nervous tissue.

11 Which tissue contains Haversian systems?
- a Compact bone.
- b Blood.
- c Simple squamous epithelium.
- d Skeletal muscle.

12 Where are platelets found?
- **a** Compact bone.
- **b** Blood.
- **c** Skeletal muscle.
- **d** Nerve cells.

13 Krebs citric acid cycle is part of:
- **a** A lemon.
- **b** Glycolysis.
- **c** Anaerobic respiration.
- **d** Aerobic respiration.

14 Anaerobic respiration produces:
- **a** Glucose.
- **b** Citric acid.
- **c** Lactic acid.
- **d** Amino acid.

15 Glycolysis is the:
- **a** Production of glucose.
- **b** Anaerobic stage of respiration.
- **c** Aerobic stage of respiration.
- **d** Stage following Krebs cycle.

16 ADP is a:
- **a** Low energy compound.
- **b** High energy compound.
- **c** Product of aerobic respiration.
- **d** Product of anaerobic respiration.

17 Which of the following represents anaerobic respiration?
- **a** Lots of ATP formed and lactic acid produced.
- **b** Little ATP formed and lactic acid produced.
- **c** Lots of ATP formed and no lactic acid produced.
- **d** Little ATP formed and no lactic acid produced.

18 Which of the following cell organelles does not have a surrounding membrane?
- **a** Mitochondrion.
- **b** Nucleus.
- **c** Ribosome.
- **d** Endoplasmic reticulum.

19 Diffusion is important in the human body. Which type of whole tissue can be adapted to allow diffusion to occur?
- **a** Epithelium.
- **b** Connective tissue.
- **c** Nervous tissue.
- **d** Muscle.

20 Which of the following represents the overall equation for respiration?
- **a** Glucose + carbon dioxide = oxygen + water + energy
- **b** Water + carbon dioxide = oxygen + glucose + energy
- **c** Glucose + water = energy + oxygen + carbon dioxide
- **d** Glucose + oxygen = energy + carbon dioxide + water

21 Which of the following is an organ of excretion?
- **a** Nose.
- **b** Bowel.
- **c** Liver.
- **d** Heart.

22 Which of the blood cells listed below produces antibodies?
- **a** Red blood cells.
- **b** Lymphocytes.
- **c** Platelets.
- **d** Phagocytes.

23 Insulin is produced by:
- **a** Pituitary gland.
- **b** Pancreas.
- **c** Adrenal gland.
- **d** Ovary/Testis.

24 Glucose is one end product of digestion. Which of the following dietary components would be the source of glucose?
- **a** Fats or lipids.
- **b** Vitamins.
- **c** Proteins.
- **d** Carbohydrates.

25 Which of the following describes a sensory neurone?
- **a** Long dendrons, short axons.
- **b** Long dendrons, long axons.
- **c** Short dendrons, long axons.
- **d** Short dendrons, short axons.

26 Which of the chemical constituents listed below, form the correct combination for the pulmonary artery?
- **a** High oxygen, low carbon dioxide, low water.
- **b** Low oxygen, high carbon dioxide, high water.
- **c** High oxygen, high carbon dioxide, low water.
- **d** Low oxygen, low carbon dioxide, low water.

27 The superior vena cava is a blood vessel which:
- **a** Delivers oxygenated blood to the tissues.
- **b** Delivers dexoygenated blood to the tissues.
- **c** Delivers deoxygenated blood to the heart.
- **d** Delivers oxygenated blood to the heart.

28 When the weather is extremely hot:
- **a** Sweating is reduced and the level of antidiuretic hormone is high.
- **b** Sweating is increased and the level of antidiuretic hormone is high.
- **c** Sweating is reduced and the level of antidiuretic hormone is low.
- **d** Sweating is increased and the level of antidiuretic hormone is low.

29 Blood sugar is increased by the effects of two hormones. These are:
- **a** Insulin and glucagon.
- **b** Insulin and adrenaline.
- **c** Glucagon and adrenaline.
- **d** Glucagon and ADH.

30 Which of the following becomes roughened and worn in osteoarthritis?
- **a** Articular cartilage.
- **b** Ligaments.
- **c** Synovial membrane.
- **d** Fibrous capsule.

31 If the body temperature is increased, which of the following will help to reduce body temperature?
- **a** Vasodilatation, increased radiation and increased sweating.
- **b** Vasodilatation, decreased radiation and increased sweating.
- **c** Vasoconstriction, decreased radiation and decreased sweating.
- **d** Vasoconstriction, decreased radiation and increased sweating.

32 Which one of the following is the pathway by which blood passes from the liver to the lungs?
- **a** Hepatic portal vein – vena cava – right atrium – right ventricle – pulmonary vein.
- **b** Hepatic vein – vena cava – right atrium – right ventricle – pulmonary artery.
- **c** Hepatic portal vein – vena cava – left atrium – left ventricle – pulmonary vein.
- **d** Hepatic vein – vena cava – left atrium – left ventricle – pulmonary artery.

33 Most of the urea entering the bloodstream is produced by the:
- **a** Kidneys.
- **b** Lungs.
- **c** Muscles.
- **d** Liver.

34 Which of the following will not pass through capillary walls?
- **a** Amino acids.
- **b** White blood cells.
- **c** Glucose.
- **d** Red blood cells.

35 Oestrogen is produced by the:
- **a** Pituitary gland.
- **b** Uterus.
- **c** Fallopian tube.
- **d** Ovaries.

36 Which of the following is not in lymph?
- **a** Lymphocytes.
- **b** Water.
- **c** Red blood cells.
- **d** Lipids.

37 An action potential is a:
- **a** Nerve impulse.
- **b** Heart beat.
- **c** Muscle contraction.
- **d** Breath.

38 Which of the following would represent hypothermia?
- **a** 37°C.
- **b** 35°C.
- **c** 36.5°C.
- **d** 37.5°C.

39 Bacteria are hindered from entering the human body by the:
- **a** Acid nature of urine.
- **b** Outermost part of skin comprising layers of dead cells.
- **c** Body temperature being regulated within narrow limits.
- **d** Body openings being usually moist.

40 Glycogen is stored in the largest amounts in:
- **a** Heart and lungs.
- **b** Skin and kidneys.
- **c** Liver and muscles.
- **d** Nerves and muscles.

41 A pulse rate lower than normal might indicate that the client is:
- **a** Frightened.
- **b** Very fit.
- **c** Anaemic.
- **d** Feverish.

42 Normal breathing rate in breaths per minute for an adult at rest is:
- **a** 8–10.
- **b** 65–75.
- **c** 16–20.
- **d** 30–40.

43 In an emergency, pulse rate is usually taken at the:
- **a** Foot.
- **b** Neck.
- **c** Wrist.
- **d** Thumb.

44 A baby's pulse rate compared to an adult's is:
- **a** Higher than normal.
- **b** Lower than normal.
- **c** The same as normal.
- **d** Irregular.

45 Blood pressure is usually shown as:
- **a** Diastolic minus systolic.
- **b** Systolic minus diastolic.
- **c** Diastolic over systolic.
- **d** Systolic over diastolic.

46 A young healthy adult has a blood pressure in the region of:
- **a** 160/140.
- **b** 80/120.
- **c** 120/80.
- **d** 120/160.

47 Tidal volume is:
- **a** The biggest breath you can take.
- **b** The smallest breath ever taken.
- **c** A normal sized breath.
- **d** The biggest breath breathed out.

48 Which of the following represents a normal ECG trace?

a

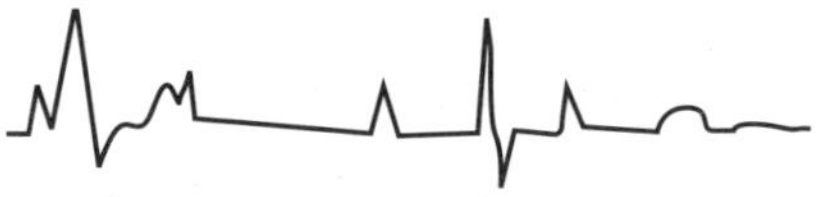

b

c

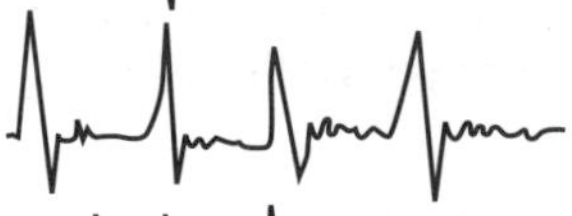

d

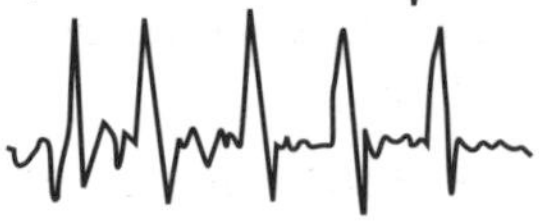

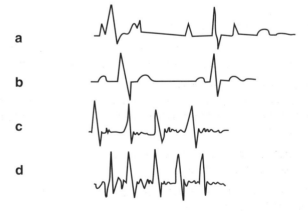

49 Jane's latest blood count reveals:
RBCs: 4.8 million per mm^3 blood
WBCs: 9000 per mm^3 blood
Platelets: 100 000 per mm^3 blood
What is the most likely condition that Jane is suffering from?
- **a** A form of anaemia.
- **b** A form of leukaemia.
- **c** An allergy.
- **d** A bleeding disorder.

50 An increase in the number of white blood cells generally might indicate:
- **a** Anaemia.
- **b** Allergy.
- **c** Infection.
- **d** Bleeding disorder.

51 Peak flow measurement is important for monitoring:
- **a** Asthma.
- **b** Angina.
- **c** Renal failure.
- **d** Hepatitis.

52 The diagram below shows a spirometer trace. The volume labelled X is:

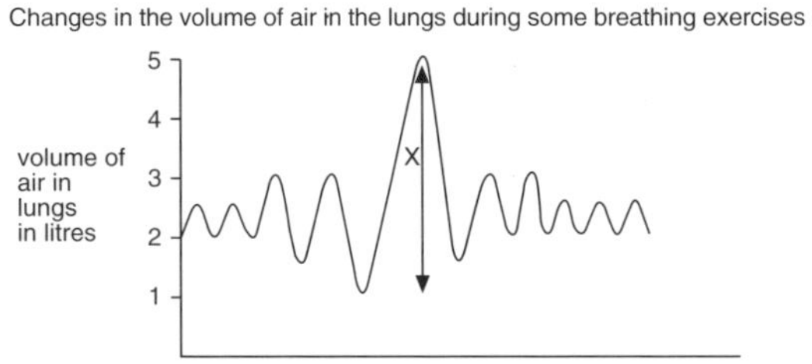

- **a** Peak flow.
- **b** Tidal volume.
- **c** Vital capacity.
- **d** Total lung volume.

53 Muscular cramps are a feature of a disordered electrolyte concentration. This is:
- **a** Low sodium.
- **b** High sodium.
- **c** Low calcium.
- **d** High calcium.

54 The imaging technique most suitable and cost-effective for detecting a bone fracture is:
- **a** Ultrasound.
- **b** Plain X-ray.
- **c** X-ray with contrast media.
- **d** CT scan.

55 It is suspected that a client might have secondary tumours in his liver. Which imaging technique would be cost-effective and suitable to use in the investigation?
a MRI.
b X-ray with contrast media.
c CT scan.
d Ultrasound.

56 The exact positioning of a brain tumour is required by a neurosurgeon. He or she particularly needs to know whether the tumour is in the grey matter of the brain. Which technique would be the most suitable?
a MRI.
b CT scan.
c Ultrasound.
d X-ray.

57 A medical consultant is trying to locate a stomach ulcer by the use of imaging techniques. Which of the following techniques would he or she employ?
a Barium swallow.
b Barium meal.
c Barium follow through.
d Barium enema.

58 During which of the following measurements should you have a trained person present? (Assuming you are not trained yourself)
a Pulse rate.
b Vital capacity.
c Blood pressure.
d Peak flow.

59 During exercise, which of the following would occur:
a Pulse rate rises, breathing rate falls.
b Pulse rate falls, breathing rate rises.
c Pulse rate falls, breathing rate falls.
d Pulse rate rises, breathing rate rises.

60 Which imaging technique is shown below?

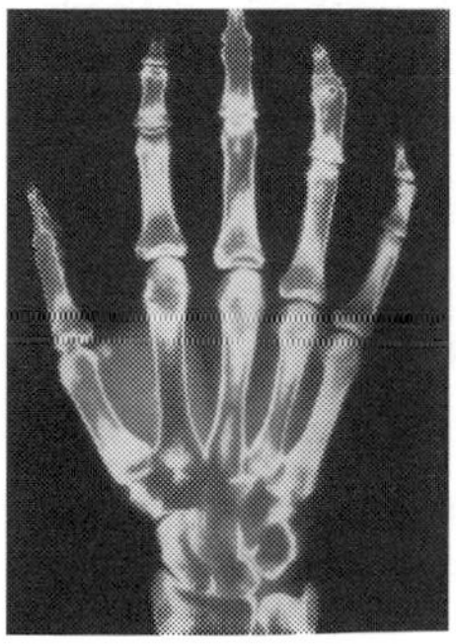

a MRI.
b Ultrasound.
c Plain X-ray.
d X-ray with contrast media.

Fast Facts

Action potential An alternative name for the electrical phenomenon usually called a nerve impulse.

ADH – antidiuretic hormone Hormone produced from the posterior pituitary gland which causes increased reabsorption of water in the last part of the renal tubules.

ADP – adenosine diphosphate A compound of adenine which is formed when energy is released from ATP.

Adrenaline Hormone produced from the medulla of the adrenal gland when the sympathetic nervous system is stimulated. It causes the body to respond physiologically to the effects of stress.

Aerobic respiration The release of energy from the breakdown of glucose in the presence of sufficient oxygen.

Anaerobic respiration A smaller release of energy from the partial breakdown of glucose, when there is insufficient oxygen.

Antibodies Substances released from lymphocyctes in response to antigens entering the body.

Antigens Foreign substances which cause the production of antibodies.

Aortic body Swelling containing chemoreceptors monitoring chemical changes in the blood. They are located close to the aortic arch.

ATP – adenosine triphosphate An energy rich compound inside mitochondria.

Autonomic system Part of the nervous system which controls internal organ activity including homoeostasis.

Bile, bilirubin, biliverdin Juice produced by the liver which contains two bile pigments, bilirubin and biliverdin, remnants of the breakdown of haemoglobin from old red blood cells.

Blood count The number of the different blood cells in a given volume of blood.

Blood pressure The force the blood exerts on the walls of the blood vessels.

Bone – compact Hard connective tissue consisting mainly of a matrix of collagen and salts of calcium built into Haversian systems or osteones.

Carotid body Similar to aortic bodies but found near the carotid arteries.

Chromatin network A network of chromatin seen in the nucleus of non-dividing cells.

Chromosomes Gene carrying bodies found in the nucleus of dividing cells. They consist of DNA and protein.

Cilia Microscopic hairlike protoplasmic projections from the cell membranes usually associated with the secretion of mucus. They have a whip-like motion which carries the stream of mucus and any trapped foreign particles to the exterior.

CNS – central nervous system The brain and spinal cord.

Collagen Insoluble protein fibres found in connective tissues such as tendons and bone.

Connective tissues Tissues which lie beneath epithelia and connect parts of the body. They consist of cells and fibres which lie in matrix e.g. bone, blood.

Corpus luteum Tiny endocrine gland in the ovary developed from the ruptured follicle after ovulation.

Cristae Shelf-like projections inside mitochondria containing the sites of enzymes for the final oxidation of glucose.

CT scan Special X-ray sensitive devices which together with a computer produces detailed images of the human body as 'slices'.

Cytoplasm The jelly-like material between the nuclear and cell membranes.

Diastolic Referring to the cardiac phase when the ventricles are not contracting.

DNA – deoxyribonucleic acid Double-stranded coiled material found in cell nuclei and responsible for hereditary units or genes.

ECG – electrocardiogram The tracing made by an electrocardiograph.

Electrocardiograph Instrument which measures the electrical potential differences occurring just prior to a heartbeat.

Electrolyte A chemical which dissociates to form ions when in solution.

Endoplasmic reticulum *Smooth* – a network of channels which form the intracellular transport system. Concerned with packaging materials for export from the cell. *Rough* – Intracellular transport system with small studded granules at intervals along its length – ribosomes.

Epithelium Tissue which lines surfaces and body cavities. Cells sit on a basement membrane. *Simple epithelia* are one-layered tissues. *Compound epithelia* are multi-layered.

Excretion Elimination of waste products of metabolism.

Feedback *Negative* – inhibition of the input by a part of the output of a system or process. *Positive* – stimulation of the input by a part of the output of a system or process.

Flagella Larger than cilia, these filamentous projections are used to propel the organism or cell e.g. tails of spermatozoa.

FSH – follicle stimulating hormone Pituitary hormone which initiates the menstrual cycle by causing ovarian follicles to develop.

Gamete Cell produced by sexual organs which cannot develop further unless united with a gamete from the opposite gender e.g. spermatozoa or ova.

Glucagon Pancreatic hormone which increases blood glucose.

Glycolysis The first part of the oxidation of glucose which occurs in the cytoplasm of the cell.

Gonads Sexual organ which produces gametes e.g. ovary, testis.

Granulocyte White blood cell characterised by darkly staining granules in the cytoplasm e.g. phagocyte, eosinophil, basophil.

Haversian systems Series of concentric circles surrounding a central Haversian canal forming compact bone.

Homoeostasis (*also* homeostasis) Maintaining a constant internal environment around body cells.

Hypothalamus Part of the brain located above the pituitary glands responsible for several vital processes e.g. water balance.

Immunity Ability of the body to resist disease.

Insulin Pancreatic hormone which reduces blood sugar.

Involuntary muscle An alternative name for smooth muscle.

Ion A charged particle.

Islets of Langerhans Clusters of cells scattered throughout the pancreas which function as endocrine glands.

Krebs cycle The last part of aerobic respiration which occurs inside mitochondria.

Lactic acid A by-product of anaerobic respiration.

LH – luteinising hormone Pituitary hormone responsible for ovulation and the development of the corpus luteum.

Lymph Milky-coloured liquid contained within the lymphatic vessels.

Lymphocytes Agranular white blood cells responsible for the production of antibodies.

Macrophages Large cells which move through tissues engulfing foreign and dead debris.

Matrix Background substance in which cells or fibres lie.

Meiosis Type of cell division which occurs once in the formation of gametes to reduce their chromosome number to half that of the parent cell.

Mitochondria Spherical or cylindrical bodies scattered throughout the cell cytoplasm, concerned with the last part of aerobic respiration.

Mitosis Type of cell division which reproduces identical daughter cells to the parent. Occurs in all cells except neurones and mature red blood cells.

Monocyte Large white blood cell which is very efficient at engulfing foreign and dead material.

MRI – magnetic resonance imaging Vibration of particles in a magnetic field in response to radio waves of particular frequency, this produces an image.

Muscle Tissue capable of contraction or shortening: *Cardiac muscle* found in the heart walls. *Skeletal muscle* attached to the skeleton and causing movement of bones. *Smooth muscle* found in the walls of internal organs for propelling substances.

Nerves Fibres from neurones bound in connective tissue.

Neurones Excitable cells capable of transmitting electrical impulses. *Sensory neurones* take impulses from receptors to CNS. *Motor neurones* take impulses from CNS to effectors (muscles and glands). *Relay or connector neurones* connect sensory to motor neurones.

Neurotransmitter Chemical produced from synaptic knob to enable the impulse to cross the synapse.

Nucleolus A darkly-staining body found inside the nucleus composed of RNA.

Nucleus The control centre of the cell; organises the activities of the cell and contains hereditary material.

Osmoreceptor Receptor cells (modified neurones) in the hypothalamus which detect changes in the osmotic pressure of blood.

Pancreas Organ which exhibits both digestive and endocrine functions.

Parasympathetic nervous system Part of the autonomic nervous system active in resting and nonstressful conditions.

Peak flow Maximum speed at which air can be forced out of the lungs.

Phagocytosis Process by which certain cells like phagocytes and monocytes engulf and destroy foreign and dead material.

Pituitary gland Endocrine gland lying below the hypothalamus of the brain which produces numerous hormones, many of which control other endocrine glands.

Pulse Shock waves transmitted along the walls of arteries when the ventricles in the heart contract.

RNA – ribonucleic acid Similar to DNA but single stranded; found in the nucleus, cytoplasm and ribosomes. Takes coded messages from the nucleus to other parts of the cell.

Ribosomes Small darkly-staining bodies found freely in the cytoplasm and on the rough endoplasmic reticulum. Concerned with the manufacture of cell proteins.

Spirometer Apparatus used for measuring lung volumes.

Striped or striated muscle Alternative names for skeletal muscle.

Sympathetic nervous system Part of the autonomic nervous system which is active in stressful conditions.

Synapse A tiny gap between two neurones.

Synaptic knob Swollen end of neuronal axons capable of secreting neurotransmitter.

Synovial fluid, membrane Part of the lining and fluid in joint cavities.

Systolic Referring to the cardiac phase when the ventricles are contracting.

Tidal volume Normal ebb and flow of air into and out of the chest during breathing.

Tissues Groups of similar cells carrying out the same function, e.g. epithelia, connective tissues, muscle, nervous tissues.

Ultrasound Image produced by high-frequency sound waves on soft tissue.

Unstriped or unstriated muscle Alternative names for involuntary muscle.

Urea Metabolic waste product from surplus amino acids produced by the liver.

Urine Watery solution of urea and salts made by the kidneys and eliminated from the bladder via the urethra.

Vital capacity Maximum volume of air which can be exhaled after a maximum inhalation.

Voluntary muscle Alternative name for skeletal muscle.

X-ray image Image produced from a photograph of extremely short wavelength electromagnetic radiation passing through the body.

References and further reading

Fullick, A., 1994, *Biology,* Heinemann Educational
Nave and Nave, 1985, *Physics for the Health Services,* Saunders
Pickering, W. R., 1994, *Advanced Biology,* Oxford University Press
Rowett, H. G. Q., 1988, *Basic Anatomy and Physiology,* John Murray (3rd ed.)
Tortora and Grabowski, 1993, *Principles of Anatomy and Physiology,* HarperCollins (7th ed.)
Vander, Sherman and Luciano, 1990, *Human Physiology,* McGraw-Hill (5th ed.)

Chapter 10

Human growth and development

This chapter investigates a wide range of issues associated with human growth and development, these include:

- **physical development**
- **language development**
- **cognitive development**
- **emotional development**
- **social and cultural influences on self-awareness**
- **personality, temperament and trait theories, environmental theories, early learning theories and humanistic theories**
- **the influence of inherited and environmental factors, genetics, determinism and interaction**
- **transition and change in life – expected and unexpected change**
- **methods of support for coping with transition and change.**

Life involves moving through a pattern of physical, mental and emotional changes. We start life as small, somewhat helpless babies with limited knowledge. As we grow in size, so we grow in our understanding of ourselves and our surroundings. We hope to spend a long time as adults enjoying our physical, intellectual, social and emotional achievements. Later life may be a time of wisdom and fulfilment, or a time of despair.

An advanced investigation into life changes raises some very deep and sometimes controversial questions. This chapter therefore covers questions about *how* and *why* people develop the cognitive abilities and personal qualities that they do. In fact, Chapters 10, 11 and 12 (which cover Unit 4) explore some key influences on people's lives.

Think it over

In the film, *Forrest Gump,* Forrest Gump is a fictional character who has superhuman abilities, but very little intelligence. At one point he wonders what life is all about – do we just float about like a feather on a breeze or are our lives guided by destiny? This question has taxed the minds of religious leaders, philosophers, writers and poets for the last 7000 years or more. Forrest Gump decides that the answer is – a bit of both. Chapters 10, 11 and 12 do not provide a final answer to the question of destiny, but they do provide an overview of the issues involved.

Physical development

Every individual has a unique pattern of growth and development. This is because there are so many factors influencing our progress. It would be logical to say that each one us begins from the moment a sperm nucleus from the father joins with the nucleus from the mother's ovum, but the exact time of this process, known as *fertilisation,* is usually unknown. To obtain a more recognisable starting date, doctors will ask a pregnant woman for the starting date of her last period and add on two weeks. The period when the ovum is available for fertilising by the sperm is halfway between menstruations.

There is, however, a great deal of controversy over when an embryo becomes a human being. This has largely arisen from discussions about abortion. In Britain, the Abortion Act (1967) allowed termination of pregnancy up to the 28th week of gestation, but after lengthy debates in Parliament, the limit was reduced to the 24th week. The debate continues, however, as babies can now survive if born at 24 weeks, due to the great advances made in modern techniques. Many groups think that the limit should be reduced even further. Some pressure groups (such as Life) and many individuals consider that all abortion is wrong and human life is sacred from the date of fertilisation.

The fertilised ovum, now known as a *zygote,* is one of the larger cells in humans and is just visible to the naked eye. Imagine the smallest dot you can make with a very sharp pencil and this is about the right size. After a short rest period it begins to divide, first into two cells, then four, eight and so on. Quickly the tiny structure becomes a ball of smaller cells – a *morula.* These cells begin to become organised into different areas. Some will be destined to form the new human being, but for a while the majority of the cells are preparing to become its coverings and developing placenta. It is important that these parts are ready to secure the food supply for the developing being as soon as the structure enters the womb, or uterus, of the mother. All the time so far has been spent in travelling down the Fallopian tube leading from the ovary into the uterus. At about a week old, the tiny structure, a hollow ball of cells known as a *blastocyst,* arrives in the uterus. The next few days are vital to the embryo. It must bury itself in the *endometrium,* the thickened lining of the mother's uterus and secure a food supply before the mother's next menstruation is due. If this does not happen, the blastocyst will be swept out of the mother's body with the products of menstruation and will die. Once embedded in this way, a process called *implantation*, the tiny embryo releases a hormone into the mother's blood which prevents the next menstruation.

Never again will growth be so rapid. By the third week after fertilisation (week 5 of the pregnancy calculation), the embryo has grown to be 0.5 cm long and has started to develop a brain, eyes, ears and limbs. Some individuals might class the development of the brain as being significant in the date of becoming a human being. There is even a tiny heart pumping blood to the newly-formed placenta to obtain nutrients and oxygen from the mother's blood.

The embryo continues to grow and develop at a fantastic rate until at week 8 all major organs have formed. Then there is a human-looking face with eyes, ears, nose and mouth. Limbs have formed fingers and toes, and the body length has increased to 3 cm (Figure 10.1). The name changes again – from now until birth it is called a *foetus*.

Growth and development of internal organs continues and the next main stage is at 20 weeks. The mother will begin to feel movements of the foetus, weak at first but getting stronger as the pregnancy progresses. The midwife can hear the heart beats through a trumpet-shaped instrument called a *foetal stethoscope*. The heart beats are very fast and difficult to count without experience.

The foetus is clearly male or female because the external sex organs have developed and the total length is now around 24 cm. The weight of the foetus is close to 0.5 kg already.

Try it

1 Using Figure 10.2, draw two graphs to show the changes in length and weight up to birth.

Time in months of pregnancy	Length in centimetres	Weight in kilograms
1	0.35	Almost none
2	3.5	0.05
3	8.5	0.1
4	15	0.2
5	23	0.4
6	30	0.75
7	38	1.5
8	45	2.0
9	51	3.5

Figure 10.2

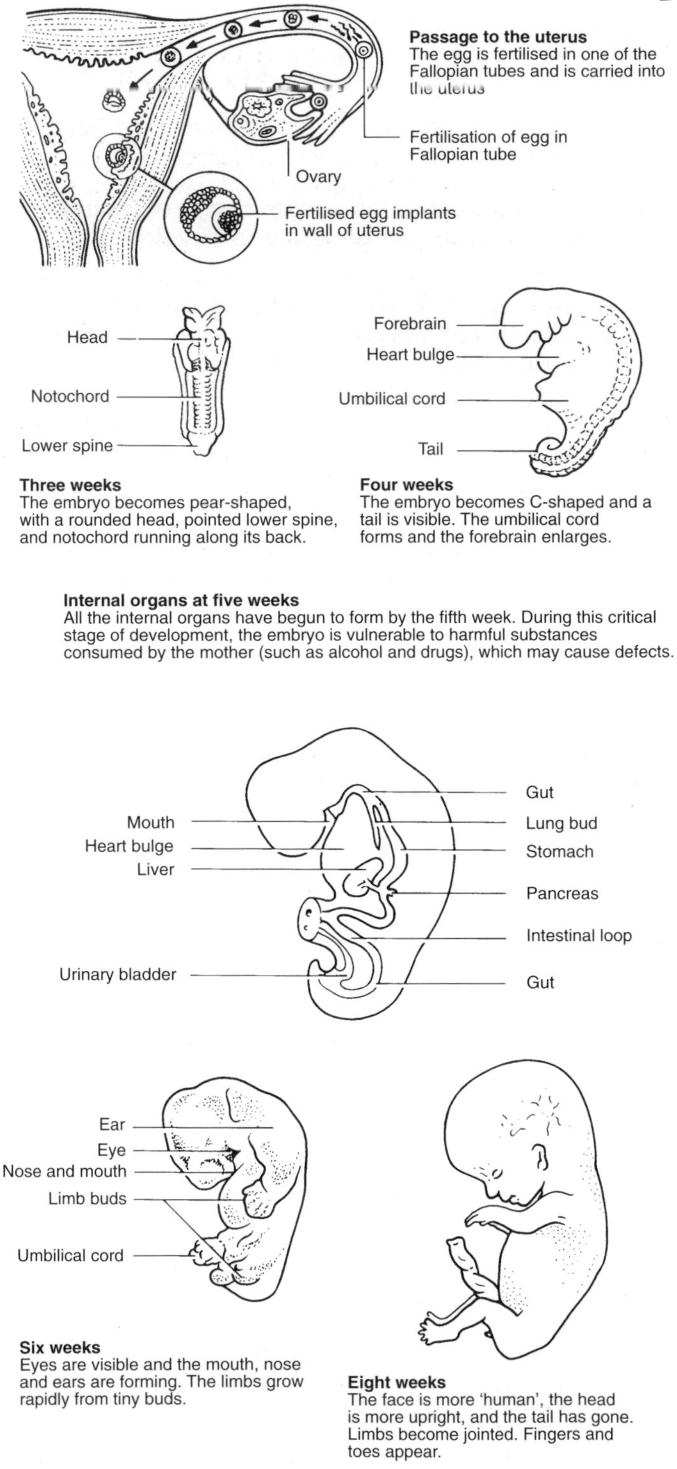
Passage to the uterus
The egg is fertilised in one of the Fallopian tubes and is carried into the uterus
Fertilisation of egg in Fallopian tube
Ovary
Fertilised egg implants in wall of uterus
Head
Notochord
Lower spine
Three weeks
The embryo becomes pear-shaped, with a rounded head, pointed lower spine, and notochord running along its back.
Forebrain
Heart bulge
Umbilical cord
Tail
Four weeks
The embryo becomes C-shaped and a tail is visible. The umbilical cord forms and the forebrain enlarges.
Internal organs at five weeks
All the internal organs have begun to form by the fifth week. During this critical stage of development, the embryo is vulnerable to harmful substances consumed by the mother (such as alcohol and drugs), which may cause defects.
Mouth
Heart bulge
Liver
Urinary bladder
Gut
Lung bud
Stomach
Pancreas
Intestinal loop
Gut
Ear
Eye
Nose and mouth
Limb buds
Umbilical cord
Six weeks
Eyes are visible and the mouth, nose and ears are forming. The limbs grow rapidly from tiny buds.
Eight weeks
The face is more 'human', the head is more upright, and the tail has gone. Limbs become jointed. Fingers and toes appear.

Figure 10.1 Embryo development

2 Find out the length and weight of a typical 6-month-old foetus.

As you can see from your graph and the table, at 9 months (40 weeks) the foetus is ready to be born. It is about 50 cm long and weighs around 3.5 kg.

A newborn infant, often called a *neonate,* is a helpless individual and needs care and protection of parents or others to survive. The nervous system which co-ordinates many bodily functions is immature and needs time to develop. The digestive system is unable to take food that is not in an easily digestible form such as milk. Other body systems, such as the circulatory and respiratory systems, have undergone major changes as a result of birth – the change to air breathing and physical separation from the mother. A few weeks later, the baby's temperature regulating system is able to function properly and fat is deposited beneath the skin as an insulating layer.

For the first three months of a baby's life, movements are unco-ordinated and many *primitive reflexes* are present. These are gradually replaced by *learned responses.*

Primitive reflexes

The main reflexes are:

- rooting
- grasp
- moro
- walking.

They are used to test the functioning of the baby's nervous system.

Rooting reflex

The baby turns its head in response to a touch on the cheek. This enables the baby to find the mother's breast and nipple. The sucking reflex occurs when the baby finds the nipple. A finger placed close to the corner of the mouth will cause this sort of response.

Grasp reflex

Any object put into the palm of the baby's hand will be grasped strongly. Often the grasp is so strong that the baby's weight can be supported.

Moro, or startle, reflex

When a baby is startled, its hands and arms are thrown outwards and the legs straightened. The baby often cries and then pulls the arms, hands and fingers inwards as if trying to catch hold of something. This is one of the first reflexes to disappear.

Walking reflex

During the first two months, when a baby is held upright with feet touching the ground, forward movements are made by the legs as if the baby is walking.

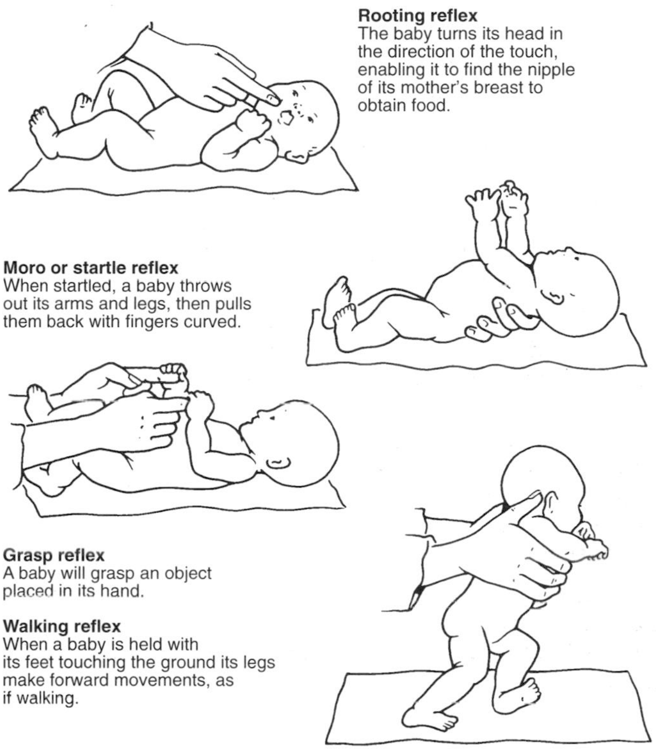

Rooting reflex
The baby turns its head in the direction of the touch, enabling it to find the nipple of its mother's breast to obtain food.
Moro or startle reflex
When startled, a baby throws out its arms and legs, then pulls them back with fingers curved.
Grasp reflex
A baby will grasp an object placed in its hand.
Walking reflex
When a baby is held with its feet touching the ground its legs make forward movements, as if walking.

Figure 10.3 The primitive reflexes of a newborn baby

Try it

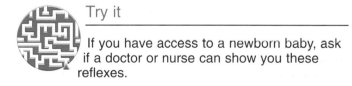

If you have access to a newborn baby, ask if a doctor or nurse can show you these reflexes.

Myelination

Nerve fibres attached to nerve cells gradually acquire a fatty sheath during the first years of life. This is known as *myelination.* Nerve impulses travel a lot faster when they are insulated in this way. Many nerve cells have to 'connect up' with each other and these two processes mean that both muscle and nerve co-ordination slowly increase.

Muscle co-ordination

Motor development is the term given to the development of muscle co-ordination. Its rate depends on the maturity of the child's nervous system. Figure 10.4 gives *average* rates for motor development. Many children will be slower or faster than those given.

Age in months	Stage of motor development
Birth	Primitive reflexes only
1	Lifts up chin
2	Lifts chest up
3	Reaches for but does not grasp objects
4	Sits supported
5	Grasps objects
6	Sits on chair, reaches for and grasps objects
7	Stands with support
9	Stands alone but holding on
10	Crawls quickly
11	Walks holding one hand
12	Pulls up on furniture to stand
13	Crawls up stairs
14	Stands alone unsupported
15	Walks alone
24	Runs, picks things up without falling over
30	Stands on toes, jumps
36	Stands on one leg
48	Walks downstairs with one foot on each step

Figure 10.4 Average rates of motor development

Hand movement

Manipulation, or hand movement, is an aspect of motor development that is easy to see and measure. Professional carers take notice of these fine movements in assessing development.

At 6 months, children can reach for and grasp objects in their hands and transfer objects from one hand to another. Two months later, things are held between fingers and the thumb, while around the first birthday tiny objects can be picked up between the thumb and the first finger. A 2-year-old child can hold a pencil like an adult does and unscrew a top from a container.

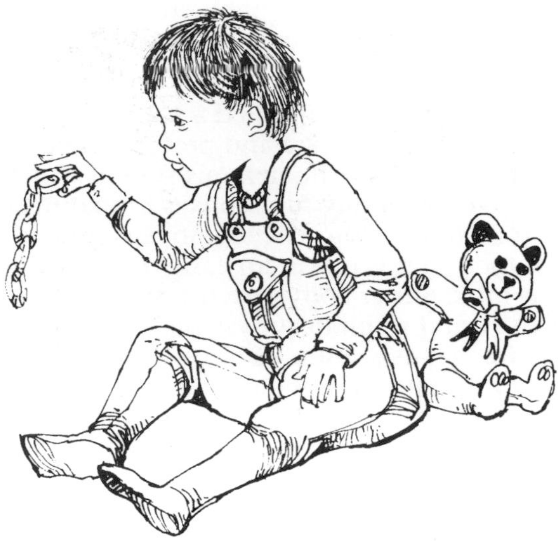

Growth rates

During childhood, different parts of the body grow at different rates.

The nervous system, sense organs and head grow very rapidly from birth to 6 years. A 6-year-old's head is 90 per cent of the adult size, and he or she can wear a parent's hat!

The reproductive organs remain small and undeveloped until the onset of *puberty* (between 11 and 16 years), and then they grow rapidly to reach adult size.

General body growth is more steady, reaching adult size at around 18–20 years, but with three 'growth spurts' at 1, 5–7 years, and puberty. Puberty is the period of hormone regulated development when physical and secondary characteristics appear. Girls generally start puberty earlier than boys, at 11–13 years, with boys being two years later. The puberty

Male	Female
1 Enlargement of testes and penis	Enlargement of breasts and nipples
2 Pubic, facial, underarm hair growth	Pubic and underarm hair growth
3 Increased muscle and bone size leads to increased strength	Increased fat deposited under skin leads to increased curvy shape
4 Voice deepens (breaks)	Onset of menstruation

Figure 10.5 Secondary sexual characteristics

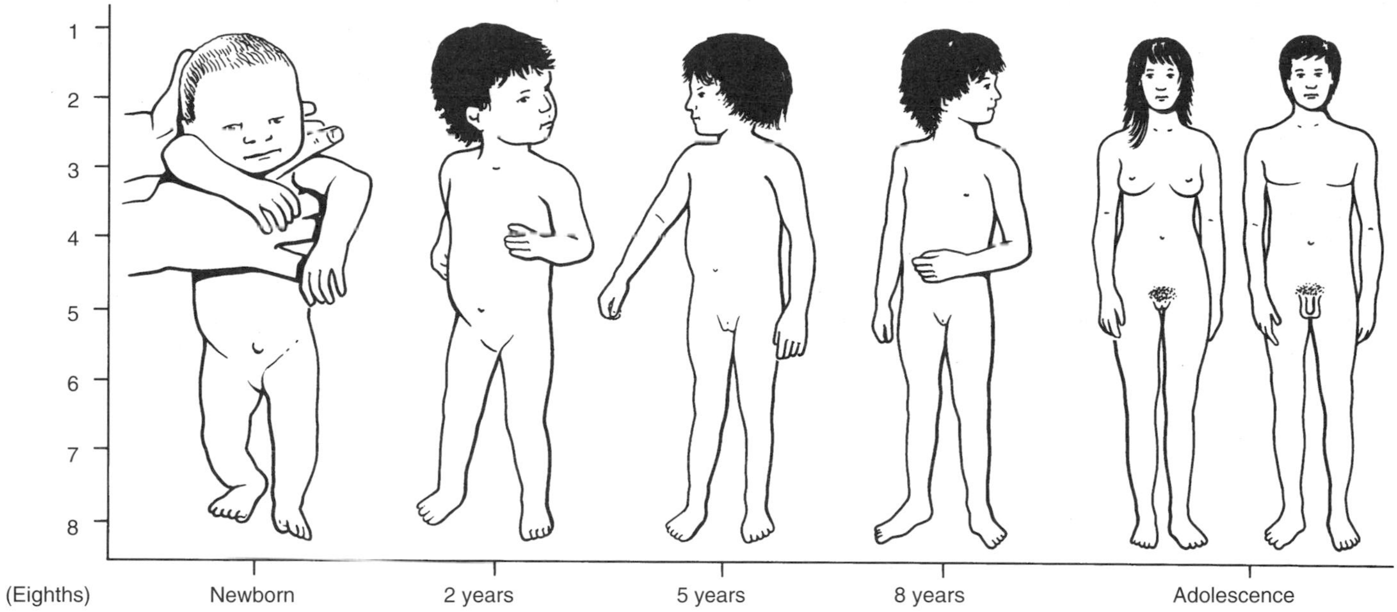

Figure 10.6 Growth profiles from birth to adolescence

'spurt' is caused by the secretion of sex hormones, oestrogen in girls and testosterone in boys. These hormones are responsible for the other changes which turn the body of a child into that of an adult. These changes are known as the secondary *sexual characteristics.*

Try it

Study Fig 10.6. Write a report of the changes you can see.

Bone development

When the skeleton first forms it is made of a flexible material called *cartilage*. This is slowly replaced by bone which is visible on X-rays. Each bone passes through the same sequence of changes of shape as it reaches maturity in a healthy adult. Bone age is, therefore, a useful measure of physical development. Height and weight standards are often associated with age, but are less useful because of the enormous differences which can occur in different individuals.

Teeth

Babies develop their first set of teeth from the age of 6 months up to 3 years. They are often known as milk teeth, or *deciduous teeth*. From about 6-years-old, these teeth are gradually replaced by the permanent teeth. There are wide variations in dates of both the eruption of milk teeth and their replacement by permanent teeth and, therefore, only average dates can be given.

Try it

Research the eruption of milk teeth and replacement by permanent teeth and present your findings as two illustrated diagrams.

Factors influencing growth and development

As mentioned earlier, every individual has a different pattern of growth and development because so many influences affect the rate of progress. A few to consider are:

- inherited characteristics from parents
- health and disease of mother and child
- hormone balance, for example the growth hormone, thyroxine
- environmental factors, such as parents who smoke or drink alcohol
- nutrition of mother and child

- stimulation and activity, for example a child will not hold a pencil correctly if he or she has never been given the opportunity.

Try it

Research one of the factors listed above. Write a report about how that factor may influence growth and development.

Adolescence

Adolescence is the stage between childhood and adulthood, roughly interpreted as the teenage years. It begins with puberty and overlaps it, but it is not the same as puberty. An adolescent has to come to terms with physical changes in the body, an increased sex drive, and mental and emotional changes.

Adulthood

During adult life, no major changes take place physically until women reach the end of their reproductive life. This is known as the *menopause* and usually takes place between 45 and 55 years of age. The ovaries stop producing ova (eggs) and, as a result, less of the female hormone oestrogen is produced. This produces physical changes and sometimes psychological changes occur as well, though this is less clear.

When menstruation stops, the reproductive organs shrink. Many women complain of hot flushes and night sweats, and body chemistry is altered. Bones become less dense and *osteoporosis* may develop later. (Osteoporosis causes bones to become more brittle and liable to fracture. It can occur in men who are ageing, but is much more common in women.) In recent years, hormone replacement therapy has become more widespread as a treatment for women, to reduce the effects of oestrogen deficiency.

Men may continue to produce sperm until well into their seventies or later.

Loss of hair may affect both sexes in the middle years of life, but it is much more common in men. Hair loss in men occurs first from the temples, then the crown of the head, with a gradual widening of the bald area to the sides of the head.

Older people are usually less active than younger people, but still continue to take in the same amount of food. This often results in a gradual thickening of the trunk, arms and legs, often called 'middle age spread'. Many people regard this as an inevitable stage in getting older, but it generally is a result of not matching food (and therefore energy) intake with energy output.

Older people

Physical and mental changes occur as time passes. Not many people live to be over a hundred years old – the average life span is around 85 years of age.

Sexual activity may decline only a little or a lot, very often depending on the usual life pattern of the individual. Elastic tissue, present in many organs, degenerates with age and this is most readily seen in wrinkled skin. Blood capillaries are more fragile so bruising occurs from relatively small injuries.

The number of nerve cells in the central nervous system steadily decreases from quite a young age because they are irreplaceable. This loss, unnoticed at first, begins to show as one gets older. It results in poorer memory, difficulty in learning new skills quickly and slower reaction times. Senses are less acute, particularly taste, smell and hearing.

The progressive loss of hearing which can come with age is known as *presbyacusis* – sounds are less clear and high tones less audible. It occurs with the degeneration of the sensory hair cells of the cochlea (in the inner ear) and of nerve cells.

The focusing power of the eye weakens with age, beginning at around 45. Often after the age of 65 there is little focusing power left. Large print can usually be seen, but smaller print needs to be held at arm's length, until eventually all focusing is replaced

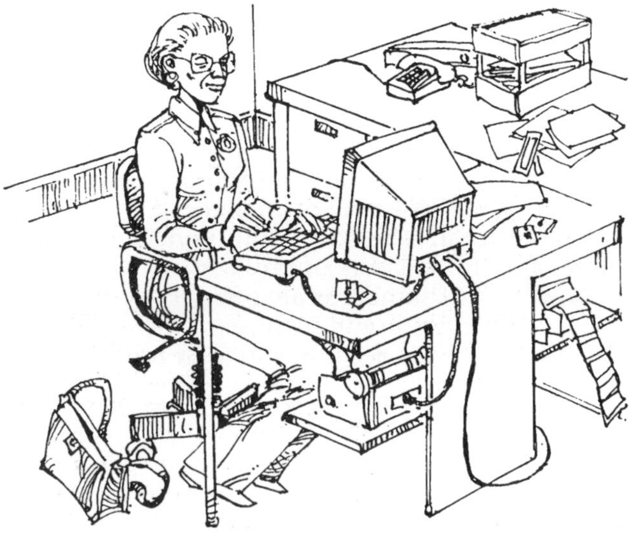

by spectacle lenses. Almost everyone over the age of 65 has some degree of cataract, where the lens in the eye has started to become opaque. The condition tends to progress with advancing years and most people have some loss of vision due to cataract formation at around 75 years.

As the body ages it gradually loses it sensitivity to cold, so when body temperature drops an old person may not feel the cold. With age there is a lowered ability to reverse a fall in body temperature, which is why older people are more likely to develop *hypothermia* in cold weather.

Heart, breathing and circulation all become less efficient, causing difficulty with climbing stairs and hills, and with strenuous exercise. A healthy young adult has a blood pressure around 110/75 mm of mercury, but around the age of 60 years this is 130/90 or higher.

Muscle thins and weakens, while joints become less mobile and total height shrinks. Wound healing and resistance to infection decline with age. Functions of organs like the kidneys and the liver slowly decline.

However, there are positive aspects to growing older. Despite the decline of physical systems, a combination of tolerance, wisdom and experience built up over the years enables older people to avoid the mistakes made by younger, inexperienced people.

Healthy older people may have greater emotional control and a more developed understanding of their self-concept than younger people. Socially, older people may have more time to appreciate people and their environment.

Dementia

In the 1950s, many people believed that intellectual ability declined with age. Research on intelligence in the 1940s was interpreted to mean that older people become less intellectually able as they grew older. In the late 1940s and 1950s there were claims that people achieved a peak mental ability at 20 or 25 years of age. However, research since then has revealed quite a different story. Many individuals who use their mental abilities and 'exercise their minds' seem to continue to increase their intellectual abilities. An increase in ability might even continue into a person's eighties. Older people may slow down in terms of the speed at which they react, and they may experience increasing irritation with poorer recent memory. But on average, older people can expect to keep the quality of their thinking at least at the level achieved by adulthood. It is important to maintain the level of mental activity. There is evidence that people who do not do much mental reasoning may lose some of their mental skills as they age. The belief that mental ability declines with age was linked with an old stereotype – that people's brains 'wore out' so that they became demented during their old age.

Dementia is *not* caused by the slow wearing out of the body. Nor is it part of any general ageing process. Dementia is a pattern of symptoms probably caused by a variety of different influences. Two types of dementia are:

- that caused by the breakdown of the blood supply to the brain
- Alzheimer's-type dementia, which involves a loss of brain tissue and the shrinkage of the brain, although the blood supply may be healthy.

Dementia can cause a range of disabilities. These include a loss of ability to control emotion, difficulties in understanding other people, difficulties in communicating and expressing thoughts, serious loss of memory, disorientation in time and place, difficulties in recognising people and places, and difficulties in performing everyday living activities, such as getting dressed.

People with severe dementia may lose the ability to swallow or even walk. Eventually dementia may result in the death of the individual.

Some types of dementia can develop in young adults and even adolescents. But in general, dementing illness is uncommon before 65 years of age. Brayne and Ames (1988) provide statistics which include all organic (brain-related) illnesses. The statistics suggest that as many as 20 per cent of people over the age of 85 years may experience symptoms associated with dementia.

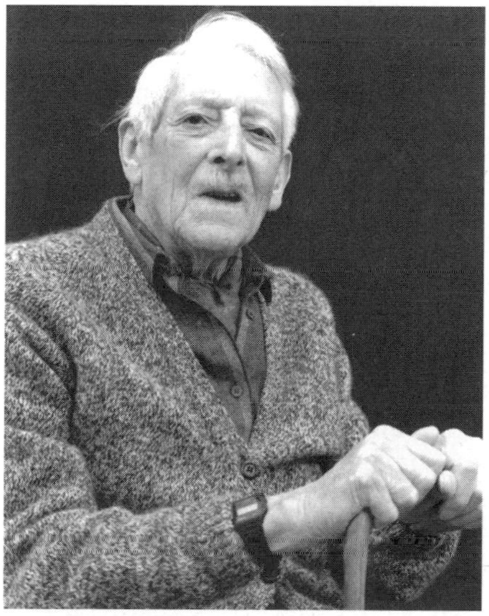

Figure 10.7 The majority of people over 85 years of age do not experience dementia

It is important to note that these statistics still imply that 80 per cent of people over 85 do not show signs of dementing illness. Although older people may be more at risk of dementia than younger people, dementia is not a normal part of the life cycle. As Edgar Milar (1977) argues, dementia represents 'abnormal ageing'.

Language development

Pre-language

On average, children do not usually start to use words until they are about 12 months old, and they start to use two words together at about 18 months of age. The first 18 months of life are referred to as 'infancy', which originally meant 'incapable of speech'. Language abilities develop gradually and infants may be able to use words to name experiences. However, infancy is still considered as a 'pre-language' stage of development.

Babies can make crying sounds from birth. During the first two months of life, they will tend to cry if they are upset or in pain. From about the third month of life, they may make 'cooing' sounds if they are content and happy. The range of sounds that babies make develops gradually, and at about 4–9 months of age babies will begin to 'babble'. Babbling might involve making sounds like 'dadada' or 'mamamama'. It involves experimenting with sounds and it is possible to interpret this stage as an in-built or 'innate' developmental stage. It may be that babies are building their ability to use sounds ready for language. Zimbardo (1992) quotes research from Petitto and Marentette. These two researchers analysed recordings of hearing-impaired infants who were cared for by hearing-impaired parents. It seems that hearing-impaired infants go through a stage of babbling with hand movements in response to the sign language used by carers. Petitto and Marentette believe that 'babbling' is not confined to learning to make sounds, but that it is a stage for learning to use language, whether that language is spoken or sign language. The pre-language stage of babbling may have something to do with organising an infant's abilities ready for language.

Infants listen to a wide range of sounds that might be used in language. It seems that they start to focus on the sounds that a particular language used by 8 months of age. It may be that infants 'lock' on to a particular range of sounds and then lose the ability to distinguish the fine detail of sounds used in other languages.

Zimbardo (1992) quotes research from Janet Werker, who studied the ability of children and adults to hear the different sounds (or phonemes) used in English and in Hindi. Infants under 8 months could hear all the differences, regardless of whether they were exposed to English or Hindi as their language. After 8 months this ability seemed to be lost. Only Hindi-speaking children could hear and distinguish the fine detail of sounds in their language. 'Thus, infants start with sensitivities to sounds that they lose if these contrasts are not used in their language.' (Zimbardo [1992], page 155.)

The first 12 months of life, therefore, are a time when infants may begin to build their ability to make signs or sounds ready for language. But it may be quite wrong to suppose that because the young infant does not use language, adults and infants do not communicate.

Infants pay particular attention to faces. Studies in the 1950s suggested that babies tend to smile at human faces. Robert Fantz (1961) found that babies between 1 and 15 weeks of age would spend longer looking at diagrams that looked like a human face than at other patterns. Julia Berryman *et al.* (1991) quote studies which suggest that babies start to recognise faces at between the sixth and ninth weeks of life. It is likely that babies are born with a readiness to smile at human faces. As learning develops, an infant may be able to pick out his or her own mother's face and respond to expressions.

Research by Arlene Walker-Andrews (1986) suggests that 7-month-old babies can recognise happy or angry voice tones. The babies were shown two films side by side, one film showing a face with a happy expression, and one film showing a face with an angry expression. The babies then heard an angry voice or a happy voice. The infants looked more at the happy face when they could hear the happy voice and more at the angry face when the angry voice was played.

Infants communicate with gaze and with facial expressions and sounds. Adults seem to have a set way of communicating with infants. They often talk more slowly and in a higher pitched voice when talking to infants. Adults may also use exaggerated facial expressions and sounds. This type of communication is called 'baby-talk'. A father might use slow, gentle sounds to comfort an infant, 'There...there...all...right...go...to...sleep...now'. And higher rising sounds catch the baby's attention,

'Hello, what's this…what's this then…look at this.' Research by Anne Fernald (quoted in Zimbardo, 1992) suggests that parents use baby-talk in many different cultures. Babies appear to respond to the baby-talk style even if it is in a language they are not used to.

Parent/infant games like 'peek-a-boo' may also help infants to learn the idea of social relationships and turn-taking in communication.

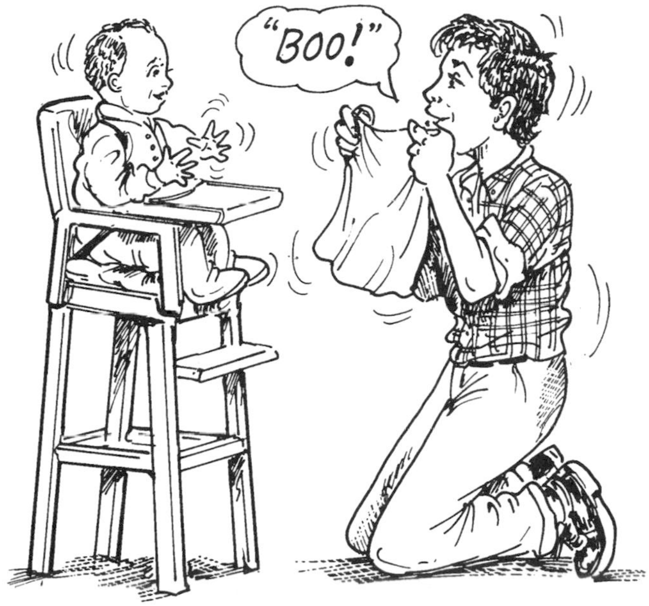

Children may begin to produce their first words between 9 and 16 months of age. Richard Gross (1992) states the average for first words as 12 months.

The rate at which children learn to use words will depend on their social context and their cognitive development. Social interaction with brothers, sisters or other carers may help a child to speak. Piaget (1896–1980) believed that cognitive development had to reach the necessary stage before language would develop. He believed that thought processes lead the development of language. Another famous theorist, Lev Vygotsky (1894–1934), believed that language development was motivated by the experience of communicating with others. Vygotsky believed that social interaction, or social relationships, provided the basis for both the development of thinking and the development of language ability. A child might want a toy that he or she cannot reach. The child's father might point at the toy and say 'Is this what you want?' The child might then copy the idea of pointing. The child learns to point because of his or her social experience.

Later the child will be able to use language in order to meet his or her social needs, as well as using ideas like pointing.

Think it over

If you live or work with young children, what can you do to help them develop language?

If social relationships are important, then an infant's development may be supported with high quality play and interaction. Speaking to the child and playing with the child using lots of clear facial expression and gesture may be useful.

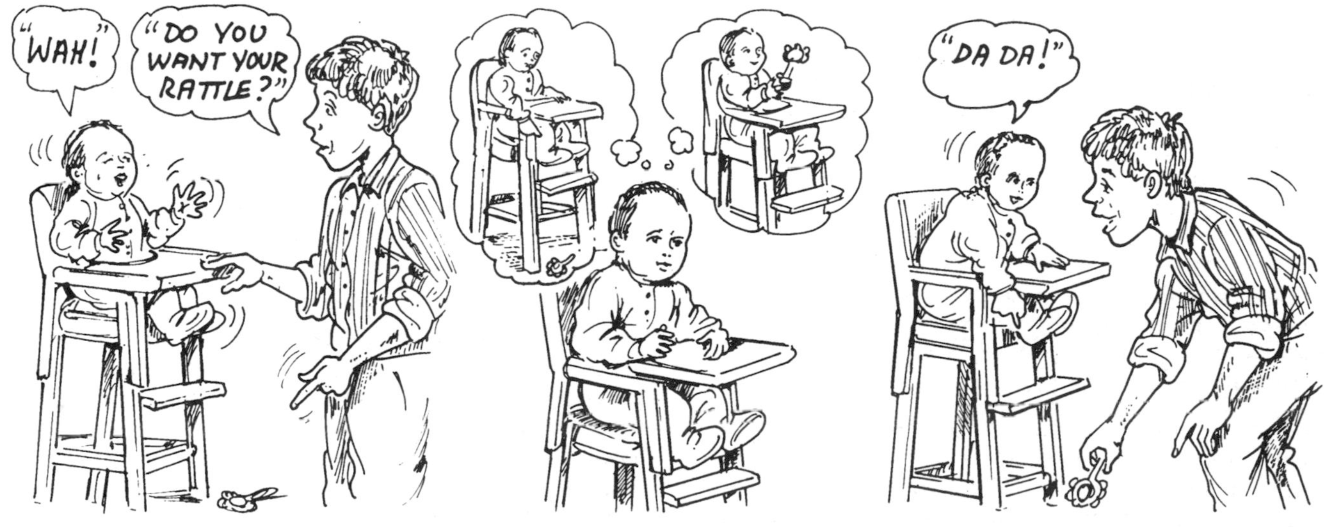

Figure 10.8 Social interaction influences learning

Whatever the balance between social and cognitive explanations for language, young children are astonishingly good at learning words. Between the ages of 1½ and 6, children may develop a 14 000-word vocabulary. This works out as almost one word for each hour that the child is awake (Zimbardo, 1992).

To begin with children will use a single word – the 'One word stage' (Gross, 1992). They may use a single word to name an experience or an object which they have seen, such as 'dadda', which can be used to mean 'Look, I can see my father (daddy), or 'I want daddy to come here', or 'Where is daddy?' A carer may be able to tell what the child means because of the setting or context in which the word is used, or the way that the child says it.

Language

Language development involves a gradual shift from babbling to the proper use of words, and so children will often continue to use nonsense sounds as well as single words during the 'One word stage'. These nonsense words are sometimes called 'jargon'. The single words that a child uses are usually linked to objects or experiences with which the child is in frequent contact.

Between about 18 months and 2½ years of age, children begin to communicate with two-word phrases. They might make up phrases like:

'Want drink' meaning 'I want a drink'.
'Nicky sleep' meaning 'Nicky wants to go to sleep'.
'Cat goed' meaning 'The cat has gone out'.

Brown (1973) described these short phrases as a kind of telegraphic speech. The child is sending a message as if by telegram where words have to be cut down to a minimum. The young child doesn't know many words and seems to concentrate on sending a message.

Brown (1973) describes the development of language in terms of five stages:

1. telegraphic two-word statements
2. the beginnings of grammar. (Grammar means the way in which language is structured or used. During Brown's second stage the child might start to structure what he or she says, for example 'I want drink', 'The cat goed'.)
3. asking questions, such as 'What that?', 'Where is cat?', 'When we see doggy?'
4. the use of sentences with more than one clause, for example 'The cat come in and the doggy come in.'
5. sentences used in an adult way.

As children learn to ask questions and make sentences they appear to follow their own rules of grammar. For example, they will invent their own idea of plurals. 'Gooses' sounds like a logical way of describing more than one goose. As adults, we know that the word for more than one goose is 'geese' – but young children may not accept this idea.

Carer: 'Where have you been today?'
Child: 'We went to feed the **gooses.'**
Carer: 'What did you feed the **geese** with?'
Child: 'Can't know.'
Carer: 'Did you enjoy it?'
Child: 'Yes the **geeses** splashed!'

The young child still puts an 's' on the end of geese as this fits his or her idea of grammar.

Gross (1992) quotes research by Braine (1971) and Tizard *et al.* (1972) which suggests that trying to teach young children grammar has little effect. Instead, there is evidence that trying to correct children's speech might actually slow their development of vocabulary. It appears that children may 'learn grammatical rules despite their parents.' (Gross, 1992, page 784.) Research by Slobin suggests that parents pay little attention to grammatical correctness, 'and even if they did, it would have little effect.' (Page 784.)

Although children appear to establish adult grammar and a reasonable vocabulary of words by the age of 5 or 6 years, Berryman *et al.* (1991) caution that children between 5 and 10 years of age still have trouble interpreting the meaning of complex sentences. Berryman *et al.* quote a study by Carol Chomsky, where children were shown a blindfolded doll and asked 'Is the doll hard to see or easy to see?' Younger children said 'that the doll was hard to see, because it was blindfolded.' The younger children appear to have interpreted the sentence to mean that the doll was doing the seeing. Berryman *et al.* provide further evidence that 5–6-year-olds have difficulty in understanding complex sentences and state: 'It is misleading, then, to think of language development as something which is more or less over by the time a child is about four or five. Important language learning continues throughout much of childhood.' (Page 101.)

Although adolescents and adults may have advanced language competence, changing demands in employment or social life may mean that communication skills have to be constantly refined and developed. Adults may continually improve their social skills and their ability to listen to and understand others' viewpoints. Vocabulary for technical terms is constantly changing. Language learning may never 'finish' until an individual dies.

The influence of inherited and environmental factors on language

In 1957, Burrhus F. Skinner put forward the idea that children learn language because of the influence of the environment. Skinner believed that parents would provide more attention and pleasurable reactions when an infant made 'correct' sounds or utterances. In this way a child would gradually learn to speak and use language. The child would respond to the smiles and approval of carers. By trial and error, a child could work out how to communicate with others The child would repeat verbal behaviour that was rewarded (or reinforced) and drop sounds or speech that did not work in terms of getting a pleasurable response.

Very few people now believe that this completely explains how language is learned. Children learn language with very little teaching (one word per hour between 1½ and 6 years). Children do not respond to being taught grammar. Children in totally different cultures across the world seem to pick up the complexities of language development at the same age. This points to the possibility that children may have an in-built ability to learn language.

Noam Chomsky argued that children are born with a 'language acquisition device'. This means that humans have an in-built mechanism to help them recognise language and speak languages. Chomsky believed that children simply need to hear language in order to begin to develop language. The language acquisition device would enable them to understand the 'deep structure' which all languages follow. Individual languages use different sounds and have special rules of grammar. Chomsky called these individual rules a surface structure. All languages have the same underlying rules or structures and these deep structures are something that babies are born to recognise.

Recently, Professor Steven Pinker has gone further than Chomsky and claimed that human ability to use language is not only inherited, but that language was produced as a result of evolutionary pressures. According to Pinker, language ability will be built into each person's genetic code. The language acquisition device is genetic and has come about because good communication skills would have given our ancestors increased advantages in terms of reproduction and survival.

Pinker claims that most successful species develop special abilities. Hawks can see a mouse move from great distances. Bats can navigate by using sonar sound waves. Many species of birds migrate across whole continents without losing their way. Pinker's idea is that language is a special ability which has enabled the human species to become so successful. Because it is so important and valuable to human survival, language has evolved as part of the human nature (our brains may be pre-wired to develop language). This genetic potential might be similar to the potential that enables birds to fly. Flight is a special ability that birds are born with. Language is perhaps our 'special act'.

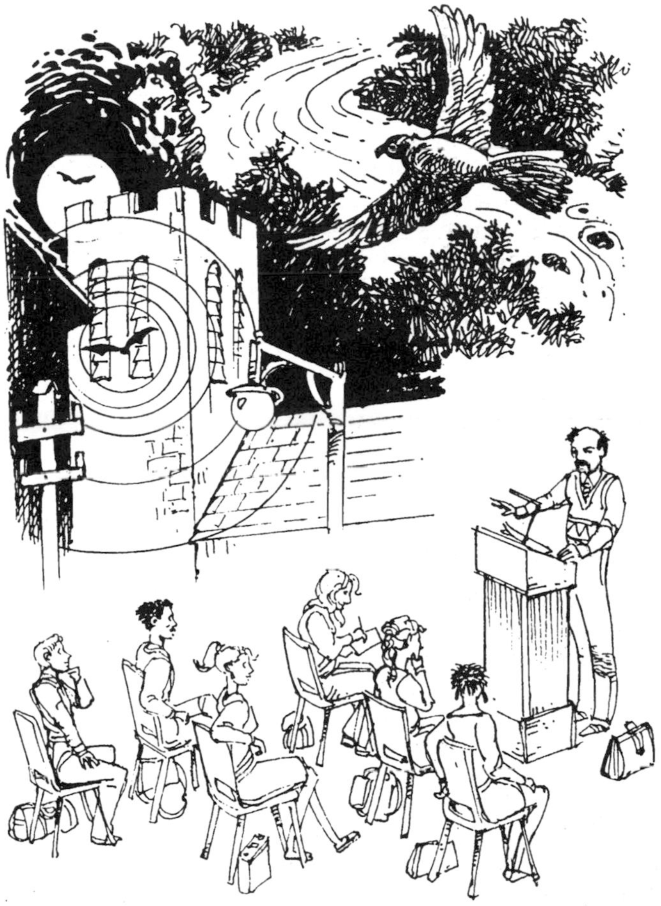

Whether language developed because of evolution or not, there is now a widespread expectation that a genetic basis for human language ability will be discovered. Professor Myrna Gopnik claims to have evidence for a genetic component for language. Her studies focus on a language disorder which 'runs in' families and which reduces individuals to learning language by rules, rather than quickly and easily.

Gopnik may have evidence of the existence of a genetic failure in the human language acquisition device, evidence that would suggest a genetic component to language (report in *Times Higher Educational Supplement*, 7 April 1995).

If the broad theories of Chomsky, Pinker and Gopnik are correct, it would only suggest that the underlying ability to learn language is influenced by an in-built or genetic factor. The actual sounds, words and grammar that children learn will depend on their environment. The speed at which children learn will also be influenced by their environment.

Cognitive development

Cognitive development covers the development of knowledge, perception and thinking. Over the past 40 years the study of cognitive development has been dominated by the work of Jean Piaget (1896–1980) and his colleagues. The study of 'object permanence' and 'conservation' refer to aspects of Piaget's theory of development. Piaget originally developed his theories of cognitive development by observing and questioning young children. When his own children, Jacqueline, Laurent and Lucienne were born, Piaget was able to illustrate his theory by observing their actions.

Piaget's theory of cognitive development specifies that children progress through four stages:

1. the sensorimotor stage – learning to use senses and muscles (birth–2 years)
2. the pre-operations stage, or pre-logical stage (2–7 years)
3. the concrete operations stage, or limited logic stage (7–11 years)
4. the formal operations stage – formal logic/adult reasoning (from 11 years).

Piaget believed that the four stages were caused by an in-built pattern of development that all humans went through. This idea and the linking of the stages to age-groups are now disputed. There is some agreement that Piaget's theory may describe some of the processes by which thinking skills develop.

Sensorimotor stage

Throughout life we have to learn to adapt to the circumstances and puzzles that we come across. This process starts soon after birth.

To begin with, a baby will rely on in-built behaviours for sucking, crawling and watching. But babies are active learners. Being able to suck is biologically necessary so that the baby can get milk from its mother's breast. The baby will adapt this behaviour to explore the wider range of objects by sucking toys, fingers, clothes, and so on. If the baby is bottle-fed, he or she will be able to transfer this sucking response to the teat on the end of the feeding bottle. Learning to respond to a new situation, using previous knowledge is called *assimilation.* The baby can assimilate the bottle into his or her knowledge of feeding. Later when the infant has to learn to drink from a cup, he or she will have to learn a whole new set of skills that will change the knowledge of feeding. This idea of changed internal knowledge is called *accommodation.* People learn to cope with life using a mixture, or balance, of assimilation and accommodation as their internal knowledge changes.

During the sensorimotor stage, the infant is slowly adapting to the world by developing his or her own motor actions. At first, the infant learns to co-ordinate tongue and lip movements to feed. By 3 months of age, an infant might start to reach for things and grasp things to suck. By 9 months, the infant might crawl towards an object that could be grasped. In all these actions the child is slowly building a knowledge of how to cope with the environment.

Spatial awareness

Young infants do not have adult eyesight. Their brains and nervous systems are still developing and their eyes are smaller in proportion to their bodies. They are effectively short-sighted, able to see close detail better than more distant objects. Piaget's observations convinced him that infants were unable to make sense of what they saw. If a 6-month-old child was grasping for a rattle and the rattle was covered with a cloth, then the child would act as if the object had now ceased to exist. It was as if the object had been absorbed into the cloth!

Piaget believed that young infants would have great difficulty making sense of objects and that they were unable to use mental images of objects in order to remember them.

Think it over

The world for the infant might be a very strange place. If we close our eyes we will

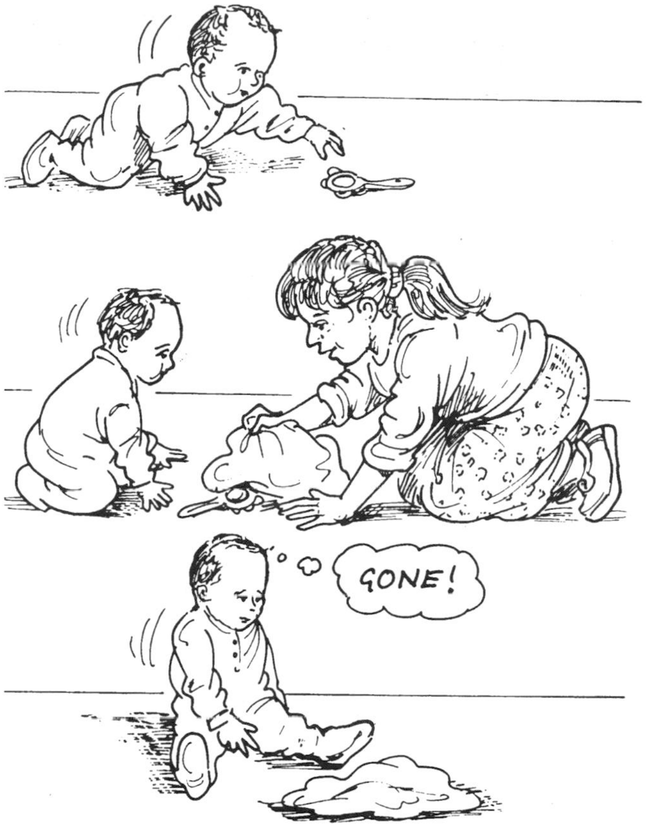

be able to use our memory for spaces, 'our spatial awareness', to walk around a room with our eyes shut. According to Piaget, young infants have no memory of visual objects when they close their eyes. If they can't see an object, it no longer exists.

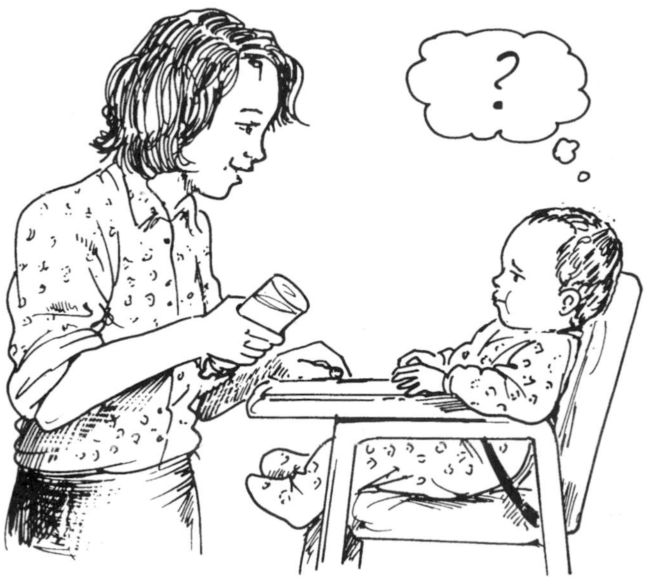

Infants will also have great difficulty in making sense of objects.

If a feeding bottle is presented the wrong way round, the young infant will be unlikely to make sense of it. The infant may not see a bottle as we would – they will see an unusual shape.

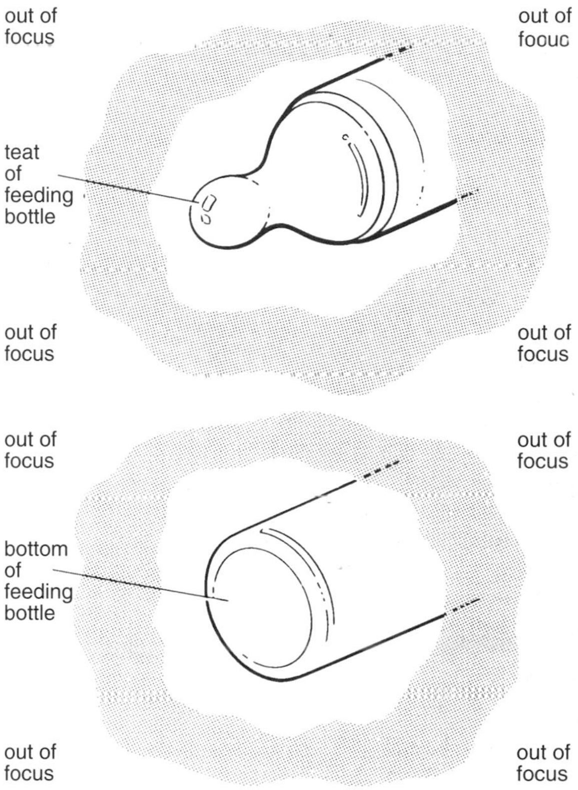

As adults, we have a vast visual or spatial memory for objects – but something of the sensorimotor experience might be imagined by looking at illusions.

Think it over

Look at the diagram on the next page. What do you see? Can you see a picture of both an old and a young woman? If not, it may be because you are not familiar with the visual patterns involved. Try to get a friend or colleague to help you see both images.

Piaget guessed that the young infant may unfamiliar with almost everything that surrounds him or her. An infant would be unable to interpret what objects like feeding bottles were, or even to know that their own body ended and that there was an outside world.

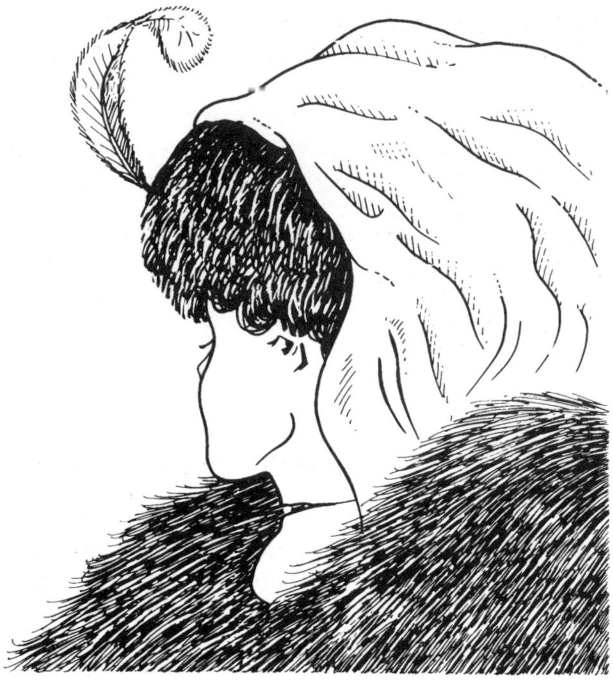

Toward the end of the sensorimotor period, children would begin to internalise picture memories in their minds. Piaget noticed this in his daughter, Jacqueline, at 14 months of age. Jacqueline had seen an 18-month-old child stamping his feet and having a temper tantrum. The next day, Jacqueline imitated this behaviour. Jacqueline must have been able to picture the behaviour in her mind in order to copy it later.

At the end of the sensorimotor period, children are regarded as being able to remember images and to make sense of objects that they see.

Object permanence

The sensorimotor period ends when the child can understand that objects have a permanent existence. The child knows that objects still exist even if he or she is not looking at them.

At the end of the sensorimotor period, children will know that their father and mother still exist even if they are not to be seen. If the child loses a toy he or she will start to search for it, because it can be pictured and because the child has learnt how objects work. If an object can't be seen, it will have gone somewhere – not just 'gone'.

The end of the sensorimotor period is also a time when the child is beginning to use one- and two-word utterances to recognise and describe things.

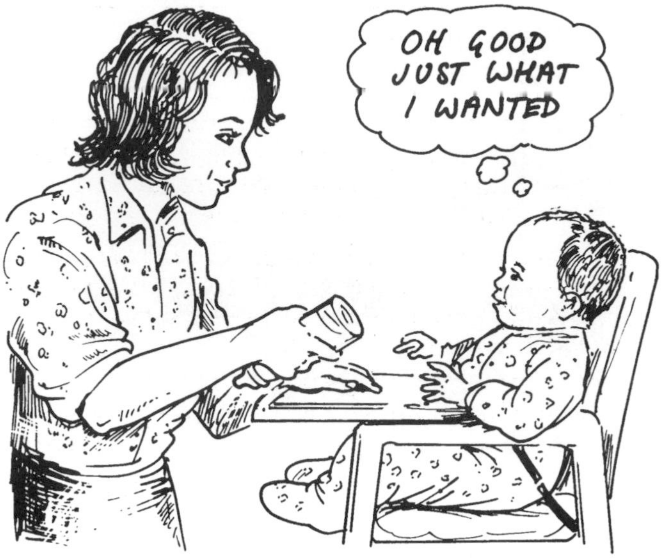

Piaget believed that language was a powerful tool that a child could use to help organise his or her knowledge of the world.

Pre-operational stage

Pre-operational means pre-logical. During this stage Piaget believed that children could not operate in a logical or rational way. Between 2 and 4 years of age, children were pre-conceptual – they could use words and communicate with adults, but they might not really understand what they were saying. For example, a 2-year-old might use the word 'cat' to mean any animal that he or she sees, and might not really have the same idea of cat that an adult has. By 5 years of age a child might name objects correctly, but still not understand the logic behind things that he or she says. Pre-operational children don't always understand how *meaning* works in language.

The classic demonstration of pre-logical thinking involves studies of children's thinking about number, mass and volume. Pre-operational children do not *conserve* these qualities. Conservation means that you know that a line of 10 buttons has the same number of buttons as a pile of 10 buttons. A young child might say there were more buttons in the line than in the pile, 'because it's longer'. The child is not conserving number. The child appears to not understand that 10 buttons in one place is the same as 10 somewhere else. The child can count to 10, but not understand what he or she is doing.

Conservation experiments

Try it: Weight

Show a 5-year-old child a pair of weighing scales and get the child to make two balls of plasticine that weigh exactly the same.

Check that the child agrees that the two balls are equal in weight (mass). Then roll one ball out into a sausage shape. Ask the child if he or she thinks the two balls will still weigh the same.

A 5-year-old might answer 'no' – the long one will weigh more now! This statement is illogical. If only the shape and not the mass have changed, then it should weigh the same. Young children don't understand mass (or weight) in the way adults do. Their judgements can be influenced by the way things look, rather than by the concept of 'weight'. Young children may not *conserve* mass – if the shape changes, they may believe that the weight can change too.

Try it: Number

Set out ten buttons in each of two lines. Ask a child to count the lines. Ask if there are the same number of buttons in one line as in the other. The child will agree that they are equal, there are ten buttons in each line. Now take one button away from one line, but space them so that the two lines still look the same length.

Ask the child if there are more buttons in one line than the other.

A 5-year-old might tell you that there are the same number. So nine buttons is the same as 10 buttons if the lines still look the same! The child is not conserving number. Once again, as in the experiment on weight, children's judgement seems to be dominated by the way things look. The child's attention is centred on visual appearance rather than logical understanding of the way number works.

Try it: Volume

Fill two glass jars to the same level with water. Ask a young child to judge if there is the same water in both jars.

Then take one jar and pour the water from it into a taller, thinner glass cylinder. Ask if all the water has gone in. Hopefully the child will agree that it has. Now ask the child if there is the same amount of water in the first jar and the tall jar.

The child will probably say there is more water in the tall jar! The child is not conserving volume. If the two amounts of water were the same in the beginning, how can there now be more water in the taller jar? Where would this extra water have come from? The child is making a judgement centred on appearance rather than logic.

Egocentricity

The pre-operational child is not only pre-logical, but according to Piaget, the child is also unable to imagine other people's perceptions. In a now famous experiment, Piaget showed 4–6-year-old children a model of three mountains. Piaget moved a little doll around the model and asked the children to guess what the little doll could see. Piaget gave the children photographs which showed different views of the mountain. The children had to pick out the photograph that would show what the doll saw. Children were also invited to try using boxes to show the outline of the mountains that the doll could see.

The young children couldn't cope with this problem. They chose pictures which showed what *they* could see of the model mountains. Piaget concluded that children could not understand other people's perspectives. Children were centred on their own way of seeing things – they were *egocentric.* Egocentric means believing that everyone will see or feel the same as you do. To understand that other people can see things from a different view, a child would need to de-centre his or her thoughts. Piaget believed that pre-operational children could not think flexibly enough to imagine the experiences of other people.

The pre-operational period is a time when children begin to develop an understanding of their world but where thinking is limited. A 3-year-old child has the spatial ability to remember how to find his or her way round a room or house, but cannot explain what he or she does. A 4-year-old cannot copy simple diagrams that he or she is shown. A child's drawings of people may suggest that he or she doesn't really conceptualise how people's bodies are made up of arms, hands, fingers, and so on.

Observations of play might suggest that Piaget's view of egocentric thought is correct. Young children might speak with other children when they play, but they do not always seem to listen to others or watch others for their reactions. Piaget believed that emotional and social development were strongly influenced by cognition. The child's ability to reason and use concepts would lead the development of social skills and emotional development. Children might learn to de-centre and understand others' viewpoints when they could use concepts and make mental operations that would free them from being dominated by the way things look. This freedom from egocentricity and the ability to think logically come with the development of concrete operations.

Concrete operations stage

Children in the concrete operations stage can think logically provided the issues are 'down to earth' or concrete. Children can solve logical puzzles provided they can see examples of the problem that they are working with. The concrete stage implies an ability to think things through and 'reverse ideas'. Very young children have problems with verbal puzzles like 'If Kelly is Mark's sister, who is Kelly's brother?' At the concrete stage, children can work out the logic of the relationship – Mark must be Kelly's brother if she is his sister. They can explore relationships in their minds. In terms of spatial ability, 7–11-year-old children are likely to be able to imagine objects as they would look from various directions. Drawing ability suggests that mental images are much more complex and complete.

Children in the 'concrete' stage still cannot cope with abstract thought or with formulating theories and hypotheses to explain the world. Although children may be able to imagine objects from different viewpoints, they may still not be able to explain their ideas using language. If a problem become too abstract, then it will prove difficult for a child in the concrete period. For example, if you ask a question like 'Samira is taller than Corrine, but Samira is smaller than Lesley, so who is the tallest?', an 8-year-old child may not be able to cope. An 8-year-old child may not be able to imagine all this information in a way that will enable him or her to answer the question. If 8-year-olds can see Samira, Corrine and Lesley, then they will be able to point to the tallest.

Children of 8–11 years may tend to concentrate on collecting facts about topics that interest them. But their real understanding may still be limited compared to older children and adolescents.

Formal operations stage

When children and adolescents develop formal logical operations they have the ability to use their imagination to go beyond the limitations of everyday reality. Formal operations enable an adolescent or adult to see new possibilities in everything. Piaget stressed the ability of children to use formal deductive logic and scientific method in their thought. With formal logic, an adult can develop hypotheses about the puzzles that life sets. The adult with formal operations can reason as to why a car won't start. Adults can check their hypotheses out. Perhaps the car won't start because there is an electrical fault. Perhaps the fuel isn't getting into the engine. Is the air getting in as it's supposed to? Each hypothesis can be tested in turn until the problem is solved.

Hypothetical constructs and abstract thinking

The adolescent or adult with abstract concepts and formal logic is free of the 'here and now'. They can predict the future and live in a world of possibilities.

Although Piaget originally emphasised logic; the ability to 'invent the future' may be the real issue of interest for many adolescents. For example, an 8-year-old will understand how mirrors work and even understand that people can dress differently, change the way they look, and so on. The 8-year-old is likely to accept that the way they look is just 'how it is',

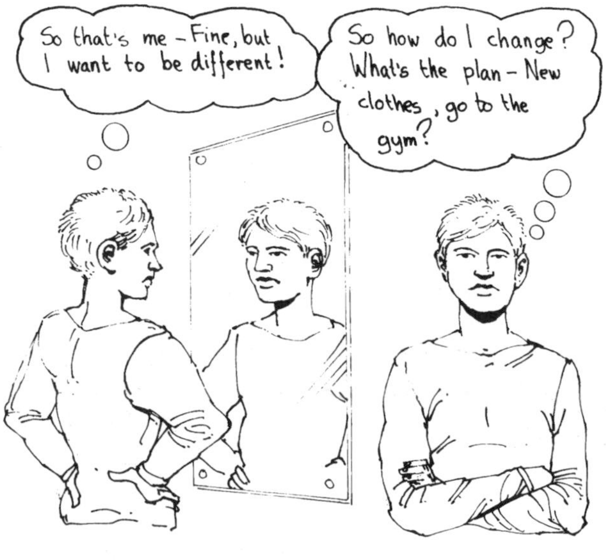
So that's me – Fine, but I want to be different!
So how do I change? What's the plan – New clothes, go to the gym?

… but adolescents see themselves differently

and is very unlikely to start planning for a change of future image. With hypothetical constructs an adolescent can plan to change his or her appearance and future.

Many adolescents will have theories or concepts about the way people in their social group should look. In order to make relationships, it will be important to present themselves in the right way, to be seen as being attractive. Adolescents and adults may spend time planning their image. Body-building, diets, new clothes, new jewellery, new hairstyles might be chosen to create the desired appearance. People build or construct an idea of the person they want to be. Because they have the mental power to think through various possibilities, they are able to re-design the way they look.

Think it over

Hypothetical constructs and abstract thinking may play an important part in care work. Each person that a carer works with will have a range of social, emotional, intellectual and physical needs. People's needs are not always 'concrete'. People don't usually just need a bus pass, a walking aid, or food and shelter. Understanding the emotional needs of a bereaved person will require a carer to understand abstract concepts like denial and acceptance. Understanding the social and emotional needs of an adolescent might involve understanding relationships and self-concept. All these concepts are abstract. It is easy to see how the breakdown of relationship can cause pain, or the success of a relationship can cause joy, but the word 'relationship' is abstract. We can see the effects of relationships but we can't see relationships as if they were concrete objects.

Being able to build interpretations or construct hypotheses about emotional needs may be an important skill in care work.

Was Piaget's view of cognitive development the whole story?

Over the past 25 years a range of research has built up which suggests that human development is not as straightforward as Piaget's theory of stages suggest.

Object permanence

Berryman *et al.* (1991) quote research by Bower (1982), which suggests that 8-month-old infants have begun to understand that objects have a permanent existence. Bower monitored the heart beat of infants who were watching an object. A screen was then moved across so that the infant couldn't see the object for a short while. When the screen was removed, sometimes the object was still there and sometimes it had gone. Infants appeared to be more surprised when the object had disappeared. This shouldn't happen if 8-month-old infants have no notion of object permanence.

Bower suggests that infants can begin to understand that their mothers are permanent from the age of 5 months. Infants begin to understand that their mothers move and exist separately from other events. Berryman *et al.* (1991) state: 'It seems that Piaget may well have underestimated the perceptual capabilities of the infant, and that some sensorimotor developments take place at an earlier age than he suggested'. (Page 116.)

Conservation

The reason why children got 'logical' tasks wrong may not be that they are completely illogical or egocentric. Part of the reason why children got the tasks wrong may be that they did not fully understand the instructions they were given. Another reason may be that Piaget was right and that young children do centre on perception. They judge things by the way they look. Even so, this may not mean that they have no understanding of conservation.

Jerome Bruner (1974) quotes a study by Nair which used the water and jars problem. This time the experiment used language and ideas that would be familiar to the child. The adult experimenter started with the two full, clear plastic tanks and got children to agree that there was the same water in each.

The adult then floated a small plastic duck on one tank of water, explaining that this was now the duck's water.

Children could now cope with the change. Many children would now say that the two amounts of water were the same because the duck kept his water.

Children may be able to make logical judgements if the problems are made simple and put in language that they can understand. Bruner believed that in the original jars problem, young children may have centred their attention on the way the jars looked. Young children might have understood that water stayed the same, but they became confused because their picture (or iconic) memory suggested that height should make volume bigger.

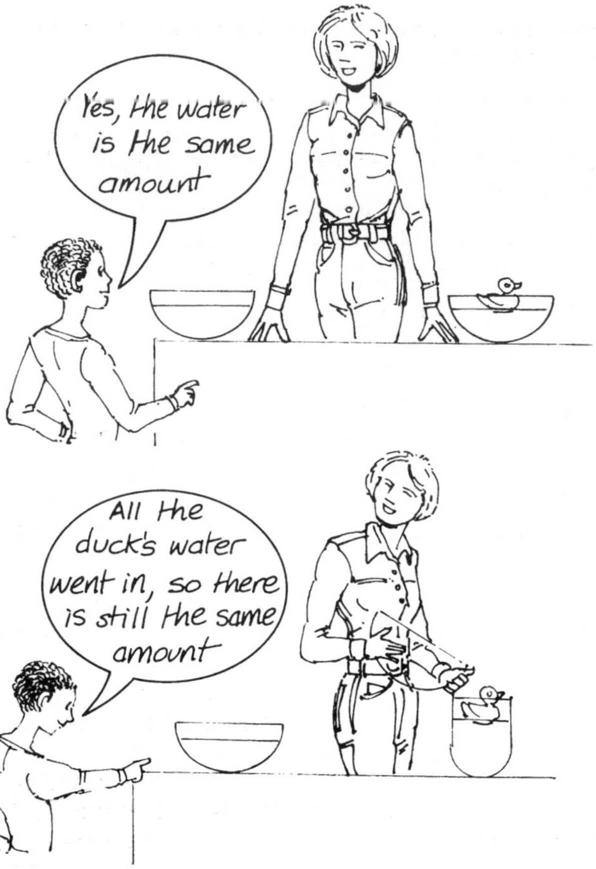
Yes, the water is the same amount
All the duck's water went in, so there is still the same amount

Figure 10.9 Pre-operational children can be logical

McGarrigle and Donaldson (1975) repeated the counters task. This time a 'naughty teddy' would make one line longer. Children of 5 and 6 were now more able to understand that there were still the same number of counters. In a play-type setting, children may not be so fixed on the 'look' of a line,

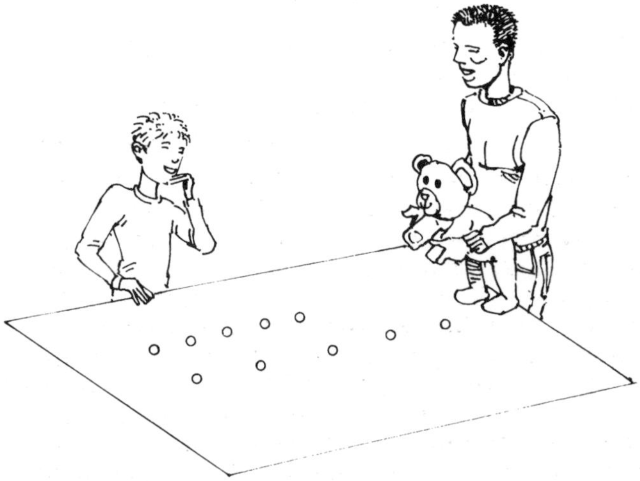

and may be able to use their developing knowledge of conservation.

It is clear that very young children take time to understand how to use concepts and that 4–7-year-olds can easily make illogical judgements. It is likely that children do develop an understanding of the logic in language at between 4 and 7 years. Piaget may have underestimated children's thinking ability.

Just because children get a problem wrong, it doesn't necessarily mean that they have no idea of the issues involved.

Egocentricity

Piaget believed that young children were unable to de-centre their perception from the way things looked, to be able to understand logical relationships. Pre-operational children were supposed to be egocentric to the point where they could not imagine that anyone could see or experience things differently from themselves. Paul Harris (1989) reports that children as young as 3 years of age do understand others' perspectives and do try to comfort others even though they are not distressed. Nicky Hayes and Sue Orrell (1993) quote research from Barke (1975) who found that 4-year-old children could choose a view that a *Sesame Street* character could see – and from different positions. Hayes also quotes research from Hughes (1975) who found that young children were able to hide a doll from another doll using partitions. The children could imagine who would see things at different angles.

Why did children fail at the 'three mountains' task if nowadays children seem to be able to understand others' perspectives? One possibility is that the task may have been too formal and too complicated for young children. In Piaget's experiment, children had to work out which photos went with perspectives, or work with complicated systems of boxes. In the studies reported by Hayes and Orrell, children were playing with characters that they understood in 'safe', informal settings. Children may not always display their full potential for reasoning in formal test settings.

Piaget's belief that pre-operational children are completely egocentric may not be safe. Modern research does not confirm his original findings.

Hypothetical constructs and abstract thinking

David Cohen (1981) is scathing in his criticism of Piaget's focus on logic:

> Furthermore, outside the domain of science, there are realms like art, music and literature which, while not illogical, hardly involve the kind of narrow logic that Piaget harped on. Perhaps even higher education – outside certain disciplines such as philosophy and mathematics – does not require that deep skill in formal logical thinking. (Page 185.)

Cohen quotes research by Watson and Johnson-Laird (1972) which suggests that at that time 92 per cent of London undergraduates did not use formal operations or hypothetical thinking to solve what was a logical problem. The majority of the population may not use formal logic as Piaget originally suggested that they would. Later in his career, Piaget claimed that it was the ability to use formal logic which developed at perhaps 11 or 12 years of age. He acknowledged that many individuals might never actually use that ability. Even so, the finding that many university students may not think in a generally logical and scientific way does throw doubt on the importance of formal operations as a general developmental stage. Segall *et al.* (1990) report a number of cross-cultural studies which may suggest that formal operational logic is dependent on education and training rather than being some natural capability that simply unfolds in humans.

Cohen (1981) devotes a chapter to his critique of Piaget's theory entitled 'cross-cultural flaws'. Within the chapter, he raises a range of difficulties and paradoxes which have occurred when Piaget's theories are tested outside of European and North American cultures. Cohen reports that one piece of work in Algeria suggested that 7-year-olds could conserve volume, 8-year-olds could not, but once again 10-year-olds could – a 'zig-zag' pattern. It may be that cultural systems of meaning can influence children's judgement and that even conservation can be strongly influenced by cultural beliefs and norms.

Think it over

Piaget's experiments with conservation of volume, mass and number do often work in the way that he originally discovered. If you work or live with children you may be able to try them out. The story of cognitive development will not be a simple story showing that Piaget's ideas are absolutely correct in discovering the nature of the human mind, or that his theories are hopelessly wrong. Understanding of human nature grows and develops as time moves on. Piaget's observations and theories may still be useful in helping us to remember the limitations of children's understanding.

In summary, it may be that Piaget's four stages underestimate the capabilities of young children and overestimate the capabilities of the average adolescent and adult.

The influence of inherited and environmental factors on cognitive development

Piaget believed that cognitive development was due to an *interaction* between environmental learning and genetic influences. He understood that genetic influences and environmental influences combined to create a new system, on which development depended.

The system which enables a person to learn and understand involves the regulation of knowledge through *assimilation* and *accommodation*. For example, consider the experience of learning to swim. Learning to float to begin with is not easy – you have to get the feeling of how it works. Once you've got the idea, then it's easy. This learning comes in a kind of automatic way. You may not be able to remember how you did it. Piaget thought that learning to float was 'regulated' by an automatic correcting and 'fine tuning' action. He called this *autonomous regulation* – you gradually get the 'feel' of how to do something.

If you are going to swim, you will have to experiment with arm and body movements. At first you may get it wrong and take in mouthfuls of water. Eventually you may get the actions right. You learn by activity or by what Piaget called *active regulation* – trial and error type of learning.

A lot of skills, such as listening or non-verbal communication, are learned by active trial and error and fine tuning of our behaviour. We don't learn them by thinking about them but through practice.

If you want to be a really good swimmer and enter swimming competitions, you will probably need *conscious regulation* of your learning. This is where you do work out and conceptualise what you are doing. You will need to work out a training routine, you will need the right diet, you may need to improve the way you turn your body and use arms and legs to swim. To get it right you may need to get your mind involved. The same applies to learning to listen, to communicate with people in social care, or to reassure people who are upset. Basic skills might

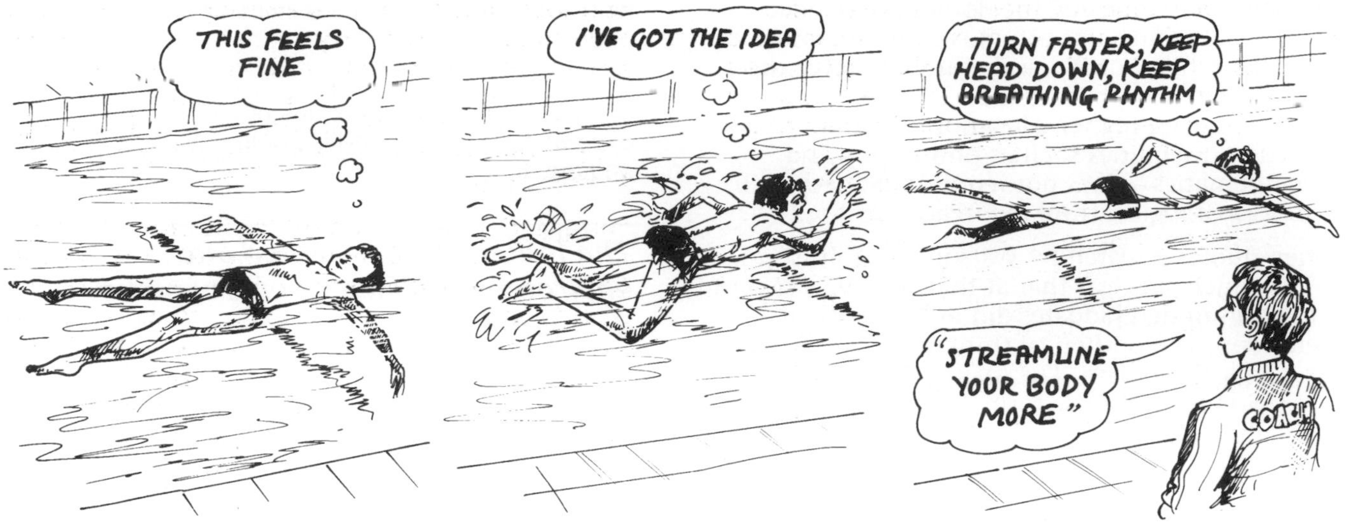
THIS FEELS FINE
I'VE GOT THE IDEA
TURN FASTER, KEEP HEAD DOWN, KEEP BREATHING RHYTHM
"STREAMLINE YOUR BODY MORE"
COACH

be developed naturally or unconsciously, but advanced skills require the ability to analyse or to evaluate what you are doing using concepts.

Piaget believed that people often started to learn from practical action. Skills could be dramatically improved by learning to use concepts to analyse action, and then autonomous, active and conscious regulation systems could be used together. With the ability to use concepts, mature learners can imagine a situation or skill that they want to improve. Imagination may even help competitive swimmers to improve their skills.

It may be that children do learn skills by learning practised actions and only later being able to conceptualise them. Some adults may be able to learn by using concepts before they try practical activities.

Think it over

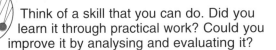

Think of a skill that you can do. Did you learn it through practical work? Could you improve it by analysing and evaluating it?

Intellectual development during adulthood and later life

Many adults will need to continue to develop their mental skills. Adults who work in professional jobs may develop special mental skills where they control and monitor their own thought processes. This ability is sometimes called *metacognition*. Many adults will specialise in particular styles or areas of mental reasoning.

Zimbardo (1992) suggests that adulthood may involve learning to cope with continual uncertainties, inconsistencies and contradictions. Logic alone, and even theories, may not be sufficient to cope with life. Skilled judgement and flexible thinking are needed. Some psychologists have gone on to call this adult stage of advanced thinking a *post-formal stage* – adding a fifth stage to Piaget's theory. As people grow older, happiness may depend on thinking skills that many cultures have referred to as wisdom.

In general, mental abilities increase with age, provided they are constantly used. There is evidence that mental ability declines if it is not used. This may be particularly important in later life. Mental exercise may be as important as physical exercise for many older people.

Emotional development

The role of interaction

Piaget's studies of infants suggested that they are unaware of an outside world and may not understand that the world exists when they are not looking at it. During the pre-operational period, children were said to be egocentric – incapable of imagining different thoughts and feelings or viewpoints from their own. Only as development progressed to logical thought were children seen as able to free themselves and de-centre their imagination

Paul Harris' study of children and emotion (1989) casts serious doubt on these assumptions. As already mentioned, babies seem capable of recognising voices and emotional tone at 7 months of age (Walker-Andrews, 1986). Harris quotes cross-cultural studies by Paul Elkman *et al.,* which suggest that there are set facial expressions for happiness, distress or anger. There is much evidence in Paul Harris' 1989 review that babies can recognise these basic, perhaps universal, emotional expressions. Emotional development may not be dependent on cognitive development as Piaget's stages suggest. Instead, children may come to imagine and understand others' feelings and reactions long before they can conceptualise or describe these issues with language. David Cohen (1981) claims that Piaget mainly studied babies' motor reflexes and movements, and that he may have gained a different view of early life if he had only studied facial expression.

Can infants respond to adult emotional expression? Paul Harris' review of research suggests they can. A study by Mary Klinnert (1984) involved 1- and 1½-year-olds being shown new toys. The infants' mothers would smile or look worried when certain toys were presented. If the mothers looked fearful their infants would tend to return to them and stay close by them.

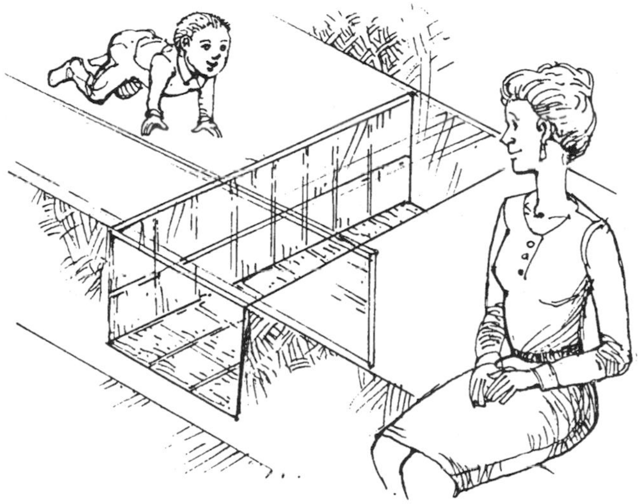

Harris states, 'By 12 months, we can conclude that infants not only react within a social dialogue in an appropriate manner to an emotional expression, they are also guided by an adult's emotion in their behaviour toward objects or events in the environment'. (Page 21.)

A study by Sorce *et al.* (1985) explored how a mother's expression would influence her baby's confidence to crawl across a 'visual cliff'. A visual cliff looks like a drop, but a strong sheet of glass is used to make sure a baby cannot come to any harm. Usually babies will not crawl across what looks like a serious drop. This may be an in-built survival reaction. The cliff was adjusted to look like a slight drop – so that the baby would be uncertain whether to cross or not.

Sorce *et al.* found that most babies crossed if their mothers smiled, but none of the babies crossed if their mothers looked fearful. Harris concludes that infants' exploratory behaviour is influenced by adult emotional reactions. 'The evidence described so far shows that quite early in the first year of life, babies adjust their social behaviour to the emotion expressed by their caretaker.' (Page 23.)

Egocentricity

Harris (1989) describes a range of research which demonstrates that 2-year-old children can recognise distress in others and will often seek to comfort them. There are instances of children under 2 years of age trying to comfort a parent who has hurt his or her foot. Although individual children vary enormously, in general, 'Young children begin to try to alleviate distress in another person; they comfort their parents and siblings at home, and later they comfort other children in the nursery school, particularly if they are hurt'. (Page 32.)

Research by Stewart and Marvin (1984) suggests that 3- and 4-year-old children who comfort younger brothers and sisters were good at taking the emotional perspective of their brothers or sisters. So a 3-year-old who is not upset by his or her mother leaving the room can provide comfort to a younger child who is upset. Harris claims that young children actively try to alter the emotional state that others are in. Children are not just imitating or copying behaviours that they have seen. If younger children were egocentric, they would not be able to understand the emotional needs of their brothers and sisters. This research on emotional development casts doubt on the idea that young children cannot de-centre and see others' viewpoints.

Research by Dennie Wolf *et al.* (1984) documents how children use their imagination of other people. Wolf explored how children play with dolls. At around 1½ years of age, children just pretend to look after their dolls. They might pretend to feed, wash or put them to bed. Between 2 and 2½ children begin to imagine dolls as talking, and as having desires and emotions. Between 3½ and 4 years, children can imagine their dolls as characters who make plans and interact with other characters. Harris believes that young children can and do imagine emotional states and can guess how real life events might lead to emotional reactions in others.

It seems that children have powerful imaginations and that they can understand the reactions and needs of others. In many ways this contradicts the picture of child development put forward by Piaget. It would appear that children do have difficulty in using concepts to describe or own their own emotions, however. A 3-year-old may feel jealousy at the arrival of a new baby sister. He or she may want to help with the baby, but may also say such things as, 'the baby should be cut up and thrown away'. These mixed emotions are clearly demonstrated by children but Harris noted that they could only start to explain such complex feelings from the age of 10 onwards. Conceptual awareness – the ability to use language to explain complex emotions – may need to wait for the developments outlined by Piaget.

Showing emotion

The way children and adults display their feelings may have a great deal to do with the social roles, norms and values that children learn. Harris (1989) quotes cross-cultural studies which suggest that people can be trained to suppress the expression of emotion, or to develop and exaggerate emotional expression. It is probable that babies are born with the capability to recognise emotions of happiness, distress or anger. How they learn to express their emotions may depend on the social and cultural context that they find themselves in.

Social and cultural influences on self-awareness

Two-year-old children appear to be able to recognise and respond to emotions in other people. It may be that they learn to understand human relationships and the individual expression of emotion as a result of social experience. George Mead (1934) believed that self-awareness developed from children's ability to imitate adult behaviour and to imagine characters. When children play, they can copy actions that they have seen. They do not need to fully understand – they just do the action. For example, a young child might pretend to be a dog, just because the child had watched the family's pet dog.

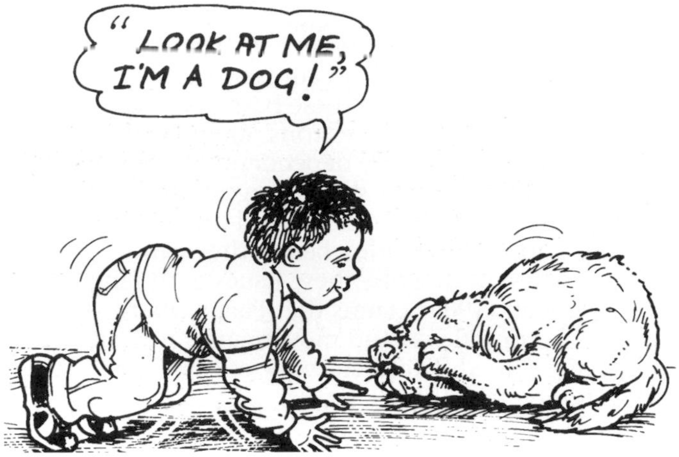
"LOOK AT ME, I'M A DOG!"

By 4 or 5 years of age, children might start to act out adult behaviour patterns. Again, children don't really need to understand adult behaviour, they just copy what they think they see. In this way, children can start to copy, or *assimilate,* adult roles. For example children might imagine that they are working together in a kitchen, cooking something for some imaginary children. As they play, they may copy behaviour that they have seen adults perform.

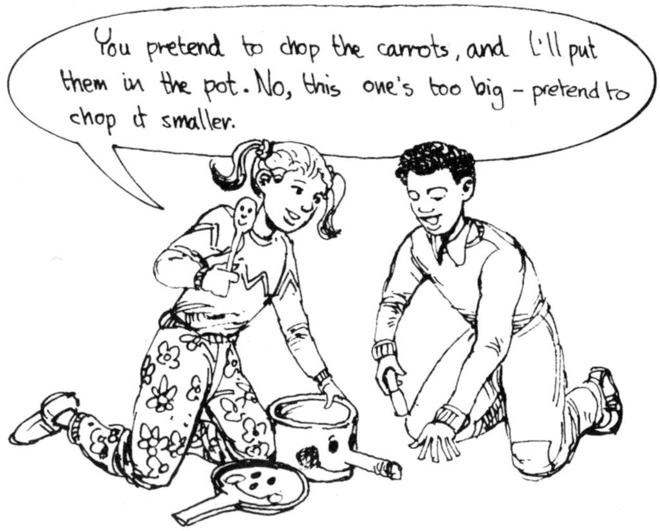
You pretend to chop the carrots, and I'll put them in the pot. No, this one's too big – pretend to chop it smaller.

As well as imitating adults, children will imitate things they have seen on TV. This might involve dramatic scenes like rescuing people, nursing people in hospital and,of course, car chases and fights. When children play, they are using imagination to create characters and to take on the roles of other people.

Mead believed that children might start to create a character for themselves – they would start to invent a 'me'. This idea of a 'me' comes about because children can understand social roles and put themselves in the place of other people.

Think it over

Have you ever watched young children inventing characters or talking to imaginary people? Have you seen the influence of TV or of family roles in what they do? Can you see what children may be imitating?

As children develop self-awareness, their idea of a 'me' will be strongly influenced by the culture that they grow up in. Culture includes the beliefs, norms and values that a specific group of people develop. Children will grow up with varying norms and values depending on the social context that they are in. The influence of culture on self-awareness is covered in detail in Chapter 11.

Children will come to be socialised into the beliefs, values and norms of their initial family or care-giving group. Later, children will be influenced by the beliefs, values and norms of the friends with whom they mix and play. Children adopt others' values and norms in order to be accepted into social groups. They will need to understand the rules of games or sports that they wish to join in. To be liked and to be popular, they have to show that they fit in with others. Mead (1934) believed that children come to learn general social rules and values at this stage. They might be able to imagine 'generalised others' or general social demands which they need to live up to.

Mead believed children might learn to display emotion as expected within the social roles and cultural context that they live in. They do not simply do what others teach them to do, however. They internalise values that are built into a sense of self. This sense of self determines what they actually do.

Think it over

A boy might imagine himself as a person who is tough and doesn't cry if he gets hurt. By adopting this gender role he may conform to the beliefs of other boys he mixes with.

Gender role might require this particular boy to suppress the emotion of distress at being wounded and to even display the emotion of being pleased. A girl living in the same neighbourhood may need to behave slightly differently in order to fit in with her friends.

These roles may become part of the child's *self-concept* and social identity. This sense of self will guide the individual to exaggerate, suppress or even substitute emotional expression. In some social class and geographical areas, boys may learn to exaggerate feelings of anger and aggression in order to achieve social status. In another social class group, boys may learn to express anger in terms of clever verbal behaviour with little hint of emotion. Some girls may learn to suppress feelings of distress in order to look 'in control'.

It is tempting just to say that society does this to people – that people develop the emotions for which society trains them. Mead's theory provides an explanation of how social influences work on an individual. It is the idea of a self, a 'me' that explains how social values influence individual behaviour.

During adolescence this sense of self becomes of central importance. Erik Erikson (1963) believed that biological pressures to become independent would force adolescents into a crisis which could only be successfully resolved if the individual developed a conscious sense of self or purpose. He wrote, 'In the social jungle of human existence, there is no feeling of being alive without a sense of ego identity'. (Page 240.) Other theorists have regarded the development of self-concept or identity as more gradual, and less centred on biological maturation. A clear sense of self may lead a person to feel worthwhile and to have a sense of purpose. A sense of self might provide a person with the confidence to cope with changes in life, and to cope with life transitions.

Emotional maturity might involve an individual feeling secure within his or her relationships with others and an understanding of his or her own self-awareness. In adulthood the expression of emotion may be strongly influenced by an adult's self-concept.

The development of personality

Personality is a wide subject area which seeks to explore human nature and behaviour. It is a difficult term to define, but Sarah Hampson (1982) chooses a definition which she claims to be acceptable to many psychologists:

> Personality refers to more or less stable internal factors that make one person's behaviour consistent from one time to another, and different from the behaviour other people would manifest in comparable situations. (Page 1.)

Personality then is about internal factors, which may have been learned and developed in relation to social influences, perhaps like the development of self-concept in Mead's theory. Internal factors could also include in-built tendencies or learned styles of reacting to situations, which have to be stable, so that we can see consistent patterns in individual behaviour. Personality is also about the study of individual differences – the way in which people vary in their individual reactions.

Personality is a very abstract concept. This section provides an overview of some of the main approaches to the study of personality.

Theories emphasising biological influences

Temperament and trait theories

The work of Thomas *et al.* (1968) documented different temperamental characteristics in babies. *Temperament* was used to refer to different behavioural styles which were readily observable. Martin Herbert (1981) points out that not only do babies show major individual differences, but that the temperament of the baby has an influence on his or her mother. Babies exert an influence on their parents. Some are more rewarding and easier to care for than others. Herbert notes that over-activity in a child 'is particularly tiring and sometimes disturbing, and leads to excessive attention-giving'. (Page 63.)

Thomas's studies looked at the activity levels in babies, their tendency to be happy or contented, their tendency to follow a routine, adaptability, and so on. The study suggested that there were some children who were 'difficult'. When they became upset they were not easily comforted. They might become upset more easily than other babies. In contrast there were babies whose temperaments appeared to make them easy to care for. In later work, a group of children who were 'slow to warm up' were identified. This 'slow to warm up' group did not respond well to changes in their environment.

The key point is that babies appear to be born with a temperament. The Thomas *et al.* studies suggest that temperament is not a result of environmental influences or learning after birth. Not only might some babies have a strong pattern of reactions but these patterns will have an influence on the parents. A mother with a difficult baby may feel less confident and competent as a carer. The mother may also find that a particular child causes her to feel increased stress because of the child's temperament.

It is possible that early behavioural styles or temperaments continue to influence a person's behaviour throughout life. Hans Eysenck (1965) developed a theory of extroversion and introversion based on the notion of different temperaments. Extroverts were thought to be people with a stimulus-hungry nervous system, while introverts were believed to possess nervous systems which would avoid excitement. Introverts might, therefore, be happy with repetitive and safe lifestyles, while extroverts would seek adventure and change. The exact expression of this need for stimulation would be different in different social contexts, but it was biological temperament which would fundamentally motivate both the introvert's and the extrovert's behaviour.

Traits are descriptions of tendencies that we see in other people. For example, a person might have a tendency to seek excitement or to avoid excitement (Figure 10.10).

Eysenck's theory of personality involves three central traits:

1 *introversion/extroversion.* An individual might be either hungry for experience and excitement (an extrovert) or eager to avoid excitement (an introvert). Most people are in the middle – neither extroverted or introverted.

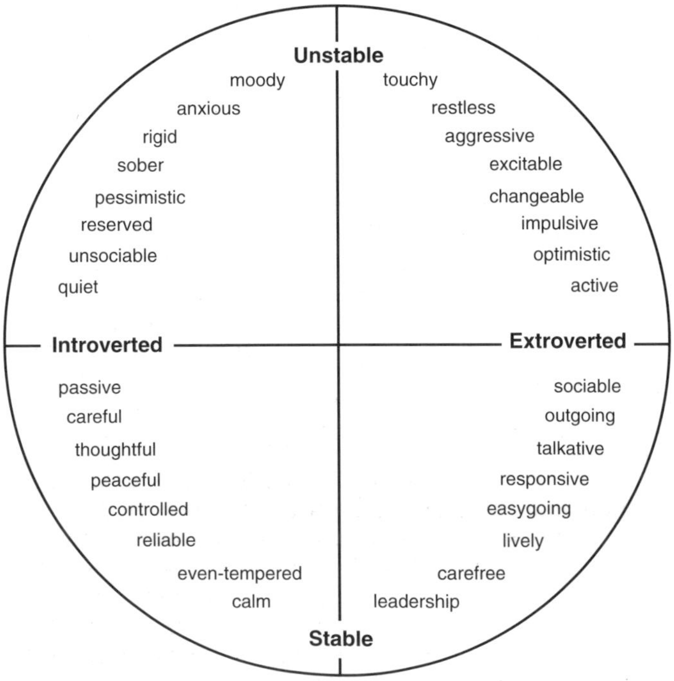

Figure 10.10 Traits of stability and extroversion

2 *stability or instability.* Again, most people's personalities would fall between the two extremes. Stability implied a calm or carefree, confident approach to life, while instability implied a neurotic, moody, changeable and restless response to living.
3 *tough- or tender-mindedness.* This trait related in particular to attitudes to people. A tough-minded person might be careless of other people's feelings, rights or needs, and might tend to believe that the 'ends justify the means'. If you need to do something and people get in your way, then they have to suffer the consequences. Tender-minded individuals would show concern for human welfare and for individual feelings. Once again, most people would not be extremely tender-minded or tough-minded.

Eysenck designed a simple test which gives a score on these three traits, the Eysenck Personality Questionnaire or EPQ. Completing the test involves giving a 'yes' or 'no' answer to a series of questions and only takes a few minutes.

Eysenck believed that extroverts would be hungry for excitement because of the way part of the mid-brain worked. In some people a part of the brain called the *reticular formation* would damp-down messages from the outside world. This would mean that these people would become easily bored. In other people, the reticular formation would boost messages so that they might soon become overwhelmed with excitement. Extroversion and introversion were, therefore, caused by the way the brain worked. Eysenck believed the other traits were also influenced by the way individuals' brains operated on a physiological level.

Eysenck's theory emphasises the biological basis for personality. Eysenck (1965) claims that criminal behaviour is associated with the traits of extroversion and instability. A final aspect to the theory is that extroverts are believed to be less likely to learn some of the subtle social rules because they are biologically less responsive to learning through conditioning (learning to associate unpleasant or pleasant outcomes with their behaviour).

So, in summary, the way a person's brain works might influence how he or she responds to conditioning. This might mean some people will be more careless about social approval. As well as this, a person might be hungry for excitement because of the way his or her brain works. This hunger for excitement might show up in response to a simple test. Some extroverts will control their behaviour because of their socialisation, but more people with unstable extrovert

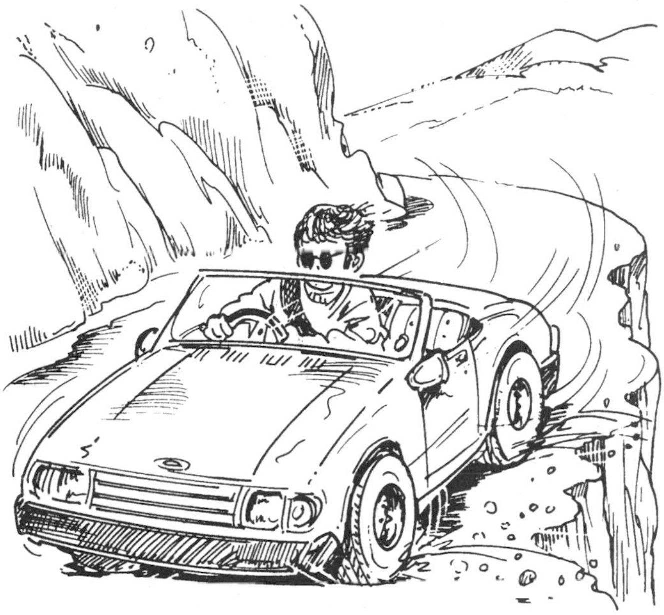

tendencies will commit crimes and engage in anti-social behaviour than 'average' people would.

Other ways of looking at traits

Raymond Cattell (1965) put forward the idea that human personality can be described as 16 *source traits.* We might label a particular person as kind, polite or rude. When we use words to describe people, we are naming what Cattell would have called *surface traits.* There may be many ways of noticing and naming other people's personalities. Cattell claimed that a mathematical technique called factor analysis could reduce all these surface traits to just 16 source traits. A person can take a test something like Eysenck's questionnaire, although rather more time is required. This test will produce a profile on the individual's personality (Figure 10.11). Cattell's theory is that personality can be summarised on the basis of a person's tendency to fit one side of a description more than another.

This 16-factor personality test (the 16 PF) is widely used in selection testing for jobs in the UK.

Eysenck and Cattell's theories have been discussed for many years. The mathematical analysis used to establish source traits can also produce other patterns. A recent controversy surrounds the idea that all descriptions can be covered with just five basic traits (Figure 10.12).

All trait theories seek to score individuals in terms of bi-polar (two-sided) dimensions of personality. Most

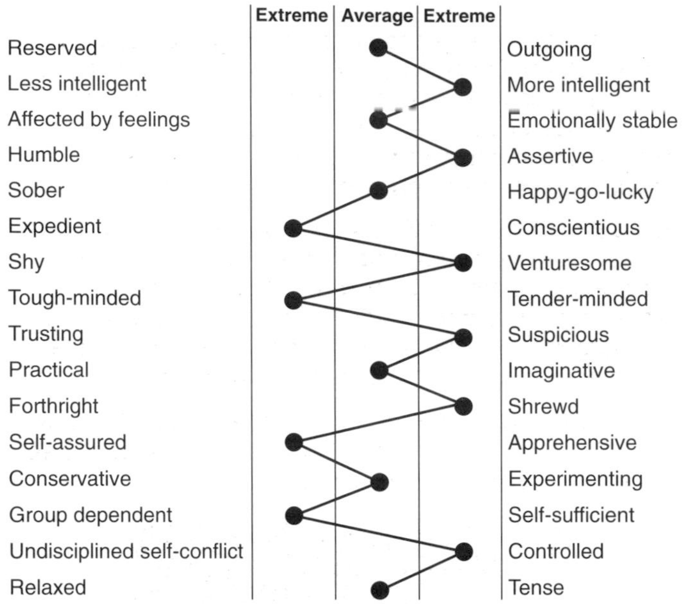

Figure 10.11 A personality profile using Cattell's 16 factors

people would come somewhere between the extreme definitions and be a bit of both (for example calm and contented most of the time but sometimes anxious). Few people would completely fit one side or the other of these trait categories.

Think it over

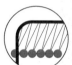

How would you rate yourself in terms of the traits described above?

Extroversion Being talkative, energetic	v	Being quiet, reserved and shy
Agreeableness Being sympathetic, kind and affectionate	v	Being cold, quarrelsome and cruel
Conscientiousness Being organised, responsible	v	Being careless, frivolous and irresponsible
Emotional stability Being stable, calm and contented	v	Being anxious, unstable and 'temperamental'
Openness to experience Being creative, intellectual and open-minded	v	Being simple, shallow and unintelligent

Figure 10.12 The five basic traits. Source: Zimbardo (1992)

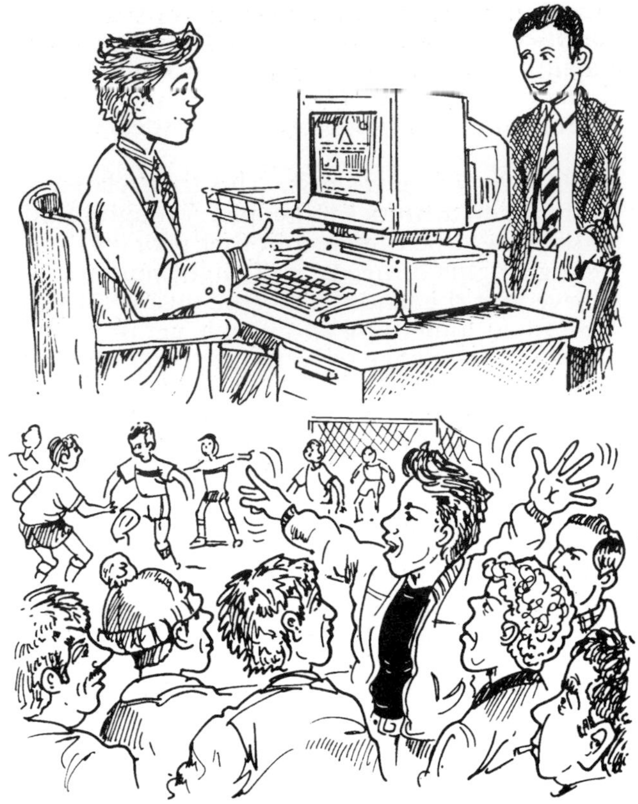

Figure 10.13 Calm, kind and intellectual at work; quarrelsome, careless, shallow and anxious at play

Although we can describe ourselves and others using trait theory, there is still a problem in that people don't always live up to the descriptions that they attribute to themselves or others, or indeed to the patterns that they score on tests. People will often change their calm, creative, conscientious behaviour to anxious, shallow and irresponsible behaviour just by moving from a work to a social context. Without knowledge of social context and the individual's perception of that context, it can be hard to predict behaviour (Figure 10.13).

Theories which emphasise environment

The social learning theory of Albert Bandura emphasises the power of the environment to influence the way people think and behave. Bandura stressed the fact that people imitate and copy other people. We adopt roles and social behaviours because of the outcomes that we expect for ourselves. If being polite and friendly helps us to get accepted into a particular group, and we want to belong to that group, then we may try to imitate the polite and friendly behaviours that we have seen others act out. Social learning theory complements the interactionist theory of George Mead – we learn to imagine and copy the reactions that will lead to pleasant outcomes for us.

Bandura's 1989 theory of *self-efficacy* may help to illustrate how social learning influences the development of personality. Albert Bandura uses the term self-efficacy to cover a person's ability to understand his or her capabilities, motivation, thought patterns and emotional reactions. Self-efficacy is how you estimate your abilities – what you believe about yourself. Self-efficacy is learned from past experiences, watching and thinking about what happens to others, copying others and from the feedback we get from other people. High self-efficacy means believing you will succeed at a task. Low self-efficacy means believing you will fail.

Once a person believes he or she is good at something, this belief will provide motivation to keep building on success. Of course, the opposite is also true. If you believe you are no good, then you will probably withdraw from the activity and avoid it.

Case study: Ashra's story

Ashra is 16 years old; she has just started a new course. She has never really thought about study before. This course seemed like the best thing to do following her studies at GCSE. Ashra has learned to value education and achievement. This was one of the values she learned from her family during the process of socialisation. Norms of doing work at home have also been learned, as Ashra's parents are in professional occupations.

Ashra does not know what to expect on her course; her first feelings are that it is very difficult and she wonders whether she should have chosen to do something else. She is asked to work with a small group and produce a piece of work which counts as evidence. The other group members are a bit unsure what to do, but Ashra is able to think up some good ideas. Ashra is pleased with her own creative thinking. She has the thought, 'I could be good at this'. Two weeks later Ashra gives an assignment in. When it comes back the work is praised as being clever and creative. Ashra is pleased. Over coffee she asks her friends how they got on. Several of her friends say they found it very difficult. Ashra feels sorry for them, but the idea comes to her that, 'I am good at this, not just average – but good'.

The idea of being good at study takes on a special feeling. Ashra starts to imagine that she is clever and creative – she will be good at everything she does in her studies. Ashra starts to use her imagination. Sometimes, when she has a chance to daydream, she thinks about ideas for assignments – books that would help her to write sections of her work. Because she uses her imagination so effectively she starts to perform very well.

Ashra now sees herself as someone who is creative and clever – someone who is good at study. These ideas become part of her *self-concept*. When the next assignment comes back with the need for extra work, Ashra does not worry. She believes she is good: if a few things don't work it doesn't matter – she will get it right.

The idea of coping and controlling the workload is now built into Ashra's personal view of herself. She now has the internal motivation to succeed.

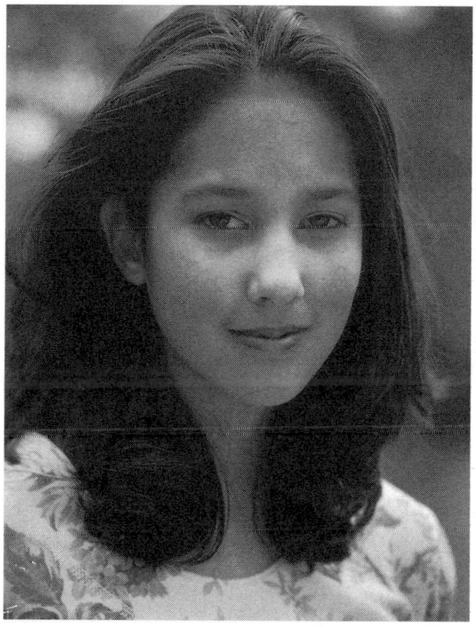

This case study provides a simplified view of the development of self-efficacy. Ashra develops appropriate norms and values during socialisation to assist her study habits. She is given positive feedback from others to support her own reflective thoughts about being good at study. When Ashra compares herself to others, she seems to be doing well. There is a lot of evidence to support the idea that she is good at study, 'not just average, but good'! At this point, Ashra evaluates herself as someone who is good at *and* enjoys study. Once people decide that they are something, the concepts they use to evaluate themselves may have a dramatic effect on their lives.

Ashra is now motivated to gain high grades and progress to further study. She may believe that she is also intelligent, creative and skilled: she is someone who will succeed in any academic area.

Self-efficacy could become a general feature of an individual's personality. It is learned from experience where an individual interacts with teachers, tests and social roles.

Some people may learn to think of themselves as capable individuals, who will be able to cope with the puzzles and problems that life holds. Others may fail to develop this view of themselves. Some people may go through life without believing they can influence what happens to them. These people may experience their lives as a series of events which just 'happen to them'. An evaluation of self as a capable decision-maker may be needed before individuals can be assertive and before they can take responsibility for their own lives.

Theories which emphasise early learning

Psychodynamic theories have developed from the work of Sigmund Freud (1856–1939) and are sometimes called Freudian theories. Psychodynamic theories accept that people are born with biological drives and patterns of behaviour. These patterns might be influenced by genetics. Psychodynamic theories also accept the importance of social learning. What makes psychodynamic theory different from trait or social learning theory is its emphasis on a particular idea of *mental structures*. These structures are thought to evolve through the interaction of in-built biological systems and the early experience of children. Early experience is thought to determine how an individual's personality will unfold. It is not the genetic potential or the environment themselves which are important, but the *interaction* between these two factors which builds the personality structure of an individual. Early development will influence later development.

Erikson's eight life stages

Freud originally believed that events in the child's first five or six years of life would determine an adult's personality. Erik Erikson extended this theory to cover the entire human life-span. Erikson believed that there were eight periods of developmental crises that an individual would have to pass through in life. How an individual succeeded or failed in each developmental stage would influence how that person's personality developed.

1. *Birth to 1½ years.* Infants have to learn a sense of basic trust or learn to mistrust the world. If children receive good quality care this may help them to develop personalities which include a sense of hope and safety. If not, they may develop a personality dominated by a sense of insecurity and anxiety.
2. *1½ to 3 years.* Children have to develop a sense of self-control or a sense of shame and doubt may predominate. They may develop a sense of will-power and control over their own bodies. If this sense of self-control does not develop, then children may feel that they cannot control events.
3. *3 to 7 years.* Children have to develop a sense of initiative which will provide a sense of purpose in life. A sense of guilt may otherwise dominate the individual's personality and lead to a feeling of lack of self-worth.
4. *Perhaps 6 to 15 years.* The individual has to develop a sense of competence, or risk the personality being dominated by feelings of inferiority and failure.
5. *Perhaps 13 to 21 years.* Adolescents or young adults need to develop a sense of personal identity or risk a sense of role confusion, with a fragmented or unclear sense of self.
6. *Perhaps 18 to 30 years.* Young adults have to develop a capability for intimacy, love and the ability to share and commit their feelings to others. The alternative personality outcome is isolation and an inability to make close, meaningful friendships.
7. *Perhaps 30s to 60s or 70s.* Mature adults have to develop a sense of being generative, leading to concern for others and concern for the future well-being of others. The alternative is to become inward-looking and self-indulgent.
8. *Later life.* Older adults have to develop a sense of wholeness or integrity within their understanding of themselves. This might lead to a sense of meaning to life or even to what could be called 'wisdom'. The alternative is a lack of meaning in life and a sense of despair.

It is important to note that all individual personalities will contain some positive and negative qualities of each life stage.

Erikson's life crises model is not accepted by all personality theorists. The notion of developmental crises may be too dramatic. Many people may experience a much more gradual development in personality. Critics have doubted that Erikson's stages would be found in all cultures. Erikson himself argued that these unfolding psycho-sexual stages were a necessary outcome of biological and social interaction.

Erikson's theory is that personality develops with each successive stage of maturity. New developments build on past learning. Early experience provides the foundation on which personality and interpersonal relationships will depend.

Bowlby's theory of bonding

John Bowlby worked within the psychodynamic perspective on personality. Bowlby (1953) states, 'What occurs in the earliest months and years of life can have deep and long-lasting effects'. (Page 17.)

Bowlby studied mothers and babies in the mid-1940s, just after the end of the Second World War. Bowlby had noticed that some baby animals would make very fixed emotional bonds with their parents. For example, baby ducklings would attach themselves to, and follow, whomever they presumed to be their mother. Wild ducklings will naturally attach themselves to the mother duck. Bowlby had studied research which showed that ducklings would attach themselves to humans if humans were all that was around during a critical period when the duckling needed to bond. Bowlby's studies of infants led him to the conclusion that human babies were similar to some types of animal, such as ducks. Bowlby believed that there was a biological need for mothers and babies to be together, and that there was a sensitive or critical period for mothers and babies to form this attachment, which is known as *bonding*. Bowlby (1953) stated, 'The absolute need of infants and toddlers for the continuous care of their mothers will be borne in on all who read this book'. (Page 18.)

If the bond of love between a baby and its mother was broken through separation, Bowlby believed, lasting psychological damage would be done to the child. If a mother left her infant to go to work every day, or just once to go into hospital, there might be a risk of damage. Bowlby believed that children who suffered separation might grow up to be unable to love or show affection. Separated children might not care about other people. Separated children might also fail to learn properly at school, and might be more likely to turn to crime when they grew up.

Some other researchers working outside of the psychodynamic perspective have doubted that babies are really affected so seriously by separation. Michael Rutter (1981) found evidence that suggests that it is the *quality* of emotional attachment between a carer and the infant that matters. Not being able to make an attachment may damage a child emotionally. But it is the making of a bond of love between the baby and a carer that matters, not whether temporary separations happen.

There is research that suggests that babies can and do make bonds with their fathers and with their brothers, sisters, or other carers. In one study (Schaffer and Emerson, 1964), almost a third of 18-month-old infants had made their main attachment to their fathers. It seems that babies give their love to the person or persons who give them the best quality affection and time.

Alan and Ann Clarke (1976) reviewed a wide range of research. They concluded that children can recover from almost any bad psychological experience provided that later experience makes up for it. It is *whole life experience* and not just the first years of an infant's life that will decide whether a child grows up to care about other people, or takes to a life of crime. Although people can recover from separation and poor relationships, it is very important that infants do have a chance to make a loving relationship or bond with carers. The first part of a person's life may set the scene for what will happen next. A lack of love in early life could be a very bad start for a child's emotional development. It would be unwise just to hope that some later quality of life could make up for it.

Theories which emphasise the personal building or 'construction' of personality (humanistic theories)

Some theorists believe that we are born with a tendency to develop certain traits of personality. Some theorists emphasise the role of culture, socialisation and social learning on personality. Psychodynamic theory accepts the importance of environmental and genetic influences, but emphasises the role of early experience in fixing a person's later personality. The humanistic perspective, however, does not see either environment, genetics or early experience as being able to fix or create human personality. Instead, personality is seen as the result of an individual's *system of thinking and/or feeling*. The humanistic approach does not question that genetic or environmental influences exist. Naturally, early experience can influence development. Self-concept may develop in the way George Mead suggested. Humanists suggest that these influences are not really important if you want to understand someone's personality. We may never unravel all the causes that make people the way they are. What matters is the system of thinking that a person is using now.

Theorists like Carl Rogers are concerned with how people seek to understand their notions of self and ideal selves. To some extent these theories focus on the way people think in the present or the way they build or construct their own self-concept. George Kelly's 1955 *theory of personal constructs* particularly emphasises the idea that individuals build or construct their own personalities.

Kelly's theory is that people have to develop a set of assumptions or theories to help them make sense of life. People need to be able to predict what will happen and how they should react. If we can predict the practical and social world we live in then we can feel confident and in control. If we can't make much sense of what happens to us then we may feel anxious and insecure. Kelly argued that individuals learn to develop their own personal theories about themselves, about other people and about the world in general. These personal theories are learned from experience.

What is important is that each individual person will invent a system of thinking that will be used to explain personality. Trait theory classifies people as extrovert, agreeable, stable, and so on. Kelly's theory was that individuals classify themselves and others on their own personal set of theories. Naturally, people will develop their theories from childhood onwards.

Kelly believed that it is personal theories built or constructed by people that create a person's personality. People who are always aggressive may be aggressive because they have come to believe that's the best way to get results from other people. People may be aggressive because they have decided that aggression works better than anything else – not because they are made to be aggressive! Kelly said that people are not controlled by their past histories, but they may be enslaved by their own interpretation of their lives. People build their own personalities and then they are at the mercy of the character they have invented.

Think it over

A 17-year-old girl says, 'You don't know what it's like where I live. It's horrible! Everyone gets by on social security and on nicking things. Just do a few cars or homes and you've got the money you need for drugs. There's no work, there's nothing in the future, like, but sex, drugs and drink make you feel better. There isn't much to life – no point in life really!'

The 17-year-old is saying that where she lives her life is horrible. This may be more than a simple conclusion about life; it may be that her thinking is *pre-emptive*. The idea of pre-emptive thinking comes from Kelly's theory. It is where a person has come to a fixed conclusion which is not open to further evaluation or reasoning. The 17-year-old has concluded that, 'There isn't much to life – no point in life really.' Her thought pattern might run like this:

Where I live = a horrible experience = life isn't worthwhile.

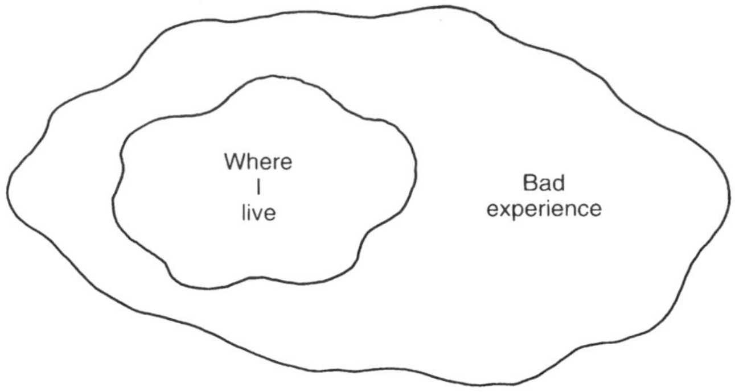

Figure 10.14 A concept map

The method of thinking is part of this person's dissatisfaction with life. No doubt life isn't good where she lives, but fixed or pre-emptive thinking will mean that she may now give up and perhaps could withdraw from trying to do anything about it.

Think it over

In hospital an adult man says, 'When I came round after the accident, I didn't believe what they told me. They said that I'd never walk again, and I thought what's the point of going on? If I can't live my life the way I want, if I can't do everything like I used to, well, I'd rather be dead!'

This person's thinking uses a network of concepts which might look like the *concept map* (Figure 10.15).

This type of concept map was called *constellatory* by Kelly because it makes a pattern rather like the constellations of stars in the sky. The idea of being disabled brings in a range of other concepts. In this map they are all negative and they have probably been learned from the discriminatory attitudes in this individual's past cultural experience. Now that he is disabled he cannot accept the conclusions that follow. Once again, the person's method of thinking (personal theories) are part of the problem.

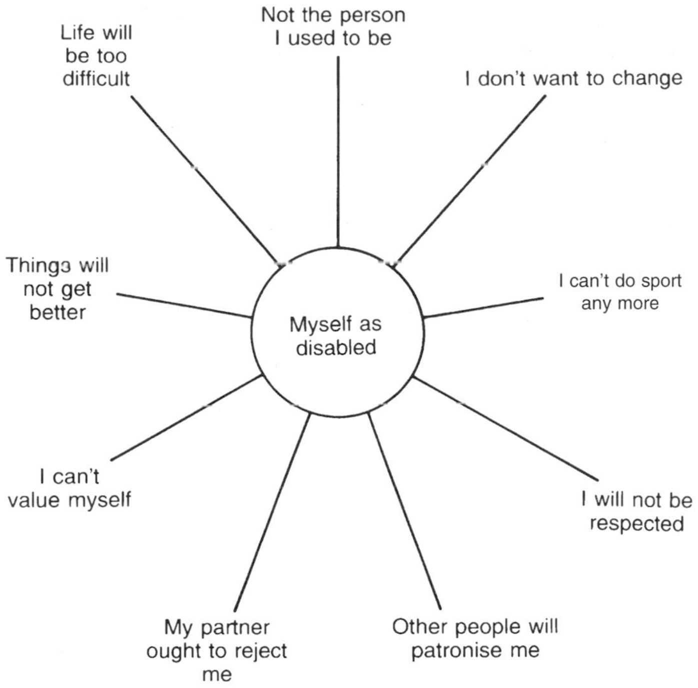
Not the person
I used to be
Life will
be too
difficult
I don't want to change
Things will
not get
better
Myself as
disabled
I can't do sport
any more
I can't
value myself
I will not be
respected
My partner
ought to reject
me
Other people will
patronise me

Figure 10.15 A constellation of thoughts based on past assumptions about disability

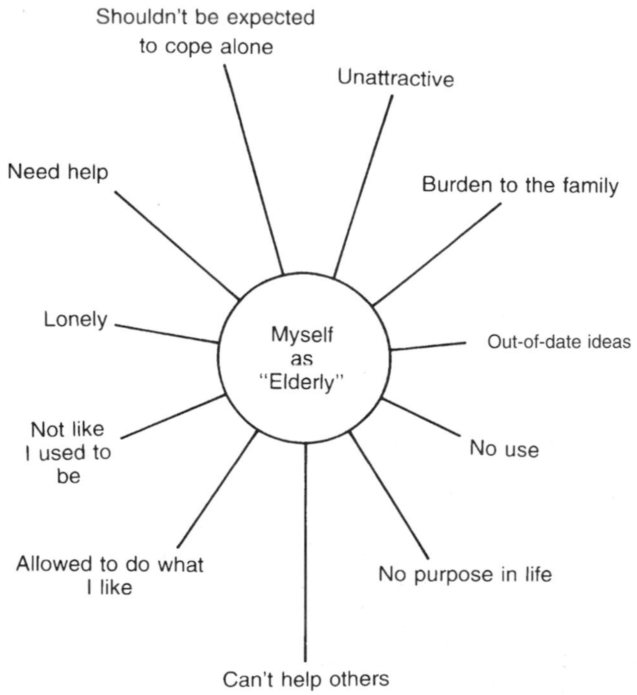

Figure 10.16 A constellation of thoughts based on past assumptions about age

Think it over

An older woman in care says, 'I don't mind you coming to talk, but do you think it will do any good? I've got nothing left to live for – what's the point? My family don't care about me, I'm no use any more!'

This third person is also thinking in a constellatory way. She has lived in a culture that does not value older people, and having adopted the concepts available in that culture, she has stopped valuing herself (Figure 10.16).

The concepts this person uses about herself means that she stereotypes and labels herself! The concept of 'elderly' causes a whole series of threatening constructs to be applied to her understanding of herself.

None of these three people can be helped by advising them that they are thinking the wrong way! Once we are fixed in our understanding and reasoning about ourselves, we will need time and fresh life experiences before we can be open to change. Kelly recommended role-play or new types of life experience in order to change these kinds of conclusions about self.

Kelly identified a third way of thinking called *propositional*. This is where our concepts or constructs are open to re-evaluation and to review in the light of new ideas. (Kelly used the term constructs because constructs are individually invented.) Thinking in an open way means that we are less likely to make false assumptions about ourselves and others. Naturally, it is best to be open to new experiences and ideas but it does cost mental time and energy. In a stressful life, not everyone can afford the effort that it takes to think in a propositional way. It's easier to label yourself and others, and risk a limited future.

Try it

How do you construct your own idea of self? Think of 15 answers to complete the phrase, 'I am...'.

Look at the answers you have given, these might show something of your own individual system of thinking about personality.

In summary some personality theories stress environmental influences, some stress biology, but others stress early experience or current thinking.

The influence of inherited and environmental factors on human development

What are genetics?

Steve Jones (1993) explains that genetics is a language, 'a set of inherited instructions passed from generation to generation'. (Page xii.) Jones argues that genes are like the words in a language. The way genes are arranged can be seen as the rules for language – a grammar. Genetics also has a literature, 'the thousands of instructions needed to make a human being.'

Genetics contain the information or 'the instructions' needed to make living organisms. At a molecular level this information is held in DNA (deoxyribonucleic acid). Each cell nucleus in a living person contains this genetic material.

Scientists are currently working very hard to understand this language system. In May 1995, Craig Venter, from the Institute for Genomic Research in Maryland, USA, announced that the research team had deciphered the whole genetic sequence for a particular bacterium, about 1.8 million sequences. By having 'read' the instructions for this life form, scientists could theoretically know how to manipulate and change it.

There is the suggestion that we could now start to create artificial life with our knowledge. The human 'book of life' is somewhat longer than a bacterium's. Steve Jones talks of 300 million letters in the DNA alphabet which go to make up a human being. Nevertheless, Jones argues that we may know the sequence by about the year 2000.

Commercial firms are extremely excited about these developments. There is the prospect of new ways of understanding illness and ways to prolong some individuals' lives. Will this new knowledge enable us to re-design or even create people? The opinion of experts is a definitive 'No!' What we are unravelling is the language of the instruction system that creates human biology. We are on the threshold of understanding the human *genotype,* the underlying pattern for making people. An individual human being is called a *phenotype*. This distinction in terminology is important because people are not simply 'caused' by underlying genetic instructions. As Nicky Hayes (1995) says, 'The genotype doesn't determine the phenotype, although it may point us in certain directions rather than others.' (Page 140.) Professors Rose, Lewontin and Kamin (1984) state, 'Genotype and environment interact in a way that makes the organism unpredictable from a knowledge of some average of effects of genotype and environment taken separately'. (Page 269.) Jones (1993) puts it very straightforwardly, 'Genetics has almost nothing to say about what makes people more than just machines driven by biology, about what makes us human'. (Page xi.)

Every individual person is a unique creation made from the inseparable and intertwined influences of genetic instructions and experience. To be alive, you will have had to have a code (genetics) to guide the construction of your body. That body could not have been built if there were no materials and no environment to build it in. Some individuals may have a genetic design or potential to grow tall, but they will not achieve this potential if they do not have enough protein in their diet as a child. The environmental and genetic influences interact. An individual, a phenotype, is the result of an interactive process, not just an example of an underlying genotype or genetic pattern.

Some very powerful genetic influences

We have known for many years that particular conditions result from genetic influences. Genes are carried on chromosomes. Usually a person has 23 pairs of chromosomes in each cell nucleus. These pairs are made up of one set of chromosomes from the mother and one set from the father. It is possible for a person to be born with three 'number 21' chromosomes, instead of two. Where this happens, the three-chromosome pattern causes 'Down's syndrome.' A person with Down's syndrome may have a learning disability and may have a physical appearance which includes a rounded face and shorter height. The extra genetic material on the additional chromosome clearly has a strong influence on the individual's development.

Richards (1993) identifies Huntingdon's disease and hereditary ovarian and breast cancer as two areas of disease which are linked to a *dominant genetic pattern*. This means that it only requires one parent to have the genetic pattern for children to inherit the illness. Other inherited diseases like beta thalassaemia and cystic fibrosis may only be passed on if both parents carry the genetic pattern responsible for these illnesses (a *recessive pattern*). Increasing knowledge has enabled tests to be designed to show whether a person is carrying one of these genetic patterns. These patterns could lead their children to develop an illness later in life. Counselling can be offered to people who are found to carry the genes for these illnesses, to enable carriers to plan their lives and avoid passing the genes on to children.

Dominant genes and chromosome abnormalities may have dramatic influences on individuals. Most genetic influences are likely to be more complex.

A rare disease which is caused when two carriers produce a baby is phenylketonuria or PKU. People with PKU cannot process phenylalanine a substance found in most diets. So in the past, babies with PKU became poisoned. They did not develop intellectually and were likely to die from their genetic defect. Nothing can be done to change the genetic make-up of people with PKU. But nowadays most babies have no problem with the illness. At birth, they are tested for PKU and a special diet can be given if the test is positive. The special diet means that the genetic inability to process phenylalanine has no effect. So people with PKU grow up to be healthy and intelligent. PKU is caused by genetics, but is made harmless by the right environment.

Think it over

Are genetic or environmental influences most important when thinking about PKU? The answer may be that it is a mistake to try to separate genetic and environmental influences. In some senses, PKU is 100 per cent genetic and 100 per cent environmental.

Jones (1993) provides a range of examples which work like PKU. Anencephaly and spina bifida are disorders which cause the spinal cord to develop incorrectly. They also appear to 'run in families'. It is now known that poor diet may sometimes influence how genes work. Vitamin supplements during later pregnancy can reduce the risk of the genes causing the illness.

Jones argues:

> Even lung cancer has a genetic component. It is, as everyone knows, most common among smokers however, smokers ... who are unfortunate enough to inherit a gene for susceptibility are far more likely to contract cancer than are those who do not. If everybody smoked, lung cancer would be a genetic disease.' (Pages 230–1.)

He then goes further and speculates;

> Most people know that smoking causes cancer and that fatty diet may lead to heart disease. Certain genes predispose their carriers to the harmful effects of smoke or fat; and some individuals may be able to drink, smoke or eat lard with impunity. Perhaps it will become possible to choose the vices best fitted to ourselves. (Page 234.)

Recent findings (June 1995) at the Patterson Institute for Cancer Research in Manchester suggest that about one person in ten inherits a general susceptibility to cancer.

Jones' point is that genetics interact with their surroundings. Some genetic diseases only happen if a person also catches a virus to trigger the disease response. Some cancers are genetic but come into operation because of diet. Some genes may cause cancer if triggered by chemicals or radioactive substances. Jones quotes the case of people who live on the island of Nauru in the Pacific. They used to eat fish and vegetables, but now that they have greatly increased their consumption of sugar and fat (a Western diet), eight out ten adults have diabetes – a susceptibility that didn't matter until they started to eat a Western diet.

Think it over

Is diabetes on the island of Nauru caused by environment or genetics?

One of the reasons for studying the human genetic code is to find answers to the puzzles of genetically inherited disease. There may be ways in which environmental influences, drugs, vitamins and so on, can influence the effects of our genetic code. The environment may often be able to 'un-cause' the consequences of our original genetic plans.

If genetics and environment are inseparable when understanding disease, then what of studies of personality and ability? Plomin (1989) reviews research on the heritability of personality and intellectual factors. Personality traits and intelligence test results provide measures which can be studied in relation to potential inheritance. This area is highly controversial, but Plomin claims evidence that traits like extroversion and ability are influenced by genetic inheritance. Plomin also finds evidence that genetic influences are inseparably linked to environmental influences. It is not simply that intelligence or personality are passed from parents to children.

There is evidence that the environment has a potential to modify genetic influences. Plomin (1989) writes, 'As the pendulum swings from environmentalism, it is important that the pendulum be caught mid-swing before its momentum carries it to biological determinism. Behavioural genetic research clearly demonstrates that both nature and nurture are important in human development.' (Page 110.)

Think it over

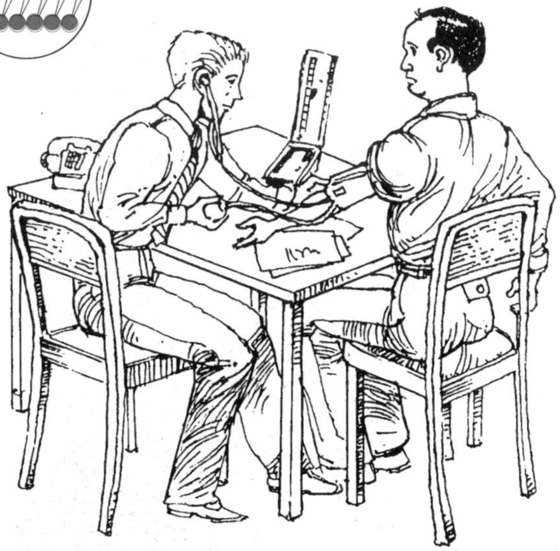

Imagine a man in his forties. He goes to his doctor with complaints of being short of breath, sometimes feeling dizzy, and being generally unfit and unwell. The doctor discovers high blood pressure. If the doctor knew a little more about the person he or she could diagnose the situation as follows:

'Well as I see it, you are an unemployed member of social class 5 (lower class). Your social habits involve excessive drinking, smoking, lack of exercise, and a poor high-fat, high-sugar diet. Your life situation provides you with little chance of changing your ways. Your family won't really support you to change your lifestyle – you are poor. Frankly you have little chance of recovery – expect to die!'

Or alternatively the doctor could have said:

'Well, tests of your genetic pattern suggest that you are at risk of developing heart disease. Some people are lucky, but I'm afraid you've inherited a tendency to heart disease – nothing I can do about that, it was all fixed before you were born – expect to die!'

Hopefully there are no doctors who would behave as in these two examples. The advice actually given would be more like:

'You have a history of heart disease in your family and it seems that you are not doing the right things to help yourself. I can't help you with money, jobs or family, but there are some things that we could do – would you take up an exercise programme if you had someone to help you? Would you follow a diet? Would you give up smoking? Can you find a sense of purpose that would make these things possible? You aren't guaranteed to live a long life if you can do these things – but at least you can try!'

The first two reactions are deterministic. The make-believe physician is interpreting the social or the genetic pressures on an individual as fixing (or determining) what will happen. Social influences do affect people – the statistics in Chapter 12 provide evidence of this. Genetic influences do affect people. But what happens to a person depends on the interplay of these factors. They also depend on the reaction of the individual. There are different levels of explanation that can be used for any area of human behaviour.

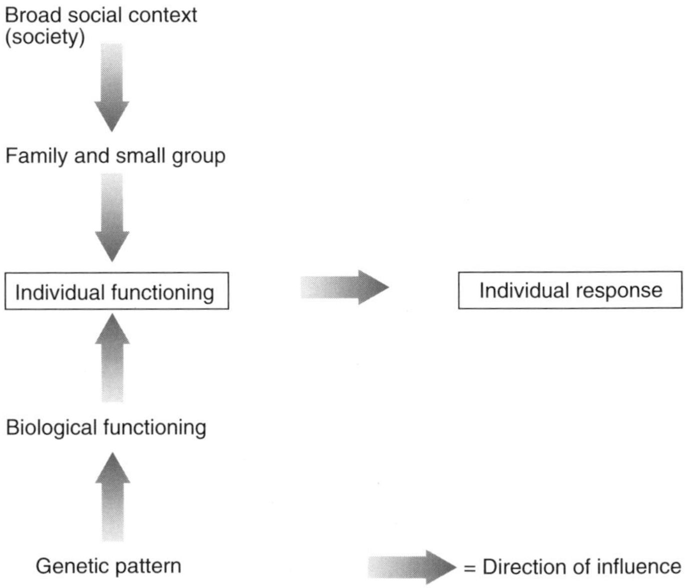

Figure 10.17 Different levels of explanation

Society, belief systems, wealth, and social roles, all have a strong influence on the way families and friendship groups behave. Individuals are socialised to behave in terms of the norms and values that they learn in these groups. Genetics also influence our biological nature. Aspects of ability, temperament and susceptibility to disease will also influence how we react. The influences of biology and social groups have been interacting in us since our birth.

Determinism

There is broad agreement amongst the majority of authors in the fields of psychology and biology that human ability, personality and susceptibility to disease result from the interaction of genetic and social influences. There are individuals who insist that human nature is the result of social influences and that genetics either do not exist or have very little influence. This view is sometimes described as *social determinism* – the idea that everything about a person is fixed by his or her social circumstances. Historically, this view has been associated with the philosopher John Locke (1632–1704). Locke believed that a newborn baby was a 'blank slate' for the environment to write on. Any baby could become anything depending on the way he or she was brought up. More recently, Karl Marx's analysis of social influences was used as a basis for a similar argument. People became what their class membership made them. Some extreme views derived from Marxism suggested that individual people were no more than representatives of particular groups. Group influences controlled or moulded what you were. So a white, middle-aged male would have to think differently from a young working-class male. A black, middle-class woman would think the way her race and class made her think. If you could control social influences, then you could control all human behaviour.

The opposite view is *genetic* or *biological determinism.* This view says that people are born to become what their inheritance dictates that they should become. There is a long history to this viewpoint in European culture. Originally a religious leader, John Calvin (1509–1564) taught that people were pre-determined to achieve salvation or not. Calvin saw human nature as fundamentally corrupt and wicked. The philosopher, Thomas Hobbes (1588–1679) took up this theme in accepting that human nature inevitably led people to be destructive. People had to be controlled in order to keep their inborn tendencies in check.

Popular views of biological determinism

At the time of the philosopher René Descartes (1596–1650), Europeans seem to have understood children as being made up from what was in their two parents. Whatever came out in a child must have in some way existed in the parents. If a child was attractive, clever or wicked, those qualities must have come from the parents. Steve Jones (1993) explains how later people believed that qualities ran 'in the blood'. In the 1800s, Europeans literally believed that it was the blood that created the abilities and personalities of children. This is the reason for terms like 'royal blood' and 'blood lines' and 'blood relatives'.

The popular understanding was that when two people had a baby, the baby would be half one parent and half the other – because of the mixing of the blood!

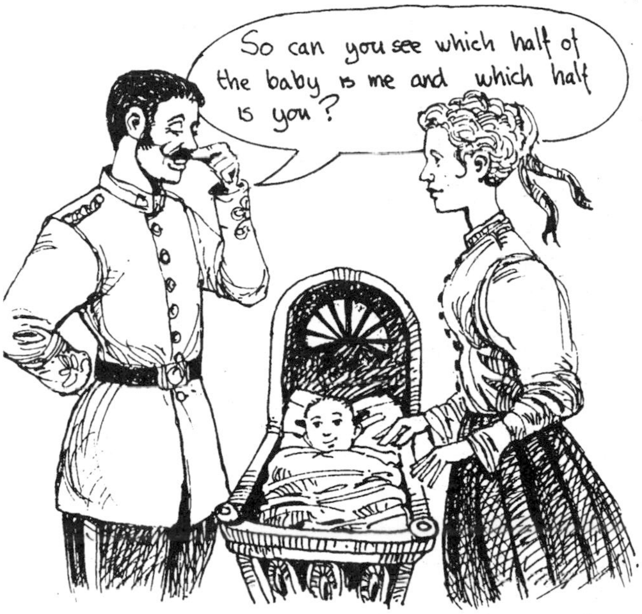
So can you see which half of the baby is me and which half is you?

Since the time of Gregor Mendel (1822–84), biologists have come to understand that genetics do not work this way. A baby is not a simple continuation of the features of his or her parents. Even the idea of dominant and recessive genes does not explain the full complexity of genetic inheritance. It may be more appropriate to think of a child as a unique outcome of the interaction of his or her mother and father's genetic patterns.

Richards (1993) provides evidence that many members of the public still think of inheritance in terms of the old Victorian idea. Some people appear to believe that if one of your parents had cancer then you will get it. If neither had cancer then you must be all right! This kind of thinking is very inaccurate and doesn't fit recent understandings of the complex way in which genetic material may work.

If people still believe the old Victorian ideas and just substitute the word 'genes' for 'blood' then no wonder many people come to believe that everything is determined by genetics. If you think that you are half your mother and half your father, then it's easy to believe that everything is fixed by genes.

Causes

Another problem people may have with understanding genes comes back to levels of explanation. Western thinking often focuses on discussing *causes*. If you are clever, attractive or wicked, there must be a cause. Looking for causes often involves very simple ideas. Rather than looking at the way things interact and interconnect, people often concentrate on ever more general ideas of cause. So a person can say, 'When I think, my thoughts are caused by all sorts of electrical messages in my brain These messages are caused by chemical reactions; the chemical reactions are caused by the biochemistry of my genes. Therefore, everything I think goes back to my genes.' Equally a person can say, 'When I think, I am thinking in patterns that I have learned. I have learned to think the way I do because of my social experiences. My social experiences have been caused by society. Therefore, everything I think is caused by society.'

Both these arguments are inaccurate – they only pick up some of the issues and ignore the complexity of human experience.

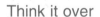

Think it over

The word 'cause' can lead people to some very strange conclusions. Imagine asking three people where they went for their holiday last year and why they chose that destination.

The first person says, 'Spain. Society and the social construction of holidays made me do it.'

The second person says, 'Spain. It was the biochemical reactions in my head that made me do it – biochemical reactions which have their origin in evolution since the beginnings of the world'.

The third person says, 'Spain. I went there because I thought I would enjoy it!'

Surely you would see the first two people as 'not fully functioning human beings' or to put it more bluntly, 'weird'. Reducing everything to distant and abstract causes can lead to explanations at the wrong level.

It would be hard to enjoy and probably hard to have a social life if you didn't think in terms of individual and personal systems of meaning. Without an

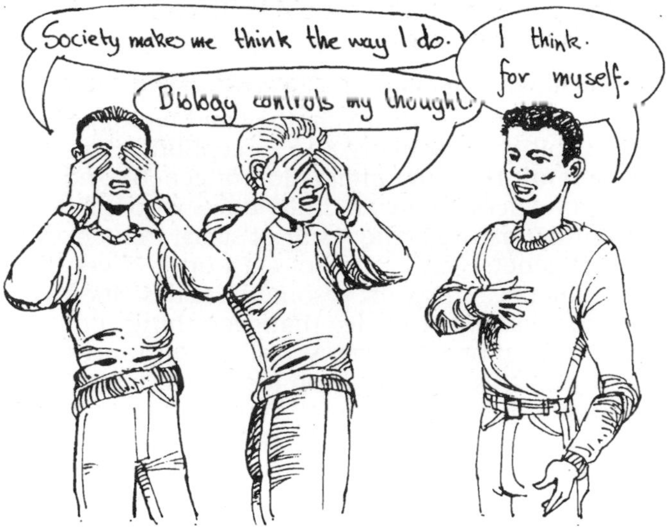
Society makes me think the way I do.
Biology controls my thought.
I think for myself.

individual level of explanation, how do you understand the skill of interpersonal communication?

All the levels of explanation have a part to play in care work and in understanding human need. It is important not to allow the word 'cause' to twist thinking into reducing everything to biochemistry. It may be equally important not to allow the idea of cause to persuade us to explain everything away in terms of 'society'.

The politics of determinism

Saying that everything is fixed by genes, or that everything is fixed by society, gives a nice simple explanation. Each is also an explanation with political consequences. If a person who visits the doctor is given the explanation he or she has a 'genetic weakness', the doctor might conclude the conversation by saying, 'we can't do anything – so go away and die quietly.' The idea of things being fixed can be used to avoid responsibility.

What's the point in spending money on cancer treatment and research, if the possibility of whether people develop cancer or not is fixed? Politically, it could be argued that tax cuts are better than spending money on people with heart disease and cancer – some people can be seen as 'no hopers' if you believe in simple genetic determinism.

Social determinism also leads to theories about political power. Once again, the individual need not matter. Individual problems can only be put right if a particular kind of government takes control. Issues about health immediately become issues about political power and who should be in control of world economic issues.

The situation becomes even more extreme if areas like wealth, intelligence, personality and crime are seen as genetically determined. It could then be possible to claim that the poor are poor because they are inferior, that crime can't be tackled socially, that education is wasted on some groups in society, and so on. Genetic determinists might be able to argue for the abolition of free health and education – they could use the argument that 'It's wasted on people who are "no hopers"'. A genetic determinist could argue, 'If people have it in them to lead prosperous, healthy, worthwhile lives, then they will. If people haven't got it in them, then why should taxpayers waste money on them?'

Professors Rose, Lewontin and Kamin (1984) state:

> Over the past decade and a half we have watched with concern the rising tide of biological determinist writing, with its increasingly grandiose claims to be able to locate the causes of the inequalities of status, wealth and power between classes, genders and races in Western society in a reductionist [everything reduces or goes back to genetics] theory of human nature. (Page ix.)

Rose *et al.* devote a whole chapter to the politics of biological determinism. Nicky Hayes (1995) reviews some of the theories of genetic determinism and states:

> These people are not purveying scientific theory, but ideology. It is a political perspective with very direct political implications: it legitimises the inequalities of society by arguing that these arise from inherited differences; and negates attempts to create a better society by implying that they are doomed to failure from the start. (Page 132.)

The interaction of nature and nurture

The debate about inherited and environmental influences is sometimes referred to as the *Nature* (inherited influences) *versus Nurture* (environmental influences) debate. This is a poetic way of putting the issues that may go back to Shakespeare. Shakespeare created the character Caliban in his play *The Tempest.* Caliban is described as a person 'upon whose nature nurture could never stick'. This means that he was fixed by inheritance. The nature/nurture debate was going on long before genes or chromosomes were discovered.

Rose *et al.* conclude,

> The contrast between biological and cultural determinism is a manifestation of the nature–nurture controversy that has plagued biology, psychology and sociology since the early part of the nineteenth century. Either nature plays a determining role in producing the similarity and differences among human beings, or it does not, in which case, what is left but nurture? We reject this dichotomy. We do assert that we cannot think of any significant human social behaviour that is built into our genes in such a way that it cannot be modified and shaped by social conditioning...yet at the same time, we deny that human beings are born tabulae rasae as [blank slate], which they evidently are not, and that individual human beings are simple mirrors of social circumstances. (Page 267.)

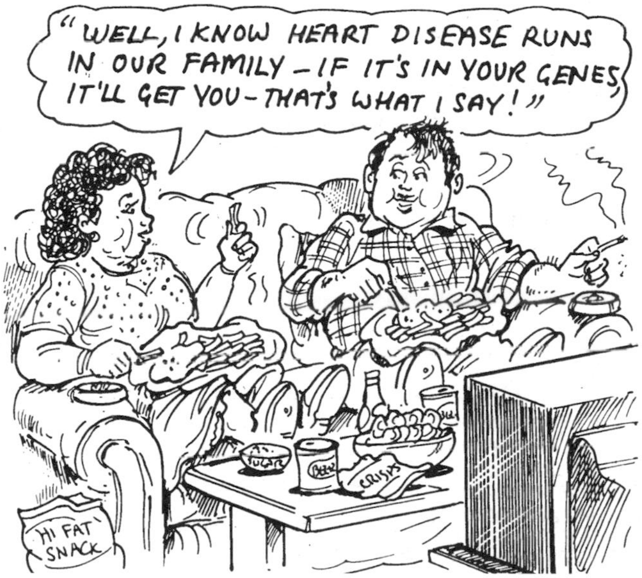
"WELL, I KNOW HEART DISEASE RUNS IN OUR FAMILY – IF IT'S IN YOUR GENES IT'LL GET YOU – THAT'S WHAT I SAY!"
SUGAR
BEER
CRISPS
HI FAT SNACK

In February 1995, there was a great deal of newspaper coverage about whether criminal behaviour could be influenced by genes. Professor Patrick Bateson, writing in *The Independent* on 18 February, commented on articles claiming that biological make-up might hold the key to criminal behaviour, or that unemployment might be the cause. He said, 'The sad thing was the determinism that accompanied the media coverage of the claims. It was obvious that, in certain quarters, the dreadful old nature–nurture debate was rampant once again'. Later, he states, 'By degrees, both sides in the nature–nurture dispute have come to appreciate that behavioural development cannot be treated as though it were wholly under the control of the genes or wholly influenced by the environment.'

It is possible to look at issues like temperament, language learning and the in-built reactions of babies and say that these are all genetic, and so, therefore, a certain proportion of language or personality is genetic. Bateson argues that this is wrong. To explain why, Bateson uses the example of baking a cake. A cake is more than the ingredients that go into it. A cake is the result of a process. When a cake is mixed and later baked, the butter, flour, milk, raisins and water all alter. The taste of the cake and the texture of the cake is different from the taste of the cake mixture. Bateson argues that human development is a process. The contribution of environment and the contribution of genetics is impossible to separate:

> You would not expect to recognise each ingredient and each action involved in cooking as a separate component in the finished cake... The development of individuals is an interplay between them and their environment. Individuals choose and change the conditions to which they are exposed; then they are themselves changed by those conditions to which they are exposed.

Rose *et al.* (1984) also use this cake metaphor.

The question as to how much human development is due to environment and how much is due to genetics could be answered by saying that it's a bit of both. But even this answer is wrong. The influence of both nature and nurture is an influence on a process. Development is a process. Jones (1993) states:

> An attribute such as intelligence is often seen as a cake which can be sliced into so much 'gene' and so much 'environment'. In fact the two are so closely blended that trying to separate them is more like trying to unbake the cake. Failure to understand this simple biological fact leads to confusion and worse. (Page 227.)

Human beings are infinitely more complex than mixing and baking a cake. The cake stays baked – it becomes a finished product. Humans are never finished. Human learning and change continue until an individual dies. Although the cake image is limited it does provide a way of understanding why it is unwise to separate the influences of nature and nurture.

Professor of genetics Steve Jones (1993) summarises the nature–nurture debate with the following paragraph:

> Most modern geneticists find queries about the relative importance of nature and nurture in controlling the normal range of human behaviour dull, for two reasons. First, they scarcely understand the inheritance of complex characters (those like height, weight or behaviour which are measured rather than counted) even in simple creatures like flies or mice, and even when studying traits like size or weight which are easy to define. Second, and more important, geneticists know that the perpetual interrogation – nature or nurture? – is largely meaningless. Its only answer is usually that there is no valid question. (Page 226.)

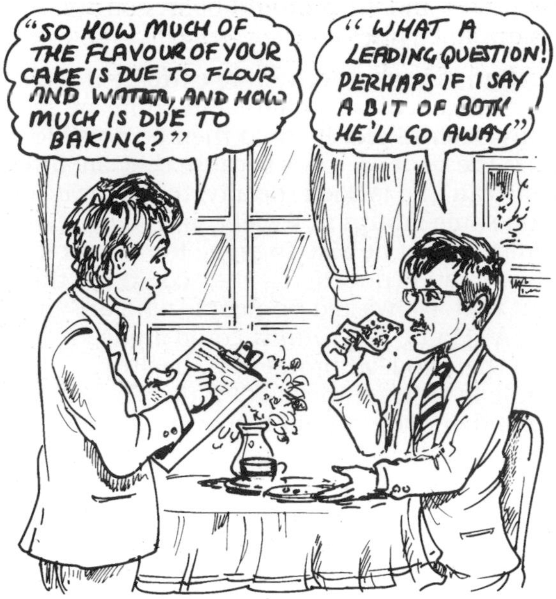
"SO HOW MUCH OF THE FLAVOUR OF YOUR CAKE IS DUE TO FLOUR AND WATER, AND HOW MUCH IS DUE TO BAKING?"
"WHAT A LEADING QUESTION! PERHAPS IF I SAY A BIT OF BOTH HE'LL GO AWAY"

A conclusion would appear to be that nature and nurture cannot be usefully abstracted from the process of development, but that nature and nurture form a process of interaction which progresses across the life-span of any organism. Environment may completely override genetic influences, as in PKU, or genetic influences may sometimes have powerful effects, depending on the environment with which they interact.

Evidence collection point

As part of a project you are asked to:

1 Explain human development in childhood, adolescence, adult and later life stages. Focus on physical development, and on language, cognition and emotional development.
2 Explain how people develop personality. This could include reference to trait, learning, early experience and humanist approaches.
3 Discuss how inherited and environmental factors interact in human development. This could include a discussion of issues such as levels of explanation,

determinism and the growing consensus that development is a process where nature and nurture cannot be seen as separate components.

Think it over

Returning to the Forrest Gump question of whether life is determined by fate or whether we just blow around on the wind like a feather, how much are you controlled by your genes and how much by social learning? How far does early learning fix your personality? Can you use your own cognitive abilities to build and develop your own self-concept?

Your view of personality and your view of levels of explanation should guide you to an answer. Many people will conclude that we are all influenced by genetics, by social context, by early learning. One idea suggests that the great thing about being human is that we get to make our own decisions – we have the last word on where our lives are going. Humans have evolved the ability to solve problems. The answers you come up with will finally determine your personality and life.

Still, if you are Forrest Gump, you might not bother with problem-solving. Then you can let your life float around on the breeze some of the time, and be fixed by events the rest of the time.

Transition and change in life

The interaction of biological and social processes may influence our individual development. Language and cognitive development enable us to become self-aware. Around the ages of 14 to 19, most people are likely to develop a concept of who they are (*self-concept*). This self-awareness is also described as an *identity* by authors who wish to emphasise the social context of self-awareness.

Although individuals develop an understanding of themselves, this understanding is always open to change and development. A range of expected and unexpected events might mean that an individual's self-concept has to change.

There is a saying, associated with Buddhism, that the only certain thing in the world is that there will always be change and something that changes. Change can be exciting and desirable. Life would become boring and stressful if you had to spend every day doing exactly what you had done the day before. Just a change in the weather – the first snow of winter, perhaps – can create a feeling of excitement. However, while some change makes life interesting, too much change can create stress. Throughout life we have to cope with changes in our social relationships, our social context and in society as a whole.

There is a range of life events, creating a need for personal change, which affect many individuals. In children and adolescents the list might include:

- coping with the arrival of a new brother or sister
- coping with changes in family structure – new step-parents
- starting at a new school
- coping with moving house
- making friends
- changing friends
- coping with new coursework and exams
- choosing a career
- making relationships; breaking up and changing relationships.

These changes may be experienced as exciting, or as things that just happen. These changes might also be experienced as upsetting, destabilising changes which destroy a person's sense of security, understanding of him- or herself and his or her social role.

Think it over

Think about the list above. Can you remember feeling stressed by any of the events? How did you cope? How did the experience influence your understanding of yourself at the time?

Many of the changes described above involve a *loss* or a letting go of some attachments. We may have liked our friends and the life at our first school. Moving to a new school takes all that away from us. Gradually losing touch with old friends; having to find new friends may involve a loss. Sometimes it may feel as if a part of ourselves is lost – the loss can cause a threat to our sense of self.

Older people who receive social care support are often very vulnerable to the threats associated with loss. Some of the life-event threats which face elders include:

- loss of partner (bereavement)
- loss of socially valued role – not being needed by children or work colleagues
- loss of health – restricting activities, illness and loss of enjoyment of life

- loss of hearing and vision, restricting satisfaction with life
- loss of mobility – restricting social contact and satisfaction with life
- loss of body image – self-labelling as unattractive
- fear of loneliness
- fear of pain
- fear of loss of control over own lifestyle and decision-making
- fear of dying

These life-event threats are not simply unpleasant or unwanted events. For some people,these events may remove any sense of capability or of being a person who can cope.

Case study: An example of loss

Mrs Kershaw is 84 years old, and her husband died two years ago. Mrs Kershaw feels that she no longer has a meaningful social role. Her children do not visit her very often and do not seem to need her. She often feels that she is just a burden, both to her children and other neighbours who collect her shopping.

Mrs Kershaw has a heart condition which means that she cannot get out easily. Because she cannot walk far, she feels that she is unable to visit her friends who live several streets away. She has cataracts on both eyes which means that reading is becoming increasingly difficult. She can no longer enjoy her books. Despite the fact that she could have an operation, she feels that everything is coming to an end. She used to have an estimation of herself as competent and capable (we could call this high 'self-efficacy'). Mrs Kershaw feels that her life has changed; she can no longer guess or understand what she is capable of and feels stressed. She no longer feels that 'she is the person she used to be'.

A combination of losses may cause older people to become threatened, or a single event may be the focus for disruption. Eric Erikson (1963) saw the main challenge for older people as being the need to keep a sense of meaning of life. In Erikson's terms, this was called *ego-integrity,* keeping a sense of self together. If this challenge was lost then a sense of despair and a lack of purpose in life might follow.

Holmes and Rahe (1967) set out to try to catalogue just how much change different life-events involved. They came up with an index of how much readjustment different life events might call for (Figure 10.18). Barrie Hopson (1986) states that this general index was found to be consistent across European countries and with the cultures of Japan, Hawaii, central America and Peru. Naturally, the amount of work needed to readjust to a life event differs for each individual. Each person has particular vulnerabilities, strengths and weaknesses. The Holmes–Rahe scale is no more than a general

Life event	Value
Death of partner	100
Divorce	73
Marital separation	65
Going to prison	63
Death of a close family member	63
Personal injury or illness	53
Marriage	50
Being dismissed at work	47
Marital reconciliation	45
Retirement	45
Change in health of family member	44
Pregnancy	40
Sexual difficulties	39
Gaining a new family member	39
Business or work adjustment	39
Change in financial state	38
Death of a close friend	37
Change to different line of work	36
Change in number of arguments with partner	35
Mortgage larger than one year's net salary	31
Foreclosure of mortgage or loan	30
Change in responsibilities at work	29
Son or daughter leaving home	29
Trouble with in-laws	29
Outstanding personal achievement	28
Partner begins or stops work	26
Begin or end school	26
Change in living conditions	25
Revision of personal habits	24
Trouble with boss	23
Change in work hours or conditions	20
Change in residence	20
Change in schools	20
Change in recreation	19
Change in religious activities	19
Change in social activities	18
Mortgage or loan less than one year's net salary	17
Change in sleeping habits	16
Change in number of family get-togethers	15
Change in eating habits	15
Holiday	13
Major festival, e.g. Christmas	12
Minor violations of the law	11

Figure 10.18 The Holmes–Rahe life-event scale

overview originally researched in the USA in the 1960s. The value scale suggests that on average the death of a partner involves ten times the change, and perhaps the threat, that being caught for speeding does. Changing to a new school is half as stressful (on average) as a new sibling being added to the family.

The Holmes–Rahe scale may be a useful list of changes and transitions which might happen to adults. But it is important to remember that few people are 'average'. In your own personal life you may rate some issues as far more or less stressful than the scale suggests.

Think it over

If the average person (in the 1960s) found being dismissed at work (sacked) half as stressful as the death of a partner, what sort of variation might exist between individuals? Could some individuals find the loss of a partner less stressful than the loss of their job? What are statistical averages or means? (See Chapter 26.)

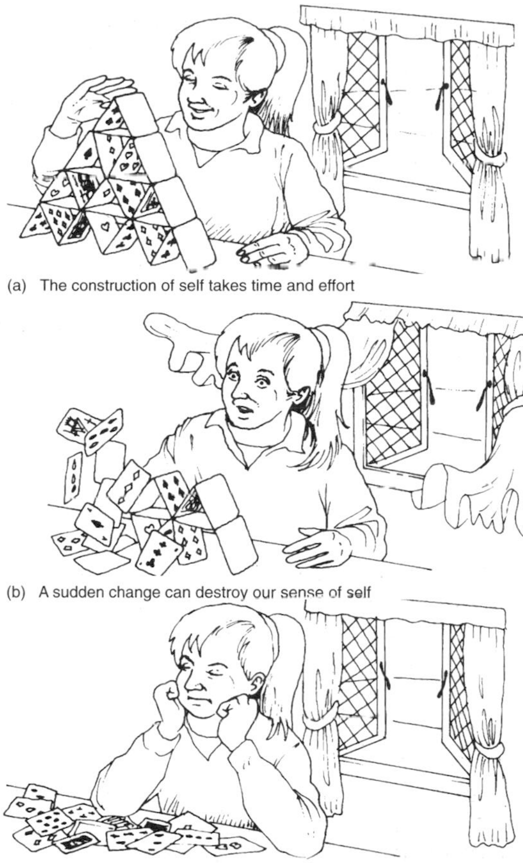

(a) The construction of self takes time and effort

(b) A sudden change can destroy our sense of self

(c) Reconstruction takes time

Figure 10.19 The construction of self may be like building a house of cards

Change and our sense of self

As we grow and develop, our learning, socialisation, group and social experiences enable us to construct a concept of self. In a perfect life, change would only happen at our own pace and it would be just the right kind of change to keep us from boredom.

As change happened we would make minor adjustments to our sense of who we were.

This construction of a personal idea of self may be like constructing a house of cards (Figure 10.19). You need a level surface with enough friction to stop the cards from falling. Bit by bit you can build your structure. If a small piece falls – that's OK, you can catch it before it does too much damage to the rest of the structure. You can start again. But suppose a breeze blows through the window, or someone knocks the table, the whole structure may collapse. It will take a bit of time to rebuild now.

Self-concept may be like a house of cards, in that it is vulnerable to sudden unwelcome changes. If it has to be rebuilt, it will be a painful and emotionally costly task. A house of cards is just a pastime. Trying to cope without an effective idea of who you are might mean that life isn't worth living.

Expected and unexpected change

Some changes such as marriage, the birth of children, or ageing, are expected and predictable. Other changes such as bereavement and facing one's own death are predictable in the loose sense that everyone understands that neither ourselves nor our friends are immortal. When bereavement or terminal illness happen, however, many people experience them as unexpected and unpredictable. Other changes, or *life events,* such as being a victim of crime, sudden disability or illness, and the breakdown of relationships are often unexpected and unpredictable.

If major life events feel under our control, then change may be exciting. If we cannot plan for or control the events, then we may become distressed. Certain unpredictable events such as redundancy, serious illness or disability, divorce and bereavement, are always likely to cause stress and insecurity to individuals who experience them. Even promotion at work and marriage can create tension in people. Why does change cause upset and tensions?

Change can:

- create uncertainty
- alter a person's self-concept
- create a need for new learning
- create a sense of loss
- use up time, money and emotional resources.

Uncertainty

When children start at a new school, they may not know what to expect. Will they get lost in the building? Will the staff be friendly? Most of all, will the other children like them? Will they get on and make friends? There are so many questions, and no one knows how the future will work out. Uncertainty can create worry.

There is uncertainty when a person decides to marry or live with a partner. Partners may think they know one another well, but how can they be sure that their partner won't change? How can they be sure they will both stay in love? How can they be sure they won't fall out – many people do fall out and one in three marriages ends in divorce!

Having children can create uncertainty. What does it take to be good parents? What does it cost to get what is needed for the children? Will the parents like their children? Will the children like their parents? Will the children strain the relationship?

Almost every form of change raises questions about the future. When we don't know the answers, it can create stress.

Self-concept

Think it over

The way we see ourselves is partly due to the way our friends, relatives and other important people see us. When we change friends, change relationships, or change jobs or school, then the people we mix with will change. New people might see us differently. New people might treat us differently. Our ideas of our skills, our social status or our importance might have to change. You may have been brilliant at a previous job, and seen yourself as clever. When you change jobs, new people might work in different ways. The new people might not see you as clever. Your concept of yourself might have to drop in value in your new job.

For example, a man may think of himself as a really sociable and outgoing person. If he and his partner start a family, they may have to stay in and care for the children. The man may have to change the way he thinks about himself. Marriage creates a partnership and so one partner (the husband, for example) cannot expect to take every decision and control every part of his life as he did when he was a single person. He may have to change his self-concept if he is to have a successful partnership.

Issues like redundancy, serious illness and bereavement may wreck an individual's self-concept.

The need for new learning

When children start at a new school, there is a vast amount to learn about the school and the people in it. New names, new places to find their way around, new customs, new teachers, and so on. Starting a new job will be similar. Having children involves a vast amount of learning; learning to care, as well as all the practical issues like feeding and bathing children. Moving home may mean learning about do-it-yourself, plumbing, decorating, finance and so on. Redundancy, serious illness or bereavement might mean learning a whole new lifestyle.

Many people enjoy learning at their own pace in their own way. Major life-event changes may not allow everyone time or the chance to go at their own pace. Individuals become stressed with the amount of learning and adapting that they have to do.

A sense of loss

Changing schools might mean losing contact with friends. Leaving home may mean an individual will not see parents, brothers and sisters so much. Having children may mean a couple has less time to spend with friends, and maybe less money to spend on themselves. Changing jobs means the loss of old work friends. Moving home means losing routines, people and views that an individual used to know. Serious changes like redundancy, sudden disability or bereavement can involve multiple losses.

Major life changes can create a serious sense of loss. A person might also feel threatened or attacked by what has happened. It takes a great deal of mental work to recover and make up for serious losses in life.

Use of time, money and emotional resources

It takes time to learn a new job, to make new relationships, to look after children, and so on. Time is a limited resource. Having children, moving home, leaving home, or getting married may also use a lot of money. These events may also be emotionally draining. Going through planned life changes can be costly on time, money and emotional commitment.

Unplanned changes such as redundancy, serious illness, divorce and bereavement may also involve extra expenditure, extra work and extra emotional involvement in order to sort things out. This time an individual is spending his or her time and money to sort out things that are unwanted!

Coping with change

The Holmes–Rahe scale places loss of partner at the top of the table of changes and transitions. Bereavement is described as a process, because it involves making sense of a loss and constructing a new sense of self. Bereavement is not just a matter of feeling sad because someone has died.

When two people have been partners for some time and one dies, what will the surviving partner have lost? Naturally, the surviving person has lost someone he or she was attached to and loved. He or she will grieve for this person. There may be a whole list of other losses as well. The surviving partner will have also perhaps lost:

- the main person he or she talked to
- the main person who gave advice
- his or her sexual partner
- the person who made social events work well
- a person to go out with
- the main person who provided emotional support
- the focus of domestic life
- a source of protection
- a source of income.

Loss of a loved one might seriously upset a person's life and lifestyle. Grief is not just about missing a person, it may also be about having to reorganise a sense of self.

Bowlby (1969) believed that humans, and indeed many animals, would form close emotional attachments during their lives. He described three phases of grief:

1. When an attachment is broken (perhaps by death), the first reaction is the pain of separation and a desperate desire to find the lost person again. During this first phase, the individual is unable to change. A person has to let go of his or her past assumptions and expectations which are focused on the lost partner before change is possible.
2. The bereaved person will experience anger and despair. This phase involves developing a degree of detachment from the dead partner. During this phase a grieving person's sense of self may become disorganised.
3. The grieving person reorganises his or her sense of self and expectations and habits, and starts to rebuild his or her life and identity. This rebuilding or reconstruction is, perhaps, like reconstructing the house of cards after it has fallen down.

Going through a bereavement involves coping with a massive amount of unwelcome change. At first, the individual cannot let go of the attachment to the lost loved one. Letting go involves coping with new ways of understanding self and lifestyle. The journey through a process of grieving ends when an individual is able to reconstruct his or her sense of self.

Colin Murry Parkes (1975) described a process of grieving based on his observations and studies of grief. He explained grief as a life crisis or a major time of transition and change for an individual. Going through a change involves a need for psychological work and this takes time and effort. Parkes wrote, 'As the old assumptions about the world prove ineffective and a fresh set of assumptions is built up, so the old identity dissolves and is replaced by a new and different one'. (Page 129.) Much of the pain and sorrow associated with loss may really be connected with our tendency to resist change. Again, Parkes wrote, 'Resistance to change, the reluctance to give up possessions, people, status, expectations – this I believe, is the basis of grief'. (Page 25.)

Naturally, each person experiences the struggle of grief differently; but there may be some general components of coping with change that can be identified.

Initially, many people experience *shock* and numbness when they are first confronted with loss. This phase may involve an inability to accept the reality of the loss, let alone trying to change.

A reaction of *searching* for the lost person may follow (sometimes literally searching faces in a crowd). Perhaps the mind can cope with the news of the loss, but not with its meaning. A feeling that, 'Yes, I know that he is dead, but that won't stop me from meeting him again.' Emotions of anger and guilt may actually help someone begin to become detached from the lost love. A phase of experimenting with defences, of beginning to try to cope with change, may occur before it is possible to gain a new identity. Parkes referred to the 'beginning to cope' phase as *mitigation.* The final phase of developing a new sense of self is called *reconstruction.*

Case study: Coping with grief

Jack had been married for 22 years when his partner unexpectedly died of a heart attack. They had been very close. When Jack was first told about the death he showed little reaction. Friends had to persuade Jack not to go to work the next day. Jack had said that it would give him something to do, take his mind off things. Later, at the funeral, Jack said that he felt frozen inside and that he did not want to eat. It was some weeks later that Jack said he felt better because he could talk to his partner, sitting in a chair late at night. Jack admitted that he never saw his partner, he just felt her presence.

As time went on, Jack said that he felt he could have done more to prevent the heart attack – if only he had noticed some signs, if only they hadn't smoked. Jack felt angry with their local doctor. His partner had seen the doctor only two months before. Surely, if the doctor was any good, she should have noticed something! On occasions, Jack just became very angry and bitter about how badly everything had gone; perhaps he was to blame?

Months later, Jack explained that he had sorted his life out a bit. Whereas his partner used to organise things, he had now learned to cope alone. He explained that he spent time with a close friend, 'a shoulder to cry on' as he put it.

After a year and a half, Jack still misses his partner but he now says that the experience has made him stronger, 'It's as if I understand more about life now. I feel – if I could cope with this loss – well, there isn't much I can't cope with.' Jack has now become involved with the local voluntary support group for people who are bereaved. He says that helping others has helped him, 'It has given me new meaning and purpose in life. I think everything in life has a purpose – things are meant to happen to you. I had a good life before and now I've got a new life to lead.' Jack says that 'life feels OK now.'

Jack's first reactions might suggest that he couldn't take in the full implications of the loss. He relied on denial to cope. The sense of his partner could be a real thing or it could be a protective fantasy. The anger and the guilt could be a sign that Jack is struggling to come to terms with the loss. He is mentally involved in trying to make sense of himself and accept some change. Jack's 'sorting out' might indicate that he has now accepted the reality of the loss. Jack is now making changes to some areas of his life and self-perception. Finally, Jack has resolved the loss. A new sense of self now gives Jack some fulfilment in life. Jack has reconstructed his sense of self. Jack still misses his partner, but can lead a fulfilled life despite those feelings.

You may have thought of other ideas: it is possible to see many different things in a real-life situation. What is important is to recognise that bereavement and change is a process. People have to find their own way through it at their own pace. There are no forms of advice or special skills which can 'cure' people or 'solve' their problems.

A general way of understanding change

Bereavement is just one example of change. Holmes and Rahe identified 43 other changes which might require some mental effort and some coping strategies. Positive life experiences, such as promotion at work, moving house or pregnancy, are included in the Holmes–Rahe scale because even positive life events require mental work and coping strategies. Just because something is welcome and exciting, it doesn't mean that there is no social readjustment. Coping with any transition or change may involve some stress. Barrie Hopson (1986) identifies a general way of understanding 'transitions' or change in life.

Hopson proposes that there are seven phases that people often go through when facing identity change (Figure 10.20). Hopson believes that these phases apply equally to situations involving a sudden shock or where there is a slow growing awareness and that change is inevitable. Whenever people have to cope with large-scale change or transition it may be possible to identify phases of:

- *Immobilisation* This first phase involves being unable to cope, so failure to respond may result. Immobilisation can include a denial that change will happen. The individual may feel 'frozen up'.
- *Minimisation* This involves denial and deflection defences. One way of trying to cope with change is to trivialise it or pretend that it won't matter.
- *Depression* When people become aware of the full need for change, depression may set in. Anger, frustration and helplessness may also occur at this time. Self-esteem may be threatened as people take the full implications of change on board.
- *Letting go* This involves accepting the need to

change, accepting a new reality. Optimism may become possible.

- *Testing* This stage of self-testing may involve trying out new behaviours and experimenting with new lifestyles. Hopson claims that this stage may involve a tendency to see life in a stereotyped way.
- *Search for meaning* This stage involves understanding the whole process of transition and change.
- *Internalisation* The seventh and final stage involves the reconstruction of expectations, ways of behaving and ways of understanding self.

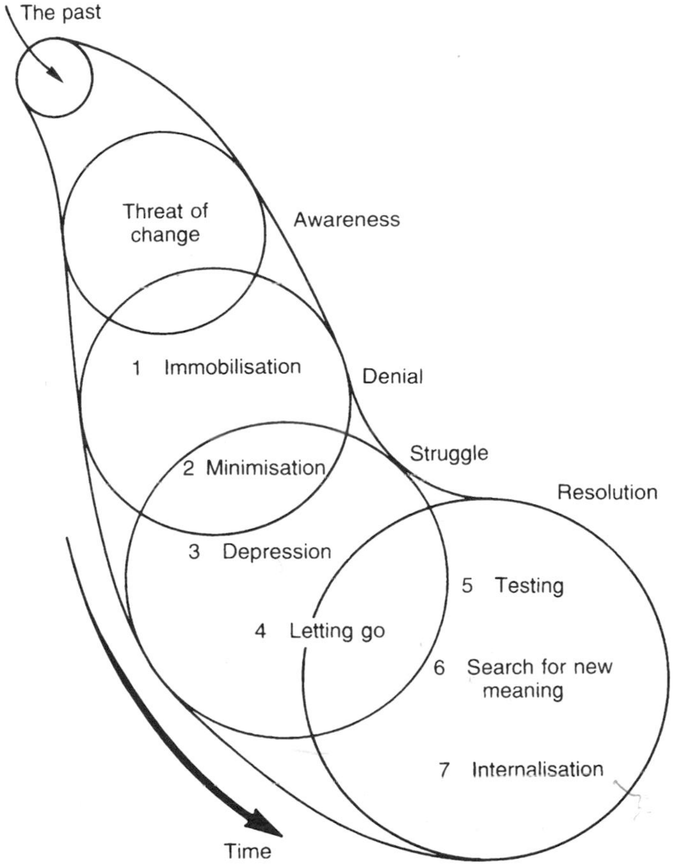

Figure 10.20 The seven phases of coping with change

Hopson sees the morale of people going through transition at its lowest point during the third stage (depression). So, going through a transition involves the feeling that things are getting worse until the light at the end of the tunnel is seen during stage four (letting go).

Methods of support for coping with change

Individuals with a clear self-concept will use their own mental and intellectual abilities to help them cope with major life change. People who choose to get married or to change job will think about planning for the change. People may sit down and check through (evaluate) their time and money resources, if they are planning on starting a family.

People faced with unexpected changes will sometimes go through a process of shock which prevents them from using planning and evaluation skills. Even so, many people will try to use their own imagination, and their own knowledge, planning and evaluation skills to cope with unexpected life changes. Few people have to struggle with major life changes entirely on their own. Most people will have family or friends they can turn to. As well as relatives, partners, people at work and other relationships, some people can turn to community figures, religious leaders, and so on. Active Christians may be able to get help from their church leaders or community. Muslims may receive support from their mosque and community. Hindu and Sikh communities will support their members. Some people live in areas where their own local neighbourhood creates a supportive community.

Where life changes involve legal, financial or medical issues, people may seek professional help. A person going through divorce might seek legal help with sharing out joint property. He or she might want medical advice for stress-related illnesses, financial advice to help plan the future or advice from specialist support groups.

Talking

Individuals may think more clearly when they can talk a problem through with other people. There is an old saying, 'A problem shared is a problem halved'. Sometimes a person may feel much better for talking something over, because people can reflect on issues and understand more when they talk to others and use others as a sounding board. Another saying is, 'I know what I think, when I hear what I say'. Talking helps some people to make sense of the changes that they are going through – 'it's good to talk!'

Carers can develop special supportive conversational skills which can help people going through major changes or difficulties with relationships. Supportive skills are explained in the Chapters 4, 5 and 6.

Networks

Many people have social networks which can provide help in times of need. In this context, a network is a range of individuals or organisations which are linked. When a person needs help, he or she may be able to contact a range of friends – an *informal network*. A formal network might involve relatives or members of the community who have an obligation to help. Within an organisation there may be a formal network of people who provide supervision or personnel services. There might also be a range of individuals who will offer informal advice and support to individuals who are facing change or transition.

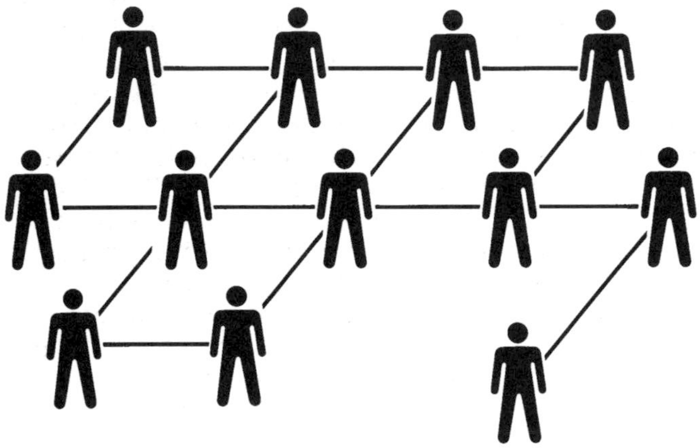

Figure 10.21 A network is like a web of contacts – people who can offer advice

Practical help

When people have to move home, they might need help to pack and unpack belongings. Friends and relatives might give this help for free. Friends might expect help in return when they need 'a hand'. People may help others with decorating, with plumbing, and so on. People who are starting a family may know others who will baby-sit for free – people they can trust. A network of friends and relatives may provide practical help. Friends might provide advice when individuals look for work. Families usually support their members in hospital. Families often provide accommodation when relationships with a partner breakdown. Family and friends usually provide support following divorce or bereavement. Family and friends might even protect individuals who are in conflict with others.

Advice

Some life changes can be planned for, for example, marriage, changing jobs or moving house.Sometimes family, friends and work colleagues can give useful advice and information which will help individuals to plan. Colleagues might tell each other about new routines at work, give advice on how to get on with a supervisor, explain how to fill in forms, and so on. Friends could give advice on, for example, where to hold a wedding reception, or purchase services for a wedding.

Improving self-concept

Other people can support individuals in feeling positive about themselves. Being with and talking to other people can create a sense of belonging – a feeling that an individual is a member of a group and is 'worth something'. Conversation may be a very important kind of help for people who are struggling to cope with redundancy, disability or bereavement. Individuals often need to feel valued and supported.

The opinions or views of other people can guide us when we have to change and develop our concept of self. Change means that a bereaved person, for example, is no longer a partner in a joint relationship. Changing back to being a single person can be a hard and painful task. Other people's support may be very important to help come to terms with bereavement.

People learn by observing how others cope. If they belong to families, social or community groups, they may have the opportunity to watch others coping with marriage, having children, moving home, becoming ill, and so on. It is possible to observe others' successes and mistakes. By imitating other people's ways of coping, it may be possible to manage change and transition. Understanding how others cope may save individuals from feeling confused or frightened.

Specialist help

Professionals and others can provide specialist help. Doctors may be able to prescribe drugs that help with stress or illness. Solicitors may provide legal solutions to problems. The Citizens' Advice Bureau can advise us on a wide range of special services in the community, such as how to obtain equipment to assist a person with a disability. Relate, the marriage guidance agency, provides guidance and counselling services for people who are having difficulties in their relationships.

Victim Support provides advice and emotional support for victims of crime.

Many individuals will get the help and support they need from support groups. These include groups like Cruse, a bereavement care group which provides counselling, advice and opportunities for social contact for all bereaved people. Many individuals can undertake the mental work needed for coping with change more easily if they have a group to talk things out with. Friendships, or social groups, may often be needed in order to work out our own understandings of life.

The National Council for Voluntary Agencies publishes the *Voluntary Agencies Directory,* which provides an up-to-date catalogue of local and national groups providing support services. Books, health education guidance notes and information leaflets on where to go for help can also provide a starting point for someone who feels the need to find a new group or individual to give support in coping with change.

The Benefits Agency may be able to provide financial support to individuals who are entitled to benefits.

Social support and health

Mildred Blaxter (1990) published the results of a national survey into health and lifestyles. She reported that, 'self-perceived stress was strongly associated with poorer health of every kind.' (Page 104.) She notes, 'Social loss or social isolation are particular forms of stress which have been shown to be particularly dangerous to health. "Life-events" such as widowhood or other bereavement, divorce, job changes, unemployment, migration, even moving from one home to another, are all associated with increased risk of morbidity (disease) or mortality (death).' (Page 103.) One key factor, which appears to be vital in protecting people from the effects of stress, is having close social support networks. Friends, family, partners and community links, all seem to act as a buffer against stress. Michael Argyle (1987) writes, 'Many studies...have found that distress is caused by stress. This effect is, however, greatly reduced or minimised if there are supportive relationships. This is known as "buffering".' (Page 25.)

So friends and supportive relationships may protect an individual against stress. They may be vital to maintain self-esteem and, perhaps, self-concept or identity when these are threatened. Relationships may be critical when our sense of self is threatened. According to Argyle, a key issue is the quality of support. See also Chapter 4, page 88.

Argyle noted that both males and females found conversations with females to be 'pleasanter, more intimate – to involve more self-disclosure' and to be more 'meaningful' than conversations with men, when this was researched in the early 1980s. This may be an interesting and important aspect of gender role socialisation.

Blaxter (1990) reported that, 'Family relationships and close bonds have been shown to be strongly protective, perhaps through effects on self-esteem and feelings of control...Certainly, the relationship between social networks and health has been found to be so strong that it can be used predictively in relation to mortality.' So it seems that people with poor social support may be at more risk of dying from an illness than those with close relationships. Argyle quotes a study of 7000 people in California during the 1970s (Berkman and Syme, 1979). Those with supportive social networks had a much lower death rate even after initial health, health practices, obesity, smoking, drinking and social class had been taken into account. In terms of support marriage produced the strongest protection, with friends and relatives then offering more protection than belonging to churches or other organisations.

A study reported by Wojtas (*Times Higher Education Supplement,* 22 October 1993) found that 'coronary patients with a wide network of friends were more likely to survive a heart attack, and that car ownership, which indicates a higher income and more likelihood of socialising, also raised the chances of survival.' This study, by staff at Nottingham University, looked at 1300 suspected heart-attack patients between 25 and 84 years of age. Those who were socially isolated (poor contact with family and friends, not members of any club or religious group) were '49 per cent more likely to die following recovery from a heart attack than those with social support'. In addition 86 per cent of car owners survived compared with 74 per cent of those without a car. The study suggests that moderate affluence (wealth) and good social support are important aspects of preventative health.

But how do relationships make a difference to a person's physical health? Argyle (1987) writes,

> One way in which stress is bad for health is that it impairs the immune system, the natural

> defence against disease... Social support could restore the immune system, by its power to replace negative emotions like anxiety and depression, and their accompanying bodily states, by positive emotions. A second way in which relationships may affect health is through the adoption of better health practices... Those who have good relationships are able to cope with stress by seeking help and social support. Those without are more likely to use other means of coping, like smoking and drinking. (Page 184.)

Blaxter's study (1990) provides evidence that there is a positive relationship between marriage, or living with a partner, as compared to being single. This relationship was particularly significant for men and, indeed, older men. For men especially, living alone was associated with more illness and poorer psychological and social well-being. The number of social roles a person had (roles like parent, worker, regular worshipper) also related to measures of good health. Although these general findings from a survey cannot be used to make predictions for individual health and happiness, it does appear that partners, friends, family and community social links help protect people from stress. People with close supportive relationships may have useful resources to fall back on when they encounter life-event threats. Socially isolated people may lack a buffer to protect themselves against the anxiety, strain and threat that change may cause.

Effects of a major life change	Methods of support (professional and informal)
Uncertainty	Friendship networks Providing information and advice. Counselling
Change to self-concept	Skilled conversation, counselling and support
A need for new learning	Guidance by learning from others' experience
A sense of loss	Supportive conversation Counselling Membership of voluntary groups
Using up of time, money and emotional resources	Providing practical help Financial help Professional advice on financial issues or entitlement to benefits

Figure 10.22 A summary of methods of support for people experiencing major life changes.

Evidence collection point

To complete Element 4.1:

1 Produce a report which broadly explains how individuals cope with both expected and unexpected change and transition in their lives. Explore both expected and unexpected change in the lives of two individuals. This may involve a small-scale piece of research or a case study exploring how two people have coped with different types of change.

2 Produce a report which explains three different methods of support used by individuals during times of transition and change. This report might link with the research for (1) above.

Chapter 11

How individuals function in and are influenced by society

This chapter explores the major influence of socialisation on individual development. The theory of 'Social Constructs' is explained and the way in which social constructs change over time is discussed.

Potential conflicts between the norms and values of different groups are analysed within the context of social construct theory. The role of different value systems which may be held by care workers and clients is discussed.

Socialisation

What is socialisation?

Socialisation can be defined as the process through which we learn the ways of behaving, and of thinking, that make us members of the groups to which we belong. Through socialisation we become aware of what is expected of us and what we can expect from others; we learn our **role** in the group. This may sound a bit like joining a football team, or learning to live in a shared flat, but socialisation has a far deeper meaning than this. Socialisation is about learning to become a social being. Without socialisation people may not even behave in ways which are recognisably human.

There are reported cases of feral (wild) children found in remote regions who have had no contact with other people for most of their lives. They have been described as behaving like wild animals, as walking on all fours and craving raw meat. Of course these children may have been abandoned in the first place because of their behaviour, but other accounts of children deprived of human interaction and stimulation bear out the crucial importance of socialisation.

Kingsley Davis (1970) described the case of Isabelle who spent her first six years in a darkened room with her deaf mute mother. She was thought at first to have serious mental disabilities because of her behaviour. She was afraid of people, especially men, and showed fear and hostility like a wild animal. She made only croaking sounds and behaved as though she was deaf. She was unable to walk properly and was described as acting like an infant. After two years of specialised training, she had developed through stages of learning that would normally take six years. Her previous behaviour was a result of lack of socialisation.

Through socialisation we learn language, customs, beliefs and behaviour – we learn the 'rules' of the game. Importantly we learn how to play our own roles. The idea of **social role** is closely linked to the concept of socialisation. We are said to be socialised into a role, and being able to play a role is an

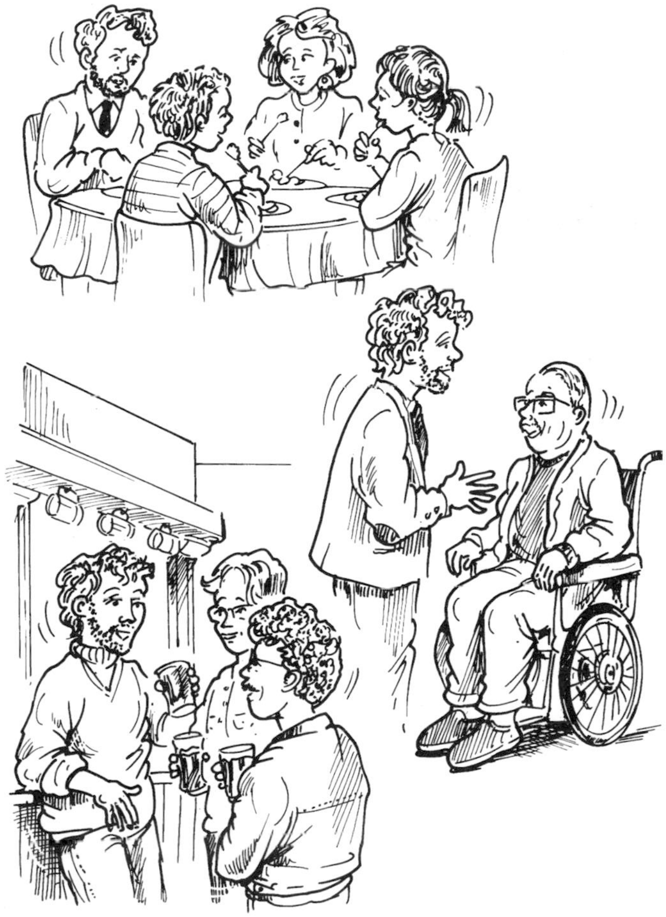

Figure 11.1 People play many different roles in their lives

outcome of the socialisation process. Each of us has a repertoire (or collection) of roles that we adopt quite naturally as the social situation demands. At home with our family we play the role of son or daughter, brother or sister. At work we play the role of carer and the role of colleague, and during our studies we play the role of student.

The influence of the family

Our first experience of socialisation is within our families. This is regarded as a crucial period which lays the foundations of our later development, and is referred to as *primary* (meaning first) *socialisation*. Chapter 10 showed that there are on-going debates about exactly how this early learning takes place, but there is general agreement about the importance of primary socialisation in making us who we are. Our experiences and observations of the interactions between those around us teach us language and behaviours that allow us to join in with the group. We see the other members acting and reacting to ourselves and to each other. The patterns of interactions become familiar and we copy them. We learn the *norms* of the group.

Norms are the customary ways of behaving within a group and describe all the behaviour patterns that are considered normal by its members. They include diet, dress, customs and ways of communicating.

Of course, each family is part of the wider society, of which we are only dimly aware at this stage in our lives. What we are learning is our family's interpretation of the *culture* that they and we belong to. Gradually, we become aware that there are views, opinions and attitudes which underlie the behavioural norms we are learning. These are known as *values* and provide a rationale and meaning for the norms of the group. Many values may be linked to the religious beliefs of our culture, and we learn about this too.

We see that group members treat each other differently, and that all are not dealt with equally. A role carries with it a level of *status* or ranking within the group. Older members usually play higher status roles, and young children are taught to respect this relationship. There may be differences in status between the roles of mother and father which suggest to us differences in the status of men and women in the wider society.

Think it over

Think about the roles played by yourself and members of your family. Remember that each person may play several roles, depending on who he or she is interacting with. Now think about the status of different members of your family in relation to each other. Can you rank the members of your family in order of status?

Now think about different situations when your family acts together. You may think of family meals, motoring trips, holidays or shopping expeditions. Do the status relationships within your family remain the same in each situation? Do you think status may vary with the circumstances?

The influence of the peer group

Primary socialisation allows us to become a social being, and provides a context for the development and demonstration of our own, individual personality. However, socialisation is a lifelong process. As we grow older, our contacts beyond the home become increasingly important. We make friends with other children who have a lot in common with us. People who we see as like ourselves, and people we feel are close to us, are known as our peers. Our membership of a *peer group* is another important socialising influence and it is here that our first relationships outside the home develop.

The influence of education

The formal education system is another agent of socialisation. Schools provide a learning experience on several levels. There is the formal level of education which is designed to teach skills and knowledge. We are taught subjects like history and science, and are helped to develop the skills needed as an adult member of our society.

We also learn how to behave towards people in authority, such as teachers, and how to relate to other pupils. We learn when it is acceptable to speak or ask questions, and how to adapt our behaviour with different teachers and pupil groups. We are also likely to find that expectations of our behaviour in one group don't fully agree with those in another. For instance, the group value of loyalty to friends may conflict with the value of honesty imposed by the school. Whether or not to 'tell' on your friends can be one of the early moral dilemmas that we face.

There are norms of behaviour towards our teachers, and others with our friends. In this situation the norms, and value systems, conflict.

Our experiences at school prepare us for the world of work. We learn how to be part of a group and how to respond to those in authority.

Think it over

We are all members of a peer group, and students are part of a group who are peers in the context of study. If you join a student group you have to learn the norms, values and behaviours associated with membership.

Think back to when you joined a course. What did it feel like at first? Were you apprehensive or confident? How did others act? What did the process of socialisation into the role of student feel like?

The influence of work

At work we are socialised into new roles and patterns of behaviour. We will probably have existing ideas about the role we are taking on at work, and will know something of what we are in for. For instance, we may have an impression of the role of care worker which might help to interest us in that career.

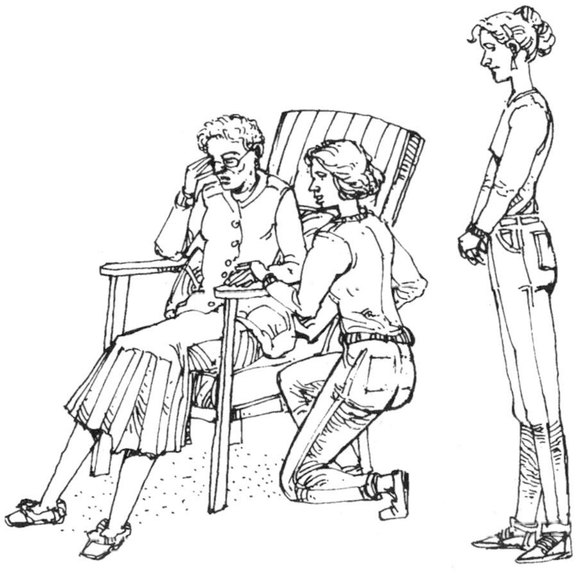

Figure 11.2 The behaviour of other carers helps us to understand our role

Socialising influences in the workplace refine and shape these impressions and we learn the norms and values of being a carer. We are influenced by the behaviour of other carers, and will get direct advice on working practices. Fellow carers are our peers and we learn their expectations of us as we work alongside them. Our role at work, and the status it has among all the other jobs and professions in society, can be an important factor in our adult development.

The influence of religion

Outside work we have other socialising influences that act upon us. Our primary socialisation will have given us the religious background of our family. We may be a believer in a particular religion throughout our lives. Religion provides a comprehensive value system that shapes the lives of most families and communities. Even if you are not brought up in an actively religious family, the broader culture you live in will have been influenced and shaped by religious ideas. Religion is associated with culture, and plays an influential part in the lives of many people. This affects beliefs and ideas, but can also influence clothing, diet, and ways of relating to other people.

The influence of the mass media

Another socialising influence on our lives is the mass media. People in the UK grow up surrounded by media images of their own and other cultures. Practically everyone watches television, listens to radio, and reads newspapers. In fact, an increasing proportion of people's time is spent receiving messages from the media. The mass media has become, for some, one of the main ways that knowledge of the broader culture is transmitted to individuals. Its messages shape our understanding of people and events, and may suggest roles, values and relationships that are outside our everyday experiences.

The influence of the media in shaping behaviour, particularly among children, is the subject of on-going debate. Are public attitudes to the Royal Family affected by press coverage of the lives of its members? Does violence on television lead to increased levels of violent behaviour among young children? There is evidence that the media are capable of affecting public opinion on issues and groups. For example, Stan Cohen (1973) looked at the media's treatment of mods and rockers in the 1960s. He concluded that the media were largely responsible for creating public concern, and even panic, over these groups which actually were a far less serious threat than they were portrayed as being. He adds that the groups themselves may shift their conduct to live up to their new reputation. Media stories of anti-social behaviour become a **self-fulfilling prophecy** as other people latch on to the image and copy the stereotypical media images. Young children are likely to be particularly vulnerable to media influence as they are at a stage when their own identity is shaping and developing rapidly. You may observe groups of children acting out the roles of the heroes and villains from television programmes. What may not be so obvious are the values that they are also picking up and which are part of the message in any media transmission.

Try it

The media portrays our culture through images which are often stereotyped and contain hidden assumptions about values and norms.

Spend some time looking at the advertisement breaks on television, at different times of day if possible. Look at the portrayal of social life in the adverts, and the stereotypes referred to. What views of social reality do the adverts offer? Are different themes and stereotypes used at different times of day? What might be the effects of these stereotypes on children in the primary socialisation stage?

Rewards and sanctions

The media may be different from other agents of socialisation in that it is a one-way communication process. There is no interaction between participants as there is in social groups. We may be able to take or leave media messages, but in groups there are sanctions to reinforce the socialisation taking place. There are consequences of breaking social rules, and rewards for upholding them. Positive sanctions may include praise, or even material reward. Children may be given sweets for behaving well, soldiers may be given medals. Negative sanctions are first experienced as parental discipline. We discover that unacceptable behaviour is met with some form of punishment.

Later we will discover that the state we live in has formal laws which punish those caught breaking them. Though laws in themselves are not an agent of socialisation, they reflect public understanding of acceptable behaviour and codify the sanctions used to enforce it. We can choose whether or not to obey the laws, and yet there is a good deal of conformity in society. This is because there are powerful **social sanctions** acting as well. A more immediate influence on our behaviour are the reactions of the people around us. Fear of ridicule, or not fitting in, may be the most powerful way that many people experience sanctions on their behaviour. The disapproval of others is enough to keep most people within the bounds of acceptable behaviour. Very few people in the UK break the social rule of forming queues, purely because it is normal behaviour here to queue. Even in crowded urban environments, people follow common codes of conduct and generally unthinkingly fit into the society around them.

Socialisation carries on throughout life. We carry on developing new roles as our situation and group membership changes. Though there is agreement that people act socially through the roles that they play, and that these roles are learned through the process of socialisation, there are different views on how the process operates and how roles become defined.

Theoretical views on socialisation

In Chapter 10 we saw that there are different views on how personality is developed, ranging from the biological determinism of Eysenck to the interactionist approach of Mead and Kelly. There are similar differences of opinion over the nature and operation of socialisation and role.

During the first half of the twentieth century, the field of sociology was dominated by a theory known as **functionalism**. There are many variants of functionalism, but they share a similar view of how society operates. Functionalists see society as a system of interdependent institutions which each contribute to the overall stability and continuity of the whole. Different parts of society have their own function in the maintenance of society, and have no existence independently of the rest of society. Society is seen as being something like the human body. Each organ and system has its own function and contribution to make to the healthy maintenance of the body. At the same time, each is dependent on the whole system for its existence and survival. These components of society are outside the direct influence of the individual human actors who comprise them. The structure of society imposes its own order and directs the lives of the people within. Because of this emphasis on structure, the theory is sometimes known as **structural functionalism.**

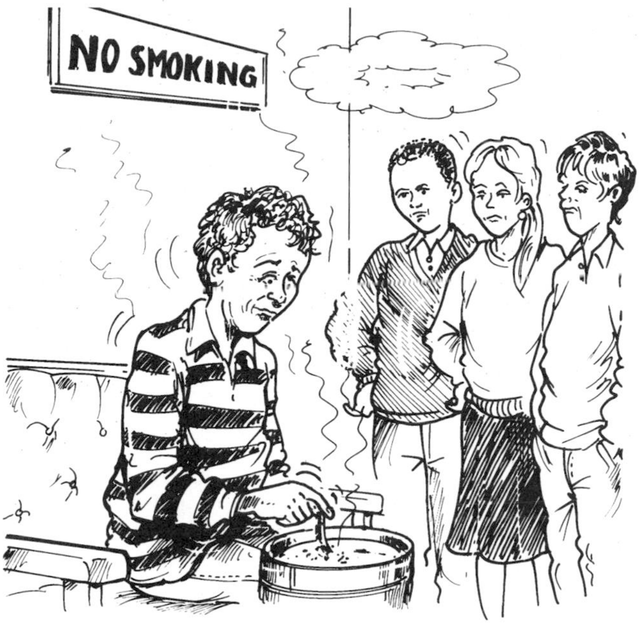

Figure 11.3 Social disapproval is a powerful sanction on unacceptable behaviour

One of the first people to describe society in this way was Emil Durkheim (1858–1917). The theory was developed by the American Talcott Parsons (1902–79) and his followers, and was extremely influential in the mid-twentieth century. An important problem for functionalists is how this order in their picture of society is brought about and sustained. Society is not held physically together like our bodies, so functionalists needed to identify the social glue that bound the parts together. For Parsons, the answer was a consensus of opinion on values. If everyone shared the same values, he argues, it followed that they would pursue common goals. This provided incentive for co-operation between people and regulated the norms of behaviour between them. Religion provides the ultimate justification for the values in the social system. For functionalists, socialisation transmits these shared values to individuals who apply them in the roles they adopt. Roles are determined by the structural components within society, and the functions that they perform for society as a whole. Individuals can choose different roles, but have minimal influence on their content which is externally defined by the needs of society.

Functionalism has been criticised for many aspects of its view on society. Some critics have complained that the emphasis on order and structure has provided no explanation of how conflicts and tensions build up in society, and that there is no explanation of how social change may take place. These critics question the assumption that there are shared values universally accepted throughout society. One such critic is David Lockwood (1978). He argued that, by emphasising the social order, Parsons and other functionalists were ignoring conflicts of interest that were built into society. Society has ways of sharing out scarce resources like food and consumer goods. In the competition for scarce resources, conflicts are built into society. Conflict is integral to the system itself.

Lockwood was strongly influenced by the ideas of Karl Marx (1818–83). Marx saw modern capitalist industrial society as being composed of two basic groups whose interests were in direct opposition: the **bourgeoisie**, who own and control the means of production, and the much more numerous **proletariat** who have only their labour to sell. Marx saw the interests of these groups as very different. The bourgeoisie were interested in maximising their profits and so were likely to attempt to get as much as possible from their workers for as little reward as possible. The proletariat were interested in survival and betterment.

For Marx, capitalist society was based on this tension created by the exploitation of the many by the few. Change would come about, he believed, when the proletariat became aware of themselves as an exploited class and rose in revolution to create an egalitarian communist state. Marx saw the individual as acting only through membership of the class to which he belongs. Roles are determined by the relationship to the means of production. Socialisation leads people to become either exploiter or exploited depending on the class they grow up in.

Although Parsons and Marx are very far apart in many aspects of their views, they have one thing in common. Both have a **deterministic** view of society. For functionalists, human beings are seen as serving the needs of the institutions in society and thus society as a whole. People are shaped to fit the system rather than the system being created by people. Through socialisation people are programmed into the norms and values which the system requires them to have. Their actions are structured within roles which fit the functional needs of the social system. For Marxists, people are shaped by their relationship to the means of production. Individuals are victims of their birthright as members of either the bourgeoisie or proletariat.

Functionalism and Marxism are both **social determinist** views since the individual members of society have no real control over their lives. People are seen as being under the controlling influence of forces in society which are greater than themselves. Both views are criticised by another approach which was described in Chapter 10, **symbolic interactionism.** George Herbert Mead (1863–1931) is regarded as the major figure in this school of thought. See page 222. Herbert Blumer, a student of Mead, developed these ideas.

Interactionists focus on the individual members of society, and their understanding of the situation they are in. Mead believed that people act on the basis of the meanings that they give to objects and events. These meanings, or symbols, are modified and developed within social interactions, and have no fixed, external definition. They are symbols that we use to make sense of the world, and we can adapt them as we interrelate with others who will have their own set of symbols, similar but not identical to our own. Here people are not simply acquiring roles but negotiating them. People may have some prior understanding of how to act in a particular situation, but will develop their own individual approach. Socialisation is a dialogue with the individual as a leading player. However commonplace the interaction may be, the personal interpretations of the actors within it will shape the outcome.

Interactionists have been criticised for putting too much emphasis on the individual's interpretation of events. Others have argued that there is regularity and pattern in social events which interactionists either ignore, or fail to account for. Although people may be interpreting an interaction in an individual and negotiated way, nurses still behave like nurses, and policemen still behave like policemen.

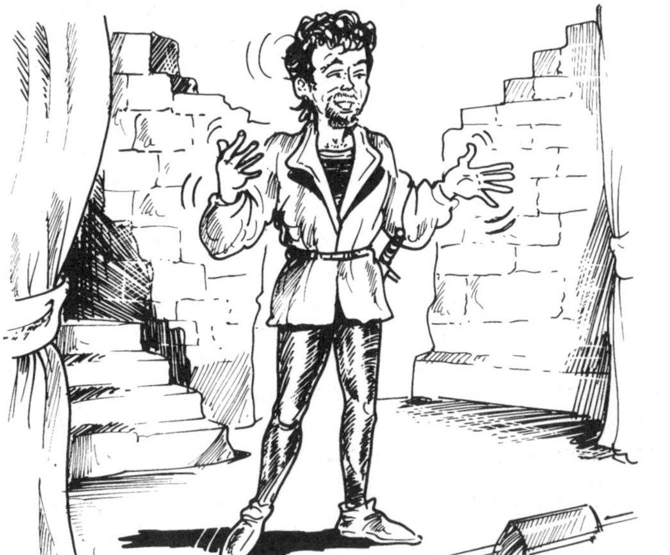

Figure 11.4 Social determinists see roles as being fixed externally, like a part in a play

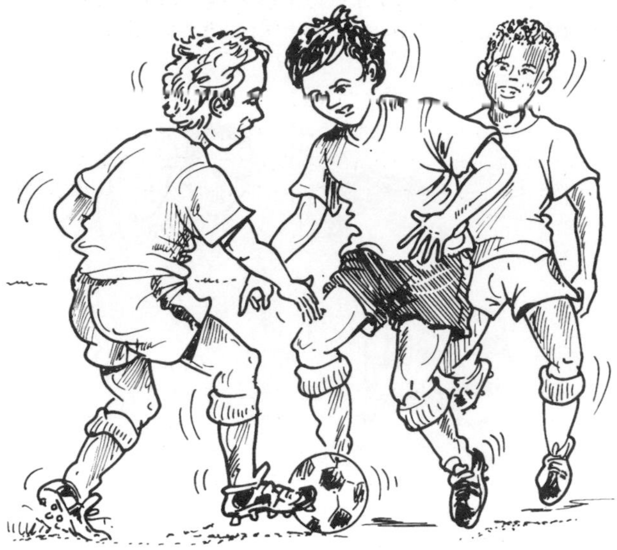

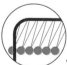

Figure 11.5 Social interactionists see roles as being negotiated. Like football players, we know the basic rules but develop our style by interacting with other players

Social determinists and interactionists have quite different views on how socialisation takes place, and roles are learned. To the determinist, it is like learning your lines in a play. Although you put your own individuality into the performance, the audience still gets Hamlet. To the interactionist it may be more like learning to play football. You share with others a knowledge of the rules of the game, but there is scope to interpret and adapt your style in a truly individual way when you interact with other players.

Socialisation is not a clear-cut concept and the different approaches to it may seem complex and theoretical. In fact, as you will see in Chapter 12, these views about the process of socialisation may be used to justify public policy and political action. If we intend to change people's behaviour, we must first have a view on how behaviour develops.

Think it over

Earlier in this chapter it was suggested that you think about your own experiences of socialisation. You may have considered the process that took place, and your own behaviour during the course of it.

Now that you have looked at some theoretical views on socialisation and roles, think again about your experience of socialisation. Which aspects of the theories we have looked at can be identified in your own experiences?

Social constructs

Whatever the mechanism behind socialisation may be, it allows us to communicate with others and understand the messages that they offer. This is possible because we share similar understandings about both the physical and the social world. When meeting a complete stranger we expect to be able to converse with him or her, taking these understandings for granted. We will both know what is meant by objects such as a chair or house, and equally we will share an understanding of ideas like family, crime or illness. Ideas like these are known as *social constructs*. Although they are not objects, and can be difficult to define precisely, we use them in conversation as though they had a reality.

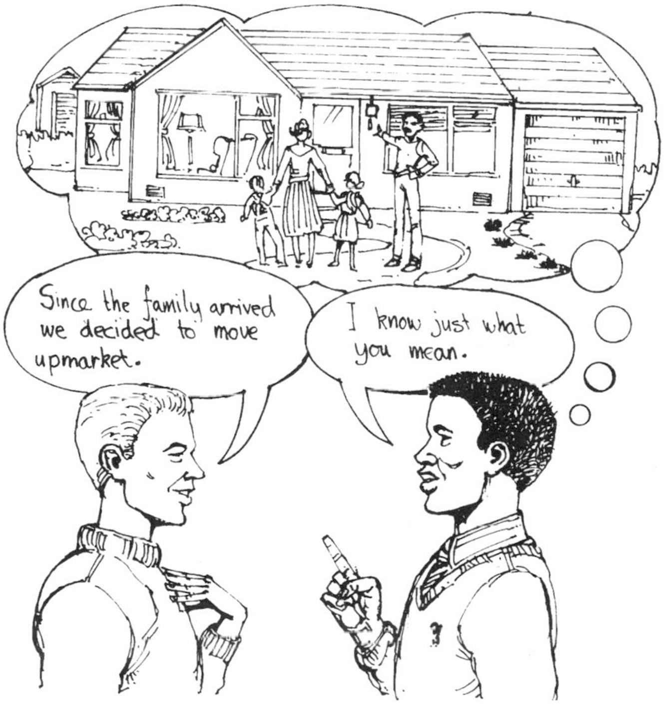
Since the family arrived we decided to move upmarket.
I know just what you mean.

Figure 11.6 Social constructs have shared meanings allowing communication to take place

Berger and Luckman (1967) describe this as the **social construction of reality**. Ideas and concepts which are socially constructed come to be seen as something with their own existence. They take on a life of their own as facts of the external social world.

Social constructs can include any commonly understood concept which describes an idea about society, or relationships within it. They have no meaning beyond that which people give to them and so they are able to change as society changes. New constructs are developed to encompass the changes and allow communication about them. For example, the term 'feminism' has a meaning to all of us nowadays. It brings to mind ideas about women's equality and the fight for their rights. In the nineteenth century women's equality was not on the public agenda. According to the dominant ideas of the day, women's rights were simply not an issue. The term 'feminism' would then have been meaningless to most people. As we saw earlier in Stan Cohen's work on mods and rockers, it is also possible that sometimes a social phenomenon can follow the media's creation and promotion of a new construct.

Think it over

We all use our knowledge of social constructs to think and talk about our experience. As much of our lives concerns people and social events we may refer to social constructs more often than we refer to physical objects like desk or door.

Listen to a brief social conversation between two of your friends. Make a tape recording if you can get their permission. Note down the subject of the conversation and try to identify the social constructs used and referred to by the participants. For instance, if the conversation concerned 'being a student' the social constructs used may include 'student', 'teacher', 'college', 'course', 'education', or 'success'. Try to list the constructs you have recognised. You might be very surprised by how much the communication made use of and relied upon social constructs.

What do the constructs used by the participants mean to you? Did both participants seem to have absolutely identical definitions of the constructs they were using, and did they agree exactly with your view? How might the conversation have gone if the participants had very little in common?

Role constructs

Some of the most important social constructs describe roles. We all have a similar idea of what a police officer is, or a politician. Roles that relate to gender and the family are particularly important to people's lives, and they are areas where changes have been taking place. These roles include man, woman, father, mother, wife and husband.

The roles of 'housewife' and 'mother' are familiar, and you may have your own understanding of what these social constructs include. These roles have a much lower status than those available to men, and carry with them less prestige and power. The laws of the state have reinforced gender inequality, and it is only in very recent history that legal equality has been approached. Ann Oakley (1974) looked at the changing status of women over the period from the beginning of the industrial revolution (the mid to late eighteenth century) to the 1970s. She charts the removal of women from the labour force during this period, and the social pressures that led to the idea that women belong in the home. Oakley concludes, 'The most important and enduring consequence of industrialisation for women has been the emergence of the modern role of housewife as the dominant mature female role.'

Ann Oakley was writing over 20 years ago and changes in the meanings of social constructs may continue to occur. The political and social struggle for women's rights has led to some shift in ideas about the role of women, and perhaps of the social constructs surrounding the roles that are available to them. However, the role 'housewife' still carries less prestige than the career roles that men usually adopt in adult life. There may be little evidence yet of the emergence of the social construct 'house husband' as a normal and valid male role.

The social construct 'family' is another case where change may be expected. There has been a marked shift in patterns of family life in the UK during the twentieth century, as Chapter 12 outlines. The number of single-parent families continues to grow, and the number of 'traditional' nuclear families with the husband as breadwinner continues to decline. This means that changes in the idea of what a family is, or can be, should be expected to occur. However, changes in social constructs don't necessarily quickly follow changes in social reality. Many children in single-parent families find themselves presented, via the media, with families comprising wife, husband and children. Images of the typical family may persist even though they are daily becoming less typical.

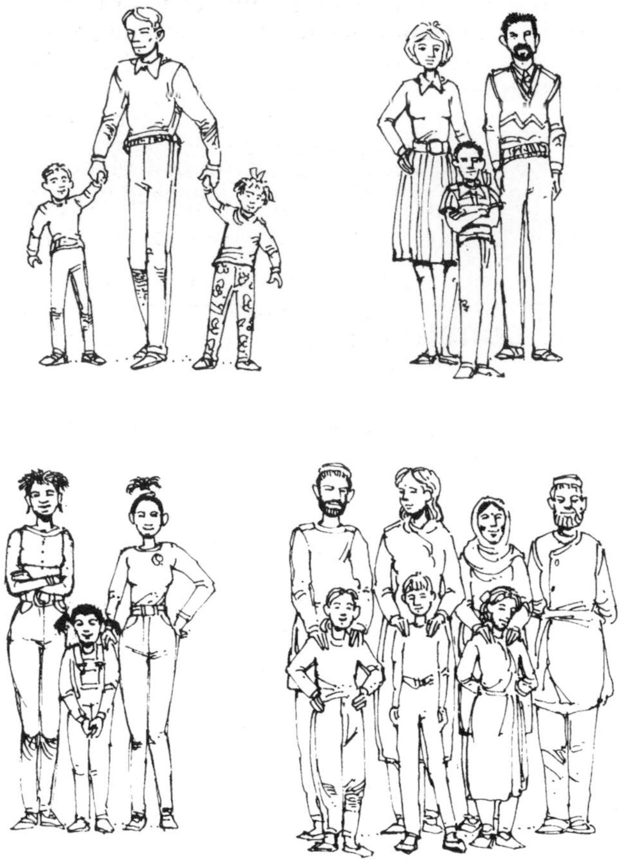

Figure 11.7 We are all families

It is possible that changes in a social construct may begin within particular groups, or age groups. Younger people may have begun to attach new connotations to the idea of family which differ from those of older people. They may have begun to attach negative connotations to the role of housewife where their mothers and grandmothers would not have done.

Power

Power is a product of social relationships, and is another example of a social construct. People only hold power when they have someone over whom to wield it. Power means **power over others**. Often, power is linked to politics where individuals have the power to make laws affecting the behaviour of others. In the UK politicians are elected by a system that people generally respect. Politicians have the authority to exercise their powers. They are not seen as forcing their will onto repressed subjects. However, power can also be gained by coercion. The playground bully has power within his limited sphere. The threat of physical violence allows him to control some aspects of the lives of other pupils.

In practice, the exercise of power may involve both authority and coercion, with coercion being resorted to if authority fails to win compliance. We may speak of the power of the police and imagine both the authority that society invests in the police, and which is usually respected and obeyed, and the physical force that the police are able to employ if the situation demands it. In fact, most of us respond to power without the feeling that there is a threat of force behind it. Through socialisation we learn about power relationships and how to respond to those in authority. Power is often linked to status, and at school we find that the head has greater status than the other teachers, and has power over them. Similarly we learn about our own position in the hierarchy of status and power that structures the school organisation. At work, we accept the authority of a manager or supervisor, and regard his or her power over us as a normal aspect of the structure of working life.

Think it over

Think about the relationship between yourself and the tutors on your course. Tutors direct your studies and have power over the learning situation. How does the power of college tutors operate? Are they using authority or coercion, or a mixture of both? Think about your own view of the consequences of resisting a tutor's directions. What threats might you face if tutors are disobeyed? How much do you think the tutor's authority relies on these threats?

Power is a social construct that has little meaning without a context within which to operate. We need to know who is exercising power, and in what circumstances. The power of a warder over prisoners in his or her charge is very different from the power a care manager has over his or her staff. Whenever someone has control over aspects of the life of other people, they have power over them. Care staff often find that they have power over aspects of the lives of those that they care for, and need to be aware that this affects the relationships between them.

Deviance

Deviance means behaviour which breaks the rules of normal conduct. This can include anything that falls outside the norms of behaviour of a particular group. If a normally respectable bank employee decided to go to work dressed only in swimming trunks, it would be regarded as deviant behaviour. If the same person dived in the pool at his local swimming club dressed in a three-piece suit, this would be deviant also. Deviance can only be understood in terms of the norms of the group being deviated from, and the expectations of people's behaviour in a particular situation. What is deviant for members of one group may be perfectly normal behaviour for members of another. To complicate matters further, actions can be deviant or not in different situations. Killing a number of people is highly deviant most of the time, but in war as part of an army it is more likely to be commended than condemned.

In UK society killing is not allowed, and is regarded as an extremely deviant act. It is against the law, as are many other behaviours regarded generally as deviant. All crimes are acts that the state regards as deviant, but some illegal behaviours tend not to be regarded as particularly deviant by the public. Many motorists break the 30-miles-per-hour speed limit. In fact, people who travel at exactly 30 may be seen as deviant by other motorists who are accustomed to traffic moving slightly faster than the limit legally allows.

The study of deviance has attracted many social theorists and researchers. Structural functionalist views on deviance began with Durkheim (1938). He felt that deviance was functional to society, and thus an inevitable aspect of it. Deviancy helped to define and reinforce the norms and values of 'normal' members of society, particularly when the deviant was caught and seen to be punished for his or her actions. This theme was developed by later structuralists who looked for the cause of deviancy in the social structures that people were shaped by. Structural functionalists see individual deviants as being directed by social forces largely outside their control. Deviancy can thus be tackled by addressing those forces that lead people to become deviant.

Interactionist views on deviance tackle the issue from quite a different angle. Instead of focusing on the deviant, the interactionists look at the process by which someone becomes described (labelled) as deviant. They see deviancy as a process of interaction. One part of the exchange involves the person performing an action, the other involves other people labelling the action as deviant. A crucial issue in this process is the relative power of the participants. By labelling someone as a thief or a junkie, the state has offered the person a definition of himself or herself that carries the weight of authority. The deviant may come to see his or her actions in the same light and regard further deviancy as normal behaviour for himself or herself.

In this way, interactionists believe, labelling reinforces the deviancy in the act of identifying it. The saying 'once a thief, always a thief' is a relic from the days when criminality was thought to be genetically determined. These ideas were discredited, and replaced by structuralist ideas about the social forces which created criminal behaviour. Interactionists said that people labelled as deviant were pushed into believing that they were a particular type of person. The old saying could now be read as 'once labelled a thief, always a thief'. It had returned as an example of a self-fulfilling prophecy.

One of the leading figures in the interactionist view of deviancy is Howard Becker (1963). He stressed that an action only becomes deviant when other, more powerful people define it as such. Once labelled as deviant, a person finds that social reactions reinforce that label. A person with a drug conviction may be rejected by friends, and family members. He or she may find it hard to get work due to the stigma of the offence, and be pushed into criminal behaviour through being denied the normal income routes open to other members of society. Such people may find that the company of other drugtakers is more comfortable since they are 'deviants like me'. This reinforces their self-image as deviants and creates a

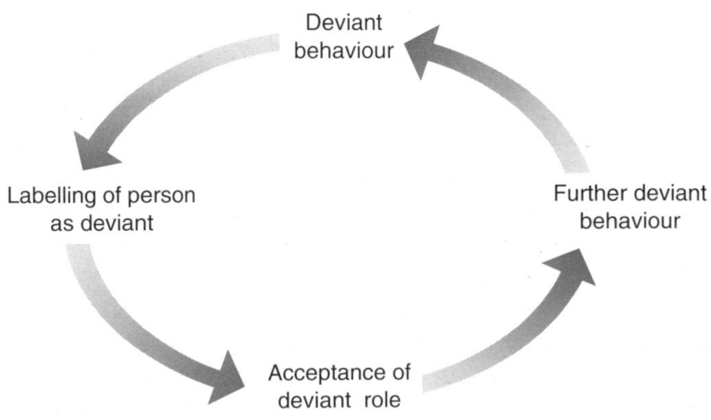

Figure 11.8 Interactionist view of a cycle of deviance

cycle of escalating criminal activity and drugtaking. In this way, Becker claimed, labelling creates further deviance. Becker rejects the functionalist idea of a value consensus which is broken by the deviant. He argues that rules reflect power, and those groups with power impose their own definitions of crime and deviance on those with less power.

Interactionists have been criticised for failing to explain the origins of deviant acts. By focusing on the act of labelling, they have ignored the process through which the labelled behaviour came about. Deviants, these critics argue, know what they are letting themselves in for. They don't suddenly become aware of their deviancy as a label is slapped on them.

The two theoretical perspectives of structural functionalism and interactionism have dominated the fields of criminology and deviance for several decades. By looking at deviance from such different viewpoints, they have been seen as opposing explanations of what deviancy is, and how it should be dealt with.

In a multicultural and diverse society like the UK, definitions of deviance may vary widely from group to group. Differences between cultural groups in diet and behaviour lead to different definitions of what constitutes deviant behaviour. Religious and cultural groups have their own norms defining what constitutes deviant behaviour for their members. For instance, it might be regarded as deviant behaviour for a Jewish person to eat pork, as this is forbidden to followers of their religion.

Ideas about deviant behaviour among the general populations may change over time. For instance, fashions in clothes and hair that were once regarded as deviant can eventually become acceptable. In the 1960s, men with long hair were seen as deviant by most of society. They would have found it difficult to establish a professional career because of the suspicion and hostility their appearance aroused. Nowadays long hair is much more acceptable and has largely lost its deviant connotations. Other fashions, such as body piercing and tattoos, have replaced it as a symbol of rebellion.

Think it over

Think about the views of yourself and members of your family. Are there areas of disagreement about whether something is deviant or not? Can you identify differences between people of different ages, or genders, in views about the deviance of some actions? For instance, all might agree that murder is wrong, but views may differ on milder areas of deviance such as lifestyle or appearance. What areas seem to reveal the greatest differences in views of deviant activity?

Health and illness

Because health concerns something very real and tangible, our body, it may be hard to think of it as a social construct. We may think of health as meaning freedom from physical and intellectual malfunction, but there are different ways in which this can be interpreted. People may believe themselves to be healthy when others would think that they were not. People may believe that they have healthy lifestyles when medical evidence seems to demonstrate otherwise. Chapter 12 deals with these issues in detail.

Evidence suggests that different social and cultural groups have different attitudes to health, and to medical practitioners. Zborowski (1969) looked at how members of different ethnic groups in New York and Boston presented their problems to the doctor. Irish-Americans tended to deny pain, and be fatalistic and accepting of the doctor's opinions. Italian and Jewish patients tended to emphasise pain; and whereas Italian patients were mainly interested in pain relief, Jewish patients were more likely to want an explanation of the problem and advice on avoiding future bouts.

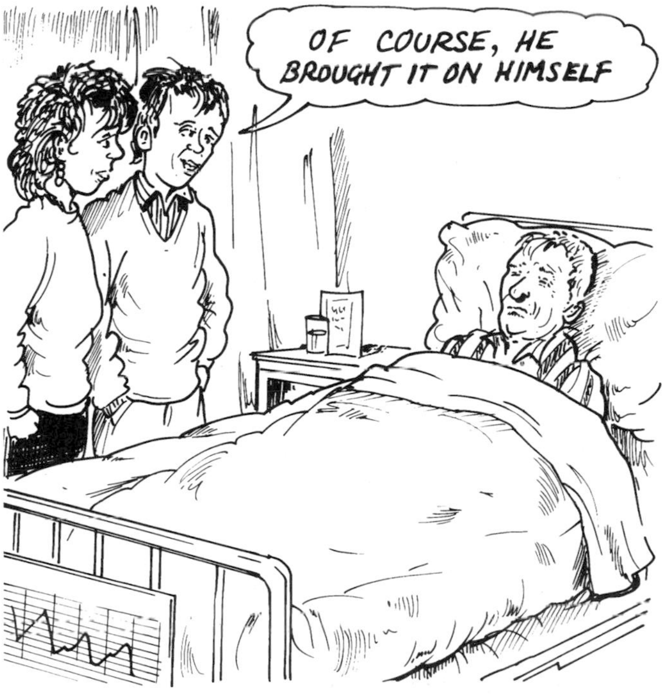

Figure 11.9 Victims may be held responsible for their own illnesses

Social constructs about health and illness have changed over time. In Europe, prior to the eighteenth century, illness was thought to be the result of sinful behaviour on the part of the victim, or of witchcraft. Since then scientific explanations of illness have generally replaced this view. Now micro-organisms, pollutants and genetic traits are usually held responsible for disease and illness. There has been a recent tendency, however, for some illnesses to be blamed on the victim, particularly where social behaviour may be a contributory factor in the development of a condition. This can be applied to many illnesses, such as HIV/AIDS, alcoholism, digestive disorders, lung cancer and heart disease.

Recently debates have arisen concerning whether heart disease sufferers who continue to smoke deserve to be treated, since they are contributing to their own ill-health. This raises deep and difficult moral issues. Should people who deliberately risk life and limb playing dangerous sports be treated when they are injured, or drivers who crash with excess alcohol in their blood? Attitudes expressed by some people towards people with AIDS have become particularly hostile. Because the disease has been associated with gay men, some people who disapprove of gays as a group have portrayed AIDS as God's retribution for sin. We have come full circle back to a medieval view of the causes of illness!

Illnesses themselves are social constructs, and recognition that they exist at all requires that they are noticed and defined. Historical records of causes of death are well known to be difficult to interpret. This is because many conditions that we now know of were unrecognised in past centuries. Death may have been described as due to 'fever' or 'a wasting sickness' for individuals suffering from quite different complaints. Scientific advances in biology and medicine now allow us to identify specifically a large number of well-defined illnesses. The public relies on information from the medical profession to identify and define the range of illnesses that we believe to exist. Social constructs about heart disease or cancer are likely to be largely based on the views of medical scientists as presented by the media and in health campaigns. In fact, the acceptance of medical findings may not be so universal, as Chapter 12 shows, but generally they are society's prime source of information about the existence and causes of different diseases.

This can mean that conditions don't become recognised until medical science decides to recognise them. Schizophrenia has only become recognised as an illness in the twentieth century. Because it came to be regarded as an illness, attempts were made to discover a biological cause. Recently social factors in the lives of sufferers have been examined, and the idea of what schizophrenia is has shifted. However, ideas about the condition amongst the general public still refer to the 'two personalities' stereotype. In fact, the split personality is a symptom of quite a different, and much rarer, condition that is not related to schizophrenia. The social construct familiar to the general public is at odds with professional medical opinion. It could be said that social constructs lag behind developments in human understanding. Unless the media pick up on new discoveries and explanations, or they are actively promoted in publicity campaigns, it is unlikely that the public at large will become aware of them. Ideas need to enter popular culture so that they can be sustained, developed and transmitted through the process of socialisation.

Evidence collection point

One way to develop some of the evidence needed towards Element 4.2 is by researching people's ideas on the meaning and content of familiar social constructs. You could use interview or self-completion questionnaire methods (see Chapters 22–24 for advice on survey methods).

You could check for differences between different groups, or age groups, in the way social constructs are defined. This may suggest ways in which social constructs change over time. You need to cover the range of social constructs defined in the GNVQ standards and this includes: role constructs associated with gender and family, power, deviance, health, and the identification of illness.

Norms and values in a multi-cultural society

The UK is an advanced, prosperous country, and like many similar states it has a diverse and complex population structure. The UK's history of international involvement and domination has led to a range of contacts with other groups and cultures, wider than that of any other nation in history. People have emigrated from the UK to other countries, and people from other countries have settled here. The modern UK is described as a multi-cultural society, where different cultural groups co-exist within the same social framework and under the same rule of law.

Culture encompasses all the behaviours, customs and beliefs that are part of the way of life of a group. It includes norms about diet, dress and decorative taste that make members of the group distinctive to the rest of society. Most of us are familiar with many aspects of the diet and style of different groups in the community. We are probably much less familiar with the roles and status structures that exist in different cultures, and with the attitudes and values that the groups hold.

Try it

Think about the different cultural groups that live in the UK. Choose three different groups and make a list of the things that you know about each culture, and its norms and values.

How did you get the information that you have written down? Was it by direct contact with the culture or through images in the media, or elsewhere?

Look again at your three lists. How many of the things you 'know' about a culture have been taken from stereotypical images of the group?

Role status, expectations and authority

There are some social roles that are common to all cultures. These roles relate to things like gender and age, which all human groups experience and must come to terms with. As animals of apparently limitless adaptability, people have developed many variants of the roles of man and woman, infant and elder. A role that seems similar between two different cultures may, in fact, be regarded very differently by members of each group. A role which has a high status in one culture may have a much lower one in another, and the expectations of behaviour associated with the role may differ. These differences may not be realised, or may be misunderstood, in situations where members of other cultures meet, and this can lead to conflicts.

In many cultures, the role of elder is awarded a high status. Elders are seen as having acquired wisdom and knowledge through a lifetime of experience. They are respected, and looked to for advice by younger people. Pre-communist Chinese society is a well-known example of this, and in that society religious beliefs sustained the status and influence of elders even after they had died. Many cultural communities in the modern UK respect elders and give high status to the role. Elders in these communities are cared for and looked up to by their family and the group as a whole.

In contrast, mainstream UK society generally regards the role of elders differently. Elders are often seen as dependent and in need. They are thought of as slower and duller than younger, fitter, people. The infirmities of old age are stressed, and the value of experience played down. Older people's ideas and opinions are devalued, and stereotyped as out-of-date or quaint. Elders are offered some sympathy, but little respect. Elders in the UK have a low-status role. People may express surprise when their stereotyped image of elders is threatened and say things such as 'She's remarkable for her age', thus demonstrating their own expectations of the role of elders.

Elders from communities where age is respected may find that they are afforded less respect in wider UK society. This can lead to clashes which are painful and confusing to the older person, and not fully understood by others who take the low status of elders for granted. Older people from minority cultural groups may come into contact with wider UK society through the health and social care services. Many cultures emphasise the family as the proper place for the care of elders, but sometimes this is not enough and people find themselves receiving regular or institutionalised care. They may be shocked to discover the low status they are given and the low self-esteem of elders from UK society who have accepted their low status role. Though health and care workers are expected to value and respect their clients, it is likely that cultural attitudes towards age will affect the experiences of elders who have other expectations.

Think it over

Think about the way older people are regarded in the UK, particularly if they become infirm or institutionalised. How does this contrast with the respect shown towards elders in other cultures?

What effects do you think the UK view of elders may have on those who are used to a higher status role within their community?

As well as differences in role status, there are differences between cultures in the behaviour that is expected to accompany the role. Some cultures see women's role as being primarily involved with domestic work and the rearing of children. Women in these cultures may be expected not to seek work, even if childless. Clashes may occur between the culture's view of a woman's role and that of wider society. Exposure to the opportunities available for women to work and develop a career in the UK may lead some women to question expectations of their behaviour within their community. They may feel that they would prefer a career to looking after the home and older relatives. Pressure to conform to cultural expectations of her role may be brought to bear and this can lead to considerable pain and disruption, both for the family and for the woman herself.

The authority given to different roles in society also differs between groups. Authority is linked to the status of a role, but includes the idea that someone has power, as well as prestige. In some cultures, authority is vested largely in the male role. Women are not expected to occupy positions of authority over men except in domestic matters. Men from these cultures may be socialised into a view of the authority which makes it hard to accept a woman in the role of manager or supervisor. This could lead to difficulties at work where women may be in more senior supervisory positions. In fact, difficulties with accepting women in positions of authority may also be fairly common amongst men from mainstream UK culture. Traditional UK views on the role of women may be less restrictive than amongst some cultural groups but tend to lead in a similar direction.

Cultural norms, pain and deviance

Norms of behaviour vary widely between cultures. There are differences in dress, diet, behaviour and religious practices. Clashes can occur when the norms of a culture conflict with those of the wider society. Norms influence behaviour that everyone takes for granted, such as body language. There are, for example, quite large variations between cultures in what is considered to be the normal distance to leave between yourself and a person that you are talking to. Many cultures socialise their members into conversing at a closer physical proximity than is usual in the UK. For instance, it is customary for people from Japan to converse at closer quarters. Conversations between people with different cultural expectations of normal

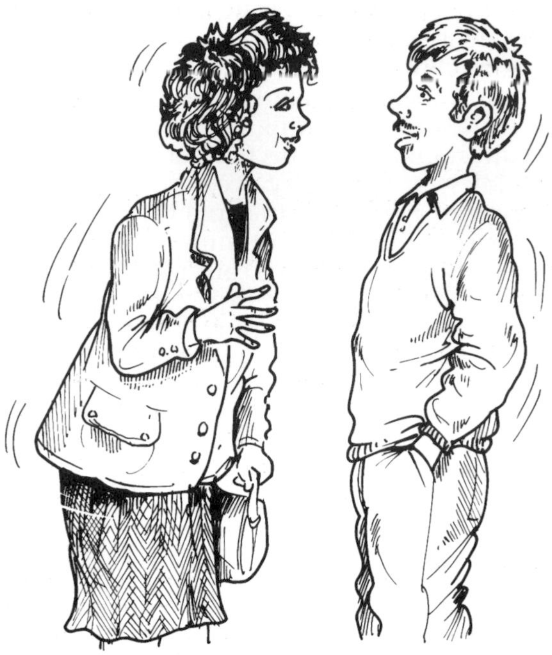

Figure 11.10 Different cultures may have different norms about personal space

personal space can be difficult and strained, without either party being aware of the reason. They may also be rather mobile, as one participant unconsciously moves backwards to his comfortable conversation distance, while the other person unconsciously pursues him so as to re-establish his own preferred distance. See, also, page 81.

Some cultures have norms of diet that are associated with religious values and practices. Jewish people eat **kosher** foods, and Muslims eat **halal** meat. In both cases, the food is prepared in strict accordance with religious requirements. Eating foods that have not been prepared correctly would be a serious breach of cultural norms. A day centre or nursery that fails to provide appropriate foods may be excluding members of some groups.

Differences in norms of religious custom can also lead to clashes in the workplace. Members of some cultural groups may be expected to observe religious festivals, and other practices such as regular prayer, at certain times of year. Some employers may be unwilling to allow them time off when they need it, or break off work to pray. The employer may see religious observance as fairly optional, as it is in mainstream UK culture, and fail to understand the significance of religion to the life of some communities.

Another area of cultural difference is attitudes to pain. In some cultures it is normal to disregard pain and play down its effects. This was the case with the Irish-Americans in Zborowski's study. Members of other cultures may learn to react differently to pain and be far quicker to seek professional help. Medical staff may not be fully aware of the effect of culture on attitudes to pain and might regard some reactions as extreme and uncalled for.

Conflicts between cultural groups can occur because of different ideas about what constitutes deviant behaviour. The norm in one group may be regarded as deviant by another. For example, the use of contraception is not allowed among Roman Catholic women. It may be deviant behaviour for them to break this ban. However, mainstream Protestant culture promotes birth control as a way of preventing unwanted pregnancies, and of avoiding sexually transmitted infections.

Serious difficulties have occurred when the norms of behaviour of cultural groups clash with the legally reinforced norms of UK society. An example of this is the experience of members of the Rastafarian community. The smoking of marijuana is part of the religious sacrament for Rastafarian believers, and yet is illegal by the laws of the state. The consequences of this clash have included the arrest of some Rastafarians for carrying out an illegal activity, and the legal testing of the Rasterfarians' claim to be a religious group.

Differences in values between carers and clients

Health and social care staff are expected to understand and promote the values associated with the caring professions. These include values associated with equal opportunities and clients' rights, and also values and norms that are associated with healthy lifestyles. However, the values that are being promoted may differ from those of clients. Clients' values may be derived from membership of a particular cultural group, or they may be associated with a particular social class. Wherever their views originate, clients should not be assumed to have the same concerns and priorities as health and social care staff.

Clients may have their own personal beliefs about illness and risks to health. They may not accept the accuracy of medical evidence which appears to contradict their ideas. For instance, some people continue to believe that the risks to health from smoking are exaggerated. They may point to people they know of who have survived a lifetime of smoking to reach great ages, and see this as proof of their point. Other may have a fatalistic view of health, believing that their health is largely outside their control. It will be difficult to promote a healthy lifestyle to those who believe that it makes no difference in the end. Chapter 12 looks at these attitudes to health in more detail.

Drug users may have come to conclusions about themselves and their fate that it is difficult to understand, or to change. Their value system may revolve around their self-image as a drug user. Ideas about long-term health are meaningless when priorities are fixed on a single aspect of their lives which dominates all others. They may accept the destructive nature of their lifestyle, but reject the idea that they can change it. Sometimes drug users refuse to accept that they have a problem at all. This is also often the case with alcohol abusers, who are much more numerous. Here the values of the health and social care profession may partly conflict with those of the wider society. Warnings about health damage and addiction are offset by the widespread acceptance of alcohol throughout society, and the general understanding that 'having a few too many' presents no real cause for concern.

Think it over

Drinking alcohol is a widespread and acceptable activity in the UK. Think about the reasons that people have for drinking. What social values promote drinking? Why do we believe that it is acceptable or even desirable?

Think about the values promoted by health and social care workers concerning healthy lifestyles. How do these two sets of values compare? Are there contradictions between the two value systems that seem difficult to resolve?

A client's cultural background may have socialised him or her into norms and values that differ from those of health and social care staff. For example, the diet that someone is accustomed to eating may be seen as unhealthy according to current medical thinking. To the client, however, this is normal food and suggestions that too much sugar or fat food are being eaten may be ignored or seen as insulting. In some cultures, cigarette smoking is far more widespread and generally accepted than it has recently become in the UK as a whole. It may be a part of the cultural identity of a client. Recommendations to stop will be offset by the pressures to conform to the norms of the client's community.

There may be differences between the views of health and social care workers and clients due to the context of the interaction. People may feel that the promotion of health is a matter to be solved in the environment and the workplace, and that the home is outside the jurisdiction of health and social care workers. Equally, people at work may feel that they are getting on with their job and health values are something to be dealt with elsewhere. Care workers need to be sensitive to people's feelings about the context of advice, and understand that people may be more responsive to receiving advice about some parts of their lives than others.

In a diverse multicultural society like the UK, there are many outlooks and viewpoints, and a range of value systems associated with them. Health and social care workers cannot learn in advance to understand the outlook of all the clients that they will meet. No amount of research and training can prepare you for the range of perspectives that you will encounter among the general public. What is possible to achieve is an awareness that different perspectives do exist, and that those of clients may be very different from your own family and friends. If you are aware that clients may be seeing the world differently from you, with different values and priorities, you will be able to work towards an understanding. You may feel that health and social care values are the right or correct values. The thing to remember is that everyone else thinks that their values are the right ones too. It is by finding out about the value systems that clients live with, and understanding their viewpoint, that health and social care workers may begin to put their own messages across successfully.

Evidence collection point

The evidence required for Element 4.2 includes two reports.

The first is an analytical report which covers two areas. Firstly you need to explain in broad terms the effects of socialisation on the development of individuals by contrasting three different influences. The influences must be chosen from the following range: the family, peer groups, work, education, religious institutions, the media. For the second part of the report, you need to explain how social constructs have changed over time.

For this section you could use data gathered by methods suggested in the Evidence Collection Point on page 200.

The second piece of work is a short report which again consists of two sections. For the first section you need to explain the potential conflicts which exist between the norms and values of two different groups in a multi-cultural society. For the second section you need to explain how values promoted by health and social care workers may differ from those of clients.

Chapter 12

The effect of socio-economic factors on health and social well-being

This chapter investigates a range of risks to health and social well-being faced by the population of the United Kingdom. Socio-economic and social policy issues relevant to health and social well-being are explored. The chapter discusses:

- demographic characteristics
- health risks
- disability and dysfunction
- risks to social well-being
- wealth and health and social well-being
- the environment
- lifestyle choices and lifestyle chances
- ways of understanding health
- social policies and their impact on health and social well-being.

Demographic characteristics

Demography is the study of population statistics. The word comes from the Greek word *demos,* which means 'people'. Demography is the science of measuring or mapping the 'people or population'.

The population of the UK was estimated to be 58.2 million people in mid-1993. This population is relatively stable – there are only 4 per cent more people than there were in 1971 (*Social Trends*, 1995, page 15.) The health of this population, the risks facing it, and the health and social care needs of the population can be explored using statistical research. Colman and Salt (1992) explain that population statistics are 'not things in themselves, rather they are visible signs of what has been happening below the surface.' (Page vi.) Statistics only show a general pattern. This pattern results from the behaviours of the 58 million individuals in the UK and the circumstances and pressures which influence them.

Population statistics are likely to become increasingly important as governments seek to reduce the health risks which face the population. Statistics are now used as a basis for understanding the major risks to health and as a basis for setting targets for general improvements in health.

Peter Aggleton (1990) argues that care should be taken when using statistics to try to understand the health of a population. Firstly, there is no clear agreement about what health includes. Aggleton argues that 'most of the measures currently used focus not on health itself but on its absence.' (Page 123.) It may be relatively straightforward to collect statistics on deaths from illnesses. However, collecting statistics on how people feel or how many minor illnesses they have had will be very much more unreliable. Judging how healthy the population is will depend on the definition of health, and on the kind of statistics which are gathered.

The World Health Organisation's (1946) definition of health is: 'A state of complete physical, mental and social well-being and not merely the absence of disease or infirmity.' Aggleton points out that some authors have criticised this definition as being idealistic – how do people achieve physical, mental and social well-being, and how should these areas be measured? Some authors have taken the concept of health to include spiritual health, environmental health and broader social health issues. There is no fixed agreement on what health is or how it could be measured.

Think it over

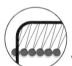

Is being healthy just 'not needing to think or worry about your body'? How wide is your own view of health?

Would you include issues like leading a balanced life in your understanding of health? You might like to review your understanding of health as you use this section.

Demographic statistics may show the *main risks* which face the population in the UK. Statistics may not provide straightforward conclusions about health. Assessing risks to health may provide a starting point for exploring the deeper issues which surround health and well-being.

Life expectancy

In the 1870s, the general population pattern for England and Wales showed a large number of children, but with fewer and fewer people in the older age groups. There were only half as many people aged 35 to 40 as there were children under 5 years of age. In the age

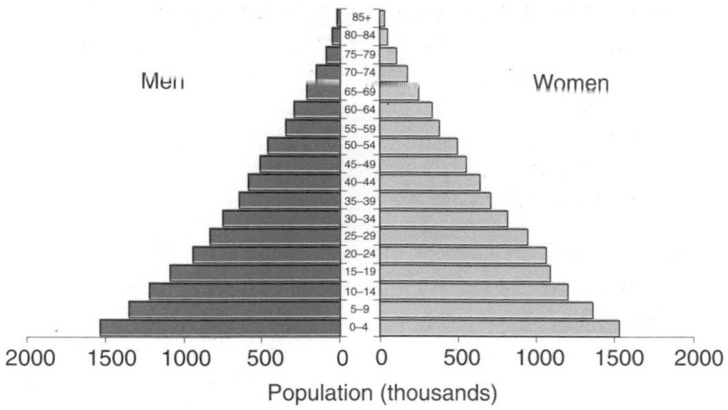

Source: Censuses of England and Wales, 1871–1971

Figure 12.1 Population pyramid showing the age structure of the population of England and Wales in 1871 (Colman and Salt, 1992)

range 65 to 70, there were only half as many people as in the 35 to 40 age group. If these figures are displayed as a population pyramid they produce a triangle pattern. (See Figure 12.1.)

The pattern in Figure 12.1 was largely due to the increasing birth rate in the population, but it was also influenced by the shorter *life expectancy* of people living at that time. *The Health of the Nation* (1992) states, 'A century ago, four out of 10 babies did not survive to adulthood. Life expectancy at birth was 44 years for

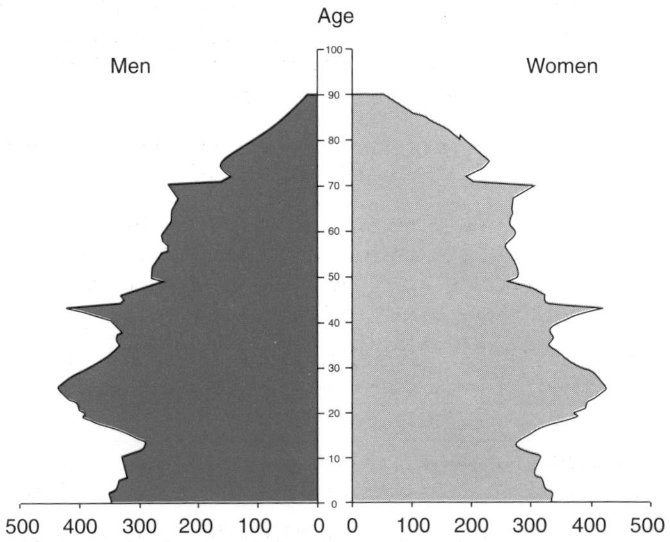

Source: Office of Population Censuses and Surveys

Figure 12.2 Age structure of the population of England and Wales in 1989 (Colman and Salt, 1992)

boys and 48 for girls ... life expectancy at birth is now 73 years for boys and 79 years for girls.' (Pages 6–7.)

The population age profile

The structure of the population for England and Wales in the 1990s is a very different pattern from that in the 1870s. The population profile looks more like a rectangle than a triangle (see Figure 12.2.) The birth rate is stable and the death rate doesn't start to show a strong influence until later in life.

Indeed, 20 per cent of the UK population were over 60 years of age in 1993 (*Social Trends*, 1995). In the last century each birthday was a real achievement. Living to 50 or 60 years of age might mean that a person had outlived their friends and other people that they had grown up with. Nowadays people often assume they will live on into their seventies and eighties. People may still be 'saving for their future' in the forties and fifties. Birthday celebrations no longer celebrate another year's survival against the risks of death – they are just social events.

Think it over

Birthday cards sometimes wish you 'many happy returns'. In the last century this was a real wish – you might not make it to the next birthday. Disease and illness killed people in all age groups. Nowadays most people under 70 years of age expect to have many more 'returns' of their birthday.

Colman and Salt (1992) state, 'Survival to early middle age is almost certain. Most people now die in old age. In 1985, 79 per cent of deaths occurred to persons aged over 64.' (Page 238.)

Life expectancy has risen so much mainly because of improved housing, improved diets, improved sanitation, and the decline in the way infectious diseases and epidemics kill people.

Causes of death

One of the greatest changes has been in the rate of infant deaths (infant mortality). As Figure 12.3 shows, deaths in the first year of life the number of infant deaths has dropped from 150 per 1000 live births in the 1890s to just eight deaths for every 1000 live births (*The Health of the Nation*, 1992).

In the last century, infants died from diseases such as dysentery and diarrhoea. Older children died from

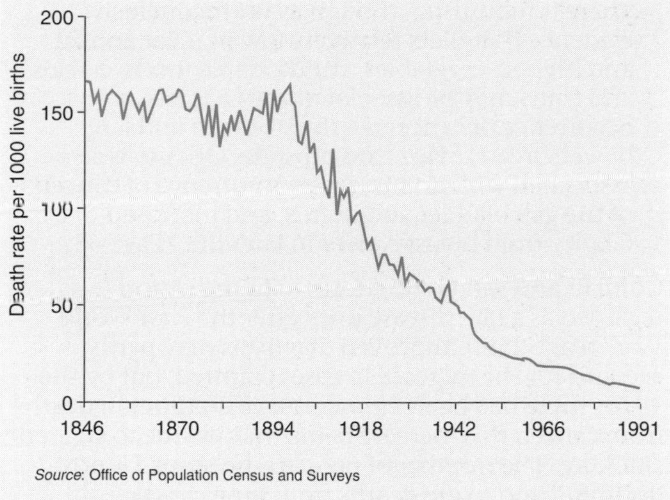

Figure 12.3 Infant mortality in England and Wales, 1846–1991 (*Health of the Nation*, 1992)

diseases such as diphtheria, scarlet fever and whooping cough. Tuberculosis (or TB) represented a serious hazard for younger adults. Colman and Salt (1992) quote the figure of 17.6 per cent of all deaths in 1839 being caused by TB, according to the Registrar-General's first national analysis of causes of death. Epidemics of typhoid and cholera, due to poor sanitation and polluted drinking water supplies, also claimed the lives of many adults.

These diseases no longer account for many deaths within the population, and the risks facing people today are dramatically different from those in the last century. New diseases like AIDS (see Chapter 19) are taking an increased number of lives. By September, 1994, 9900 cases of AIDS had been reported and 6700 people had died of AIDS in the UK since the virus was identified (*Social Trends,* 1995). However, the number of people in the general population who die from infectious diseases is likely to be very small in comparison to the numbers who die from circulatory diseases or cancers. *The Health of the Nation* (1992) contains statistics of the 566 992 deaths in 1991. Circulatory diseases caused 46 per cent of deaths and cancer caused 25 per cent of deaths. Heart and circulatory disease and cancer now represent the major causes of death for people in the UK.

Circulatory disease

'Circulatory disease is primarily a disease of middle and old age, not of childhood or adolescence.' (Colman and Salt [1992], page 253.) Circulatory disease includes:

- degeneration of the coronary arteries, the restriction of arteries as they 'fur up' called *arteriosclerosis*.
- blood clots (*embolisms* and *thrombosis*) which block the arteries and may result in a stroke where the blood supply to the brain is restricted.
- *haemorrhage,* the bursting of the blood supply system, which can result from restricted arteries and consequent high blood pressure.
  (For further details see Chapter 19.)

Like most degenerative diseases, genetic and environmental factors will interact to influence whether a person develops circulatory disease at any age. Some people may be more at risk of developing early heart problems than others. Even so, there is a lot that might be done to reduce the risk of early heart disease or circulatory disease.

The Health of the Nation (1992) states:

> 'It is generally accepted that the main risk factors for coronary heart disease and stroke are:
>
> - cigarette smoking
> - raised plasma cholesterol
> - raised blood pressure
> - lack of physical activity
>
> All the main risk factors can be influenced by changes in behaviour.' (Page 46.)

The advice is to stop or avoid smoking, to cut dietary intake of saturated fatty acids (which leads to raised plasma cholesterol levels), and to avoid excessive consumption of alcohol and salt (which contribute to raised blood pressure). Exercise helps to reduce the risk of coronary heart disease and stroke, and also helps to reduce or prevent obesity (being very overweight). 'Obesity contributes to raised plasma cholesterol levels and raised blood pressure'. (Page 47.) It is, therefore, important to avoid or reduce obesity.

People at risk of circulatory disease

Social Trends (1995) reports data from the 1991 Health Survey for England. The survey found that 'just over half of men and just over two fifths of women were overweight or obese' using the body mass index.

Around a fifth of all adults in England had taken no moderate or vigorous exercise for as long as 20 minutes in the four weeks before being interviewed.

'The survey found that over two thirds of adults had cholesterol values above the desired level.' (Page 118.)

High blood pressure is associated with increasing age. 'Only 2 per cent of men in the 16 to 24 age category had high blood pressure, but by the age of 75, nearly 60 per cent of the sample had, or were being treated for high blood pressure. A similar pattern was found for women. Over the age of 55, a fifth of both men and women had high blood pressure but were receiving no treatment.' (Page 117.)

The survey also found links with being overweight and heavy drinking in men, being overweight and being an ex-smoker, and social class and being overweight. Working-class women were more likely to be overweight than middle-class women.

Social Trends (1995) reports that 29 per cent of men and 28 per cent of women smoked in 1992. Smoking is strongly related to measures of social class. In 1992, only 14 per cent of 'professional' males and 13 per cent of 'professional' women smoked. Forty-two per cent of males in 'unskilled manual' work smoked and 35 per cent of 'unskilled manual' females smoked. Nearly a quarter of 15-year-olds smoked and 1 per cent of 11-year-olds smoked.

Reports of alcohol consumption in *Social Trends* (1995) state, 'Nearly two in five men aged 18 to 24 drank more than the sensible maximum amount compared to only one in six aged 65 and over.' On average, '27 per cent of men and 11 per cent of women drank more than the sensible maximum amount.' (Page 129.)

Survey data from the early 1990s clearly show how individual lifestyles and behaviours create a risk of circulatory disease, or of circulatory and heart disease developing earlier than might otherwise have happened.

Cancer

One in four people is expected to die of cancer. Cancer involves the uncontrolled growth of abnormal body cells. A malignant cancer involves the growth of tissue which will disrupt normal body functions. A malignant cancer might spread secondary cancers throughout the body (for further details see Chapter 19). There are many types of cancer, and cancers can occur in most parts or areas of the body. Lung, skin, breast and cervical cancer represent diseases where many deaths might be prevented.

The Health of the Nation (1992) states:

> Though the factors affecting cancer incidence are by no means fully understood, it is clear that genetic, behavioural and environmental factors all have a role.
>
> Smoking has been shown to contribute to approximately 30 per cent of all cancer deaths and is responsible for at least 80 per cent of those from lung cancer.
>
> There is mounting, though as yet inconclusive, evidence that diets relatively low in meat and fat and high in vegetables, sturdy staple foods, cereals and fruits may be associated with a lower occurrence of cancers of the stomach and large bowel, breast, ovary and prostate. Obesity is also associated with an increased occurrence of cancers of the gall bladder and uterus, and increased fatality from breast cancer in later life. (Page 65.)

Colman and Salt (1992) note that lung cancer 'was regarded as a rare disease until after the First World War.' (Page 259.) Improved diagnosis may partly account for the increase in cases counted, but by the 1970s there had been an increase of 20 times in deaths from cancer, this increase being mainly due to cigarette smoking. The number of people who smoke is now declining and so are deaths from lung cancer.

Cancers such as breast cancer, leukaemia, cancer of the oesophagus and testicular cancer have all shown an increase over the past 40 years, according to Colman and Salt (1992). *Social Trends* (1995) suggests that one person in three will develop a cancer during their lives although only one person in four dies of cancer. Malignant melanoma is a form of skin cancer. It is still relatively rare, but has increased since 1970. Fair-skinned people with a tendency to burn when their skin is exposed to sunlight are thought to be especially at risk from sunbathing.

European code against cancer, or 'Ten Commandments'

1. Do not smoke. Smokers, stop as quickly as possible and do not smoke in the presence of others.
2. Moderate your consumption of alcoholic drinks – beers, wines and spirits.
3. Avoid excessive exposure to the sun.
4. Follow health and safety instructions at work concerning production, handling or use of any substance which may cause cancer.
5. Frequently eat fresh fruit and vegetables, and cereals with a high fibre content.
6. Avoid becoming overweight, and limit your intake of fatty foods.
7. See a doctor if you notice a lump or observe a change in a mole, or abnormal bleeding.
8. See a doctor if you have persistent problems, such as a persistent cough, a persistent hoarseness, a change in bowel habits or an unexplained weight loss.
9. Have a cervical smear regularly.
10. Check your breasts regularly, and if possible undergo mammography at regular intervals above the age of 50.

Advice on prevention and the early detection of cancer is provided in the 'European code against cancer' in *The Health of the Nation* (1992), page 66.

Assessing the health of the population

Statistics for the last two centuries show that on average, people are living longer and that many serious illnesses no longer kill infants, children and young people. Yet people may still be dying from preventable diseases. The health of the nation has improved dramatically, but it could still improve further.

Nettleton (1995) quotes work by Ashton and Seymour (1988) which analyses phases in the development of public health in Europe and North America over the past two centuries. Each new phase builds on the achievements of the past phase, so that public health keeps improving.

Phase one was the development of public health measures to provide sanitation, better housing and better food hygiene. These measures helped to prevent epidemics and the transmission of disease in the overcrowded towns and cities of the industrialised world.

Phase two was a shift to educating individuals about the importance of personal hygiene and the use of immunisation to protect people from disease.

Phase three, from the 1930s on, was the 'therapeutic era' when governments concentrated health care on curing people. Cures might involve drugs or surgery and were best delivered through central hospital diagnosis and intervention systems. During this phase, disease prevention received less attention than the development of services to care for people who suffered from disease.

Phase four might date from the mid-1970s. This phase is called 'the new public health phase' because government policies have again started to address the issue of preventing illness. This new approach emphasises the interaction between biology, disease, environment, social issues and individual lifestyles.

General environmental issues like sanitation and housing are still important. Immunisation and personal hygiene are stressed. Treatment by doctors and surgeons is still vital. Any improvement in general health is seen as coming about through an analysis of the risks for the population and the *development of health strategies to reduce those risks*. These health strategies will include approaches attempting to influence individual lifestyles. Nettleton (1995) notes, 'Indeed, a central theme of both Labour and Conservative policy documents has been that individuals must take more responsibility for their own health in that they must adopt more healthy behaviour.' (Page 228.)

As part of a strategy for improving health, the government assesses the risk of disease and then publishes targets for reducing the amount of disease. The responsibility for reducing disease is shared between the government, the National Health Service, primary health services such as GP surgeries, public health services such as health education, environmental health, and individuals. Strategies focus on targets. *The Health of the Nation* (1992) targets for reducing heart disease, cancers and AIDS are:

Coronary heart disease and stroke targets

- To reduce death rates from both coronary heart disease and stroke in people under 65 by at least 40 per cent by the year 2000. (Baseline 1990)
- To reduce the death rate for coronary heart disease in people aged 65–74 by at least 30 per cent by the year 2000. (Baseline 1990)
- To reduce the death rate for stroke in people aged 65–74 by at least 40 per cent by the year 2000. (Baseline 1990)

Cancer targets

- To reduce the death rate for breast cancer in the population invited for screening by at least 25 per cent by the year 2000. (Baseline 1990)
- To reduce the incidence of invasive cervical cancer by at least 20 per cent by the year 2000. (Baseline 1986)
- To reduce the death rate for lung cancer under the age of 75 by at least 30 per cent in men and by at least 15 per cent in women by 2010. (Baseline 1990)
- To halt the year-on-year increase in the incidence of skin cancer by 2005.

HIV/AIDS and sexual health targets

- To reduce the incidence of gonorrhoea by at least 20 per cent by 1995 (Baseline 1990), as an indicator of HIV/AIDS trends.
- To reduce by at least 50 per cent the rate of conceptions amongst the under-16s by the year 2000. (Baseline 1989)

The targets for reducing risk factors are:

Smoking targets

- To reduce the prevalence of cigarette smoking to no more than 20 per cent by the year 2000 in both men and women (a reduction of a third). (Baseline 1990)
- To reduce consumption of cigarettes by at least 40 per cent by the year 2000. (Baseline 1990)
- In addition to the overall reduction in prevalence, at least 33 per cent of women smokers to stop smoking at the start of their pregnancy by the year 2000.
- To reduce smoking prevalence of 11–15-year-olds by at least 33 per cent by 1994 (to less than 6 per cent). (Baseline 1988)

Diet and nutrition targets

- To reduce the average percentage of food energy derived by the population from saturated fatty acids by at least 35 per cent by 2005 (to no more than 11 per cent of food energy). (Baseline 1990)
- To reduce the average percentage of food energy derived from total fat by the population by at least 12 per cent by 2005 (to no more than 35 per cent of total food energy). (Baseline 1990)
- To reduce the proportion of men and women aged 16–64 who are obese by at least 25 per cent and 33 per cent respectively by 2005 (to no more than 6 per cent of men and 8 per cent of women). (Baseline 1986/87)
- To reduce the proportion of men drinking more than 21 units of alcohol per week and women drinking more than 14 units per week by 30 per cent by 2005 (to 18 per cent of men and 7 per cent of women). (Baseline 1990)

Blood pressure targets

- To reduce mean systolic blood pressure in the adult population by at least 5 mm Hg by 2005. (Baseline to be derived from new national health survey.)

HIV/AIDS targets

- To reduce the percentage of injecting drug misusers who report sharing injecting equipment in the previous four weeks from 20 per cent in 1990 to no more than 10 per cent by 1997 and no more than 5 per cent by the year 2000.

Disability and dysfunction

Disability means a loss of ability. Ability always has a social side to it. A person may not be able to spell due to the disability of dyslexia. This might restrict what he or she can achieve. If the person is allowed to spell-check everything using a computer (or speak text directly into a computer) then the disability is no longer an issue. A dyslexic person can function as well as other people. Mobility problems might be similar. A person might have problems using his or her legs. The extent to which this disability will disrupt lives depends on the availability of disabled access. Are building equipped with lifts and ramps? Are transport and parking arrangements appropriate? Other people's attitudes and behaviour have a major influence on the nature and extent of disability.

Where a purely physical condition is being discussed, the term *impairment* is usually used to mean damage to a function or component of the body.

The term *dysfunction* means a loss or impairment in a function, i.e. that something is not working as it should do. Functions can be seen as purely physical or as physical and social. The amounts of disability and dysfunction are hard to assess. Stephen Moore (1993) states, 'In 1988, six million adults [in the UK] experienced some form of disability. The figure is not entirely accurate, because it is difficult to define exactly what disability means.' (Page 278.)

The General Household Survey for 1993 is reported in *Social Trends* (1995). This survey gathered information on individuals' own perception of their health. Chronic sickness which includes disability, dysfunction and long-standing illness was reported by individuals. When compared with the 1974 reports of chronic sickness, the figures suggest a substantial rise in long-term illness and disability (Figure 12.4.) These figures may not be entirely safe to use as a measure of disability and dysfunction, because they relate to individuals' expectations of their health rather than objective measures of impairment. Even so, the figures are still important because 'it can be argued that perception can have a direct relationship with the demand for health services.' (Page 121.)

Another chronic sickness, or dysfunction, which appears to be increasing is asthma. *Social Trends* (1995) states, 'Over the past decade there has been a striking increase in hospital admissions and GP consultations for asthma. This now affects over two million people in England including some half a million below the age of 16, and causes over 1600 deaths annually.' (Page 122.)

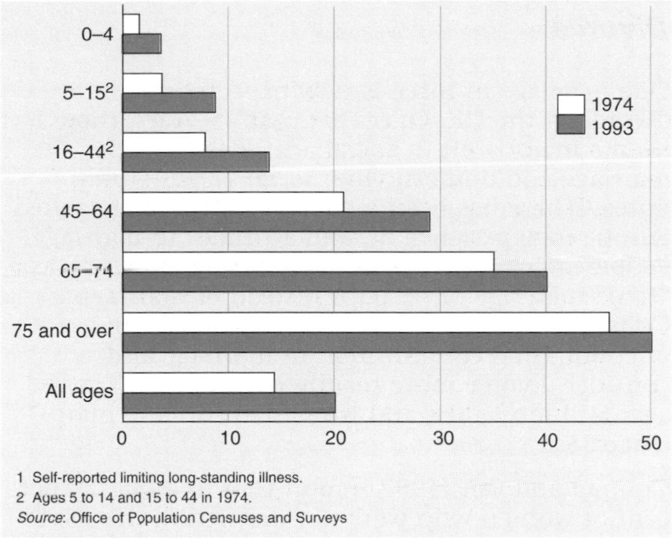

Figure 12.4 Chronic sickness[1]: by age, 1974 and 1993, Great Britain, percentages (*Social Trends*, 1995)

Many disabilities and dysfunctions are more common in later life. With more people living longer lives, it is not surprising that some disabilities have increased. *Social Trends* (1995) estimates that two out of five people over the age of 75 years have a hearing disability compared with only one in 20 people aged 16 to 44. Three per cent of the total population now wear hearing aids, although 20 per cent of men and 17 per cent of women over the age of 75 use hearing aids.

Stopford (1987) states that there are about 135 000 people in the UK who are registered as blind. Many of those people will still have some limited ability to see. A further 40 000 people were estimated to be partially sighted.

Social Trends (1995) reports the 1992 General Household Survey which showed that 'Two-thirds of the professional group wear glasses or contact lenses compared with just under half of the semi-skilled manual group.' Employment and lifestyle may exert an influence on the need to correct vision.

Moore (1993) accepts an estimate of 200 000 wheelchair users in the UK. The majority of people with chronic illness or disability are not wheelchair users.

Mental illness and suicide

Mental illness covers disabilities such as depression, anxiety, manic depression, schizophrenia and dementia. *The Health of the Nation* (1992) estimates that mental illness leads to about 14 per cent of certificated absence from work and 14 per cent of National Health Service in-patient costs.

The lifetime risks of depression are calculated as greater than 20 per cent or, in other words, one in five people may expect to experience clinical depression at some time in their lives after the age of 16. Depression can vary from mild conditions where an individual is unable to cope with daily living due to grief, through moderate depression where a person may appear to others to be irrational or self-destructive, to severe problems where an individual may appear to be seriously irrational and even deluded.

The estimated frequency of mental illness in the adult population over 16 is shown in Figure 12.5.

Mental disorder	Point prevalence (percentage of the population over 16)	Lifetime risk (percentage of the population over 16)
Schizophrenia	0.2–0.5%	0.7–0.9%
Affective psychosis	0.1–0.5%	1%
Depressive disorder	3–6%	>20%
Anxiety states	2–7%	
Dementia (over age 65)	5%	
(over age 80)	20%	

Source: The Health of the Nation, 1992, page 81

Figure 12.5 The estimated frequency of mental disorders in the adult population over 16 (*Health of the Nation*, 1992)

Mental illness leads to death from physical illnesses and from suicide. Suicide is not necessarily associated with a history of mental illness, but the *Health of the Nation* (1992) includes targets for suicide within the targets for improving mental health.

Suicide rates have historically been much higher for men than for women, and for older rather than for younger people. There may be a link between depression in old age and suicide. Recent figures (Figure 12.6) show some major changes in the pattern of suicide. Suicide is three times more common in men than in women, but *Social Trends* (1995) notes: 'Since the early 1970s, suicide rates among men have generally been rising, while rates for women have continued to fall ... However, among men aged 65 and over, the suicide rate has been falling, while the rates for men aged between 25 and 44 have risen to such an extent that they now exceed the rates for those aged 45 to 64.' (Page 132.)

Social Trends (1995) notes that younger men have been affected by high unemployment rates. Other stresses include 'exposure to armed combat,

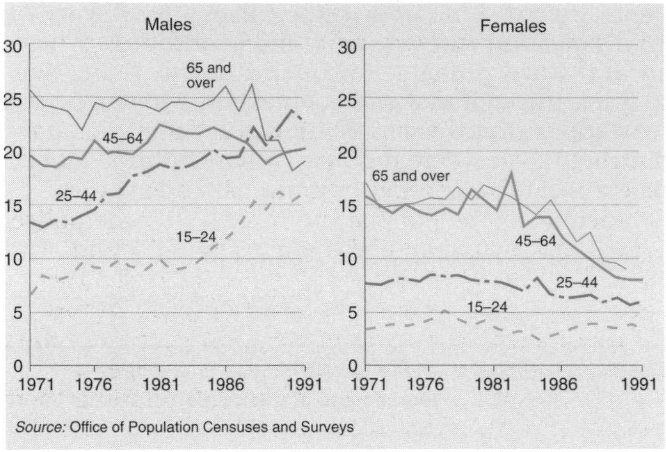

Figure 12.6 Death rates from suicide: by gender and age, England and Wales, rates per 100 000 population (*Social Trends*, 1995)

increasing risk of imprisonment, an increase in misuse of alcohol and other drugs and the HIV virus'. (Page 132.) These issues may provide an increasing range of stresses and pressures on younger men which result in depression and suicide.

Social Trends (1995) also states, 'The Office of Population Censuses and Surveys has carried out research which suggests that, particularly for young men, the increasing numbers of men remaining single or becoming divorced may explain up to half of the increase in suicides observed since the 1970s.' (Page 132.)

The Health of the Nation (1992) targets for mental health and suicide are (Page 84):

A To improve significantly the health and social functioning of mentally ill people.

B To reduce the overall suicide rate by at least 15 per cent by the year 2000 (from 11.1 per 100 000 population in 1990 to no more than 9.4).

C To reduce the suicide rate of severely mentally ill people by at least 33 per cent by the year 2000 (from the estimate of 15 per cent in 1990 to no more than 10 per cent).

Divorce

One marriage in three is now expected to end in divorce in the UK. Over that past 45 years, there has been a major shift in social attitudes towards marriage and domestic life. *Social Trends* (1995) notes, 'There has been a considerable change across Europe in experience of, and attitudes to marriage. People are choosing to cohabit before marriage, as a "trial" marriage or perhaps instead of marriage ... Couples may well place less emphasis on the unconditional commitment of marriage and consider divorce more readily than 20 or 30 years ago. Still most men and women eventually marry.' (Page 35.)

Colman and Salt (1992) report that in 1988, 29 per cent of women who were not married in the 18–49 group were cohabiting. In another study, 11 per cent of single men and 18 per cent of single women aged 20 to 24 were cohabiting. There is strong evidence that many couples choose to cohabit before becoming married.

Colman and Salt quote an estimate that as many as 50 per cent of cohabitations may not end in marriage. They also report that, 'Although the recent trend is still upward ... marriage in Britain is not yet being permanently displaced by cohabitation as it is to a marked degree in Sweden and Denmark... There, more young people aged 20 to 24 are cohabiting than are married – and about a half of babies are born outside marriage, most of them to couples rather than to single women.' (Pages 188–9.) Colman and Salt also quote estimates that as many as 20 per cent of recent generations may remain single in the future.

Social Trends (1995) charts the fall in marriage and the rise in divorce rates in Great Britain. 'Marriages fell by 24 per cent between 1971 and 1991... Divorces on the other hand increased sharply.' (Page 36.) *Social Trends* also notes that, 'Between 1977 and 1992, both the number of divorces and the number of children aged under 16 of couples divorced increased by a sixth... divorce of couples with young children is more common; the number of children aged under five affected by divorce in 1992 was... almost two thirds higher than in 1977.' (Page 37.) (See Figure 12.7).

Interpreting these statistics requires some caution. Divorce became easier in the 1970s and 1980s than it was in previous generations. It may be that couples struggled on in unhappy marriages for social and economic reasons. In the 1960s and

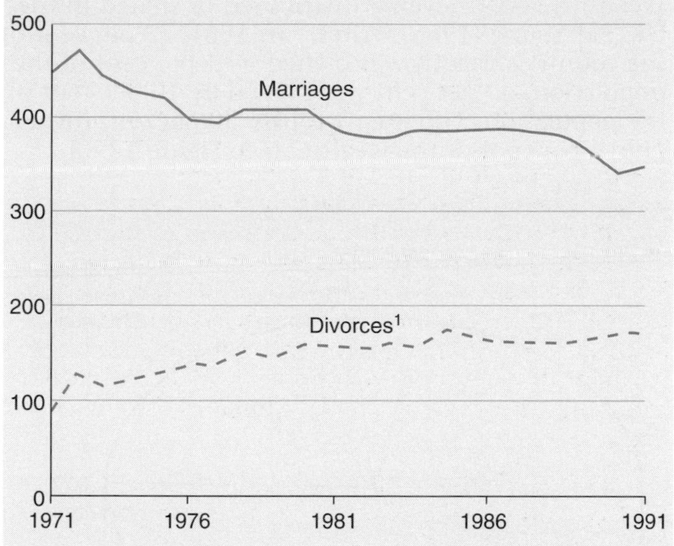

[1] Including annulments

Source: Office of Population Censuses and Surveys; General Register Office (Scotland)

Figure 12.7 Marriages and divorces, Great Britain, thousands (*Social Trends*, 1995)

1970s many women may have faced the threat of economic hardship following divorce. Divorce was often socially disapproved of 40 years ago. The ability to end an unsatisfactory partnership may be a positive development for many individuals.

According to the 1995 edition of *Social Trends,* 38 per cent of marriages in 1992 were re-marriages, and one million children lived in step-families. *Social Trends* estimates that 24 per cent of children might experience divorce in their family by the age of 16; 13 per cent might become step-children, based on the 1988–9 divorce and re-marriage rates.

The 1950s image of contented happy families may no longer be meaningful for a proportion of the population of the UK. Families may be seen as less stable than previously. It is not so easy to take family life for granted. While this may not necessarily mean that people are happier or less happy than in the past, there may be stresses and tensions around an individual's expectations and experience of his or her life. These stresses may contribute to poor health and even depression in some people.

Haralambos and Holborn (1991) note that there is a link between the divorce rate and low income. In the USA this link is very clear. In the UK, divorce is more frequent in the lower middle classes and lower income levels of the working class. People who marry in teenage or early adult years may be more likely to divorce than couples who marry later.

Divorce may represent a 'stressful transition' for adults and children which, when combined with poverty, may lead to poor health.

Crime

Crime is another 'social trend' which appears to have increased over the past 25 years. *Social Trends* (1995) reports that the number of notifiable offences per 100 people in the population, recorded by the police, tripled in England and Wales between 1971 and 1992. 'In 1993 there was one offence recorded for every 10 people.' (Page 155.) Most of these crimes (over 90 per cent) were crimes against property rather than attacks on people. Crimes against property include burglary, fraud, forgery, theft (including theft of cars) and handling stolen goods.

Social Trends (1995) also identifies poorer areas as the areas where crime is most likely to happen. Wealthy areas experienced almost a third less crime than poor areas of the country. An exception to this rule was wealthy areas in cities.

It is easy to assume that crime is committed by a small group of individuals within any community or area. Haralambos and Holborn (1991) quote a study in the USA where 91 per cent of a surveyed group of adults admitted committing crimes which were serious enough to justify a prison sentence. It is possible that most of the population have engaged in illegal behaviour of one kind or another at some time.

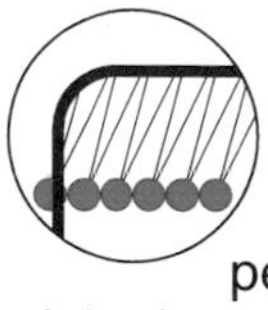

Think it over

Just because there might be more crime in poorer areas, it doesn't mean that poor people are more criminal or less moral. Why might there be more crime in poorer housing areas? Some points to think about: People who are moderately well-off are less likely to steal cars (they own cars) or break into houses or cars (they wouldn't make enough money doing so). Wealthy people are more likely to commit acts of tax fraud or other financial crimes. These 'middle-class crimes' may not be measured in terms of housing areas.

The economic stress in poor areas might mean that minor acts of theft pay off – they seem worth doing. Why would wealthy people want to steal something like a mobile phone? They can afford whatever phones they want, and they can make more money by working legally than they could by using their time to pass on stolen goods!

Crime statistics may suggest that anti-social and criminal behaviour is either increasing or being reported more often. The concentration of crime in poor areas may imply greater stress for people living in poor areas.

Stress from social factors such as crime and divorce may contribute to poor health.

Health in the sense of freedom from infectious disease has improved dramatically in recent years. Health in the sense of general physical health may be greatly improved if progress is made towards the *Health of the Nation* targets. Indicators of social well-being – crime, divorce and perhaps suicide – may suggest an increasing degree of change and stress for some people.

Evidence collection point

For Element 4.3 you will need to provide a summary of demographic characteristics and an analytical report which describes the use of three demographic characteristics in assessing the health and social well-being of the population. At this point you might choose to make notes on life expectancy, disease, disability and dysfunction, suicide, crime or divorce.

The inter-relationship between socio-economic factors, demographic characteristics and health and social well-being

While life expectancy has improved dramatically over the past century, there is evidence that not everyone stands the same chance of living a long life, or experiencing good physical health. Nettleton (1995) writes, 'Poor people die younger than people who are rich; they are more likely to suffer from chronic long-standing illnesses.' (Page 160.)

Relative wealth

Wealth refers to the value of things we own, such as a car, a home, pension rights, savings, investments or other property.

Wealth is very unevenly distributed or shared in the UK. Pat Young (1985) writes, ' In 1981, 23 per cent of the country's wealth was owned by 1 per cent of the population, 60 per cent was owned by 10 per cent of the population. The least wealthy 50 per cent owned only 6 per cent of the wealth.' (See Figure 12.8.)

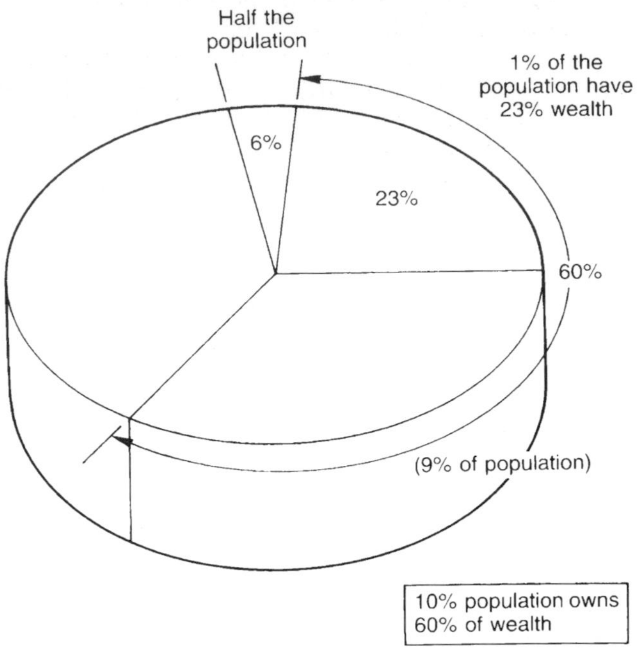

Figure 12.8 The wealth cake in Britain

An article by Robert Chote and Patricia Wynn Davis in *The Independent* (9 February 1994) suggested that 'tax changes announced since 1985 made the richest 10 per cent of the population better off by an average of £30 a week, whilst the poorest 10 per cent has lost nearly £3 a week', according to a report by the Institute of Fiscal Studies. Another *Independent* report by David Nicholson-Lord on 27 January 1994 summarised data from *Social Trends* (1994). The top 20 per cent of earners in the country saw their income grow (after housing costs) from 35 per cent to 43 per cent of total income for the country. By contrast, the bottom 20 per cent of earners saw their income drop from 10 per cent of the country's total to 6 per cent. This means that 80 per cent of people in the UK increased their real income during the 1980s, but the bottom 20 per cent have suffered a loss. People in the poorest fifth of the country's population spend half of their income on food and housing, compared with only 32 per cent (less than one third) for the other 80 per cent of people.

A second report from Nicholson-Lord (*The Independent*, 1 February 1994) quotes Mintel's 'British Lifestyles' report for 1994. The report suggested that the wealth gap will go on widening for the next five years. Mintel's head of research is quoted as saying, 'In simple terms, the well-off are getting wealthier; the poor, poorer.' He is reported to have explained that the growing polarisation had important implications for business markets. 'On the one hand there is an increasing demand for luxury goods and services, while on the other, a growing proportion of households only have sufficient income for simple products and necessities.'

In February 1995, the Joseph Rowntree Foundation published its report on income and wealth. The report found that the gap between the rich and poor had widened, 'Over the period 1979 to 1992 the poorest 20–30 per cent of the population failed to benefit from economic growth, in contrast to the rest of the post war period [1945 to 1979].' (Page 6.) The report noted the effects of unemployment, but also that there were wider differences between low- and high-paid workers. Education now has a major influence on an individual's chances of being employed and on his or her level of pay. The higher the level of education, the better the general chances of getting work and being well-paid. Families where both partners worked were generally better-off than single-earner households or no-earner households.

The Rowntree Report (1995) noted that particular groups and geographical areas have done disproportionately badly. The report states, 'It can no longer be assumed that all pensioners are poor but nor can it be assumed that there are no longer poor pensioners.' (Page 7.) Pensioners with occupational or work pensions were much better off than those who relied on state pensions.

In general, ethnic minority groups tended to be disadvantaged. 'The incomes of certain ethnic minority groups are well below the national average and a large proportion of their population live in areas ranked highly by indicators of deprivation.' (Page 7.) Whereas only 18 per cent of the population classified by survey interviews as white was in the poorest fifth of the whole population, more than a third of the 'non-white' population was in the poorest fifth. (Page 28.) In terms of geographical areas, 'The already substantial differences between deprived and affluent neighbourhoods grew further over the 1980s.' (Page 7.) The report noted that there was a strong link between council housing and low incomes. The report explains: 'In the 1960s and 1970s, fewer than half of the individuals living in council housing were in the poorest 40 per cent of the population. By 1991 the proportion was three-quarters. (Page 29.) Council housing tends to be built as estates rather than evenly spread through towns or cities, so poverty is often concentrated in particular neighbourhoods.

The Rowntree Report provides evidence that relative wealth, education, housing and employment are interlinked. Wealth and social class provide a major focus for studying the inter-relationship of socio-economic factors and health. Factors like education and housing may be hard to understand without reference to social class and wealth.

It would be very unusual for wealth and power to be distributed evenly in any society. The concept of social stratification is used to divide society into different layers (or strata) of wealth and power. In the UK, these layers or social strata are usually referred to in terms of the *class system*.

Traditionally, there has been an upper class, a middle class and a working class. Occupation is used as the basis for the Registrar-General's social classification of the middle and working classes which is widely used in research into social issues (see Figure 12.9).

	Social class	Examples of occupation in each class
Middle class	*Class 1* Professional people	Doctor, lawyer accountant, architect
	Class 2 Managerial and technical people	Manager, teacher, librarian, farmer, airline pilot
	Class 3A (non-manual) Clerical and minor supervisory people	Sales representative, office worker, policeman
Working class	*Class 3B (manual)* Skilled people	Electrician, tailor, cook, butcher, bricklayer
	Class 4 Semi-skilled people	Farm worker, postman, packer, bus conductor
	Class 5 Unskilled people	Porter, labourer, window cleaner, messenger, cleaner

Figure 12.9 The Registrar-General's social classification

The occupations given as examples for each class are chosen because they are linked to more than a level of income. They are ranked according to the general standing of the occupations within the community, which means that people in these occupations have a particular place or status in society and the behaviour and lifestyle associated with it.

This is illustrated by the way that Class 3 is divided into two, with 'non-manual' placed above 'manual' in the ranking of occupations. Although a skilled manual worker's income may be higher than a clerk's, he or she is still regarded as being in the working class. Non-manual (or 'white collar') workers are seen as tending towards the middle class and are expected to have many of the values and norms of behaviour associated with middle-class culture.

There are clearly great differences between people in terms of wealth. Those in the poorest categories may be at risk of poorer health. There is substantial evidence that lack of wealth may link with lack of health.

Jones and Moon (1987) quote evidence from the Registrar-General in 1978, showing that death rates for people are closely related to social class. In the case of still births (babies born dead) and infants, children and adults, there is far more premature death (mortality) amongst people in Social Class 5 than in Social Classes 1 and 2. In the case of infants less than 1 year old, there is more than double the amount of mortality in Social Class 5 (unskilled) than there is in Social Class 1 (professional) (Figure 12.10).

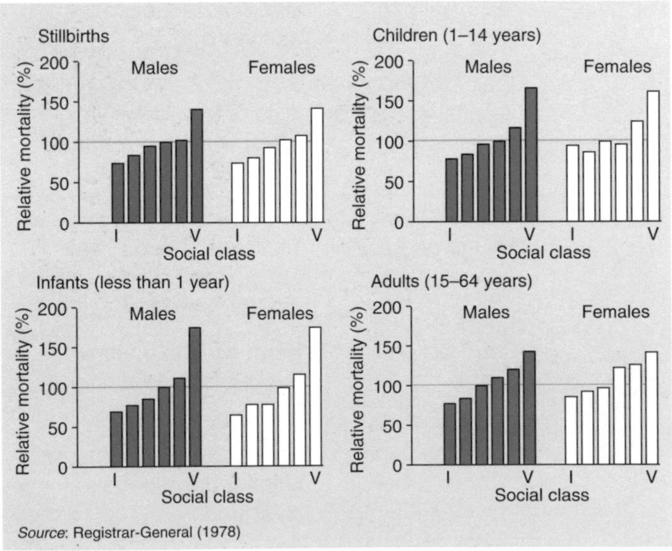

Figure 12.10 Death rate (mortality) by occupational class and age (Jones and Moon, 1987)

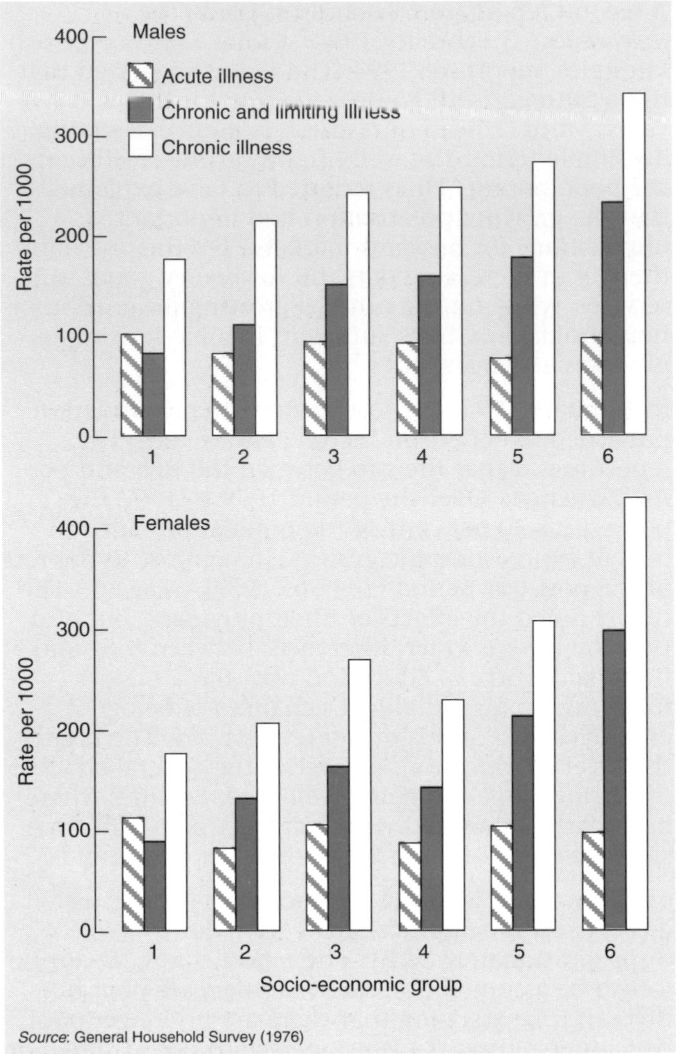

Figure 12.11 Rates of self-reported illness by socio-economic group (Jones and Moon, 1987)

Data from the General Household Survey 1976, reported by Jones and Moon (1987), shows that the amount of chronic (persistent) illness, and chronic and limiting illness, is again more than double for the unskilled class as compared with the professional class. Not only this, but there is an increase in illness for each class as you go down the scale (at least for men). Social Class 2 has more illness than Class 1, but Social Class 3 (non-manual) has more illness than Class 2. Social Class 3 (manual) has more illness than Class 3 (non-manual), and so on (Figure 12.11).

In 1980 Sir Douglas Black chaired an inquiry into health inequalities. The Black Report identified strong, class-related differences in mortality rates, very marked differences in deaths from accidents, poisonings and violence, and differences in deaths from infective and respiratory disease. Once again, the upper and middle classes experienced fewer premature deaths than the lower classes. The same pattern was found with respect to various kinds of diseases. The Black Report data has been updated by Margaret Whitehead (1988) in her work on 'The Health Divide'. She confirmed that more recent statistics still show the pattern originally evidenced by the Black Report. In addition, Whitehead notes:

> Other indirect measures of affluence and poverty, such as household-based classifications and employment status, also highlight inequalities in health. Owner-occupiers continue to have lower rates of illness and death than private tenants, who in turn have lower rates than local authority tenants. It is well known, and confirmed in recent studies, that the unemployed have much poorer health than those with jobs. (Page 263.)

Argyle (1987) states, 'The lower social classes are affected by most illness more often, take more days off from work, and die a little sooner because of them [the illnesses]. This is partly due to inequalities in the conditions of life – smaller homes, less heating, larger families, less good food, and so on.' (Page 189.) Argyle goes on to argue that middle-class people make more use of preventative health services such as antenatal clinics, vaccination programmes and cervical screening, than do working-class people. 'Doctors spend more time with middle-class patients and there is evidence that National Health Service expenditure on middle-class people is 40 per cent higher than on those in Classes 4 and 5 – because Classes 1 and 2 know how to make better use of the system.' (Page 190.) Argyle suggests that middle-class people may have responded to health education campaigns more effectively than working-class people in the past. In particular, there is evidence that middle-class people smoked less, were slimmer and took more exercise than working-class people in the past.

Mildred Blaxter's study (1990) throws some interesting light on the class issue. Her work finds a very strong relationship between low income and disease, disability, illness and poor psychological and social (psycho-social) health. But it seems that it is poverty which is associated with ill-health, rather than the case that health gets better the richer you are! Her studies show that there might be just slightly more illness and disease for the very rich than for the more moderately well-off. Money itself doesn't seem to create health; but a lack of money may be strongly associated with disease and illness. Blaxter writes, 'The apparently strong association of social class and health is primarily an association of income and health.' (Page 72.) Blaxter's study found that self-perceived stress was strongly associated with poorer health of every kind, but, 'It is notable that the relationship was particularly strong for men in manual classes, at all ages.' (Page 104.)

Environment

Gordon and Forest (1995) have produced an atlas for England based on 1991 census data. It shows that most social variables like education, class, and wealth, are not spread evenly across the country.

Long-term sickness (including disability) is mapped in ratio to the number of health care professionals (Figure 12.12). A low ratio, i.e. 9–34, suggests more care professionals in relation to need than a high

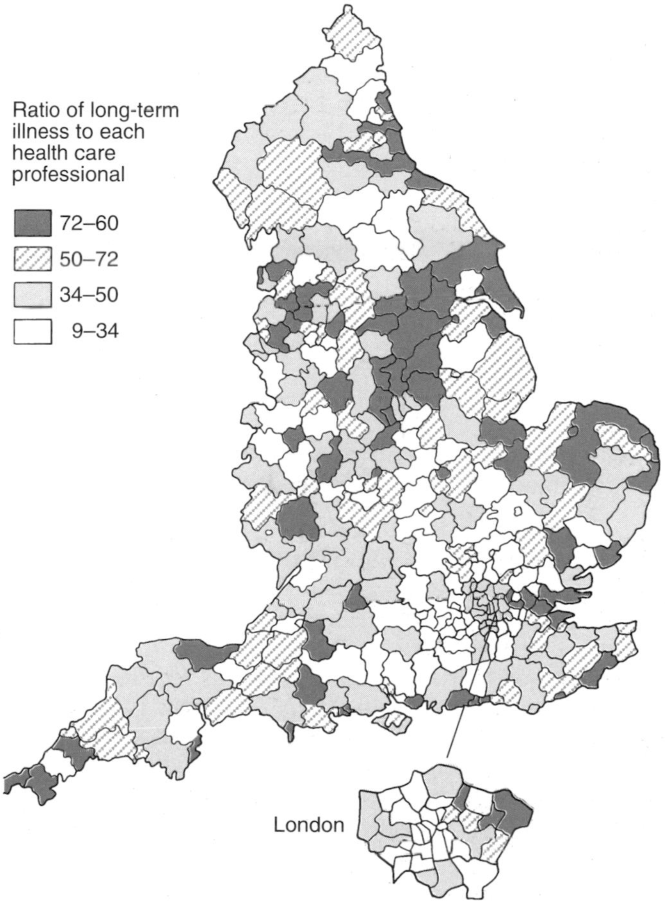

Figure 12.12 Where to be sick in England: the ratio of long-term sickness to the number of health care professionals (Gordon and Forest, 1995)

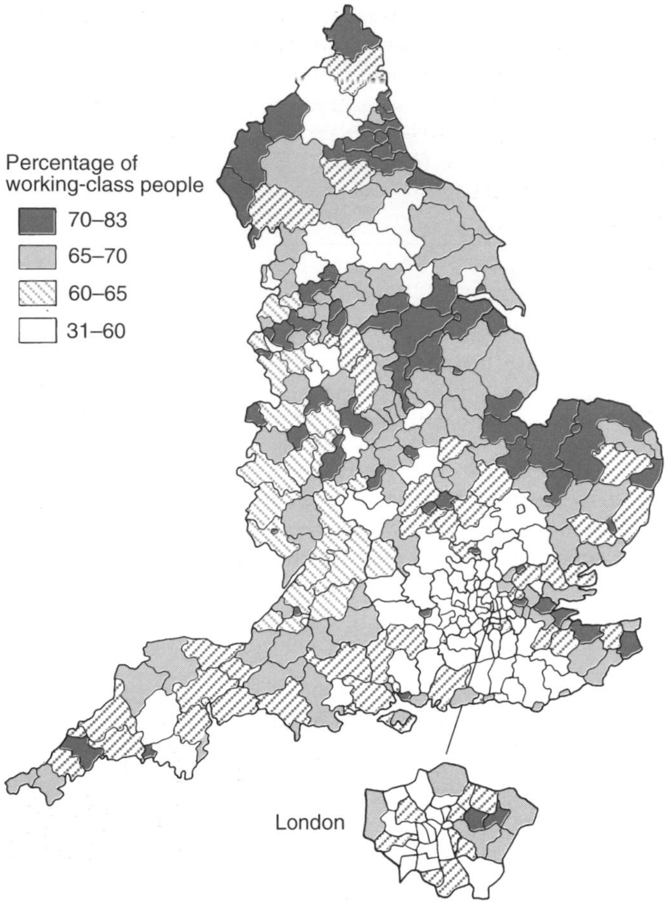

Figure 12.13 Where the working class is in England (Gordon and Forest, 1995)

ratio, such as 72–600. Some areas appear to be disadvantaged in comparison to others.

The distribution of the working class (Figure 12.13) appears to show some similarities with the high care-to-need ratios in Figure 12.12. The top three districts for density of working class also come into the top six districts with high care-to-need ratios. Corby is listed as 82.7 per cent working class and has a ratio of 598 people with long-term disability or illness to each health professional. Barnet in North London is only 51 per cent working class, well below average, and has a ratio of only 15 people with long-term illness to each health professional.

Think it over

Just because there might be a pattern which matches some working-class areas to poor care ratios, does it mean that the working class is discriminated against? The issue will be complicated. Some working-class districts may be in areas where it is difficult to site hospitals. Some hospitals may have excellent geographical links with 'working-class' districts, but not fall into the categories needed for inclusion on the map. There is no one-to-one link between areas on the two maps. It is dangerous to jump to conclusions from limited evidence. But is does appear that some geographical areas are advantaged compared with others.

Poverty and environment

Poor areas have extreme problems, according to the Rowntree Foundation (1995). The Rowntree Report states: 'Despite 15 years of major changes affecting the poorest council estates in the country – with physical regeneration, intensive management, and tenant involvement – poverty remains a major problem which threatens to overwhelm the investment which has been made in the people and fabric of the neighbourhoods.' (Page 35.) The report cites the following problems: high rates of family break-up (and divorce), large numbers of lone parents, crime and victimisation, large numbers of children on 'at risk' registers, youth unemployment, vandalism, poor education 'sometimes rejected by children as a symbol of authority', poor parenting which might be the result of parents never experiencing good parenting themselves, lack of social and family support. The Rowntree Report suggests that although residents on poor estates want to tackle these problems, they will need support from the wider community before they are likely to be successful. The report identifies three groups of people who are especially at risk in poor environments: elderly people who live alone, people with mental health problems and families with relationships in difficulty. People in these categories may fail to benefit from the kind of social provision which might be available in less stressed areas, according to the report.

Think it over

The Rowntree Report provides a list of stress factors which might reduce the 'social well-being' of people who live in poor housing areas. If people experience stress and reduced social well-being, will they be as concerned about healthy eating and exercise as people who experience less stress? Would it be more difficult to get a health education message across to people who are stressed just trying to cope with daily life?

Environment and pollution

Social Trends (1995) reports on a survey by the Department of Environment. Eighty-five per cent of people surveyed said they were quite concerned or very concerned about the environment. Concerns about chemical pollution of rivers, and toxic and radioactive waste topped the list of worries. Forty per cent of people were worried about traffic exhaust fumes, an issue that appears to be of increasing concern.

Air pollution

Air pollution has been a problem in cities for many years. In the 1950s and early 1960s, London in particular used to suffer from smog – a thick fog mixed with soot and sulphur dioxide from coal smoke. Many homes and industries burned coal for heat or power. The Clean Air Acts and new electric and gas heating systems solved that problem, and smogs disappeared. Since the 1970s the numbers of cars and other vehicles on the roads have been steadily increasing. There are fears that a new kind of invisible, or chemical, smog is affecting people's health (Figure 12.14).

Vehicle exhausts produce a range of pollutants including carbon monoxide, oxides of nitrogen, volatile organic compounds and particulates (see below). During periods of high pressure (or anticyclonic) weather, the air in cities may become relatively still. Sunlight reacts with exhaust gases to produce ground-level ozone. Ozone protects the planet when it is part of the ozone layer high up in the atmosphere. At ground level, however, it creates breathing problems for people with asthma or other respiratory illnesses. The World Health Organisation suggest a safe limit of 50 parts of ozone per billion parts of air. This limit is now often broken in cities during spells of warm, still, sunny weather.

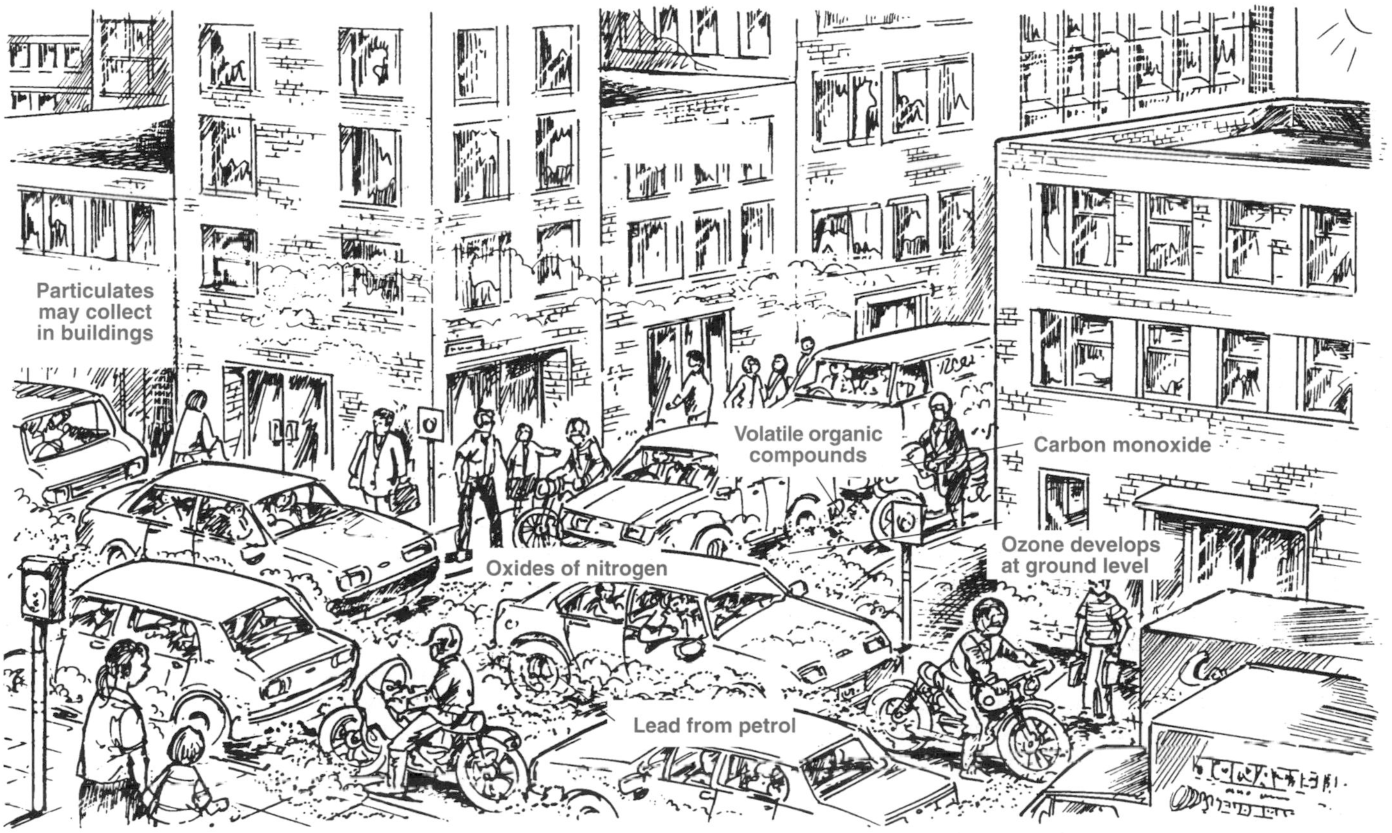

Figure 12.14 Invisible chemical smog

The effects of particulates are not fully understood. Particulates are very tiny 'soot-like' particles which are too small to see, and too small to settle in the way that dust settles. They may spread for miles and build up inside houses and rooms. Diesel engines produce a great deal of particulate exhaust. Professor Seaton of Aberdeen University has put forward the theory that some lung and heart diseases may be associated with particulate pollution. People living in polluted air may breathe in millions of these particles. The particles become stuck in the alveoli (tiny air sacs of the lungs). White blood cells attempt to 'clean' the lungs, but they become 'overwhelmed' and release 'a stream of chemicals that set-off an inflammatory reaction in the lungs and increase the stickiness of the blood so it is more likely to clot' (report by Liz Hunt, *The Independent,* 20 January 1995). Inflamed lung tissue and blood clots may increase the risk of death from heart and lung disease, particularly for older people or people who smoke.

Lead pollution, caused by vehicles which use leaded or 4-star petrol, is now decreasing due to a switch to unleaded petrol. Fifty-nine per cent of petrol sales in the autumn of 1994 were of unleaded petrol, according to *Social Trends* (1995). Lead is particularly dangerous to children. Some research has suggested that intellectual development can be damaged by lead pollution.

The UK government is reported (1995) to be considering ways of reducing air pollution from vehicles. Ideas discussed in the media include local councils being invited to draw up plans for controlling traffic, more people being encouraged to use public transport or bicycles, restricting speeds on motorways during times of high pressure weather, and better and cheaper public transport to stop the growing trend of commuting to work by car.

Catalytic converters fitted to car exhausts may reduce pollution from petrol engines. *Social Trends* (1995) estimates that pollution may fall until about 2010 because of the introduction of catalytic converters. After the year 2010, pollution may rise because of the expected increase in the number of vehicles on the road.

Noise

A study by the Building Research Establishment (1991) is reported in *Social Trends* (1995). The study found that just under a third of people said that noise spoiled their home life to some extent. Noise from people nearby or neighbours was found objectionable by almost three-quarters of those who heard it. Traffic noise was also a serious problem. Many people stated that noise caused them to feel angry, resentful, annoyed or anxious. Complaints about noise to Environmental Health Officers have almost tripled between 1980 and 1991.

Radiation

Social Trends (1995) states that 85 per cent of the radiation to which people are exposed comes from natural sources. Half of radiation is produced by radon, a gas emitted by trace amounts of uranium found in most rock. *Social Trends* estimates that about 5 to 6 per cent of deaths from lung cancer might be caused by radon. Radon can collect inside homes or other buildings. 'In Devon and Cornwall, around 12 per cent of homes have radon concentrates above the recommended level.' (Page 193.) Fall-out from the Chernobyl nuclear disaster is reported to have fallen back to a fifth of its 1986 level by 1993.

Inter-relationships between socio-economic factors, demographic characteristics and health

In general terms, the kind of work a person does and his or her ability to find work will be influenced by the education he or she received. Social class is a measure of employment status, and relative wealth and housing will be strongly linked to employment status. Whether a person lives in a high-crime area or an area with heavy traffic, air and noise pollution, is likely to be influenced by wealth and employment status. The wealth of older people – 20 per cent of the population are over 60 years of age – will be strongly influenced by past employment and pension rights. Social class is not the same as wealth, housing is not dictated by wealth, and education does not always link with later earning potentials. Even so, wealth and social class are powerful factors which influence the lifestyles and the risks that individuals face. In general terms, the poor and the working class may have more risk of disease, chronic illness and lower social well-being than people who are better off. People with good economic resources, education and social contacts can ensure that their housing and lifestyles serve their needs. People who are economically insecure may be more likely to be housed in poor environments, and more likely to have been socialised into lifestyles which may place them at greater risk of poor health.

Evidence collection point

Your report for Element 4.3 will require you to consider the inter-relationships between health and social well-being and socio-economic factors.

You might wish to make notes or establish conclusions for your report at this point.

Lifestyle choices and lifestyle chances

The new public health approach seeks to improve health by preventing disease. One key element to prevention is to convince people to choose a healthy lifestyle. This healthy lifestyle would include:

- exercise – preferably a *minimum* of 20 minutes' vigorous exercise three times a week
- healthy diet – low in saturated fat, high in fibre, vegetables and fruit
- avoidance of obesity
- moderate drinking of alcohol
- avoidance of smoking
- avoidance of drug abuse or misuse
- avoidance of stress.

Stress

A balanced lifestyle, with just the right amount of stimulation or excitement, leisure, rest and sleep, would help to prevent stress. Stress may contribute to heart disease and to mental problems, such as depression. Friedman (1975) identified a stressed lifestyle or learned behaviour pattern which was called 'Type A behaviour'.

Type A people try to achieve as much as possible in a short time. They tend to be too busy to bother listening to others and often try to do two or three things at the same time. People with Type A behaviour may be insecure; they may spend a lot of time trying to gain approval from their employers or the public. Type As may feel guilty when relaxing; they may be selfish, impatient, easily bored. They may be highly competitive, treating life as a game to be won.

Type B behaviour contrasts with Type A. Type B behaviour means being easy-going, putting just the right amount of effort into a task. Type B people are not rushed: they listen, they relax, they are not competitive. Friedman believed that Type A behaviour might be linked with the risk of heart attack. Type A people may have learned to stress themselves in order to get on in their careers or in order to cope with life pressures. Type A people create their own anxiety and their own risks to health.

Think it over

Do you know any people who behave in a Type A way? How much pressure do you see in care settings? Do any of the staff you have observed use Type A behaviour in an effort to cope?

Learning to lead a balanced life would help prevent Type A behaviours. When combined with good diet, exercise, and a health-conscious approach to substances such as alcohol, drugs and tobacco, this might reduce an individual's risk of disability and premature death. Health and happiness might improve.

Think it over

There is so much on offer – a longer and happier life – that surely everyone would follow this lifestyle advice! You will know many people, however, who do not lead healthy lifestyles. Why don't people follow the advice?

Reasons could include:

- They don't believe the advice.
- Health is not the most important thing in their lives, so people sacrifice it in pursuit of other goals.
- People *cannot* follow the advice.
- People *believe* that they cannot follow the advice.
- Unhealthy behaviours are enjoyable and difficult to give up in favour of less pleasurable activities.
- People haven't understood the lifestyle advice.

Thinking of you own or other people's lifestyles, what further reasons would you give?

Ways of understanding health

Peter Aggleton (1990) suggests four types of explanation which people use to understand health, emphasising biological factors, social and economic issues or the individual's own way of understanding his or her life.

Explanations which emphasise biology might focus on the cause and effect relationships that have been shown to exist between diet, genetics, alcohol and the development of degenerative diseases. The focus is on the technical nature of disease and how treatments or environmental factors may influence it. Aggleton calls this type of explanation *bio-medical positivism.* Positivism is the belief that logical analysis will lead to satisfactory solutions to all problems. Positivism concentrates on analysis rather than exploring patterns or relationships.

An alternative to bio-medical positivism is *social positivism.* Social positivists believe that health can be understood by analysing the lifestyles and behaviours of individuals and their immediate surroundings. Each lifestyle choice is an individual issue and the reasons for drinking alcohol or eating a high-fat diet have to be analysed on an individual, action-planning level.

Not everyone focuses on individual or biological causes. *Structuralist* explanations of health and disease study the patterns of disease in relation to the structure of society. Working-class or poorer sections of the community tend to have more serious illness than middle-class and wealthy people. There are exceptions, such as malignant melanoma (skin cancer), which is more common in the middle classes. Structuralists try to understand how issues such as race, gender, class and wealth influence health and illness. The assumption is that the way society is organised will bring about differences in the chances of individuals developing poor health.

Interactionist explanations of health emphasise the idea that people construct or build their own ideas or meaning about health. People get their ideas from other people they mix with, especially friends and partners. People develop lifestyles based on their way of understanding their situation.

The Choices v Chances debate: On a simplified level, the debate between bio-medical positivists, social positivists, structuralists and interactionists might go as follows.

The bio-medical positivist

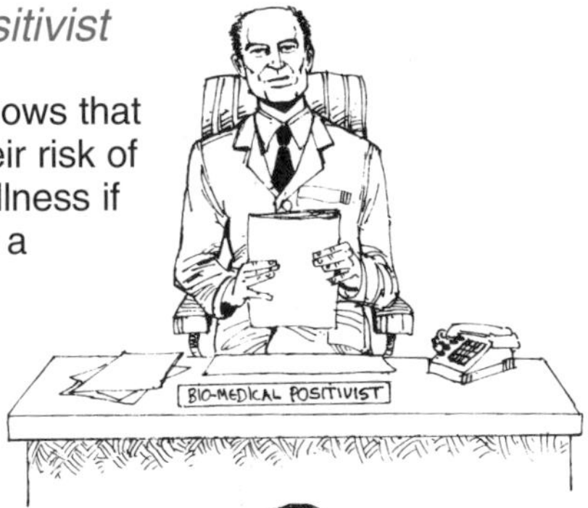

'Analysis of research shows that people could reduce their risk of disease and long-term illness if they would only choose a healthy lifestyle – we understand what is needed. People need to start listening to our message and make the right choices.'

The social positivist

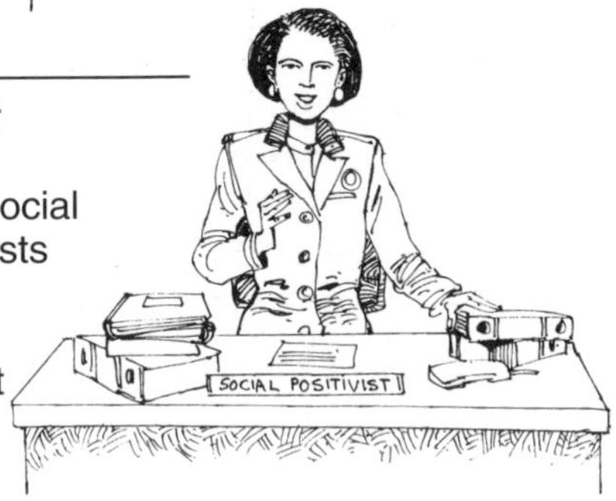

'Well, that's the point – social science research suggests that individual people have individual needs. Just telling people about medical findings isn't enough. Individuals might need their own action plan for health – they will need guidance and support to change their lifestyles or develop positive behaviours. We need to look at marketing good health – and plan media coverage to convince people in language that is appropriate to different people.'

The structuralist

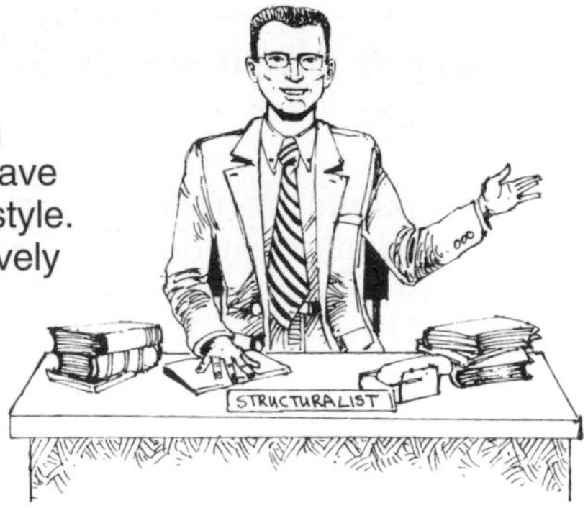

'Only a few people with resources and power have choices about their lifestyle. Most people are effectively forced to adopt the lifestyle that they have. What's the use of telling an unemployed family to eat a healthy diet? They probably can't afford to! What's the point of telling stressed and worried individuals not to smoke or take drugs? It's all they've got! Even the better off don't always have a choice about leisure and rest – they have to do two jobs just to pay the mortgage. No – people don't have choices, they have *life chances!* People get fixed into activities because of the structure of society. A lot depends on the class and groups that you are born into.'

The interactionist

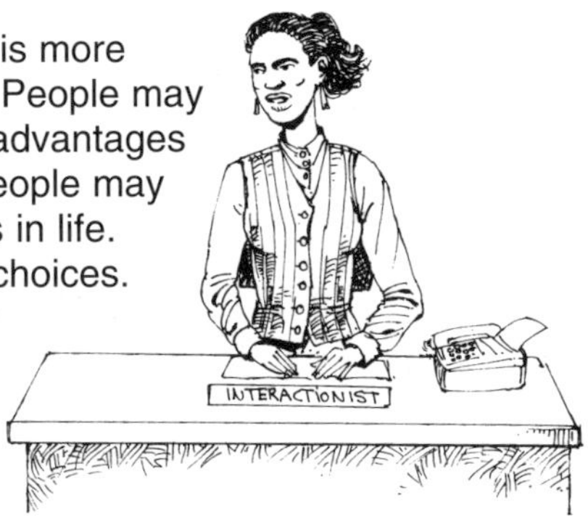

'But the whole debate is more complicated than this. People may be born with different advantages and disadvantages. People may have different chances in life. But people also have choices. Choices are limited by the way individuals learn to understand their health. The way individuals behave depends on the beliefs that they share with friends, relatives and their community. Social structure doesn't fix what happens to people, it only influences it. If you can get groups to believe in healthy lifestyles, it may be possible to improve health. The fact that people have different chances in life doesn't have to mean that individuals can't change.'

If the debate between these approaches went on for a while, we might get to the point where serious criticisms were made.

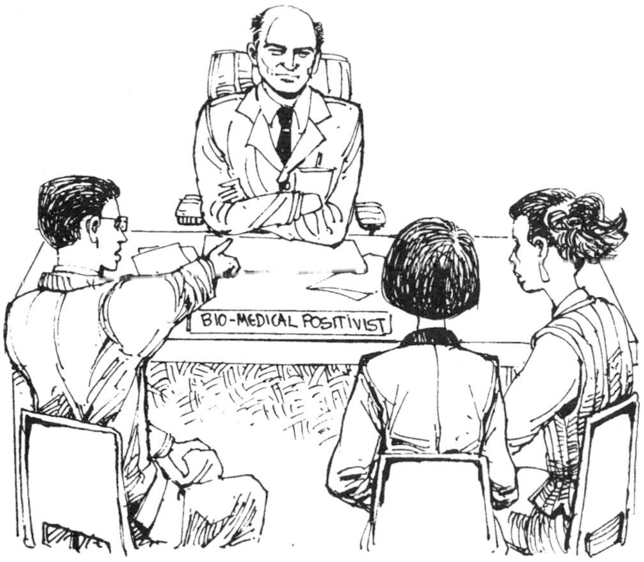

'You are trying to avoid all the social issues. You might go on to blame individuals for not taking your advice when they:

- can't understand the advice
- can't change their lifestyle
- won't necessarily believe the advice.'

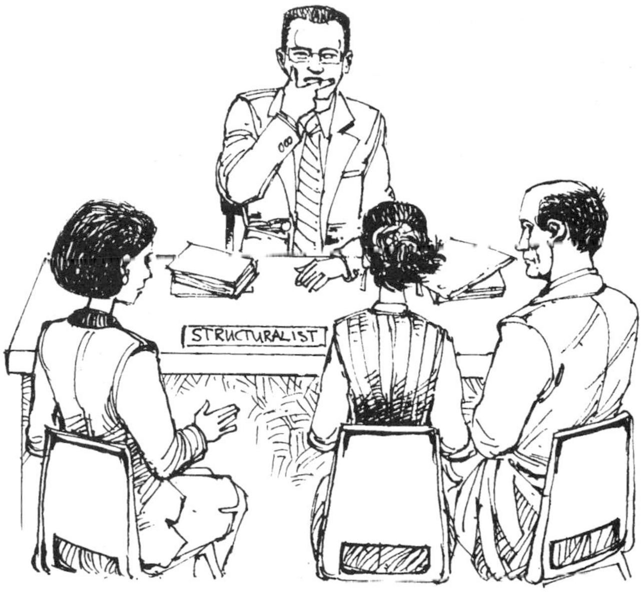

'Your analysis is too simple and too rigid. Social structure doesn't control what happens to individuals even if it might influence things. Poverty might be linked with poor health, but that doesn't prove that it causes it. The causes could be more complex. Do we really have to change society before we can reduce heart disease or cancer?'

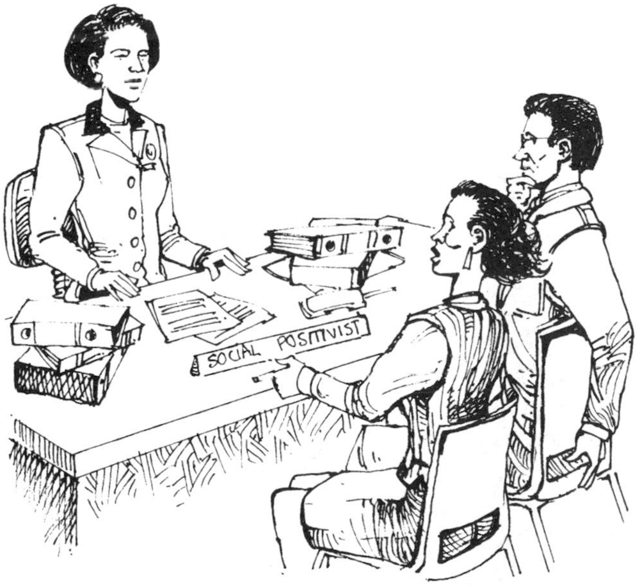

'Just like the bio-medical positivist, you are putting all the responsibility for health on individuals. Individuals don't always have the chance to develop healthy lifestyles. You might end up blaming the victim – when you find that people can't follow your advice!'

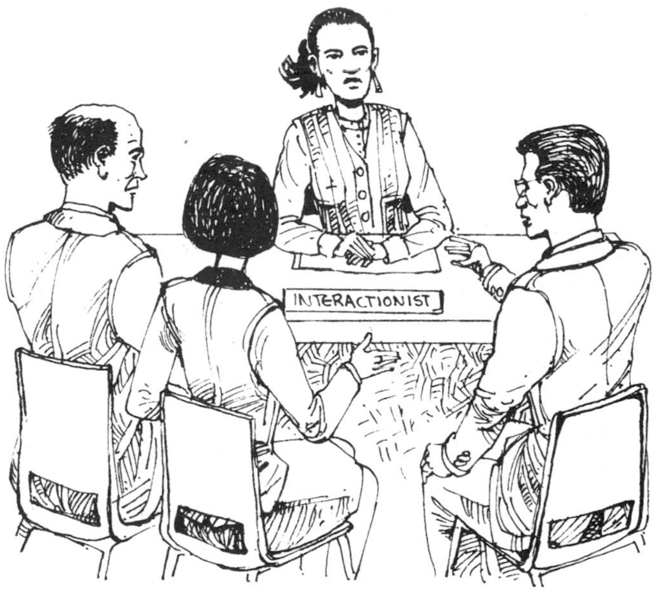

'All this stuff about beliefs and meanings – are people supposed to take responsibility for themselves or not? Aren't you just sitting on the fence? Isn't this just a soft

continued overleaf

version of the structuralist explanation? You really want to say that social structure fixes people's chances but you are disguising this with theories about beliefs. Aren't you really with the positivists? Your view under-emphasises the inequality in society and over-emphasises the responsibility of the individual. This won't help in the struggle for a fairer society.'

Think it over

Different explanations emphasise different issues. There is no easy answer as to how far socio-economic factors influence individuals in their lifestyle choices. It may be useful to keep the different types of explanation in mind when discussing lifestyle choices.

Making lifestyle choices

Although the bio-medical positivist view might not be interested in socio-economic factors, most of the other viewpoints would accept that wealth, class and associated social issues do influence the health of the population. The arguments are about how factors like poverty influence health. Structuralists might argue that poverty causes poor health. Interactionists argue that poverty only causes poor health in an indirect way, by influencing how people think. Structuralists are concerned with the inequality that exists between different groups in society. The poor have much worse health and perhaps even health services than the better off.

Ethnic communities and women may be relatively disadvantaged compared to white males in general. Interactionists do not necessarily disagree with this analysis, but they are interested in researching the complexity of the issues. Positivists may tend to ignore the health inequalities debate.

How do people understand their health? An interactionist view

In previous centuries life may have been hard. Many people had to work long hours just to survive. Disease and death were affecting people all the time. It is tempting to believe that people's lives were often simple in one respect – they could often explain their lives in forms of straightforward religious or social beliefs held in their community. At the end of the twentieth century, things are not so easy. People are aware of a great range of views. It seems that individuals often have to make their own sense of life. They have to use their own personal experience to build their own idea of what health, individuality or personal identity are. It is as if people have to make up a story to explain their lives.

Nettleton (1995) quotes research from Stainton-Rogers, who identified alternative ways in which people understand their health. Some people see their body as a machine. This machine can break down or wear out. If the machine stops working properly it will need to be fixed. Another view is that the body is under attack from all the germs and dangers that exist in the world. Health is a matter of fighting off all the attacks from outside. Some people see health as something you achieve from having the right lifestyle. Others see health as a matter of will-power. Health depends on having the emotional strength to make the right choices. Other people stressed the need for modern medicine, but were concerned that not everyone had an equal chance of getting the best treatment. Some people stressed the problems with modern medical treatments. Whatever the theories, people seem to invent their own views of health. Their own views may influence their lifestyle choices.

Think it over

What stories do you use to think about health? If you catch a cold do you think:

- I've been living an unhealthy life – I must improve my lifestyle to avoid this in future.
- The germs have broken through – I must get some treatment to help me recover.
- I don't believe in tablets – I'll use a herbal remedy to restore my balance.
- I'm not going to allow myself to be ill – I'll carry on as normal. My body will just have to cope.
- What's wrong with my body? Why is it always letting me down like this?
- I'll go to the doctor, but he or she won't help me. You have to pay to get good treatment nowadays.
- A combination of these ideas – or something different?

Many people understand their health in terms of luck. If you are forever fighting off stress and disease, then sometimes you will lose a struggle. You may be unlucky enough to lose the fight altogether. Nettleton (1995) quotes research from Blaxter (1993), where Blaxter interviewed working-class women. Many of the women believed that they had no control over their own health. Disease was believed to be caused by infection or by genetics, or by other risks in the environment. Many people believe in *determinism* – they think their health is not something they can influence with their own lifestyle choices. Nettleton also quotes a study by Cornwell in 1984, where 22 out of 24 working-class people did not believe that there was a link between smoking and lung cancer. Apparently they did not believe the health education message because their own experience did not fit with it. They knew of people who had died of cancer who didn't smoke and smokers who had suffered no problems.

It may be that people develop their own theories of what causes disease and that they then live by their own theory. People interact with others to learn about and understand health. They develop their own interpretations. When health educationalists put over a simple message, many people may not believe it because it doesn't fit with their own understanding or observations about health. The middle classes and wealthier sectors of society my find it easier to believe health education messages than many working-class people (see Argyle, 1987).

Think it over

If you want to influence people with a health education campaign, is it enough just to keep the message very simple and straightforward so that 'anyone can understand it'? Or should the campaign find out what people believe first? Should some posters give more complex information rather than just simple information in order to get people to re-think their ideas?

There is evidence that some working-class people may refuse to believe in a link between poverty and ill-health. Nettleton (1995) quotes studies by Colman (1987) and Blaxter (1993) which show that people's personal theories about health stopped them from believing statistical information. It may be that many people feel threatened by research that suggests they are vulnerable. An easy way out is to refuse to believe the information.

A study by Davidson *et al.* (1992) reported by Nettleton (1995) researched a health education campaign in Wales. Davidson reported that many individuals seemed to believe in a fixed destiny. People often believed that their health was dependent on genetics, or might be influenced by pollution or climate, or by the pressures of their work or social environment.

The idea of a lifestyle choice doesn't seem to make sense to a lot of people. Instead of lifestyle choice, many people appear to believe that health is a matter of good or bad luck. The stories that some people invent to explain their health often focus on the environment or on genetics – there is no notion of choice in the way they think.

Poverty and health

Poverty creates problems for individuals in terms of managing their daily living requirements. Poverty may remove many of the small daily satisfactions of life, such as buying small presents for friends, going out and giving yourself treats. Poverty or low income may also provide a source of stress for individuals. This stress may be linked to the self-esteem and identity of people who may not be able to keep up with the consumer values which are promoted by advertising and which are a big part of contemporary society. If you have lost the consumer race, you may be inclined to evaluate yourself as a loser. This alone could create stress.

When a person feels stressed, anything which promotes an easing of tension will be very desirable. A National Children's Home study (1994) found that, 'two-thirds of children interviewed said they smoked to "escape" their problems, while one in three said they drank, and one in six took (illegal) drugs.' Sarah Hirsh of the anti-smoking charity, Quit, is quoted as follows in *The Independent* of 9 March 1994: 'As smoking rates increased in line with poverty, it was not surprising that women found it more difficult to stop. Women who are in the lower social groups may be stuck at home with no luxuries. Many tell us on the helpline that smoking is all they have got.'

Oakley (1989) quoted in Nettleton (1995) 'found that smoking was significantly inversely related to income, housing tenure, access to a car, telephone ownership and central heating.' (Page 54.) In other words, the poorer women were, the more they were likely to smoke. Nettleton theorises that poor health 'choices' like smoking may enable people to cope with poverty. 'Thus whilst affecting women's physical health, smoking may facilitate their mental well-being.' (Page 54.)

Think it over

Health choices may not matter in the same way to different groups of people. Wealthier people may be very concerned about surviving to enjoy their future pension rights. Poorer people may just want to live for today.

For some people in some situations health may not be the most important thing in their lives.

It appears that some people choose to smoke or drink, to be lazy and not exercise, or to eat a poor diet. But it may be that many individuals feel compelled to drink excessively or to smoke because this activity helps to relieve day-to-day stress. Eating sugary snacks, crisps and chocolate may be a treat in a life that feels empty. Eating fruit or a carrot doesn't necessarily give the same rewarding feeling.

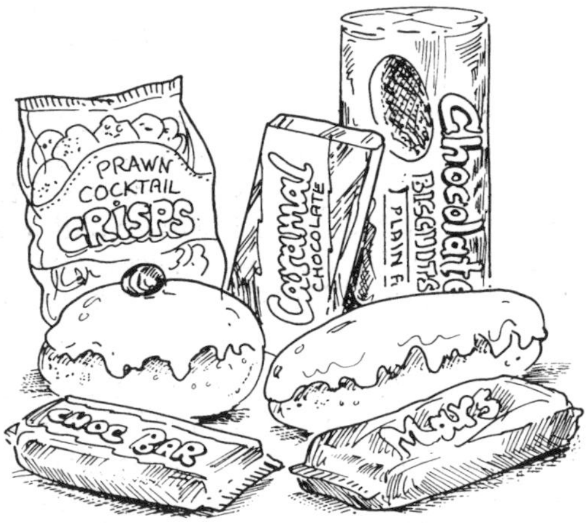
PRAWN COCKTAIL CRISPS
Caramel CHOCOLATE
Chocolate BISCUITS
CHOC BAR

People may trade-off aspects of a healthy lifestyle in order to cope with other pressures. An overworked business person may ignore exercise in order to spend more time at his or her work. In this way the person can maintain the self-concept of a successful individual and make money. Health is traded in exchange for other personal needs.

Many people may believe that they do not have health choices. Instead, they have to make compromises between a healthy lifestyle and surviving the stresses and pressures which they face. Having a balanced amount of work and leisure, sleep and rest; eating a balanced diet, taking exercise, avoiding harmful substances like tobacco – all this may be possible for people with the time and money to choose their way of life. Many people can only manage compromises between the demand on their time or other resources and the need to be healthy.

Other people may feel they have no choice at all!

Blaxter reported that only 15 per cent of people in her sample had completely healthy habits in the areas of diet, smoking, exercise and drinking, and only 5 per cent led totally 'unhealthy' lives. What was striking was that most people knew the risks they were running, but may have chosen to accept risks to their health in an attempt to control personal stress and cope with life.

Blaxter (1990) writes,

> The Health and Lifestyle Survey adds to much existing evidence that beliefs are not very good predictors of behaviour. It seems from the interviews here that the public have, in general, learned very well the lessons of health education ... it is those who indulge in unhealthy lifestyle habits who are most conscious of the links between behaviour and disease ... substantial proportions of the population did not see health as the most important thing in life – and these were more likely to be people with more, rather than less, education. (Pages 240–1.)

As a general conclusion, people appear to have believed in health and understood health; but other pressures meant that they did not necessarily act on their beliefs.

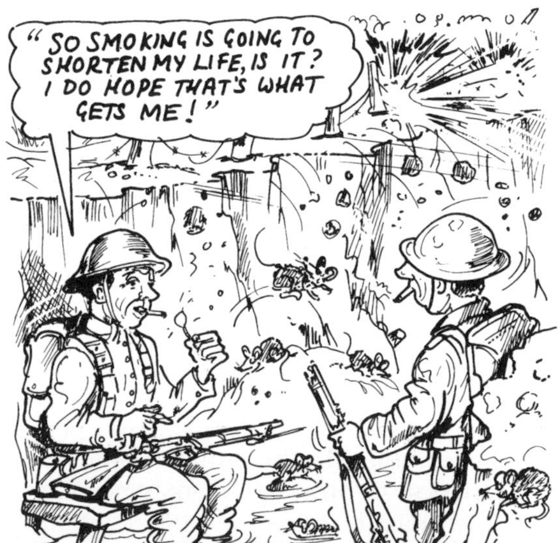
"SO SMOKING IS GOING TO SHORTEN MY LIFE, IS IT? I DO HOPE THAT'S WHAT GETS ME!"

Figure 12.15 Health education may not convince everyone

Poverty and low social class appear to be very closely linked with ill-health. A lack of income may directly cause problems with the purchase of food for a satisfactory diet and so on. The Mintel Study (*The Independent*, 1 February 1994) reports a 'strong link' between wealth and diet:

> The affluent are more likely to eat fresh fruit and vegetables regularly, to have a varied diet, and to say they try to eat healthily than those on a lower income. People who are dependent on state benefits have the least varied diet and are least concerned about healthy eating, maybe because they can't afford to be.

Poorer people were also reported to consume more snacks like crisps and sweets than higher earners.

A National Children's Home study reported by Mary Braid (*The Independent*, 9 November 1993) focused on 120 young people, aged 16 to 25 years, who had left care. One in three of this group said that they had only one or no meals in the last 24 hours. The diet of nearly all this group was reported as nutritionally very poor. Most of this group were living alone and said they were depressed, worried or anxious. The main worries were money and health.

It may be that lack of income also causes people to ignore health as a priority. Why worry about diet, exercise, a balanced lifestyle, and so on if there are other threats and stresses which take priority? Argyle (1987) quotes studies which show that lower-class people made less use of preventative and other health maintenance services. It may not be because of any restriction or lack of entitlement, but rather the issue of how they saw life's priorities.

It would appear that poverty or low income may be a source of stress and compound other stresses which an individual may face. Blaxter notes, 'People with very low incomes, the unemployed, single-handed parents, the divorced and separated, elderly widowed men living alone – all these fared badly on measures of stress and on measures of social isolation.' (Page 222.)

Social policies and their impact on health and social well-being

Nettleton (1995) states, 'According to Lalonde (1976) any effective health policy must work at four levels: health care provision; lifestyle or behavioural factors; environmental pollution and biophysical factors.' (Page 233.)

The new public health approach places great emphasis on individual decision-making. Individuals are to be encouraged to develop healthier lifestyles in order to reduce the number of early deaths from heart disease and cancer. *The Health of the Nation* strategy aims at changing the way individuals behave in order to create a healthier nation. Health care provision has been moving resources to primary health care in the community. Over the past 15 years, large general hospital care for the long-term sick, mentally ill, and old people has gradually been transferred to care in the community.

There is growing concern about environmental pollution. New policies and legislation are likely to be introduced in the future to combat air pollution. Research into medical development continues at a dramatic pace. Much medical research is undertaken within the private sector where market competition motivates research into genetics and medical drugs.

Social policy: The impact of the lifestyles and individual decision-making approach

The Health of the Nation (1992) provides a strategy for greatly reducing the risks of disease and extending the life expectancy of the average person in the UK. The strategy includes targets for reducing mental illness and suicide (see page 272). The approach relies on co-operation between individuals, communities and the government.

Specifically, *The Health of the Nation* initiative sets out the government's role as one of creating individual opportunities and healthy alliances. The issue is to encourage individuals to adopt healthier lifestyles. Healthier lifestyles are seen as the key to improving the health and well-being of the population.

Action to improve the safety of work and home environments and reduce risks from pollution are also built into the policy. Organisations work with the government and individuals to promote safety and healthy lifestyles. *The Health of the Nation* strategy involves the National Health Service, local authorities, the Health Education Authority, voluntary organisations, the media and employers all working to improve the health of individuals. Health promotion is to be targeted at schools and in the workplace.

Practical work on improving health is to be targeted on promoting healthy cities, healthy schools, healthy hospitals, healthy workplaces, healthy homes and healthy environments. *The Health of the Nation* represents a strategic approach to health. This means that the government has a strategy or a 'grand plan' to bring a range of organisations together in order to improve health. This plan will be researched and monitored by health officials who will update the strategy as they receive feedback on its effects.

On the face of it, the *Health of the Nation* policy would appear to have the answers for improving the health and well-being of the population. As was suggested in the previous section, however, there are different perspectives on health, and the lifestyle and health education approach is open to criticism.

Structuralists will criticise the approach for not taking the problems of the poorest people into account. One argument is that health education will mainly benefit the middle classes. People with money will be able to pay for healthy diets, they will be able to pay to use gyms, to buy expensive and fashionable exercise equipment and clothes. Well-educated and well-paid professionals will be able to take up stress-reduction activities, and will be able to find alternatives to alcohol and tobacco to help them relax. The poor will not have access to these privileges. One fear is that the healthy lifestyles approach will lead to improvements in the nation's health, but that all the improvement will be among the better off and the middle classes. Health inequality will therefore get worse as a result of health education.

Those who agree with the interactionist view might add that the problem is not simply about money or disadvantage. The poor and the working class may not be able to accept health education messages in the same way as middle-class people. Many working-class people seem to see health as dependent on luck. Health education campaigns, which stress the importance of diet and exercise, might not be taken seriously by people who are sure that health depends on the 'luck of the draw'. So once again, health inequalities (the fact that the wealthy enjoy better health than the poor) might get worse.

Some authors emphasise that the lifestyle strategy is a 'top down' approach. Health managers decide what they believe is necessary and then set about convincing everyone else to change. An alternative might be to try to work within specific communities to understand their beliefs and needs. Health promotion could then be focused at a community level.

The impact of the lifestyles approach

Individual responsibility and lifestyle choices are a central theme in current social policy. The idea is that individuals make informed choices about their health and social well-being.

The second progress report on the *Health of the Nation* strategy, in July 1995, suggested that some aspects of health are improving. Deaths from heart disease in people under 65 years of age fell by 11 per cent in 1994, suicides fell by 6 per cent between 1993 and 1994, and a reduction in the incidence of gonorrhoea suggests that the 'safe sex' message may be taken seriously. On the other hand, more teenagers are smoking, lung cancer among women may be rising, suicide by young men is increasing, the number of women who drink more than the safe limit of alcoholic drinks may be increasing, and the number of obese men and women is rising.

Assessing the impact of the lifestyle approach may depend on the perspective you choose. The imaginary positivist, structuralist and interactionist characters might react in a range of different ways.

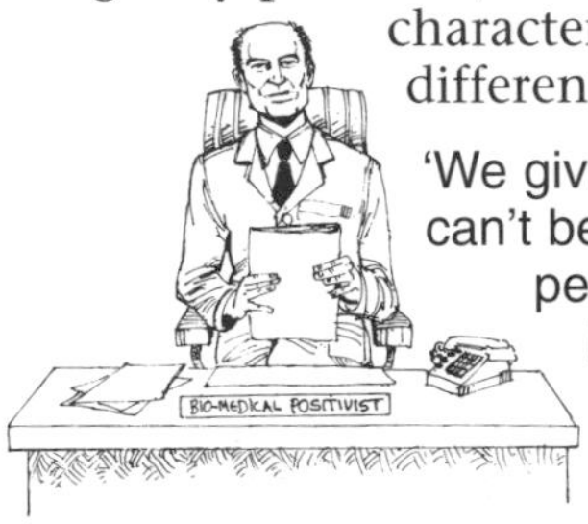

'We give people the information – we can't be responsible for the choices people make. Government and health service workers are not here to control what people do. People are free to listen to us or ignore the evidence … it's up to them. Trying to force people to be healthy would just make them angry. We tell people the truth – what else can we do? People make their own decisions.'

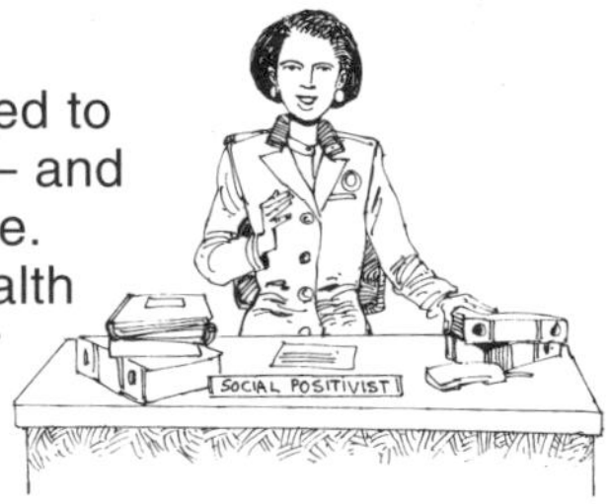

'I suppose people have listened to some of the health message – and not other parts of the message. Perhaps we could try new health education campaigns – better media coverage – to try to make sure everyone is informed in a way they can understand.'

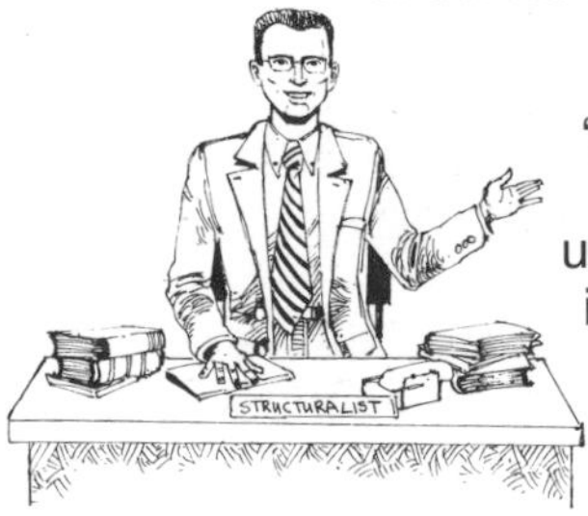

'Many people can't change their lifestyle! As poverty, unemployment and stress increase, so more people will smoke, drink, and become obese or commit suicide. People with resources, money, partners, friends, time – these people can change their lifestyles. Disadvantaged people don't have the same chance. Social policy based on individual decision-making will only really benefit middle-class people.'

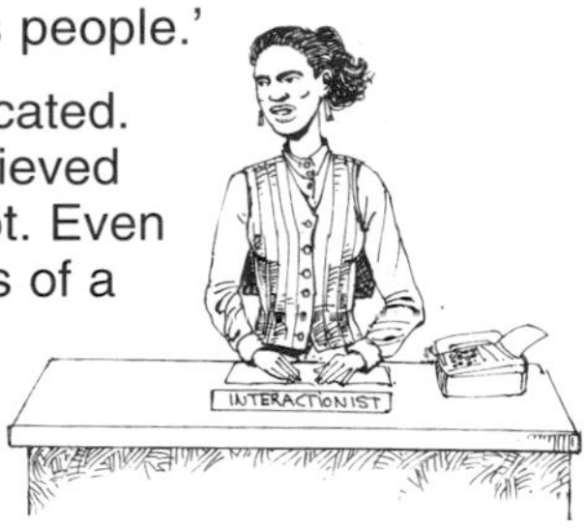

'But the situation will be complicated. Some health messages are believed and responded to, some are not. Even if people have different chances of a healthy life, there may be ways of influencing individuals and communities so that lifestyles might become healthier over time. Just informing people isn't enough, social groups would need to believe that health was important and believe that the advice in *The Health of the Nation* mattered. People would need new opportunities to practise a healthy lifestyle. Social policy based on individual decision-making might mainly benefit middle-class people to begin with. Other groups might benefit if general cultural beliefs promote healthier lifestyles.'

Evidence collection point

You will need to assess the impact of one social policy on the health and social well-being of the population using three demographic characteristics (e.g. disease, disability and dysfunction, suicide, crime, divorce, life expectancy). One idea might be to assess the impact of individual decision-making or lifestyle choices in relation to the *Health of the Nation* targets for disease, disability, life expectancy or suicide. Your assessment might include differing perspectives as well as statistical evidence.

Social policy and the environment

As well as attempting to encourage healthy lifestyles, governments have to regulate or control hazards which may affect people's health. Legislation such as the Health and Safety at Work Act (1974) is designed to protect workers from hazards. Building regulations take health into consideration. There are regulations designed to protect the safety of drinking water, a range of legislation to provide road safety and so on. The government may introduce new legislation to control air pollution and new legislation to monitor and control the general quality of the environment.

Regulation of pollution is widely accepted as a task for central or local government. Environmental pollution is not an issue which can be left up to individuals to choose or decide how to act.

Social policy and community responsibility

The new public health approach focuses on individual responsibility for lifestyle choices. Government control and regulation is necessary in order to combat pollution and maintain a healthy environment. Between individual decision-making and government control lies the idea of community responsibility. Individuals develop their personal lifestyles as a result of socialisation with family and friends. Children's attitudes to health will be influenced by what they learn in school. Attitudes and beliefs are developed during conversations with friends, neighbours, relatives and other people in the local community.

Some politicians are becoming increasingly interested in trying to strengthen the role of the family and of local communities. If families and neighbourhoods are safe, stable and supportive, then social stress and distress may be reduced for some people. So far, community responsibility policies have concentrated on reducing divorce and crime. Some politicians believe that divorce is so widespread because it has become too easy. In the future, couples seeking a divorce may be required to undertake counselling provided by the advice agency Relate before a divorce is granted. The theory is that relationship problems may be helped by counselling and that even if divorce does go ahead, perhaps the process will be managed more carefully.

Crime prevention strategies also seek to build on the role of the community. In 1993 there were 130 000 Neighbourhood Watch schemes, covering some five million households in England and Wales (*Social Trends*, 1995). There is evidence that people who belong to Neighbourhood Watch schemes are likely to be more security conscious than the average. *Social Trends* (1995) notes that Neighbourhood Watch schemes are more likely to operate in areas with a lower risk of burglary, rather than in high crime areas. However, the number of Neighbourhood Watch schemes continues to grow. It may be that community action to prevent crime will become a focus for social policy which emphasises the role of the community.

Social policy and poverty

Some politicians see poverty as a major cause of ill-health, shorter life expectancy, lower social well-being, and therefore crime. The Commission on Social Justice, a group set up by the Labour Party, reported in October 1994 that one in five people is dependent on benefit, one in five men of working age is unemployed, and one in three children lives in poverty. The gap between the highest and the lowest paid is greater than at any time since 1886. Over one million people are classed as long-term unemployed, and over one million pensioners live on income support. The Commission's proposals to reduce poverty included raising child benefit, creating a minimum wage, paying benefit to people who are in work but on low pay, and creating a guaranteed minimum pension. The belief is that a reduction in poverty would lead to improved health and well-being.

The Rowntree Report (1995) also echoes the need to reduce poverty. The report argues that too much public spending 'is directed at paying the costs of failure, rather than in promoting future success.' (Page 41.) That is, public money is used to pay benefits to people who are out of work or poor, but public money is not being used effectively to prevent unemployment and poverty.

The report argues that 'resources need to go into investment, rather than in the future paying the price of failure.' (Page 40.) The Rowntree Report suggests that new policy initiatives are needed to improve the nation's education and training schemes, to encourage people back to work, to review social security benefits, pensions, the balance of taxation, housing benefits and to provide economic support for poor neighbourhoods ('marginalised' or run-down estates and housing areas). New policies aimed at reducing poverty may give people new chances to lead healthier lifestyles, choose healthier diets, reduce chronic illness, suicide, crime and family break-up.

Social policy based on competition and the open market

The idea that reducing poverty will improve the health of the nation is disputed by 'the new right' political viewpoint in the 1990s. Many politicians within the Conservative Party argue that benefits and state pensions create a burden on individuals and businesses. Too much spending on benefits may result in increased taxation. Higher taxation is said to damage 'wealth creation' and the country's prospects for economic growth. Some 'new right' politicians argue that state hand-outs create a dependency culture where individuals stop taking responsibility for their own lives and rely on the state to provide everything. Health and social care professionals, it is said, argue for extended benefits and new services, because this provides new career opportunities for them. Their opinion may often be dismissed as self-interest.

Current government policy has been concerned with introducing market competition into the provision of health and social care services. Markets are often seen as a very good way to increase quality and save money.

Think it over

If you want to buy some apples – you could go to the market place. In the market place providers set out their stalls and you can study the price and quality of what is on offer. You can shop around for the best deal that suits you. This means that:

- the providers (stall holders) are motivated to get your business – they are likely to be helpful and polite
- as stall holders compete with each other, it should keep the price down – if one provider starts to over-charge he or she will lose business
- you will buy what you like, and providers have to try to meet customer demand – to get the kind of apples people want
- quality should be good – you will take your business elsewhere rather than pay for poor-quality produce.

If political systems where the state provided fruit for 'the people' none of these features existed. The state fixed the price, there need only be one type of fruit and the quality was decided by the state. The people 'serving' you didn't need to be helpful – they were doing you a favour! In the state system, the provider controls what you can have. In the market system, the customers control what they get.

If health and social care was as simple as buying fruit, there would be a general agreement that the state should not act as provider and that there should be a market system. But not everyone supports the market idea for health and social care. Buying hospital treatment is very different from buying fruit. Firstly, the patient may not know what he or she needs, how to get it or how to recognise quality. Because of this the purchaser is not the patient but the professional care manager. The system of purchaser–provider service is described in Chapters 13, 14 and 15.

In theory the development of a market for care services should lead to better quality, consumer satisfaction and reduced costs. But because the patient or client is not really in control, there are doubts that the market system will work so effectively. Nettleton (1995) argues that social policies based on the open market create a culture where managers have the power rather than the consumer:

> People's views are being sought ... by health managers, but there are limited mechanisms for ensuring that managers actually act upon these views. Thus there is danger that consumer satisfaction surveys may become an end in themselves. Further, the split between providers and purchasers of care requires that the needs of populations have to be assessed so that health authorities can purchase the appropriate care, and when developing their contracts, Health Service managers can acknowledge people's needs and preferences. However, these activities contribute to a further tier of management in the form of contract managers, needs assessors and quality managers. Is is they who ultimately decide what the consumers want and not the consumers themselves. (Page 250.)

The purchaser–provider system described in Chapters 13–15 is the outcome of the market-based social policy for the delivery of health and social care services. It may be argued that this new system focuses control in the hands of managers, rather than clients or professionals.

Recommendations for improving health and well-being – a summary

The Health of the Nation (1992) sets out a strategy for improving health and well-being. Much of the strategy focuses on the need to persuade individuals to choose healthy lifestyles and habits. The key problem is how individuals might be encouraged to make healthy choices. Is informing people enough? Do some people have a better chance of health than others? The positivist, structuralist and interactionist perspectives lead to different approaches for health education.

The issue of 'life chances' and the association of poverty and poor health is a key issue. People living in run-down housing estates are unlikely to be able to improve their health or well-being, according to the conclusions of the Rowntree Report. Additional financial resources may be needed to reduce poverty and crime in some sections of the community.

One policy option is to increase taxation and use the money to provide better benefits, better state pensions, and education, and to reduce unemployment. Such an approach would reduce poverty and greatly increase opportunities for everyone to enjoy a healthy lifestyle. Most people would like to see better services and better opportunities for health, but not all voters are enthusiastic about paying extra tax. One political argument is that high taxation may reduce the efficiency of the country's economy, and that if the country generally gets 'poorer', there will be less money to improve services.

The issue of pensions may turn out to be a major problem in the future. The level of state and many occupational pensions may depend on the ability and willingness of people still in work to pay towards pension provision.

New policies to support family and community living may reduce some sources of stress. Neighbourhood Watch systems could provide a focus for community action to reduce crime.

A combination of initiatives to reduce crime, support relationships, promote healthy living and reduce poverty might provide the best way forward. Government regulation of pollution and the maintenance of effective health care will continue to be important.

Evidence collection point

For Element 4.3 you must produce an analytical report which describes the use of three demographic characteristics in assessing the health and social well-being of the population, and a summary of how other demographic characteristics are used. The report has to:

- consider the inter-relationships between health and social well-being and socio-economic factors
- assess the impact of one social policy on the health and social well-being of the population using three demographic characteristics in the range
- make at least two reasoned recommendations for possible ways of improving the health and social well-being of the population.

Self-assessment test

1 All major organs of the embryo should have formed by:
  a 2 weeks.
  b 1 week.
  c 20 weeks.
  d 8 weeks.

2 A human from the eighth week of pregnancy until birth is called a:
  a Neonate.
  b Embryo.
  c Foetus.
  d Baby.

3 The stopping of monthly bleeding in females is known as:
  a Menarche
  b Menopause.
  c Menstruation.
  d Menses.

4 The Moro reflex is demonstrated when a baby:
  a Grasps someone's finger strongly.
  b Throws arms and legs out when startled.
  c Turns head towards a touch on the cheek.
  d Makes stepping movements when held upright.

5 Myelination is the process by which:
  a Nerve cells acquire fatty sheaths.
  b Eyes begin to focus.
  c Muscle co-ordination develops.
  d Fat cells begin to form.

6 The hormone responsible for the development of sexual changes during puberty in males is:
  a Oestrogen.
  b Testosterone.
  c Thyroxine.
  d Growth hormone.

7 Babbling is a stage in infant language development when:
  a The baby first learns to use words.
  b The infant starts to organise his or her ability ready to use language.
  c Infants copy the sounds they hear others make.
  d Carers working with infants use baby talk.

8 Which of the following statements is correct?
  a Children have to be taught the grammatical rules of language directly by their carers.
  b Children develop their own grammatical use of language.
  c Children complete their understanding of language by 5 years of age and develop their vocabulary only after this age.
  d Children learn to use language and grammar only by trial and error learning, where other people correct their mistakes.

9 Conservation means that:
  a A child understands how objects, mass,. volume or number work. They can conserve the meaning of the number 10 or understanding that volume doesn't change when water is moved from one container to another.
  b A child conserves his or her intelligence by not trying to use advanced language to describe practical things.
  c A person can improve his or her skills by using concepts to improve performance.
  d Children make appropriate reactions when their reflexes are tested.

10 Egocentric means:
  a That a child is selfish.
  b That a child is unable to imagine other people's views or perceptions if they are different from the child's.
  c That a child is stuck in his or her emotional development and will need professional guidance.
  d That a child is centred in the sensorimotor phase of development.

11 Evidence in the past 20 years suggests that:
  a All children are completely egocentric during the pre-operational period of development.
  b The idea of sensorimotor, pre-operational and concrete periods of cognitive development is totally untrue.
  c Nearly all people develop and use formal logical thought soon after 12 years of age.
  d Many children are not necessarily egocentric and can avoid egocentric behaviours and egocentric answers to questions in the right settings.

12 Which of the following statements best describes the development of self-concept?
  a Parents teach their children how to understand themselves.
  b Children copy the behaviours they see, and start to learn social roles. A sense of self-awareness develops in the context of social roles.

c Self-concept is genetically determined.
d The development of self-concept depends on formal operations.

13 Temperament refers to:
a Types of behaviour to which a person may be pre-disposed from birth.
b A person's general personality.
c The things a person is taught during childhood.
d The genetic inheritance of patterns of behaviour which are invariably inherited from one generation to the next.

14 Traits are:
a Descriptions of general features of an individual's personality.
b Terms which describe the individual's own perception of their character.
c Descriptions of early experience and the influence of early experience on personality.
d Descriptions of negative or problem behaviours which an individual is likely to perform.

15 Humanistic theories of personality:
a Emphasise ethical approaches to understanding personality.
b Emphasise individual perception and thinking systems in interpreting human behaviour.
c Emphasise human genetics and biological influences.
d Emphasise the influence of society and social learning.

16 Psychodynamic theories are theories which:
a Emphasise the struggle between different class groups within society.
b Emphasise the importance of early learning in influencing the development and working of human personality.
c Emphasise the role of genetics and biology in the development of personality.
d Emphasise the importance of self-perception and individual construction of self in understanding personality.

17 Which statement best describes the role of genetics and environment in influencing human development?
a Human development is mainly controlled by the genetic code that a person inherits.
b Genetics has nothing to do with personality, social or emotional development because these things are controlled by society.
c Human development involves both genetics and environment – it's a bit of both.
d Human development is a process where both genetic instructions and environmental influences interact. The two influences are fundamentally inseparable.

18 Which statement best describes how people cope with life transitions?
a People are likely to experience emotional stress and need time to work through a process of adapting to change.
b People usually cope on their own and do not really need help.
c People usually need counselling to cope with major transitions in life.
d People can always cope with change provided they have friends.

19 Which of the following might describe a successful process for coping with transitions in life?
a Denial, projection, acceptance, testing, immobilisation, letting go, internalisation.
b Immobilisation, search, denial, re-evaluation, depression, acceptance.
c Immobilisation, depression, search for meaning, internalisation, testing, letting go, minimisation.
d Immobilisation, minimisation, depression, letting go, testing, search for meaning, internalisation.

20 Which of the following statements is false?
a Changes in life can cause problems for people because change creates uncertainty.
b Major life events can change a person's self-concept and this change can cause stress.
c Major life changes use up time, money and emotional resources.
d Major life changes only cause stress to people who were not expecting them.

21 People learn the ways of thinking and behaving that make them members of the groups that they belong to. This process is known as:
a Acclimatisation.
b Learning.
c Socialising.
d Socialisation.

22 People play many different roles during their lives. A role can be defined as:
a An individual's personality.
b The prestige a person has within a group.
c A socially defined idea of the way a person is expected to behave.
d An artificial way of behaving that people may decide to adopt.

23 People learn language and customs of behaviour during their early years within their family. This is known as:
- **a** Primary socialisation.
- **b** Infancy.
- **c** Early learning.
- **d** Personality development.

24 Through socialisation, people learn the norms of the groups they belong to. Norms can be defined as:
- **a** Ideas about what is right and wrong.
- **b** The ranking of different members of a group.
- **c** A list of what is legal and what is illegal behaviour.
- **d** The customary ways of behaving within a group.

25 Though socialisation, we learn ideas about right and wrong. These ideas are called:
- **a** Values.
- **b** Morals.
- **c** Religious beliefs.
- **d** Norms.

26 Group members have a different rank and level of prestige within a group. This is known as:
- **a** Leadership.
- **b** Role.
- **c** Status.
- **d** Hierarchy.

27 People are socialised by membership of a peer group. A peer group is:
- **a** People who live in the same neighbourhood as ourselves.
- **b** Other members of our family.
- **c** People of the same gender as ourselves.
- **d** People with whom we have a lot in common, and whom we regard as friends.

28 Most people attend compulsory schooling during childhood and early adolescence. Which of the following statements is true of this period in people's lives?
- **a** Socialisation takes place at many levels during schooling.
- **b** Socialisation takes place only through the influence other pupils.
- **c** The formal educational aims of the school are the only significant socialising influence at school.
- **d** People do not experience socialisation at school.

29 The mass media are a part of the lives of everyone in modern Britain. Which of the following statements is true of the media?
- **a** Only young children are socialised through the media.
- **b** The media has no socialising influence on members of society.
- **c** The media can be a socialising influence on anyone who receives its messages.
- **d** The media is only a socialising influence if people are not strong enough to think for themselves.

30 People tend to follow group norms of behaviour, even in crowded and culturally mixed urban environments. This is because:
- **a** People are afraid of facing legal penalties if they don't.
- **b** Fear of ridicule and appearing out of place makes people conform, often without realising that they are doing so.
- **c** People are afraid of being assaulted by others if they don't conform.
- **d** People feel that they will be more successful if they conform to group norms.

31 Structural functionalism is a theory which suggests how roles are defined and acquired by individuals. Which of the following statements describes a functionalist view of social role?
- **a** People learn to be members of either the bourgeoisie or the proletariat.
- **b** People learn roles which are defined by society and support its stability and development.
- **c** People learn roles by negotiation during interaction with others.
- **d** People adapt roles to suit their own needs and inclinations.

32 Some social theorists believe that roles are negotiated through exchanges of ideas and understandings when people communicate with each other. These theorists are known as:
- **a** Social determinists.
- **b** Marxists.
- **c** Structural functionalists.
- **d** Symbolic interactionists.

33 A social construct is:
- **a** A socially defined idea about human life which has no material reality.
- **b** A fact about society.

c A set of ideas about the right way to behave in society.
d A social fact that is part of the experience of every human society.

34 Which of the following statements is true of social constructs?
a Social constructs are fixed and do not change over time.
b Social constructs change only when people's behaviour changes.
c Social constructs change immediately when people's behaviour changes.
d Social constructs may not always change quickly in response to changes in society.

35 Role constructs are one form of social construct. Which of the following is true of role constructs?
a Changes in role constructs always lead to greater equality in society.
b Role constructs are little influenced by changes in the economic structure of society.
c Role constructs can be a major influence on the opportunities open to some members of society.
d Role constructs change rapidly in response to changes in patterns of family life.

36 Power is a social construct that influences many interactions in society. Which of the following statements applies to power?
a Power rests entirely on the capacity to coerce others into submission.
b Power is usually exercised through a combination of authority and the ultimate capacity to coerce.
c Power is usually dependent entirely on the authority an individual commands.
d Power can be exercised by an individual without anyone else being involved.

37 Deviant behaviour may be defined as:
a Behaviour which falls outside the accepted norms of a particular group.
b Behaviour which is dangerous to other people.
c Behaviour which is against the law.
d Behaviour which is morally wrong.

38 Some interactionists believe that labelling someone as deviant may lead him or her to commit further acts of deviancy. This is because:
a All deviants have a tendency to re-offend.
b People may accept the label deviant and begin to live up to it.
c People may want to get back at society for labelling them.
d People are driven by social circumstances to carry out further deviant acts.

39 Differences in cultural background can lead to conflicts in a multi-cultural society. This is because:
a People with different cultural backgrounds have different levels of income.
b Some cultures have values that are right whilst others have values which are wrong.
c People often don't understand the languages used in other cultures.
d Different cultures may have different values and norms of behaviour associated with particular issues and situations.

40 Different cultures have different norms defining deviant behaviour. Which of the following is a likely outcome of this?
a The norms of minority cultures change to fit those of broader society.
b Conflicts occur occasionally between the expectations of members of different groups.
c The norms of the broader society change to accept the behaviour of members of minority cultures.
d People are not concerned with the behaviour of members of other groups in society.

41 Demography is:
a The study of democratic institutions.
b The geography of a country.
c The study of population characteristics.
d Local or small-scale geography.

42 Health is:
a A concept which is always understood as meaning that people are free from disease and illness.
b A concept that means that people feel they are all right.
c A concept which means that people have enough money to be healthy.
d A concept with different meanings for different people and where there is no general agreement as to how it can be measured.

43 Between 1971 and 1995 the population of the UK grew by:
a 75 per cent
b 40 per cent
c 14 per cent
d 4 per cent

44 The main single cause of death in the UK today is:
- **a** Heart and circulatory disease.
- **b** AIDS.
- **c** Lung cancer.
- **d** Tuberculosis.

45 In 1991, deaths in the UK from all types of cancer accounted for:
- **a** 50 per cent of all deaths.
- **b** 25 per cent of all deaths.
- **c** 15 per cent of all deaths.
- **d** 5 per cent of all deaths.

46 Which of the following activities does not increase the risk of circulatory disease?
- **a** Smoking.
- **b** Heavy drinking, i.e. high consumption of alcohol.
- **c** A high-fat diet.
- **d** Regular exercise.

47 Three of the following statements can be justified by the recent Health Survey for England. One statement is untrue. Identify the false statement.
- **a** One in five adults takes no serious exercise.
- **b** Two-thirds of adults have cholesterol values above the desired level.
- **c** Working-class women were more likely to be overweight than middle-class women.
- **d** Only a small group of men in the 18 to 25 category drink more alcohol than the recommended maximum amount.

48 Three of the following statements can be justified by evidence published in *Social Trends* (1995). One statement is false. Identify the false statement.
- **a** Smoking is strongly related to social class; far more working-class people smoke than middle-class people.
- **b** In England, half of men and two in every five women are overweight or obese.
- **c** High blood pressure is a serious problem for younger people.
- **d** Almost one in four 15-year-old children smoke.

49 Three of the following statements can be justified by evidence published in *The Health of the Nation* (1992). One statement is false. Identify the false statement.
- **a** Smoking contributes to 80 per cent of deaths from lung cancer and 30 per cent of all deaths from cancer.
- **b** Most people get cancer at some time in their life.
- **c** Obesity (being very overweight) is associated with certain types of cancer.
- **d** It is a good idea to avoid excessive consumption of alcohol in order to avoid cancer.

50 Current government policy as set out in *The Health of the Nation* strategy is sometimes called the 'new public health' approach. What is the main focus of this policy?
- **a** To spend more on treating people in clinics and hospitals.
- **b** To try to influence people to lead healthier lifestyles.
- **c** To provide better sanitation and food hygiene.
- **d** To boost immunisation programmes to protect people from disease.

51 Three of the following statements can be justified by evidence reported in *Social Trends* (1995). One statement is false. Identify the false statement.
- **a** People generally live much happier and healthier lives than 25 years ago.
- **b** Long-term illness and disability may have increased in the last 25 years.
- **c** Over the last 10 years there appears to have been a major increase in the amount of asthma in the population.
- **d** Suicide rates for younger males have more than doubled since 1971 in England and Wales.

52 General demographic evidence may be used to justify three of the following statements. One statement is false. Identify the false statement.
- **a** One in three marriages now ends in divorce.
- **b** Almost one in four children might expect their parents to divorce before the child's sixteenth birthday.
- **c** One child in eight might expect to become part of a step-family in the UK in the 1990s.
- **d** People are getting married earlier than in previous generations.

53 Which statement is false?
- **a** The number of notifiable offences recorded by the police tripled in England and Wales between 1971 and 1992.
- **b** Over 90 per cent of notifiable offences in 1993 were crimes against property rather than attacks on people.
- **c** The majority of crimes against property are committed in wealthy areas.
- **d** Neighbourhood Watch schemes are more likely to operate in areas with a lower risk of burglary, rather than in high crime areas.

54 Which statement best describes the distribution of wealth in the UK today?

- **a** Wealth is shared evenly between everyone.
- **b** The richest 10 per cent of the population owns well over half the country's wealth whilst the poorest 50 per cent of people own less than 10 per cent of the country's wealth.
- **c** Although wealth is not spread evenly, the poorer section of society is rapidly increasing its share of the country's wealth.
- **d** The richest 10 per cent of the population owns 25 per cent of the country's wealth whilst the poorest 50 per cent owns 40 per cent of the country's wealth.

55 Which statement best describes the links between social class and health?

- **a** Working-class people and poor people are more likely to die at a younger age than middle- and upper-class people, and working-class people are likely to have more long-term illnesses in their life than middle-class people.
- **b** Class and wealth have nothing to do with health. Health is just a matter of luck.
- **c** Working-class people suffer more respiratory illnesses, but middle-class people suffer more effects from smoking and excessive drinking because they can afford these habits.
- **d** Working-class people suffer more physical illness, but middle-class people have more stress-related illness and mental illness because of mental pressures.

56 Which of the following air pollutants is not seen as an issue of major concern nowadays?

- **a** Low-level ozone
- **b** Oxides of nitrogen and volatile organic compounds.
- **c** Soot and sulphur dioxide.
- **d** Particulate – exhaust particles.

57 Which of the following best describes the links between poverty and environmental stress?

- **a** People living in poverty are more likely to be exposed to crime, to stressed relationships, to poor housing and to poor employment opportunities and lifestyles which place their health at risk, as compared to others.
- **b** People living in poverty have trouble making ends meet, but they are more likely to enjoy a fulfilling community life because of their close links with others.
- **c** People living in poverty learn to cope with stress because they are brought up to cope.
- **d** People who live in poverty cannot afford bad habits and so they tend to live healthier and more stress-free lives than middle-class people.

58 Which statement would most closely fit structuralist interpretation of health issues?

- **a** People's health mainly depends on their genetic inheritance and making the right life choices.
- **b** People's health is a matter of their life chances. People don't really have choices. Middle-class people have better chances of health than poor people.
- **c** People's health is strongly influenced by the way people come to understand their health and what matters in life. People have different chances, but they also have choices.
- **d** People's health would improve dramatically if only we could get health education messages across effectively.

59 From an interactionist viewpoint, what would be the most important issue when preparing a health education campaign?

- **a** To find out what the target group believe about health issues at the moment; before organising a campaign.
- **b** To ensure that the information was simple and to the point.
- **c** To give people the facts and warn people of the dangers they face.
- **d** To think of clever ways to catch people's attention and keep them interested.

60 The market model in Health and Social Care means that:

- **a** People in need can choose exactly what services they want.
- **b** The state enables people to be given a fixed service if they can prove they deserve or need it.
- **c** People's needs are assessed and there is a managerial role to find the right services within budget constraints to meet individual need.
- **d** People can shop around to get the best service for themselves.

Fast Facts

Accommodation A process which happens when existing knowledge is changed to fit with new learning.

Assimilation Learning to link a new piece of knowledge to what you already know.

Asthma A rapidly increasing long-term (chronic) illness which now affects over 2 million people in the UK and causes over 1600 deaths a year.

Babbling A stage infants go through before they can use language. The infant makes sounds which may later help him or her to use words.

Baby talk Adults use a high-pitched voice and slow down their speech when talking to infants. Adults may also use exaggerated facial expressions. Baby talk may help to keep an infant's attention.

Belonging A feeling of identifying with a particular group of people. Feeling safe and supported by a particular group.

Bereavement and loss A process of transition or coping with change following a loss. Loss of a loved person is usually called bereavement. But the process may be similar in any loss, such as loss of a limb. The process may involve phases of shock, searching, using defences, anger and guilt, before final reconstruction of identity is possible.

Bio-medical positivism The view that logical analysis using biological science and knowledge will explain the causes of health and ill-health without reference to broader viewpoints.

Bonding Making an emotional attachment to a person. Babies usually make an attachment to carers during the first year of life.

Buffering Partners, friends and family may protect a person from the full stress of life changes and conflicts. Michael Argyle called this protection buffering.

Cancer The uncontrolled growth of abnormal body cells. Malignant cancer will disrupt normal body functions. In 1991, 25 per cent of all deaths in the UK were caused by cancer. One in four people might be expected to die from cancer, and one in three might develop cancer in their lifetime.

Change Life involves coping with a wide variety of change – some of which is welcome and some not. Change can also be classified as predictable or unpredictable.

Circulatory disease Disease of the heart and blood circulatory system. It was the cause of 46 per cent of all deaths in the UK in 1991. It is the major cause of death in the UK.

Cognition A term which covers the mental processes involved in understanding and knowing.

Concepts Linguistic (language) terms used to classify, predict and explain physical and social reality. They are probably dependent on experience of events, usefulness in terms of simplifying experience and ability to be shared with others.

Concrete operations The third stage of intellectual development in Piaget's theory. At this stage, individuals can solve logical problems provided they can see or sense the objects with which they are working. At this stage, children cannot cope with abstract problems.

Conservation The ability to understand the logical principles involved in the way number, volume, mass and objects work.

Construction Construction means to build or develop. Beliefs about self and others are often built or 'constructed' from our experience within a social context.

Constructs Individual concepts which don't have to be shareable. Constructs are private ways of evaluating ourselves, others and things. They can be used in patterns to create pre-emptive, constellatory or propositional evaluations.

Culture The collection of values, norms, customs and behaviours that make a group distinct from other groups. Cultures have their own system of values which may be linked to religious beliefs. The culture we are raised in may be one of the biggest influences in our lives.

Cycle of deviance Part of the theory of labelling that was developed by interactionists in their work on deviant behaviour. People who are labelled as deviant by society are said to be pushed by this into further deviance, thus entering a cycle of deviant behaviour.

De-centring The ability to use concepts and mental processes to free judgement from the way things look.

Dementia A term which covers a range of illnesses involving the degeneration (or wasting) of the brain. Dementia is not part of normal ageing. Most very old people shown no sign of dementing illness.

Demography The science of measuring the population characteristics of a country.

Depression Used as a clinical term, depression indicates a loss of social and emotional functioning. One in five people may be expected to experience clinical depression at some stage of their lives.

Determinism The view that human behaviour is determined or caused either by the environment (social determinism) or by genetics (biological determinism).

Differential growth rates The nervous system grows rapidly in the first few years of life, the reproductive organs hardly grow until puberty, while general bodily growth occurs fairly steadily throughout childhood.

Disability The loss of ability. Ability is socially constructed, i.e. it depends on the perceptions of social groups.

Dysfunction The loss or impairment of a function, something not working so as to fulfil its function.

Egocentricity An inability to understand that other people's perceptions or feelings could be different from your own. Piaget believed that pre-operational children were egocentric. More recent evidence casts some doubt on this theory.

Embryo The developing child during the first eight weeks of life in the womb.

Emotional development A focus on the feelings that individuals may have in association with expected relationship patterns in their culture.

Emotional maturity The development of a stable self-concept, or identity, which enables an individual to become independent and take responsibility for his or her own actions.

Environment The surroundings that a person or people function in. Environment includes air quality, water quality, landscape, housing, noise, physical and social context – everything that affects people.

Expected life events Changes which upset people's normal life routines. Expected life events can be welcome or unwanted. Emotional reactions may have more to do with the desirability of the change than with its predictability.

Extroversion In Eysenck's theory of temperament, extroverted people are hungry for stimulation. Extroverts might seek adventure and change.

Fertilisation The point in time when a sperm nucleus from the father joins with an egg nucleus from the mother. This can begin the process which will lead to new life.

Foetus The name given to the developing life within the mother's womb from week 8 to week 40 (birth).

Formal operations The fourth and final stage in Piaget's theory of intellectual development. People with formal logical operations can solve abstract problems.

Functionalism Also called structural functionalism. A theory about the structure and workings of society. Emil Durkheim and Talcott Parsons were leading functionalist thinkers. Functionalists see society as made up of interdependent sections which work together to fulfil the functions necessary for the survival of society as a whole. People are socialised into roles and behaviours which fulfil the needs of society.

Genetic code A set of instructions passed from one generation to another for building a living organism.

Grammar The rules for organising or using a language.

Group A collection of individuals who are seen as being linked by common characteristics such as appearance, interests or behaviour.

Health The World Health Organisation's definition of health is, 'A state of complete physical, mental and social well-being, and not the absence of disease or infirmity.'

Health of the Nation targets Goals the government has set for improving the health of the population.

Holmes–Rahe scale A scale of life events which may put pressure on individuals to make a social readjustment. The scale was researched in the USA in the 1960s by Holmes and Rahe. The scale may be a useful starting point for cataloguing life-event threats.

Humanistic theory A perspective on human personality and behaviour which regards personality as resulting from an individual's system of thinking and feeling.

Hypothesis A theory or idea which can be tested out in practice.

Hypothetical constructs Theoretical ideas which can be helpful when trying to solve abstract problems. Part of intelligent adult problem-solving.

Identity Put simply, a person's identity is how she understands herself and make sense of her life in relation to other people and society.

Impairment Damage to, or loss of, a physical function of the body.

Income Money that an individual or household gets from work, from investments and other sources. Income is usually thought of as income per week or income per month. For statistical purposes, income per year may be recorded.

Independence Being able to function without being dependent on others. Adolescence is seen as a time of growing independence in Western culture.

Infancy A term used to cover the first 18 months of life.

Interactionist perspectives The view that people construct their own view of social reality during their interaction with others. People also build their own ideas as to what causes health or ill-health.

Introversion In Eysenck's theory of temperament, introverted people try to avoid stimulation. Introverts might try to avoid excitement.

Language acquisition device Noam Chomsky theorised that people had an in-built ability to learn, think and communicate using language. The language acquisition device enabled children to understand the deep structure which all languages follow.

Life chances The view that people are born with different advantages or disadvantages with respect to wealth and health. Some people have a better chance of being socialised into healthy habits than others. Some people will experience less stress than others. Some people may be exposed to poorer housing and poorer diets than others from birth.

Life crises Eight developmental stages which influence personality in Erikson's theory of personality.

Lifestyle choice The view that people are free to choose their way of life. For example, people may be free to choose a healthy diet, a healthy balance of rest and exercise, healthy habits such as only moderate drinking of alcohol and not smoking.

Maternal deprivation Bowlby's theory that children would become emotionally damaged if separated from their mother during a critical period of their early life.

Media All the methods of mass transmission of information within society. It includes television, radio and newspapers.

Menopause Cessation of menstruation, usually occurring naturally between the ages of 45 and 55.

Mental illness A loose term, used to cover social and emotional disability. Categories include schizophrenia, affective or emotional illness (psychosis), depression and anxiety. Sometimes the term is also used to include dementia.

Metacognition Understanding or knowledge of your own knowledge.

Motor development How muscles co-ordinate and pull together to enable more and more complicated movements to occur.

Nature–nurture debate A debate that has gone on for hundreds of years as to whether inheritance (nature) or environment (nurture) are most important in making people what they are. A modern view claims nature and nurture cannot be meaningfully separated.

New public health care The most recent stages of health care philosophy, according to Ashton and Seymour. Governments seek to improve public health by influencing the habits and lifestyles of the population, rather than by concentrating on curing illness or offering therapy. This approach is seen as starting from the mid-1970s.

Norms Patterns of behaviour that are expected to be followed by the members of a particular group. Different groups have their own sets of norms to which members are expected to conform. Society as a whole has norms which all are expected to follow, and some of which are backed by legal sanctions.

Object permanence The understanding that objects exist whether they can be seen or not. Piaget theorised that infants would develop object permanence only at the end of the sensorimotor period.

Oestrogen A female sex hormone (actually a group of hormones) responsible for secondary sexual characteristics.

Peer group A group of people who share common characteristics or circumstances, and feel themselves to be like one another. We are all members of peer groups, and may join several different peer groups during our lives. Peer groups are an agent of socialisation. We learn our role, and the norms and values of the group, as we become a member.

Power A relationship where one person is able to influence or control aspects of the life of another. Power is an aspect of many social relationships. It may be exerted through coercion or authority, or through a combination of the two.

Pre-conceptual A period when children can communicate, but do not necessarily understand the meaning of the terms they use.

Pre-operational The second stage of Piaget's theory of intellectual development. pre-operational children are understood as being pre-logical. They cannot reason logically.

Primary socialisation The socialisation that takes place during early childhood. The language, values and norms of the society the child has been born into are acquired. Through primary socialisation in the family the child learns how to be an accepted member of the group. (See also **Socialisation**.)

Primitive reflexes Reflexes which are present in the newborn, but disappear after a few months to be replaced by learned responses.

Psychodynamic A perspective on human personality and behaviour which emphasises the importance of early learning.

Puberty The period of change leading towards being capable of sexual reproduction.

Registrar-General's social classification A method of stratifying the population along the lines of class. Occupational groups are used as the basis for deciding class membership, and there are five class groups in the scale.

Regulation The monitoring and control something. In Piaget's theory the development of knowledge is regulated by a balance of assimilation and accommodation. Autonomous, active and conscious regulation systems may explain how skills are learned and developed.

Risk factors Physical states or behaviours or lifestyles that create a risk of illness or disease.

Role The behaviour adopted by individuals when they are interacting in social situations. People learn their roles through the socialisation process, and may play many different roles during their lives.

Self-concept The use of many concepts to describe, understand and perhaps predict what we are like. Understanding of self.

Self-confidence An individual's confidence in his or her own ability to achieve something or cope with a situation. Self-confidence may influence and be influenced by self-esteem.

Self-efficacy An individual's ability to understand and perhaps predict his or her own abilities in relation to any tasks or challenge. High self-efficacy involves the belief that you will succeed at a given task. Self-efficacy may become a general feature of a person's identity.

Self-esteem How well or badly a person feels about himself or herself. High self-esteem may help a person to feel happy and confident. Low self-esteem may lead to depression and unhappiness.

Sensorimotor The first stage in Piaget's theory of intellectual development. Infants learn to co-ordinate their muscle movements in relation to things that they sense.

Sexual maturity A stage of physical development that results in the ability of males and females to reproduce.

Smog A fog mixed with soot and sulphur dioxide from coal smoke. Smog affected cities in the UK in the 1950s and early 1960s. Chemical or invisible smog may create a serious air pollution problem nowadays. This new air pollution problem is caused by motor vehicles.

Social class A social group who share a common degree of power or wealth in society. Class membership is linked to occupation, income, wealth, beliefs and lifestyle.

Social construct A feature of society about which people share a common understanding. Ideas like 'housewife', 'crime' and 'health' are examples of social constructs. Social constructs have no concrete existence, but they are such an integral part of social interaction that they may seem as though they have.

Social context The setting for group and social influences or individual learning.

Social development A focus on the way groups may influence relationship patterns within a culture.

Social learning theory A perspective on human personality and behaviour which emphasises the importance of the environment and the ability of individuals to learn from, and copy, the behaviour of others.

Social networks Where people are linked to each other like the links in a net. Social networks may provide help and support during times of need.

Social positivism The view that logical analysis using biological and social science knowledge will explain the causes of health or ill-health.

Social stratification The outcome of dividing the population up into layers or strata. Society can be stratified on the basis of class, income, race, age, or any other characteristic by which people can be separated into groups.

Social support networks Partners, friends, family and relatives, membership of community groups which provide a source of support for own self-esteem. Support may often be provided in the context of conversation which permits self-disclosure (talking about oneself).

Socialisation The process by which we learn the norms, values and behaviour that makes us a member of a particular group. We learn the roles that we are expected to play as a group member.

Spatial awareness The ability to make sense and respond appropriately to objects in space.

Status A measure of the rank and prestige of a person or a group of people. Status helps to define how people are treated by others, and how they see themselves. Status is linked to role, and different roles in a group have different levels of status attached to them.

Stress response A physical reaction that helps a person to fight or run away. The stress response may create problems when a person cannot fight or run or such a reaction is inappropriate. A person may become 'stressed' because he or she cannot escape from an emotional problem.

Stress-related illnesses Many illnesses may be made worse by stress. Illnesses particularly associated with stress are heart disease, strokes, diabetes, digestive disorders, skin problems and extra vulnerability to colds and flu. Migraines, headaches, aches and pains, anxiety, insomnia and obsessional behaviour may all be caused or made worse by stress.

Structuralism The view that society is structured in terms of economic power, with different groups having very different advantages and disadvantages when it comes to understanding health and illness.

Telegraphic speech A kind of early speech where a child sends a message using only a few words, for example 'Cat goed' meaning 'The cat has gone away'.

Temperament The behaviour style or styles that an individual develops as a result of biological influences. Behaviour patterns in babies and infants are thought to influence their care-givers. As well as early reactions, traits like introversion and extroversion have been thought to be due to temperament.

Therapeutic era A stage in the development of public health, according to the authors Ashton and Seymour. From the 1930s to 1970s, governments concentrated health care policy on the idea of curing individuals or intervening in their problems or illnesses (giving therapy). Secondary health care services, such as hospitals and clinics, were seen as the focus for improving the nation's health.

Threat Something which is understood as a danger to physical, social or emotional well-being.

Trait A description of a person's characteristics. A person might be perceived as extroverted, sympathetic, stable, creative, and so on.

Transitions Changes in a person's life which may require a process of readjustment. Transition is a wide term which can include changes in work patterns and work culture, as well as issues like life-event threats.

Type 'A' behaviour A stress-inducing behaviour pattern which people may learn. 'Type A' behaviour is associated with heart disease. Key features include being hurried, competitive, aggressive, selfish, impatient and easily bored.

Unexpected life events Changes which upset people's normal life routines and expectations. Unexpected life events may be welcome or unwelcome. Unwelcome events may create a range of problems for an individual to cope with.

Values Beliefs about what is good and bad, right and wrong, worthless or worth striving for. Group values help to explain and define group norms of behaviour.

Wealth The value of the property owned by a person. Wealth includes the value of houses, cars, savings and any other personal possessions.

References and further reading

* Recommended further reading

* Aggleton, P., 1990, *Health,* Routledge

* Argyle, M., 1987, *The Psychology of Happiness,* Methuen

Bandura, A., 1989, 'Perceived self-efficiency in the exercise of personal agency' in *The Psychologist,* 2 (10), 411–24

Becker, H., 1963, *Outsiders: Studies in the Sociology of Deviance,* Free Press

Berger, P. and Luckman, T., 1967, *The Social Construction of Reality,* Penguin

* Berryman, J. *et al.*, 1991, *Developmental Psychology and You,* BPS books and Routledge

*Bilton, T., *et al.*, 1987, *Introductory Sociology,* Macmillan

Black, D., *et al.*, 1980, 'The Black Report' in Townsend, P., *et al.*, 1988, *Inequalities in Health,* Penguin

* Blaxter, M., 1990, *Health and Lifestyles,* Routledge

Bowlby, J., 1953, *Child Care and the Growth of Love,* Penguin

Bowlby, J., 1969, *Attachment and Loss,* Vol. 1, Hogarth Press

Brayne, C. and Ames, D., 1988, 'The epidemiology of mental disorders in old age' in Gearing, B. *et al.*, 1988, *Mental Health Problems in Old Age,* John Wiley & Sons

Brown, R., 1973, *A First Language: The Early Stages,* Harvard University Press

Bruner, J., 1974, *Beyond the Information Given*, George Allen & Unwin

Cattell, R.B., 1965 *The Scientific Study of Personality,* Penguin

Clarke, A.M. and Clarke, A.D.B. (eds), 1976, *Early Experience: Myth and Evidence,* Open Books

Cohen, D., 1981, *Piaget : Critique and Reassessment,* Croom Helm

Cohen, S., 1973, *Folk Devils and Moral Panics : The Creation of the Mods and Rockers*, Paladin

Colman, D. and Salt, J., 1992, T*he British Population,* Oxford University Press

Davis, K., 1970, *Human Society,* Macmillan

Durkheim, E., 1938, *The Rules of Sociological Method,* Free Press

Erikson, E., 1963, *Childhood and Society,* Norton

Eysenck, H.J., 1965, *Fact and Fiction in Psychology,* Pelican

Fantz, R., 1961, 'The origin of form perception' in *Scientific American,* 204, 1097–104

Friedman, M and Roseman, R., 1975, *Type A Behaviour and Your Heart,* Wildwood House

Gordon, D. and Forest, R., 1995, *People and Places 2: Social and Economic Distinctions in England,* School for Advanced Urban Studies, University of Bristol

Gross, R., 1992, *Psychology* (2nd edition), Hodder & Stoughton

Hampson, S., 1982, *The Construction of Personality,* Routledge and Kegan Paul

* Haralambos, M., 1985, *Sociology Themes and Perspectives,* Unwin Hyman

Haralambos, M. and Holborn, M., 1991, *Sociology Themes and Perspectives* (3rd edition), Collins Educational.

* Harris, P., 1989, *Children and Emotion,* Basil Blackwell

* Hayes, N. and Orrell, S., 1993, *Psychology: An Introduction*, (2nd edition), Longman

Hayes, N., 1995, *Psychology in Perspective,* Macmillan

Herbert, M., 1981, *Behavioural Treatment of Problem Children,* Academic Press

Holmes, T.H. and Rahe, R.H., 1967, 'The social readjustment rating scale' in *Journal of Psychosomatic Research,* 11, 213–18.

* Hopson, B., 1986, 'Transition: Understanding and managing personal change' in Herbert, M. (ed), 1986, *Psychology for Social Workers,* The British Psychological Society and Macmillan

Jones, K. and Moon, G., 1987 *Health, Disease and Society,* Routledge.

* Jones, S., 1993, *The Language of the Genes,* Flamingo/HarperCollins

Joseph Rowntree Foundation, 1995, *Inquiry into Income and Wealth*, The Joseph Rowntree Foundation

Kelly, G.A., 1955, *A Theory of Personality*, Norton (Norton Edition, 1963)

Klinnert, M., 1984, 'The regulation of infant behaviour by maternal facial expression' in *Infant Behaviour and Development,* 7, 447–65.

Lockwood, D., 1978, 'Some remarks on "The social system"' in Worsley, P. (ed.), 1978, *Modern Sociology,* Penguin

McGarrigle, J. and Donaldson, M., 1975, 'Conservation accidents' in *Cognition,* 3, 341–50

Mead, G.H., 1934, *Mind, Self and Society* (ed. Morris, C.), University of Chicago Press

Millar, E., 1977, *Abnormal Ageing,* John Wiley

* Moore, S., 1993, *Social Welfare Alive,* Stanley Thornes

* National Council for Voluntary Agencies, 1991, *The Voluntary Agencies Directory* (12th edition), Bedford Square Press

* Nettleton, S., 1995, *The Sociology of Health and Illness,* Polity Press

Oakley, A., 1974, *Housewife,* Allen Lane

Parkes, C.M., 1975, *Bereavement,* Penguin

Pinker, S., 1995, *Language Instinct,* Penguin

Plomin, 1989, 'Environment and genes' in *American Psychologist,* 44 (2), 105–11

Richards, M.P.M., 1993, 'The new genetics: Some issues for social scientists' in *Sociology of Health and Illness,* 15 (5)

Rose, S., Lewontin, R.C. and Kamin, L.J., 1984, *Not in our Genes,* Penguin

Rowntree Report – See Joseph Rowntree Foundation

Rutter, M., 1981, *Maternal Deprivation Reassessed* (2nd edition), Penguin

Schaffer, H.R. and Emerson, P.E., 1964, 'The development of social attainments in infancy' in *Monographs of Social Research in Child Development,* 29 (94)

Segall *et al.*, 1990, Human *Behaviour in Global Perspective,* Pergamon Press

Skinner, B.F., 1957, *Verbal Behaviour,* Appleton Century-Crofts

* *Social Trends 24,* 1994, HMSO

* *Social Trends 25,* 1995, HMSO

Sorce, J.F. Emde, R.N., Campos, J.J. and Klinnert, M.D., 1985, 'Maternal emotional signalling' in *Developmental Psychology,* 21, 195–200

Stewart, R.B. and Marvin, R.S., 1984, 'Sibling relations' in *Child Development,* 55, 1322–32

Stopford, V., 1987, *Understanding Disability*, Edward Arnold

The Health of the Nation, 1992, HMSO

Thomas, A., Chess, S. and Birch, H.G., 1968, *Temperament and Behaviour Disorders in Children,* University of London Press

Townsend, P.,*et al.*, 1988, *Inequalities in Health,* Penguin

Walker-Andrews, A., 1986, 'Intermodel perception of expressive behaviours: Relation of eye and voice?' in *Developmental Psychology,* 22, 373–7

Watson, P. and Johnson-Laird, N.J., 1972, *Psychology of Reasoning: Structure and Content,* Batsford

Whitehead, M., 1988, 'The health divide' in Townsend, P., *et al.*, 1988, *Inequalities in Health,* Penguin

Wolf, D., Rygh, J. and Altshuler, J., 1984, 'Agency and experience: Actions and states in play narratives' in Brehterton, I. (ed.), 1984, *Symbolic Play,* Academic Press

World Health Organisation, 1946, Constitution, Geneva

* Worsley, P. (ed.), 1992, *The New Introducing Sociology,* Penguin

Young, P. (ed.), 1985, *Mastering Social Welfare,* Macmillan

Zborowski, M., 1969, *People in Pain,* Jossey-Bass

* Zimbardo, P.G. *et al.*, 1992 *Psychology and Life,* HarperCollins

Chapter 13

The provision of health and social care services and facilities

Health and social care has, for a long time, been provided by a mixture of statutory, private and voluntary agencies and informal carers. Who provides what proportion of care at any one time depends on a number of factors. These will include:

- **the attitude of the public towards state intervention**
- **the ability of the state to finance the services that are required**
- **the ability of individuals to contribute towards either the practical aspects of caring, or financially towards the cost of care services.**

The two main statutory organisations which organise the provision of health and social care in Britain are the National Health Service and local authority social services departments (Figure 13.1).

This chapter deals with:

- **the legal framework for the provision of services, including statutory services**
- **the role of the private and voluntary sectors in the provision of health and social care**
- **informal care provision**
- **how services may be classified**
- **how health and social care is resourced**
- **how health and social care services may be accessed.**

The legal framework for the provision of care

Care services operate within a legal framework. The powers and duties of the services, in particular social services, are set out in various Acts of Parliament. The difference between powers and duties is quite straightforward. Where the law imposes a duty on a person or an organisation, then they *have* to carry out that duty – they have no choice. Where the law gives a person or an organisation the power to do something, then they may *choose* to exercise that power, but they do not have to. Statutory services are those services set out in Acts of Parliament that organisations have a duty to provide.

The principal Acts of Parliament which set out the powers and duties of the health and social care services are:

- the National Health Service Act 1946
- the National Assistance Act 1948
- the Health Services and Public Health Act 1968
- the Local Authority Social Services Act 1970
- the Chronically Sick and Disabled Persons Act 1970
- the Mental Health Act 1983
- the Disabled Persons (Consultation and Representation) Act 1986
- the Children Act 1989
- the National Health Service and Community Care Act 1990.

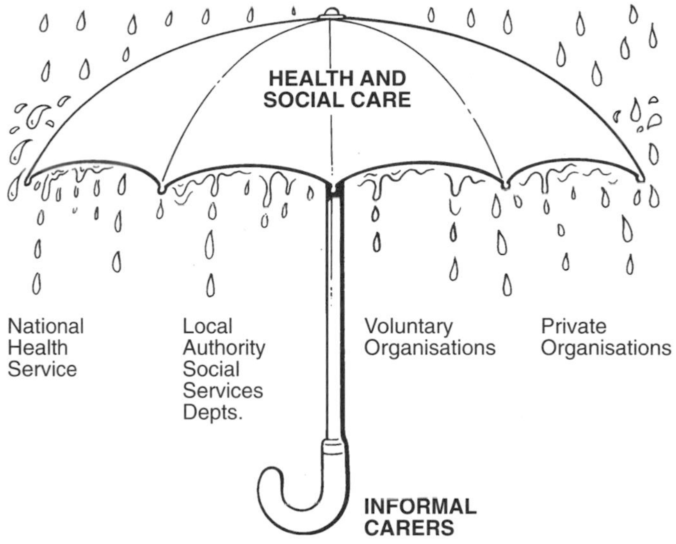

Figure 13.1 The providers of health and social care services

Historical background

The Poor Law system, introduced in 1572, was the beginning of the concept that there should be legislation to provide a basic 'safety net' that would prevent people from literally finding themselves in the gutter. From 1834 it was reorganised with boards of guardians elected by local ratepayers. At that time it was considered that people were totally responsible for their own misfortune and therefore they were only given very basic help, and they had to work for it (i.e. in workhouses). Initially, it was the responsibility of the local parish council to administer the Poor Law. The job was then taken over by the national government in order to ensure a uniform, national level of subsistence benefit. Social services functions are derived from the original role of the parish council. Additionally, the drive for public health, through the supply of adequate water supplies and drainage, led to the development of a public health service.

The National Health Service Act 1946

The basic principle of this Act was that a universal health service should be available to everyone. It set out to provide a comprehensive health and rehabilitation service available to everyone through a tripartite system of hospitals, medical and local health services and welfare services. Local authority and voluntary hospitals were nationalised. Local health and welfare services included maternity and childcare, vaccination and immunisation, health visiting, domestic help, home nursing and ambulances (Figure 13.2).

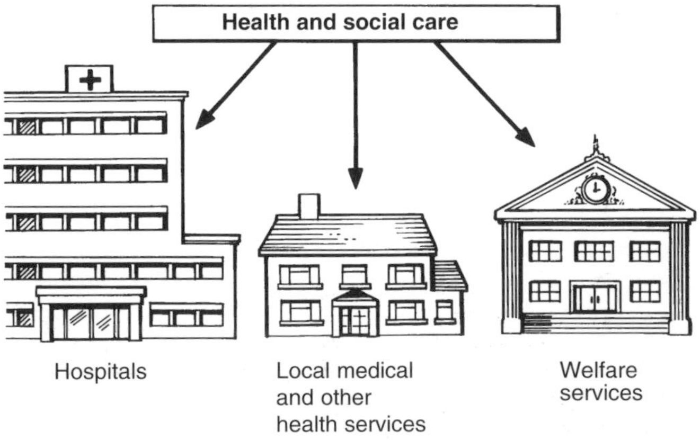

Figure 13.2 The organisation of health and social care services under the National Health Service Act 1946

The National Assistance Act 1948

The National Assistance Act was designed to replace the old Poor Law, which had given an outdated and punitive form of poverty relief. It was designed to complement the National Assistance Acts of 1946, providing financial assistance to people in need.

Part three of the Act empowered local authorities to provide many services designed to improve the quality of lives for people who were disabled. It imposed on local authorities the *duty* to provide homes and hostels for older people and people with disabilities, who were unable to care for themselves and who had no one to look after them. Local authorities were also *empowered* to charge residents according to their means, leaving some part of their pension for personal expenses.

The Act made it a *duty* for local authorities to inspect and to register the private residential establishments for older people and people with disabilities. Section 29 of the Act gave the *power* to local authorities to promote the welfare of all people with disabilities, such as those with a mental disability. Use of these powers varied greatly from authority to authority.

The Act also made it a *duty* for the authorities to arrange general social work support and advice in the home and elsewhere; facilities for rehabilitation and adjustment, and for occupational and recreational activities; as well as ensuring the protection of property of people while in hospital or in residential care.

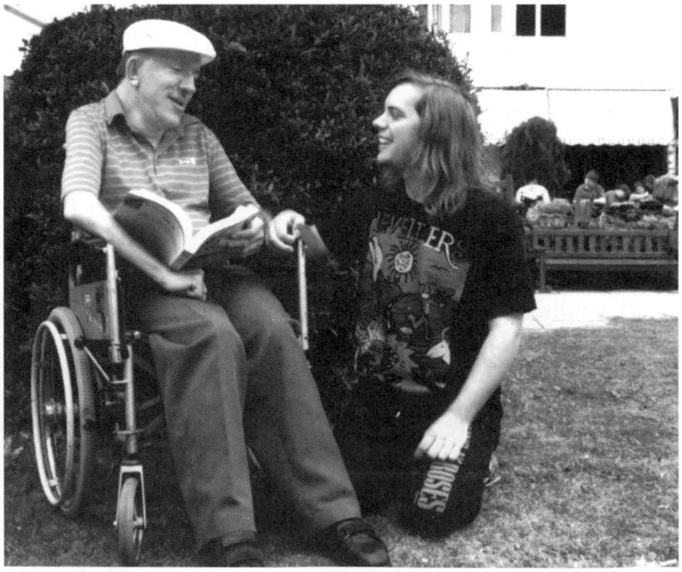

(*Photo courtesy of Winged Fellowship Trust*)

The Health Services and Public Health Act 1968

Section 45 of this Act provided local authorities with the *general power* to promote the welfare of older people. Subsequently the provision of meals-on-wheels, home care, day care (including transport to day centres), adaptations to property and the provision of warden-controlled property (with Housing departments usually having responsibility for this), have been developed. However, local authorities do not have a duty to provide any of these services.

The Local Authority Social Services Act 1970

Following the Seebohm Report and the subsequent Local Authority Social Services Act 1970, social services departments developed into the form that we know them today. The Act requires local authorities to set up Social Services Committees who administer all of the functions carried out by the social services departments. The Act sets out the framework for social services provision, however it is not specific about the way in which this is to be organised.

The Chronically Sick and Disabled Persons Act 1970

This Act makes further provision for the welfare of people with disabilities. It gives local authorities a positive *duty* to provide amenities and services recommended under the Act. These duties include:

- the duty to establish the numbers of disabled people in their area, to determine their needs and publicise services
- the duty to provide the following services (but only where they are satisfied there is a need):
  - practical assistance in the home
  - help with radio and television
  - library and recreational facilities
  - help to take up facilities outside the home
  - assistance with travel
  - meals
  - telephones
  - aids and adaptations.

Today many of these services are provided by the local authority social services departments, with the exception of library and recreational facilities, which are usually the responsibility of a different local authority department.

Although the above services may be widely available, each authority is able to decide whether there is a need for them to be provided in their area. They are also able to set the criteria for their provision. For example, in one area people may be entitled to assistance with paying for their telephone rental charges if they are over a certain age and registered as being disabled. In another area, however, people may also have to be living alone and have a medical condition that might necessitate instant help, such as chronic heart disease, before they qualify for such assistance.

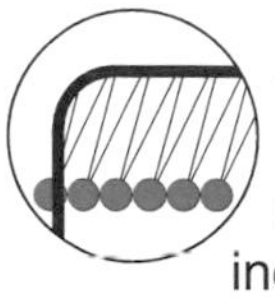

Think it over

What help is there in your area to assist disabled people with travel? Schemes may include travel permits, dial-a-ride schemes, orange badge schemes (which make parking easier for disabled people), or free local authority transport (usually to day centres, etc.).

The Chronically Sick and Disabled Persons Act also made it a duty of local authorities (and others) to provide access for disabled people in certain buildings to which the public have access.

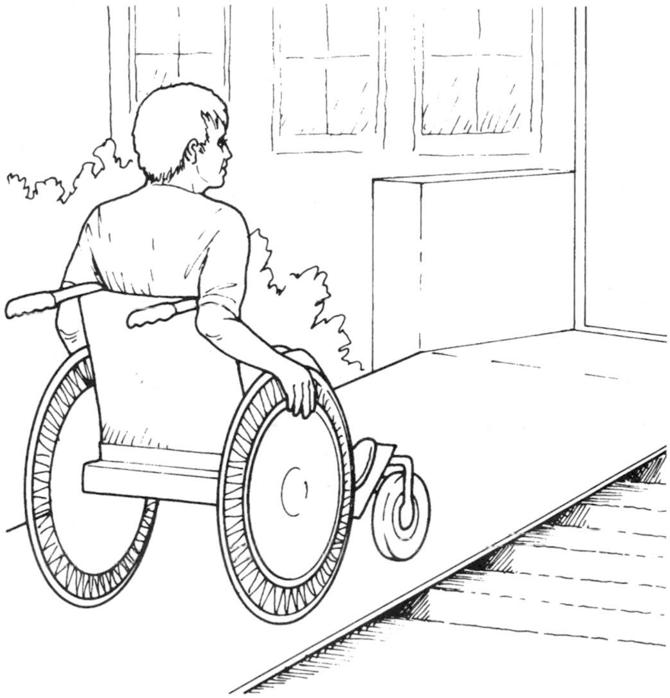

This Act is also very important for older people, since people over the age of 60 comprise approximately 60 per cent of the disabled population as a whole.

The Mental Health Act 1983

This Act deals with the rights of people who have a mental disorder, and the procedure that must be followed in order to provide them with appropriate care. It relates to a person's welfare when that person, due to a mental disorder, is not able to make decisions regarding his or her own welfare. Under the Act, local authorities must appoint approved social workers (ASWs), who have a duty to assess people for hospital admission. The approved social worker must interview the person in a suitable manner and make application for hospital admission, or guardianship, where appropriate. Other duties of the approved social worker include:

- a duty to respond to a 'nearest relative's' request for assessment, and to inform the nearest relative in writing if no application is made for admission to hospital
- a duty to inform the nearest relative of application for admission to hospital, and to consult with him or her if the patient is to be admitted for treatment, or if guardianship is to be sought
- a duty to inform the nearest relative of his or her rights to make application for admission to hospital, and to discharge the patient.

The Social Services Department also has the duty to arrange for a social worker (not necessarily an ASW) to provide reports to the hospital managers when a person is admitted, and to provide social circumstances reports for mental health tribunals.

The definition of the term 'mental disorder' is central to the functioning of the Act. Section 12 of the Act refers to four specific forms of mental disorder:

1 mental illness
2 arrested or incomplete development of the mind
3 psychopathic disorder
4 'any other disorder or disability of the mind'.

This definition means that people with learning difficulties may come within some sections of the Mental Health Act. However, sexual deviancy and dependency on drugs or alcohol do not constitute a mental disorder and do not come within the scope of the Act.

Although the local authority has the responsibility for providing approved social workers to assess the need for admission to hospital, and more recently to supervise people returning to the community from psychiatric hospital care, it is the health authority which has the responsibility for developing services within the community for people with mental health problems. These services may include *community psychiatric nurses* (CPNs), who visit people in their own homes, or who give support to their clients on an individual basis, or in groups, in clinics. They may also include out-patient or clinic consultations with a psychiatrist, short-term residential accommodation, and resource centres (which may be similar to a clinic).

Evidence collection point

Find out if there is a resource centre or clinic in your area, specifically for people with mental health problems. Write a report which includes the following information:

a what services are provided and whether they are statutory or non-statutory services
b how the services are classified within the NHS
c how the centre or clinic is funded
d how people gain access to the services that are offered.

The Disabled Persons (Consultation and Representation) Act 1986

The Act requires local authorities to provide information not only about their own services, but also about those services provided by other statutory and voluntary agencies concerned with people with disabilities. The Act also requires that the needs of carers be taken into consideration when the need for services is being assessed. Sections 1 to 3 of the Act provide for the appointment of *advocates,* or representatives, to be appointed, to speak on behalf of those clients who are unable to express themselves directly. Section 3 also requires the local authority to provide a written statement setting out the assessment of need.

The Children Act 1989

Under Section 17 of the Children Act, local authorities have a *general duty* to safeguard and promote the welfare of children in need. They must also promote the upbringing of such children by their families and to do this must provide services appropriate to the individual child's needs. Some of the main duties are:

- a duty to provide and publicise services including day care for under-5s, family centres, services aimed at helping children while living with their families
- a duty to take reasonable steps to prevent ill-treatment or neglect of children, to prevent the need for children being placed in care or in secure accommodation and to encourage children not to commit crime
- a duty to provide accommodation to children in need. This is a voluntary agreement where those with parental responsibility for the child, and who are unable to provide suitable care and accommodation, may request the local authority to provide accommodation and care. There is an additional duty on the local authority to consider the child's views and feelings, depending on the child's age and ability to understand
- a duty to children looked after by the local authority, to safeguard and promote their welfare, to consider their wishes and those of parents and relevant others, and have regard for the religious, racial and cultural background of individual children
- a duty to provide aftercare for young people leaving the care of the local authority

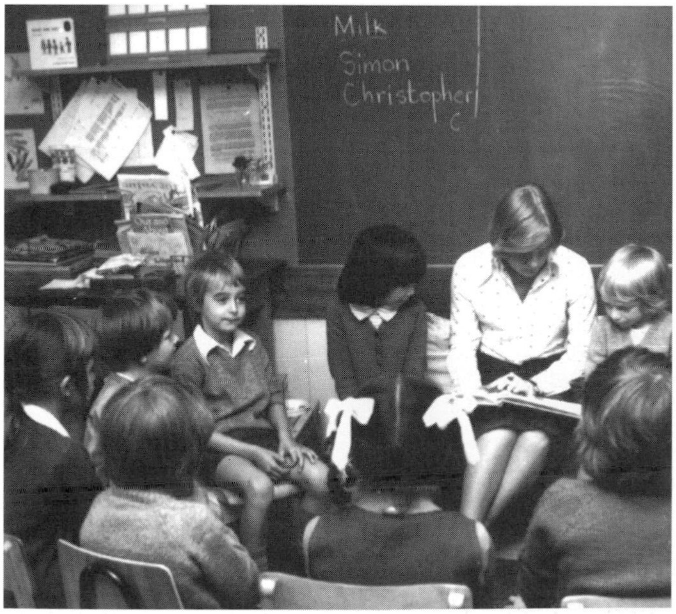

- a duty to provide secure accommodation where children have a history of absconding and are likely to abscond, may suffer some form of harm, or may cause injury to themselves or others
- a duty to have a complaints procedure for children in care, parents, those with parental responsibility and others with an interest in a child's welfare
- a duty to investigate where a child in their area is suffering, or likely to suffer, significant harm and to decide what action to take to safeguard or protect the welfare of the child.

Through this Act, local authorities are given wide-ranging responsibilities towards children in need. It highlights the rights, duties, powers and responsibilities of people with parental responsibility, but above all confirms that the welfare of the child is paramount.

Evidence collection point

Find out from your local Social Services Department what services they provide for children under 5 years of age. These may include nurseries, family centres, family aids to help the family at home, fostering and adoption facilities, child protection teams. Note which of these services are statutory and which are non-statutory. Write a report on your findings, including an explanation of how the Social Services Children and Families section receive funding for the services they provide. Also explain how children and families may gain access, or be referred, to these services. Who may provide informal care for children?

The National Health Service and Community Care Act 1990

The NHS and Community Care Act incorporates the proposals set out in the Government White Papers 'Working for Patients' (on reforming the NHS) and 'Caring for People' (on community care).

There are six key objectives:

- to promote the development of home care, day care and short stays in residential units, to enable people to stay in their own homes for as long as possible
- to ensure that the needs of the carers are also taken into consideration by service providers

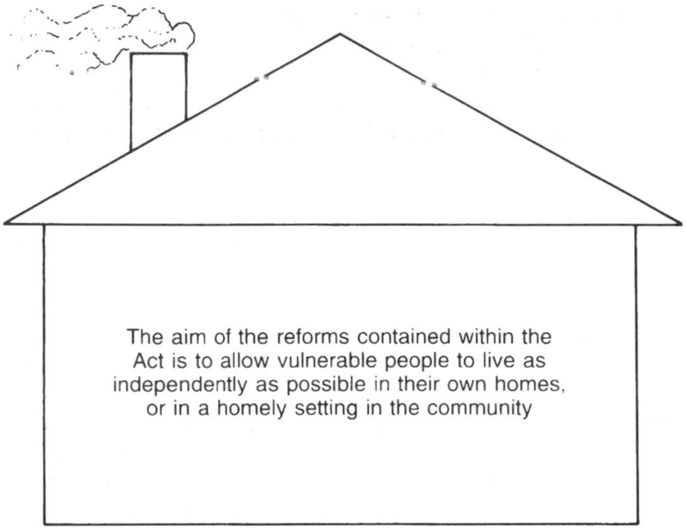

The aim of the reforms contained within the Act is to allow vulnerable people to live as independently as possible in their own homes, or in a homely setting in the community

- to make full assessments of the needs of the individual and to promote good case management to ensure a high quality of care
- to encourage the development of the independent sector alongside good-quality public provision
- to clarify the responsibilities of both the social services and health authorities and to hold them accountable for their performance
- to secure better value for taxpayers' money by introducing a new funding structure for social care and health care.

The Act is very significant in that it incorporates important developments in the philosophy of community care and in the delivery of services called for in other legislation. The Act emphasises a care management approach, (see Chapter 16) based on the assessment of individual need and the designing of tailor-made packages of care. It also introduces a split between the purchasing and providing of care. In addition to this, the Act encourages more involvement of the private and voluntary sectors in the provision of services.

The Act places an obligation on health authorities to ensure that:

- health service staff contribute towards needs-led assessments
- appropriate health care is provided
- reviews of individual health care needs take place and service provisions are revised accordingly.

Local authorities should also:

- communicate assessments and decisions regarding service provision to the individual
- regularly review social care needs and adjust service provision accordingly
- feed back information regarding changing community care needs into a planning system
- publish information to all service users on the range of community services available.

Duties[1]	Powers[2]
Health and social care services have a duty to: ■ provide homes and hostels for older people and people with disabilities ■ inspect and register private residential establishments ■ arrange general social work support ■ provide facilities for rehabilitational, occupational and recreational activities ■ protect the property of people who are in hospital ■ establish the number of disabled people in their area ■ provide access for disabled people to certain buildings ■ appoint approved social workers ■ provide services for children under the age of 5 ■ prevent the neglect and ill-treatment of children ■ provide accommodation and secure units for children in need	Health and social care services have the power to: ■ charge for residential care ■ promote the welfare of older people, which may include the provision of: – meals-on-wheels – home care – day care – adaptations to the home – warden-controlled homes ■ promote the welfare of all people with disabilities and provide (where there is a need): – library facilities – recreational facilities – meals – help with telephones – aids and adaptations
Notes: 1 Duties are *statutory* – they *must* be provided.	2 Powers are *non-statutory* – they *may* be provided or exercised.

Figure 13.3 A summary of the duties and powers of statutory health and social care service providers

Provision of care in the private and voluntary sectors

The work of voluntary and private organisations in health and social care has always been of great importance. Some services to which people are statutorily entitled are provided by this independent sector, especially by voluntary organisations, although they may be commissioned by the National Health Service or by local authorities. Services may be commissioned either by awarding grants to certain organisations, or by contracting with the organisation to provide certain services. For example, local authorities may delegate their duty of inspecting and monitoring the facilities for children to the National Society for the Prevention of Cruelty to Children (NSPCC).

The voluntary sector has been established over a long period of time and is by far the largest provider of care within the independent sector, and the past 30 years has seen a major growth in this area. The range of activities of voluntary organisations is very wide and may include self-help groups (such as Alcoholics Anonymous), pressure groups (such as the Child Poverty Action Group), advocacy groups (such as Release, which works with drug users), specific support groups (such as the Multiple Sclerosis Society), or umbrella organisations that help to co-ordinate a number of other agencies (such as the Organisation Development Unit, which acts as a development agency for black voluntary groups).

The private sector has also grown in the recent past and may continue to grow. However, it is always susceptible to fluctuations in the economic state of the country and of individuals.

The move away from a Welfare State to a *mixed economy* of health and social care will mean an increased role in care provision for the independent sector.

Evidence collection point

1 Create a directory of all the voluntary organisations in your area. (Information may be obtained from the library, from directories, and from your local Social Services Departments.)

2 Visit one of these organisations and find out:

- **a** what services they provide and for whom
- **b** whether any of these services are statutory services
- **c** how the organisation classifies its services
- **d** where the organisation gets its funding from
- **e** how people gain access to the organisation and its services
- **f** whether any of the service users are helped by informal carers and what kind of help the informal carers give.

Informal care provision

In recent years, the term *carer* has come to be used to describe anyone other than a paid worker who is looking after an ill or disabled person. The carer may be an adult looking after an ageing parent, a husband or wife looking after a sick partner, an adult looking after a child who has a physical or mental disability, or even a child who is helping to look after a sick or disabled parent. A friend or neighbour may also fulfil this informal caring role.

Many people do not like the term 'carer'. However, using this term does help in acknowledging that the carer is doing a job of work, and it is a job that can be very difficult and demanding.

Informal carers provide all sorts of care:

- helping people get up from and return to bed
- helping them to get washed and dressed
- helping them to bathe or shower
- helping them with toileting
- preparing meals and refreshments
- monitoring and dispensing medicines
- providing transport for social and medical purposes
- providing leisure activities
- ensuring general safety and well-being.

People who give up full-time work in order to care for someone at home may be entitled to some financial assistance. The Invalid Care Allowance is a taxable benefit for people if they are looking after someone for at least 35 hours a week.

Informal care may also be provided by people who belong to a local group, such as a church or other religious group, or by a group especially formed to help, advise and support carers. Usually no charge is made for this help and the people that provide the help give their services on a voluntary basis.

Try it

Write to the Carers National Association head office at 20/25 Glasshouse Yard,

London EC1A 4JS and ask if there is a branch of the association in your area. Find out what sort of support your local branch is able to provide.

Evidence collection point

Either contact a religious centre in your area, or speak to someone you know who provides care on an informal basis. Find out what sort of help and support they provide and to whom.

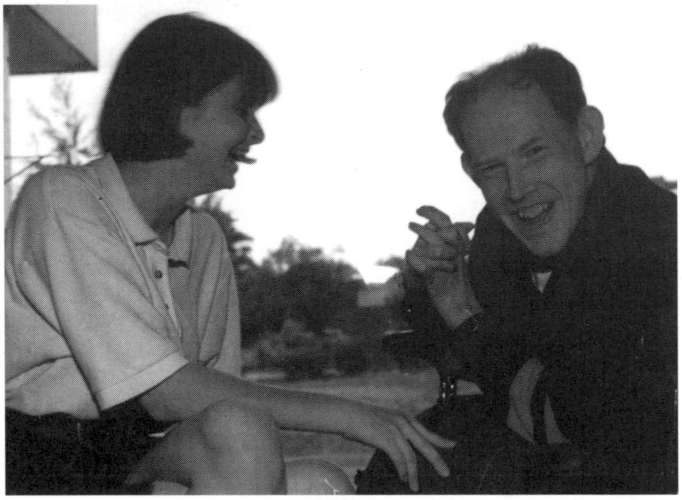

(*Photo courtesy of Winged Fellowship Trust*)

Classification of services

There is no single straightforward way of classifying health and social care services. Classifications differ according to the different perspectives that are taken, such as: care setting (Figure 13.4), client group or age (Figure 13.5), client need (Figure 13.6).

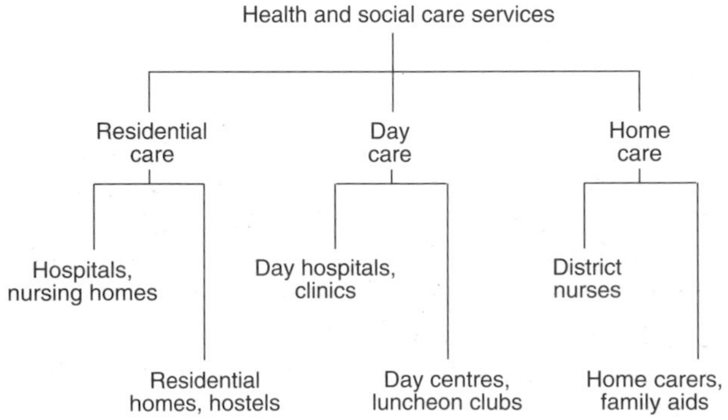

Figure 13.4 Services organised according to care setting

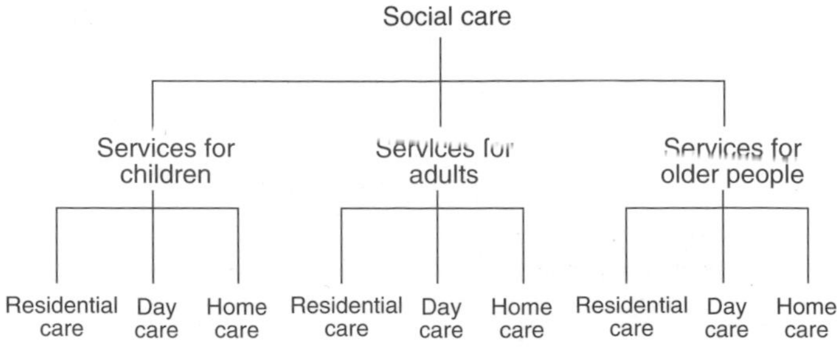

Figure 13.5 Services classified according to a client-centred perspective and age

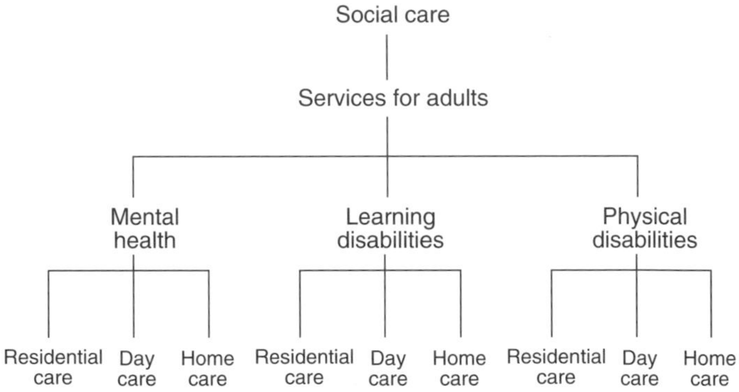

Figure 13.6 Classification of services by need of the client

Many social services departments use a combination of age, client group and client need perspectives. This makes the organisation of services far more complicated but much more client specific (see Figure 13.7).

Think it over

What are the classifications being used in Figure 13.7?

Another way of classifying services is by the level of care that is needed. A good example of this is seen in the National Health Service (Figure 13.8).

Primary care refers to the first contact that people have with health care services, which can be through a GP, practice nurse, dentist or clinic nurse. The sort of care that is offered is often preventative or the treatment of minor ailments. *Secondary care* often follows a referral from the primary care worker. It is often curative in nature and is given in hospitals, day surgeries and out-patient clinics. Tertiary care may be

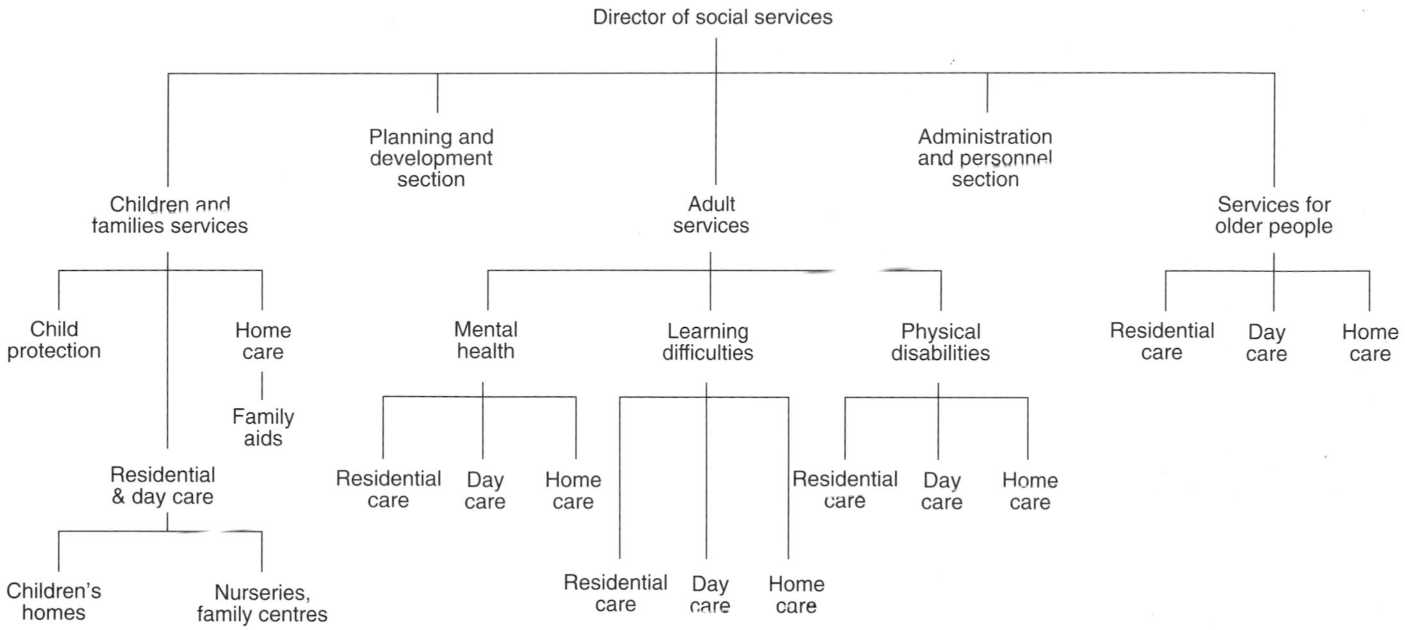

Figure 13.7 A social services department using a combination of classifications for the organisation of services

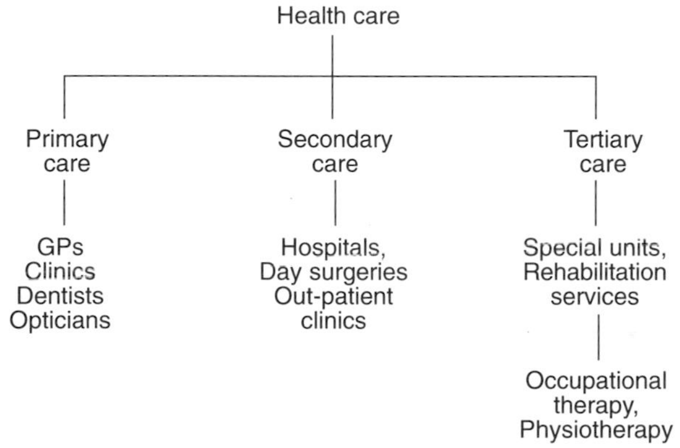

Figure 13.8 Classification of services in the NHS by level of care

provided in specialist units and is often rehabilitative in nature.

A broader way of classifying services to to define the service which is being supplied. This will more easily cover all health and social care services that are available, whether they are provided by the statutory organisations (the National Health Service and social services departments) or by voluntary and private organisations. These services include:

- physiotherapy
- occupational therapy
- aromatherapy
- osteopathy
- psychotherapy
- services for drug abuse
- services for alcohol abuse
- support services by religious organisations
- self-support groups
- counselling.

No matter how services are classified, it is important to remember that individuals may be in receipt of more than one service at any one time. Classifications are therefore not mutually exclusive, but will overlap in order to provide for the total health and social need of the individual, as the following case study shows.

Case study: overlap of services

Margaret Whittaker is a 78-year-old lady who has severe arthritis and who lives alone, although her son and daughter visit her daily and provide her with meals at the weekends. The services that Margaret receives include:

- monthly check-ups by her GP
- a yearly visit to the arthritis out-patient clinic at the hospital
- daily help from a home-carer in getting up, washed and dressed
- meals-on-wheels five days per week

- attendance at a day centre once a week
- residential care when her family are on holiday.

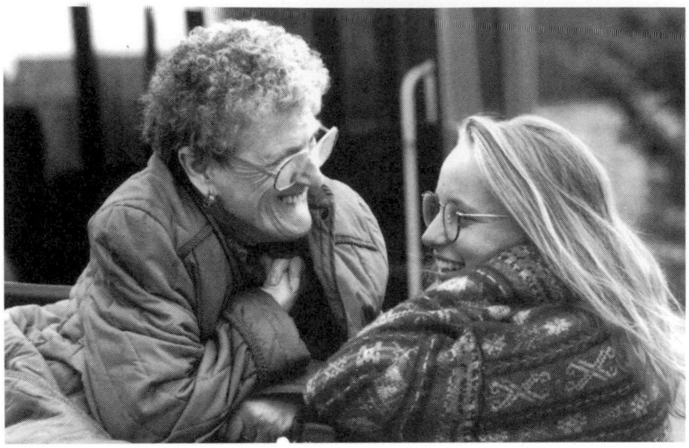

Think it over

Consider the differences in circumstances of two older people who are known to you. What services do they receive from health and social services? What additional services do you think they would benefit from?

In summary, services may be classified in many different ways. Examples of the variations are:

- *care setting:* residential, day or home care
- *age:* child, adult, older person
- *needs:* mental health, learning difficulty, physical disability
- *level of care:* primary, secondary, tertiary
- *service being supplied:* physiotherapy, aromatherapy, services for drug or alcohol abuse, general support services, etc.

Evidence collection point

Visit a local health centre.

1 Find out what services they are able to provide for adults and older people. Which of these services are statutory and which are non-statutory?
2 Describe how the services are classified within the National Health Service.
3 Find out where the clinic obtains its funding.
4 Find out how people are referred to the clinic and to the services that the clinic provides.

The way that services are classified depends largely on the way that the organisation is structured and therefore managed. The two main things that influence the structure of the National Health Service and social service departments are legislation (together with government guidelines) and the way the organisation has developed historically

For example, the NHS and Community Care Act 1990 has resulted in both the NHS and social services departments dividing the purchasing and providing functions. However, the tripartite structure (family practitioner services, community health services and environmental health and social care) has remained. So there are still three separate agencies involved in the provision of statutory health care. The structure is based on the original tripartite structure of the NHS, as it was set up in 1948.

Patterns of service provision often reflect the way that Acts of Parliament focus on certain groups of people within the community, for example children in the Children Act 1989, people with disabilities in the Chronically Sick and Disabled Persons 1970, and people with mental problems in the Mental Health Act 1983. Service provision within social services departments tends to mirror this.

Resourcing health and social care services

Health and social care may be resourced by:

- by central government
- by local government
- by charity
- by private insurance schemes
- by direct payment
- by the individual or client.

The cost of welfare provision (including education, housing and benefit costs) has continued to grow steadily over the years. The total cost of welfare stood in excess of £120 billion in 1990, having risen from around £90 billion in 1973 (Figure 13.9).

Gross government expenditure on personal social services rose from £1900 million in 1980–1 to an expenditure of £2950 million in 1988–9. Expenditure on the NHS increased from £444 million in 1949 to £29 billion in 1990.

Funding the NHS

Money for the NHS comes from three main sources:

1 central and local government tax revenues
2 National Insurance contributions
3 charges paid by users of the service and income generation.

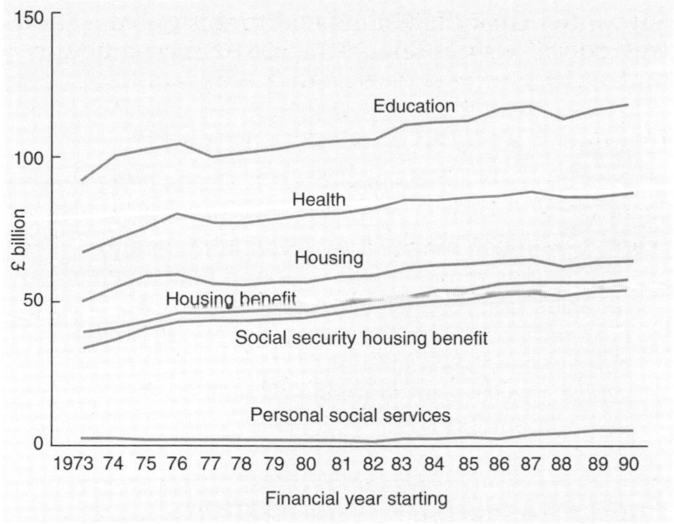

Figure 13.9 Public spending on welfare in the UK, 1973–90 (1990–1 prices)

Public services are funded by local and national taxes – income tax, value added tax (VAT) and National Insurance contributions paid by individuals and organisations. The main source of income from 'charges' are from prescriptions issued by GPs and dentists for treatment and examinations.

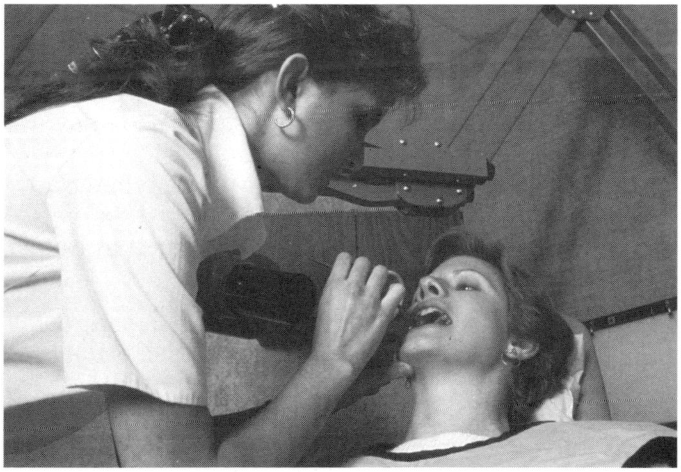

The amount of money spent on the NHS each year is decided between the Department of Health and the Treasury. The Department of Health then allocates money to the Regional Health Authorities (RHAs), according to a formula based on the size, age and health of their resident population.

The Regional Health Authority then allocates money to the District Health Authority (DHA) in its area, who will then purchase services to meet the needs of its

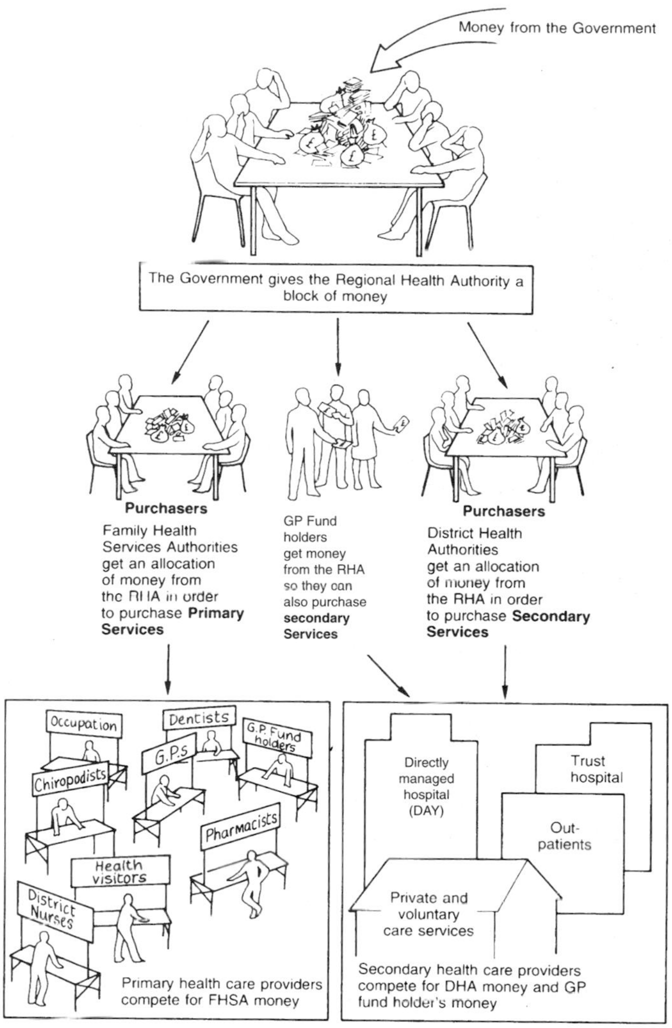

Figure 13.10 Funding the NHS

residents. The Regional Health Authorities are also responsible for allocating funds to the Family Health Service Authorities (FHSAs) so that they are able to purchase primary health care services.

A fund-holding GP also receives money directly from the Regional Health Authority in order to purchase services for patients.

Funding social services

Each district and local council has responsibility for maintaining certain services, which include:

- social services
- education (excluding grant-maintained and private schools)

- leisure and recreation facilities
- housing – general funds
- highways and car parking facilities
- refuse collection and waste disposal
- planning and economic development within their area
- contributions to police, fire, water and other services.

Funding for these services comes from two main sources – a yearly allocation of money from the government and from council taxes. Each year the government allocates money to local authorities to help meet the cost of services. How much it gives is based on a formula called the 'Standard Spending Assessment' (SSA). The formula takes into account such things as the number of old people living in the area, the percentage of rented accommodation, the number of single-parent families, the percentage of people from ethnic minority backgrounds, and the density of population. Local council taxes are levied on each household and business in the area and the level of taxation is based on the value of the property.

The local authority allocates money to the various services which it must maintain. For many authorities their biggest expenditure is on education, with social services taking the next largest amount (Figure 13.11).

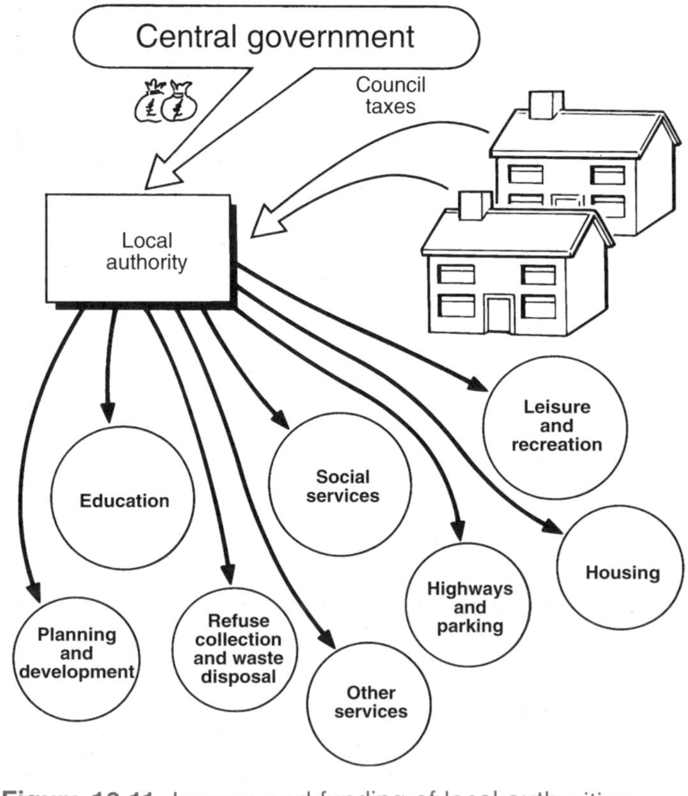

Figure 13.11 Income and funding of local authorities

Try it

1. Find out from your local authority how much money it receives from central government each year and how much it receives from council taxes.
2. Find out how much the authority spends on the various services each year.
3. Which services are financed directly from government funding?

Funding voluntary organisations

Funding for voluntary organisations comes from four main sources:

- grants direct from central government, in order to carry out specific projects
- grants from local authorities, usually to provide non-statutory services
- grants from organisations and businesses
- contracts with health authorities or social services departments, who contract the voluntary organisation to provide statutory or non-statutory services.

For example, a local authority may give some funds to the local Age Concern group, who provide day centre facilities and luncheon clubs for older people in its area. A District Health Authority may have a contract with a local hospice to provide palliative care for people with a terminal illness, such as cancer or AIDS.

The remainder of a voluntary organisation's funds (and this sometimes constitutes more than 50 per cent of the total running costs) will be raised through fund-raising events and charitable donations from individuals or groups of people (Figure 13.12).

Income for the voluntary sector appears to be dropping, with grants from local authorities decreasing. Although the 'contracting' culture may provide more financial security for some voluntary organisations, others may not be able to survive. Many voluntary organisations may only have short-term contracts with health authorities and local authorities, making future planning very difficult and making workers in the organisations feel very insecure.

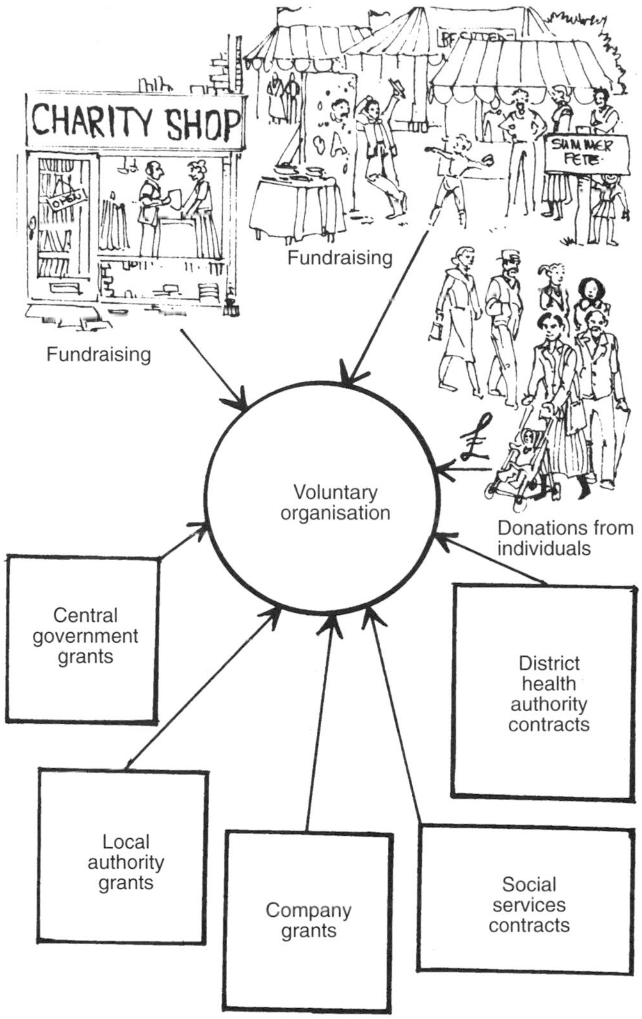

Figure 13.12 Financing voluntary organisations

Funding private care services

Private organisations, run on business lines, are self-financing. Individuals may pay directly to these organisations for the services they receive. However, individuals may belong to private insurance schemes that will cover the cost of private care when it is needed. Private health care insurances have been available for many years, but increasingly people are taking out private insurance that covers services they previously received from the NHS. For example, there has been a marked increase in the number of people taking out dental insurance over the past few years. Also, in the future it may be possible to take out insurance to guard against the need for residential or nursing home care.

In addition to the money that they receive from individuals, private organisations may have contracts with health or social services purchasers, to provide certain services on their behalf. For example a local authority social services department may contract with a private residential home for older people to provide a number of places in the home for social services clients.

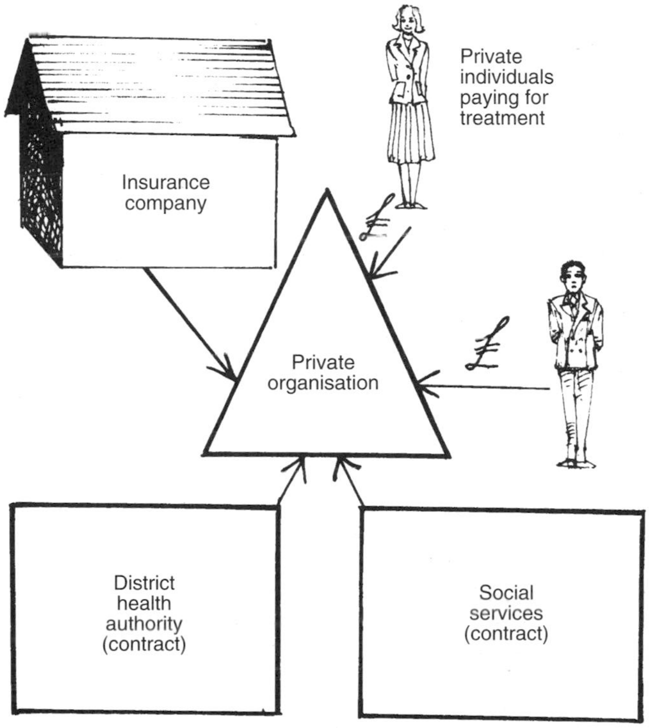

Figure 13.13 Financing private organisations

Access to services

Access to health and social care services can be achieved in one of four ways:

- through self-referral
- by referral by a third party, such as a relative or friend
- by recommendation of a professional
- by recall.

Self-referral

For a person to refer themselves to a service, they must first know of its existence (Figure 13.14). People gain information about the services that are available in various ways:

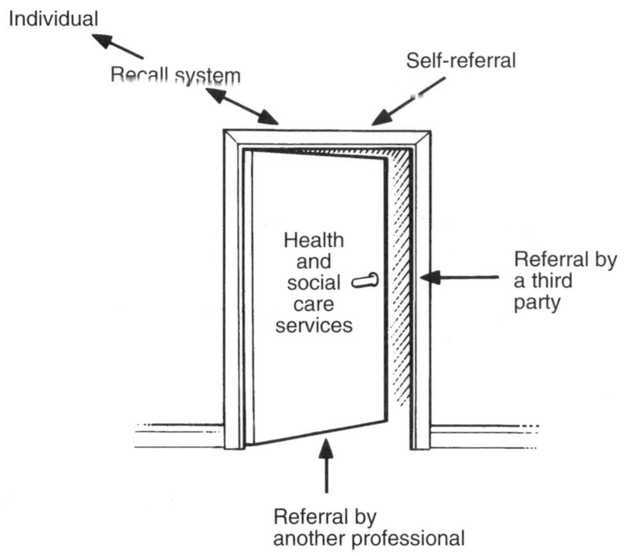

Figure 13.14 Opening the door to health and social care services

- from general publicity in the media, for example television and newspapers
- from leaflets and posters in public places
- by word of mouth from relatives, friends and neighbours.

The health care services to which people are able to refer themselves are the NHS primary care services – the GPs, dentists and opticians, or services for which they pay privately. People can refer themselves to social services departments. However, they will then be assessed as to whether they are in need of any specific service, before it can be provided. People wishing to obtain social care through private agencies are able to refer themselves.

Referral by a third party

People may be referred to either the primary health care services or social services by a third party. In particular, referrals in respect of services for children are often made through a third party.

Recommendation of a professional

Some services are accessible only through the recommendation of another professional. This applies particularly to secondary health care services. For example, a GP will refer a patient to specialist hospital services, a teacher will refer a child to the Educational Welfare Officer or Educational Psychologist.

Recall

For many services there may be a 'recall' system operating. For example, once an individual has registered with a dentist or an optician, following the first visit a follow-up appointment may be sent automatically after a certain period of time. Other services which often have a recall system are screening services, such as breast cancer screening campaigns.

Think it over

Can you think of any other services where there is an automatic recall system?

Evidence collection point

To provide evidence for Element 5.1, write a report on *five* local health and social care services and facilities, covering statutory and non-statutory and informal provision. This report must:

- describe the extent to which there is statutory entitlement to the services
- describe variations in classification and explain any difficulties in classification
- describe the major forms of resourcing and relate these forms of resourcing to the classification of services
- explain how clients might access services and what access routes exist for different services.

You may wish to go back to pages for ideas of how to obtain the information that you require in order to do this:

- *page 308:* Services provided by a local resource centre for people with mental health problems
- *page 309:* Social services provision for children under 5
- *page 311:* Making a directory of local voluntary organisations and the services provided by one of them
- *page 311:* The provision of care on an informal basis
- *page 313:* Health care services provided by a local clinic for adults and older people.

Chapter 14

The development of health and social care provision

This chapter looks at why health and social care provision develops and changes. It covers:

- **The origins and development of health and social care in the UK**
  - **the historical background 1300–1939. The Beveridge Report, the NHS 1948–79, Care in the community, 1980 onwards, developments in technology**
- **Government policy, structures and funding – approaches to care, focus of responsibility and intervention, funding and resourcing health and social care, payment for health and social care services**
- **demographic characteristics – the diminishing labour force, the ageing population, the incidence of disability, disease and mental illness, geographical variations**
- **The role of the independent sector – origins and development, government policies and funding, demographic influences, additional roles.**

The origins and development of health and social care

Historical background 1300–1939

Between 1348 and 1350 an epidemic known as the Black Death raged through Europe, reaching England in late 1348 and Scotland a year later. In England at this time one in three people died from 'the plague'. This sudden and drastic reduction of the number of working people encouraged labourers to leave their masters and sell their services to the highest bidders. This was viewed as a dangerous threat to the social order and resulted in the first of what became known as the Poor Laws being introduced in England in 1389. The new law fixed a legal maximum wage and made it illegal for labourers to leave the manor to which they belonged.

However, the first Poor Law did not prevent the number of itinerant (travelling) labourers and homeless people from growing during the next two centuries. The population also rose rapidly during this time, adding to the homelessness problems, which also increased following the Wars of the Roses. Before their dissolution (closure) in 1540, the monasteries had provided some food and shelter to the poor and sick. In the sixteenth century various laws were introduced to allow parishes to collect money (the start of today's council tax system) to provide relief (food and shelter) for the old, sick, disabled, children and able-bodied poor. The able-bodied poor were required to work to earn their relief.

In 1601, a new comprehensive Poor Law Act was introduced, replacing the earlier laws. The government decided that each parish should look after its own poor and unemployed. These people were divided into three groups: the 'impotent' (helpless) poor; the able-bodied poor; and 'rogues and vagabonds'. Each group was treated in a different way. The helpless (the old, sick, crippled, and children) were viewed as deserving relief, with children being 'apprenticed' at the parish's expense. The able-bodied, who could not find a job, were admitted to workhouses, given tasks to do and paid from the poor rate, until they could find work. 'Rogues and vagabonds', who preferred to beg, steal or scrounge, were flogged and sent to 'the house of correction' (prison). Persistent offenders were hanged.

By the end of the 1700s, the population had increased again, but the after-effects of war and bad harvests resulted in shortages in food. Food prices rose and even people in work found themselves living below the poverty line. In response to this, many parishes supplemented low-paid workers' wages from the poor rate (similar to today's Family Income Supplement).

The first part of the nineteenth century brought concerns about the increasing costs of poor relief (from £1.5 million in 1776 to £7 million in 1831). The laws at that time were not performing their social control functions effectively. So, in 1834 the Poor Law Amendment Act was introduced. This Act created a government body to supervise poor relief, elected Boards of Guardians to run each of the new poor law unions and infirmaries (hospitals), oversaw relief to the old, sick and disabled and ensured that only those able-bodied people who were prepared to suffer the hardships of the workhouse received relief.

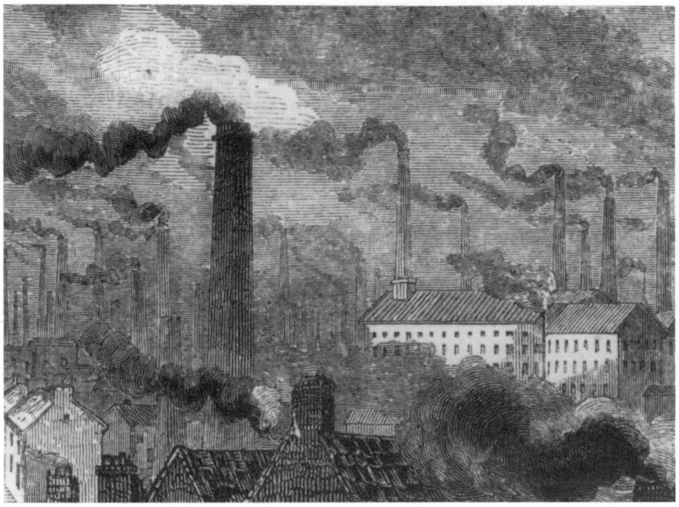

Figure 14.1 The Industrial Revolution brought the growth of an urban industrial society

The poor were held responsible for their own poverty.

The Industrial Revolution (roughly 1760–1840) resulted in a complete change in society, replacing a rural society with an urban industrial society. It was the massive move of people from the countryside, to towns and cities which created public health problems. (A combination of preventative medicine, civil engineering and community administration and legal resources was known by the generic term of 'public health'.) Although public health legislation was set by central government, it was up to local government to implement it and to develop public health services. These health-related services included water supplies, sanitation, food and hygiene inspection and pollution control. Later it also included housing, personal and community health services.

By 1861 workhouses had become part of the public hospital system, providing approximately 65 000 hospital beds in England and Wales. Eighty-one per cent of hospital beds were provided by workhouse sick wards, the rest were provided by voluntary hospitals.

Try it

Find out if there are any buildings in your area that were originally built as workhouses. They were often converted into general hospitals. What are these buildings used for today?

The Boer War (1899–1902) raised concern about the condition of the working classes, as the defeat of the British army by a relatively small number of Boer farmers was attributed to the poor physical condition of many of the soldiers. From 1870 onwards, reforms implemented by successive Liberal governments gradually chipped away at the old Poor Laws. This programme of new initiatives provided the basis for the introduction of the Welfare State system. State intervention began to be an accepted notion.

In 1909 members of a Royal Commission on the Poor Laws produced a report which recommended a unified state health service to be run by local authorities. It also sought to introduce the principle of free health care for the poor, as a right.

Following the First World War (1914–18), there was little co-ordination of health and social care for the most vulnerable people such as children and the elderly. Although a National Insurance scheme had been introduced, it did not provide for dependants, the long-term unemployed, or those people needing specialist services. Also, massive unemployment undermined the National Insurance system. Many people exhausted their entitlement to assistance through long-term unemployment.

The government's intervention in health services during the Second World War (1939–45), through the emergency medical services, is often thought to be the major reason for the creation of the National Health Service. However, in the years before the war, there had been considerable thought given to the setting up of a National Health Service. In 1942,

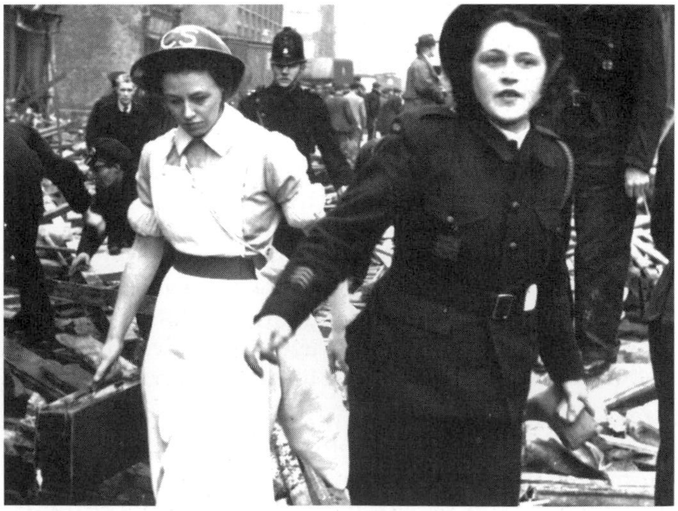

Figure 14.2 The emergency medical services in the Second World War

the Beveridge Report set out the broad framework for the welfare state of post-war Britain.

The Beveridge Report, 1942

The report aimed to tackle five major areas of concern: want, disease, ignorance, squalor and idleness – and it covered the whole population.

The plan envisaged a compulsory insurance scheme where a single, weekly contribution would provide a 'cradle-to-the-grave' provision of care. This contribution was to cover sickness, medical, unemployment, widows', orphans', old-age, maternity, industrial injury and funeral benefits. The scheme had six components: flat-rate subsistence benefits, flat-rate contributions, unification of administrative responsibility, adequacy of benefits, comprehensiveness and classification. It promised universal social security, without means tests, uniformly administered by a Ministry of Social Security. The report was considered very radical, even by Beveridge himself. It was based on a redistribution of income, i.e. the philosophy that wealth should be shared more evenly.

Although there was broad agreement by all political parties on the need for a comprehensive health service, there were many different opinions as to how this should be organised and financed. An amended plan was put forward (called the Brown Plan), but this too had many opponents, including GPs, local authorities and voluntary hospitals. So the government revised its proposals and in 1944 a White Paper was published which detailed these revisions.

Under the revisions, health services would be comprehensive and free of charge at the point of delivery, GPs would come under the control of a central medical board, be salaried and work from health centres, and hospital services would be overseen by joint local authority boards. Again, these revisions were rejected.

Another White Paper containing further revisions was planned, but not published prior to the 1945 General Election, which was won by the Labour Party. The Labour Party's Aneurin Bevan became Minister for Health. Despite the Labour Party's support for a comprehensive health service, based on local authority control, Bevan preferred a tripartite system of health care provision (see Figure 14.3).

Bevan has often been called the father of the National Health Service, although the service has its roots in the reforms previously set out, in a very modified manner, in the Beveridge Report.

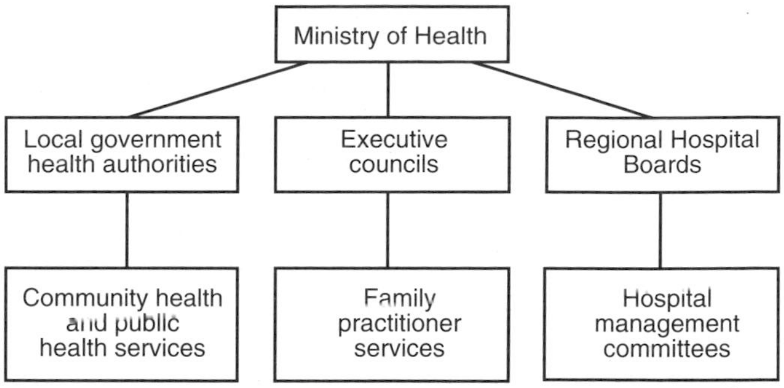

Figure 14.3 The structure of the NHS, 1948–74 (England and Wales)

Health and Social Services 1948–79

The National Health Service provided a comprehensive health care system which was open to all and free at the point of delivery. Also, being a national service it had the potential to ensure a high standard of health care throughout the UK. The bringing together of a range of health and social care services under a Minister of Health meant that it would be possible to provide a more coherent, planned and integrated range of services, especially within the health care system.

In the mid-1940s, the Ministry of Health appointed welfare officers, mainly to deal with the problems of evacuation and, later, with housing problems. By 1945, 70 local authorities had appointed social workers to help develop the provision of social care. In addition to the Ministry of Health's welfare and social workers, the Provisional Council for Mental Health was also providing social care for people with mental health problems.

When the NHS came into existence in 1948, the provision of care by local authorities for old and disabled people, homeless families and, most importantly, for children was extended. The Children Act 1948 instituted a unified service for all children deprived of a 'normal' home life. Local authorities created children's departments and employed child care officers. For the first time, social workers were employed in large numbers by local authorities.

During the 1960s, the demand for a family service in social care arose and in 1968 the Seebohm Report on personal social services was published. This resulted in the amalgamation of the children's departments and welfare services, within local authorities. Following the Seebohm Report, the subsequent Local Authority Social Services Act 1970 required local

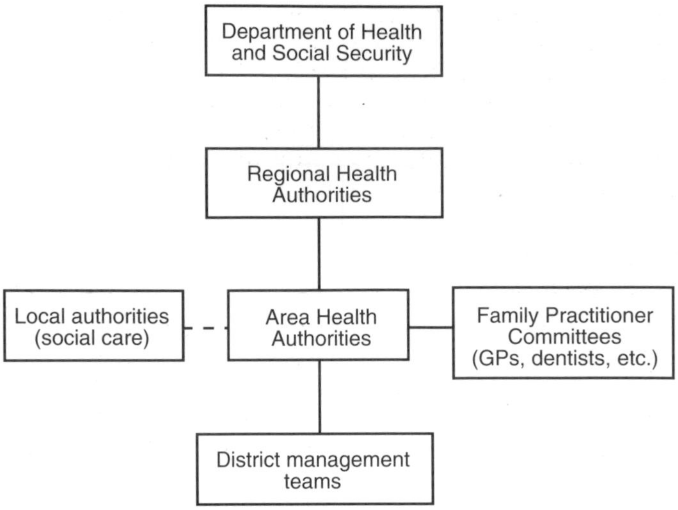

Figure 14.4 The structure of the NHS, 1974–89

authorities to set up Social Services Committees and set out a framework for social care provision.

The 1960s showed up problems in the structure of the NHS, with overlaps, duplication and lack of co-ordination of services. This eventually resulted in a reorganisation of the NHS in 1974, with three tiers of health service management being introduced, at regional, area and district levels. This structure was criticised as being bureaucratic, having too many tiers of management and needing too many administrators (see Figure 14.4).

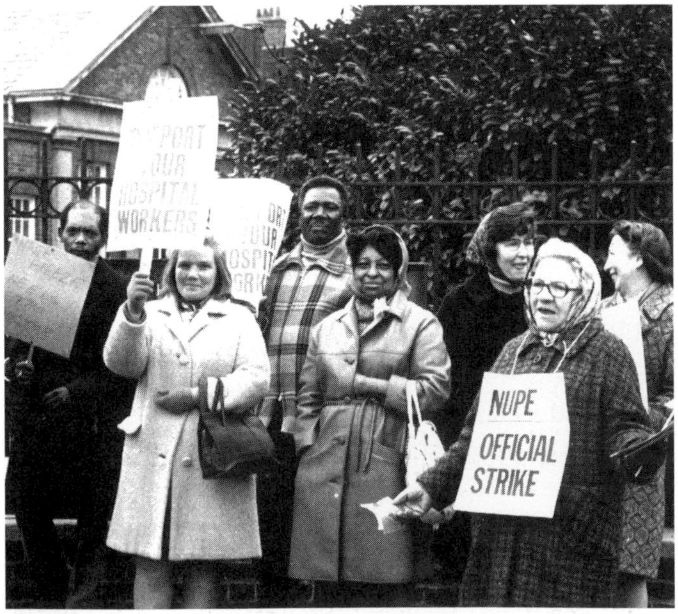

Figure 14.5 NHS workers on strike in the 1970s

The 1970s saw a deterioration in industrial relations throughout the UK including the health care services. Disputes involved nurses, doctors and ancillary staff. The disruption to services, resulting in long waiting lists and occasional malpractice scandals, affected the general public's support of the NHS. Some people (those who could afford it) began to turn to the private sector for their health care.

In 1973 Parliament created the post of Health Service Commissioner to look at maladministration in the NHS. The Royal Commission report set out seven key objectives:

- to encourage people to remain healthy
- to ensure equality of entitlement to health services
- to provide equality of access to services
- to provide a high-quality range of services
- to provide a free service at the time of use
- to satisfy the expectations of users
- to maintain a national service responsive to local need.

Not all of the report's recommendations found favour with the subsequent Conservative government.

Try it

Ask three people, one aged over 65 years, one aged between 40 and 50 years and one aged between 20 and 30 years of age, what their expectations of the health and social care services are. Compare the responses you receive.

Care in the community, 1980 onwards

In May 1979 a Conservative government was elected to Parliament and this proved to be a watershed as far as the welfare services were concerned. Although support for care in the community can be traced back to the 1960s, it wasn't until the mid-1970s that moves were made to promote and support this. In 1974 joint consultative committees, consisting mainly of health authority and local authority representatives, were formed. Joint finance also became available so that community-based schemes, involving health and social care, could be established.

The new Conservative government was keen to encourage care in the community for several reasons, and it was seen as a way of saving public money in health and social care. In order to do this it meant that:

- people needed to be transferred from long-term hospital care back into the community
- there needed to be more involvement of the private and voluntary sector in the provision of care
- informal care by relatives, friends and neighbours needed to be encouraged
- more efficient use of existing resources needed to be made.

However, in addition to this, the government wanted to ensure that a high quality of care standards was also developed and maintained (see Chapter 15).

In March 1987, Sir Roy Griffiths was appointed to examine the problems involved in the implementation of care in the community. His report set out three main principles on which he felt community care should be based:

- that the right services should be provided early enough and to the people who needed them most
- that people should have more choice and a greater say about how they were helped
- that people would be cared for in their own homes wherever possible, or in a homely environment within the community.

Although there were various concerns about the content of the Griffiths Report, eventually the government published its response to it in 1989 in the form of a White Paper called 'Caring for People'. The White Paper generally upheld the recommendations of the report, especially that local authorities should have the main responsibility for community care and that 'care management' should be one of the underlying principles for the provision of social services (see Chapter 16).

Also in 1989, the White Paper 'Working for Patients' was published. The main proposals within this paper included:

- formation of a new policy board responsible for strategic planning
- clarification in the responsibilities of the various health authorities
- the introduction on the notion of internal markets (see Chapter 15)
- changes in the terms and conditions of service for consultants
- more emphasis of the quality and monitoring of the quality of services
- tax relief for people age 60 and over on private health insurance
- encouragement for the use of private health facilities.

Implementation of care in the community has taken longer than first envisaged, with progress being even slower in Scotland, but faster in Wales. The effects of the reforms are likely to be spread over many years, although some consequences, especially in the field of mental health services, have already had an impact.

Think it over

There have been several highly publicised reports regarding the care of mentally ill offenders who have returned to live in the community. What have been the main issues and concerns raised by people re-offending when they have been discharged from institutional care?

Developments in technology

In addition to the changes brought about by government policies and ideology, and by social and economic changes, technology has also brought about massive changes in health and social care provision.

The computer age has brought many changes in the way that information is communicated. Information technology (IT) has revolutionised the way that information is kept and distributed. Now patient and client case notes can be kept on computer and easily accessed. For example, a person visiting an out-patient clinic, then going for a blood test and then for a chest X-ray, no longer has to carry his or her file around the different departments. A patient's case history notes can be accessed in any of the hospital departments through the computer system.

In health care, the development of technology has resulted in the use of complex machines and techniques, in the diagnosis and treatment of patients. Examples of this include:

- ultrasound, used to disperse stones in the kidney and gall bladder.
- endoscopic surgery where a small instrument is passed into the body through a natural orifice (such as the mouth), or through a small incision in the skin ('keyhole' surgery)
- radiotherapy and chemotherapy, used in the treatment of diseases such as cancer
- scanners, machines used in the diagnosis of illnesses, for example for detecting growths in the body

- laser surgery, which can be used in a number of ways, from the treatment of cancer to delicate eye surgery.

The results of the use of advanced technology include quicker and more accurate diagnosis of illnesses and other medical conditions and the ability to carry out more complicated treatments, such as organ transplants. Also, in some instances advanced technology reduces the cost of traditional treatments. For example, using ultrasound to disperse kidney stones reduces the patient's length of stay in hospital by about a third.

The use of these technologies does, however, raise various issues.

- In many instances the capital and running costs can be very high. (For example, heart transplants cost approximately £26 000.)
- The use of machines in diagnosis could cause doctors' interpersonal and diagnostic skills to become less expert.
- The use of technology raises ethical dilemmas. (For example, to what extent should genetic engineering be used to alter the characteristics of unborn babies?)

The use of advanced technology has yet to be evaluated fully, taking into account not only cost-effectiveness, but also how it affects the doctor – patient relationship, its effect on the skills of doctors, and all the ethical issues that it raises.

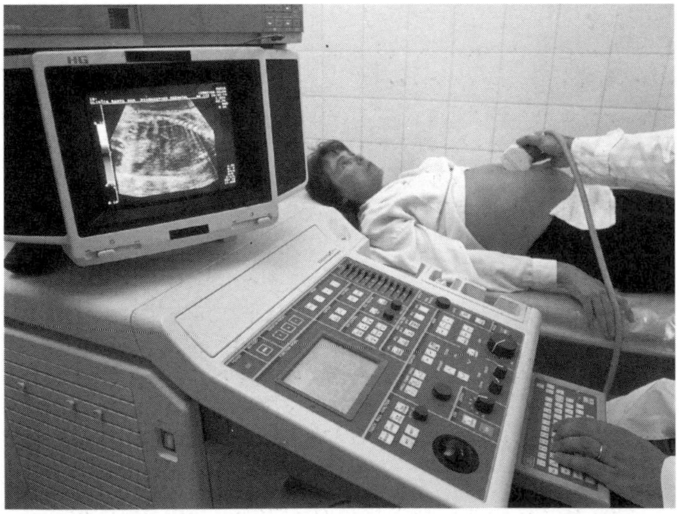

Figure 14.6 Ultrasound is often used in pregnancy to monitor the health of mother and child

Evidence collection point

Write a short report about how health and social care services have developed and changed in your area. To do this you may wish to contact:

- your local Social Services department, to ask about any new projects that have been developed in the past five years – think about services for people under these headings: children and families, people with physical and mental disabilities, people with mental health problems, older people.
- your District Health Authority to ask about services that have become available in the past ten years – think about services under the headings of: hospital services, community services, GP services, dental services.

Government policy, structures and funding

Approaches to care

The term 'approach', in relation to health and social care, refers to the formal arrangements that are made by society in dealing with illness, disability, premature death, prevention of illnesses, rehabilitation following an illness or accident, and other health-related issues, such as epidemics. These arrangements may take into account contributing factors such as poverty, the environment and individual lifestyles. The formal arrangements for dealing with health and social care will include regulating access to the care available, financing the services, and organising the delivery of care.

A number of contemporary health care systems have been developed throughout industrialised countries of the world. Field (1989) provides a useful overview of health care systems. Field identifies the various approaches mainly by the way the services are allocated, and identifies five main types of health care approaches:

- emergent
- pluralistic (USA)
- insurance/social security (France)
- National Health Service (UK)
- socialised (former Soviet Union).

(See Figure 14.7.) It has been suggested that the health care policies of different countries are gradually moving closer together and so becoming

Emergent	■ Health care viewed as item of personal consumption ■ Physician operates as solo entrepreneur ■ Professional associations powerful ■ Private ownership of facilities ■ Direct payments to physicians ■ Minimal role in health care for the state
Pluralistic	■ Health care viewed mainly as a consumer good ■ Physician operates as solo entrepreneur and in organised groups ■ Professional organisations very powerful ■ Private and public ownership of facilities ■ Payments for services direct and indirect ■ State's role in health care minimal and indirect
Insurance/social security	■ Health care as an insured/guaranteed consumer good or service ■ Physicians operate as solo entrepreneurs and as members of medical organisations ■ Professional organisations strong ■ Private and public ownership of facilities ■ Payment for services mostly indirect ■ State's role in health care central but indirect
National Health Service	■ Health care as a state-supported service ■ Physicians operates as solo entrepreneurs and as members of medical organisations ■ Professional organisations fairly strong ■ Facilities mainly publicly owned ■ Payment for services indirect ■ State's role in health care central and direct
Socialised	■ Health care a state-provided public service ■ Physicians are state-employed ■ Professional organisations weak or non-existent ■ Facilities wholly publicly owned ■ Payments for services entirely indirect ■ State's role in health care is total

Source: Field (1989)

Figure 14.7 Types of health care approach

increasingly similar. For example, the UK government is moving towards a 'market-place' (or pluralistic) approach to health care, while the US government is moving towards a more universal (or national) health scheme.

Focus of responsibility

The concept of the Welfare State is a relatively recent one in the UK. The Welfare State requires a high level of state intervention in the provision of health and social care services.

Although the provision of welfare has become one of the functions expected of all modern states, it is the level of intervention that is debatable. Alongside this is the question of individual responsibility, i.e. how much responsibility each individual should take in ensuring and providing for his or her own health and social welfare.

There have been great shifts in thinking in the UK about the required balance between state and individual responsibility. Before the Welfare State was established there was a greater emphasis on the individual's responsibility to provide for his or her own care, although for centuries the church and voluntary groups, together with some state provision, had made substantial contributions to this.

From the 1870s onwards, successive Liberal governments expanded the functions of the state and the state's role in the provision of welfare services. This began to raise various issues, such as the need for efficient operation of state functions versus the need for wider involvement of its citizens, and the definition of individual rights.

Socialist proposals for state-provided health and social care can be traced back to the early 1900s, but it wasn't until the introduction of the National Health Service in 1948 that the Welfare State came into being in the UK. The socialist perspective dominated government policy in respect of health and social care from the end of the Second World War to the mid-1970s. During this time, policies were underpinned by the principle of a free, comprehensive, universal and state-provided welfare system.

Since 1979 and the election of the Conservative government, there has been an emphasis on promoting self-reliance, the build-up of an informal sector of care, the promotion of an independent sector, the elimination of waste and, even more vigorously pursued, a reduction in public expenditure.

Government policies have, therefore, focused on state responsibility for assessment of health and social care needs, and for the organisation of services to meet those needs, rather than the actual provision of services by the state. Arguably this gives individuals more choice and more personal responsibility for their own health and social care. It is also argued by some that 'families owe responsibilities to each other, and for humanitarian and religious reasons the duty of charity to others. State welfare it is claimed, undermines both kinds of obligation' (Ranade, 1994).

Focus of intervention

Although the NHS created a 'medical service', some people feel that it did not create a 'health service'. The medical service model tends to focus on curing illness and disease and restoring health following injury or trauma, rather than preventing ill-health. Health policies have, to one degree or another, tried to restore the balance between prevention, cure and care, ever since the introduction of the NHS.

Both the Conservative government and the previous Labour government placed emphasis on preventative medicine. The government's national health strategy targets the reduction of illnesses such as heart disease, and the promotion of good health, for example with government health warnings in respect of cigarette smoking (see Chapter 19).

Although there is now widespread acknowledgement of the advantages of preventative medicine, especially where the treatment of illness requires expensive and prolonged intervention, there may also be opposition to a health promotion strategy. Opposition may come from industrial interests, such as the tobacco and alcohol industries whose existence depends upon consumption of their products, or from industries based on curative medicine, such as medical equipment manufacturers or pharamceutical companies. The government also receives considerable revenue from these industries through taxation.

However, the main reasons for the thrust towards presentative medicine comes from the belief that it will be more cost effective and will enable health care costs to be reduced. The government has not acknowledged that poor social and economic conditions lead to ill-health, though in the late 1980s it did begin to accept that environmental factors, such as pollution, cause illness.

Evidence collection point

Contact your local Family Health Service Authority and find out what health promotion project it is currently undortaking. How do these projects fit in with the trend towards preventative medicine? Write about this in a short report.

Funding health and social care

The NHS is mainly funded from taxation and National Insurance contributions. Although many of the services appear to be free, we pay for them in an indirect way. Public services are funded by local and national taxes (income tax, VAT) and National Insurance contributions paid by individuals and organisations. Approximately 86 per cent of all health care is publicly funded. (See Figure 14.8.)

The NHS and local authority social services have to compete for funding against other national expenses, such as defence, housing, highways, education and social security. How much each of these receives is decided by the annual setting of public expenditure.

Until recently each department would bargain with the Treasury for money for specific projects. This has now changed, and the government sets an overall level of expenditure for a three-year period. Each department then negotiates with the Treasury for a share of this. Conservative governments since 1979 have placed great emphasis on controlling public expenditure, which has an effect on NHS and local authority spending on social services. However, the NHS budge has increased from 10 per cent of the total

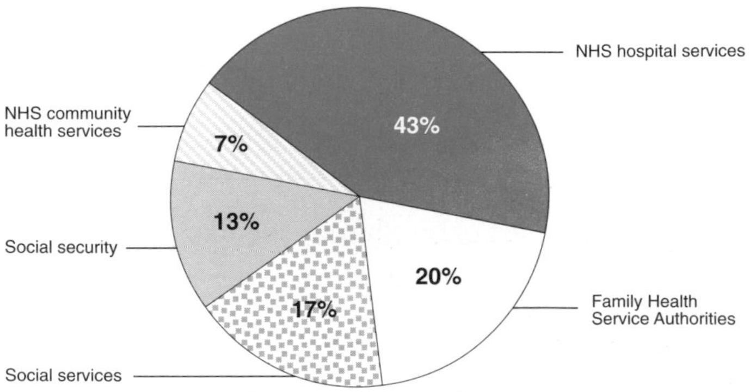

Figure 14.8 Expenditure on health and social care in England 1989–90

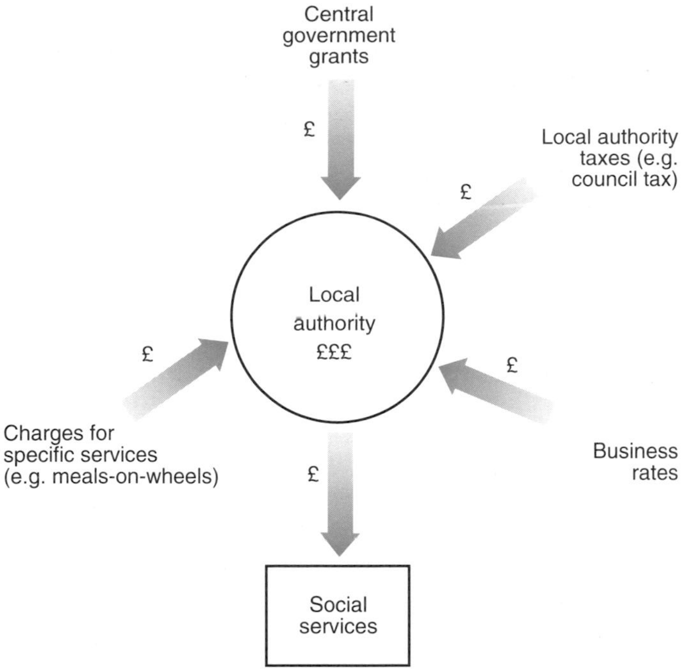

Figure 14.9 Sources of funding for social services

public expenditure in the 1960s to 14 per cent in 1990. In 1990, more that £29 billion was spent on the NHS.

Funding for social services is obtained in various ways: central government grants, local council taxes, business rates, and charges made for some of the services (see Figure 14.9).

Resourcing services

State intervention in the provision of health and social care ensures that essential resources are available for people who otherwise would not be able to afford them.

In 1989–90, 43 per cent of the total expenditure for welfare services was spent on hospital services, Family Health Services Authorities received 20 per cent and social services received 17 per cent, Social security spending accounted for 13 per cent and the remaining 7 per cent was spent on NHS community health services.

At present, bearing in mind the move towards care in the community, there seems to be an imbalance between the amounts spent on hospitals and community care. However, this does seem to be gradually changing – compare the proportion spent on hospital services in 1989–90 (43 per cent) with the proportion spent in 1979–80 (52 per cent).

Health care

In 1977, the Labour government set up a Resource Allocation Working Party to introduce a formula for the allocation of resources within the health service (RAWP). This formula sought to allocate resources on the basis of each health region's relative health care needs. It took into account issues such as the size of the population in that area, how the population was made up (the number of older people, etc.), and mortality rates in respect of specific conditions and illnesses (standardised mortality rates). The introduction of RAWP resulted in the redistribution of resources to areas of the UK which previously had been less well resourced. Resources were also moved away from the London health authorities, and resulted in a cutback of acute services in London during the 1980s.

In 1986 another initiative aimed at ensuring the management of resources at a more local level was introduced. This programme was called the Resource Management Initiative (RMI). It also sought to increase the involvement of doctors in the decision-making process regarding resources, and to give them the responsibility for budgets. This programme has been slow to get under way, but it is becoming more important as the marketplace approach to care increases.

Social care

Each year the government allocates money to local authorities to help meet the cost of the services they organise and provide. Again, there is a formula which is used to decide how much each authority will receive. This is called the Standard Spending Assessment (SSA). The formula takes into account such things as the number of older people living in the area, the percentage of rented accommodation, the number of people from ethnic minority backgrounds, the number of single-parent families, and the density of population.

The local authority allocates money from all its sources to its various departments – housing, education, leisure, refuse collection, environmental health, etc. In many authorities, the biggest

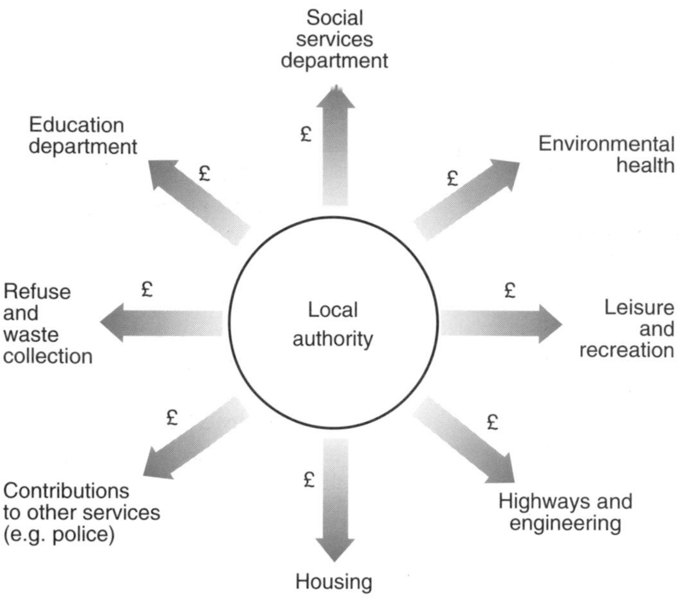

Figure 14.10 Resourcing the social services

expenditure is on education, with social services taking the next largest amount (see Figure 14.10).

Try it

Find out from your local authority how much it spends on the various services for which it is responsible. This information is usually sent out with each year's council tax demands.

Payment for social care services

The National Assistance Act of 1948 imposed a duty on local authorities to provide residential establishments for older people and people with disabilities. It also empowered them to charge residents, according to their means, for residential care. Local authorities also have the power to make charges for other services that they provide, such as meals-on-wheels and home care services. Many authorities chose not to make a charge for home care services until very recently, but with the greater demands on services (as a result of the emphasis on people remaining in their own homes wherever possible) and the greater restrictions on public spending, many have now begun to make charges for previously 'free' services.

Evidence collection point

Contact your local Social Services department and find out what services it organises that are financially assessed and to which clients make a contribution. Which of these services were previously provided free of charge? Write up your findings in a brief report.

Payment for health care services

The majority of secondary health care, including accident and emergency services, treatment for acute medical conditions (for example, following a stroke or the onset of an acute illness) and planned treatment (for example, eye surgery such as the removal of cataracts or hip replacement surgery), is free of charge at the time that the care is required. However, other medical care, particularly primary health services, still require the user to make a payment towards the cost at the time they require the service. These include:

- NHS prescriptions
- NHS dental treatment
- glasses and sight tests
- NHS wigs.

Some people are exempt from these charges. These include women over the age of 60 and men over 65, pregnant women and women who have had a baby in the past 12 months, children under 16 and young people under 19 who are in full-time education. Other people who are on low incomes can also obtain help with these charges. Assistance with travel costs to hospital for treatment is also available to people on low incomes.

Benefits

An individual's health and care problems may be linked to his or her social and financial situation.

With the exception of Housing Benefit (which is dealt with by the local authority), financial matters are dealt with by the Department of Social Security (DSS) via the Benefits Agency. The DSS produces a number of leaflets which set out people's rights and entitlements to benefits.

Benefits can be the same for everyone (such as child benefit), or they may be 'means tested' (i.e. take account of the individual's income and savings before the benefit is awarded). Some benefits are payable only if the person has made contributions to

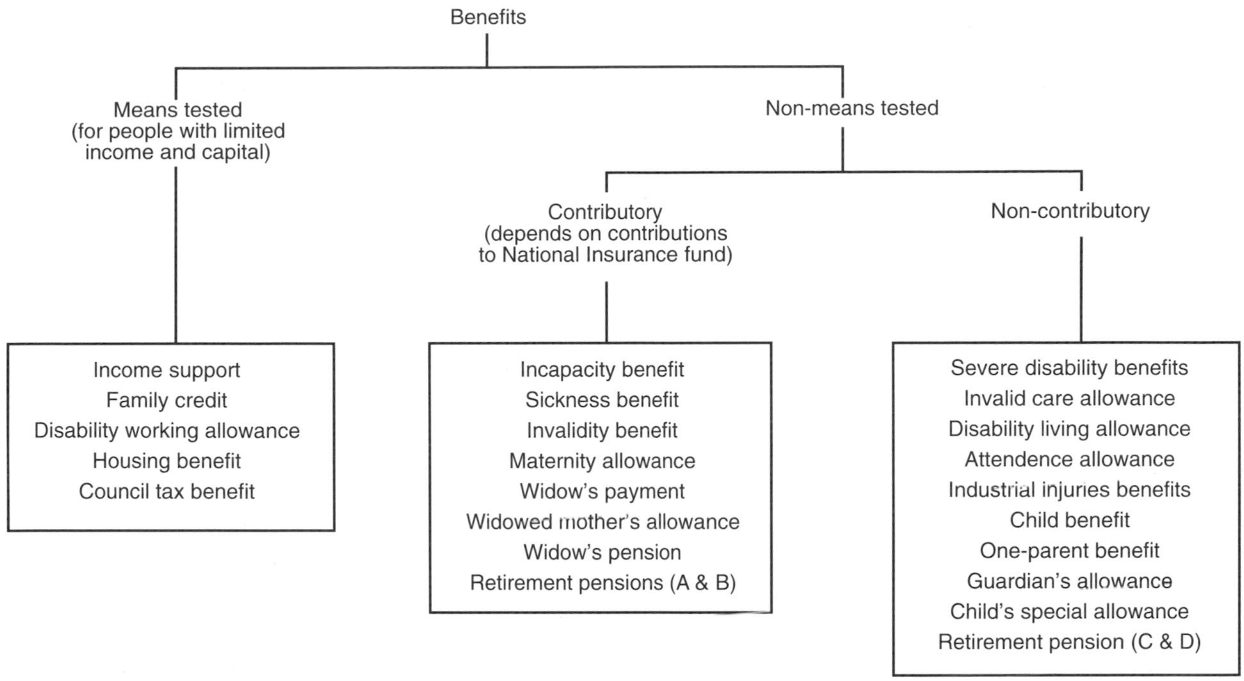

Figure 14.11 Types of benefit

the National Insurance scheme. These include incapacity benefit, sick pay, maternity payments and pensions. (See Figure 14.11.)

Evidence collection point

Collect a range of leaflets from your local DSS office. Use this information to write a short report on benefits that are means tested and benefits that are non-means tested.

Private health care

Increasingly, people are taking out private health care insurance or paying privately for health care. Insurance may cover such things as routine dental treatment, payments for hospital admissions, or maternity care. Even more recently, insurance cover has become available for such things as residential and nursing home care.

Try it

Undertake a mini-survey of all your family members to see who would have to apply for an eye test and who wouldn't. Is there anyone in the family who receives home care from the local authority? Is he or she required to contribute towards the cost of this? How is this charge worked out?

Demographic characteristics

Demographic changes in the population affect the need for health and social care. For example, when there is an increase in the numbers of older people, more resources are required to meet their needs. Government policies therefore need to reflect actual and projected demographic changes. Recent government policies, such as care in the community, a mixed economy of care and the move towards preventative medicine, have all been responses aimed to cope with demographic changes. This section sets out to explore some of the demographic trends that are currently of concern to health and social care.

The diminishing labour force

As we have already seen (page 319) the number of people available for work compared with the number

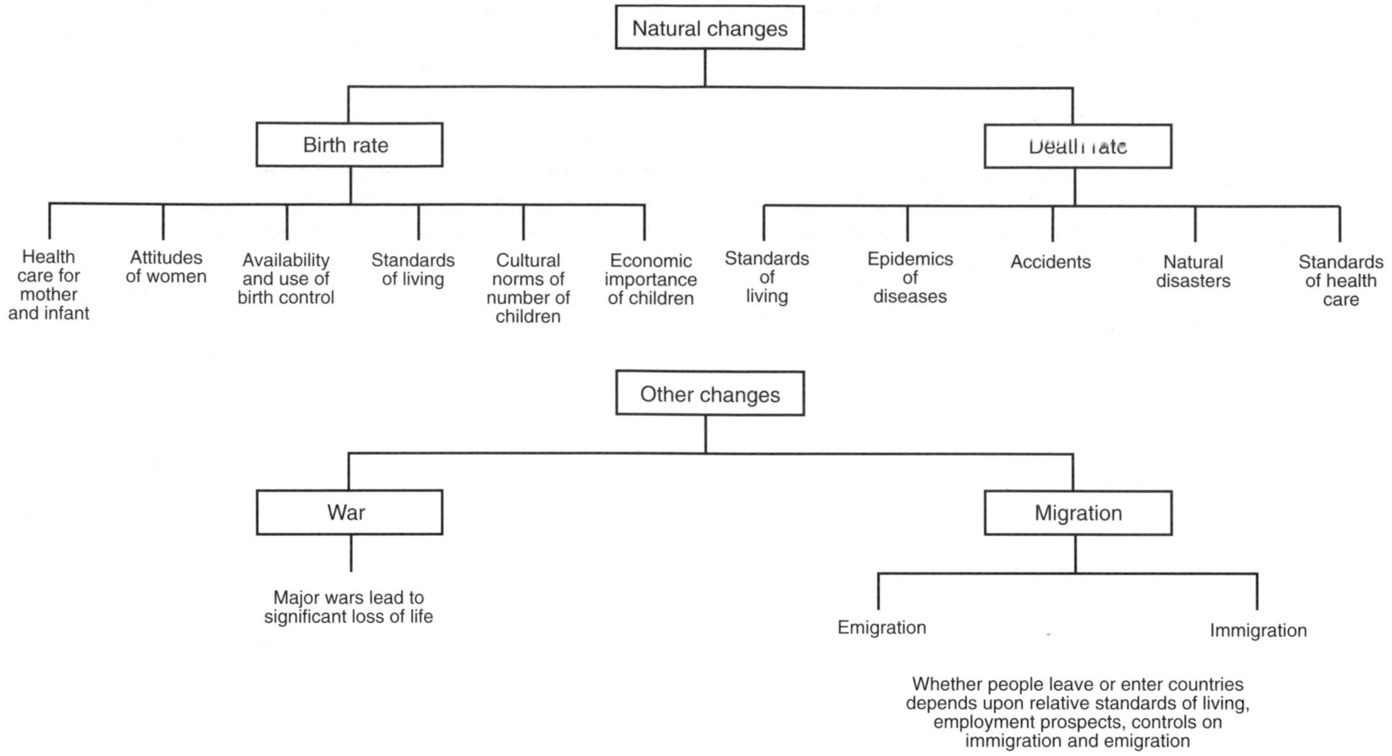

Figure 14.12 Factors which influence population size

of people required for jobs has a major influence on welfare policy.

In recent years there has been considerable concern about the labour force in the future. It is predicted that there will be a shortage of skilled and educated staff.

A number of factors influence population size, including birth rates, death rates, war and migration (see Figure 14.12). Until the nineteenth century, births and deaths were in rough balance. As industrialisation and medical advances progressed, so there was a rapid increase in the population. In the early part of this century, people began to limit the number of children they had.

Between 1984 and 1994 there was a 35 per cent decline in the number of 18-year-olds, and an average 1.8 births per woman (i.e. below the population replacement rate). This reduction may continue as more women enter the workforce. Research has shown that higher earnings for women depress the birth rate, while higher earnings for men raise it.

The ageing population

Life expectancy has increased greatly in the twentieth century and the number of elderly people is likely to continue to grow in the foreseeable future, with nearly a fifth of the total population

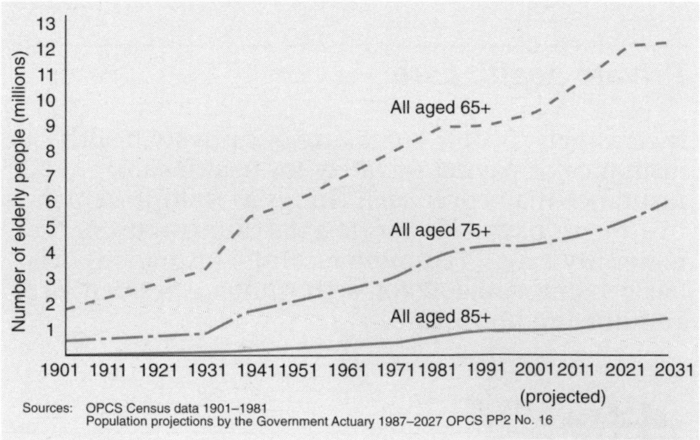

Figure 14.13 The elderly population in Britain, 1901–2031 (projected)

being aged 65 and over by the year 2030. Also by the year 2030, one in 20 people will be aged over 80 (see Figure 14.13).

For many older people, their ability to remain independent will be determined by the level of support and practical help provided by relatives, friends and by organised services (voluntary, private or state provided). However, as the population ages, so do the people who would formerly have been carers. Also, as more women enter the work force, so there will be fewer people available to be 'informal' carers.

The growing number of older people is not a problem in itself. However, the consequences of increased need for health and social care services could be problematic. Compared to other age groups, people aged over 75 years are heavy users of health care services (see Figure 14.14). Expenditure on pensions and health care for older people will soon become the largest single budget expense, according to the International Labour Organisation's 1995 World Labour Report.

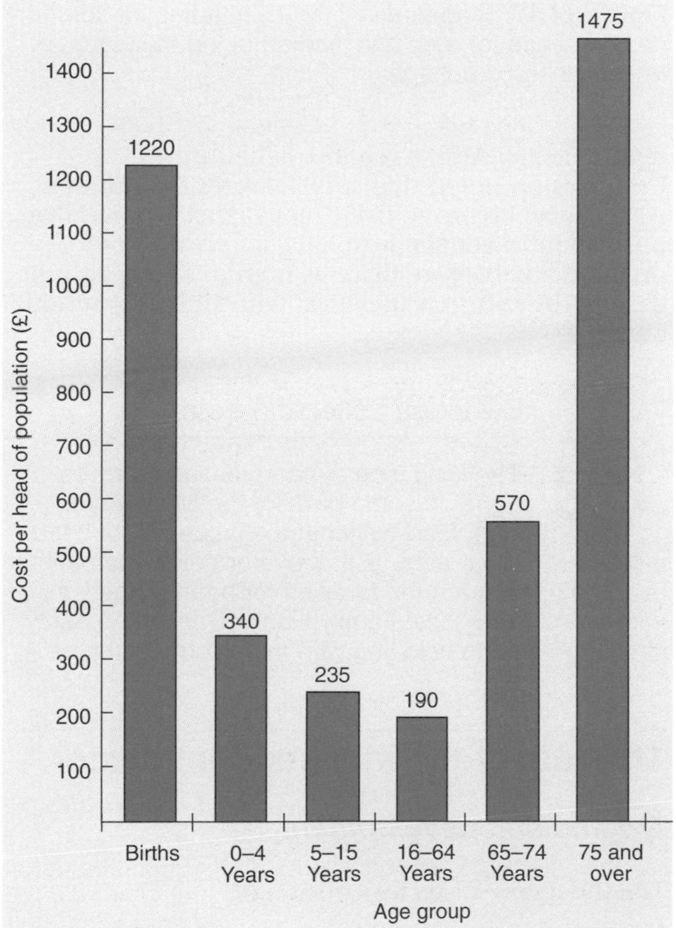

Source: HM Treasury (1988).

Figure 14.14 Health and social care costs per head by age group, England (1988)

The working population faces an increasingly heavy burden of providing the resources necessary for the care of older people. In 1961 there were approximately six people of working age for every person over the age of 65. By 2011 there will be fewer than four working age people to every person over 65.

Evidence collection point

The number of older people in the UK is rising. What changes did the NHS and Community Care Act 1990 introduce to try to cope with the increased demand for resources to meet their needs?

Incidence of disability, disease and mental illness

The decline of many major infectious diseases (such as measles, poliomyelitis and typhoid) has been offset by the increase in degenerative disease (such as cancer, heart disease and strokes).

Many of today's degenerative diseases, and other chronic diseases and dysfunctions, may be associated with modern lifestyles and environments. Lifestyle factors include smoking, alcohol abuse, poor diet, stress and lack of exercise. Almost 90 per cent of adults have at least one risk factor for heart disease and stroke according to the Department of Health.

Levels of infectious disease have also risen again recently. These include the incidence of tuberculosis, hepatitis and meningitis. The notification of food poisoning quadrupled during the 1980s.

It has been estimated that there are more than six million adults in the UK who have at least one form of disability, i.e. 15 per cent of the adult population.

Mental illness is another aspect of health care that may give cause for concern. In recent years there has been an increased call upon mental health services and in the use of antidepressants. Fourteen per cent of all GP consultations are concerned with mental health issues and at least 3 per cent of the adult population suffer from a depressive illness and 2 per cent from anxiety states.

Evidence collection point

Write a brief report about how immunisation programmes have helped to reduce the spread of infectious diseases, such as measles and whooping cough. Why is it felt that immunisation programmes should be a priority in health care?

Geographical variations

As can be seen by the effect of the Industrial Revolution on public health, there are important variations in health and illness within industrial countries. For example, within the UK, variations can be seen in infant mortality rates – mortality is lower in England than in the rest of the UK. Scotland and Northern Ireland also have higher rates of coronary heart disease and diseases of the circulatory system.

Within England itself there are also regional differences. In broad terms, there seems to be a north–south divide, with general health in the north being worse than in the south. However, there is evidence that the local environment is more significant than living north or south, with pockets of 'good' health and 'bad' health being found in both.

Since the Black Report was published in 1980, there has been wider acceptance that social and economic circumstances affect health. The report concluded that causes of ill-health include:

- the physical environment – housing, working conditions and air pollution
- social and economic influences – income and wealth and levels of employment
- behavioural factors and barriers to adopting a healthier lifestyle
- access to appropriate and effective health and social services.

Although one of the principles underpinning the NHS was to provide a universal health care service, it is a local health service, with widely differing standards of care and level of provision, that has been developed around the country. For example, people with heart disease living in Huntingdon are three times more likely to receive surgery than those living in Great Yarmouth according to a Clinical Standards Advisory Group report. Death rates from breast cancer are 23 per cent above the national average in Hartlepool, but are 38 per cent below the national average in Darlington (*Woman and Home* report, 1995). Also, a report by the Audit Commission noted that survival rates for children with cancer are up to five times higher in specialist units than in general hospitals. Survival rates for premature babies are twice as high in specialist units, despite the fact that they deal with the most serious cases.

	Men*	**Women***
Scotland	119	123
Northern Ireland	118	123
North West	117	116
North	116	124
Yorkshire and Humberside	111	110
Wales	111	106
West Midlands	103	104
East Midlands	99	102
South West	91	88
South East	89	87
East Anglia	86	89

* all UK = 100

Source: Newcastle DHA, *CHD Prevention Policy,* 3 November 1988. Crown ©, Reproduced with the permission of the Controller of Her Majesty's Stationery Office

Figure 14.15 Standardised mortality ratios for coronary heart disease for men and women in the standard UK regions in 1985 (all ages).

Evidence collection point

The incidence of heart disease may be higher in some parts of the UK than in others. Find out what the incidence of heart disease is in your area. Is it above or below the national average? What are the facilities for heart surgery in your area? (Your local Family Health Service Authority should be able to help you with this information.)

The role of the independent sector

Origins and development

The independent sector consists of:

- voluntary organisations (non-profit-making)
- private organisations (profit-making)
- informal care, provided by relatives, friends, neighbours or groups (such as church groups).

The extent of the independent sector's role in the provision of care has always varied from one area of care to another. Within health care, the private organisations have always played a major role in the provision of routine, non-emergency surgery, and abortions. More recently they have also become increasingly involved in the long-term care of older people and in health-screening facilities.

Prior to the establishment of the NHS, GPs were private practitioners who charged for their services In Victorian times, working-class people began to subscribe to clubs, and friendly societies who would hire the services of GPs for their members. With the introduction of the National Insurance Act in 1913 came the provision of sickness benefits and free GP services for employed working-class people.

Voluntary organisations range from very small groups of people within a locality providing specific help to a limited number of people (such as church groups providing practical and emotional support to their members) to large national charities (such as Age Concern).

Historically the voluntary sector has always had a great deal of involvement in the provision of health and social care. For example, during the eighteenth and nineteenth centuries, many voluntary hospitals were established by philanthropic individuals or by groups of caring people. The number of voluntary hospitals also increased between 1911 and 1938. Voluntary hospitals provided care free of charge, and often doctors, who felt it a privilege to be associated with the voluntary hospital, waived their fees. Organisations came into being following the Industrial Revolution and the urbanisation of communities, which brought with them the associated problems of overcrowding, poverty, squalor, drunkenness and child labour. These include: Dr Barnardo's (founded in 1866 and now known simply as Barnardo's), the Church of England Children's Society (founded in 1881 and now called The Children's Society) and the NSPCC (National Society for the Prevention of Cruelty to Children founded in 1889).

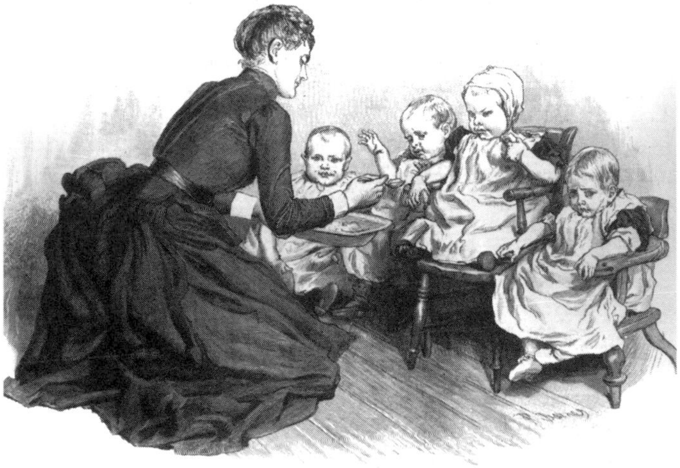

Figure 14.16 The NSPCC began its work with disadvantaged children over one hundred years ago

In 1869, because there were so many charitable organisations all overlapping in the services that they provided, the Charity Organisation Society (COS) was set up to co-ordinate the various organisations. In the 1900s this became the Family Welfare Association and became directly involved in the relief of poverty and in the promotion of mental health. There are now three organisations which have 'umbrella roles': the Council for Voluntary Service, the National Council for Voluntary Organisations and the National Council for Social Services.

Since 1945, various organisations have been formed to meet specific needs as they have become of concern to the public, for example, MIND (the National Association for Mental Health) and Gingerbread (support for single parents).

Evidence collection point

Contact a voluntary agency in your area. Find out how and why it developed within the area, what its role is and whether it is changing.

Government policies and funding

A major development in government policy over the past decade has been to reduce state responsibility for the direct provision of health and social care.

Voluntary and private organisations

The Beveridge Report referred to voluntary groups as being 'society's conscience', being able to defend and champion the interests of minorities in society, and being able to respond to changing needs as they arose. However, since the introduction of the Welfare State, voluntary organisations have had close links with statutory provision, with many organisations being concerned with the provision of services, rather than being focused on other roles (see the next page).

More recently the introduction of a market-style system of care provision has placed greater emphasis on competition between statutory agencies and independent (private and voluntary) agencies. In 1984, private and voluntary hospitals and nursing homes provided 7.5 per cent of hospital-based treatment in the UK. By 1990 this had increased to 15 per cent. Voluntary organisations are also increasingly working with local authorities in care provision in areas such as child welfare, maternity, aftercare of offenders, community nursing, and mental and physical handicap. There are an estimated 400 000 voluntary organisations in the UK (1995 figures), many of which are involved in health and social care.

Informal care

Before the introduction of the Welfare State and before industrial and economic need led the labour force to becoming more mobile, the extended family and the local community played a vital part in the provision of care. This decreased to some extent with the introduction of the NHS and the government's increased participation in the provision of health and social care services during this century. However, especially with the policies of recent years, informal carers are again increasingly shouldering the burden of caring for sick, disabled and older people.

Recent changes in government policy have brought about a shift from state responsibility for welfare to the **mixed economy** (or pluralistic) approach to welfare provision. Private health care is encouraged, as is the use of private organisations in social care. Social Service departments are given transitional grants to enable them to set up community care arrangements, but the government insists that a large proportion of these grants be used to buy in care from the independent sector.

The role of informal carers is likely to increase. Currently there are over six million informal carers in the UK with a quarter of them spending at least 20 hours per week caring for someone. Fifty-eight per cent of carers are women and a quarter of women in the age group 45–64 years are carers.

Funding

Funding for voluntary organisations may come from various sources – the government, local authorities, grant-giving organisations and trusts, groups of people or individuals.

At a time when public expenditure is falling, the UK government is putting more and more resources into the voluntary sector. This happens in a number of ways:

- contractual agreements via health and social service authorities
- local and central tax exemptions
- tax incentives – covenants and donations are tax-deductible
- grants via local authority Social Services departments

The estimated total income of the voluntary sector is about £17 billion per year. The government provides approximately £2 billion of this, with about £50 million being allocated to voluntary agencies in the field of health and social care. Most of this is funded by the Department of Health, but voluntary agencies also receive funding from the NHS, local authorities and the general public (see Chapter 13).

However, government funding for voluntary organisations has been reduced in recent years and is likely to decrease further. Local authority funding is also decreasing. Throughout 1991–2 the National Council for Voluntary Organisations (NCVO) reported, voluntary agencies lost almost £30 million in local authority funding and the projected loss for 1992–3 was £43 million.

Evidence collection point

Contact a voluntary organisation in your area and find out how it is funded. This will assist you in writing your report on the role of the independent sector (see the next page)

Funding for private organisations comes mainly from direct payments by the customer, or a third party. This 'third party' may be a relative or friend, a purchasing agency, such as a health or social services authority, or a private insurance scheme.

While some people are turning more towards the use of private insurance to meet their health and social care needs, many companies and employees are cancelling health insurance plans due to business failures and redundancies.

Demographic influences

Some of the strengths of voluntary organisations include:

- flexibility and the ability to respond quickly to changing needs
- a capacity to innovate, experiment and test new ideas
- good communication links with the community
- the ability to take risks
- cost-effectiveness
- the capacity to promote change.

All of these characteristics are needed if services are to be able to adapt quickly to demographic changes in the community. For although national trends are helpful in the planning of future services, local variations may require a more rapid response.

Private organisations may also be able to respond in a similar way. For example, many private residential homes are now offering day-care services. This initiative has been taken up as a response to the emphasis on providing more care in the community and the increasing numbers of older people requiring care. The number of private facilities may also increase for similar reasons.

Evidence collection point

Find out how many private residential homes for older people there are in your area compared with ten years ago. Have any of these homes now increased the range of services that they offer? What are these? These findings will assist you in producing your report on the independent sector.

Additional roles of the independent sector

What voluntary agencies actually do varies a great deal from organisation to organisation. They are not all involved in the direct provision of services. Examples of their other roles include:

- self-help groups, which provide mutual help based on a common need or problem, for example Gamblers Anonymous (GA)
- advocacy groups, which speak for, or represent, the interests and views of particular groups of people, for example Release (for drug users)
- pressure groups which campaign for a particular group or interest, for example Child Poverty Action Group (CPAG)
- co-ordinating groups, for example the National Council for Voluntary Organisations
- joint planning – in 1986 voluntary agencies were given a role in the joint planning of services, together with the NHS and local authorities.

Evidence collection point

The evidence required for Element 5.2 is a report which outlines how services and facilities have changed in your country; describes three effects of recent government policy on the structure and funding of health and social care services; and gives three examples of ways in which demographic characteristics affect priorities for health and social care. The report should also include a detailed explanation of the role of the independent sector in influencing provision.

Chapter 15

The organisation of health and social care planning and provision

This chapter deals with:

- **the structure of the National Health Service (NHS)**
- **the structure of social services**
- **the market for care**
- **the purchasers of care**
- **the role of the purchasers**
- **the role of the providers**
- **the changes that the providers have had to make**
- **the future of health and social care.**

The structure of the NHS

The structure of the NHS is complex. While this chapter mainly focuses on the health care system in England, there are some differences in the structure of the NHS in Wales, Scotland and Northern Ireland. There are four main tiers to the health care system in the UK:

- central government, including the NHS Policy Board and NHS Management Executive
- Regional Health Authorities and Special Health Authorities
- District Health Authorities and Family Health Service Authorities
- the service provision tier, which includes GPs (both *fund-holders* and non-fund-holders), hospitals (both *directly managed units* and *self-governing trusts*), and other community-based services, such as district nursing services, dentists, opticians and chiropodists. (See Figure 15.1.)

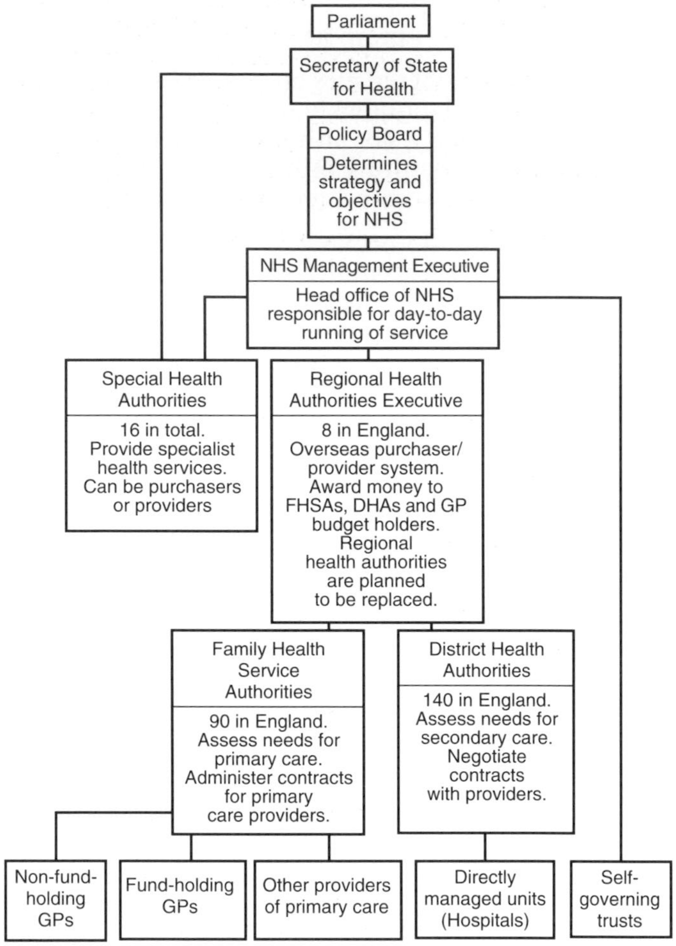

Source: Adapted from *NHS Made Easy* (Department of Health 1993)

Figure 15.1 The National Health Service

Central government

The *Secretary of State for Health* is responsible for the provision of services in both health and social care. The Department of Health (DoH) has the responsibility for determining policy and priorities, circulating advice to NHS authorities, reviewing the performance of the NHS authorities and allocating resources to them. The Secretary of State is accountable for the financial resources spent on the Department of Health and the NHS. He or she also has a general responsibility for promoting the health of all people.

The *NHS Policy Board* is responsible for the overall policy and strategy of the NHS. The *NHS Management Executive* has the responsibility for implementing policies and strategies formulated by the Policy Board. Both these departments were formed in 1989 in an attempt to separate policy-making and the management of the NHS.

(The Secretaries of State for Scotland, Wales and Northern Ireland are responsible for the health policy and services in each of their areas of the UK.)

Regional Health Authorities

There are eight *Regional Health Authorities* (RHAs) in England (see Figure 15.2). The role of the RHAs is primarily strategic. They are responsible for planning services, within national guidelines, within their areas, allocating resources to District Health Authorities and GP fund-holders, overseeing the work of the District Health Authorities and Family Health Service Authorities, providing services that are needed on a regional basis rather than a more local district basis, and managing the internal market. This includes sorting out disputes that may arise between purchasers of health care, (District Health Authorities and fund-holding GPs) and providers of health care (self-governing trusts and directly managed units).

(There are separate Regional Health Authorities in Scotland, Wales and Northern Ireland.)

District Health Authorities

District Health Authorities (DHAs) are responsible for assessing the health needs of people living in their area. They are the *purchasers* of services to meet those health needs, with the exception of services provided by GPs (see page 388). They arrange contracts with the providers of services and set the standards for the carrying out of these services. DHAs are expected to work closely with Family Health Service Authorities and GP fund-holders to draw up plans for the purchasing of services. These plans should include a statement of the priorities of services needed, an outline of how services are to be improved, guidelines for how the services and the improvements are to be monitored, and the range of services to be funded.

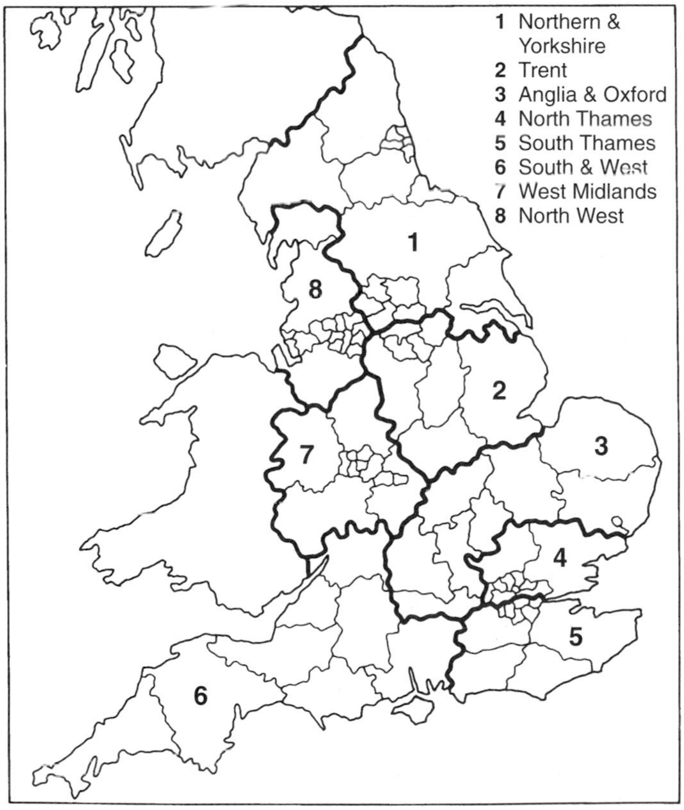

Figure 15.2 Regional Health Authorities in England

In 1995 there were 140 DHAs in England, compared with 190 in 1991. In APRIL 1996 The DHAs and the Family Health Service Authorities will merge. In many areas the merged authorities will be called the 'Commissioning Health Authority'.

DHAs are responsible for:

- assessing the population's needs for health care
- evaluating the effectiveness of services
- drawing up service specifications
- negotiating contracts with providers
- building in quality standards
- monitoring contract performance

Source: *NHS Made Easy* (Department of Health, 1993).

Family Health Service Authorities

Family Health Service Authorities (FHSAs) have the responsibility for managing family practitioner services within their areas. These services include GPs, dentists, pharmacists and opticians, who are contracted to provide services and not directly employed by the FHSAs. The FHSAs also have a role in providing information about services, as well as developing and monitoring the quality of the

FHSAs are responsible for:

- the administration of the new contracts for GPs, dentists, pharmacists and opticians
- identifying primary health needs of the population
- developing services to meet those needs
- managing funds for GP practice team development and premises improvement
- making services responsive to consumers' wishes.

Source: NHS Made Easy (Department of Health, 1993).

services. In addition to this, the FHSAs manage complaints procedures which investigate complaints against family practitioners.

Try it

Write to the Family Health Service Authority in your area and ask for information about the services it provides and for a copy of its complaints procedure.

Special Health Authorities

There are a number of health authorities outside of the structure described above, They are called the Special Health Authorities (SHAs) and they report directly to either the Department of Health in London, or the NHS Management Executive. There are three types:

1. Non-hospital SHAs: these provide a service for the whole NHS which needs some coordination at national level. Examples are the NHS Supplies Authority and the Health Education Authority.
2. Hospital SHAs: a number of specialist post-graduate teaching and research hospitals in London have SHA status. Examples are the Hammersmith, the National Heart and Chest Hospitals and the Royal Marsden.
3. Special Hospitals: Special Hospitals are those dealing with the care of seriously disturbed offenders (Rampton, Ashworth and Broadmoor are the English Special Hospitals). They form an SHA in their own right – but not all SHAs are Special Hospitals.

Source: NHS Made Easy (Department of Health, 1993).

GP fund-holders

GP fund-holders receive a budget from Family Health Service Authorities which is used to cover the costs of running the practice, buying drugs and for buying some non-emergency hospital services and some community health services.

Originally only GP practices with more than 9000 registered patients could apply to become fund-holding. Now practices with 7000 registered patients can become fund-holders. In the future, it is likely that even smaller practices will be eligible to apply to become fund-holders. By the end of the 1990s, it is expected that about 50 per cent of the population will be patients of GP fund-holders.

Fund-holding GPs can buy services direct from a range of providers of services, but the ordinary GP has to place patients on a waiting list for District Health Authority funded services. Some people claim that this creates a two-tier system. However, both fund-holders and non-fund-holders are working within limited budgets.

Try it

How aware are people of the distinction between fund-holding and non-fund-holding GPs? Devise a simple questionnaire and research the opinions of the people on your course.

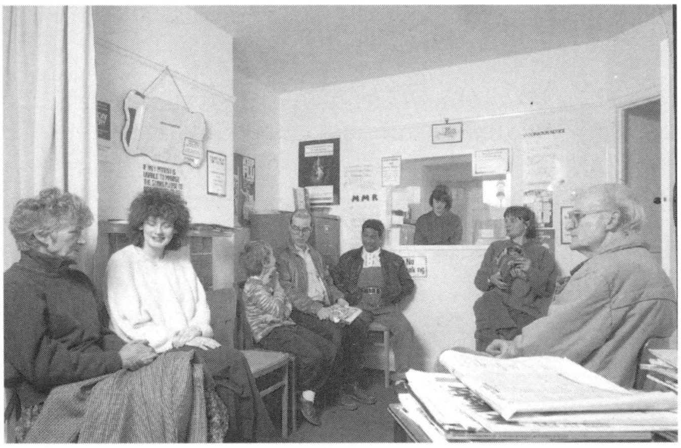

Evidence collection point

Find out which GP practices in your area are GP fund-holders (this may be done through the local FHSA). You could make an appointment to see someone in the practice, perhaps a senior GP partner or the practice administrator, and ask for a description of his or her role as a purchaser of services. Or you could use some secondary research on the nature of a fund-holding practice as a purchaser of health care services.

Self-governing trusts and directly managed units

Within the NHS there are two kinds of organisations *providing* services: *self-governing trusts* and *directly managed units* (DMUs). They provide hospital and community health care services. These services are purchased by GP fund-holders and the District Health Authorities. The majority of providers are now self-governing trusts, and it is probable that by the mid-1990s 95 per cent of NHS hospital and community health services will have trust status.

Self-governing trusts have greater freedom to determine their own management structures. They are able to negotiate the terms and conditions of service of their staff, and have greater control over their own investments, borrowing and assets.

> NHS Trusts are self-governing units within the National Health Service. They are run by boards of directors and are accountable directly to the centre. Major acute hospitals are the obvious candidates for this status but trusts can cover a range of services including community services, services for patient groups such as people with mental illness, and ambulance services.
>
> By being trusts these organisations can:
>
> - determine their own management structures
> - employ their own staff using their own terms and conditions of service
> - acquire, own and sell their assets
> - retain surpluses and borrow money (subject to annual limits).
>
> Each trust has a board of directors with complete responsibility for managing the trust's affairs. Each year they prepare a business plan, setting out proposals for service developments and capital investment. At the end of the year they prepare and publish an annual report and accounts.
>
> *Source:* Adapted form *NHS Made Easy* (Department of Health, 1993).

Think it over

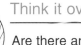

Are there any hospital or community trusts that operate in your area? What are they called and what services do they provide?

Directly managed units are primarily hospitals that are still under the authority of the District Health Authorities. Although they do not have the same freedoms as the hospital trusts, the DHAs are delegating more responsibility to them for managing their own affairs.

As the availability of long-term care in hospitals diminishes, the role of community services increases. In some areas the management structures which previously had responsibility for long-term hospital care and rehabilitation services have become increasingly involved in the provision of community services. These services include district nursing, chiropody services, bathing services, a range of services provided from clinic settings, and may also involve services for children. These units may also have become self-governing trusts. They are often referred to as *community trusts*.

The structure of social services

The Secretary of State for Health is responsible for the *provision* of social services. However, it is local authorities that administer them. Local authority social service departments have responsibility for the coordination of all forms of social care in the community (see Figure 15.3).

Each local authority has a Social Services Committee which has responsibility for the social services within its area. It must appoint a Director of Social Services. The director is in charge of the department which administers the services. Social service departments are often organised into area offices from which the services for that area are operated.

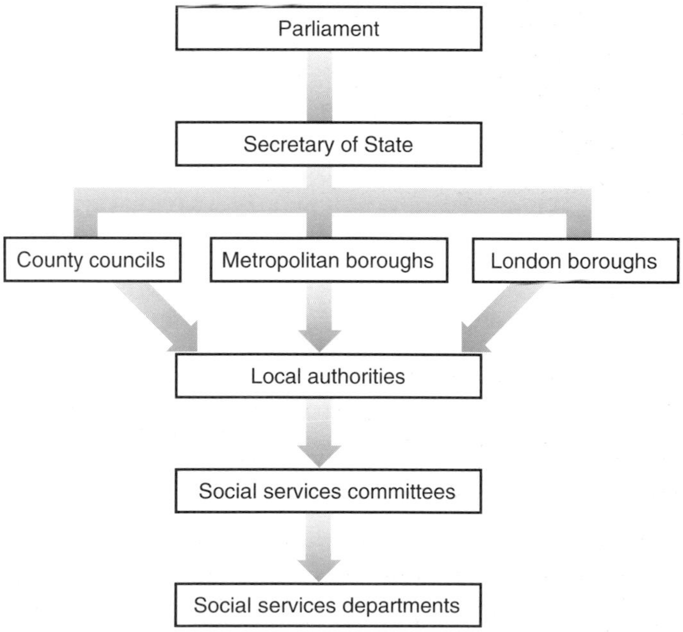

Figure 15.3 The structure of social services

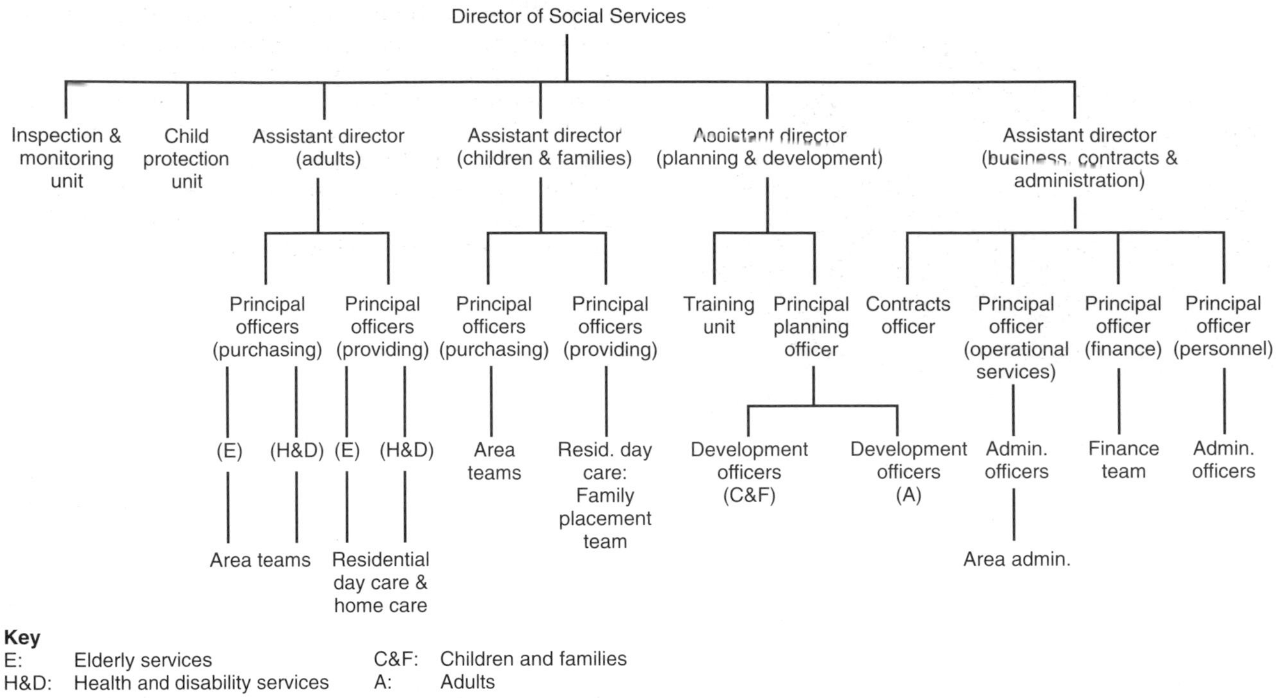

Figure 15.4 An example of a social services department structure

Organisational structures within the local authority social services departments have changed considerably in recent years to enable the departments to carry out their new roles, as required by new legislation, in particular, the National Health Service and Community Care Act 1990.

Many social services departments have new sections within them, such as inspection and monitoring sections (which often also have the responsibility for dealing with complaints procedures). Planning and development sections have taken on increased importance now that the authorities are required to work more closely with their health service planning colleagues, as well as with the private and voluntary sectors. Additionally, some local authorities have sections which are specifically responsible for contracting with service providers. Many social services departments have also re-organised their staffing structures to reflect a clear division between the purchasing and providing responsibilities (see Figure 15.4).

County councils run local authority services in England and Wales, as do metropolitan councils and the London boroughs.

In Northern Ireland there are four boards set up to administer social and health services. This unified structure is outside political control. In Scotland, regional local authorities control social work departments.

Social services should not be confused with the Department of Social Security (DSS), which administers benefits and pays out money. Apart from an occasional small sum in an emergency, the social services do not hand out money. Their main function is to offer advice, to provide access to services and to provide a number of services themselves. They provide access to community and residential services for all client groups, such as children, people with mental health problems, people with mental or physical disabilities and older people.

Try it

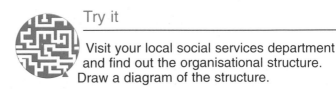

Visit your local social services department and find out the organisational structure. Draw a diagram of the structure.

The market for care

The UK government has been concerned to create a *market system* for the delivery of health care.

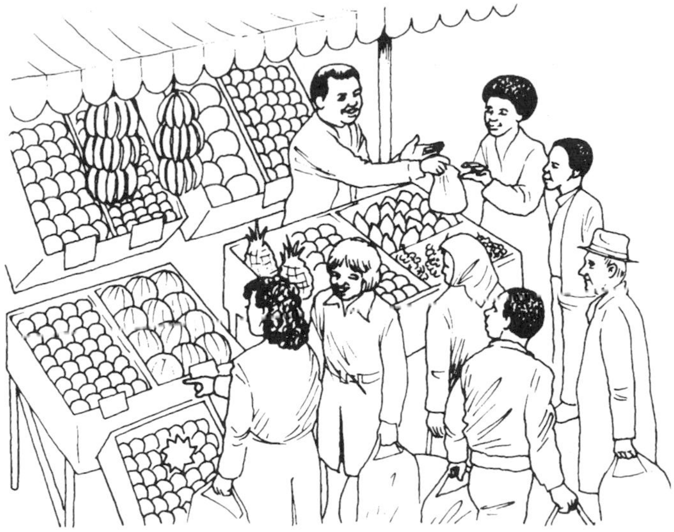

A marketplace is where people sell things to consumers. In health and social care, the sellers are called *providers* and the buyers of services are called *purchasers*. So, in order to create a market for health care provision, the National Health Service is divided into a system of purchasers and providers. Providers offer the direct care a person receives when he or she attends a doctor's surgery or hospital. Purchasers organise and plan the types and levels of care provision that are needed.

In a marketplace, providers set out their stalls, while purchasers work out what they need to but. Market-places often encourage cheaper prices for things like fruit and vegetables. There might be competition between providers, for example more than one stall selling fruit. Providers have to work hard to try to provide good quality at the most competitive prices if they are to attract purchasers and stay in business. The government has transferred this idea of a marketplace into both health and social care provision.

Supporters of the market idea argue that it will lead to good quality care for patients. Patients will be treated more like customers – they will be seen as vital for the maintenance of staff jobs. Supporters of the market idea also argue that competition will lead to greater efficiency and that services will improve at no extra cost to the tax payer.

However, not everyone supports the market idea for health care. One argument against it is that a complex service like medicine will not respond to the simple ideas which work when selling fruit and vegetables (see Chapter 12, page 290). Some opponents of the market idea claim that certain individuals may be disadvantaged because *their* purchasers are not in such a powerful position as other purchasers. Some opponents of the market system believe that the market will eventually lead to a privatisation of services. This would mean that certain types of care will only be available to individuals who can afford to pay privately. These issues are open to political debate.

The purchasers of care

The NHS and Community Care Act 1990 separated the functions of purchaser and provider of services both within the National Health Service and within social services authorities.

Purchasers in the social services

Social services departments are no longer the major providers of services. They are gradually decreasing their function as providers of services and becoming assessors and purchasers of services (see Chapter 16 on Assessment and Care Planning). A local authority's commitment to the provision of social services is closely related to which political party is in control. Generally, Labour councils have, in the past, been more prepared to spend on developing social services. As not all provision is statutory, local authorities have a choice about which services are developed. However, services will be developed depending on the amount of money available.

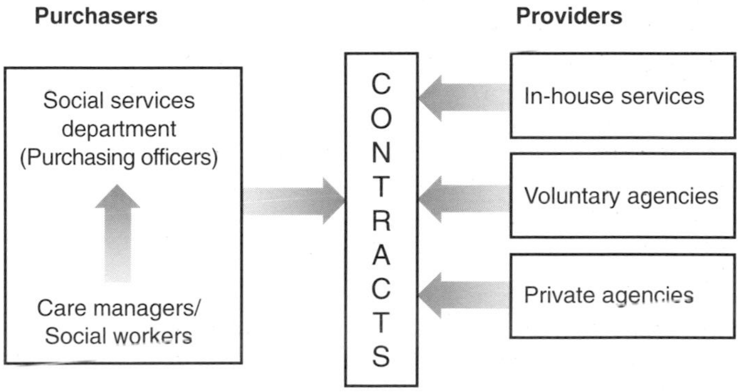

Figure 15.5 Social care purchasers and providers

Purchasers in the NHS

The purchaser and provider roles for health care are held at different levels within the NHS, although sometimes these do overlap, for example GP fund-holders.

GP fund-holders are both providers of primary health care and purchasers of secondary health care. They are small purchasing authorities in their own right. They contract with other service providers, such as community and hospital trusts, directly managed hospitals and independent hospitals, to provide services for their patients. Many individuals argue that being able to buy secondary health care services directly gives the patients of GP fund-holders an advantage compared to patients of non-fund-holding GPs, who may have to wait much longer for treatment, may have a more limited choice of where they get their treatment, or may even find that they are denied some treatments that GP fund-holders are able to purchase.

Primary care services, such as doctors' surgeries, are organised and paid for by the Family Health Services Authorities (FHSAs) which act as purchasers of primary care (see page 337). Secondary care services, such as hospital provision, are organised and 'bought' by District Health Authorities (see page 337) or by GP fund-holders. From April 1996 the merged FHSAs and DHAs are responsible for purchasing both primary and secondary health care.

The role of the purchasers

The role of the purchasers of care include:

- assessing the health and social care needs of the population of their area
- planning how to meet health and social care needs
- stimulating service provision where it is missing
- assessing service providers' ability to deliver services
- contracting with service providers
- monitoring and evaluating services against the terms and conditions of the contract.

Assessing needs

In some instances, the major purchasers of health and social social care (DHAs, FHAs and social services departments) will work independently in assessing a particular need within their area. For example, a social services department may assess the need for the provision of hot meals for elderly and disabled people within the area without involving the District Health Authority. The District Health Authority may assess the need for chiropody services within the area together, without involving the social services department. However, at other times both they, and the FHSA, may decide to assess the needs of the people living in their area especially where the need cannot be easily and clearly defined as either a health or a social care need. An example of this could be a special team of home carers who provide an intensive short-term service for someone being discharged from hospital.

Case study

Every week, Mabel Green Hospital discharges approximately ten people who have had various sorts of orthopaedic operations such as hip replacements, knee-joint replacements or surgery following the fracture of a bone in the arm. Within a few days of the operation, the patient is well enough to be able to go home. However, if the patient lives alone or lives with someone who is elderly or disabled, he or she may not be able to manage at home without additional help until fully recovered.

Mabel Green District Health Authority and Mabel Green Social Services Department together decided that the kind of help that the people would benefit from most would be a specialist team of home carers who would not only carry out the practical household tasks (cleaning, shopping, etc.) and help with personal care needs (getting washed, dressed, etc.), but who would also help people to regain their confidence in performing these tasks, and help rehabilitate them back into their daily routines.

The special Home From Hospital Care Team was commissioned to provide intensive, short-term care of people being discharged to their homes.

Ways of assessing needs

Health and social care needs can be assessed in a number of ways.

- Local authorities are already required to find out the numbers of people in their area who have disabilities. They are also required to keep a register of children in need.
- Both social services and health authorities are able to use the local census information to find out how many older there are in their area, and to predict the number of older people who will be living in the area in the future.
- Previous health need trends are also useful indicators of future health care needs.

- Current trends can also be monitored through the collection of statistical information either from people who already use the services, or from surveys carried out within the general population of the area.

Planning services

Although District Health Authorities have the responsibility of assessing the health care needs of people in their area, and planning services to meet those needs, the Department of Health has continued to specify areas of service provision. Previously they set targets for such things as surgical procedures, including hip replacements, operations to remove cataracts, bone marrow transplants and coronary artery bypass grafts.

There is now a movement away from specific targets towards broad areas of development. The NHS operates within the guidelines laid down by the Department of Health, in the government White Paper, *The Health of the Nation* (1992). This prioritises five areas of health care: cancer, coronary heart disease and strokes, mental health, HIV/AIDS and sexual health, and accidents.

Although local authorities have been given the lead responsibility relating to assessing the social care needs of people in their area, they also work within a legal framework. The gives them various powers and duties with respect to the provision of services (see Chapter 13).

So, although both health and social care purchasers and planners are required to assess and meet the specific needs of the people within their areas, they are still required to work within the guidelines set out by government and the Department of Health.

Joint planning

Various governments have tried to encourage the joint planning of services between health authorities and local authorities but this was made difficult because of the differences in the ways that the authorities were structured. For example, in health care terms, the care of elderly, mentally-ill people has been the responsibility of the mental health services; in social care terms, the same people have come under the responsibility of services for older people.

Other problems are caused by the different timescales to which the two types of authority work, the different management structures and the fact that

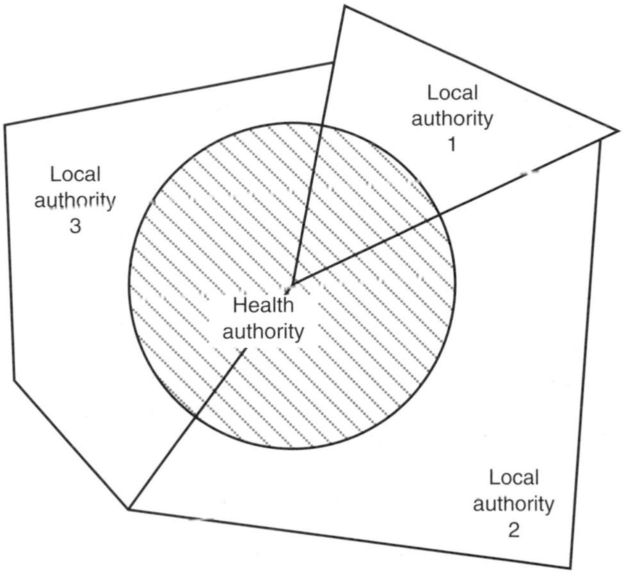

Figure 15.6 One health authority may cover all, or part, of a number of local authority areas

health authorities and local authorities do not have co-terminous boundaries (for example, one health authority area may cover all or part of a number of local authority areas, see Figure 15.6). Alternatively one local authority area may involve negotiating with a number of health authorities (see Figure 15.7).

The advantage of joint planning is that, in instances where the care required cannot easily be defined as either health or social care, services need not be duplicated or neglected altogether. Poor joint

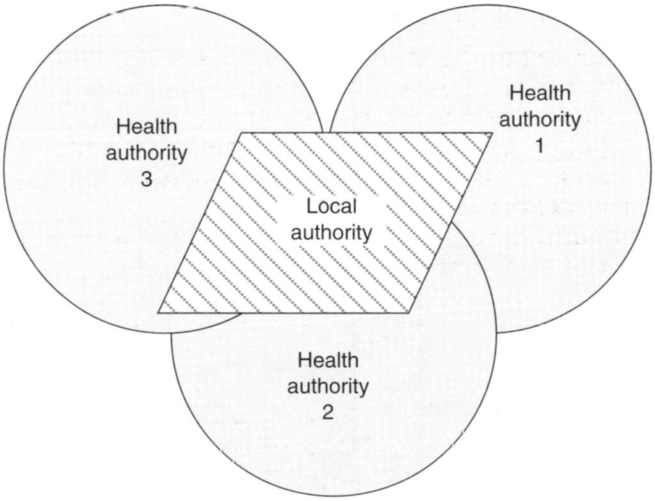

Figure 15.7 One local authority may negotiate with a number of health authorities

planning results in poor coordination of services and inefficient use of resources.

Stimulating service provision

The NHS and Community Care Act 1990 imposed a duty on local authorities to develop a *mixed economy of care*. This means more emphasis is being placed on the contribution of the private and voluntary sectors in the provision of social care. The purchaser–provider split has enabled this to happen, with the purchasing (or commissioning) of services being separated from the provision of services. Local authorities are also required to stimulate the development of services in the private and voluntary sectors. To ensure that local authorities do this, the government requires that local authorities spend 85 per cent of all funds on care provision from the independent sector.

Supporters of the notion of a mixed economy of care argue that better value for money can be obtained, as a competitive market would improve quality, efficiency and economy of services. It is also hoped that the competitive market will result in the cost of care being kept down. It is argued that individuals will have more choice in how and where their care is obtained.

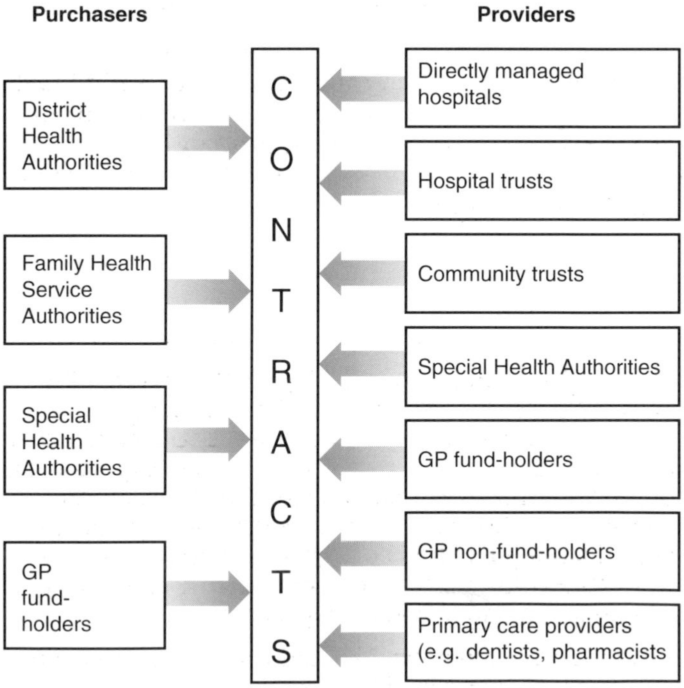

Figure 15.8 The internal market – purchasers and providers of NHS services

Within the NHS an *internal market* is being developed. This means that, in future, hospitals will compete with one another in attracting contracts with the purchasers of health care. The providers of other health care services will also be in competition with each other. (See Figure 15.8.)

Opponents of the internal market system feel that it does not always deliver services effectively. In some instances, such as where there are a small number of specialist providers, where there are technical complexities, where purchasers are tied to long-term contracts and where there is uncertainty about the cost of the service, costs could be very high, off-setting the advantages of a market economy. Also, it is felt that providers could become obsessed with pursuing their own interests, rather than working within an overall strategic plan. Many feel that the market system does not work in the best interests of the individual service user. This can be resolved by ensuring that contracts include service specifications (see opposite), and that the individual's needs will be met through the assessment and care management process (see Chapter 16).

Purchasers are responsible for stimulating new forms of service (such as peripatetic night care services, which provide a 'pop-in' service at regular times throughout the night for people with disabilities or for older people who have senile dementia). Purchasers may also decide that some services, that are already provided, are not needed, or that demand for them has decreased. For example, working towards the principle of 'care in the community', the number of hospital beds is gradually diminishing, while the provision of nursing home care is increasing. The contraction of one service may allow for the expansion of others, but this must still be in relation to meeting the needs of the population.

There has often been some confusion about the terms 'purchasing' and 'commissioning'. Purchasing can be described as going to a supermarket and buying what is on the shelves. Commissioning can be described as deciding what is to be put on the shelves in the first place. Purchasers have a major role to play in commissioning services, through the planning process as well as in the buying in of services.

Try it

Find out from your local District Health Authority the number of hospital beds that it had ten years ago, and how they intend to provided nursing care for people now. Also find out how many private nursing homes were registered in your area ten years ago, and how many there are registered with the health authority now.

Contracting and assessing the provider's ability to deliver services

Together with the introduction of the market system for the provision of health and social care, and the purchaser–provider split, came the need for formal agreements to be set between the purchaser of the service and the provider of the service. These *contracts* specify what services are to be delivered, the minimum quality requirements (known as *service specifications*) and how services should be monitored.

Contracts

There are three main types of contract:

- *Individual contracts* (sometimes called 'Cost per case' contracts). The providers receive an agreed price for services given to an individual person. For example, a place in a nursing home may be purchased for an individual person. The sum agreed may not include constant attention throughout the night. If this late-night service becomes necessary, an additional sum may be paid over and above the original cost.
- *Cost and volume contracts.* This is where the provider receives a fixed sum for an agreed basic level of service, but may then receive an extra payment for care given over and above the minimum level.
- *Block contracts.* The provider receives a fixed sum for providing specified services. For example, a local authority may have a block contract with a nursing home to provide four beds. When any of the four beds are not occupied, the local authority is likely to have to pay part or all of the cost, in order to retain the use of the bed.

The contracting process begins once purchasers have decided what their overall aims and objectives are (*strategic framework and planning*). Service specifications will then be developed, which will set out the *quality standards* that the purchasers expect.

Service specifications

There are usually two levels of service specifications:

- general service specifications which apply to all contracts
- individual service specifications for particular services.

Quality issues that come under the heading of general service specifications might include:

- the appropriateness of the care to be delivered
- an attitude that treats all clients with dignity and respect
- procedures and an environment that are conducive to the clients' safety and well-being
- involvement of clients in their own care
- taking into account clients' cultural and religious needs
- speed of response to clients' needs.

The contracting process enables the purchasers to assess the provider's ability to deliver the required service, and contracts would not be awarded to providers unable to meet the minimum service specifications required by the purchasers.

In many instances just one purchaser will be involved in the purchasing of care for an individual or group of people. However, at other times multi-agency purchasing, using joint funding arrangements, may be used to pay for the care of an individual or group.

Case study: Mr Pardeza

Mr Pardeza is a 75-year-old man who has severe arthritis in his knees, wrists and shoulders. He is a widower and lives alone in a council house. He requires help with washing, bathing, dressing and carrying out household tasks including cooking and shopping. He finds it difficult to get up the stairs and to get in and out of the bath. Since his wife died, Mr Pardeza has been very lonely, so recently he has begun to attend a local day care centre.

All of the equipment that Mr Pardeza requires, together with services regarding his personal, social and domestic care, is purchased through the local authority social services department.

Case study: Mrs Cusack

Mrs Cusack is 29-years-old and recently gave birth to a healthy baby boy. This is her second child. Following the birth of her son, Mrs Cusack became very depressed and has been diagnosed as having post-natal depression. Mrs Cusack needs help looking after her 2-year-old daughter and her baby son while her husband is at work. This is provided by a Family Aid Worker. She also receives help and advice about the management of her depression. This is provided by a Community Psychiatric Nurse.

Mrs Cusack's care is funded partly by the social services and partly through the NHS.

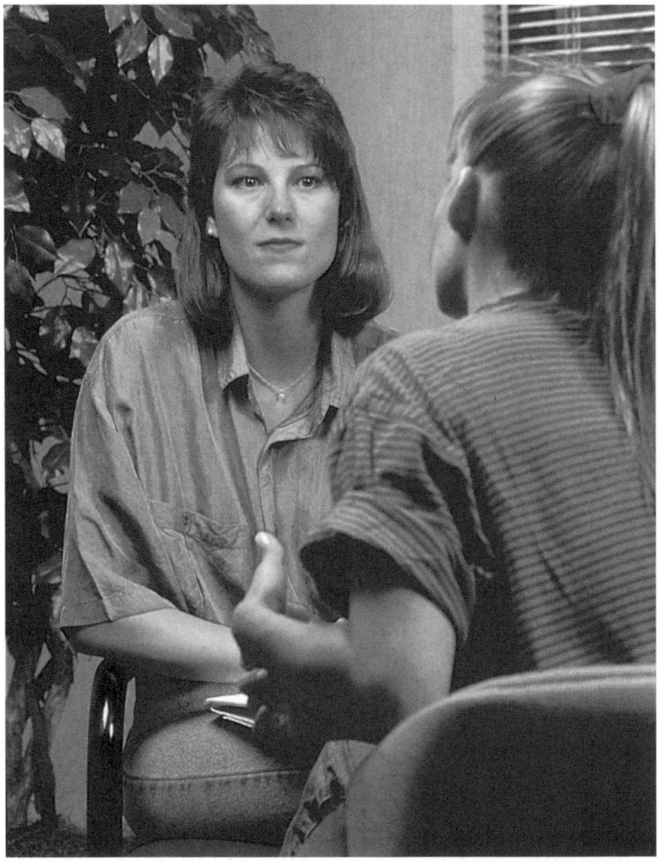

Services for groups of people may also be jointly funded by health and social services authorities. For example, a day centre for people with mental health problems may provide medical treatment, psychiatric services and social care services including a team of home care workers and social workers. The centre therefore may be jointly set up and financed by health and social services. Developing services in this way is known as *joint commissioning*.

Monitoring and evaluating services

The contract may also specify how the quality of services is to be monitored and evaluated. Both purchasers and providers maintain statistical information regarding services that are provided. Providers are often required to report back to the purchasers on their performance. For instance, a District Health Authority may contract with a hospice to provide a minimum number of admissions for people from their area during a one-year period. The hospice would have to monitor the admissions from that health authority area and provide quarterly reports on whether they are meeting the targets for those admissions.

Increasingly, service users are becoming involved in the monitoring and reviewing of the quality of services. This seems mainly to be happening in the following ways:

- consumer representation on planning and steering groups
- client/public surveys
- feedback from service users and their carers
- regular meetings between purchasers and users of specific services and their carers (and may include the providers).

The role of the providers

Health and social care in the UK are developing and extending along community care principles. *Community care* is believed to be an appropriate response to the growing and more complex health and social care needs of people. It is also thought by many that community care is a better way of using scarce resources, making services more cost-effective.

For a long time it has been recognised that there are specific groups of people whose needs make more demands on health and social care services than others. These groups include people who are mentally ill, people with physical or learning disabilities, older people and children. Individuals within these groups often have many health and social care needs.

Within the NHS, services have traditionally been focused on acute services (treatment of acute illnesses, surgery, treatment following accidents, etc.). Similarly, within the social care field, services have traditionally been perceived to concentrate on child-care. Services for people with mental health

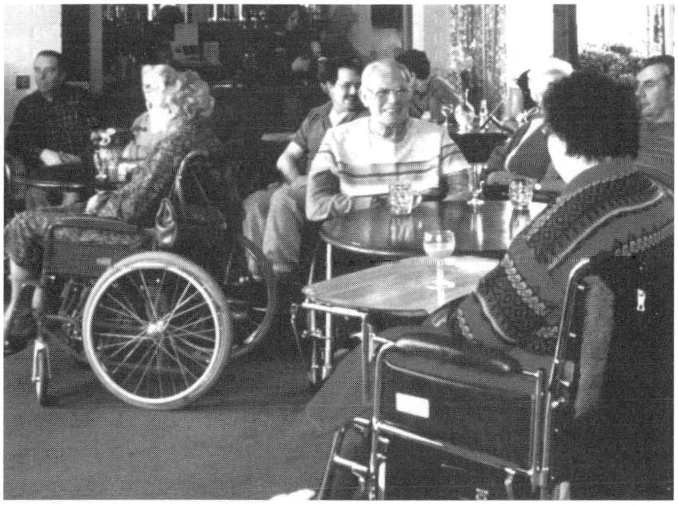

(*Photo courtesy of Winged Fellowship Trust*)

problems, people with learning disabilities and older people have been regarded as the 'Cinderella services' – services which receive fewer resources and lower priority than childcare.

Governments since the 1960s have been concerned to develop services for people with mental health problems, people with learning disabilities and older people. Government policies have therefore had three main aims:

- to shift resources towards the care of these groups
- to improve the co-ordination of health services, social services and private and voluntary provision
- to develop services in the community (rather than in hospitals).

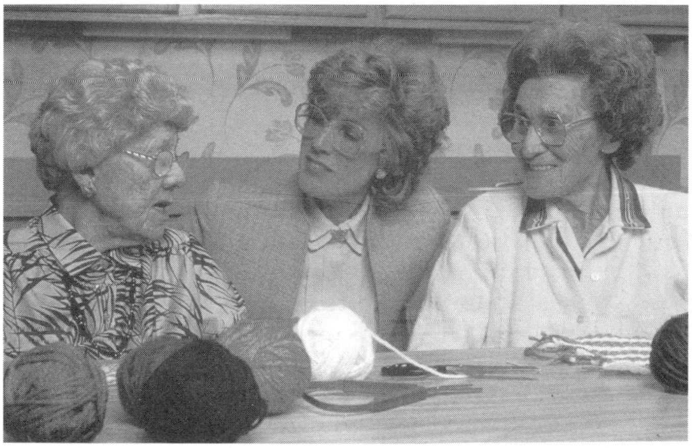

(*Photo courtesy of Winged Fellowship Trust*)

The move towards community care has its roots in the early part of the century and arose mainly as a response to criticisms of institutional forms of care. By the 1980s the demand for care, especially among very elderly people, combined with budgetary and resource constraints, made cost effectiveness much more important than ever before. It is from this that the notion of a *mixed economy of care* began to be developed.

The Griffiths Report, published in 1988, has often been regarded as a landmark in the provision of health and social care. At the centre of the report is a key statement which defines the role of the public sector: 'The role of the public sector is essentially to ensure that care is provided.' For local authorities this would mean that their role would be to *manage* care, not necessarily to provide it. In health services it meant a split of the purchasing and providing functions between the different authority levels.

Following the Griffiths Report, the NHS and Community Care Act 1990 set out the framework for the changes in the way that health and social services are to be delivered in the future.

The role of the providers of care includes:

- providing directly to individuals services that are contracted by the purchaser
- ensuring that the services meet the standards set by the purchaser
- ensuring the quality of services.

The notion of 'contracting' is quite new for many service providers, as is the idea of monitoring the standard of services against set criteria. However, ensuring the quality of services has been part of service provision for some time, although it has not been undertaken very systematically in many instances. Also, the involvement of service users in the monitoring and evaluation of the quality of services has only recently become accepted practice.

Changes that the providers have had to make

Changes that the providers of services have needed to make can be described under four main headings:

- structures
- accountability
- contracts
- client involvement.

Structures

The new market-style provision of care, together with the need for all service providers to ensure 'value for money', means that all service providers must now work within a business culture, even if their agency is non-profit-making. In order to obtain contracts, or attract grants, the service provider must operate in a businesslike manner.

For the majority of people in the UK the term 'welfare' is synonymous with state provision – health care being provided by the NHS and social care by the social services departments of the local authority. With the introduction of the mixe-+ economy of care this will inevitably change. It must be said, however, that the private and voluntary sectors have always played their part in the provision of care and their contribution will become increasingly important in the years to come. In 1984, private and voluntary hospitals and nursing homes supplied only 7.5 per cent of UK hospital-based treatment and care. By 1990 this had grown to 15 per cent.

Voluntary agencies, increasingly large-scale and professional in their organisation, are relatively cheap (though not cost-free) and flexible in their way of delivering services. They too will need to be able to operate within the business and contract culture which surrounds the provision of care.

Accountability

The formal separation of policy-making, at central government level, and purchasing and providing functions means that there is less likely to be ministerial involvement at local levels of health and social care provision. However, this also means that there could be a reduction in public accountability of these services. Also, there no longer have to be local representatives on health authority boards, or on the boards of self-governing trusts.

The government's view in the 1990s is that public accountability can best be achieved through the mixed economy of care, which, it is stated, gives individuals more freedom of choice. The Citizen's and Patient's Charters also lay down consumer rights and entitlements. However, these charters have yet to ensure that services are responsive to the changing needs of service users.

Many service providers are trying to involve service users more closely in monitoring the quality of services, as previously described in this chapter. However, this does not ensure that the services are accountable to the service user.

Contracts

As well as tendering for contracts with the purchasers, providers will have their own development plans, and will try to convince purchasers of their merit, in order to attract longer term contracts. Many providers, having more control over their own resources, are often able to be more creative, suggesting new services or new patterns of care.

One of the most significant developments reported by many providers is the monitoring of service specifications against the terms and conditions of the contract. This calls for the development of new skills in setting up ways of measuring the quality of the services provided. Gathering quantitative and qualitative information is necessary and often required by the purchaser as proof that the terms of the contract have been adhered to.

Evidence collection point.

Contact your local social services department and find out what changes the home care department has had to make in its structure since the implementation of the NHS and Community Care Act 1990. Gather information regarding the service specifications that the department now works to and how it monitors the quality of the services it provides. Also contact a private home care agency and find out how it monitors services.

Client involvement

The service user's experience is often a good measure for looking at the quality of services. Service users judge quality by comparing the service they receive against the expectations they have of the service. However, the disadvantage of this is that perceptions and expectations are not objective and are therefore difficult to measure properly. For example, someone waiting to see a GP, knowing beforehand that there is likely to be a 30-minute wait, may be happier than someone waiting for 30 minutes but not knowing how long they may have to wait.

The introduction of clear and well-publicised complaints procedures ensures that services users and their carers have a way of making heard their concerns and grievances regarding the delivery and quality of services.

There are various models of ways in which service users can increase their influence on the quality of services:

- service users are represented by an organisation which monitors local services on their behalf and which takes up individual cases (for example, Community Health Councils)
- service users elect representatives to the bodies which manage local services
- service users decide for themselves the care they require
- service users and the professionals come together to decide what action to take. This can work on an individual basis (between a client and a social worker) or at an organisational level (between health agencies and patient representatives). This is sometimes referred to as *working in partnership*.

The future of health and social care

The reforms within the health and social care services have the potential for creating more dynamic, responsive and efficient services in the future. Welfare in the UK is likely to continue to develop according to the broad principles that have been identified through the 1980s. These include:

- a commitment to competition through a marketplace system for the provision of care
- separation of the responsibility for a service from direct provision (the purchaser–provider split)
- more involvement of private, voluntary and informal provision (the mixed economy of care)
- a commitment to greater consumer choice
- the operation of all agencies and organisations in a businesslike manner
- the development of new forms of accountability and new methods of monitoring services
- the development of care in the community
- a commitment to close co-operation between both health and social care purchasers and providers.

The funding of health and social care remains a major issue. Resource constraints, in terms of both people and money, continue to be of great concern.

Although both the Labour Party and the Liberal Democrats set out plans to abolish the internal market system prior to the General Election in 1992, both now support the idea of the split between purchasers and providers of care. Further reforms, to plan and regulate the market for health and social care, are a possibility.

Evidence collection point

To complete Element 5.3, you will need to provide a short report which:

- describes the role of a local purchaser of health or social care services
- explains the changes required of a local provider in meeting the needs of the purchaser
- explains the overall structure of health and social care provisions, including examples of the different agencies involved.

Self-assessment test

1 Which are the two main statutory organisations responsible for the provision of health and social care?
  - **a** The Family Health Service Authority and the local authority.
  - **b** The Regional Health Authority and Social Services department of the local authority.
  - **c** The District Health Authority and Social Services department of the local authority.
  - **d** The National Health Service and Social Services department of the local authority.

2 Acts of Parliament give a legal framework for the provision of health and social care. These Acts of Parliament give 'powers' and 'duties' within which care providers work. Having the 'power' to provide certain types of care means:
  - **a** That the service must be provided.
  - **b** That the service is only provided in exceptional circumstances.
  - **c** That the service may be provided at the discretion of the providing organisation.
  - **d** That the service must be provided, but only to a limited number of people.

3 The National Assistance Act 1948 was a piece of legislation that:
  - **a** Replaced the Poor Law and made it a duty for local authorities to provide homes and hostels for older people and people with disabilities.
  - **b** Amended the Poor Law and empowered local authorities to provide accommodation for anyone in need.

- **c** Replaced the Poor Law and required local authorities to set up social services committees.
- **d** Amended the Poor Law and made sure that every local authority provided exactly the same services to everyone throughout the UK.

4 One of the most important pieces of legislation for people with disabilities is:
- **a** The Health Services and Public Health Act 1968.
- **b** The Local Authority Social Services Act 1970.
- **c** The Chronically Sick and Disabled Person's Act 1970.
- **d** The Mental Health Act 1983.

5 The Mental Health Act 1983 made it a duty for local authorities to appoint 'Approved Social Workers'. The main duty of the Approved Social Worker is:
- **a** To ensure the safety of children.
- **b** To make sure that people with mental disorders take their medication.
- **c** To find accommodation and work for people with mental illnesses.
- **d** To assess people for admission to hospital.

6 The definition of the term 'mental disorder' includes the following:
- **a** Mental illness and psychopathic disorders only.
- **b** Mental illness, arrested or incomplete development of the mind, psychopathic disorders and any other disorder of the mind.
- **c** Mental illness and learning disabilities.
- **d** Mental illness; learning disability and any other disability of the mind.

7 Which of the following statements most accurately describes the Children Act 1989?
- **a** A piece of legislation which gives limited powers to local authorities in relation to all children.
- **b** A piece of legislation which gives general powers and duties to local authorities in relation to all children and their families.
- **c** A piece of legislation which gives wide-ranging responsibilities to local authorities in respect of children in need.
- **d** A piece of legislation which gives some additional powers and duties to local authorities in respect of children in need.

8 The term 'accommodation', in relating to the Children Act 1989, means:
- **a** A voluntary agreement between the local authority and parents to provide accommodation and care for a child.
- **b** The place where a child may be required to live.
- **c** The right of the local authority to take a child into its care.
- **d** A children's home as opposed to a foster home.

9 'Care management' is a term used in the NHS and Community Care Act 1990. It relates to:
- **a** A system for assessing and organising the provision of health and social care for an individual.
- **b** A new approach in nursing techniques.
- **c** A new name for local authority Social Services departments.
- **d** A system which ensures that everyone receives the same sort of care as everyone else.

10 The term 'provider', in relation to the NHS and Community Care Act 1990, refers to:
- **a** An individual person who gives a service free of charge to a patient or client.
- **b** An organisation that sells care services to a purchaser.
- **c** An organisation that buys care for an individual patient or client.
- **d** An individual who gives money towards the cost of care services.

11 The term 'purchaser', in relation to the NHS and Community Care Act 1990, means:
- **a** An individual who buys in care services for a relative.
- **b** An organisation that gives health or social care direct to an individual.
- **c** An organisation that buys in necessary health or social care services.
- **d** A patient or client who contributes towards the cost of the care that he or she receives.

12 The term 'voluntary organisation' refers to agencies which:
- **a** Are non-profit-making but make a charge for their services.
- **b** Are statutory and non-profit-making.
- **c** Are non-statutory, non-profit-making and do not make a charge for their services.
- **d** Make a charge for their services and aim to make a profit.

13 The move away from a state-provided health and social care direct provision of services is likely to result in:
- **a** Less care being provided by the independent sector.

b More people being in need of health and social care services.
c A decrease in the need for relatives to be involved with the care of family members.
d An increase in the role of the independent sector in the provision of health and social care.

14 The independent sector is made up of:
a Informal carers, private organisations and voluntary organisations.
b Private and voluntary organisations.
c The National Health Service and voluntary agencies.
d Social Services departments and private organisations.

15 Secondary health care refers to:
a Services provided by GPs, dentists and opticians.
b Services provided at hospitals, clinics and out-patient departments.
c Services that are given in order to prevent illnesses and disease.
d Services such as occupational therapy, speech therapy and physiotherapy.

16 Health and social care services are classified mainly by:
a How they are funded.
b Who uses the service.
c What service is being provided.
d The way that they are structured and managed.

17 Funding for Social Services comes mainly from:
a Central government and council taxes.
b Payments made by individuals for services.
c National Insurance contributions and council taxes.
d Council taxes only.

18 The funding for voluntary organisations may include the contributions from:
a Fund-raising activities by groups only.
b Individuals only.
c A mixture of central government, local authority and district health authority grants and contracts only.
d A mixture of grants from central government, local authorities and other grant-giving organisations; district health authority and local authority contracts; individuals and groups of people; and fund-raising activities.

19 Private organisations are funded through:
a Central government grants and council taxes.
b Direct payments by individuals, private insurances, district health authority and social services contracts.
c National Insurance contributions and charges made to users.
d Local government contributions and individual donations.

20 Access to health and social care services may be achieved in the following ways:
a Referral by a professional only.
b Self-referral only.
c Self-referral, referral by a third party, recommendation by a professional, by recall.
d Self-referral and recommendation by a professional only.

21 The 1601 Poor Law Act divided people in need of health and social care into three groups. These were:
a Deserving people, undeserving people, the in-betweens.
b Helpless people, able-bodied poor people, rogues and vagabonds.
c Disabled and sick people, children, elderly people.
d Sick people, poor people, children.

22 The first National Health Insurance scheme (1918) did not provide relief for:
a Children, widows, people with a mental handicap.
b People who were blind or deaf, the unemployed people, sick people.
c Dependents, long-term unemployed people, people needing special services.
d Unemployed people, children, elderly people.

23 The Beveridge Report (1942) was aimed at tackling the following major areas of concern:
a Want, disease, ignorance, squalor and idleness.
b Crime, poor sanitation, injustice.
c Illness, disease, disabilities and crime.
d Single-parent families, illness, poor housing.

24 The Ministry of Health began appointing Welfare officers in —— and social workers by ——
a 1918 and 1928.
b 1934 and 1948.
c 1940 and 1945.
d 1957 and 1960.

25 The implementation of the Seebohm Report in 1968 resulted in the amalgamation of the following local authority departments:
 a Welfare and housing.
 b Children and education.
 c Mental health and welfare
 d Children and welfare.

26 In 1989 two government White Papers were published which made proposals for the revision of health and social care in the UK. These were:
 a *Social Service Reforms* and *Health Care Changes.*
 b *Caring for People* and *Working for Patients.*
 c *The Griffiths Report* and *The Health Care Report.*
 d *Community Care* and *Hospital Care.*

27 The use of advanced technology in health care has resulted in:
 a Fewer doctors being needed.
 b Doctors and nurses needing longer training courses.
 c More operations being carried out each year.
 d Quicker and more accurate diagnosis of illnesses and more complicated treatment.

28 The term 'pluralistic', in regard to approaches to care, means:
 a Health care as an insured service, with private and public ownership of facilities
 b State-supported health care, with facilities mainly publicly owned.
 c Minimal and indirect role of the state in health care, with private and public ownership of facilities.
 d The state's role in health care is total, and facilities are wholly publicly owned.

29 Health care in the UK seems to be gradually moving towards which of the following approaches to care?
 a Socialised.
 b Insurance/social security.
 c Pluralistic.
 d National Health Service.

30 The National Health Service was founded on the principle of:
 a A free, comprehensive, universal and state-provided welfare system.
 b A localised welfare system, paid for by local taxes.
 c A private health care system, funded by private payments and insurances.
 d State-managed facilities, but treatment paid for by insurances and benefits.

31 The National Health service created a health care system based mainly on:
 a Preventative medicine and health education.
 b 'Alternative' medical treatment (e.g. acupuncture).
 c Prevention, cure and care – in equal parts.
 d Curing illness and disease, and restoring health following injury and trauma.

32 The NHS is funded mainly by:
 a National Insurance contributions, national taxes and payments for some services.
 b National Insurance contributions only
 c Mainly national and local taxes.
 d Local taxes and National Insurance contributions.

33 For which of the following types of service may people be required to contribute towards the cost?
 a Accident and emergency treatment at hospital.
 b NHS prescriptions, dental treatment, residential care and meal-on-wheels.
 c Ear, nose and throat operations.
 d Maternity and ante-natal care.

34 Which of the following factors influences the population size and thus the numbers of people available for work?
 a Percentage of men v. women.
 b Attitudes towards work and leisure.
 c Number of people aged 65 years and over.
 d Birth rates, death rates, war, migration.

35 The cost of health and social care per head is highest in the following age group:
 a 0–4 years.
 b 16–64 years
 c 65–74 years.
 d 75 and over.

36 Health may be affected by the following factors:
 a The length of the working week.
 b The number of people per household.
 c The physical environment, social and economic influences, lifestyle, appropriate and effective health and social care.
 d The benefits that are available.

37 Prior to the establishment of the NHS, GPs were:
 a Employed by the government.
 b Employed by hospitals.
 c Employed by private companies.
 d Private practitioners – self-employed.

38 The independent sector is made up of the following types of organisations and care providers:
- **a** Private agencies and statutory agencies.
- **b** Private agencies, voluntary organisations and informal carers.
- **c** Statutory agencies and informal carers.
- **d** Voluntary and private agencies.

39 Voluntary agencies have various functions in addition to service provision. These may include:
- **a** Co-ordinating groups of organisations, advocacy, acting as a pressure group, working as a self-help group.
- **b** Supervising social security benefits.
- **c** Writing government policies.
- **d** Making a profit from the services they provide.

40 Which of the following are means-tested benefits?
- **a** Incapacity benefit, sickness benefit, invalidity benefit.
- **b** Widow's payment, widowed mother's allowance, widow's pension.
- **c** Income support, disability working allowance, family credit.
- **d** Disability living allowance, attendance allowance, one-parent benefit.

41 The health authority responsible for non-fund-holding GP services, dental services and ophthalmic services is:
- **a** The Regional Health Authority.
- **b** The District Health Authority.
- **c** The Family Health Services Authority.
- **d** The Special Health Authorities.

42 The health authority responsible for assessing the health care needs of people, and for purchasing services to meet those needs is:
- **a** The Regional Health Authority.
- **b** The District Health Authority.
- **c** The Family Health Services Authority.
- **d** The Special Health Authorities.

43 GP fund-holders receive a budget which is used to provide:
- **a** Emergency treatment at hospitals for their patients.
- **b** Dental and ophthalmic treatment for their patients.
- **c** Social care services for their patients.
- **d** Practice running costs, drugs, non-emergency treatment and community health services for their patients.

44 Self-governing trusts are responsible to:
- **a** The NHS Management Executive.
- **b** The Regional Health Authority
- **c** The District Health Authority.
- **d** The Family Health Services Authority.

45 Although the Secretary of State for Health is responsible for the provision of social services, they are administered by:
- **a** The National Health Service.
- **b** Regional Health Authorities.
- **c** Private consultative agencies.
- **d** Local authorities.

46 The role of purchasers of care services is to:
- **a** Plan services, stimulate service provision, contract services and monitor the quality of services.
- **b** Give direct provision of services.
- **c** Register and inspect various service provisions.
- **d** Collect national statistics for service planning.

47 Local authorities are required to keep the following registers:
- **a** Single-parent families.
- **b** Children in need and disabled people.
- **c** People with mental health problems.
- **d** Families receiving income support benefit.

48 The Government White Paper *Health of the Nation* provides guidelines relating to the following health care priorities:
- **a** Maternity and ante-natal care.
- **b** Infectious diseases, such as whooping cough and typhoid.
- **c** Cancer, coronary heart disease, strokes, mental health, sexually transmitted disease and accidents.
- **d** Respiratory diseases, neurological illnesses, rheumatic illnesses and congenital illnesses.

49 A mixed economy of care means:
- **a** The service is paid for by the service user and from contributions to National Insurance benefit.
- **b** Services are provided from various sources, e.g. statutory agencies, private and voluntary agencies, and informal carers.
- **c** Staff of different levels, e.g. student nurse, qualified nurse and special nursing sister, provide the necessary care.
- **d** Staff from different statutory agencies, e.g. NHS and social services and private services, provide the necessary care.

50 The term 'internal market' means that:
- **a** Providers of health care services will be in competition with one another in attracting contracts with purchasers of care.
- **b** Purchasers will only be able to buy in services from providers in their immediate area.
- **c** GPs will only be able to send their patients to hospitals in their immediate area.
- **d** Patients will have vouchers with which to purchase health care services.

51 The term 'commissioning' means:
- **a** Buying in existing services.
- **b** Buying in consultants to find out what services will be needed in the future.
- **c** Deciding which services will be needed in the future and ensuring their development.
- **d** Monitoring and evaluating existing services.

52 What are the three main types of contract used by purchasers of services?
- **a** Fixed-term contracts.
- **b** Individual, cost and volume and block contracts.
- **c** Short-term and long-term contracts.
- **d** Non-specific contracts.

53 Service specifications are:
- **a** The quality standards that the purchasers expect the providers to meet when they are awarded a contract.
- **b** The detailed guidelines for recruitment and training of staff.
- **c** The contract between an employing agency and a member of staff.
- **d** The contract between a provider of services and the person receiving the service.

54 Monitoring and evaluating services is carried out by:
- **a** Purchasers of services.
- **b** Providers of services.
- **c** Users of services.
- **d** A combination of all three above.

55 Services previously regard as 'Cinderella services' have included:
- **a** Acute hospital services, including surgery.
- **b** Services for people with mental health problems, people with learning disabilities, older people.
- **c** Services for children and families.
- **d** Accident and emergency services.

56 The Griffiths Report (1987) is often regarded as:
- **a** Insignificant and out-dated.
- **b** Important in the development of specialist services.
- **c** A landmark in the provision of health and social care.
- **d** Unimportant and lacking in insight.

57 The role of providers includes:
- **a** Buying in services to meet an individual's care needs.
- **b** Direct provision of services, monitoring service quality.
- **c** Planning and developing services.
- **d** Researching and assessing future service needs.

58 There have been two government charters: The Citizen's Charter and the Patient's Charter. The purposes of these are to:
- **a** Set out people's responsibilities regarding their own health and social care.
- **b** Set out people's rights and entitlements in respect of public services and health care.
- **c** Set out people's responsibilities in respect of one another.
- **d** Set out people's rights in respect of caring for their children.

59 Services users can help to monitor the quality of services by:
- **a** Telling their neighbours if they are unhappy with the service.
- **b** Telling their GPs about the quality of any of the services that they receive.
- **c** Writing to their MPs.
- **d** Using the complaints procedures of the purchasing authority and of the service provider, in order to voice their concerns and grievances.

60 Health and social care service are likely to develop in the following way:
- **a** With a division of purchasing and the provision of services, more involvement of the independent sector and more care in the community.
- **b** More state involvement in the direct provision of care.
- **c** Less involvement of voluntary and private agencies, and informal carers.
- **d** More long-term hospital, nursing home and residential home provision.

Fast Facts

Access Gaining entry to services.

Accommodation A term used in the Children Act 1989 to describe a voluntary agreement whereby the local authority provides accommodation and care for a child.

Approved Social Worker (ASW) A social worker especially appointed under the Mental Health Act 1983 to assess the need for admission to hospital.

Beveridge Report Published in 1942. The report set out the broad framework for the setting up of the Welfare State in the UK. The working party was chaired by William Beveridge.

Care management A system for assessing and organising the provision of care for an individual.

Carer Anyone who is looking after someone who is ill or disabled.

Caring for People Government White Paper published in 1989 as a response to the Griffiths Report. It set out the proposals for care in the community, giving social service departments the lead responsibility.

Children Act An Act of Parliament passed in 1989 which supersedes many previous Acts relating to the welfare and protection of children.

Chronically Sick and Disabled Person's Act An Act of Parliament which makes provision for people with disabilities, passed in 1970.

Classification A way of arranging services into groups.

Commission An agreement to provide a service for which a financial contribution is made.

Contract A formal legal agreement to ensure the delivery of services.

Demographic changes Statistical changes that occur in the population and that can be used for planning services.

Department of Health A central government body which administers health and social care.

Directly managed units (DMUs) Hospitals which are controlled by District Health Authorities.

Disabled Persons (Consultation and Representation) Act An Act of Parliament, passed in 1986, which requires local authorities to provide information about services that are available. It also requires them to assess the needs of people requesting services.

District Health Authorities (DHAs) Purchasers of health care.

Duties Services and other provisions that individuals or organisations are required to provide or carry out by law.

Family Health Service Authorities (FHSAs) Employ the services of GPs, dentists, opticians and pharmacists. They share the same geographical boundaries as District Health Authorities and have strong links with them.

GP fund-holders GP practices which receive a budget from FHSAs. The budget is used to cover the running costs of the practice, to buy drugs and for buying some non-emergency and some community health services.

Griffiths Report Published in 1988. The report set out the main principles for the provision of care in the community. The working party was chaired by Sir Roy Griffiths.

Health Services and Public Health Act An Act of Parliament, passed in 1968, which provides local authorities with the power to promote the welfare of older people.

Independent sector Organisations providing health and social care other than statutory organisations.

Informal care Care provided by people and groups who are not paid for their services.

Local authority Social Services These departments are responsible for ensuring clients' social care needs are met in the community.

Local Authority Social Services Act An Act of Parliament, passed in 1970, which sets out the framework for social services provision.

Joint consultative committees Committees set up in 1974, consisting mainly of health authority and local authority representatives, to plan health and social care services.

Marketplace economy An approach to health and social care where the responsibility for purchasing care and providing care is separated. It also puts providers of care in competition with one another in providing effective and efficient services.

Mental Health Act An Act of Parliament, passed in 1983, which sets out the framework for the provision of care for people with mental health problems.

Mixed economy of care An approach to health and social care which involves the public and independent sectors in the provision of care.

National Assistance Act An Act of Parliament, passed in 1948, which replaced the Poor Law and gave local authorities the duty to provide accommodation for elders, people with disabilities and children who were in need.

National Health Service In England, the Secretary of State for Health has the overall responsibility for the National Health Service. The NHS is responsible for ensuring the provision of health care.

National Health Service Act An Act of Parliament, passed in 1946, which sets out the basic principles of health and welfare services.

National Health Service and Community Care Act An Act of Parliament, passed in 1990, which aims to allow vulnerable people to live as independently as possible, within their own homes or in a homely setting in the community.

Need A need is an essential requirement which must be met in order to ensure that an individual reaches a state of health and social well-being.

Packages of care A variety of integrated services that have been put together in order to meet an individual's assessed needs.

Poor Law Act of Parliament passed in 1389 which fixed a legal maximum wage and made it illegal for labourers to leave the manor to which they belonged.

Poor Law Act Act of Parliament passed in 1601 which placed a duty on parishes to provide relief for their own poor and unemployed parishioners.

Poor Law Amendment Act Act of Parliament passed in 1834 which created a government body to supervise poor relief and elected Boards of Guardians to run each of the poor law unions and the infirmaries.

Powers The permission for authorities to provide services according to perceived needs.

Primary care Health care provided in the community, often preventative in nature. Accessed by self-referral.

Private organisations Agencies run on business lines, which provide services for which a charge is made.

Provider An organisation that sells services to a purchaser.

Purchaser An organisation that buys in necessary services.

Resource Allocation Working Party (RAWP) Formula introduced by the Labour government in 1977, used in deciding the allocation of resources to each regional health authority.

Resource Management Initiative (RMI) Initiative introduced in 1986 aimed at increasing the involvement of doctors in the decision-making process regarding resources and giving them the responsibility for budgets.

Royal Commission Report Report published in 1973. Commissioned by the government to look at maladministration in the NHS.

Secondary care Health care that is often curative in nature and is given in hospitals, clinics and surgeries.

Seebohm Report Government report published in 1968 which resulted in the amalgamation of the children's department and the welfare departments within local authorities.

Service specifications Statements describing the nature of the services that the purchaser expects to buy.

Special Health Authorities (SHAs) Specialist health services which operate at a national level, postgraduate and research hospitals, or which provide care for seriously disturbed offenders.

Standard Spending Assessment (SSA) Formula used by the government in deciding how much each local authority will receive towards the cost of services that they are responsible for.

Statutory organisations Health and care organisations providing care that must be given by law (statute). The National Health Service and local authority Social Services departments form two main branches of the health and social care industry.

Tertiary care Health care often provided in specialist units and rehabilitative in nature.

Trusts Self-governing units within the NHS. They are run by boards of governors and are accountable directly to the NHS Management Executive.

Voluntary organisations Non-profit-making organisations which provide services, usually free of charge.

Welfare State Where the state's role in health and social care is central and direct in the provision of services, with many facilities being publicly owned.

Working with Patients Government White Paper published in 1989 as a response to the Griffiths Report. It set out proposals for the health authorities' responsibilities for care in the community.

References and further reading

*Recommended further reading

* Baggott, R., 1994, *Health and Health Care in Britain,* St Martin's Press.

Carter, P., Jeffs, A. and Smith, M.K. (eds), 1992, *Changing Social Work and Welfare,* Open University Press

Deaking, N., 1994, *The Politics of Welfare,* Harvester Wheatsheaf

Department of Health, 1991, *Care Management and Assessment: The Manager's Guide*, HMSO.

DSS, 1981, *Care in Action,* HMSO

DSS, 1981, *Community Care,* HMSO

Field, M.G., 1989, *Success and Crisis in National Health Systems*, Macmillan

Griffiths, K., 1988, *Community Care: Agenda for Action,* HMSO

* Ham, C. and Higginbotham, C., 1991, *Purchasing Together,* Kings Fund

Harrison, S. and Wistow, G., 1992, 'The purchaser/provider split in English health care' in *Policy and Politics,* 20 (2), 123–30

* Leadbeater, P., 1990, *Partners in Health: The NHS and the Voluntary Sector,* National Association of Health Authorities and Trusts

* Meredith, B., 1993, *The Community Care Handbook: The New Systems Explained,* Age Concern.

Pettigrew, A. *et al.,* 1991, *Research in Action: Authorities in the NHS,* University of Warwick.

* Ranade, V., 1994, *A Future for the NHS? Health Care in the 1990s,* Longman

* Reading, P., 1993, *Community Care and the Voluntary Sector,* Venture Press

Report of the Royal Commission on the NHS (The Merrison Commission), 1979, Cmnd 9716, HMSO

*Strong, P. and Robinson, J., 1990, *The NHS Under New Management,* Open University Press

Titmuss, R., 1968, *Commitment to Welfare,* Allen & Unwin

Whitefield, D., 1992, *The Welfare State,* Pluto Press

Wistow, G., *et al.*, 1993, *Social Care in a Mixed Economy,* Open University Press

Chapter 16

The planning of care and interventions for individual clients

This chapter provides an in-depth explanation of the care planning process and its role in meeting client needs. Key practitioners who may be involved in care planning are described. The role of enabling, caring and treatment interventions is discussed in the context of the care planning process. A number of case studies are used to explain how care may be organised and delivered. The rationale for a care planning process to guide intervention is explained. The importance of empowering clients and their carers, and the role of multidisciplinary working, is emphasised throughout the chapter.

The care planning cycle

The care planning cycle comprises seven stages, as outlined in Figure 16.1 below.

The term 'care management' is used to cover all seven stages of the care planning cycle. Assessment and care management constitute one integrated process for identifying and addressing the needs of individuals, recognising that those needs are unique to the people concerned. Care management is the process of tailoring services to individual needs. Assessment is an integral part of care management, but it is only one of the seven core tasks that make up the whole process.

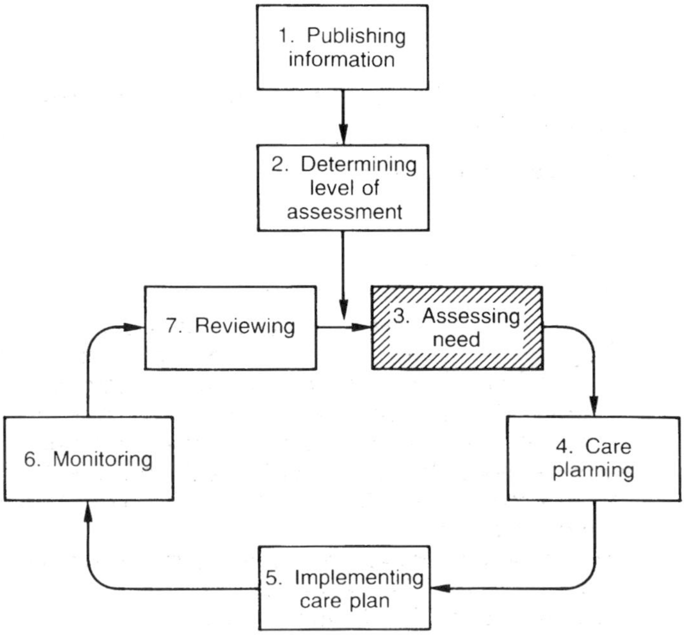

Figure 16.1 The process of care management

Core tasks

The seven core tasks of the assessment and care management process are as follows:

1. *Publishing information*
   Clients and their carers are given information about the needs for which care agencies accept responsibility and the range of services available.
2. *Determining the level of assessment*
   An enquirer requests more than just information; sufficient details are obtained in order to determine the type of assessment that is required, e.g. a simple assessment or a complex assessment.
3. *Assessing need*
   The needs of individuals are assessed in a way that recognises their strengths and aspirations as well as those of their carers. The purpose of the assessment is to define the individual's needs in the context of local policies.
4. *Care planning*
   The role of the assessor is to assist clients in making choices from statutory, private or community sources that best meet their needs.
5. *Implementing care plans*
   This means securing the necessary finance or other resources. It may involve negotiating with a variety of service providers and ensuring that services are co-ordinated with one another.
6. *Monitoring*
   Because circumstances change, the care plan has to be monitored continuously and adjustments made where necessary.
7. *Reviewing*
   At specified intervals, the progress of the care plan has to be reviewed with the client, carers and service providers to ensure that the service remains relevant to needs and to evaluate services as part of the continuing quest for service improvement.

For the purpose of this chapter we are concentrating on the core tasks of:

- assessment
- care planning
- implementation of care plans
- monitoring
- reviewing

How assessment works

Under the NHS and Community Care Act 1990, all assessments must be focused on the actual *needs* of clients and of their carers, irrespective of what resources are available. A *needs-led* assessment fits resources to people – not people into services.

Client need

The term *need* is used as shorthand for the requirements of individuals to enable them to achieve, maintain or restore an acceptable level of social independence or quality of life.

Individuals may perceive their needs in different ways, therefore the assessor must understand the viewpoints of clients and what is important to them. This will determine the scope of the assessment and the degree of detail required in order to complete the assessment. Needs may be categorised in different ways.

- personal and social care
- physical health
- cultural and religious needs
- accommodation
- transport/access
- finance
- education/employment/leisure
- needs of carers

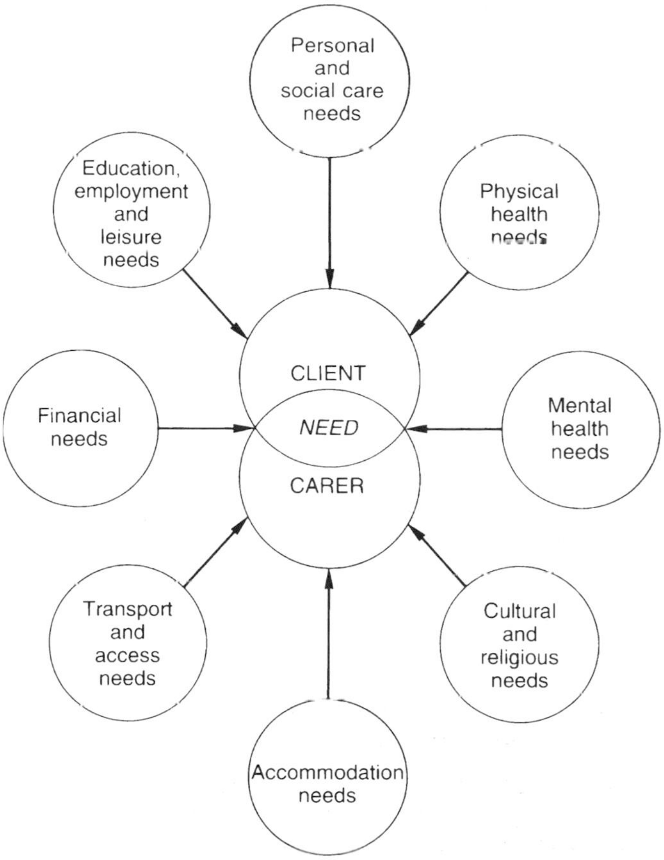

Figure 16.2 Determining 'need'

The assessor, who could be a social worker, occupational therapist, home-care manager, community psychiatric nurse, district nurse etc., carries out the assessment through discussion with the client and his or her carer. The assessment takes into account the whole range of needs and wishes. The assessment may involve further meetings and discussions with others (with the permission of the client), including other professionals and possible service providers. However, only in a minority of cases will there be any kind of formal panel meeting or conference.

Read Case Study A below.

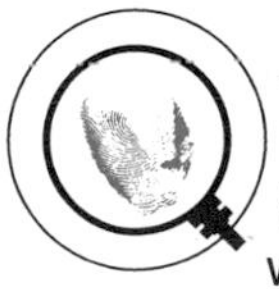

Case Study A

Mr Andrews is 68 years old. He is currently in hospital following a serious chest infection which caused him to become extremely confused. He has recovered from the chest infection, but has other problems related to multiple sclerosis which he has suffered from for the last ten years. He has become less mobile and is finding it difficult to walk, even using sticks.

Mr and Mrs Andrews are a white couple who have been married for thirty years and live in council accommodation. They have no children.

Mrs Andrews is happy to care for her husband, but this has put her under great emotional and physical strain. Mrs Andrews weighs only eight stone; her husband weighs sixteen stone. Mrs Andrews needs support and time for herself. She would like to be able to go out shopping without having to worry about her husband. She would also like to be able to visit a friend who lives many miles away, once or twice a year.

Mr Andrews has reluctantly agreed that he needs to use a wheelchair. This means that some adaptations are needed to their home.The bedroom has currently had to be moved downstairs, to be on the same level as the toilet and kitchen; but it would be difficult to get a wheelchair into the toilet. Mr Andrews enjoys the company of other people and likes to play cards occasionally.

Mr Andrews is keen to get home. His wife is also keen for him to leave hospital but is anxious about how the care package will work out. In the past she has only had contact with the District Nurse, and more recently has had some support from Age Concern. Neither are sure what help could be available to them.

Think it over

Who is the client? How would a care plan help Mr and Mrs Andrews? What are the main concerns of Mr Andrews? Mrs Andrews?

Care plan assessment

Assessment of need checklist

It is suggested that this checklist is not printed as a form as such, but as a set of headings and pointers with spaces, so that people can use it as a note pad or aid to memory, etc. The intention is to gain information for the care management and assessment process, so as to enter appropriate needs information on the care planning and assessment form. It is important to avoid collecting too much information or intruding on clients' privacy.

1 Environment and housing

1.1 Any problems with the heating or the person's ability to control it? Any problems with access or issues for providing services? Can the person use the telephone, hear/answer front door? What about handles, switches, taps etc.? Emergency contact?

1.2 Is the housing suitable? Problems? Type of housing (owner occupier, council, private, rented, sheltered, shared, house, flat etc. if relevant)

1.3 Access to transport?

2 Communication

Do we have a problem in communicating – i.e. do we need to supply an interpreter? Does the person have any problems with sight, hearing, speech that cause difficulty? Equipment used/needed?

3 Personal care

Dressing/undressing – difficulty? help needed?
Washing –
Continence –
Mobility (indoors and out), transfers (chair, bed, toilet)

4 Housework

Prepare meals? Feed selves? Equipment/help?
Shopping
Laundry
Cleaning

5 Physical and emotional health

Any concerns about the person's health?
Any disability? Relevant doctor's diagnosis?
Been contacted?
How does this affect daily living? Any problems with e.g. forgetfulness, sense of direction etc.?
Bereavement, loss, other major changes?
Sleep pattern?
Can the person manage medication? (What is it, if relevant?)

6 Abilities, aptitudes, social life
What does the person enjoy, do well, want to do?
Any difficulties in their doing it?
Who do they like to be with?
Live alone? With whom?

7 Employment, educational needs/wishes

8 Financial information
Is income sufficient for needs? Are they receiving a benefit?

9 Other agencies
Are other agencies involved? What help are they giving? Any problems around this? Any key people?

10 Carer/care network
Is there a carer/care network? Who is able and willing to help? Stresses? Gaps? Long term?

Case Study B

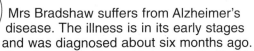

Mrs Bradshaw suffers from Alzheimer's disease. The illness is in its early stages and was diagnosed about six months ago. She also suffers from arthritis and takes medication for this. There is some evidence of an alcohol problem, but details about this are not clear.

Family background
Mrs Bradshaw is 71 years old. She is married and lives with her husband in a ground-floor flat. Mr and Mrs Bradshaw migrated from the Caribbean to England in 1955. They have four children, who live away from home. They have seven grandchildren. Mr and Mrs Bradshaw have close links with their children and grandchildren. Both Mr and Mrs Bradshaw have retired from paid work.

Services involved and current situation
Mrs Bradshaw attends an Afro-Caribbean lunch club one day a week to give her husband a break. Staff there say she often seems worried and agitated on arrival, but is in a better state by the time she leaves.
Mr Bradshaw has contacted you (a social worker at the local Social Services office) through the staff at the lunch club. He would like a longer break from caring for his wife and wonders if something residential could be arranged, so that he could visit relatives on his own. He says that he is finding his wife's behaviour hard to handle. She doesn't sleep well, is often up during the night, and her memory is deteriorating. For example, she often decides to do something, like go to the kitchen, and when she gets there, she can't remember why she's there. She likes to have a drink and, now that her memory is so bad, he worries that she is drinking too much, because she can't remember if she's had one already. She is becoming difficult with him when she mislays things and accuses him of hiding things from her.

Think it over

Who is the client? What are Mr Bradshaw's main areas of concern? What do you think are the key needs of: Mrs Bradshaw? Mr Bradshaw? How would you begin to assess the needs of Mr and Mrs Bradshaw?

Practitioners involved in care planning

Social workers

Social workers, who are usually organised in teams, aim to provide a co-ordinated services to families and individuals with a wide range of social problems, including personal, practical and financial difficulties. Some social workers specialise in child care, others in working with people with mental illness, learning difficulties, physical disability or with elders.

Most 'field' social workers (the name given to those who work in the community) are based in area offices. However, some may be based in hospitals, although they remain employed by the Social

Services Department. Occasionally social workers may be attached to general practices or health clinics. They can act as a useful link between health and social services.

A social worker may be the 'gatekeeper' to many service provisions, such as:

- home care services
- night care services
- meals on wheels
- laundry services
- equipment for daily living
- adaptations to the home
- day care facilities for adults and older people
- residential homes for short stays or permanent care for adults and older people
- nursing home placements
- nursery or playgroup placements
- short- or long-term fostering placements
- short- or long-term residential care for children.

These services may be directly provided by the local authority, or may be commissioned by them from the independent sector (i.e. private or voluntary agencies).

Social workers can be either *care managers* (purchasing role) or providers of care to a client. If acting as care managers their role is to ensure that the needs of the client have been properly assessed. They will be responsible for ensuring that the care plan developed from the assessment is implemented and properly addresses the identified needs. This will involve liaising closely with the client, carers, and all the professionals concerned with the implementing the care plan.

If the social worker is a provider of care, he or she may work as part of a team to implement the care plan. However, if the only need is for social work provision, he or she will work alone with the client and family.

It is important to remember that social workers are regularly supervised by their line manager. This ensures their work is supported and guided appropriately.

District nurses

District nurses, sometimes called 'community nurses', provide the full range of nursing care in people's own homes. District Nursing Sisters are RGNs (Registered General Nurses), with an additional qualification, who may head a small team of ENs (Enrolled Nurses) and health support care workers. Support workers may have an NVQ in Care. District nurses are usually based at a GP's premises or at health centres.

District nurses may be able to arrange some of the following equipment: bed rails or a raised bed; special mattresses; sheepskin underblankets; hoists of various kinds; bath seats and boards; incontinence pads or sheets; access to bathing services; and access to a night nurse. However, this might depend on what is available locally.

District nurses can also be care managers (purchasing role) or providers of care. Their role as a care manager is as described above for social workers. As providers of care they will visit the customer for medical provision. This will often involve working closely with the general practitioner.

Try it

Contact your local District Nursing service and find out how district nurses are involved in care plans in your area.

Occupational therapists

Occupational therapists (OTs) may work in the community, in hospitals or in private establishments. Those working in the community will usually be employed by the local authority and be based in the Social Services department.

The role of the OT is to work with people who have a disability: to promote independent living skills, such as dressing, washing, toileting. They ensure that capabilities are maximised and disability minimised. OTs use a number of therapeutic activities.

OTs can also advise on what equipment or home adaptations might help the individual, and they may help to arrange for the provision of these. Equipment for everyday living may include: washing aids; dressing aids; a commode; chairs with high seats; adapted cutlery; play equipment; and adaptations including widening doors, installing stairlifts etc.

Occupational therapists can be care managers or providers of care. As providers they work closely with the customer to ensure that capabilities are maximised. OTs will work closely with other professionals involved in the client's care plan.

Home care workers

Home care staff go by different names in different parts of the country. They be called 'home carers', 'home helps', 'domiciliary care workers' or 'community care aides or assistants'. They provide support in a number of ways according to the individual needs of the service user. Most home care staff work with elders, although they can work with any client group. Home carers may be holders of NVQs in care or other care qualifications.

Home carers can provide physical care, including help with personal hygiene and everyday activities, as well as domestic chores, such as housework, cooking and shopping, which may be provided as part of a package of care.

Think it over

What are the main differences between home care workers and care workers?

Residential and day care staff

Some social care staff provide physical and emotional care on a daily basis for the full range of clients in either day care or residential care settings – including, for example, older people in residential homes and day centres.

Community psychiatric nurses

Community psychiatric nurses are a relatively small group of nurses who have all undergone a basic psychiatric nurse training, studying various aspects of people's behaviour, emotions and relationships. Some CPNs have training in counselling, family therapy and hold the CPN Diploma.

A CPN will see people with a whole range of problems relating to life events, for example, bereavement, divorce, marriage, having children, unemployment, retirement, etc. CPNs can also offer help in dealing with anxiety states, depression or serious mental illness, such as schizophrenia.

CPNs work with people helping them to find solutions to their difficulties, by taking them through problems or by learning skills such as communication, relaxation and assertiveness skills. They explore areas of life which may be worrying, confusing or painful, so that they can build a picture of the client as a person, rather than as a set of problems.

The assessment process as a basis for interventions

When referrals come into the agency they are allocated to the appropriate client group. For example: in Social Services – physical disabilities, learning disability, mental illness, children and families, or elderly services; in health settings – acute or community services. After allocation a person will be identified to assess the client's needs, but also to take into account the needs of the client's carer.

The assessment of need should broadly follow this sequence (see Figure 16.3):

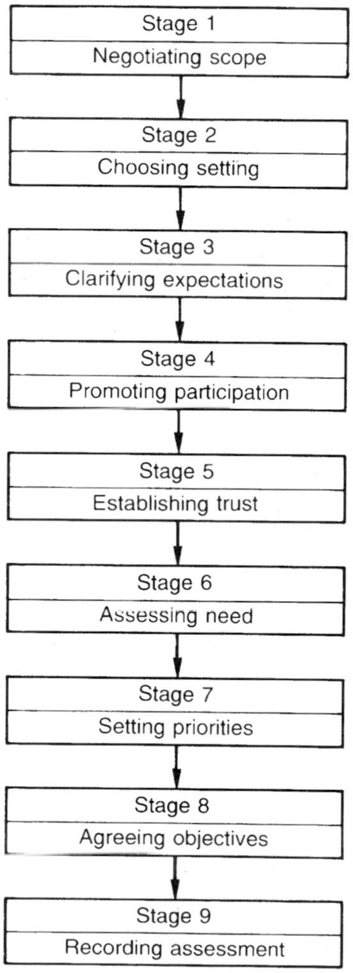

Figure 16.3 9-stage assessment process

- negotiate scope of the assessment
- choose setting for assessment
- clarify expectations with clients
- promote participation with clients
- establish relationship of trust between yourself and clients
- assess need
- set priorities
- agree objectives with clients
- record the assessment

1 *Negotiating the scope of assessment*
Simple needs will require less investigation than complex ones. The assessment should be as simple, speedy and as informal as possible.

Procedures for assessment should be based on the principle of what is the *least* that it is necessary to know. It follows therefore that the assessor must be trained to use his or her discretion and to target the relevant areas of need. The scope of the assessment has to be individually negotiated.

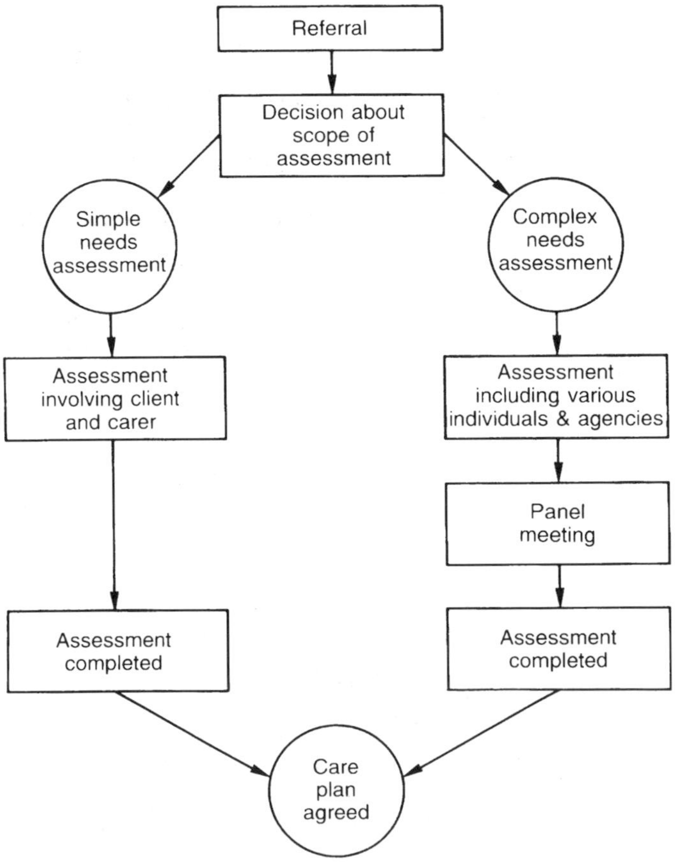

Figure 16.4 Deciding scope of assessment

Assessment is a two-way process between the assessor and the client. However, it may be necessary to involve other people and other agencies in the process. This will generally be in more complex assessments and must be subject to the consent of the client. A minority of clients will have complex needs. (See Figure 16.4.)

2 *Agreeing the setting*

The assessor carries out the assessment through discussion with the client (and carer, where appropriate), at a prearranged place and time. In order for the client and carer to participate as fully as possible it is often better to use an informal place for the interview, such as the client's home, rather than the formal setting of an office. This should encourage the client to relax and thus give a fuller picture of his or her needs and wishes.

If clients are considering admission to a residential or nursing home, involving the irreversible loss of their homes, they should always be given the opportunity of experiencing that setting before making their final decision.

It may be necessary for some part of the assessment to be undertaken away from their homes, for example, at a day centre or residential care setting, which enables the assessor to work more closely with clients and for longer periods. It is therefore important to look flexibly at the setting to be used when completing the assessment. However, care must be taken to avoid causing unnecessary disruption to clients.

3 *Clarifying expectations*
The assessor must ensure that clients understand.

- what is involved in the assessment
- the likely timescale for completing the assessment
- the possible outcomes
- their entitlement to information, participation and representation
- their right to withdraw from the process at any time

4 *Promoting participation*
The assessor must judge how clients and/or their carers can be actively involved in the process. Some clients will have a clear understanding of their own needs. Some clients will confuse 'wants' with 'needs'. For example, a person who feels isolated due to lack of mobility, and difficulties in getting up and down stairs, may *want* alternative accommodation. What he or she *needs* may be an adaptation to the home, such as moving the bedroom downstairs or the installation of a stairlift. Others will need the support

of representatives (or advocates) in order to be able to make their needs known. Where clients and carers are unable, for any reason, to be able to speak for themselves, it is important that they are given information regarding any advocacy schemes funded by the local authority or run locally. For example, the local branch of Age Concern may have volunteers who will work with individuals by helping them express their views in discussions with others.

If the assessor can focus on the client's strengths at the beginning of the assessment process, then this will encourage the client to contribute to the whole assessment procedure.

An assessment should help the assessor and the client to balance both the positives and negatives in a given situation. In so doing, clients are helped to feel that they are being regarded as whole persons. The assessor will be enabled to place the client's needs in perspective. Clients and carers should receive every help to speak and act for themselves by ensuring that:

- staff have, wherever possible, the appropriate communication skills (e.g. language, cultural understanding or technical skills, including signing).
- clients and carers have ready access to communication equipment and to interpreters or communicators, where assessment staff do not possess such skills
- the use of interpreters or communicators in no way disqualifies clients and carers from also having an independent representative if that is what they wish.

5 *Establishing a relationship of trust*
The assessor has to establish a relationship of trust with the clients and their carers. Listening, observing and understanding are of paramount importance. Assessment involves considerable skills in **interpersonal relations.** Assessors should be aware of their limitations and know when to involve others with more specialist expertise or cultural understanding.

If clients are dissatisfied by either the process or the outcome of the assessment, they should be supported in making representation under the complaints procedures. This will encourage trust.

6 *Assessing need*
The assessor has to define as precisely as possible the cause of any difficulty; for example, someone with learning disabilities may be under-functioning through lack of knowledge, loss of confidence or depression, or as a consequence of some breakdown in relationships. The proper identification of the cause is the basis for the selection of the appropriate service response. Everybody involved in the assessment process is likely to perceive the need in a different way. The assessor must aim for a degree of consensus; however, wherever clients are competent, and capable of expressing their wishes, their views must carry most weight. Where differences between the views of the client and the assessor are irreconcilable, these views should be acknowledged and recorded as this may help in the understanding of the client's needs over time. The assessment process must ultimately define the *client's* need.

7 *Setting priorities*
The assessor and the client must now agree on their relative priorities. It will be comparatively easy to distinguish between:

- immediate needs, e.g. health crisis or breakdown of care
- acute short-term needs, e.g. home care following a fractured hip
- chronic long-term needs, e.g. continuing support for personal care.

However, the assessor will first wish to identify:

- those needs that most concern the client
- those needs that most concern the carer
- those needs that the client/carer is most motivated to address
- those needs on which intervention is acceptable to the client/carer.

8 *Agreeing objectives*
The final stage of the assessment of need consists of agreeing the objectives to be met for each of the

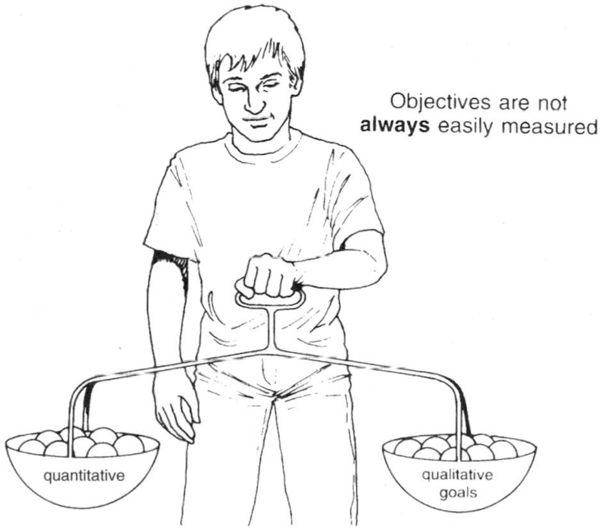

prioritised needs. As far as care agencies are concerned, objectives fall into four main categories:

- promoting or restoring independent functioning
- maintaining care for the client
- providing substitute care
- arranging support for carers.

To have any value, objectives must be capable of being measured. This is easy when it relates to quantitative goals, like the speed or frequency of completing self-care tasks; but it can be more difficult for qualitative goals where, for example, social well-being may have to be measured by indicators such as contact time with friends.

9 *Recording the assessment*
All assessments must be recorded and most agencies will have some type of proforma. This is a pre-designed form which can be used with each client. In many instances the Local Authority and Health Authority will use a form that has been designed jointly.

Although it is the assessor's responsibility to ensure that the form is completed appropriately, there is no reason why the client (or their carer) should not complete part, or all, of his or her own assessment form. Again, this encourages full participation in the assessment process. Assessment forms should therefore be easily understandable and in clear language. This must distinguish between fact and opinion, 'needs' and 'wants'.

The client, carer, any representative of the client and all the people who are to provide a service to the client, including other agencies, should receive a copy of the assessment form. This record will normally be accompanied by a written care plan (the next stage of the care management process). The care plan will set out how the needs of the client and their carer are to be addressed.

Try it

Think about either Case Study A or B, then write out possible answers to the assessment checklist questions below. Alternatively, think about a real person you have worked with and answer the checklist questions.

Interventions in relation to client need

There are two forms of care plan, known as **macro** and **micro** care plans.

Assessment checklist

Assessors can use this list to check that they have covered all the key points.

1. Has the assessment been negotiated with the client and their carer?
2. Has the appropriate setting been chosen?
3. Has the client (and the carer) understood how the assessment will be done, what this will involve and how long it will take?
4. Has the client (and carer) been involved in making the assessment? Have ethnic, cultural and communication needs been taken into account?
5. Have clients and carers had access to advocacy support where appropriate?
6. Have different perceptions of need been reconciled? If not, have they been recorded?
7. Have the needs been prioritised?
8. Have the objectives been agreed and has the way that they are to be measured been decided?
9. Has a record of the assessment been shared with the client, carer and relevant service providers?

(Adapted from *Care Management and Assessment – Practitioners' Guide* HMSO, 1991.

- The **macro care plan** is the overall identification of needs and lists all the agencies who will be involved in providing services.
- The **micro care plan** is the plan which the individual service provider will use to describe the action plan within their own agency.

For example, below are the care plans for Mrs Banerjee:

Macro care plan

Needs	Action	Provider
Help with personal hygiene	(i) daily wash (ii) weekly bath	Home carer Bath service

Micro care plan (home care)

Needs	Action	By whom
(i) daily wash	■ assist to bathroom ■ wash face, neck, hands, arms ■ assist to dress after drying	Home carer

Micro care plan (bath service)

Needs	Action	By whom
(i) weekly bath	Wednesday a.m. ■ seated bath ■ hair wash ■ nails cut	Bath attendant

Care planning is a tool which provides direction for all those working to meet clients' needs. It:

- ensures continuity/responsibility/commitment
- should be realistic/practical/workable
- recognises client's choice/carer's needs
- gives consistency – linking all appropriate services
- has flexibility.

It is the role of the care manager or assessor (purchaser) to develop a care plan. A care plan is a clearly defined document of needs designed for the client, bringing together all the agencies involved and indicating what services are provided and by whom. An assessor may be a social worker, occupational therapist or home care purchasing officer.

The care manager carried out the assessment though discussion with the client (and carer if appropriate) at a prearranged place and time. The assessment takes account of the whole range of needs and wishes.

An assessment is a purchasing function, it is important that the care manager has an understanding of the financial resources available and is able to discuss these and the client's own financial situation with the client and carer if appropriate. This is an integrated assessment of need and financial situation, rather than a specific assessment for a particular service.

The outcome of the assessment will normally be a clear statement of needs and realistic options for meeting them.

A needs-led assessment must:

- share and agree information and inter-agency assessments of needs
- define clients'/carers' needs
- agree and plan options for packages of care.

The plan agreed after this process is the *macro* care plan.

Types of intervention

Intervention means to 'come between and alter the course of events'. Many clients have problems and needs which mean that their quality of life will not be as good as it could be. Health and social care services can intervene in a client's life so that the client's future is altered (hopefully for the better!). Sometimes health and social care services intervene by trying to help clients to help themselves. These interventions might be seen as 'enabling'. Miss Smith is a client with learning disability, who has complex mental health needs. A care plan and detailed programme of intervention are shown on page 368. The plan covers Miss Smith's social, intellectual, emotional and communication needs. As well as trying to enable Miss Smith to learn independent living and shopping skills, the plan also provides for caring services to support her. Miss Smith receives medication. This treatment is provided by the Community Psychiatric Nurse.

> Most clients who receive planned care will have multiple types of need and many will receive a combination of enabling, caring and treatment-focused intervention.

The case study described below in Figure 16.5 shows how the care planning cycle is able to meet the needs of Miss Smith. A full needs-led assessment has been completed, which involved Miss Smith, her mother (who has been the main carer), the Community Psychiatric Nurse, doctor and social worker.

The social worker has to discuss in detail, with the staff in the community home, how Miss Smith's weekly care plan will be implemented. The result of their discussion is reflected in Figure 16.6 which is the weekly care plan.

Care planning

Definition of 'care plan'

One definition could be as follows: 'To identify the most appropriate ways of achieving the objectives identified by the assessment of need and incorporate them into an individual care plan'.

Process

First, the assessor should, having identified the needs, link into the appropriate resource to meet those needs. Care planning is then a series of linked activities: determining the type of plan; setting priorities, and so on.

Customer Miss Smith
Care Manager
Key worker To be agreed after placement
Review date 6 weeks after placement

Needs	How needs are to be met	Action
a *Accommodation* Supportive environment in which to develop independent daily living skills	Social worker to discuss proposed placement with social services management to obtain funding	Social worker to discuss proposed placement with Social Services Management to obtain funding
b *Tasks of daily living* (i) Assistance/guidance with undertaking co-ordinated household routine (ii) Assistance/guidance with budgeting/finance (iii) Assistance to build independent shopping skills (iv) Assistance to build confidence when travelling alone	Social worker to discuss the needs with staff in the community home and agree to daily plan to meet all identified needs.	Social worker to discuss the needs with staff in the community home and agree a daily plan to meet all the identified needs
c *Personal care* Reminding to maintain a regular personal care routine	Staffed community accommodation	
d *Emotional support* (i) Reassurance, particularly when agitated and fearful at night	Staffed community accommodation	
(ii) Encouragement when demotivated by mental state	All agencies involved with care plan	
e *Social contact/occupation* (i) Social contact/leisure activity in a community setting	Day social project	Social worker to liaise with day social project manager
(ii) Structured occupation	Day centre	Social worker to liaise with centre manager
f *Medication* Monitoring and reviewing	Local health clinic	Community Psychiatric Nurse

Figure 16.5 Needs assessment for Miss Smith

Determining the type of plan

Care plans will vary according to the complexity of need. If it is a simple need which can be met by a single service, the care planning will be swiftly accomplished. All people who receive a service should have a care plan which defines the user's needs and the objectives to be met by any services from a number of different agencies. For example, see Case Study A of Mr Andrews (page 359) and the care plan on page 369.

Set priorities

The assessment should have prioritised the client's needs so they should be tackled in priority order. Care planning should be flexible and able to adjust priorities as the needs of the client changes. For example, Mr Andrews may need more residential respite care as his condition changes.

Client's name Miss Smith **Address**	**Dr** .... **Tel no**	**Key holder** ....
Special instructions: 5 weeks' trial **Next review**	**Other agencies involved:** Day centre Day social project	**Liaison:**

Monday a.m.	*Tuesday a.m.*	*Wednesday a.m.*	*Thursday a.m.*	*Friday a.m.*	*Saturday a.m.*	*Sunday a.m.*
Change bed & washing	Day centre 9.30 am–15.30 pm 1 hour computer study	Clean lounge and dining area & kitchen duties	Day centre 9.30 am	Day social project 10.00 am	Visit parents all day	
Lunch	*Lunch*	*Lunch*	*Lunch*	*Lunch*	*Lunch*	*Lunch*
Clean toilets and bathrooms	Day centre 15.30 pm	2 pm till 4 pm visit parents 4 pm cooking	Day centre 15.30 pm	Day social project 16.00		Menu planning
p.m.	*p.m.*	*p.m.*	*p.m.*	*p.m.*	*p.m.*	*p.m.*
	Ironing		Clean bedroom landing and stairs	Extra chore	Return to community home	Community meeting

Figure 16.6 Care plan for Miss Smith

Complete definition of service requirements

Once the client's needs are defined, and the services identified to meet those needs, the macro care plan must be precise as to how the service will meet those needs. For example, times of the day that care will be needed.

Explore the resources of clients and carers

For the majority of clients the aim will be to promote their independence, and care planning should enable clients and carers to make the most of their own resources and abilities, i.e. the things that they can do well.

Review existing services

Existing services should be reviewed in the light of the needs-led assessment and new services introduced appropriately.

Consider alternatives

In taking a fresh look at users' needs, it is essential that practitioners have a comprehensive knowledge of services available across the statutory and independent sector. Care planning is an opportunity to be creative and innovative in designing packages of care to meet the user's needs.

Discuss options

Once identified, these options should be fully discussed with the client and relevant carers only.

Establish preferences

Wherever possible, clients should be offered a choice of service options appropriate to their ethnic and cultural background. For example, Mrs Bradshaw (page 361) attends an Afro/Caribbean club.

Cost care plan

It is vital the care plan be costed. Clients should always know the estimated cost to themselves of any options under active consideration.

Assess financial means

If charges are to be levied in respect of any services, care planning will involve an assessment of the client's financial means and ability to pay. Clients should not agree a care plan before they have been advised in writing of any charges involved.

Reconcile preferences and resources

Having established the wishes of the client, and the cost of the selected options, these may have to be checked against the available resources. This may be done by the care manager alone, if this person holds delegated budgets, or in conjunction with other relevant management.

Agree service objectives

Having confirmed the service options that can be resourced, the next stage is to finalise the agreements with all the agencies and individuals who are to contribute to care plans. This will include the contribution of the clients and carers themselves. The objectives of their inputs should be made clear to all contributors. These should be consistent with the objectives agreed with the client during the initial assessment stage. There should also be a common understanding of how these objectives will be measured.

Co-ordinate plan

Care managers and other workers must integrate the parts of a care plan into a coherent whole that makes sense to the client and their carers. All contributors to a care plan should be aware of the overall objectives of the plan and be mutually supportive to one another. A care plan must be flexible.

Fix review

The client should be told the name of the worker (or key worker) who will be responsible for the

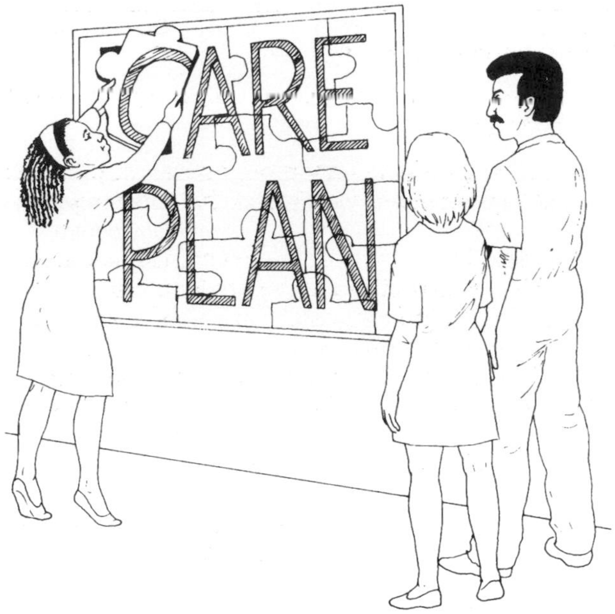

implementation, monitoring and review of the care plan. A date should be set for the first review of the care plan. The key worker (a named person with special responsibilities toward the client) should undertake an earlier review should circumstances require this.

Identify unmet need

Having completed the care plan, the worker should identify any assessed need which it has not been possible to address and identify for whatever reason. This information should be fed back for service planning and quality assurance.

Record the care plan

Care plans should be set out in concise written form linked with the assessment of need. A care plan should be a blueprint for action.

Try it

Using Case Study A or B, or a real-life situation, check if the care plan contains the components suggested in the checklist (see opposite).

Care planning: checklist

Practitioners can use this list to check that key points are covered:

1 Is the care plan based on the needs, priorities and objectives identified at the assessment stage?
2 Does it have a clear overall objective, with specific objectives for all contributors, including the means of measuring their performance?
3 Does it set out the services to be supplied?
4 Does it make maximum use of the client's and carer's own resources?
5 Was the user offered a genuine choice of options?
6 Does it make co-ordinated and cost-effective use of the resources available to the client and agencies across the statutory and independent sectors?
7 Has it been costed?
8 Does it identify any unmet need?
9 Does it record any points of difference?
10 Have the practitioner(s) responsible for implementation, monitoring and review been decided?
11 Has a date for the first review been set?
12 Has a copy been given to the client and other contributors?

(Adapted from *Care Management and Assessment – Practitioners' Guide* HMSO, 1991)

Implementing the macro care plan

The guiding principle of implementation should be to achieve the stated objectives of the care plan with the minimum of intervention necessary. It should therefore seek to minimise the number of service-providers involved (see Figures 16.7 and 16.8).

Process of implementation

The person responsible for devising the care plane should carry the responsibility for its implementation.

The tasks of implementation will include the following:

- determine the client/carer participation
- agree pace of implementation
- confirm budget
- check service availability
- renegotiate existing services
- contract new services
- test options
- revise care plan and costing
- establish monitoring arrangements.

Encouraging involvement of client and carers in care planning

The starting point for implementation should be the clients and their carers, because all other inputs should be geared to supporting their contribution. Clients and carers should be encouraged to play as active a part in the implementation of their care plan as their abilities and motivation allow. Clients may require considerable reassurance and persuasion to accept help, as may carers who feel threatened by such intrusion. All clients should be included in the decision-making associated with the implementation of their care plans.

Agree pace of implementation

Work on implementation should commence as soon as the care plan has been finalised, but the pace at which it is implemented should be carefully negotiated with the clients and their carers.

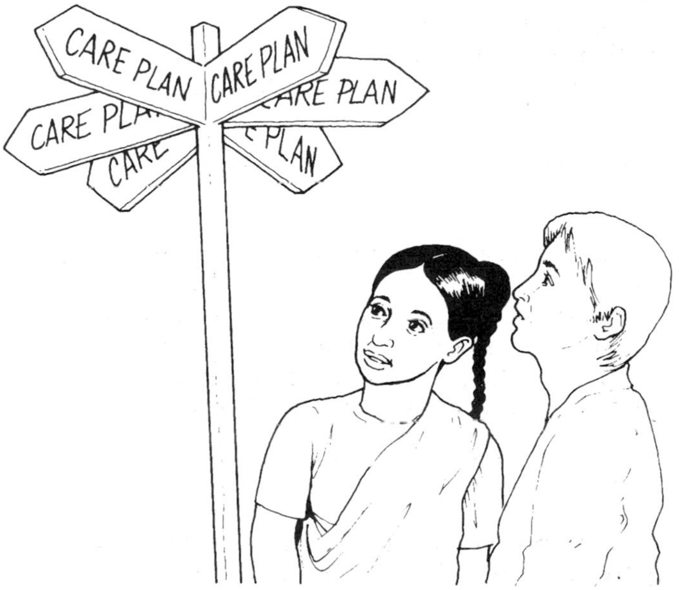

Assessment by Care Manager (Health and Social Services)
Customer Mr Andrews
Key worker

Date
Care Manager
Review date

Needs	How needs are to be met	Action by
1 Personal care to assist Mr Andrews get up, go to bed and use toilet	1a Personal care service daily, morning and evening as part of care package	1a Care manager to negotiate Home Care Service
2 Regular breaks/respite, so that Mr and Mrs Andrews have more personal space	2a Mr Andrews to have day care 4 times a week, and to have a bath while there	2a Care manager to negotiate with Day Centre/key worker
	b Mr Andrews to have short stays in residential respite care for 2 weeks twice a year	b Care manager to negotiate with residential home
	c Mrs Andrews to attend carers' group – once every fortnight	c Care manager to negotiate with Age Concern
	d Person to sit with Mr Andrews while Mrs Andrews goes to carers' group	d Care manager to negotiate with Cross Roads
	e Transport needed to enable these breaks/respite to occur	e Care manager to negotiate with Day Centre/key worker
3 Emotional needs – both Mr and Mrs Andrews need somebody to talk through their situation	3a Mr Andrews needs to be met by Day Centre worker – key worker	3a Care manager to negotiate with Day Centre/key worker
	b Mrs Andrews will attend carers' group	b Care manager to negotiate with Age Concern
4 Mr Andrews feels he needs broader interests and hobbies	4a Day Centre worker – key worker – to discuss and pursue with Mr Andrews	4a Care manager to negotiate with Day Centre/key worker
5 Mrs Andrews wants to know more about her husband's condition and how she can help as a carer	5a Support for Mrs Andrews through carers' group	5a Care manager to set up. Key worker to link with chair of carers' group
	b Care manager will ask GP to discuss with Mrs Andrews	b Care manager to activate
6 Continuing assessment of Mr Andrews' ability to perform tasks in his home	6a Occupational therapy assessment to be updated once has moved home	6a Care manager to negotiate with occupational therapist
7 Adaptation of home to ease access problems	7a Door to be widened if possible	7a Care manager to request and liaise with occupational therapist and Housing Department
	b Possibility of lift to be considered	

Figure 16.7 Example of a care plan (Case Study A)

Assessment by Care Manager (Health and Social Services)
Customer Mrs Bradshaw
Key worker

Date
Care Manager
Review date

Needs	How needs are to be met	Action by
1 Mrs Bradshaw needs assessors who respect cultural background	1a Contact Afro/Caribbean agency and request person from same cultural background	1a Care manager
2 Mrs Bradshaw needs to be able to continue with friends/sports/other activities	2a Involving her children, grandchildren and friends in her care whenever possible	2a Care manager
3 Mrs Bradshaw needs to be able to express fears about her condition/change of role	3a Weekly meetings with Community Psychiatric Nurse	3a Care manager
4 Mrs Bradshaw needs to be able to sustain relationships with family	4a Encouraging family visits and outings	4a Care manager
5 Mrs Bradshaw needs to establish a regular sleep pattern	5a Involve GP	5a Care manager
6 Mrs Bradshaw needs to keep as much in touch with reality as possible	6a Lifestyle needs to be reality/orientation-centred	6a Specialist home carer for dementia
7 Mrs Bradshaw needs system to monitor her alcohol	7a Set up a system of recording alcohol intake	7a Home carer and husband
8 Mr Bradshaw needs a break regularly	8a Arrange regular short-stay breaks for Mrs Bradshaw	8a Care manager
9 Mr Bradshaw needs to be able to sustain relationships with family	9a Point 8 would assist Mr Bradshaw to do this	9a Care manager
10 Mr Bradshaw needs to understand diagnosis and prognosis	10a Regular meetings with Community Psychiatric Nurse and Carers' Support Group	10a Care manager
11 Mr Bradshaw needs to be able to talk about his fears and frustrations	11a Regular meetings with Community Psychiatric Nurse and Carers' Support Group	11a Care manager
12 The whole family need to be enabled to meet to solve problems.	12a Regular meetings of family with care manager	12a Care manager

Figure 16.8 Example of a care plan (Case Study B)

Confirm budget

It is essential to confirm that relevant finance is available.

Check service availability

The practitioners must check on the availability of preferred services and confirm with the client whether he or she is prepared to wait for a particular service or settle for another option. If services are unavailable it is essential that the service planning system is informed.

Renegotiate existing services

It may be that the existing pattern of services may have to be renegotiated, either to accommodate changing needs or simply to achieve the desired objectives more effectively.

Contract new services

In assessing new services, practitioners will have to adjust to the contracting arrangements that authorities and agencies are developing as part of the community care changes. Practitioners will have to acquire skills in devising service specifications and quality standards, and in negotiating and monitoring contracts. The aim is to produce a quality service as cost effectively as possible within the agreed timescale.

Establish monitoring arrangements

It is essential to establish monitoring arrangements to ensure that the care plan remains on course.

Implementing the care plan: checklist
Practitioners can use this list to check that key points are covered:

1. Has the client been involved to the limit of his or her capacity in the implementation process?
2. Have the inputs of clients and carers been maximised and have formal service inputs been geared to their support?
3. Has the pace of implementation been agreed with the client?
4. Has the budget for implementation been clearly defined, together with the responsibility for allocating that budget?
5. Have deficiencies in service availability and quality been notified to service planning and quality assurance/inspection respectively?
6. Have existing services been renegotiated to meet the care plan objectives more effectively?
7. Has the care plan been delivered to time and to quality?
8. Have resources been co-ordinated in a cost-effective way?
9. Have the reasons for any departure from the original plan been recorded?
10. Have arrangements been established to monitor the ongoing implementation?

(Adapted from *Care Management and Assessment – Practitioners' Guide* HMSO, 1991)

Try it

Using Case Studies A or B, check whether the key points are covered from the 'implementing the care plan: checklist' (see opposite).

Case Study C

Mr Collins has a severe physical disability. He is 47 years of age. Following a road traffic accident at age 15, he is a wheelchair user with legs extended in spasms and he cannot raise his arms above shoulder level. His speech is very slurred. Cognitively he is very alert.

Referral
Mr Collins lived with his father who is 84 years old and his main carer. Following a dispute which neither wished to resolve, Mr Collins decided he wished to live independently in the community.

Outcome
Mr Collins was admitted to an assessment centre to take part in the independence training programme to acquire new skills in independence, He submitted an application form for a purpose-built flat. A multi-disciplinary assessment was undertaken to identity his needs. He applied to the Independent Living Fund (prior to April 1993) and was awarded £465.00 per week towards purchasing the care and assistance he needed.

A multi-disciplinary Assessment Panel was held and Mr Collins' needs were identified as: 1) personal care;

2) domestic; 3) equipment; 4) transport;
5) accommodation. A social worker was allocated as his care manager, to work jointly with an occupational therapist.

Mr Collins was allocated a purpose-built flat by a Housing Association. Mr Collins assisted in the design of the package of care he felt he required. He employed four private carers, through contacts made by staff at the local assessment centre and private agencies and other customers in a similar situation to himself. Independently, he: 1) worked out a rota for his private carers, carefully timetabling the support he required;
2) decided how much the hourly rate of pay would be by seeking advice from the Disability Action Group;
3) found out about paying his carers' tax and National Insurance through an information pack obtained from the Inland Revenue and further advice from a Disability Action Group.

Through advice from his social worker, Mr Collins selected the appropriate household contents, personal accident and professional liability insurances.

Conclusion
Mr Collins will be living independently in the community with the support of a care package he assisted in designing. Mr Collins has been able to organise his own care, although physically unable to care for himself. He applied to the DSS Social Fund for a Community Care Grant, which he used to furnish and equip his own flat.

This, along with his Independent Living Fund Award, support from Social Services Staff (social worker, OT, assessment centre staff) and local Disability Action Group, has: 1) enabled him to achieve his aims to live independently in the community; and 2) empowered him to mobilise community resources to meet his needs.

See page 375 for the macro and micro care plans for Mr Collins.

Clients' rights

Clients come from all sections of the community and will differ in many aspects from one another, such as age, ethnic and cultural background, gender, disability/ability. Their needs will be different and their preferences as to how these needs are to be met will be different. Whatever the personal characteristics and needs of the individual, *everyone* has the same rights as a client. Equality of care is a central value to all the caring professions and is written into codes of practice, and in the government's Patient's Charter. There are also laws

CLIENT RESPONSE TO FIELDWORK ASSESSMENT

Mr Collins is in agreement with the assessment shown and is very keen to achieve independent living in the community.

Client: ______________________

Assessing Social Worker: ______________________

Team Manager
Physical Disabilities Team: ______________________

Date: ______________________

Figure 16.9 Example of Client Agreement Form

designed to protect vulnerable groups from discrimination in employment, education and other areas of life.

Clients have a right to expect certain standards, or codes of practice, to be followed by those assessing their needs, and those providing a service to meet the needs. These rights include:

- freedom from discrimination
- confidentiality of information
- independence – as far as possible
- power of choice
- dignity in the care received.

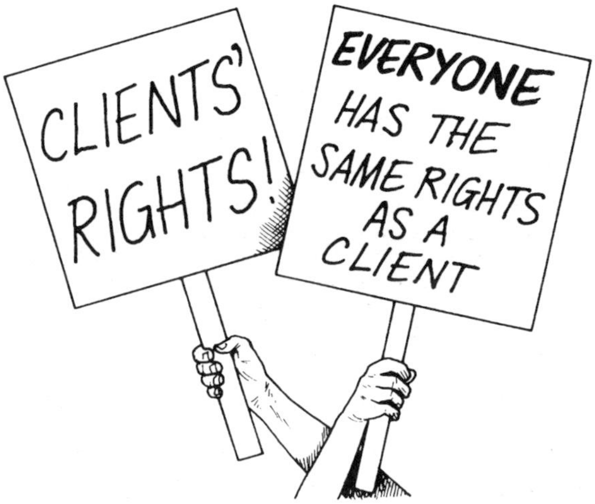

Macro Care Plan – Mr Collins

Needs		How needs are to be met		Action by	
1a	Assistance with personal tasks, e.g. dressing and undressing, bathing, hair washing and care of feet	1a	Personal care service to be arranged	1a	Social worker to liaise with providers
b	A suitable toilet facility	b	Closomat toilet to be installed in new property	b	Social worker and occupational therapist
c	Assistance with transferring on and off bed, toilet, and in and out of wheelchair	c	Rails to be fitted and personal carer to assist with transfers	c	Social worker and occupational therapist
2a	Assistance with all domestic tasks, some food preparation, shopping, bed making and ironing	2a	Domestic service and home carer to assist	2a	Social worker to liaise with providers
3a	To be able to summon help quickly in an emergency situation, to open front door, to operate TV and switch on lights	3a	Environmental Control Unit at previous address to be reassessed to accommodate all these functions	3a	Occupational therapist
b	To have access to a telephone and assistance with handset and speaking on the phone	b	British Telecom to be approached	b	Occupational therapist
4a	Various items of furniture, household equipment and furnishings. Where possible materials should be fire resistant	4a	To be purchased with Community Care Grant when obtained from DSS Social Fund	4a	Mr Collins
5a	Certain domestic appliances and work should be height adjusted.	5a	Kitchen units in new property are adjustable and work surfaces at wheelchair height	5a	Occupational therapist
b	Items of equipment such as grabrail, shower chair, cutlery, non-slip mats and other kitchen equipment	b	OT assessment	b	Occupational therapist
6a	Assistance with collecting benefits and paying bills	6a	To collect benefits with escort and pay bills by standing order	6a	Mr Collins to organise standing orders and pay bills
7a	To go shopping weekly	7a	To be escorted	7a	Social worker to liaise with possible provider and/or volunteers
b	To be able to visit his father	b	To be escorted	7b	Social worker to liaise with possible provider and/or volunteers
8a	Assistance with booking dial-a-ride and taxis	8a	To plan ahead and make booking with help from Local Assessment Unit	8a	Assessment unit
9a	Regular support to be able to live independently in the community	9a	Regular pattern of respite care at local respite facility	9a	Social worker to liaise with local respite facility
10a	To be able to accommodate a large outdoor electric wheelchair	10a	New property has space under stairs with power point for battery to be recharged	10a	Provision exists in new property
b	To be able to charge wheelchair battery overnight	b	Carer would need help to plug in	b	Social worker to liaise with provider

Micro Care Plan – Mr Collins

The micro plan for Mr Collins contains the detail needed to ensure Mr Collins is able to live independently.

Needs	Needs
1 Personal care The care manager, who is a social worker, arranges for a home carer to visit every morning and every evening to assist Mr Collins to dress and undress. The home carer will also assist Mr Collins with personal hygiene. The care manager arranges a bathing service to visit twice weekly, and a chiropodist to visit weekly	**4 Visits to his father** The care manager will arrange for a volunteer to accompany Mr Collins when visiting his father
2 Domestic tasks Care manager to liaise with domestic services and home carer. The care manager will ensure that help is available three times a day for the preparation, and cooking of food, plus time to set aside daily to complete other household tasks. The home carer will accompany Mr Collins on shopping trips twice weekly	**5 Respite care** The care manager will book this on a regular basis with the local assessment centre
3 Collecting benefits Care manager will arrange an escort to accompany Mr Collins when he needs to collect his benefits	**6 Charging wheelchair battery** The care manager would arrange for the home carer to plug in the charger every evening

The staff involved with Mr Collins will need to monitor the effectiveness of the micro care plan and suggest alterations to his care plan as time goes by.

Freedom from discrimination

All people have a right to expect to be treated fairly. People should not be discriminated against for any reason; for example, because of age, gender, ethnic, racial, cultural or religious backgrounds, disability or sexual orientation.

Discrimination may take many different forms. It ranges from physical and verbal abuse to judgements made about people based on stereotypes with which they have been labelled.

Discrimination may also appear in other ways, such as information regarding what services are available, or how an assessment and care plan is to be carried out, not being accessible to everyone. Information may not be available in appropriate languages, or in Braille, or on tapes for those who cannot hear. Interpreters, including signers, may not be available either at the assessment stage, or through service delivery. Another example of discrimination could be that a day centre, or residential establishment, may not take account of the dietary needs required by the religion and culture of some clients. Managers need to make sure that all groups are equally catered for.

Confidentiality

Clients have to right to know that information about themselves will not be repeated to others. When any information is to be shared with another person or agency, the worker should explain to the client this needs to be done. For example, there may be times when the worker needs to share information with another professional in order to get the care that the person needs. Confidentiality ensures that clients continue to trust the worker and will talk freely about their situation and their needs.

Independence

Clients have the right to remain as independent as possible whilst receiving care. There is a danger of clients losing their independence because of the care they receive. For example, older people may find that they have all their personal care, such as dressing, done for them, instead of workers encouraging clients to find alternative ways of coping and allowing clients to take their own time to do things. In a care situation, where the client is reliant on others for assistance, the client is vulnerable to loss of independence. Clients must be helped to do as much for themselves as they possibly can.

Information and choice

In order to be and feel independent, it is important that the client is able to maintain choice. Traditionally, services have offered clients little choice and clients have not been aware of the choices open to them. It is important that clients have as much information as possible regarding services available to them, and that assessors and care workers fully involve the client in any decision-making.

Dignity

All clients should be treated with respect, and their feelings and wishes given due consideration. All clients should expect assessors and care workers to treat them with courtesy and to pay due regard to their dignity. Some people, such as those requiring help with personal tasks, e.g. bathing, are particularly vulnerable. The effect of not respecting or taking account of a client's feelings will be to lower their self-esteem. Maintaining the dignity of a client, in situations where people are very dependent on

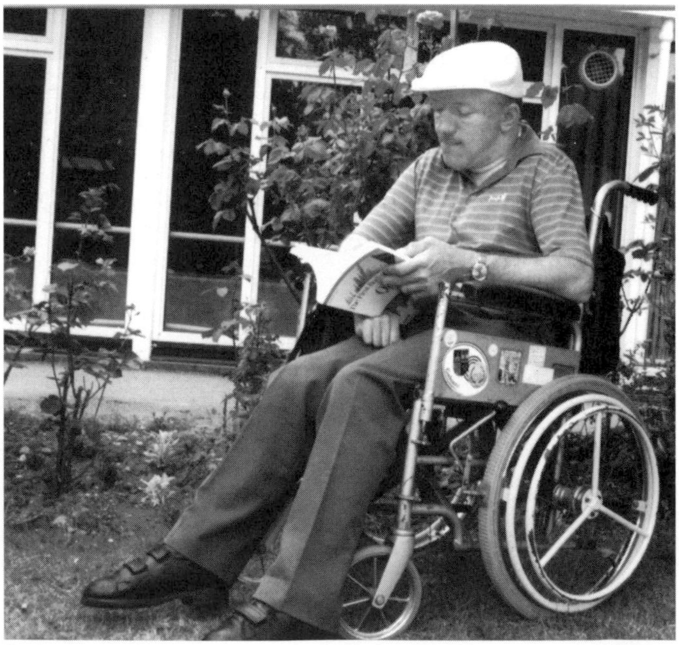

Figure 16.10 Care workers must ensure that the client's dignity is preserved
Photo courtesy of Winged Fellowship Trust

others, is a skill that care workers must develop in order for clients to have their dignity respected.

Think it over

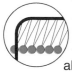

Think about clients' rights. Write down five ways (i.e. one for each of the rights listed above) that clients could have their rights violated.

Monitoring

What is the purpose of monitoring?

The purpose of monitoring is to:

- check the achievement of care plan objectives
- co-ordinate all services
- ensure that services are delivered according to laid-down specifications
- oversee the quality of care
- manage the budget
- support users, carers and service providers
- fine-tune the care plan and contribute to the review.

1 Care plan objectives

The first purpose of monitoring is to ensure that the objectives set out in the care plan are being achieved. The person monitoring the care plan has to check that each agency providing a service is on track in terms of delivering their specific objectives.

2 Co-ordinating services

The more contributors there are to the care plan, then the more important becomes the role of co-ordination. The person with the responsibility for monitoring must ensure that the services complement each other and that all necessary information is shared. They must also play a key role in managing any changes that are made in the way in which services are delivered, so that continuity of care is maintained.

3 Service delivery

The contributions of all the people and agencies participating in the care plan, including the contributions of the client and their carer, must be written into the original care plan. It is important that all contributors continue to fulfil their commitments to the care plan, or all of the care arrangements could be jeopardised. It should be remembered that unpaid carers, such as a husband, wife, partner, other relation, neighbour or friend, may also be contributing to the care plan. For example, a neighbour may be providing the client with a light meal each weekday evening, a relation may be providing personal care and meals at the weekend.

4 Overseeing the quality of care

Each of the service providers, and participants in the care plan, has a responsibility for the quality of their own contribution. However, the standards for the quality of each service should be specified in contracts between the monitoring worker (*purchaser*) and the service provider. These agreements are called *service specifications*.

Quality lies in the attention to detail that matters to each individual. The care manager or monitoring worker, therefore, has a responsibility to ensure that contributors take account of the personal requirements of the client – for example, the way a person with a disability likes to be lifted.

5 Managing the budget

The monitoring worker may have responsibility for the budget and may be required to oversee the budget. This will become more important where financial responsibilities are developed from senior managers to individual care managers.

6 Support to clients, carers and service providers

Support to clients, carers and service providers may take different forms:

- counselling
- progress-chasing
- resolving conflicts.

7 Fine-tuning the care plan

Changes in the needs of the client and carer need to be taken into account in the care plan; therefore as the needs change so the care plan must be adjusted in order to reflect those needs. However, adjustment to the care plan can only take into account minor changes in need. Any major changes in need will be sanctioned (agreed) by a *review*.

Reviews will normally be held at regular intervals but they can also be triggered should anyone involved in the provision of care perceive any difficulties. Where a client's capabilities are diminishing, monitoring has to identify when a review is required so that the increased needs of the individual can be reassessed.

The monitoring process

Wherever possible, the person responsible for assessment, care planning and implementation should continue to hold the responsibility for monitoring. This person will co-ordinate the monitoring process, although various other people should be involved in it. For example:

- clients, carers – as contributors as well as service users
- service providers – as monitors of their own service
- managers – to oversee the quality of services
- purchasing agents – as monitors of contracts
- inspection units – as monitors of quality standards in residential care.

Approaches to monitoring

Care management stresses the importance of monitoring in ensuring that objectives are being met and in adapting the care plan to the changing needs of the clients. Monitoring can be achieved in a variety of ways, depending on the complexity of the care plan. For example:

- home visits
- telephone calls
- letters
- questionnaires
- observation.

Try it

Using Case Study C, write out how you would monitor the care plan, using the following checklist as a guide.

Draft a simple questionnaire to be used for testing client satisfaction.

Monitoring questionnaire for a bathing service

1. Are all referrals assessed within 5 working days?
2. Has feedback been given to the referrer regarding the outcome of the referral?
3. Has a key worker (person with special responsibility for the client) been identified?
4. Have joint assessments and visits been undertaken where appropriate?
5. Is training provided to all staff on an ongoing basis?
6. Have systems been introduced to assess client satisfaction?
7. Is there a clear complaints procedure in place?
8. Has a care plan been devised for each client?
9. Does each client have a copy of his or her care plan?
10. Are service specifications being met?
11. Is the service being delivered within budget?
12. Are procedures in place so that reviews can be called if necessary?

Monitoring checklist

Monitoring workers can use this list to check that they have covered all the key points:

1. Is the type of monitoring appropriate to the care plan?
2. Are clients and carers actively involved?
3. Is the monitoring of objectives regularly undertaken?
4. Does the monitoring worker continue to co-ordinate all the contributions to the care plan?
5. Are services regularly checked against service specifications?
6. Is the care plan being delivered within the budget?
7. How regular is the support to clients, carers and service providers?
8. Are the reasons for minor changes recorded?
9. Is monitoring systematically recorded?
10. Are all contributors aware of the procedures for calling a review?

(Adapted from *Care Management and Assessment – Practitioners' Guide* HMSO, 1991)

Reviewing

What is the purpose of a review?

A review fulfils a variety of different purposes. It might be needed to:

- check that care plan objectives have been achieved
- evaluate reasons for failure or success
- evaluate quality and cost of care provided
- reassess current needs
- revise objectives of the care plan
- revise services that are required
- reassess costs
- note any unmet need
- record results of review
- set date of next review.

1 Care plan objectives

It is important that each review should first consider the views of the client and carer as to what progress has been made in achieving the care plan objectives. The views of the service providers should also be obtained. The realism of the original objectives and their continuing relevance can then be determined.

2 Reasons for failure or success

An evaluation of why objectives may – or may not – have been met should help to determine any future action and future care plans.

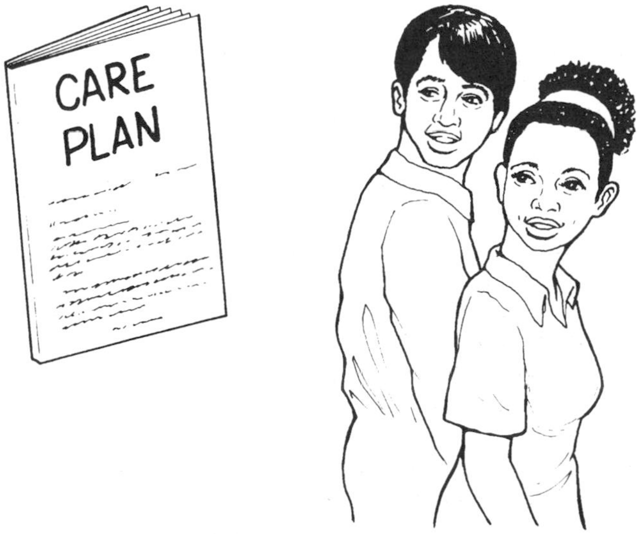

3 Quality and cost of care

By using the evidence gained through the monitoring process, the review will be able to check that services have maintained the required standards of quality and are being provided within the budget limits. A judgement regarding the cost-effectiveness of the care package, to date, should be taken into account when adjustments or changes are made to the care plan.

4 Reassessing current need

A review should not repeat the original assessment. It should pick up any needs that were previously not identified and any new needs that have developed since the previous review. It should also take into account any changes in the preferences of the client and carer for how the needs are to be met.

5 Revising care objectives

The original care objectives should be reviewed and adjusted to meet changing needs. The short-term objectives of each provider should also be reviewed and new targets should build on past achievements.

6 Revising service requirements

Changes to the care plan may result in the renegotiation of services contracts, including the level of service and/or the way the way in which the services are to be provided.

7 Reassessing cost

Changes in service levels may result in a financial change – how much the package will cost. A new budget may have to be agreed.

8 Unmet needs

Either the required quality of service, or ways to meet identified needs, may not be available. Any short-comings should be noted and this information should be passed to those responsible for planning services.

9 Recording results of review

The finding of the review should be recorded and a copy given to the client and all contributors to the review (Figure 16.11). The recording of the review should include:

- evaluation of achievement of objectives, with reasons for success or failure
- evaluation of the quality and cost of services provided
- reassessment of current needs
- revision of care plan objectives
- note of changes required in service provision
- revision of cost of care package
- identification of any unmet need
- date of next review; name of person who is to carry out the monitoring until next review; name of person who is to co-ordinate the next review.

10 Date of next review

Agencies should set a minimum frequency for reviews. However, intervals between each review should reflect the complexity of the care package and/or the anticipated pace of change in the needs of the client. For example, where a client has a rapidly deteriorating illness, then it may be necessary to review the situation every eight weeks. Additionally, it must be possible to hold reviews sooner than the specified date should the need arise.

REVIEW FORM		
NAME OF CLIENT: REVIEW HELD ON: FIRST\SECOND\THIRD REVIEW (delete) AT:		
PRESENT		
APOLOGIES		
REVIEW OF DECISIONS MADE AT PREVIOUS REVIEW	*Action*	*By*
VIEW OF CLIENT RE CARE PLAN		
VIEW OF CARER RE CARE PLAN		
VIEW OF KEY WORKER		
VIEW OF SERVICE PROVIDER		
REASONS FOR SUCCESS/FAILURE OF CARE PLAN		
REVISED SERVICE REQUIREMENTS		
REVISED COST OF CARE PACKAGE		
UNMET NEEDS		
DATE OF NEXT REVIEW		

Figure 16.11 A sample review form

The review process

Scope

As for the assessment, the scope of the review will depend on the complexity of need and the frequency on how quickly the needs are subject to change. Also, like the assessment, reviewing should be **needs-led.** Not everyone contributing to service provision is required to attend every review. However, all those involved in the original care plan, or previous review, should be consulted either by telephone, letter or direct meetings (Figure 16.12).

Venue

The venue should be decided by what is judged to be the most effective way of involving the client and carer. It may, therefore, be appropriate to hold at least part of the review in the client's home, or at any venue where they receive some of the services, for example at a day centre.

Review worker

In order to maintain continuity both in the processes and in understanding the client's needs over a period of time, there are advantages in the assessment, monitoring and reviewing processes being the responsibility of one person.

Review checklist

Reviewing workers can use this list to check that they have covered all the key points:

1. Is the review taking place on the scheduled date?
2. Is the review centred on the needs and preferences of the client?
3. Are all the service providers involved?
4. Has the client (and the carer) been able to participate, and have their wishes been taken into account?
5. Has the review addressed both the positive and negative aspects of the care plan?
6. Has the evaluation taken into account both the quality and cost of services?
7. Have all changes in the services to be provided, and any changes in how they are to be provided, been noted?
8. Has the review been recorded and the date of the next review set?

(Adapted from *Care Management and Assessment – Practitioners' Guide* HMSO, 1991)

c.c. Mr Jacob (client)
Miss Jacob (client's sister)
Social worker
Occupational therapist
Psychologist
Home care manager

Date: 21.11.95
Customer Mr Jacob
Care Manager: Social Worker
Review date To be arranged

	Needs	Now needs are to be met	Action by
a	*Personal care* Prompting and guidance for all personal hygiene tasks (i.e. washing, shaving, dressing, care of clothes)	Home carers' services within group home setting	Social worker to liaise with home care manager
b	*Tasks of daily living*		
	Household/domestic assistance	Home care services	Social worker to liaise with home care manager
	shopping assistance	Home care services	Social worker to liaise with home care manager
	budgeting assistance	Community care worker	Social worker to liaise with home carers and day centre managers
	cooking meals assistance	Home care services/day centres	
	co-ordinating personal/household routine	Social worker/community care worker	Social worker to liaise with community support worker
c	*Finance* Assistance with financial affairs	Social worker/family	Social worker to liaise with Miss Jacob (sister)
	Social contact	Day care/sheltered workshop scheme (SWS)	Social worker to liaise with day centre manager, SWS
	Ongoing assessment	Occupational therapist/psychologist	Social worker to liaise with occupational therapist and psychologist

Figure 16.12 Needs assessment for Mr Jacob

Think it over

Using Case Study C, think about who you would ask to make contributions to a review. Consider how frequently a review for a client might need to take place.

Involving clients

Various research studies have shown that clients generally hold the following views:

1 Most people prefer to stay in their own homes
2 Most people want to have control over what happens to them
3 Most people want choice and flexibility in the services that are offered to them
4 Most people want to be assured of the level and quality of services that they receive

An example of a care plan involving the client and his family, NHS Trust hospital staff and Social Services staff is shown in Figure 16.13. Mr Jacob is a vulnerable person with complex mental health needs. As part of the care planning cycle, Mr Jacob's mental and social needs have been assessed, and a meeting has been called to identify clearly his needs and how these needs are to be met.

The care plan involves input from Mr Jacob's family, medical staff and social services staff. Figure 16.13 shows a programme where Mr Jacob's needs have been broken down by activity. It is an example of one week's activity in Mr Jacob's care plan.

Changes in care planning and interaction

Historically, health and care services concentrated on

Client's name Mr Jacob **Dr** .... **Tel no** .... **Key holder** ....

Address ....

Special instructions: Would all carers please use Mr Jacob's wipeclean board for prompting memory jog.

Other agencies involved:
Social worker
Community carer/home carer
Sheltered workshop scheme (SWS)

Care manager:

Monday a.m.	*Tuesday a.m.*	*Wednesday a.m.*	*Thursday a.m.*	*Friday a.m.*	*Saturday a.m.*	*Sunday a.m.*
Wash, shave, dress, clean teeth, clean clothes, make bed and breakfast	Wash, shave, dress clean teeth, clean clothes, make bed and breakfast, OT unit	Wash, shave, dress, clean teeth, clean clothes, make bed and breakfast, SWS	Wash, shave, dress, clean teeth, clean clothes, make bed and breakfast, pay rent, community support worker arrives	Wash, shave, dress clean teeth, clean clothes, make bed and breakfast, SWS	Wash. shave, dress clean teeth, clean clothes, make bed and breakfast	Wash, shave, dress clean teeth, clean clothes, make bed and breakfast
Lunch	*Lunch*	*Lunch*	*Lunch*	*Lunch*	*Lunch*	*Lunch*
Market garden	OT Unit of local hospital	SWS. Market garden	Budget with GIRO, CNS; any other shopping needed	SWS. Market garden		
p.m.	*p.m.*	*p.m.*	*p.m.*	*p.m.*	*p.m.*	*p.m.*
Chores Evening meal; ensure room tidy	Household chores Evening meal; ensure room tidy	Household chores Evening meal; ensure room tidy	Household chores Evening meal; ensure room tidy	Chores Evening meal; ensure room tidy		

Figure 16.13 Care plan for Mr Jacob

the idea of treating people in need. This is referred to as the 'therapeutic era' of health and social care (see Chapter 12). When people could not cope with daily life they were offered a service. If an older person could not cope with housework or shopping, they were 'given' a home-help service. If they were lonely and depressed an older person might be 'given' residential care. People with learning difficulties might be 'sent' to an adult training centre. People with needs were allocated a service or treatment, to deal with their need. Sometimes the services were very caring and many clients may have been content with the help they received. However, from the early 1980s onwards the idea of allocating people to a service was seen as an inefficient way of meeting need. It was understood to be inefficient because:

- people often received a level of service that they didn't need, whilst other people's needs were not met by the services they were given
- people were not treated as individuals – people often got the same service regardless of their gender, race, culture, or even their physical, emotional or social needs.
- some people believed that care services had become service-centred rather than client-centred. This means that the staff 'treated' people in terms of the needs of the organisation, rather than in terms of personal need.

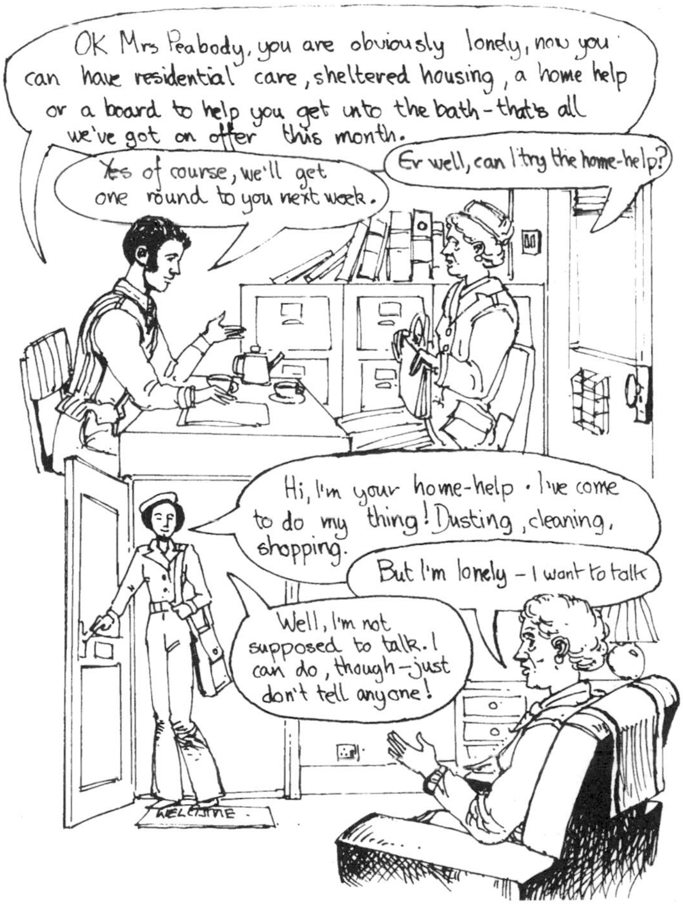
OK Mrs Peabody, you are obviously lonely, now you can have residential care, sheltered housing, a home help or a board to help you get unto the bath – that's all we've got on offer this month.
Er well, can I try the home-help?
Yes of course, we'll get one round to you next week.
Hi, I'm your home-help. I've come to do my thing! Dusting, cleaning, shopping.
But I'm lonely – I want to talk
Well, I'm not supposed to talk. I can do, though – just don't tell anyone!
WELCOME

The cartoon, below left, helps to summarise graphically the problem that some people saw in the 1970s services.

Whilst the cartoon is not a fair overall summary of the operation of services, there were examples of allocation to service involving problems like this.

Care planning was developed to avoid problems associated with 'putting people into a service'. The focus on assessment, planning, monitoring and reviewing is designed to meet individual needs with efficient and effective services; the ideal is to involve the client and/or carer completely in checking that the care plan meets their needs. The provision of care should be adapted to meet precise personal needs rather than giving a general service. Clients have to be provided with accurate information, advice and opportunities for skills development. Most importantly, clients and their carers (or network or friends and carers) must be involved in every step of the care plan process. Interventions are negotiated with clients and carers.

The key issue is that clients and their carers should be empowered to make their own choices, and be in control of the services provided as far as is

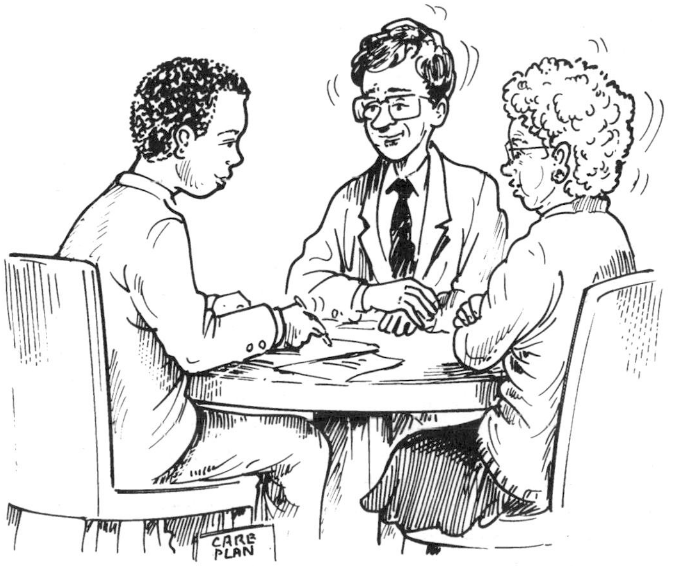
CARE PLAN

appropriate and possible – within resource constraints. The process of care planning described in this chapter describes how clients are involved and how services might be co-ordinated to meet a wide range of needs. Recent care planning services aim to assess, plan, monitor and review interventions so as to empower clients and provide a service which meets individual needs.

Evidence collection point

For this element you need to produce a report which describes the care planning cycle and illustrates how it works by reference to one client's needs, identifying five different practitioners who may be involved in care planning and the extent to which they may work alone, with other professionals or with the client. The report should explain two interventions (approaches to enable, care or treatment of clients) and relate these interventions to client needs, giving two examples of each intervention. The report should also explain ways of encouraging client and carer involvement in care planning and describe two recent changes in the practice of care planning and interventions.

Chapter 17

Methods for promoting and protecting health and social well-being

This chapter describes the range of practitioners involved in promoting health and creating environments conducive to health and well-being. Services and legislation designed to protect the public are considered, together with some discussion of the ethical issues associated with individual liberty.

Health promotion

Health promotion is essentially an 'umbrella term', covering health education as well as environmental and legal issues. The following definitions can be used:

- Health promotion can be defined as a programme of 'health-enhancing activities'. These health-enhancing activities are used to promote the overall health of individuals. These activities use education, prevention and protection spread across whole communities. Health promotion endeavours to create an environment in which people may make a positive change to a healthier lifestyle.
- Health education can be defined as programmes aimed at enhancing well-being and preventing or diminishing ill health in individuals and groups.

To some extent, everyone is involved in health promotion in some form or other as everyone, at some point, has offered advice to others about health-related issues (Figure 17.1). This may have been on an informal basis, i.e. a friend asking advice, or a parent teaching a child good personal hygiene routines. Healthier behaviour can also be promoted in other hidden ways, such as a supermarket reducing the cost of low-fat, low sugar foods, so encouraging the customer to purchase them rather than foods with higher fat or sugar content.

Think it over

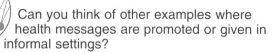

Can you think of other examples where health messages are promoted or given in informal settings?

How important do you think informal sources of health promotion are in improving health and changing habits?

This section is mainly concerned with professional practitioners who have a role in promoting health. This role could form part of their job or be their main purpose. Essentially, this chapter concentrates on people who deliberately promote health in a planned way.

Practitioners promoting health

Health promotion aims to make people aware of issues that affect their health, to give information on ways to improve health and, ultimately, empower

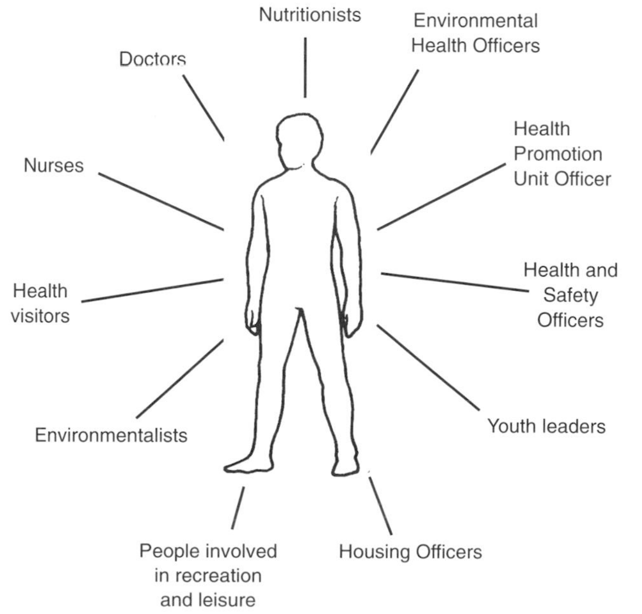

Figure 17.1 People involved in health promotion

people to make informed decisions about the choices open to them which can affect health. These choices can be related to the behaviour of the individuals themselves, for example, smoking or food choice, or factors which affect their immediate environment, such as petrol and its effect on air quality, or the use of pesticides which may cause water pollution. Information on these areas comes from a number of sources. There are also professionals who are concerned with campaigning for and ensuring healthy social and work environments.

International organisations (World Health Organisation, European Union)

Government (Department of Health, Department of Social Security, Ministry of Agriculture, Fisheries and Food, Department for Education and Employment, Central Office of Information, Department of the Environment, Department of Transport)

National Health Service

- Health Education Authority
- Health Education Board for Scotland
- Health Promotion Authority for Wales
- Northern Ireland Health Promotion Unit
- NHS Training Directorate
- NHS Trusts
- Health Authorities and Health Boards
- Family Health Services Authorities
- Community Health Councils
- Health Promotion education officers
- Health professionals: doctors, dentists, nurses, health vistitors, dieticians, chiropodists, etc.

Local Government

- Teachers
- Planning officers
- Environmental Health officers
- Social Services staff
- Housing officers
- Leisure officers

Training

- Training & Enterprise Councils
- Lecturers

Other National Organisations

- National voluntary organisations and pressure groups e.g. RoSPA
- Professional organisations
- Trade Unions
- Churches and religious organisations
- National organisations and local branches e.g. MIND, Citizens' Advice Bureaux
- National Health practitioners
- Manufacturers and retailers
- Industrial and commercial organisations
- Private preventative medical services
- National media – TV, radio, newspapers etc.
- Local media
- Police
- Institutions of higher education
- The informal network – family, friends and neighbours, etc.
- Health and Safety Executive
- Local community and voluntary groups, e.g. youth groups, self-help groups
- Workplace employees, occupational health services, personnel officer managers

Figure 17.2 Practitioners and agencies involved in promoting health and social well-being

It is worth remembering that messages about promotion and protection of health and well-being may come via individuals who represent bodies or groups of people, for example a government officer or a pressure-group spokesperson as well as individuals operating in a professional capacity, such as a GP, health visitor or practice nurse.

Some practitioners have health promotion as their main job, such as those who work for the Health Promotion Unit. Others have health promotion as part of their tasks, for example, the GP who is involved in curative and preventative activities as well as promoting healthy choices to patients.

A more exhaustive list of practitioners and agencies involved in promoting health and social well-being might be laid out as in Figure 17.2.

The government

There are various individuals within the government who have a responsibility for health through its various departments, such as the Department of Health and the Ministry of Agriculture, Food and Fisheries. They are particularly involved through the impact of legislation and matters which affect government finances, for example, prescription charges and VAT on cigarettes and alcohol.

In addition to this, in 1991, the government published the 'Health of The Nation' White Paper which appraised five key areas of health:

- coronary heart disease
- cancers
- mental illness
- accidents
- HIV/AIDS and sexual health.

Its overall aims were to 'add years to life and life to years'. The papers set targets for improvement in all five areas and provided suggestions on how these might be achieved. (See Chapter 12.)

The government also influences health promotion practices by those in direct contact with the public, eg. GPs have to meet targets which affect the funding they receive.

The way in which services are structured and organised can influence health. An example of this is the NHS and Community Care Act 1990, which brought about change in the running of the caring services. One result is that GPs are required to provide health checks and are given incentives to provide health promotion clinics. This in turn could help to ensure that there is movement towards the targets published in the *Health of the Nation* document.

National voluntary groups and pressure groups

There are numerous national organisations involved with health promotion in some form. Some only operate on a national level, for example, TACADE (The Advisory Council on Alcohol and Drug Education), however, many of these have local offices, such as Age Concern, MIND (National Association for Mental Health) and the NCT (National Childbirth Trust). These groups offer advice to the public through educational materials and talks which are concerned with promoting the health of their members, as well as making others aware of their members' lifestyles and needs.

Some voluntary groups also act as pressure groups, which attempt to bring the issues of concern to their particular members to the attention of the government and/or those in authority. They aim to bring about change which is of benefit to their members.

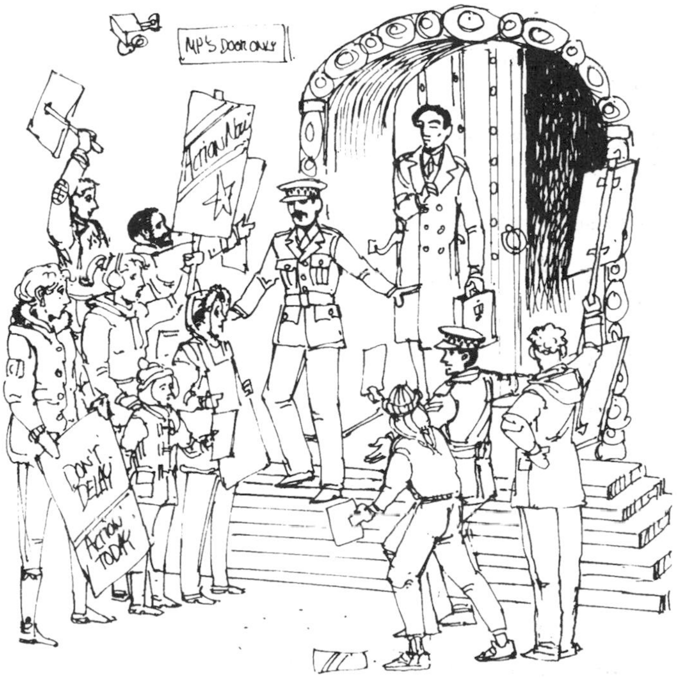

Health Education Authority

The HEA was established in 1987 and is required to provide information and advice about health directly to members of the public. Its objective by the year 2000 is to enable the population to be more knowledgeable, better motivated and more able to acquire and maintain good health. It also supports other organisations and people who provide advice. The HEA advises the Secretary of State for Health and so has an input into broader areas of public health.

District Health Authorities

As explained in Chapter 13, the NHS and Community Care Act 1990 established the purchaser/provider relationship in health-care provision. The District Health Authority is a purchaser and so has responsibility for purchasing the services required to meet the needs of the population. DHAs also have a facilitative role to play in health promotion.

Health promotion/education units

Many areas of Britain have health promotion/education services as part of the NHS provision. Their role is to provide advice, training and resources to support health promotion within the local area. They hold a range of materials, including leaflets, videos and posters, which cover the broad spectrum of health promotion and will also provide speakers/trainers on different health issues.

Health professionals and health promotion

Nurses

Nurses make up the largest proportion of the workforce in hospitals. They are the primary carers of patients and, although operating under instruction and guidance from doctors, are primarily responsible for the care and well-being of the patient. Through this role, they carry out many health promotion tasks, including physical and emotional care.

GPs

General practitioners (GPs), or 'family doctors', work from their own premises or from health centres. The role of the GP is to provide consultation and physical examination, as appropriate, in order to prevent, identify or treat illness, disease or injury. Providing immunisation and vaccination against infectious diseases such as measles, mumps and rubella (German measles) and polio, as well as more unusual diseases which can be contracted whilst travelling abroad, is also part of the doctor's role. When necessary, the GP can refer patients to other service providers such as hospital consultants, social workers, community nurses and midwives, and to providers in the private and voluntary sectors.

Their role in health promotion comes through the advice they offer patients or the services they provide, such as well-man/woman clinics, screening for cancers etc. It could be suggested that everything a doctor does has some relationship to health promotion.

Think it over

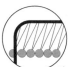

What health promotion services does your own GP surgery provide? Who accesses these services?

Practice nurses

Practice nurses are employed by GPs to carry out a range of nursing functions, usually in the doctor's premises or 'practice'. Practice nurses give routine injections and screen elders to prevent, or identify at the earliest stage, those medical conditions that are treatable. Practice nurses also take part in health promotion through clinics they run, such as well-man/woman clinics, asthma clinics and so on.

District nurses

District nurses, sometimes called 'community nurses', provide the full range of nursing care in people's own homes, including health promotion. District nurses are usually based at GPs' premises or at health centres.

Besides physical and preventative care of the client, they are also involved in promoting their quality of life by ensuring they have aids and equipment which may help them.

District nurses may be able to arrange some of the following equipment: bed rails or a raised bed; special mattresses; sheepskin underblankets; hoists of various kinds; bath seats and boards; incontinence pads or sheets; access to bathing services; and access to a night nurse. However, this might depend on the resources available locally.

Midwives

Today most babies are born in hospital, although some are born at home. Midwives provide ante-natal and post-natal care as well as delivering babies. Community midwives, who work with GPs and hospital doctors, may be based in clinics, doctors' surgeries and health centres; or they may work from home. Hospital midwives work within a hospital setting.

Midwives have a very important role in promoting the health of the pregnant woman. They monitor progress through pregnancy, in conjunction with the GP, and can help to identify early signs of problems, such as pre-eclampsia, i.e. very high blood-pressure, which can be very serious for the woman and her baby.

They also have a vital role in the first five to ten days of a baby's life, where they are responsible for the baby's care. They offer advice as well as taking physiological measurements to ensure the child is developing appropriately.

Health visitors

The role of the health visitor is to provide advice and guidance on health matters across the age ranges. The promotion of good health and the prevention of ill-health is the health visitor's main function.

However, the bulk of their work is usually related to babies and children under five. They take over responsibility for the health of the baby and mother from the midwife at about ten days post-partum. They are responsible for running health clinics which monitor the child's development and also administer part of the developmental checks, for example the 18-month check. They offer advice on feeding, sleeping, eating and any other concerns a parent may have. Their role in health promotion is extremely important.

Health visitors work from clinics or a health centre and visit people in their own homes. The health visitor also teaches health education in schools and a variety of other settings.

Occupational health nurses

Occupational health nurses are concerned with the effects of work on health and the effects of health on work. They aim to promote the highest possible standard of health for all employees.

Occupational health nurses provide: pre-employment screening to ensure the individual is medically fit for the job; visits to work environments to ensure the job is fit for the worker, i.e. it does not adversely affect health. They advise on medical aspects of a job – such as health policies, procedures and practices, in conjunction with the Occupational Safety Office. They also offer advice to employees and help regarding return to work, following long-term sickness.

Occupational health nurses can also provide general health checks, i.e. blood pressure, pulse, height, weight, urine tests, lung function and eye tests. They are involved in health promotion by giving advice on diet, exercise, stress, weight, smoking and regarding what specialist organisations can do to help people to help themselves.

Occupational health nurses can offer: advice regarding reputable sources of alternative medicine; counselling regarding any matter which affects health, including hospital treatment; emergency first-aid training; and immunisation of certain groups, who many be put at risk through their work, and also immunisation advice can be given to travellers.

Try it

Enquire at your local GP's practice and find out:

1 the role of the practice nurse in health promotion; and
2 the difference between the role of the district nurse and the health visitor.

Dentists

The role of the dentist is concerned with promoting dental health and hygiene, as well as identifying and treating conditions of the teeth and gums. Many are contracted to the National Health Service through Family Health Service Authorities. Other dentists are in private practice, or offer a combination of these services. Some dentists will visit people in their own homes.

Opticians

Opticians usually work through dispensaries or clinics. They offer regular eye tests which monitor the health of the eyes. They can identify not only changes in vision, such as short- or long-sightedness, but also potential eye problems such as glaucoma, which can lead to blindness.

Opticians offer advice on eye care and promote eye health for all ages. Many people have to pay for this service but exemptions are made for those under 16 or with a history of glaucoma in the family.

There are different therapists who also promote people's health through the work they do. However, individuals will normally attend a therapist to improve or rectify an existing problem.

Occupational therapists

Occupational therapists (OTs) may work in the community, in hospitals or in private establishments. Those working in the community will usually be employed by the local authority and be based in the Social Services department.

The role of the OT is to work with people who have a disability; to promote independent living skills, such as dressing, washing, toileting. They ensure that capabilities are maximised and disability minimised. OTs use therapeutic activities including craft work.

OTs can also advise on what equipment or home adaptions might help the individual, and they may help to arrange for the provision of these. Equipment for everyday living may include: washing aids; dressing aids; a commode; chairs with high seats; adapted cutlery; play equipment; and adaptations including widening doors, installing stairlifts etc.

Speech therapists

Speech therapists can help adults or children who have speech difficulties. Speech problems may arise as a result of disability, an illness such as a stroke, or through damage such as a head injury caused by a road traffic accident. Speech therapists may also be able to assist where a person has swallowing difficulties.

Speech therapists can be based in schools, clinics, health centres or in hospitals. They may sometimes visit people in their own homes.

Physiotherapists

Physiotherapists help to relieve pain and provide treatment for, and advice on, restoring and maintaining mobility through the use of physical activity and exercise. They may be based in hospitals, in the community, in voluntary organisations or might be in private practice.

Some physiotherapists specialise in certain areas of treatment, for example, in sports injuries. Community physiotherapists will visit people in their own homes to give advice and treatment in relation to mobility and fitness. They can use various kinds of therapies; for example, play therapy with a child who has a physical or mental disability. Physiotherapists may also be able to arrange for the provision of some equipment, such as: walking aids, e.g. a walking stick or ZImmer frame; or a wheelchair.

Chiropodists

Chiropodists are qualified professionals who specialise in foot care. This can be essential for older people, or people with a disability, in helping them to remain mobile. However, they provide a service for people of all ages. Even a minor foot injury or condition, such as a corn, can lead to difficulty in walking.

Chiropodists hold surgeries in hospitals, health centres and clinics; some are self-employed and work from private practices. Community chiropodists visit people in their own homes' however, in some areas this service is very limited. GPs can arrange an appointment with a chiropodist or individuals may refer themselves for a private appointment.

Environmental health officers

Public health has been a key issue since 1848. Originally, officials were mainly concerned with issues such as inadequate sewerage and water supplies. Polluted food supplies caused much ill-health in the last century. To combat ill-health caused by the environment, inspectors of sanitation and public health were appointed. Nowadays the role of the environment in influencing health is monitored by environmental health officers.

Most environmental health officers are employed by local councils. Generalist environmental health officers may be responsible for all aspects of the environment which may affect health in a particular area. Specialist environmental health officers can work alone or as part of a team. Specialists officers might concentrate on issues such as air pollution or food safety.

Some environmental health officers may work for private companies, where their work may focus on enabling the company to meet legal requirements and standards. Environmental health officers may also be employed by the Crown services such as the military services and the Civil Service. As in many professions, some environmental health officers may work as consultants; providing consultancy to the public or private sectors.

Evidence collection point

Think of the geographical 'patch' where you live. Identify its boundaries as clearly as you can, for example, an area serviced by a GP practice or the catchment area served by your local hospital.

Identify as many health promotion agents and agencies on your 'patch' as you can.

The professionals described above are clearly identifiable, but they are not the only ones who have a responsibility for health promotion. In recent years, an increasing number of people and agencies are recognising that they have a role to play in promoting health and ensuring a healthy environment. For example, employers are liable for the illness/injuries which employees might develop as a result of working for them. There have been cases of employers being found liable for cases of lung cancer in non-smokers, where a non-smoking environment has not been provided, and nervous breakdown as result of stress, where the employer has not provided adequate support in the work situation. These help to highlight the responsibility we all have for providing a healthy environment for others; however, there are also professionals with a role to play in creating a healthy environment.

The creation of healthy environments

The term 'environment' means the external conditions or surroundings in which people live or work, including the natural environment, such as air, water; socio-economic conditions, such as housing; and social conditions, such as the quality of the social environment in which people live and their working conditions. There is wide evidence to show how the environment can affect an individual's health and behaviour.

Natural environments

The natural environment can be seen as being under attack from the daily activities of individuals and the way people choose to live. Essentially people are damaging land, water and air. Some of this damage could be irreversible. Figure 17.3 shows some sources of pollution.

Think it over

Think of examples of how day-care provision, such as a nursery or a day centre for the elderly, might contribute to pollution of water and air.

Inspection and enforcement agencies

There are four main inspection and enforcement agencies who oversee air and water pollution.

HM Inspectorate of Pollution

This is a statutory body which covers air pollution, hazardous waste and radiochemical waste. It provides an integrated approach to pollution control as it recognises that pollution in one area can well affect another. It exercises statutory legal powers; and monitors the effectiveness and efficiency with which waste-disposal authorities and waste regulation authorities exercise their powers. The inspectorate develops economical and sound ways of disposing waste and offers independent advice on pollution control practices.

Local authorities

Environmental health departments have a wide range of responsibilities – they may be the first point of contact when people have a complaint.

The environmental health departments in local authorities are involved in health education, for example through educating caterers about food handling in the kitchen. They are also involved in environmental measures, for example, control of air pollution, and they 'have important duties related' to

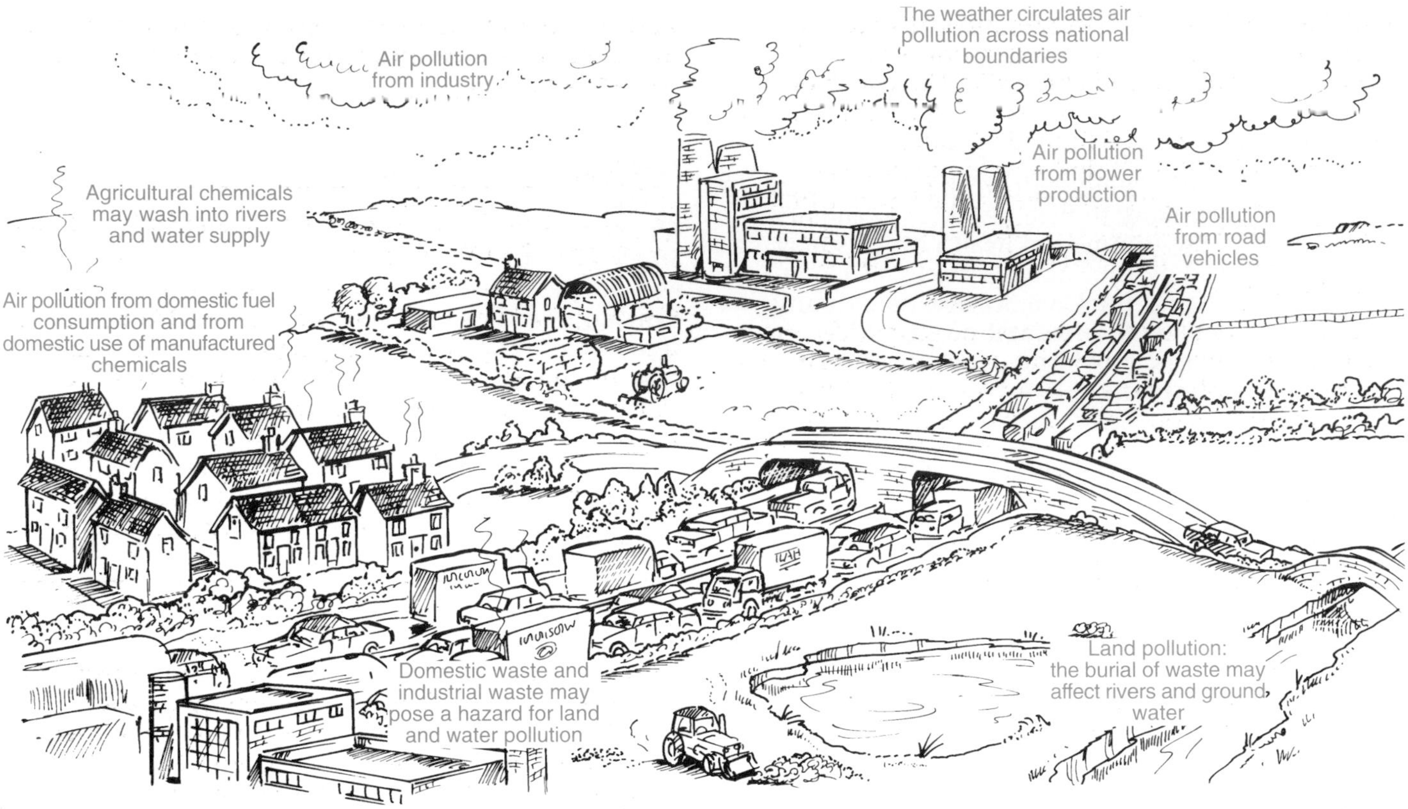

Figure 17.3 Some sources of pollution

the enforcement of certain laws; for example, food hygiene regulations and health and safety at work legislation.

National Rivers Authority

Under the Water Resources Act 1991, the National Rivers Authority is responsible for the control of water pollution. The NRA ensures water quality objectives are met, and is responsible for pollution control and issuing discharge consents and conserving water resources.

Health and Safety Executive

The Health and Safety Executive enforces health and safety law for industrial premises and protects the workforce and general public.

Socio-economic conditions

The provision of a healthy living environment is of special concern to all involved. It is widely agreed that

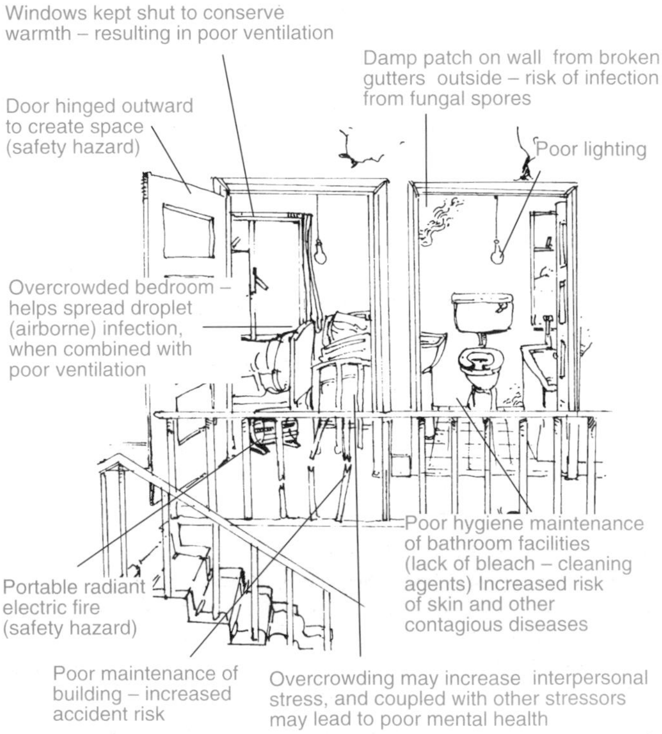

Figure 17.4 Poor housing may contribute to a wide range of hazards to health and social well-being

individuals who live in deprived inner city areas are likely to suffer from a number of interrelated deprivations (Turton and Orr, 1985). These include poor housing, limited employment opportunities, poor health-care facilities and limited educational and recreational facilities, including open spaces. The environment may be poorly maintained, with a high proportion of vandalism, and crime rates can be high, which increases individual isolation as people do not want to venture out alone.

The Black Report (1980) also provides support for the relationship between poverty and poor health. There is a close relationship between housing and health as poor housing not only affects physical health, such as respiratory infections due to overcrowding and inadequate heating and ventilation, but also creates psychological problems, such as stress due to lack of space for privacy caused by overcrowding.

Because of this connection, the primary health care team (in particular) are interested in the social conditions in which a family lives. They can help to put pressure on local authorities to rehouse people who are in poor local authority housing or help individuals obtain grants for house improvements (Figure 17.4).

Each local authority has a housing department which is particularly responsible for providing rented accommodation. If a family or individual is living in poor conditions they can apply for rehousing and are then assessed by a Housing Officer. The Housing Officer will allocate points to the case, which determine the urgency and priority with which alternative accommodation is to be found.

Try it

Contact your local housing department and find out which circumstances attract how many points. Explore how the Housing Officer can help people living in poor housing conditions, both in rented and private housing, and which other professionals they may work with to improve the situation.

Social workers can also help in cases of poor social conditions by offering supported places in playgroups for children, to help give respite for the family – so relieving stress and also giving the child social contact with peers in a learning environment which will help development.

If an elder is also living with the family, Social Services may be able to assist in finding day-care places to help to relieve family stress. A family centre may also help to support a family. Social workers are available at such centres to offer support and advice to family members.

Try it

Visit a local family centre and find out about the work they do.

Shelter (The National Campaign for the Homeless) is a pressure group which campaigns for better-quality housing for all. They argue that everyone has the right to a decent home. This does not mean just having a roof over someone's head but housing which is secure and not over-crowded, damp or lacking in basic amenities. Shelter also provides Housing Aid Centres which offer advice and help.

Working environments

Healthy working environments are the responsibility of every employer. This is a requirement of the Health and Safety at Work Act 1974 and supported by other regulations such as the Control of Substances Hazardous to Health (COSHH) regulations. Such regulations are enforced by a range of practitioners.

Health and Safety at Work Act 1974

This Act brought together a range of legislation covering health and safety since the first Safety Act was introduced in 1802. It covers almost everyone in a work situation except the armed forces and domestic employment. Although the Act emphasises how important it is that everyone plays a part in health and safety, it places most of the responsibility on the employer – including the provision of somebody with responsibility for health and safety.

The HASAW Act is enforced by two main bodies:

a *Environmental Health Officers* dealing with health and safety in smaller areas such as nursing homes, shops, restaurants etc.
b *Health and Safety Executive* whose inspectors deal with health and safety in other settings such as factories, hospitals, etc.

Representatives from these two bodies are able to enter premises at any reasonable time to carry out an inspection of the workplace and activities. They could take photographs as evidence of what they see, take samples or even remove equipment. They can ask to see documents, such as evidence of risk assessments made under COSHH. If unhappy about arrangements they could:

- provide *advice* to help improve safety
- serve an *improvement notice,* which give a time limit within which any requirement for improving health and safety must be made
- serve a *prohibition notice,* which immediately stops the unsafe piece of equipment/practice being used until it is made safe.

Employers can be prosecuted under the Health and Safety at Work Act and may be fined or imprisoned.

COSHH regulations

The COSHH regulations require employers to complete a risk assessment of all hazardous substances used in the workplace. This must be recorded for inspection if necessary (Institute of Environmental Health Officers, 1993). In a care establishment this will range from the correction fluid used in the administration department to the disinfectant used for cleaning and sterilisation. Steps must then be taken to protect employees exposed to the substance through **risk assessment.**

> **Hazard** = anything with the potential to cause harm.
>
> **Risk** = how likely it is that the hazard will cause harm.

The stages of risk assessment are as follows:

1 Identify any hazardous substance that is used in the workplace.
2 Identify who is at risk by assessing who uses or comes into contact with the substance.
3 Evaluate the risk by assessing how it might cause damage to health. Potential accidents should be assessed in terms of how likely they are to happen and how serious they might be.
4 Decide on a control measure. This might entail changing the substance for another which does the same job but is less hazardous, if that is possible, or introducing strict controls for use.
5 The assessment must be recorded.
6 The assessment should be reviewed regularly and, additionally, every time there is a change in the circumstances such as new staff or equipment.

All employees must be informed of any substance which may be hazardous to their health and receive appropriate training in their usage. Some substances may be hazardous but the risk that a hazard may occur may be small on assessment; therefore the establishment may be prepared to take the risk, with appropriate guidelines in place.

Practitioners who protect the public

Many of the practitioners already discussed have some role in protecting the public from potential risks through the work that they do.

Immunisation programmes

The role of immunisation is outlined in Chapter 20. Immunisation programmes are administered by the GP who keeps records and informs patients when they are due for immunisation. GPs will also chase clients who do not take up their immunisation to ensure they are fully aware of the risk they are taking if they choose not to be immunised or do not have members of their family immunised.

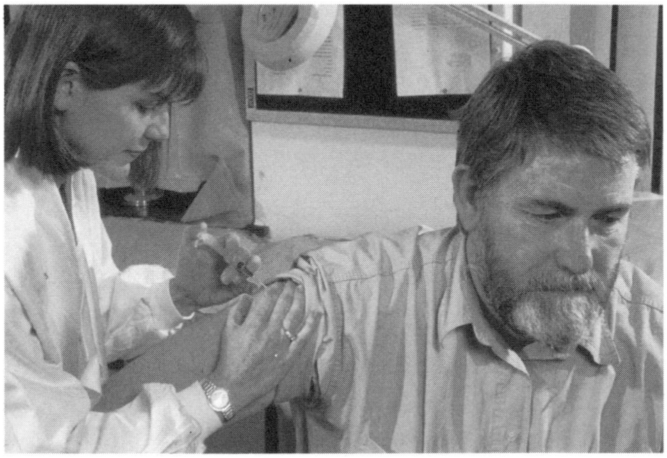

The actual immunisation is usually given by the practice nurse, with the doctor on hand for advice if needed.

Screening and contact tracing

Screening programmes and contact tracing occur for a range of infectious conditions including TB, sexually transmitted diseases (STDs) and HIV and AIDS. With any condition, the process is similar.

Taking HIV as an example: a client will initially be seen by a doctor to establish if there is any infection or cause for concern and what it might be. Consultations on the NHS are free and confidential and will offer both advice and treatment. If necessary, the doctor will ask clients to advise any sexual partners over a period to see their GP or attend the clinic. This is because they may be infecting others without realising it.

Health advisers at a clinic will help clients to decide how a partner should be contacted. Some people may prefer not to do it themselves and prefer an anonymous letter or a contact from the clinic itself. Contact tracing can be a complex process as one individual may have had many contacts. They may have only one partner, but that partner may have other partners, and those themselves may have others and so on.

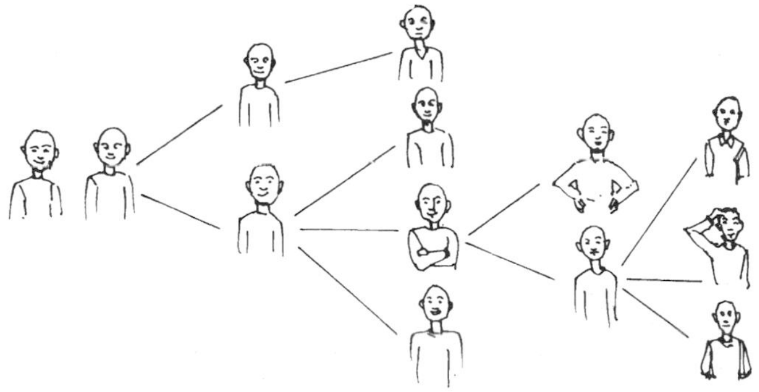

Child protection legislation and practitioners

The practitioners involved with child protection are a direct result of the Children Act 1989. An understanding of this law will give some insight into the role of practitioners who operate in this complex area.

The Children Act 1989

The Children Act 1989 is a major piece of legislation in that it supersedes many previously existing pieces of legislation that had built up in a piecemeal fashion over the years. The aim of the Act is to clarify the law relating to children. However it also introduces new duties and responsibilities for the courts, Social Services departments and, to a certain degree, parents. Three main principles guide the Act:

i the welfare principle
ii the non-delay principle
iii the non-intervention principle

The *welfare principle* requires the courts to treat the welfare of the child as paramount. Although the courts still have to balance the rights of the child and the rights of the parents, ultimately they must do what they consider to be in the best interest of the child.

The *non-delay principle* is a response to the recognition that delays in settling issues are not usually in the best interest of the child. For many reasons there are often delays within the legal system. The section of the Act relating to this principle requires that in any proceedings involving children, courts must: (i) draw up a timetable for the proceedings; (ii) give directions so that the timetable is adhered to.

The *non-intervention principle* states that the court should not make an order unless it considers, 'that doing so would be better for the child than making no order at all'.

Duties of the local authority

The Act outlines the duties of the **local authority** in relation to children, such as responsibilities relating to child protection (section 47), and general safeguarding and welfare of children (section 27). Additionally, section 17 itemises a comprehensive list of powers and duties, which include:

- identification of children in need and the provision of information
- maintenance of a register of disabled children
- assessment of children's needs
- prevention of neglect and abuse
- provision of accommodation in order to protect a child
- provision for disabled children
- provision to reduce the need for care proceedings
- provision for children living with their families (e.g. family aides)
- family centres (to provide guidance for children and their parents)
- maintenance of the family home (to enable children to continue to live with their family, or to maintain contact with them)
- duty to consider racial groups to which children in need belong. (This has implications when selecting day centres, foster parents etc. for a child.)

This work would be carried out by specially trained **social workers.**

Orders that can be made under the Children Act include:

i Care Order (section 33).
The main function of a care order is to give the **local authority** parental responsibility, it makes the local authority the child's 'parent'.

ii Interim Care Order (section 37).
Most interim orders are made in the situation where, for one reason or another, the full hearing cannot take place.

iii Supervision Order (section 34).
A supervision order is an alternative to a care order. In the Act there is no guidance given as to when a supervision order should be made rather than a care order.

iv Interim Supervision Order (section 38).
Just as there are specific provisions for interim care orders, so there are provisions for interim supervision orders.

v Child Assessment Order (section 46).
This provision allows the compulsory assessment of the state of the child's health and development, if need be by the removal of the child from the home.

vi Emergency Protection Order (section 41).
This is a new order that is designed to remove the criticisms of the former place of safety order. It is a short-term order that removes the child from the home, for an initial period of seven days, extendable to fifteen days for medical reports.

vii Removal by **police** to accommodation (section 46).
The police, in the course of their duties, may come across children at risk who need protection. As there may be the need for immediate action, they are given the powers, under the Children Act, to take them into police protection.

There were four new orders under section 8:

a Residence Order.
This is an order 'settling the arrangements to be made as to the person with whom the child is to live'.

b Contact Order.
This order requires the person with whom the child is to live to allow the child to have contact with specified others. Contacts may be by letter, phone or visits, which may be supervised. It may provide contact with any other person, e.g. parent, sibling, grandparent, friend.

c Prohibited Steps Order.
This is an order that would be used where it is necessary for the court to play a continuing role. The court may specify matters which have to be referred back to the court, e.g. it could prohibit a child's removal from the UK.

d Specific Issues Order.
These may be made on their own or in conjunction with residence or contact orders.

Children at risk

The legal framework suggests three possibilities for action when a child is considered to be at risk:

- leaving the child at home and providing support
- removing the child from the home on a temporary basis
- removing the child on a permanent basis.

A social worker who is concerned about the safety of a child has five ways in which a child may be removed from the home on a temporary basis:

i by obtaining a child assessment order (section 43)
ii by obtaining an emergency protection order (EPO) (section 44)
iii by the police removing the child to suitable accommodation (section 46)
iv by obtaining an interim care order (section 38)
v by obtaining a care order (section 33).

When a child is removed from home on a temporary basis, they may be 'accommodated' by being placed with a relative or other suitable person (such as a foster parent), or by placing them in a children's home or in secure accommodation.

In order for a child to be removed from home on a permanent basis a care order must be obtained. However, the Act envisages that this step should only be taken as a last resort. Unless a care order is discharged (or ended) earlier, it remains in force until the child is 18.

Supervision orders

Additionally, as an alternative to a care order, the court can make a supervision order (section 34). The duties of the supervisor include:

a to advise, assist and befriend the supervised child
b to take such steps as are reasonably necessary to ensure that the order is carried out
c to request variations to, or discharge of, the order when it is not complied with, or when it is no longer necessary.

Adoption

In certain circumstances it is clear that some children will never be able to return to their parents or any other family member. In these cases the local authority must seek an alternative permanent substitute family. (Exceptions can be made if the child would benefit from remaining in some form of children's home.) Adoption is governed by the Adoption Act 1976, but has been modified by the Children Act. Section 12 of the Adoption Act defines 'adoption'. The main effect of the new Children Act on existing legislation is that, following adoption, the child now has the right to retain contact with its family of origin whereas, previously, all ties were severed. Social workers have a vital role to play in the whole range of processes which are involved in adoption.

Parental responsibility

The Children Act uses the concept of 'parental responsibility' to replace the notion of 'parental rights and duties', which was used in earlier legislation. The phrase emphasises the fact that, legally, parenthood is a matter of responsibility rather than rights. The extent of responsibilities varies according to the age of the child. For example, parents are required to sign forms consenting to medical treatment for a child until the child reaches the age of 16.

Mental health services

Practitioners involved in protecting the public from potential risks in terms of mental health can be seen as practitioners who make decisions about a person's welfare due to their mental state under the Mental Health Act 1983. These practitioners may be protecting the public from an individual and possibly protecting the individual from harming themselves or harming those who provide care for clients with mental health illnesses.

Mental health services include day care and residential accommodation. Care of individuals with mental health problems usually involves a multi-disciplinary approach. Personnel involved will include social workers, who will support the client with their key worker in the establishment. Together they will promote the health and well-being of the client in the choices they support them in making.

Day centres will help to promote an individual's health by teaching life skills and, through this, healthy life choices. They also encourage independent living, which can promote health through developing a positive self-image. Day centres provide mental stimulation and social contact as well – again important for maintaining individual health and social well-being. The GP will also have a central role in providing any medication that may be required.

Criminal justice service

This involves the provision of services to support young offenders such as the probation service. This service has the aim of helping offenders to re-establish themselves in society and not reoffend.

Legislation

Legislation may restrict the liberty of individuals for their own or others' health and social well-being. The Mental Health Act (1983), the Children Act (1989) and Criminal Justice Act (1994) are examples of such legislation.

The Mental Health Act 1983

This Act provides professionals with the power to make decisions about a person's welfare when that person, due to a mental disorder, is not able to make decisions regarding his or her own welfare. The Act is supported by the Code of Practice, which is a guide to good practice in the interpretation of the Act. It lays down procedures that try to ensure that abuse of power does not occur, while necessary treatment and containment is still provided. It aims to find a balance between maintaining the basic civil liberties of the individual and the need to impose interventions. However, section 131 of the Act makes it clear that, for anyone over the age of 16, capable of expressing his or her own wishes, then an informal admission to hospital should be the norm 'and should be used whenever a patient is not unwilling to be admitted and can be treated without the use of compulsory powers'.

Admission to hospital can be made under the Act in various ways:

- *Section 1 – Compulsory Admission*
  Applications for admission under this section can

be made either by an Approved Social Worker or by the person's nearest relative.

- *Section 2 – Admission for Assessment*
  Applications must be founded on the recommendations of two medical practitioners and allows the person to be detained for a limited period of up to 23 days.
- *Section 3 – Admission for Treatment*
  This allows for admission to hospital and also involves the power to give treatment to the person without his or her consent.
- *Section 4 – Emergency Admission*
  This allows for admission for assessment on the grounds that admission is urgently required and that compliance with all the procedural formalities under section 2 would cause undesirable delay.

This definition of the term 'mental disorder' is central to the functioning of the Act. Section 12 refers to four specific forms of mental disorder: mental illness; arrested or incomplete development of mind; psychopathic disorder; and 'any other disorder or disability of mind'. This definition means that people with learning difficulties may come within some sections of the Mental Health Act. Sexual deviancy or dependence on drugs or alcohol do not constitute a mental disorder and do not come within the scope of this Act.

Try it

Contact your local Social Services department to find out more about the role of an Approved Social Worker.

Mental Health (Patients in the Community) Bill

This Bill proposes that where a person is detained under the Mental Health Act 1983 for treatment in hospital on the grounds of 'mental disorder', his or her discharge from hospital can be made subject to certain conditions.

The Bill is the measure announced in the Secretary of State for Health's ten-point plan in August 1993 and was then called 'Supervised discharge'. The Mental Health (Patients in the Community) Bill now refers to 'after-care under supervision'.

A 'patient subject to after-care under supervision' can be required to live at a specified place and attend at specified times for medical treatment, occupation, training or education. The 'supervisor' – who is likely to be a health-care professional – can either 'take or convey' a patient to a place where he or she is required to attend, or authorise anyone else to do so.

After-care under supervision can be applied for only by a detained patient's responsible medical officer (RMO) in respect of patients detained in hospital for treatment (under sections 3 or 37 of the Mental Health Act), and it would come into effect when they left hospital.

The RMO is supposed to consult with the patient and with professional and other carers before making the application, but he or she does not have to obtain the patient's consent to the proposed arrangements for after-care. The application is made to the health authority, who has the power to accept it after consulting the social services authority. The grounds on which the RMO may make the application are that:

- the patient is suffering from a mental disorder
- there would be a substantial risk of serious harm to the health or safety of the patient, or of the patient being seriously exploited, if he or she were not to receive after-care services
- being subject to after-care under supervision 'is likely to help to ensure that he receives the after-care services to be provided'.

After-care under supervision would last for six months, may be renewed for a further six months and then for a year at a time. A patient has the right to appeal to a Mental Health Review Tribunal.

Health and Social Services have the duty to keep the supervised after-care under review, which includes modifying the requirements, informing the person's doctor (the 'community responsible medical officer') if they think it should end and informing an approved social worker if they think the person should be admitted to hospital. Supervised after-care can be ended by the patient's doctor or by the Mental Health Review Tribunal. It also ends if the patient is admitted to hospital.

The Mental Health Act Commission

The Mental Health Act Commission is a Special Health Authority which acts as a public watchdog over the rights and interests of patients detained under the Mental Health Act. It visits hospitals without warning and can deal with complaints from detained patients.

The Mental Health Review Tribunal

The patient may apply to the Mental Health Review Tribunal, which has the power to order discharge. Patients may be legally represented at these hearings.

Supervision Register

In December 1993 the Secretary of State for Health announced a requirement for all health authorities to ensure that mental health service providers establish and maintain supervision registers for people with a serious mental illness, who are a risk to themselves or others. This requirement built upon the after-care arrangements of the Care Programme Approach and followed concern about instances where people with a serious mental illness being managed in the community fell through the net of care with serious consequences to themselves and others.

Background to and purpose of Supervision Registers

NHS Trusts and other provider units were required to set up Supervision Registers for categories of mentally ill people.

This requirement builds upon an original suggestion for the introduction of Supervision Registers, which was made in the White Paper, 'Caring for People'.

Supervision Registers are intended to reinforce the support and care for vulnerable mentally ill people in the community embodied in the **Care Programme Approach** (CPA).

Supervision Registers aim to identify a smaller, more vulnerable group than the total client group covered by the CPA, and, through the inclusion of these patients on the Register, to alert professional staff involved in their care to the need for vigilance in maintaining contact with and providing support for them.

Supervision Registers are distinct from, and should therefore not be confused with, the proposed Supervised Discharges. There may be an overlap between those included on the Register and those subject to Supervised Discharge but they are separate procedures and those included within the Supervised Registers should not be seen as being subject to the restrictions of the Supervised Discharge regulations.

Criteria for inclusion on Supervision Registers

The categories of people who should be included on Supervision Registers are identified as follows: people who are over 16, have a mental illness, live in the community and fall in one of the three at-risk groups:

a significant risk of suicide
b significant risk of serious violence to others
c significant risk of severe self-neglect.

Notification to patient of inclusion on Supervision Register

Whenever possible people should be informed when they are placed on the Supervision Register, of:

- the broad reasons why they have been placed on it
- how the information on the Register will be used
- to whom the information may be disclosed
- the procedure for review.

This notification should normally be made orally during the multidisciplinary meeting. It should be reinforced in writing.

The only time when it is not appropriate to tell the patient are when there are clinical reasons, for example when informing the patient may cause serious harm to his or her physical or mental health. In some instances it may be appropriate not to tell patients straightaway (for example, while still in hospital) but to tell them at a later date when they are no longer judged to be at risk of harm.

Reviews of patient on Supervision Register

A patient's continued inclusion on the Register should be considered at every review under the CPA. CPA reviews should take place at least every six months.

The patient's views should be considered at the review, as should those of relatives, advocate, carer or other person that a patient chooses to accompany them to a review. However, ultimately the decision whether a patient continues on the Register or not is not the patient's.

Any of the professionals involved in the CPA may request that a special review meeting be held to consider withdrawal of the patient from the Register. Patients themselves or their carers may request a review to consider their withdrawal from the Register.

The decision to withdraw a patient from the Register is ultimately a matter for the responsible consultant, taking into account the views of the other professionals involved and of the patients. Withdrawal of a patient from the Register will be appropriate if he or she is no longer considered to be at significant risk of serious violence, suicide, or severe self-neglect. The decision to withdraw a patient from the Register can be taken only after a review.

Criminal Justice and Public Order Act 1994

This Act covers the areas listed below:

1. Young offenders
2. Bail
3. Evidence and court procedure
4. Police powers
5. Public order
6. Prevention of terrorism
7. Obscenity and video recordings
8. Prisons
9. Sexual offences

1 Young offenders

The Act creates a new sentence (the **secure training order**) for persistent juvenile offenders. It will apply to both boys and girls. It will be made available to the courts as soon as the new secure training centres are ready.

- Under *Section 1,* a Youth Court or the Crown Court will be empowered to impose a secure training order when a child or young person is aged between 12 and 14 years and:
  - is convicted of an imprisonable offence committed when at least 12 years old; and
  - has been convicted of at least three imprisonable offences (not necessarily on separate occasions); and
  - has been convicted of an imprisonable offence committed whilst subject to, or has failed to comply with, the requirements of a supervision order made in criminal proceedings.
- The court will also need to be satisfied that the offending is so serious that only a custodial sentence can be justified or, in the case of a violent or sexual office, that the public need to be protected from serious harm.
- The first half of the order will be served in detention in a secure training centre, the second under compulsory supervision in the community. If no place is available at the secure training centre designated for the use of the court, the Home Secretary will direct that the offender should be held in alternative accommodation. In exceptional circumstances the Home Secretary may also transfer an offender to alternative accommodation once the sentence is under way.
- The maximum length of the order is two years and the minimum length is six months. If a person subject to a secure training order fails to comply with the requirements of his or her supervision in the community the court may order the offender to be further detained in a secure training centre for up to three months or it may impose a fine. Supervision may be provided by a probation officer, local authority social worker or any other person designated by the Home Secretary (e.g. employees of voluntary organisations or of the secure training centres themselves). Each trainee will have a supervision notice drawn up specifying requirements with which he or she must comply. Rules and National Standards will be drawn up regulating the supervision of trainees.

2 Bail

Restriction on the grant of bail: The general scheme of the Bail Act 1976 is that people charged with an offence (or convicted of one but not yet sentenced for it) have in some circumstances a **right** to bail, and in other circumstances may be granted bail. The Act amends these provisions so as to restrict the grant of bail by comparison with the 1976 Act:

- No bail for defendants charged with or convicted of homicide or rape with a previous conviction for such an offence.
- No right to bail for persons accused or convicted of committing an offence while on bail.
- There will be new powers for the police to attach conditions to bail once a person has been charged.
- Where a person charged with an indictable offence has been given bail, a court may now reconsider this decision at any time if information comes to light which was not available to the police when the original bail decision was taken.

3 Evidence and court procedure

Imputations on character: *Section 31* of the Act amends Section 1 of the Criminal Evidence Act 1898 concerning the admissibility of evidence of the previous misconduct of the accused. Under the 1989 Act, the accused may be cross-examined on his or her previous misconduct if he or she attacks the character of the prosecutor or any prosecution witness including the victim.

- Under Section 31, where the victim of an alleged crime has died, the accused may be cross-examined on his or her previous misconduct if he or she attacks the character of the dead person, in the same way as he or she attacks the character of the prosecutor or of a prosecution witness.

Corroboration:

- *Section 32* abolishes the current common law requirement that the jury must be warned in sexual cases of the danger of convicting on the uncorroborated evidence of the complainant. It also abolishes the requirement on the judge to give a warning in a case where uncorroborated evidence is given against the accused by an accomplice. The removal of these mandatory requirements allows judges to sum up as the facts of each particular case demand.
- *Section 33* repeals those provisions of the Sexual Offences Act 1956 under which a court is prevented from convicting any person of the offence of procuration on the sole basis of the uncorroborated evidence of a single witness.

Inferences from silence:

- *Sections 34 to 39* set out circumstances in which a court or jury may draw proper inferences from the fact that accused persons do not give evidence at their trial or answer questions put to them by the police. These sections do not make failure to give answers or information a criminal offence, nor do they compel people to incriminate themselves.
- *Section 41* inserts a new Section 9B in the Juries Act 1974 to clarify the position of physically disabled people summoned by the jury service. New section 9B makes it clear that if potential jurors are physically disabled and there are doubts as to their capacity to serve, the judge should allow the persons to serve unless he or she is of the opinion that the disability means that they could not act effectively as jurors. This does not affect existing arrangements whereby disabled persons may apply for and be granted excusal if there is good reason why they should not serve.
- *Section 42* concerns the right to be excused jury service. It adds to the list of people who may be excused as of right (in Part III of Schedule 1 to the Juries Act 1974) practising members of religious societies in orders, the tenets of beliefs of which are incompatible with jury service.
- *Section 43* substitutes a new section 13 in the Juries Act 1974 (under which a jury may be allowed to separate at any time *before* they consider their verdict). The revised section 13 extends the court's discretion so that a jury may be permitted to separate at any time, whether before *or after* they have been directed to consider their verdict.

Juries:

- *Section 40* provides that a person who is on police or court bail in proceedings is disqualified from serving as a juror in the Crown Court.

Sentencing penalties: There is new legislation which includes powers to:

- review unduly lenient sentences
- make curfew orders.

There will be trials of electronically monitored curfew orders. The three trial areas are the City of Manchester, the Borough of Reading and the County of Norfolk. The trials will be conducted during 1995 and are expected to last for about nine months.

Child evidence: There is new legislation relating to video recordings of testimony from child witnesses.

4 Police powers

The Police and Criminal Evidence Act 1984 which deals, amongst other things, with fingerprints and body samples, has been amended. The purpose is to implement, with certain modifications, recommendations of the Royal Commission on Criminal Justice that wider and more effective use should be able to be made of DNA profiling in the investigation of offences, and that legislation should allow DNA profiles to be taken from certain classes of suspects and retained on a database if the suspect is convicted. The scheme which is implemented in sections 54–58 broadly puts powers to take body samples – principally for the purposes of DNA profiling – on the same basis as powers to take fingerprints.

5 Public order

The new legislation covers trespass and 'raves' where there is a gathering in the open air of 100 or more people at which amplified music is played during the night. The music must be likely to cause serious distress to the inhabitants of the locality. *Section 63* empowers a police officer of the rank of superintendent or above to direct people to leave. It also gives powers of entry and seizure.

There is also legislation on squatting and unauthorised camping.

6 Prevention of terrorism

The Act extends the powers of the courts and police to deal with terrorism.

7 Obscenity and video recordings

The Act updates and expands the law concerning indecent photographs of children so as to take account of the use of computer technology.

Section 90 establishes in statute for the first time certain of the criteria on which the designated authority (i.e. the British Board of Film Classification) is to base its decisions on the classification of video works.

8 Prisons

The Act extends and improves the existing arrangements for contracting out within the prison service including prisoner escort arrangements. It also gives new powers for drug testing of prisoners and new powers to search prisoners.

9 Sexual offences

The Act covers: rape, buggery and homosexual acts; homosexual acts in the armed forces and merchant navy; and anonymity of victims of sexual offences.

The Carers (Recognition of Services) Act 1995

This new Act is to be implemented on 1 April 1996.

According to the Act, where: (a) a local authority carries out an assessment under section 47(1)(a) of the National Health Service and Community Care Act 1990 of the needs of a person ('the relevant person') for community care services: and (b) an individual ('the carer') provides or intends to provide a substantial amount of care on a regular basis for the relevant person, the carer may request the local authority, before making a decision as to whether the needs of the relevant person call for the provision of any services, to carry out an assessment of his or her ability to continue to provide care for the relevant person.

If a carer requests an assessment: 'the local authority shall carry out such an assessment and shall take into account the results of that assessment in making the decision as to whether the needs of the relevant person call for provision of services.'

The Act covers not only adult carers but young carers also. Children and young people who are carers would therefore be entitled to an assessment on request.

There are similar provisions for carers who provide regular and substantial care for disabled children, whose needs are assessed by the local authority for the purposes of Part III of the Children Act 1989 or section 2 of the Chronically Sick and Disabled Persons Act 1970. Those who provide care as part of their job, or as volunteers for a voluntary organisation, are specifically excluded from the Act's provisions.

Ethical dilemmas

The protection of individuals, and protection of the public, can raise many serious problems or dilemmas. Professional decision-making skills are slowly developed over years of experience by practitioners. These skills enable practitioners to use their knowledge of law, social and psychological principles and ethical principles to make appropriate and balanced decisions about individual situations.

Practitioners must always seek to balance the interests of their clients with the interests and safety of society as a whole. Practitioners must assess the potential risks inherent in any decision that they make. These include risks to the client, risks for the public and risks for the practitioner themselves. These can involve physical risks, such as injury, and emotional risks, such as damage to self-esteem or self-concept. Restricting a person's liberty can involve a wide range of potential deprivations and harm for an individual. Professionals are responsible for the decisions that they take and legal action may be taken against them if they make inappropriate or incompetent decisions. Poor decisions can also be the focus for media attention. The past few years have seen several examples of individual social workers being criticised in the press for poor decisions with respect to child protection. Failure to assess correctly the risks a child faces could lead to the death of a child. However, an over-protective decision can lead to children being separated from their parents with possible emotional damage as a result.

The complexity of professional and ethical decision-making might be illustrated with the examples of the following case studies.

Case Study 1

Mrs Pugh is an older person with dementia; she is a wheelchair user and receives day care. Her main carer is her husband.

An incident occurred when Mrs Pugh went to use the toilet unassisted. She fell and bruising was evident. Mrs Pugh's husband was angry and complained over the lack of care which resulted in Mrs Pugh's fall.

On examination, as well as the new bruising it was noted that Mrs Pugh had extensive old bruising, particularly evident on her upper legs. The social worker contacted Mrs Pugh's doctor (GP) to discuss this bruising. The GP said he had always had concerns as Mrs Pugh often has unexplained bruises on her body. The GP had never recorded this on the medical notes, however.

The GP was asked to attend to examine Mrs Pugh. He refused to do this.

This case study raises a number of issues:

- Should the social worker proceed with the investigation? Does Mrs Pugh need residential care for her own protection? What can the social worker do?
- Should the GP's practice be investigated?
- Should the carer be questioned in more detail?
- Should Mr Pugh be questioned in more detail?

Initially the social worker should investigate the cause of Mrs Pugh's bruising. For example, could the bruising be caused by her falling or could it be caused by abuse? If bruising is evident high up on her legs or under her arms it is unlikely to be caused by falls.

The needs of the carer should be looked at: is he receiving sufficient support? There may be a need for the carer to receive respite care. There are organisations, e.g. Crossroads, who would assist the carer to care.

The social worker could encourage the GP to become more involved in his patient's care. A joint visit involving the social worker and GP could be arranged. Any decision about suggesting residential care could only be made when the outcome of these steps is known.

Case Study 2

Mr Roberts is a young man who lives with his parents and older brother in the family home.

A request is made to the Approved Social Worker (ASW) to visit Mr Roberts with a view to assessing him under the Mental Health Act.

Mr Roberts' General Practitioner (GP) is a family friend of many years standing. He has been approached by Mr Roberts' father to activate the sectioning process and remove Mr Roberts from the home situation.

On visiting to assess Mr Roberts, the ASW feels that the application for sectioning is not appropriate. The GP insists that because of the relationship with the family he would like the section to be implemented. The GP cites Mr Roberts' behaviour as distracting his brother who is unable to study for his exams.

The issues in this study are:

- Does the ASW ignore the situation?
- Does the ASW talk to Mr Roberts regarding the issues and determine from his point of view how he would like the situation handled?

An Approved Social Worker (ASW) is legally bound to respond to a request for an assessment under the Mental Health Act, made by a GP.

If the ASW is aware of the social relationship between the GP and the family, it could be appropriate to discuss the dilemmas this may cause before commencing the assessment. A final decision cannot be made until all the issues have been clarified.

Case Study 3

Mr Lee is a 65-year-old man with dementia. He is married with a daughter. Mr Lee owns a number of houses and a substantial number of stocks and shares.

The onset of Mr Lee's dementia began five years ago. At that time his daughter was given *power of attorney*. She therefore managed Mr Lee's financial affairs.

Mr Lee was admitted to hospital but is now ready to be discharged. Following a needs-led assessment, Mr Lee was identified as requiring nursing home care. As the family has considerable means, they would have to fund Mr Lee's placement in a nursing home. Miss Lee, who had the power of attorney, refused to allow this to be paid for.

Mrs Lee was the main carer for her husband and wanted him to come home. But it was evident that Mrs Lee's health was deteriorating due to the demands of caring for her husband.

Mr Lee was discharged from hospital back to the family home. An extensive package of care was put in place and a nominal charge for this was made by the local authority.

The dilemmas raised in this case are as follows:

- Despite the need for a nursing home placement being identified, because Miss Lee has power of attorney, this could not be pursued.
- Can you legally pursue the daughter who has enduring powers of attorney?
- Can you prove that the daughter's decision is financially based and not needs-led?
- Mr Lee has transferred the management of his finances to his daughter and not his wife. He did this because he knew his daughter would be more hard-headed than his wife in managing his affairs.
- Do you ignore what he said when he was able to make informed decisions?
- Do you make decisions based on his current needs?

A needs-led assessment has identified that Mr Lee requires nursing home care. Despite the power of attorney now held by his daughter, and her refusal to agree to Mr Lee going to a nursing home, the social worker – who is likely to be the care manager – still has a duty to ensure that Mr Lee is in receipt of appropriate care and support. The resolution of this problem is still not straightforward, but some sort of care plan to meet Mr Lee's needs will have to be negotiated.

Case Study 4

Fiona is eighteen months old. She is seriously brain damaged, and in constant pain. Her parents have two other children. They have been told by the doctors that Fiona's chances of survival are not good. The only way to continue Fiona's life is by feeding her through a tube.

Family life has been seriously disrupted since Fiona was born. The psychological and physical impact of Fiona's needs has overwhelmed the family.

The dilemmas identified in this case study are:

- Should Fiona's condition be allowed to run its course with no interventions?
- Should tube feeding commence, which may help to prolong Fiona's life?

There are complex legal issues surrounding Fiona's case. These are principally between the medical staff and the parents. It would be the duty of a social worker to ensure the family were being assisted appropriately when making any decisions. It may be that Fiona could be voluntarily received into care. There could also be a role for the social worker – working in the child protection team – to support Fiona's parents and the other two children.

Evidence collection point

For Element 6.2, you need to produce a report which discusses two ethical dilemmas practitioners may face when they are balancing the needs of individuals and groups. The report should contain a summary description of the way in which legislation may restrict the liberty of individuals. The report should also provide a summary describing at least three practitioners who work in services which promote health and social well-being, and at least three practitioners who are involved in creating environments conducive to health and social well-being. The report should also provide at least three examples of practitioners who seek to protect individuals from risk.

Chapter 18

Clients' perception of health and social care services

This chapter provides an overview of the general issues surrounding clients' perceptions of services, the continuity of care, the assessment and management of care; and also the way in which clients may take control of and be involved in the services they receive.

Perceptions

Many people with a variety of needs may never enter into the health and social care services. Their needs may be met through an 'informal' network of friends, neighbours or relatives. This network often provides the bulk of their care in the community.

It is necessary to ensure that when clients enter the health and social care services they understand what is available to meet their needs within these organisations. It is important to use language that is straightforward and sensitive to issues of race, gender and disability. Jargon may cause clients to perceive themselves as lacking in awareness if they do not understand the terms that carers use. Terms like assessment review need to be explained clearly.

Modern care in the community should give priority to:

- extending choices for users
- creating a real partnership between users of the service and providers of the service
- securing better joint working between health and social care organisations.

It is important that clients feel valued; this includes:

- feeling they have control over the process of their care
- feeling they are respected
- feeling they are in receipt of proper information to include services and facilities.

The approach of your local health and social care services should ensure that people are enabled to:

- live a full life in the community with equal opportunity for privacy and dignity
- be in charge of their own lives and make their own decisions, including decisions to take risks
- have their cultural, ethnic, religious, sexual and emotional needs recognised and respected
- be fully informed of the purpose of an assessment
- have clear information about what is available and how things happen
- see what information is written about them and have this explained to them in a form of language they can understand
- have a named person as a point of contact and a named substitute when required
- have a person to speak or act on their behalf when necessary
- enjoy confidentiality in all their dealing with community care services
- comment on, challenge or complain about services or service delivery.

Continuum of care

The principles of good service delivery and a 'seamless service' apply equally to Social Services Departments, all council departments, National Health Service bodies and private and voluntary organisations. Working together is often a difficult process.

Evidence collection point

Look at your local community care plan and identify areas of care where joint working is evident.

It is essential that all agencies should work together to provide the best social and health care. Agencies should:

- be committed to joint planning and common ownership of good practice principles
- be committed to equal opportunity, anti-discriminatory practices
- have users involved in the planning and delivery of their services
- ensure that available resources are used effectively, innovatively and to the benefit of people using services

- show willingness to respect the decisions made by organisations and people who are working collaboratively on assessment and service provision
- develop means of linking information and publicity services and, where possible, share common styles and service leaflets
- ensure such leaflets are fully accessible to people whose first language is not English
- develop compatible information technology and recording systems where appropriate
- have straightforward entry to services, to avoid unnecessary referrals to different departments
- establish a single transferable assessment procedure
- have agreed arrangements for multi-disciplinary assessment where appropriate
- ensure there are ways of checking that there is no overlap of service provisions, or confusion about the responsibilities of those arranging services
- ensure that discussion and decisions about arrangements are not carried out by any one body in isolation from others involved in service delivery to the same person
- make sure that information is transferred between organisations with the consent of the person concerned so that people do not have to repeat it
- develop a complaints system that is agreed between organisations providing services
- develop arrangements for sharing and interchanging staff who have similar roles and skills
- create and establish opportunities for staff from different professions and departments to train together.

Think it over

Look at the report on page 407 of a meeting held to identify the needs of a patient with a physical disability, who is ready to be discharged from hospital to his home.

Try it

Write a short evaluation of the meeting called to identify Mr Anwar's needs. Focus your evaluation on the seamless service being offered to meet these needs.

Support and empowerment

Smale *et al* (1993) review the idea of empowering clients. In the past there may have been a tendency for professionals to act as experts. The experts would meet the adult client and try to assess the client's physical, financial, social or emotional needs. The expert practitioner would try to make this assessment by using skilled questioning techniques to obtain information from a client. The expert then made his or her decision as to what assistance the client needed, based on the information he or she had been able to extract.

Smale *et al.* (1993) contrast this 'expert' approach with the idea of an 'exchange model' of working with the client. This new approach is based on the idea that the client is the expert on the client! The client is likely to have a better understanding of his or her own needs than a professional. The idea of an exchange is that the professional tries to build a shared understanding of need with the client. People live in 'different worlds of meaning'; the idea is that the professional has to understand the client's world.

Support can only be provided in relation to a shared understanding of the client's perception of his or her own need. Knowledge of the client's needs will only come about through an exchange of meaning, through discussion and enquiry.

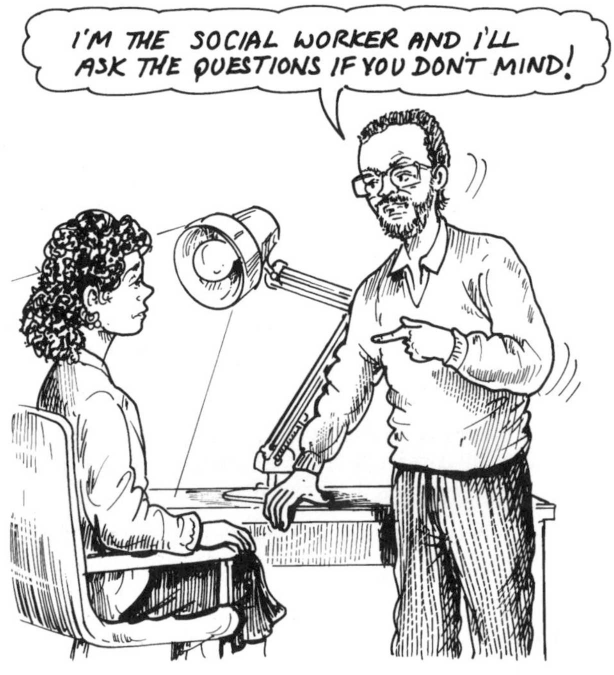
I'M THE SOCIAL WORKER AND I'LL ASK THE QUESTIONS IF YOU DON'T MIND!

Figure 18.1 The 'expert' approach to assessment

Report of meeting held on Mr Anwar

Attended by:

Mr Anwar (customer)	Mrs Anwar (wife)
Doctor (hospital-based)	Occupational therapist (hospital-based)
Ward sister	Physiotherapist (hospital-based)
Occupational therapist (community-based)	Social worker (community-based) who is also care manager

Needs:	How to be met:	Action by:
Needs two people for all personal care tasks , i.e. washing, dressing, bathing, showering	Two carers will be needed in the home situation to minimise the risk of Mr Anwar falling. Occasionally, hospital staff have managed with one carer but Mr Anwar's ability to help is very unpredictable	Social worker to liaise with District Nursing Service and Care Agency
	Strasbourg Test (a test of physical and psychological dependency) to be carried out to determine the level of care needed	Ward sister
Needs two people for all transfers, i.e. bed, commode, chair	As above	As above
Tray for wheelchair	Mr Anwar has a suitable wheelchair which he can manoeuvre with prompting and encouragement	Occupational therapist (hospital)
	Wheelchair tray to be applied for	
Requires pressure area care, emptying of catheter bag, fit night-time catheter bags. A bladder wash out may be required in order to prevent urinary infections. Bowel care with the use of regular enemas is also required	District Nursing Service to be approached to meet these needs	Social worker to liaise with Clinical Manager for District Nursing Service
Medication to be administered	To be included in care plan	Ward sister to liaise with Mrs Anwar
Someone to provide supervision for Mr Anwar to allow Mrs. Anwar to go out. He cannot be left unattended at anytime	Mr Anwar is unable to recognise the risk of falling and frequently attempts to climb out of his wheelchair or bed. His communication skills are limited. A suitable sitting service will be needed for the times when Mrs Anwar or a carer are not in attendance	Social worker to liaise with relevant agencies
Provision of suitable equipment to prevent pressure sores i.e. bed, chair. There is a danger of Mr Anwar falling out of bed	Suitable bed with cot sides and suitable mattress to be provided	Social worker to liaise with District Nursing Service
Need for regular respite care throughout the year to alleviate stress for Mrs Anwar	Community social worker to apply for respite	Social worker
Provision of toileting/showering/bathing once a week. (Referral for assessment of long-term toileting/ bathing requirements have been made)	Community occupational therapist to carry out home assessment. Temporary measures to be met by bed and commode to be moved to downstairs room in Mr and Mrs Anwar's home	Social worker to liaise with community occupational therapist
Provision of suitable day care to give social contacts and mental stimulation	Community social worker to apply for suitable day care	Social worker
To continue with physiotherapy exercises	Referral to be made to community physiotherapist	Physiotherapist at hospital
Speech therapy to continue	Referral to be made to community speech therapist	Speech and language therapist at hospital

Mrs Anwar's needs:

- to receive support maintaining Mr Anwar's care and safety at home
- to be able to take a break from caring for her husband
- to be involved with drawing up a care plan prior to Mr Anwar's discharge from hospital
- to be kept informed of her husband's medical condition and needs
- to receive continued support from community social worker.

Agreed needs prior to hospital discharge:

- Strasbourg Test to be carried out by hospital staff
- Community social worker to liaise with clinical manager for District Nursing Service
- Care plan to be drawn up by nursing staff on ward
- Community OT to check that ramp is in place
- Hospital OT to arrange provision of commode.

Review date to be set up after discharge

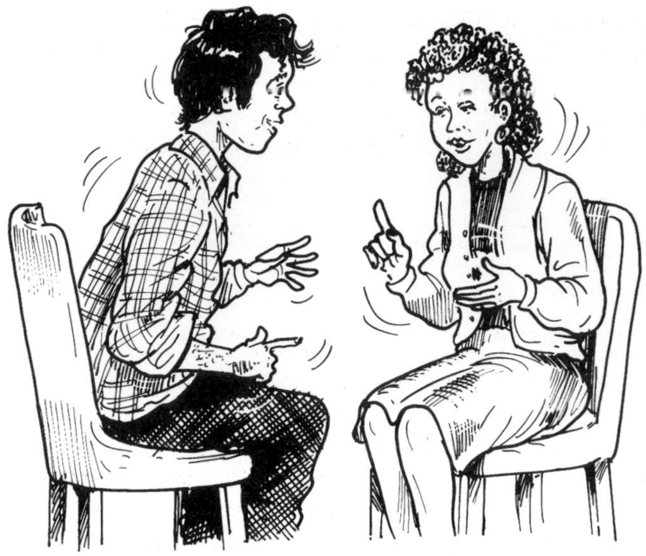

Figure 18.2 An empowering approach to care involves an exchange of ideas and meaning – not an expert dictating to a less powerful recipient of services

Building an understanding of client need will require social workers to have supportive skills of understanding, warmth and sincerity, as described in Chapter 6. These skills are more complex and require more time to use than simple questioning skills. However, if the social worker or carer can really understand the client, then they will be able to work together to exchange ideas. Both client and carer may be able to work on solving problems together. This is very different from care workers or social workers solving clients' problems for them – perhaps by simply allocating them to a service.

The client is given respect and power when working with a carer in the exchange model. The client remains responsible for resolving his or her needs and for working with others to clarify the support needed. The carer or social worker works *with* the client – not *on* him or her! It is an empowering approach to care.

Smale *et al.* (1993) state:

> The essence of empowerment, of working in partnership, is to work with people, not to take over what responsibility or control that they do have, but to bring new resources to their situation to build on and add to what they do and the choice they have in how care in the community works for them. (Page 24)

Not all clients receive empowering support. Sometimes clients may only need advice. Sometimes they may only need some guidance such as how to take a particular medicine or what remedy they might try. Some clients may need a day centre to provide the opportunity for social interaction. Some clients may have straightforward financial needs. Many adolescents and adults will have more complex needs which are unlikely to be met without a process of assessment. The idea of an empowering 'exchange' approach to assessment and the provision of resources will be important for these clients.

Involvement of clients

Clients may be involved in health and social care in a number of ways. The National Health Service (NHS) launched the Patient's Charter, which puts the Citizen's Charter into practice. It helps the NHS to:

- listen to and act on people's views and needs
- set clear standards of service
- provide services which meet those standards.

The Patient's Charter refers to rights and expectations across the NHS, including in addition private services, hospital services, community services, ambulance services, dental, optical and pharmaceutical services.

Rights can be defined as entitlements to a quality of service which all patients can expect to receive all the time.

Expectations are standards of service which the NHS is aiming to achieve. Exceptional circumstances may sometimes mean these standards are not met.

The government has published their special charter for pregnant women and new mothers. This explains their rights and the standards of service they can expect to receive during pregnancy, the baby's birth and post-natal care.

Try it

Obtain a copy of the Patient's Charter and list the ten rights identified.

The Community Health Council (CHC) is a body set up by the government to represent the interests of the public in each Health District. It is independent from the management of the local Health Service and is the consumers' 'watchdog'.

The aims of the CHC are to 'improve the local health services' and 'reflect public opinion'. The CHC Joint

Chief Officers also act as the 'patient's friend'. They will help someone with an enquiry or lend support and advice if a person wishes to complain.

The main policy aims of the Community Health Council are:

1 To form a representative view of the health needs of the population and the wishes of the public.
2 To monitor the operation of local health services and make relevant comparisons; to formulate a measure of local achievement, gaps and problem areas and quality of services.
3 To represent the public's interest and recommend improvements in order to influence the nature and quality of services.
4 To respond in a representative manner to consultation exercises, planning documents and proposals for change.
5 To inform and involve the public regarding the standard of local health services, the performance of the Health Authorities and activities of the CHC in order to facilitate an informed and participative community.
6 To support individual users and voluntary groups in their dealings with the Health Authorities, especially regarding problem areas and complaints to help increase user input and the improvement of services.

(*Source:* Winchester and Central Hampshire Community Health Council – Annual Report, 1993/94.)

Clients have to become involved in their care nowadays through the care management process. This is explained in detail in Chapter 16.

Supporting carers

In order to help people stay in their own homes, attention must focus on needs for support of carers, particularly close relatives, and the role played (or not played) by people in the wider community. This has been a major influence on community care reforms and, specifically, the aim to ensure that providers make practical support for carers a high priority. Assessment of care needs should always take account of the needs of caring family, friends and neighbours.

Thus social services and social work intervention are a response to the nature of a person's social relationships. In many situations it is the relationship between the 'client', their immediate 'carer' and other people in the support network, and how the situation can be maintained by supporting all of these people, that are of central concern.

Taking control of care

To enable clients and carers to exercise more control over their care, it is essential that information produced by health and social care agencies is in clear simple language which describes what that department can and cannot provide. The tone, detail and openness of information can indicate to the public whether their search for services is being received with understanding. honesty and enthusiasm.

It is essential to consult with all groups, including black and minority ethnic communities, before information systems are established. Particular attention should be paid to any potential barriers to communication due to disability, deprivation or different culture or language.

The people who know whether the content, style or presentation of information is suitable are those who receive it.

Therefore information systems should:

- ensure that people have information that is straightforward, relevant, accurate and sufficient, so that they can make informed choices
- ensure that everyone has access to this information in a variety of forms appropriate to their needs
- be regularly reviewed and up-dated.

They should take special account of those people who:

- have different cultures and languages
- have sensory impairment
- have restricted mobility
- are isolated within their communities
- have difficulty with reading or writing
- are not motivated to seek or use information.

This can be done by:

- consulting users, their carers, community groups and those who provide services, about the content and style of the information
- building information networks on existing

patterns of community life, e.g. libraries, religious and community centres, post offices and surgeries; including key community leaders and spokespeople
- being open about what people can and cannot have and the constraints of their choices
- using the expertise and experience of others to define the content and presentation of information
- giving better information to callers. The role of receptionists should be considered in relation to this.

Information for users whose needs make them eligible for services, and the types of services available, should be brief and clear. It should say:

- for whom the service is intended
- what it does
- what its availability is
- what it costs
- how to apply for it.

Assessment and review

The assessment of needs and review of the package of care is another means whereby clients and carers are able to exercise more control over their care.

Assessment is a participative process. It necessarily involves establishing mutual trust and understanding if meaningful information is to be obtained. The most effective way of achieving understanding may be to enable people to describe their situation in their own words, using their preferred language and at their own pace. Assessment should be a process of working alongside people.

Assessment should:

- recognise that some users may be the best assessors of their own needs and solutions
- consider the needs and strengths of individuals in the context of their everyday lives (Beardshaw and Towell, 1990)
- be separate from the decision about allocation of services
- strike a balance between invading privacy and obtaining sufficient information to gain an understanding of need
- recognise the rights of carers to a separate assessment where necessary
- be ethnically and culturally sensitive.

The Social Services Inspectorate summarise client involvement during assessment as follows

A review procedure should:

- enable users or their representatives to ask for reviews
- ensure care plans are regularly re-examined and formal review dates set
- provide open and honest information about all stages of the review process.

People who use services might be apprehensive about review and reassessment and fear these are ways of putting a good face on unpleasant decisions to stop or change services without good reason.

To minimise this unease you should:

- inform people that assessment agreements will be looked at periodically in partnership with them
- advise people that they can request a new assessment if they believe their circumstances have changed
- explain how reviews help services to remain in touch by giving people a chance to state their needs and opinions and by giving all service providers a chance to look again at what they are doing
- ensure your staff and all other organisations and consumer groups understand the purposes of review.

(From *Getting the Message Across*, HMSO Page 17)

Finding out about clients' views

This part of the chapter is intended to help you to collect the evidence needed for Element 6.3, 'Evaluate how clients experience and influence health and social care provision'. This element has a very practical focus. The work you need to do, and the activities it will involve, link closely with the research skills that are the subject of Unit 8. You will need to gather data from clients of the health and social care services, and from some of those involved in service delivery, in order to satisfy the evidence indicators. You will find that this chapter is much easier to understand if you have already looked at the chapters in this book on research methods. Without some knowledge of research the recommendations and advice will be impossible to put into practice.

Try it

Read Chapters 22, 23 and 24 if you have not already done so. If you follow this guidance you will get a lot more from your reading of this chapter.

Putting research into practice

For Element 6.3 you need to produce a project report to the following specifications: *A report comparing at least two clients with health and social care needs, dealing with how they experience care and how they feel able to influence the provision.*

The report should look at:

- their perceptions of their care
- the extent to which they perceive a continuum of care
- the support which has been offered compared with what is potentially available
- whether the clients feel that they have been in control of the care which is available.

The report needs to include a summary of how one health and social care service in your local area is attempting to improve its service, and your own recommendations on how it could be improved on a day-to-day basis.

Your report therefore needs to be based around a primary research project. You will be gathering data from a small sample of subjects to evaluate their experience. You can use one or more of the research methods that are discussed in Chapters 22 and 23, and may gather quantitative or qualitative data, or a combination of both. Like all researchers you need to follow the stages of the research process. This begins with defining the research question, and the population it applies to.

The research question

The overall research aims cover every possible type of client and service. This leaves room for you to focus on people that you can easily reach, and who you believe will be willing to provide the information you need. Your research question can address a population which is accessible. There is nothing necessarily unscientific about choosing to study people you have easy access to, provided that you accept the limitations which may result. You may have good contacts with a particular group of service users, or with several individuals who have care needs. For a small project like this it may be sensible to consider using your existing contacts. They could be fellow students, neighbours, family or friends. The 'clients' referred to in the element title could mean any service users, so you could choose to look at people you already know.

However, you need to be sure you are comfortable about using people close to you, like family and friends, for a research project. You also need to be confident that your prospective subjects will have no reservations about this. If you have any doubts then you should choose subjects with whom you don't have a close personal relationship.

Another issue is the suitability to your research aims of people you already know. If you want to link your recommendations for service improvement with the experiences of users, it will help to get data from people who are using similar services. Your personal contacts may have little in common with each other; they may have different needs and use a different range of services. This will make it hard to recommend improvements, except in general terms. If each of your subjects uses a different service your results cannot claim wider applicability.

You may have contacts with a group of service users through work placement, or because of your own

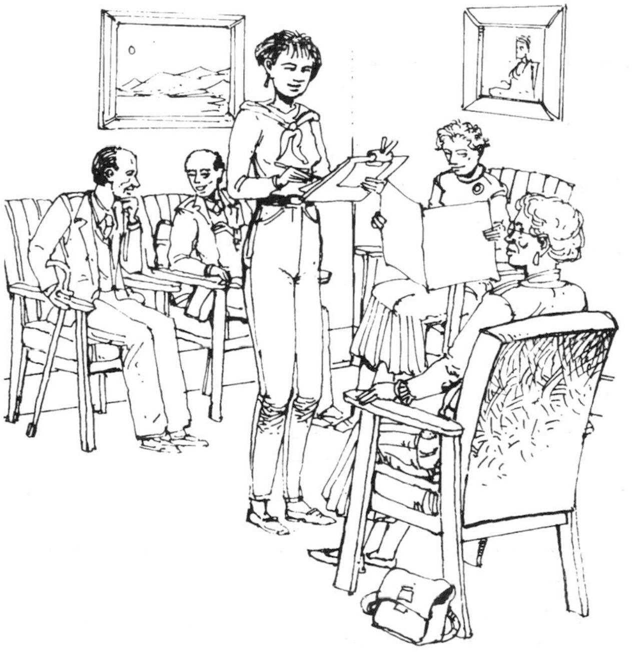

Figure 18.3 Research may be easier where you have professional rather than personal relationships with clients

voluntary activities. A group like this may provide good data because members use a similar range of services, and have some needs in common. Also, your relationship with members of the group may be more professional than personal, making it easier to carry out research amongst them.

If all else fails it is possible that you could try to contact a group of service users through other means. One way may be to make contact with groups through 'user forums', or other local service-user groups. You could find them through your local Community Health Council, or perhaps via advice from tutors or fellow students. Alternatively, you could look at people using local residential or day-care provision. Here you would also need to check that the centre staff are happy to co-operate with your research.

When you have chosen a group from whom to seek data, you have identified the **population** that your research is about. You will also have narrowed down the services that you are investigating to ones that your subjects use.

Sampling

To gather the information in your report you will need to choose particular clients and find out how they feel about the issues identified in the evidence indicators. Deciding which people to ask is, in research terms, choosing a **sample.** The evidence indicators specify that the experiences of at least two clients need to be compared. This is a very small sample indeed, and you may feel that a larger sample is needed if you want to try to apply your results convincingly to others in a similar position. Some research methods, particularly those which aim to gather mainly *quantitative* data, will probably be fairly easy to use on a larger sample. However, if you are thinking about collecting *qualitative* data using in-depth interviewing techniques you will need to keep your sample small.

Whatever research methods you intend to use, your sample can be chosen using **random** methods. The chapters on research explain the importance of this, and describe methods that can be used. Since the size of sample that you can handle is related to the data collection methods you intend to use, decisions on this need to be made.

Research methods

The aims of your research project allow a good deal of freedom in the choice of research method. You may collect either quantitative or qualitative data, or both. You could use in-depth interviews, structured interviews, semi-structured interviews, or self-completion questionnaires. The decision of which methods to employ should be made in the light of the information that you need to get.

What data do you need to collect?

You know that your research centres on clients' experiences, and their perceived level of influence over their care. Your research needs to meet the specifications outlined in the performance criteria by collecting data on all the areas that are listed below.

1 You need to find out the clients' perceptions of health and social care services on:

- control of the process
- respect they are shown as individuals
- care received
- information given
- services and facilities they use.

2 You need to discover the extent to which they perceive there to be a continuum of care. This relates to:

- seamlessness of service
- continuity of provision
- the smoothness of the transition from one care setting to another
- the smoothness of transition from one care worker to another
- smoothness of flow of information.

3 You need to find out the support that they have been offered. Types of support include:

- physical
- financial
- emotional
- knowledge
- understanding
- social.

4 You need to discover the extent to which clients feel that they have been in control of the care which they are receiving. Taking control refers to:

- obtaining information
- obtaining advice
- development of skills

- deciding how resources should be used
- deciding how care should be planned and delivered
- client and carer networks and forums
- clients managing their own care.

This is a fairly comprehensive list of the factors which affect clients' experience of care, and your research must cover each of them. In addition, you may wish to collect some factual, or demographic, data about your sample. This will include things like gender, age group, services used, and perhaps personal factors which affect care needs, such as a registered disability.

One danger with relying on less structured research methods is that you will have less control over the data that you collect than if you use a fixed set of questions. In-depth and semi-structured interviews could give you a mass of views and opinions, but this data is under the subjects' control. You may find that areas you need to find out about don't come up in the interview. Another issue is the ease with which data can be analysed and compared. It is often hard to put together the views of different respondents if in-depth interviews are used, because they may approach a topic from different viewpoints.

Tightly structured questionnaire methods, which use only fixed-response questions, can be guaranteed to cover each area. However, the danger now is that, because your subjects are restricted to the options available in the questions, they will not be able to explain the details of their views, or the reasons behind them. Now it is easy to compare answers, as this simply means comparing responses given on a fixed scale, but these comparisons may be shallow or even misleading.

Good research uses a variety of methods to minimise the effects of these problems. Questionnaires often contain a mixture of fixed-response and open questions, sometimes linked together so that the reasons behind a fixed-response choice are probed. For instance, a question might ask, 'Do you feel that you have been shown respect as an individual whilst receiving care?' The scale of fixed responses available might range from 'Shown great respect' to 'Shown no respect'. A follow-up open question such as 'Can you explain your answer in more detail?' will help you to pick up the range of views behind answers to your fixed-response question.

Another approach could be to use more than one method. You could carry out structured interviews, or use self-completion questionnaires, to get mostly quantitative data which can be analysed and compared. Some open questions could be included to add depth and background to the fixed responses. In addition to this, you could carry out in-depth or semi-structured interviews with a much smaller number of people. This tactic allows you to measure people's opinions on the health and social care services and also explore the thinking behind those opinions.

Think it over

Consider the population you are interested in and the range of services that they use. Which research methods do you think you could use to collect the data that you need from this population?

Consider the issues surrounding the use of each method, particularly the difficulties that you may have in implementing it. Remember that this is a small-scale project and be prepared to compromise on scientific accuracy for the sake of collecting the complete range of data that you need.

An important factor in your choice of research method is the time available to you for the work. Don't make ambitious plans for a multi-tiered research project that you will be unable to complete properly.

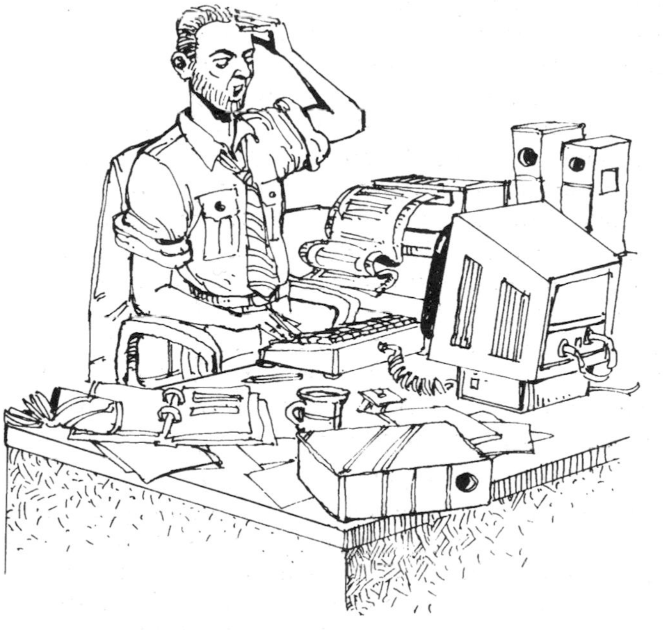

Figure 18.4 Don't make your research too ambitious to complete

You then need to plan the questions you intend to ask. This means structuring your questions towards the areas you need to investigate. This will only be possible if you have an understanding of the areas that you are enquiring into, and the kind of issues that are raised. There are different ways to ask questions, and some are better at dealing with particular types of data needs. You need enough understanding to be able to pose your questions in the most appropriate way.

Understanding the issues

Clients' perceptions of health and social care services

There is a range of issues associated with clients' perceptions of their care, all of which need to be dealt with in your questionnaire or interview schedule. This means looking at each in turn and trying to choose the best way of obtaining data about it.

The first aspect of client perceptions that you need to find out about is their **control** of the process of care. We will look at this in detail later.

Clients' perceptions of the **respect** that they are shown as an individual need to be discovered. Different people will have different standards by which they judge whether respect has been shown. If you simply ask, 'In your contacts with the health and social care services do you feel that you are shown respect as an individual?' it would be hard to imagine what each person was thinking about when he or she answered. You could introduce a scale of possible answers from 'Great respect shown' to 'No respect shown' to get more precise measurement of views. However, you are still relying on people having similar ideas about what constitutes respect if your scale is to be meaningful for comparison between different respondents.

One way of dealing with this problem is to explain what you mean by respect in the question, or in a preamble to a set of questions. This way you have given each respondent a frame of reference for their answers and you might expect to get more comparable answers. For example, your questionnaire could state, 'People may feel that they have been shown respect as an individual if their personal needs, ideas, and lifestyle choices are supported, and are not criticised or commented on negatively'. Now you can follow this up with questions about the respect people feel that they have been shown, with the hope that there is some common understanding about the dimensions of the concept 'respect'.

Another issue is that people may well feel that they have been shown respect on some occasions, but not on others. Also, they may feel that different individual carers show different levels of respect, or that some services show more or less respect in general than other services. Asking 'Do you feel that you are shown respect as an individual?' may invite the answer, 'It depends.'

There are several ways to deal with this problem. One way is simply to ask people to explain their answers in more detail with an open question. However, here you are likely to receive different types of answer making data analysis difficult. Another way is to try to predict the range of situations where respect shown could be judged and ask separate questions to cover each possibility. But this is likely to be extremely difficult to get right , and could lead to such a mass of questions that the idea becomes unworkable.

A compromise might be to ask a small group of fixed-response questions to establish general opinion, and then to follow up with open questions on specific aspects of that opinion. The fixed-response questions could ask about some of the variables that we have considered. For example, you could ask, 'Do you think that, in general, the health and social care services you use show similar levels of respect for you as an individual?' This could be followed up with a question asking people to rank the services they receive in order or the level of respect that they feel they are shown. A follow-up open question could also ask people to outline the reasons for their feelings. Similar combinations of fixed-response and open questions could be constructed to probe feelings about respect shown by different carers, or in different care settings.

The basic point is that you need to construct questions which minimise the ambiguity in the idea of 'respect as an individual'. Your solution to the problem must be one that you, and your respondents, find manageable and understandable.

Think it over

Think about ways of tackling the issues raised above. How do you think you would go about getting useful data on people's perceptions of the respect they are shown?

The methods you use could be applied to other areas of your research where definitions and common understandings may be problematic. It is best to design survey instruments that have a consistent style of data collection. Regular patterns in the question style help respondents to relax and minimise confusion. This is a good reason for thinking hard about which approach you are happy with. You may be designing several sets of questions using that method.

You need to seek clients' perceptions on the **quality of the care** they receive. This raises similar issues concerning the subjective definition of 'quality', and you could use methods like those described above to overcome these difficulties. Here it will be important to identify the services that each client is receiving, since perceptions of quality may vary widely between different services. Possible differences between different carers, and different care settings, may also have to be considered. Can you think of a definition of quality that could introduce the questions and provide a common frame of reference? With regard to clients' perceptions of the **quality** of health and social care services and **facilities,** you may think about issues like overall quality, accessibility, fitness for their intended purpose and staffing levels. Facilities may also be judged on their state of repair, and their general attractiveness to users. You could frame a set of fixed-response questions to cover these issues, and some follow-up open questions to probe for the individual reasons behind these views.

Clients' perceptions of **information** that they have been given also need to be looked at. This may present an opportunity to find out what information is potentially available to clients, and what the service aims to ensure that they receive. This will allow you to draw up a checklist which can be used in your research into clients' perceptions. You could simply present a list of information categories and ask respondents to tick which have been received. Other aspects of the issue of information could be how well it was explained, how clearly it was presented, and whether there have been contradictions between information from different sources.

A point to be aware of is that you need to look at issues associated with obtaining information as an aspect of the control which clients have over their care. So be careful not to ask the same thing twice. You may find that one question, or set of questions, can cover more than one of your research areas.

Perceptions of a continuum of care

Your enquiries also need to explore the extent to which clients perceive there is a continuum of care. Some clients may not have considered this issue, or may not feel that it is important. Questions need to focus on the details which are specified in the range, concerning specific issues.

The first aspect is **seamlessness of service.** Here again you need to think about your questions so that respondents have a common understanding of 'seamlessness', and so that you have covered differences between perceptions of different services and situations. **Continuity of provision** is another aspect of a continuum of care. Clients could be asked whether they have experience of gaps in provision using a fixed-response question. Those answering 'Yes' could be asked to identify the gaps in more detail using an open question.

Another aspect of continuity is the smoothness of **transition** from one care setting to another. The questions you come up with here may depend on the population that you are researching. If you know that all of your subjects are likely to have had particular transitions in common then you could focus your questions specifically on these. For example, you may be interviewing people in a day-care setting who also receive care at home, many of whom have received residential care at some time. You could design questions about the smoothness of transition between these specific care settings. This will help respondents to give much more accurate answers than questions that are posed in general terms.

Smoothness of transition could involve issues like the transfer of information about clients in advance of their arrival. It could also involve the extent to which the ethos and practice of different care settings are similar, so that clients find it easy to move between them.

A related issue is the smooth transition from one care worker to another. Clients' perceptions here may be affected by their personal relationships with individual carers. It is important to design questions that steer away from considerations of personality, and which focus instead on the process of the transition between care workers. What you want to find out is whether clients feel that each care worker is working in the same way, with the same aims, skills and information available.

The smoothness of the **flow of information** is another aspect of a continuum of care. This could involve information being passed between care settings, or between care workers. It could also involve the smoothness with which information flows to and from the clients themselves. Again, beware of duplicating your questioning. Obtaining information is an aspect of clients' control of the care they receive and you may want to cover information in your questions on this.

An important issue in connection with a continuum of care is the extent to which clients think that it matters. You may find that some aspects of a continuum of care are seen as important, whereas others are not. You could cover this by adding a question like, 'How important do you consider ... to be ?' after questions about each aspect of a continuum of care. You could round off the whole section by stating that the previous set of questions have been about experiences of a continuum of care, and then ask people how important they think this is. This method serves to define a continuum of care for the respondents, and may help them to give an accurate general opinion on it.

Think it over

In this section you have been focusing on the idea of a continuum of care, and you need to report on clients' perceptions of this continuum. Look at the question ideas you have developed to address this data need.

Do you think that these questions, when put together in a survey document, will give you the data that you need? You may think that you have too many questions, or too few, when they are looked at together. Can you adjust the number of questions you are planning to ask so that they are both adequate and manageable?

Do your questions on a continuum of care have a consistent pattern so that respondents will find the research approach easy to follow? If not, can you develop a consistent pattern and style at this stage?

Do you think that, when put together, your questions form a clearly distinct section of your research? Can you improve the coherence of your questions so that the idea of a continuum is clearly addressed throughout?

Support

Your research needs to find out the support that clients have been offered, and compare this with what is potentially available. This means that you need to link your findings from clients with your findings from the services themselves so that comparisons can be made.

There are several categories of support that clients may have been offered. **Physical support** could include any form of practical help that has been provided. Clients may have a clear statement of the physical support that they can expect in their care plan. Make sure to ask direct questions to establish the actual physical support that clients receive, and the frequency with which they receive it. You could also look at clients' views on the quality and suitability of the physical support.

Another area is **financial support.** Be careful here, because money is a sensitive issue for most people. Direct questions about the level of financial support received are likely to offend your respondents. Look at the advice in Chapter 23 on asking questions about sensitive subjects. There are usually ways to obtain data without causing offence.

Emotional support could involve subjective ideas about the amount of understanding people feel that they have been shown. They may see this as having a shoulder to cry on, or someone to share problems with. They may need to feel that carers have time and room to provide support like this. Perceptions about emotional support may be even more dependent on the relationship between client and carer. Try to create questions that probe the level of support offered without the issue of the personalities concerned overwhelming the accuracy of the answers.

Think it over

Sometimes people may be less aware of having received emotional support than they are of receiving physical help. How can you find out what may actually have been offered in this situation? Can you present respondents with a view of emotional support that will help them to identify it in their experience of care?

Support concerning **knowledge** relates to questions about information which are likely to occur elsewhere. Here, however, the emphasis could be on face-to-face explanations, and on ways that services and workers respond to more personal and individual knowledge needs. You could ask questions around particular pieces of knowledge that respondents feel that they have needed.

Understanding may be interpreted as a client's understanding of issues surrounding their care, or as the understanding that they are shown in the course of their care. The first interpretation may duplicate questions that look at how clients obtain information, so you could focus on the second. Here you may be dealing with issues that link with emotional support, so be careful that the questions asked give distinctly different data. This time you are looking at whether clients feel that their situation and view of the world has been appreciated during their care. Feelings here may crucially affect whether clients feel that carers 'see things their way'.

Lastly, you need to look at **social support.** This could take a variety of forms, and here again you may have particular knowledge of your population and the services that they use, which can help. You may expect to find particular types of social support offered to the people you are researching, and can thus ask specific questions about them. You could present a list of the different ways that social support may be offered and ask respondents to identify those which have been received. Comments on quality and suitability can be obtained through follow-up open questions.

Taking control of care

The extent to which clients feel that they are in control of the care that they receive is at the heart of the issue of **empowerment.** There are several areas of enquiry within the notion of control, and you need to obtain data on each of them.

First, there is the ease with which **information** is obtained. There are many types of information that may be held about an individual, and some may be shared between services whereas others are not, perhaps for reasons of confidentiality. The extent to which clients have access to information held about them will depend partly on their awareness that it *is* being held. Clients themselves may not be in a good position to judge how well informed they are. However, clients' experiences of getting information that they have sought might easily be discovered. You could, again, develop a checklist of categories of information and ask clients which they had been given. Alternatively, you could ask open questions concerning how clients go about finding things out and how easy they have found it to be.

Think it over

There are references to information throughout your research. You need to look at 'information' in terms of a continuum of care, in terms of clients' control over the care they receive, and in terms of clients' general perceptions of the care that they receive.

You may be able to deal with information as a section of enquiry in its own right. A set of questions could address each of your research needs whilst seeming to respondents to be related and coherent.

Look through the list of areas you need to gather data about and identify those items in different sections which relate to information. List them, noting the different emphasis that needs to be taken because of the differences in focus between sections. Can you write a set of questions that form a distinct section concerning information? How easy will it be to apply the results gained to different sections of your research when you are analysing the data?

Obtaining advice could be tackled in a similar way. Some clients may see advice as a form of support similar to obtaining knowledge. Others may think of advice as very similar to information. They may think that you are repeating yourself, so be careful to word your questions carefully to avoid this. You could use a scene-setting statement which makes it clear what advice refers to, and stresses its practical nature.

Questions on the **development of skills** may get more accurate responses if you encourage people to think about the issue first. Skill development can be a subtle process. Unless a person has taken a course, or received a structured and defined programme of training, they may not believe that it has taken place at all. To get accurate information you could first ask respondents to think about the sorts of things they are able to do. This could lead to questions about the guidance that they may have been given in developing these skills. You could also probe areas where people feel that they lack skills, and enquire about their efforts to obtain help to improve them.

Another area is clients' involvement in decisions about how **resources** should be used. This may have happened in several ways. Clients may have been asked their views in an informal and unstructured way during the course of their care. Alternatively, people's opinions could have been canvassed through questionnaires or other forms of enquiry organised by the service providers.

People's perceptions of their involvement in the decision-making process may not be realistically related to the actual influence they have. You should link your enquiries to the ideas which the services themselves have about how clients are able to influence decisions.

Clients' control in decisions about the **planning and delivery** of their care needs to be investigated. You are trying to find out the level of influence that clients themselves feel they have over an important area of their lives. This is an area that you must deal with sensitively. It is related to a client's rights to choice, and your questions could look at alternative methods of care delivery that may have been suggested.

Clients' feelings about who made the final decisions on the care plan are also relevant here. Do they feel that it was a process that they really have control of? Some clients may feel that they should not be in control of these issues, and that decisions on care are best left to experts. This may be because they have low levels of self-esteem, perhaps owing to their personal experiences, or it could reflect attitudes associated with their cultural background. You could try to establish the level of involvement that was offered, even if it was rejected or seen as inappropriate by some clients.

Another area to consider is clients' awareness of, and involvement in, **client and carer networks** and forums. Here again you may want to present a list of the local opportunities that are available and ask respondents to indicate those that they know of, and those that they are part of. You will need to research local networks and groups to use this approach. Alternatively, you could simply ask people to list groups they know about, and indicate those in which they participate. Follow-up questions could explore the nature and extent of their involvement in more detail.

A final area of enquiry is clients' control of the overall **management** of their care. To some extent this brings together the other dimensions of empowerment that this section of your research deals with. Management implies informed and effective control and you could ask questions which allow respondents to sum up their feelings about control of their care.

Finding out about services

Getting information

You research needs to deal with the services themselves, as well as clients' experiences of them. You may feel that it would be best to carry out this part of the investigation first. You can get an overview of the service and the care that it provides, and you can get specific information that will help you to develop questions to put to clients. This is your opportunity to find out what the services consider themselves to be doing. You need to find this out so that you can compare and contrast it with the clients' experiences and perceptions.

You cannot look at all services, so you need to choose the most relevant for the client group you are interested in. This may be obvious, or you may have to choose between alternatives. It may be best to pick a service that you have some knowledge of, or involvement with. This will help you to identify potential sources of information, and may make it easier to arrange interviews with relevant staff. The services chosen should be used by all or most of your population, and be services that you are able to research easily.

The approach you take needs to be well organised. You must identify the things on which you want to gather information and establish the best way to collect this information. In the previous section, several areas were mentioned where prior knowledge of the intentions of the services themselves will help you to frame relevant questions. For instance, a service may have expectations of the range of information that should be offered to clients; this would help you to ask direct questions of clients about which types of information they have received.

You could get data through leaflets and other informative publications produced by the service. But you may find that not all the areas you need information about are covered. This will allow you to generate a list of things that you need to make enquiries about. Rather than writing for information, it is probably better to speak to someone within the service who has direct knowledge of these points.

You need to be as professional as possible when seeking information from care organisations. Find out who you want to speak to and make an appointment to see them. You could explain the purpose of the meeting, and outline the things you need to find out about, by sending a covering letter confirming the appointment. This will help to improve the information you get as the people involved have time to prepare for the meeting. Take paper and pen with you and be sure to make sufficient notes.

As well as information which supports your design of questions to put to clients, there are specific issues concerning clients' involvement that you need to find out about. This part of your research report will look at how health and social care services are trying to involve clients in improving services. There are several dimensions to this and you need to get information on each one.

Involving clients

One way that clients can be involved in service improvements is in relation to **physical** aspects of care. This could include consultation over the design and improvement of buildings and other facilities. Services may have established a process to involve their clients in this. There may also be procedures to ensure that clients are able to influence things like decoration and furnishings. This may be particularly important in residential or day-care settings and there should be policies and procedures to help clients' views influence decisions.

Services should also be seeking to improve the **emotional** support offered to clients. This could mean that care staff are given guidance and training to help meet the emotional needs of clients. There may be policies designed to ensure that staff have the time, and flexibility of work routines, which allow them to listen to clients and offer support. An issue here also is the extent of clients' involvement and influence over the process. You need to find out how the service is attempting to involve clients in improving the emotional support they receive.

Another area to be looked at is how services are improving their response to the **social needs** of clients. This may be through the provision of facilities or activities which are appropriate to their client group. Find out what is available and how clients are involved in their development.

Finally, you need to look at how services facilitate the exchange of **information** between themselves and their clients. Putting information out might involve charters of service, the publication of eligibility criteria, and the production of a variety of other publications which aim to inform people about the aims and practices of the service. You may have collected examples of this information during your initial enquiries into the service. The other side of the exchange involves obtaining information, views and opinions from the users of the service. This could be through forums, or the local Community Health Council. Some services may have developed other ways of seeking the views of their clients. They may, for example, carry out some form of survey using questionnaire methods.

You need to discover what the service you are looking at is doing to involve clients in improving their work in all these areas. Find out what you can from the literature available, and then work out a schedule of questions to get information on the areas you still need to find out about. Your meeting with a member of the service staff can address these points and fill in the gaps.

Try it

Make a list of the information that you need to collect about health and care services. Your list should include the specific points described in the research specifications, and other information that you think would help you to ask better questions of clients.

Collect all the published information about the service, and note how easily you were able to obtain it. Now make a list of the areas of information that you have not been able to cover through the published literature. Arrange to contact suitable members of the service staff and try to collect the data you need from them. Follow the advice given above on preparation and professionalism.

Drawing conclusions from your research

When you have completed your research you need to analyse the data and begin to draw conclusions. The methods of data analysis you use will depend on the type of data you have collected, and the type of comparisons you wish to make. Chapter 24 examines different ways of dealing with data analysis, and Chapter 27 (on information technology) looks at ways of making it easier by using computer-based methods. The important issue in data analysis is the specific aim of your research project.

You are trying to establish the relationship between clients' experiences of their care and the aims and intentions of the services themselves. This suggests that comparisons need to be made between what services *claim* to do and what clients *say* they experience. You can compare data in all the areas of enquiry that we have looked at, to draw conclusions about the match between service aims and client experience. If you have collected qualitative data you can look for the feelings that clients have about their role in the care process. You may get good indications of their feelings of involvement and empowerment, or otherwise.

Your goal in this part of your work is to be able to make recommendations about how service to clients might be improved on a day-to-day basis. Your recommendations should be based on your findings about clients' perceptions of their experience of care. You should make recommendations that are justified by the data collected from clients, and that are realistic in terms of the aims of the service and the resources available to it. Don't disguise negative criticism as recommendations. You need to suggest positive and constructive improvements.

Finally, prepare your report. Look at Chapter 24 for advice on presentation. Remember that your report should be primarily about clients' experience of the health and social care services. Don't spend too long detailing your research methods and the difficulties you encountered, except where these might have affected the results.

Evidence collection point

The evidence needed towards Element 6.3 has been specified in detail in this chapter. You need to plan and carry out your research, and complete your report. Look at Chapter 24 on presenting your results, and use information technology resources wherever possible to help you in your work.

Remember that your work towards this element can also be used as evidence of your use of research, and you may use it towards elements in Unit 8.

Self-assessment test

1 A care plan is:
- **a** A review of existing services.
- **b** An assessment of financial means.
- **c** A written document which outlines how the needs of an individual are to be met.
- **d** A financial assessment.

2 The general process of which care planning is a part is called:
- **a** Home care process.
- **b** Nursing process.
- **c** Review process.
- **d** Assessment of care management process.

3 A person's 'needs' are:
- **a** What a person wants.
- **b** A local resource a person can visit.
- **c** A requirement to enable a person to live at an acceptable level of social independence.
- **d** What a relative thinks a person wants.

4 An assessor could be:
- **a** A social worker.
- **b** A relative.
- **c** A neighbour.
- **d** A home carer.

5 Which of the following describes an assessment?
- **a** A chat over coffee.
- **b** A two-way process between the assessor and the client.
- **c** A conversation with the main carer.
- **d** An assessor fitting a client into existing resources.

6 Assessment may be described as:
- **a** A providing function.
- **b** An identification function.
- **c** A purchasing function.
- **d** A purchasing/providing function.

7 Three of the following are core tasks of assessment and care management. Which task is not?
- **a** Publishing information.
- **b** Assessing need.
- **c** Fitting people into resources.
- **d** Monitoring.

8 Three of the following identify ways in which needs can be categorised. Which is not a category of needs?
- **a** Personal and social care.
- **b** What a person wants.
- **c** Physical health.
- **d** Cultural and religious needs.

9 Three of the following must occur when implementing a macro care plan. Which should not occur?
- **a** Clients must not be aware of their care plan.
- **b** Budgets must be confirmed.
- **c** Service availability must be identified.
- **d** Pace of implementation must be agreed.

10 Clients have a right to expect certain standards. Three of the following describe those rights. Which does not?
- **a** Freedom from discrimination.
- **b** Power of choice.
- **c** Information need not be confidential.
- **d** Dignity.

11 The following statements describe the purpose of a review. One statement is false.
Identify the false statement:
- a A review should determine if care plan objectives have been achieved.
- b A review should evaluate reasons for failure or success.
- c A review should reassess current needs.
- d A review should be an opportunity to cut services.

12 Which statement is false when discussing discrimination?
- a People should be encouraged to make their own choices.
- b Information regarding services should be printed in appropriate languages.
- c People should eat the same food, regardless of religion or culture.
- d Interpreters and signers should be made available when necessary.

13 Three of the following statements can be justified when discussing the purpose of monitoring. Which statement cannot be justified?
- a Care plan objectives must be monitored.
- b The co-ordination of services should be monitored.
- c The role of unpaid carers need not be monitored.
- d Service specifications should be monitored.

14 Confidentiality means:
- a Professionals can share information freely about a client.
- b Clients have no access to their records.
- c Information can be passed freely across agencies.
- d Clients have the right to know that information about themselves will not be repeated to others without their permission.

15 Which of the following activities does not promote independence?
- a Involving clients in their own care as much as possible.
- b Empowering people to take control of their lives.
- c Not involving the clients and their carers in the discussion process regarding their care.
- d Encouraging clients to do things for themselves.

16 Self-advocacy is not:
- a Helping people to speak for themselves.
- b Telling people what to say.
- c Promoting advocacy through the care plan.
- d Helping people to understand their rights.

17 How soon should the first review be held after the agreement of the care plan?
- a 6 weeks.
- b 3 months.
- c 6 months.
- d 12 months.

18 Whose responsibility is it to co-ordinate the first review?
- a Key worker.
- b Care manager.
- c GP.
- d Service manager.

19 Who should assess a client's financial means?
- a GP.
- b Consultant.
- c Care manager.
- d Key worker.

20 Which of the following should not be contained in a macro plan?
- a Personal care needs.
- b Physical and emotional care needs.
- c Details of times that providers will visit.
- d Mental health needs.

21 Which of the following is an area of work not covered by occupational health nurses?
- a Visiting work environments.
- b Health screening.
- c Working in GPs' surgeries.
- d Health education and promotion.

22 Three of the following are areas of work covered by environmental health officers. Which is not among their areas of work?
- a Helping people to improve living conditions in unfit or old housing.
- b Monitoring and controlling levels of pollution.
- c Checking standards in premises producing food.
- d Providing general health checks.

23 Health screening can be defined as:
- a General health checks, i.e. taking blood pressure, pulse etc.
- b X-rays.
- c Surgical operations
- d Home visits by district nurses.

24 Which of the following functions is not covered in the Mental Health Act 1983?
- **a** Compulsory admission to hospital.
- **b** Arresting a person.
- **c** 'Guardianship' of those suffering a mental disorder.
- **d** Managing the property and financial affairs of someone who is judged incapable of doing so.

25 Section 2 of the Mental Health Act allows someone suffering from a mental disorder to be detained for up to:
- **a** 6 months.
- **b** 31 days.
- **c** 3 months.
- **d** 28 days.

26 Section 3 of the Mental Health Act provides the power for long-term admission, in the first instance, of up to:
- **a** 12 months.
- **b** 3 months.
- **c** 6 months
- **d** 8 months.

27 Which of the following is not part of the role of the Mental Health Act Commission?
- **a** It acts in accordance with the rights and interests of detained patients.
- **b** It arranges inspection visits to hospitals without prior appointments.
- **c** It represents hospital staff's views.
- **d** It deals with complaints from detained patients.

28 The date of implementation for the Carers (Recognition of Services) Act is:
- **a** 1 April 1996.
- **b** 1 January 1997.
- **c** 1 September 1996.
- **d** 1 April 1997.

29 Which of the following is not a priority for community care?
- **a** Extending choices for clients.
- **b** Giving clients everything they want.
- **c** Better joint working between health and social care organisations.
- **d** Ensuring that clients feel they are respected.

30 Which of the following does not help clients to feel valued?
- **a** Having their cultural, ethnic, religious, sexual and emotional needs recognised and respected.
- **b** Being fully informed of the purpose of an assessment.
- **c** Having a care manager take charge of their lives.
- **d** Having a person to speak or act on their behalf when necessary.

31 'Seamless service' can be described as:
- **a** Council departments, National Health Service bodies, private and voluntary agencies working independently of each other.
- **b** Working in a disjointed way.
- **c** Having a difference of opinion in the way services are delivered.
- **d** Services working together in harmony.

32 Three of the following describe the ways in which the Patient's Charter puts the Citizen's Charter into practice in the National Health Service. Which is the false statement?
- **a** The NHS listens to and acts on people's views and needs.
- **b** The NHS decides what is best for its clients.
- **c** The NHS sets clear standards of service.
- **d** The NHS provides services that meet established standards.

33 Which of the following is responsible for setting up Community Health Councils?
- **a** The National Health Service.
- **b** Local authorities.
- **c** Voluntary organisations.
- **d** Central government.

34 Which of the following is not a main policy aim of the Community Health Council?
- **a** To form a representative view of the health needs of the population.
- **b** To monitor the operation of local health services.
- **c** Always to support health authorities.
- **d** To inform and involve the public in the setting of standards for local health services.

35 Three of the following describe ways in which information produced by health and social care agencies can be made clear. Which does not?
- **a** Using jargon.
- **b** Using clear, simple language.
- **c** Paying attention to any potential barriers to communication.
- **d** Paying attention to the tone and detail of information.

36 Which of the following does not describe a way in which information for carers and clients should be presented?

a Information should say for whom a service is intended.
b Information should use technical and scientific words.
c Information should say what the service provides.
d Information should describe availability of the service.

37 Which group of people should not be taken into special account when producing information about services?
a People from different cultural backgrounds.
b People with restricted mobility.
c People who have no communication problems.
d People who have difficulty in reading.

38 Which of the following describes the assessment process most accurately?
a Assessment is carried out by a care manager.
b Assessment is a participative process.
c Assessment is concerned only with money.
d Assessment should exclude the client and carer.

39 The word 'rights' in the Patient's Charter refers to:
a What the NHS says it can afford to offer to patients.
b What a patients wants.
c Entitlement to a certain quality of service that patients can expect to receive all of the time.
d The services a carer wants for a patient who is his or her relative.

40 The word 'expectation' in the Patient's Charter refers to:
a Standards of service that the NHS is aiming to achieve.
b What NHS staff expect to do in their work.
c What patients expect from services
d What the community as a whole expects from services.

41 If you are researching into the experiences and perceptions of users of the health and social care services, your research population could be defined as:
a Everyone living in Britain.
b All users of the health and social care services.
c People who need regular care.
d Disabled people.

42 When choosing a sample for a small research project you should:
a Always choose people with whom you have a close personal relationship.
b Never choose people with whom you have a strong personal relationship.
c Choose people who have little in common with one another.
d Choose people who have similar care needs and have no objection to being studied.

43 You will need to choose a sample of people to ask questions. Which of the following is true of sampling?
a Sampling methods are unimportant to a small-scale research project.
b Researchers should always try to use a random sampling method.
c Quota sampling methods are likely to give the best results.
d Sampling errors should always be calculated mathematically.

44 Which of the following research methods is likely to be most useful in investigating people's views on the health and social care services?
a Experiments.
b Participant observation.
c Direct observation.
d In-depth interviews.

45 All research collects data. Which of the following statements best describes the data to be collected in an investigation of people's views about the health and care services?
a There will be a mixture of quantitative and qualitative data.
b Only quantitative data will be collected.
c Only qualitative data will be collected.
d No demographic data need to be collected.

46 Researchers often use more than one method of data collection in their work. This is because:
a They may be unsure which is the best method to use.
b It helps them to practise methods that they don't use very often.
c Results from one method can complement and illuminate results from another.
d Results obtained from only one method are likely to be untrustworthy.

47 Clients may have different views on what respect means. Which of the following does this suggest?

a You may need to offer a common definition of respect in your questionnaire.
b You should avoid asking questions about respect.
c Clients may be confused about what respect means.
d Qualitative methods should always be used.

48 Clients' views on the quality of care that they receive may be influenced by the personalities of themselves and their carers. Which of the following is most likely to help the research to avoid this problem?
a Avoid asking questions about quality of care.
b Set out a definition of quality for respondents which avoids personality issues.
c Ask only open questions about quality.
d Instruct respondents not to involve personalities in their answers.

49 A continuum of care may be defined as:
a A care service which caters for all needs.
b The need for care from more than one service.
c People needing care throughout their lives.
d A care service where the parts are not seen as separate but as part of an overall caring service.

50 A service that is seamless may be defined as:
a One having smooth administrative procedures.
b One which emphasises the individuality of clients.
c One which has no perceptible breaks in service delivery.
d One which employs caring staff.

51 Clients may have views on the smoothness of transition from one care service to another. Which of the following may be an important aspect of this transition?
a Whether information about their needs has been transferred between services.
b Whether they like the care workers in the new service.
c A client's level of need.
b The age of the client.

52 Clients may not feel that a continuum of care matters to them. What should you do about this as a researcher?
a Try to persuade respondents that it does matter so that your results are improved.
b Ignore the issue and carry on with your research.
c Try to find out the nature and strength of clients' views on the issue.
d Warn carers of clients' views.

53 A researcher wants to assess whether clients feel that they receive the levels and types of physical support that services claim to offer. Which of the following approaches may give the best results?
a Ask clients to evaluate the physical support that they receive using a single open question.
b Ask clients to choose a single option in answer to a fixed-response question about physical support.
c Use in-depth interviews methods to find out clients' views on the support that they receive.
d Compile a list of the physical supports that services claim to offer and ask clients to indicate which they receive, and at what level.

54 Some clients may see financial support as a personal matter. Which of the following methods could you use to get information about this?
a Explain to clients that it is important that they answer questions about financial support.
b Offer clients a pre-coded prompt card to choose an answer so that they only need to indicate a code number.
c Try to spring the question on clients so that they answer spontaneously.
d Tell clients that others have revealed their financial needs to you in detail.

55 Control of care is related to the concept of empowerment. Empowerment means:
a Carers have power over clients.
b Clients have full control over the behaviour of carers.
c Clients have control and influence over their care.
d Clients have control over financial aspects of their care.

56 The ease with which information may be obtained by clients is an aspect of the control they have over their care. Which of the following may be true of this information?
a Clients may not be aware of information that is held about them.
b Clients should not need to have access to a lot of the information held about them.
c Carers should protect clients from knowing too much about their cases.
d Services are likely to routinely send to clients copies of all information held about them.

57 Clients may have been helped to develop skills during their care. Which of the following approaches may collect the best data on this issue?
- **a** Asking clients a single open question about skills they have developed.
- **b** Asking carers what skills clients have developed.
- **c** Asking clients a single fixed-response question.
- **d** Asking clients a series of questions about skills that they have, and a follow-up question about how the skills were developed.

58 Some clients may feel that they should not be in control of the planning and delivery of their care, believing that it is best left to experts. How could you find out the level of involvement that these clients have been offered?
- **a** By asking carers.
- **b** By insisting to clients that they should have control.
- **c** By exploring the clients' experience of care to assess what involvement may have been offered.
- **d** By asking care service managers what level of involvement clients are offered.

59 When designing questions for a research project, which of the following is it important to consider?
- **a** Questions should have a variety of formats to keep respondents' interest.
- **b** Questions should be mainly of the fixed-response type.
- **c** Questions should be mainly open.
- **d** Question style should be similar throughout.

60 Finding out how services themselves see their work is important if clients' views are to be compared with this. Which of the following is good advice to follow in this research?
- **a** Don't give service staff prior warning of your information needs to avoid prejudicing their responses.
- **b** Accept that what service staff tell you is likely to be true.
- **c** Structure your research so that you have clear ideas of what you want to find out.
- **d** Don't waste time studying publications produced by the service.

Fast Facts

Acceptability Services should satisfy the reasonable expectations of users.

Accessibility Services should be easily available to users in terms of time, distance and ethos.

Advocacy Speaking for another person and representing their interests on their behalf.

Appropriateness A service should be that which the users require.

Assessment and care management The process of assessing, co-ordination and implementing services to meet an individual's needs.

Assessor The person undertaking the assessment of need of an individual. (It may be the same person as the care manager.)

Care manager The person undertaking the care management process in order to address the needs of the individual.

Care package A combination of services designed to meet the assessed needs of a person requiring care.

Care plan (macro) A care plan is a written document which outlines how the needs on an individual are to be met. It lists all the agencies which will be involved.

Care plan (micro) The plan which the individual service provider will use to describe the action plan for a client within his or her own care setting.

Care planning The process of negotiation between assessor, client, carers and other agencies on the most appropriate ways of meeting assessed needs, within available resources and incorporating them into an individual's care plan.

Children Act 1989 A major piece of legislation which aims to clarify the law relating to children.

Choice The right of clients to be able to make choices about the care they receive.

Client rights The rights of clients to particular standards of treatment.

Code of practice A guide to good practice in the interpretation of the Mental Health Act.

Community Health Councils These monitor the services commissioned by District Health Authorities (DHAs). They represent the views of health service clients (service users).

Confidentiality The right of clients to have private information about themselves kept secret.

Continuum of care Continuum of care refers to the idea of a care service which is continuous, with each part blending smoothly with others. Clients experiencing a continuum of care should feel that each service works together as part of a coherent whole.

Data Data refers to the facts and information that are collected by research. Data can be qualitative and expressed verbally, or quantitative and expressed numerically.

Department of Health A central government body which administers health and social care.

Dignity Being worthy of respect and possessing pride and self-esteem.

Discrimination Treating some people less well than others.

Effectiveness Services should achieve the intended objectives.

Efficiency Services should achieve maximum benefit for minimum cost.

Environmental Health Officers They have the task of protecting people living or working in their area.

Equity The principle that users have equal access to and/or benefit from services.

Expectations In the Patient's Charter these are standards of service which the NHS is aiming to achieve.

Health education Programmes aimed at enhancing well-being and preventing or diminishing ill health in individuals and groups.

Health promotion A programme of health-enhancing activities.

Health protection The use of traditional preventative public health activities.

Independence The right of clients to be free of control by others, and to be able to help attend to their own needs.

In-depth interview In-depth interviewing is a research method which involves an unstructured conversation between the interviewer and the respondent. In-depth interviews collect qualitative data.

Inspection The process of external examination intended to establish whether a service is managed and provided to stated quality standards.

Key worker The service-providing practitioner who has most contact with the client. (May undertake similar co-ordinating function as care manager.)

Local Authority Social Services Social Services Departments (SSDs) are responsible for ensuring that clients' social care needs are met in the community.

Mental Health Act 1983 This Act provides professionals with the power to make decisions about a person's welfare when that person, due to a mental disorder, is not able to make decisions regarding his or her own welfare.

Mental Health (Patients in the Community) Bill This refers to 'after-care under supervision'.

Monitoring The process by which the implementation of the care plan is evaluated. It also supports clients, carers and service providers in delivering quality services.

Monitoring worker The person who undertakes the monitoring process. (It may be the same person as the assessor and care manager.)

Need A need is an essential requirement which must be satisfied to ensure that an individual reaches a state of health and social well-being.

Patient's Charter This refers to the rights and expectations of users of the health service.

Population The whole group that a survey or research project is concerned with. A population usually consists of people, though it can be other things such as households.

Provider Any person, group of persons or organisation that sells a community care service to a purchaser.

Purchaser An organisation that holds the budget to buy in necessary services.

Qualitative data Data which cannot be expressed in numerical form. Qualitative data is descriptive, and is often about attitudes, opinions and values. Qualitative research methods seek to collect this type of data.

Quantitative data Data which is expressed in numerical form. Quantitative research methods seek to collect this type of data.

Questionnaire A list of questions designed to collect primary data. Questionnaires are filled in by the respondents themselves, without an interviewer being present.

Research The process of findings things out in an organised and thoughtful way.

Respondent A person who provides data for a social investigation.

Review A formal meeting attended by the client, carer and service providers in order to reassess the needs of the individual and revise the care plan as necessary.

Reviewing The process by which the needs of the individual are reassessed with a view to revising the care plan. Reviewing is undertaken at specified intervals.

Sample A group chosen from the population on which research is conducted directly. Samples are intended to be representative of the population as a whole.

Seamless service Working across all agencies to provide the best care.

Service specifications Statements describing the requirements of the services which the purchaser expects to buy.

Statutory organisations Health and care services are provided by statutory, voluntary and private organisations. Statutory organisations must be set up by law (statute) to provide a service or range of services. The National Health Service and local authority Social Service Departments form the two main branches of the health and social care industry.

Structured interviewing A method of social research which uses tightly controlled interviews to collect data. Structured interviewing aims to minimise differences between each interview to help eliminate bias.

Supervision Registers These are intended to reinforce the support and care for vulnerable mentally ill people in the community embodied in the care programme approach.

Voluntary organisations Voluntary organisations provide a vast network of services to bridge gaps in statutory provision. Their services are often provided free of charge. Voluntary organisations are non-profit making.

References and further reading

Beardshaw, V. and Towell, D., 1990 'Assessment and Case Management' in *Briefing Paper No. 10,* King's Fund

British Association of Social Workers, 1990, *Managing Care,* BASW

NHS, *The Patient's Charter*

Seymour, J., and Girardet, H., 1987, *Blueprint for a Green Planet,* Dorling Kindersley

Smale, P., Tuson, G., Biehal, N., and Marsh, P., 1993, *Empowerment, Assessment, Care Management and the Skilled Worker*

Social Services Inspectorate, 1991, *Care Management and Assessment – Practitioners' Guide,* HMSO

Social Services Inspectorate, *Getting the Message Across,* HMSO Guidance document

Turton, P., and Orr, J., 1985, *Learning to Care in the Community,* Hodder and Stoughton

Chapter 19

Health education campaigns

Health has been at the forefront of the news in recent years with the government producing documents such as *The Health of the Nation* (1992) in an attempt to set targets for the nation's health and to initiate ways of implementing these targets and monitoring their success.

This chapter explores health education and investigates the different aspects that health education campaigns focus on. It investigates the concepts of health, health education and the different levels of health education. This includes different types of campaigns and how messages are affected by factors such as age, gender and activity.

Before looking in detail at health education, it is worth defining the terms *health and well-being.*

What is health?

Being healthy means different things to different people. It is very much a personal issue. An individual may be very well aware of the risks to health connected to a habit such as smoking, but he or she may still do it – for example, a doctor or nurse may smoke.

Some habits create a dependency which is hard to break. This, can prevent an individual breaking the habit despite the fact that he or she is aware of the risks to health.

Think it over

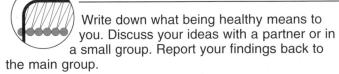

Write down what being healthy means to you. Discuss your ideas with a partner or in a small group. Report your findings back to the main group.

Comment on how the ideas are similar or differ.

The World Health Organisation defines health as 'a state of complete physical, mental and social well-being, and not merely the absence of disease or infirmity'.

- *Physical health* covers the normal functioning of the body.
- *Mental health* covers the health of the mind and being able to think clearly and carry out intellectual processes. It can also include being able to express emotions appropriately and cope with demands on the mind, such as stress and worry.
- *Social health* covers being able to form and keep relationships, both on a personal and professional level. As much of modern life involves contact with others, this is an important aspect of health and it is often said that loneliness can be a major contributor to ill-health.

The World Health Organisation definition provides a starting point for looking at the idea of being healthy. It might be suggested that this definition is somewhat unrealistic as complete physical, mental and social well-being is hard to achieve, but the definition does emphasise a holistic view of health. It highlights that being healthy is not just a physical matter. For example, an individual who has suffered a bereavement may be physically healthy, but for a while at least may not be in full mental health.

It is also important to remember that each of the 'categories' often links with another. A physical illness can have an effect on the mental health of an individual. For example, a pregnant woman whose pregnancy is in danger due to high blood pressure may have to spend a considerable time in hospital. She may become depressed because she cannot do much and is away from her family. So mental, social and physical health cannot be seen in isolation from each other. A health education programme should reflect this.

Think it over

Go back to your ideas on what being healthy means. How do your ideas fit within the categories of physical, mental and social well-being?

An individual's state of health can have an effect on everything else that they do. Health can affect a person's ability to work and consequently his or her earning potential, which in turn has an effect on lifestyle.

Health is also something that changes, more often for some people than others. An individual who suffers from migraines may have days when he or she is not healthy and cannot function as normal, but other days when no symptoms are present. Alternatively, an individual with progressive AIDS may be physically ill all of the time compared with someone who does not have the illness, but will have some days which are better than others. Such times may be considered times of health by the individual.

The definition of health changes, therefore, depending on what you compare it to. People with physical disabilities may always be regarded as physically ill by others, but in their own eyes they live to their potential and become 'ill' only when they are unable to function to their own accepted levels.

In short, the definition of health is not an easy or clear one. It covers may facets of an individual, varies according to circumstances, and is constantly changing.

What factors affect health?

It is difficult to look at what health is without considering the factors that affect an individual's health. These are more complex than many people think. It is useful to look at them on three levels – the individual, the family and the society or environment. Each of these levels interlink and have an effect on each other, which should be reflected in any health education campaign. For example, a middle-aged man may want to change a habit which is proving to be a risk to his health, such as eating a high-fat, high-sugar diet. This is especially important if he is obese and is running the risk of a heart attack. However, he needs the support of his family to do this and if he relies on his wife to shop and cook food for him and she does not appreciate the need to change, he will not succeed. Equally, he may need his workplace to support him by providing healthier food for working lunches. Both of these situations have a direct effect on his ability to change, but he may have little control over them.

What is health education?

There is often confusion between the terms 'health promotion' and 'health education'. *Health education* focuses on the individual and aims to make him or her aware of factors that affect health. It provides information on ways to improve health. Essentially it empowers people to make informed decisions about the choices they make in their lives which affect their health. It can involve changing habits but this is not always its main aim.

Health promotion is a much broader term. The World Health Organisation's 1984 definition of health promotion is 'the process of enabling people to increase control over, and to improve, their health'. Health promotion involves not only improving personal health, but also the wider health issues such as protecting the environment, food safety, and personal safety in the workplace – issues that affect wider society.

However, you can provide people with the evidence and all the facts, but *they* have to make the decision to act upon it. See Chapter 12 for a full discussion of these issues.

Who provides health education?

Health education occurs in a number of different ways and through a range of different people. The common factor is that people and methods all aim to improve health either through education or prevention (Figure 19.1).

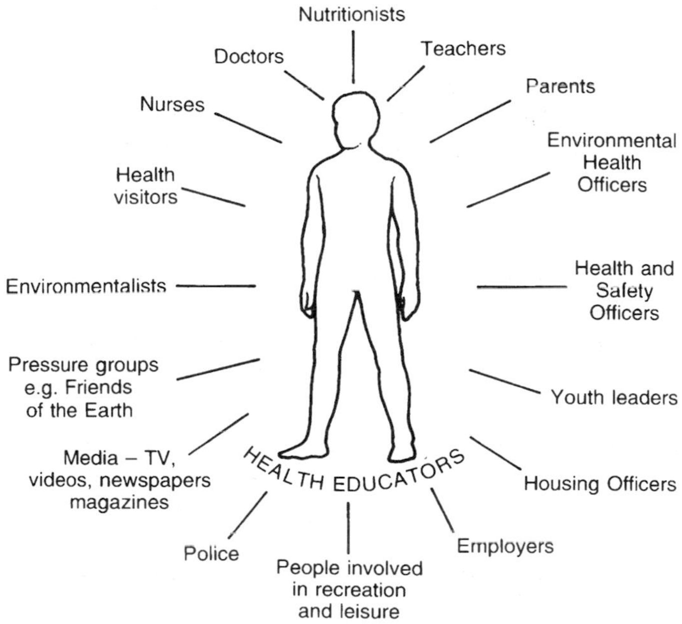

Figure 19.1 People and agencies involved in health education

Think it over

Make a list of all the people and agencies:

a you have had contact with in terms of health education

b who have had an effect on your health in an indirect way.

Levels of health education

Health education occurs on different levels. Ewles and Simnet (1992) suggested three levels:

- *Primary health education* (prevention) Health promotion aimed at informing different groups about health-related issues with the aim of prevention, for example telling children about the risks related to smoking in the hope that they will not take up the habit.
- *Secondary health education* (curative) Health advice which encourages people to change the habits they already have. This may be a result of symptoms and/or illnesses connected with a habit where an individual needs to ensure it does not get worse. For example, an overweight individual may receive health promotion advice on healthy eating, weight loss and how to eat a diet to prevent him or her becoming obese. Obesity is associated with heart attacks, varicose veins and breathlessness.
- *Tertiary health education* (adjustment) This involves educating the individual to get the most out of life when he or she has an irreversible or chronic illness or condition. For example, rehabilitating an individual who has had a heart bypass operation and advising him or her on necessary changes in lifestyle, such as diet and exercise.

Whatever the intended outcome, every health education campaign will need to consider the *target group,* as this can affect the approach and level of information provided. It is important to remember that all groups may need to be educated, but their stage of development and their needs will vary. A target group may be defined by:

- age, for example children, older people, adolescents
- activity, for example, smokers or non-smokers, drug users or non-users
- gender – male or female
- specific needs, which may be temporary, such as pregnancy, or permanent, such as people with learning difficulties.

Working with a group can be complex as groups often have a social identity, part of which may include certain behaviours or activities. Therefore, campaigns could be attempting to change aspects of a sub-culture within a society and these may be well rooted in the ethos of the group and difficult to change. The scale of the required change can sometimes be large. Groups form an important part of people's individual identity and change may require people to question who they are. As health education campaigns aim at the individual, a situation may be created where an individual is in conflict with the ethos of his or her group. The strength of the group can be a powerful factor and so the choice may not always be the healthy one.

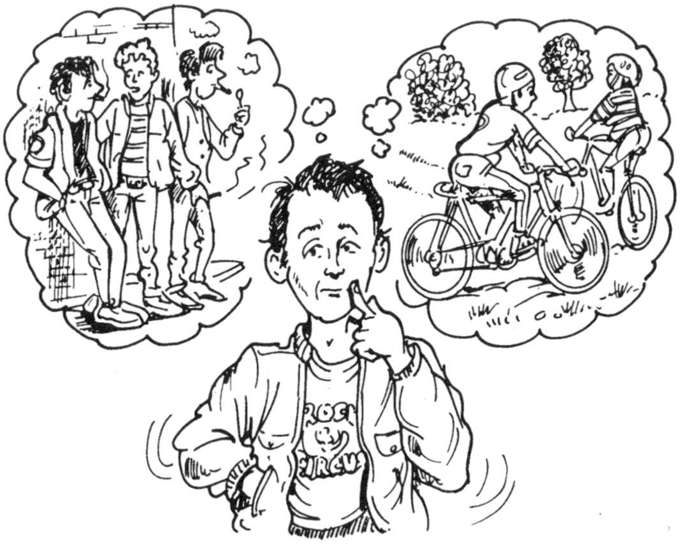

The target group will affect:

- the language used
- the presentation of the information
- the emphasis of the information
- the content of the information.

Language

The complexity of the language used will differ according to the target group. A promotion aimed at children will use simpler language than one aimed at adults. Equally, a promotion aimed at professionals in a particular field is likely to use professional jargon, whereas one aimed at the 'average' man or woman in the street is more likely to use straightforward language. Language can be a means of reaching a client group. Certain sub-cultures are known to have their own set of expressions which may be exploited in a promotion to make the message more credible. For example, a drugs awareness promotion aimed at adolescents may use the slang names for the drugs to make the message seem more relevant to the target group.

Presentation

The way in which a message is presented can often influence whether the recipient gives it a second thought. There may be situations where a large amount of dense continuous writing will be guaranteed to discourage the target group from reading it, and then the message will be lost. In promotions aimed at children and adolescents, the use of pictures, diagrams and cartoons to support any text may make it more readable, and so more effective.

Equally in a live presentation, a high proportion of lecturing from the front may not be as effective as audience participation through group work. Less factual knowledge may be covered in group work, but what is covered may be more memorable.

Think it over

Think of a learning situation which was successful for you. What was it about the situation that made it successful? Was the situation suitable for one target group, or could it be used with other target groups?

Emphasis of the message

Some aspects of health education, such as the risks of smoking, are relevant to many target groups. However, the emphasis of a message will change according to the target group's characteristics. For example, to a group of non-smokers, the emphasis might be on giving hard facts aiming to prevent them taking up the habit. To a group of smokers, however, the emphasis might be on pointing out the positive aspects of not smoking and encouraging them to give up the habit. Even with non-smokers there will be differences. The message to a group of non-smoking children could be less complex and hard-hitting than one to adult non-smokers.

Content of the message

Some health education campaigns are aimed at specific target groups, such as male or female. For example, health education material focusing on breast and testicular cancer will be aimed at women and men respectively. 'Well Woman' and 'Well Man' clinics will be promoted to each gender as appropriate – they are not open to both.

Some campaigns are aimed at groups with specific needs. An example of this may be the promotion of regular eye tests for people with diabetes because of the increased risk of glaucoma. Material might be produced in different languages for groups for whom English is a second language. There are many examples of general health promotion material being packaged for a specific group. For example, the campaign for the use of condoms as protection against unwanted pregnancies and AIDS is aimed at both males and females, but there are specific campaigns for the gay community who have a specific need.

Areas of health education advice

Health education can be given on a range of topics from personal health to personal safety. However, before being able to comment on the effectiveness of any campaign, it is important for you to be aware of the issues that surround a topic. Aims and objectives should also be identified. Only then is it possible to make valid judgements on factors such as the accuracy of the message, its impact and possible effects, and the extent to which it achieves its aims and objectives.

Background understanding may also help to identify which aspects of any health risk might best be used as the focus message for different client groups.

Aims and objectives

The aims and objectives of health education programmes may include:

- *self-empowerment,* which involves giving the individual the knowledge and understanding to be able to make an informed choice about something
- *to change behaviour/attitude,* the aim being to bring about change in some way
- *to provide knowledge,* to increase understanding about a topic
- *to raise awareness,* which might not involve a behaviour change as such, but is an attempt to increase a person's awareness of a topic, for example in AIDS education health professionals aim to inform people who may be at risk of

contracting the HIV virus about how they can protect themselves
- *to meet national or local targets* (funding for services may depend on these)
- *to promote the interests of a particular group,* for example to raise support for charities who research into cancer
- *to promote a hidden message,* to further commercial interests or engage in product competition.

Aims are broad statements about what the campaign hopes to achieve from a programme or session. They often begin with a verb, for example:

- to explore the issue of smoking and health
- to appreciate the role of diet in coronary heart disease.

There may be one or several aims to a programme and this might cover an hour's work or a year's campaign. Aims are broken down into objectives.

Objectives develop from the aims and the two are therefore linked together. Objectives are more specific and often include measurable targets. They may also state intentions of how to achieve the aim they are connected to. Objectives should be attainable and if possible measurable, for example:

- to reduce the percentage of fat in the average diet by raising the profile of low-fat products via taste tests
- to provide the audience with information on the effect excessive fat in a diet may have on the arteries.

The aims represent long-term goals and the objectives explain how they will be achieved.

Issues in health education campaigns

Common issues which health education campaigns have focused on include:

- promotion of healthy-living practices, such as a healthy diet, the need to increase exercise, the role of contraception
- campaigns to reduce disease, such as immunisation programmes
- minimising the risk from potentially harmful living practices, such as substance abuse, smoking, alcohol, unsafe sexual practices and sexually transmitted diseases
- promoting personal safety and security, for example home security, road safety, safe use of electricity/gas and appliances.

Promoting healthy-living practices

Diet

One aspect of everyone's lives which has been connected with health is the diet the individual chooses to eat. Every individual needs a *balanced diet* appropriate to his or her age and stage of life. This diet should contain all the nutrients in the appropriate quantities for the body to grow and function efficiently. However, the *type and source* of food providing these nutrients has been the focus of a number of health education campaigns. It has been shown that diet can have a marked effect on health (Figure 19.2).

In 1983, the National Advisory Committee for Nutrition Education (NACNE) published a report of findings and recommendations for improving the diet. Essentially they found that many conditions such as obesity, cancer, high blood pressure and coronary heart disease were connected with diet. Therefore, they produced recommendations for change. These were to:

- reduce the total proportion of energy in the diet which comes from fat, but also to obtain more of that energy from vegetable sources of fat rather than animal sources

A diet high in	**Contributes to**	**Change from**	**Change to**
Total fat and saturated fat	Heart disease Obesity	Animal fat	Vegetable fats
Refined carbohydrate e.g. sugar	High calories Obesity Tooth decay	Sugar Cakes and biscuits	Sweeteners Fruit
Salt	High blood pressure	Salt Salty foods	No salt, herbs Salt-free foods
Alcohol	High calories Obesity Organ damage	Alcohol levels above recommended units	Low alcohol drinks Alcohol-free drinks Soft drinks
A diet low in	**Contributes to**	**Change from**	**Change to**
Unrefined carbohydrate e.g. fibre	Constipation Colon cancer	White products e.g. bread, rice	Brown'/ wholemeal products More fresh fruit and vegetables

Figure 19.2 The health benefits of changing your diet

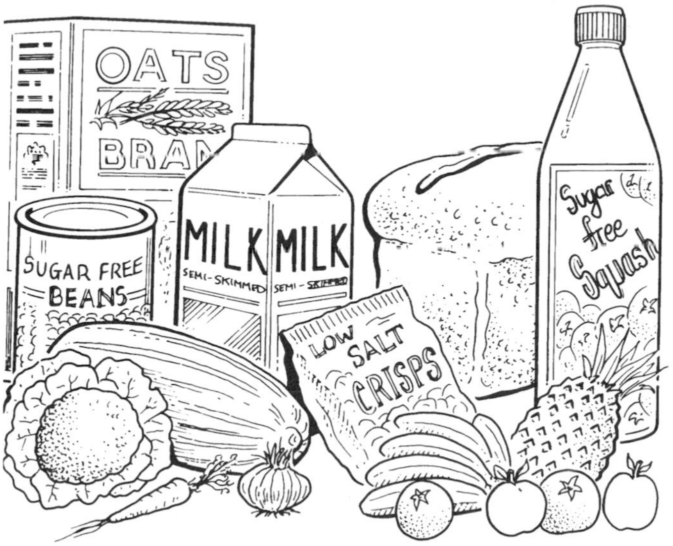

- increase intake of non-starch polysaccharides or dietary fibre
- decrease intake of refined sugar
- decrease intake of salt
- decrease intake of alcohol.

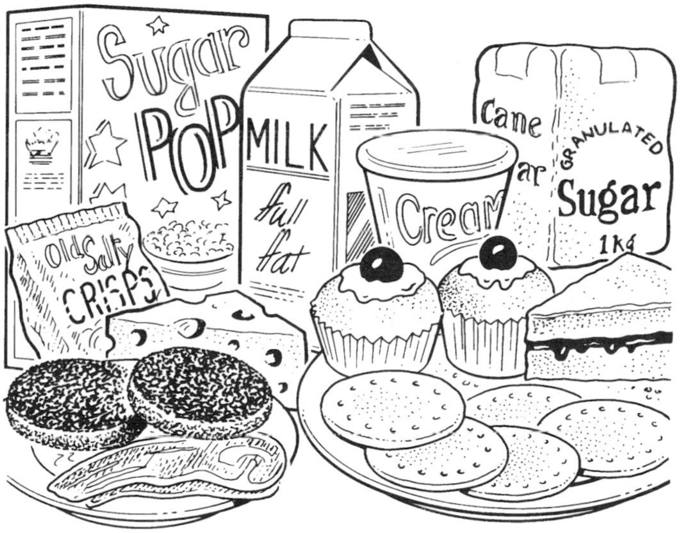

The committee suggested 15 years as the timescale for their recommendations to be adopted because the changes would require a considerable change in people's diets. Thus they gave targets for 1990 and the year 2000 (Figure 19.3).

One example of a health education campaign around general dietary change was the Traffic Light System, aimed at simplifying the message particularly for school children. Red was linked to foods to avoid,

Area	1983 levels of intake	Recommended changes by 1990	2000
Total fat (% of diet)	38%	34%	30%
Sucrose (kg/head/yr)	39 kg	34 kg	20 kg
Dietary fibre (g/head/day)	20 g	25 g	30 g
Salt (mg/head/day)	12 mg	11 mg	9 mg
Alcohol (% of total energy)	6%	5%	4%

Figure 19.3 A summary of the NACNE recommendations

amber to foods to eat cautiously and green to those which could be eaten without concern.

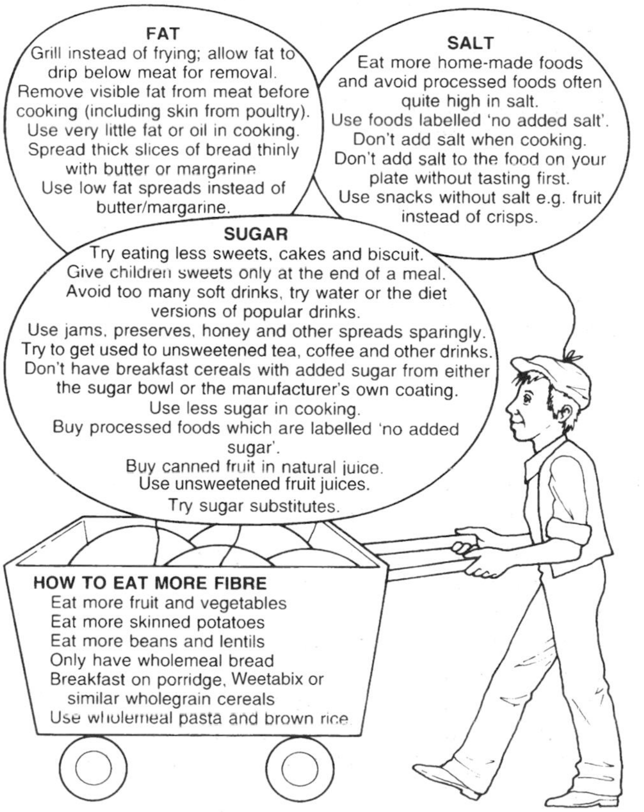
FAT
Grill instead of frying; allow fat to drip below meat for removal.
Remove visible fat from meat before cooking (including skin from poultry).
Use very little fat or oil in cooking.
Spread thick slices of bread thinly with butter or margarine.
Use low fat spreads instead of butter/margarine.
SALT
Eat more home-made foods and avoid processed foods often quite high in salt.
Use foods labelled 'no added salt'.
Don't add salt when cooking.
Don't add salt to the food on your plate without tasting first.
Use snacks without salt e.g. fruit instead of crisps.
SUGAR
Try eating less sweets, cakes and biscuit.
Give children sweets only at the end of a meal.
Avoid too many soft drinks, try water or the diet versions of popular drinks.
Use jams, preserves, honey and other spreads sparingly.
Try to get used to unsweetened tea, coffee and other drinks.
Don't have breakfast cereals with added sugar from either the sugar bowl or the manufacturer's own coating.
Use less sugar in cooking.
Buy processed foods which are labelled 'no added sugar'.
Buy canned fruit in natural juice.
Use unsweetened fruit juices.
Try sugar substitutes.
HOW TO EAT MORE FIBRE
Eat more fruit and vegetables
Eat more skinned potatoes
Eat more beans and lentils
Only have wholemeal bread
Breakfast on porridge, Weetabix or similar wholegrain cereals
Use wholemeal pasta and brown rice

Figure 19.4 Eating a healthier diet

Think it over

The *Health of the Nation* document published in 1992 touched on dietary issues with regard to coronary heart disease, obesity and cancer. The statistics showed that the targets devised by NACNE ten years before had not been met and this new document repeated the same advice. Why do you think people have not made the necessary changes?

Exercise

Exercise is an important aspect of both physical and mental fitness. It can also help reduce the stress of modern life. It is suggested that an individual should aim to do 20 minutes of exercise, three times a week to achieve fitness. This exercise can range from gentle walking to strenuous swimming.

There are many different ways to exercise. But whatever the exercise is, it should work the heart, lungs and muscles. Most exercise is a combination of *anaerobic* (which stretches muscles) and *aerobic* (which works the heart and lungs). Above all, it must suit the individual's circumstances.

Exercise will develop:

- stamina – the heart's ability to work under strain
- suppleness – the body's ability to bend without damage
- strength – the body's physical power.

It will also improve muscle tone and body shape.

Campaigns to promote sport have include 'Sport for All' which aimed to emphasise sport's all-round appeal.

Reducing the likelihood of disease

This area covers education programmes aimed at raising awareness of the preventative medicine available, such as immunisation programmes, 'Well Man' and 'Well Woman' clinics, child health clinics.

Immunisation

Immunisation is the process of using a vaccine to protect people from a disease. Vaccines contain either small parts of the bacteria which cause the disease or small amounts of the chemical they produce. Vaccines are administered by mouth or injection and stimulate the body the produce antibodies which will protect the person against the disease in future should they come into contact with it. This will mean that the infection will not develop or it will be less serious.

Common infections for which immunisation is available include:

- meningitis (Hib form)
- diphtheria
- whooping cough
- tetanus
- polio
- tuberculosis
- measles
- mumps
- rubella.

Immunisations are given at various times – many in the first year of life with boosters at later dates. They are given so early because some diseases, such as whooping cough, are very dangerous for young babies. It is believed that babies have some natural immunity at birth which lasts for a short time, about two or three months. Figure 19.5 sets out the timetable for immunisations.

When due	Immunisations		Type
At 2 months	Hib		One injection
	Diphtheria Whooping cough Tetanus	DTP	One injection
	Polio		By mouth
At 3 months	Hib		One injection
	Diphtheria Whooping cough Tetanus	DTP	One injection
	Polio		By mouth
At 4 months	Hib		One injection
	Diphtheria Whooping cough Tetanus	DTP	One injection
	Polio		By mouth
At 12–15 months	Measles Mumps Rubella	MMR	One injection
3–5 years (around school entry)	Diphtheria Tetanus Polio		Booster Injection Booster by mouth
Girls 10–14 years	Rubella		One injection
Girls/boys 13 years	Tuberculosis		One injection (BCG)
School leavers 15–19 years	Tetanus Polio		One injection Booster by mouth

Source: Based on a leaflet issued by the Health Education Authority and the Department of Health

Figure 19.5 Timetable for immunisations

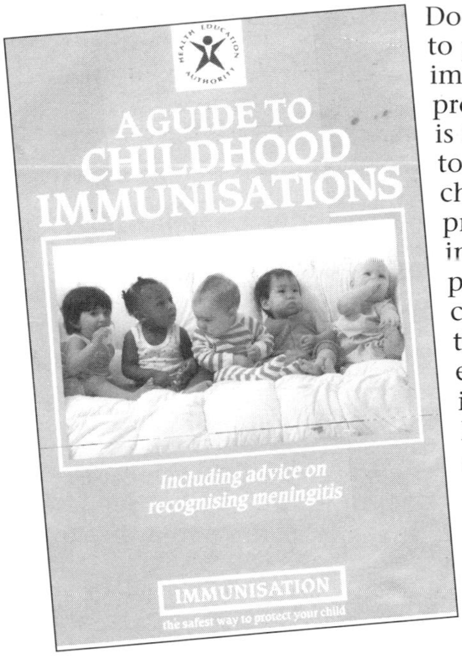

Doctors are funded to promote immunisation programmes and it is in their interests to ensure all children in their practice are immunised. Some parents are concerned about the possible side effects of immunisation. However, the risk of lasting complications is small compared to the potential effect of contracting the disease itself.

Education about immunisation programmes begins at ante-natal classes for expectant mothers. Once registered with a GP, the child is automatically put onto the immunisation programme and is routinely called for the immunisations. Doctors cannot force parents to bring their children to have the immunisation but they try to follow up every parent who does not.

In times of concern, other ways have been used to promote immunisation. In 1995, it was believed that a particularly strong strain of the measles virus was developing, which could cause severe illness and even death in the UK. There was a large media campaign on TV, in newspapers and magazines and in schools to try to ensure that every teenage child had access to an immunisation programme.

Heart disease

Coronary heart disease is a condition which has increased with modern living. It is currently estimated that around 465 people may die from heart disease each day. One in four victims are women and death rates in the north of England are twice those in the south-east.

Heart disease may result from the build up of fatty patches on the lining of the arteries. This is known as atheroma. We are not aware of these changes until the atheromatous patch has narrowed the blood vessel so much that the part of the body it serves begins to suffer. For example atheroma in:

- the heart leads to pain on exertion (known as *angina pectoris*)
- the brain causes periods of confusion and poor memory (called by doctors *transient ischaemic attacks*)
- skeletal muscle causes pain on walking short distances (called *intermittent claudication*). The Roman emperor Claudius suffered from this!

After many years, when atheroma has become extensive, the previously smooth inner arterial lining may be roughened and the usually streamlined blood flow turbulent. These two factors possibly influence the next stage of the disease process (see Figure 19.6). A clot or thrombus forms on and within the atheromateous plaque until the whole vessel becomes blocked. Blood flow is suddenly cut off to that part of the organ. If this is a small vessel, the area served might be quite small and after a period of illness the individual will return to normal physical health or near to it. However, this attack should serve as a warning that the circulation is in a poor state and a change of lifestyle will be strongly recommended by medical advisers. If, on the other hand, the vessel is medium to large in diameter, then severe disablement or even death may occur.

Atheroma occurring in the heart or brain is most likely to result in death; in other less vital organs survival is more likely. Such a blockage in the heart is

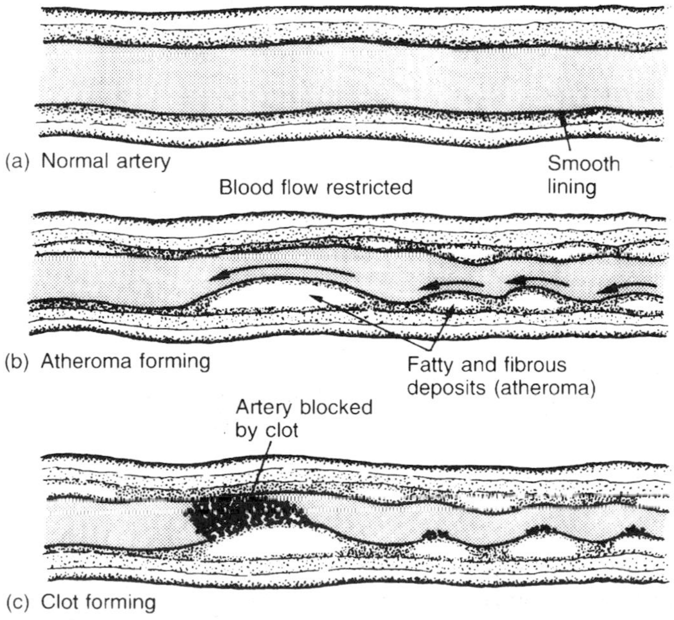

Figure 19.6 Atheroma and clot formation

known as *coronary thrombosis* or heart attack, whereas in the brain it is a *cerebral thombosis* or stroke.

Heart disease tends to run in families so it is described as having *familial tendency,* but families also tend to eat the same foods. As western countries have become richer so the incidence of heart disease has risen. People with diets high in animal fats tend to be at greater risk of developing heart disease. More recently, larger numbers of people have been having their blood cholesterol levels measured, and it has been found that some families have what is considered to be abnormally high levels of blood fats (*hyperlipidaemia*). Such families are being advised to consume diets low in cholesterol, i.e. cutting down on foods such as dairy fats, fat meat and meat products.

Many commercial companies have had business successes in food manufacture by using vegetable fat sources in their products and claiming the product is healthy eating on the label (see Figure 19.7).

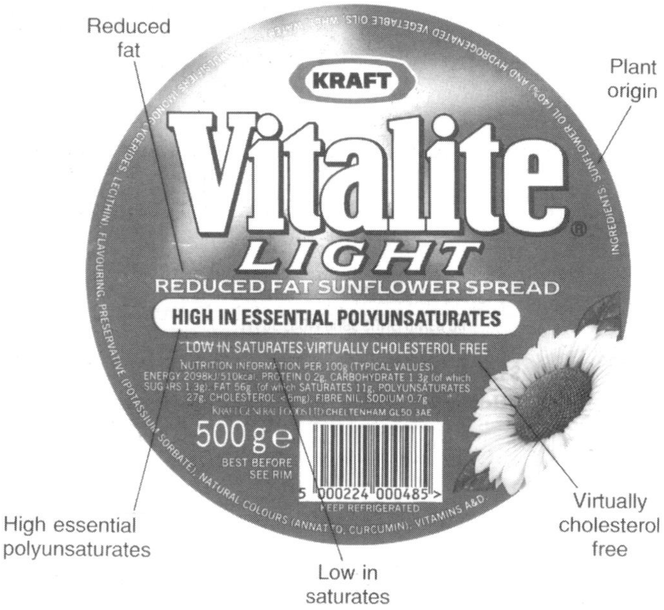

Figure 19.7 Example of a 'healthy' spread

Think it over

What advice would you give to a friend or relative about dietary changes to reduce the incidence of heart disease or stroke with increasing age?

Other risk factors in heart disease are considered to be:

- smoking
- obesity
- stress
- lack of exercise.

Heredity, and ageing may account for approximately 50 per cent of cardio-vascular deaths. Lifestyle choices such as smoking, diet and drug treatment account for the remainder.

Heart attack

This is known as a *coronary* or *coronary thrombosis.* Study Figure 19.8, which shows all the possible symptoms of a heart attack. A victim may suffer from some or all of them.

The role of diet, smoking, and 'lifestyle' are discussed in Chapter 12.

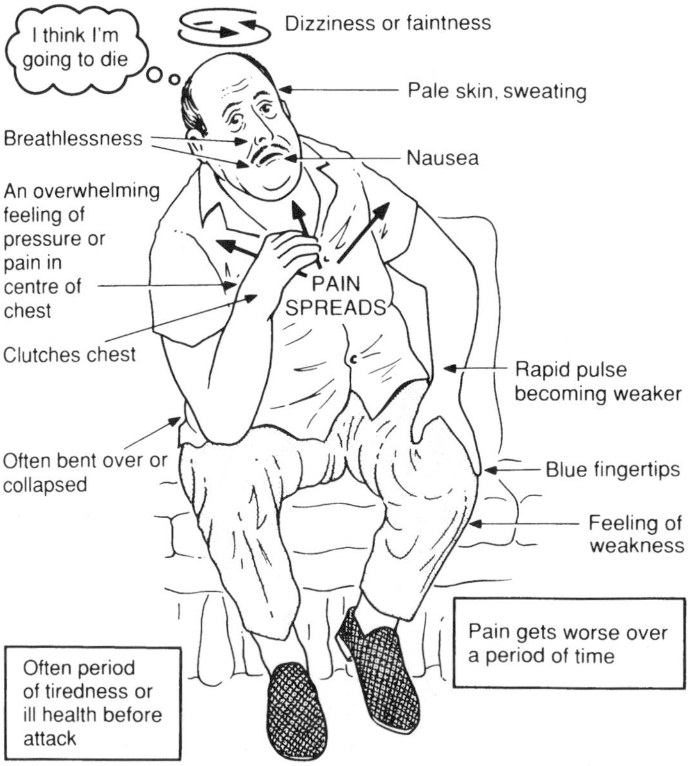

Figure 19.8 The possible symptoms of a heart attack

Campaigns aimed at raising awareness of heart disease address the many factors which contribute to the condition. An example is shown below.

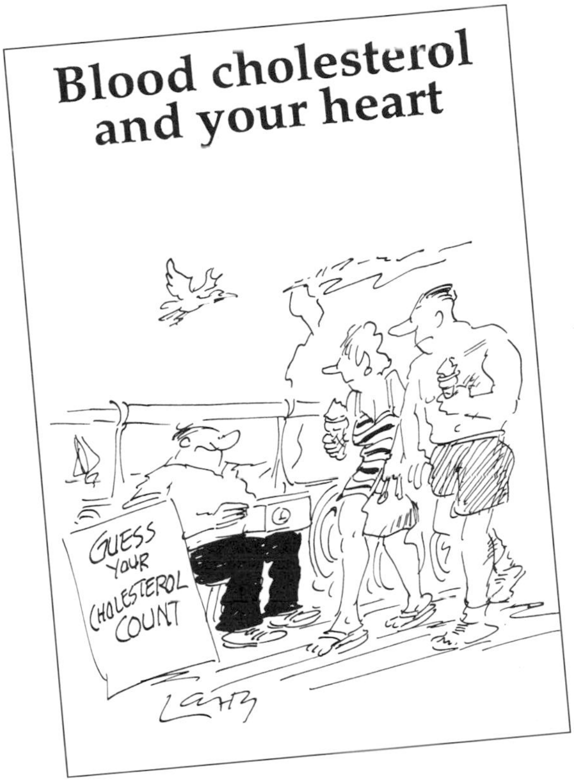

It is interesting to note that a budget of £4.6 million was spent on heart disease prevention programmes through the Health Educational Authority in 1993. This seems a lot of money, but is small compared to the £32 million spent on AIDS prevention programmes.

Cancer

Cancer is another disease which has increased with modern living. After coronary heart disease, cancer is the most common cause of death in the UK. This includes breast, skin, cervical, colon and lung cancers. Cancer is responsible for approximately one quarter of all deaths per year.

Cancer is the term given to any one of a group of diseases where symptoms are caused by the unrestrained growth of cells. Malignant tumours often develop in the major organs such as lungs, skin, breasts and pancreas, but they can also develop in the testes, ovaries and on the tongue. As cancer grows, it spreads into the tissues around it. It can destroy nerves and eat away at bones. Cancer cells also spread to other parts of the body via the blood stream and lymphatic system, forming secondary tumours in other parts of the body.

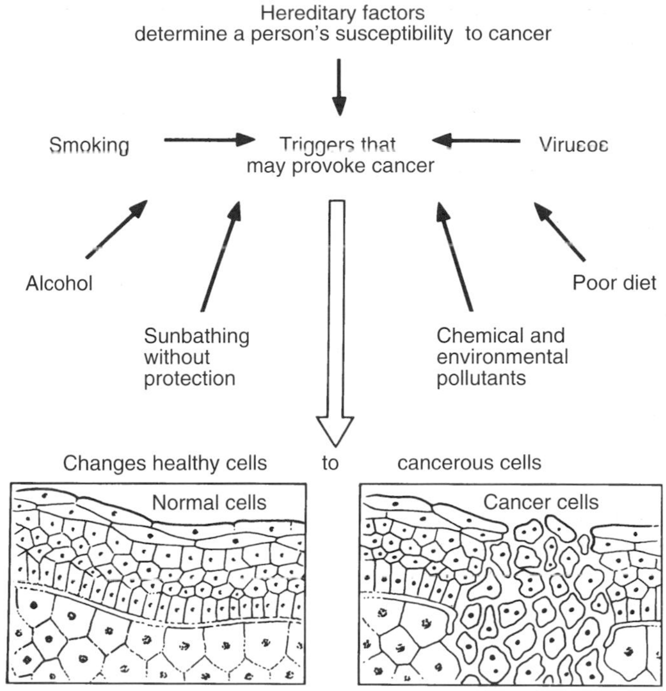

Figure 19.9 Contributory factors in cancer

Two or three or more factors may interact to cause cancers in the skin or body organs (Figure 19.9).

The earlier a cancerous growth is detected, the better the chance of a cure. There are several general symptoms which could indicate the risk of cancer, and they should be checked by a doctor. These include:

- rapid weight loss for no apparent reason
- coughing up phlegm
- a mark or mole which changes appearance and/or bleeds
- coughing up blood
- difficulty swallowing or recurring hoarseness in the throat
- blood in the urine without pain on urination
- lumps or changes in shape of testes or breasts
- bleeding or spotting between periods.

The risk of developing cancer can be reduced by making choices such as not smoking, eating a low-fat, high-fibre diet and consuming only sensible amounts of alcohol. Undertaking all the appropriate screening tests, such as cervical smears and mammograms, can also reduce risk. Undertaking regular self-examination of the testes or breasts, and generally being vigilant about skin changes on the body can also help to detect cancer in the early stages.

Health education campaigns have focused on all of these factors contributing to cancer and on promoting healthy life choices. They have promoted both self-examinations and screening under the NHS for the relevant target groups. The *Health of the Nation* targets for cervical and breast cancers include increasing the number of people who are screened for cancer. Some Regional Health Authorities have built targets into their contracts with the District Health Authorities and Family Health Services Associations. These targets have to be achieved for full funding (*Health of the Nation: One Year On*, 1993).

Sexual practices

Sex is a natural part of life. It offers a way for people to express their feelings for one another and it is also the way humanity reproduces itself. However, being sexually active does carry risks, such as unwanted pregnancy and sexually transmitted diseases, including HIV and AIDS. The current advice is to practise 'safer sex' to minimise risks.

Contraception

Unless they wish to conceive a child, contraception is an extremely important issue for any sexually active couple. However, contraceptive methods can also have a secondary function of preventing the spread of sexually transmitted diseases – including HIV. It is important, therefore, that contraception is seen as a joint responsibility and not just that of the female.

Contraception aims to prevent conception. Therefore a review of the male and female reproductive systems, including how conception occurs, will ensure a better understanding of how each method of contraception is designed to work. An understanding of the reproductive system may also assist in understanding how the spread of STDs may be prevented. A knowledge of contraception is also important in the light of the *Health of the Nation* document (1992) where two of the aims are connected to contraception and sexual health. These are:

- to reduce the incidence of gonorrhea by 20 per cent
- to reduce the number of conceptions in the under-16 age group by at least 50 per cent by the year 2000.

Reproductive systems

From the age of puberty, girls become fertile, this is marked by the start of monthly periods (menstruation). Each ovary produces an egg alternatively on a monthly basis. The egg, once released, travels down the Fallopian tubes to the womb (uterus). In the first part of the monthly cycle the womb lining builds up to become receptive to

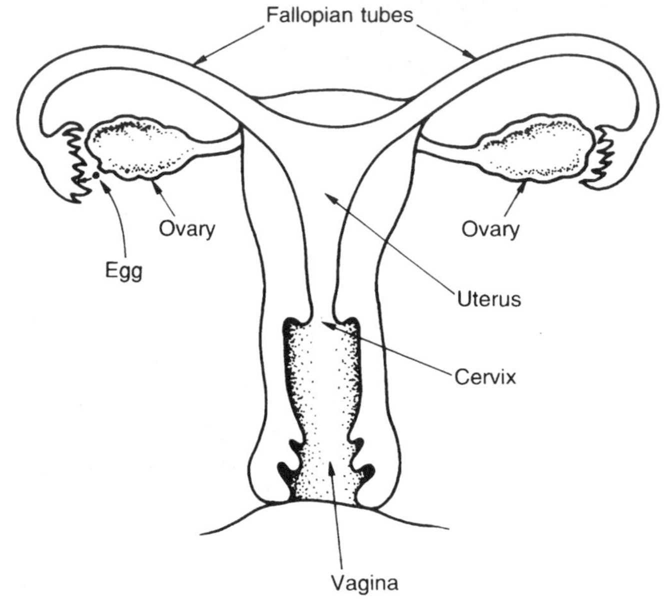

Figure 19.10 Female reproductive system

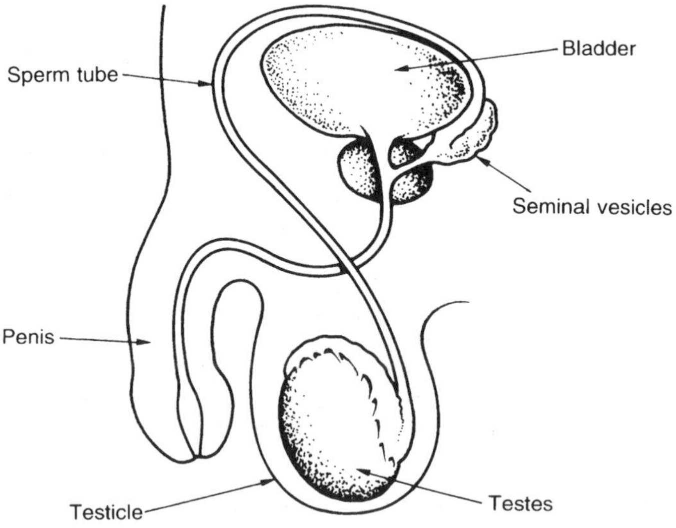

Figure 19.11 Male reproductive system

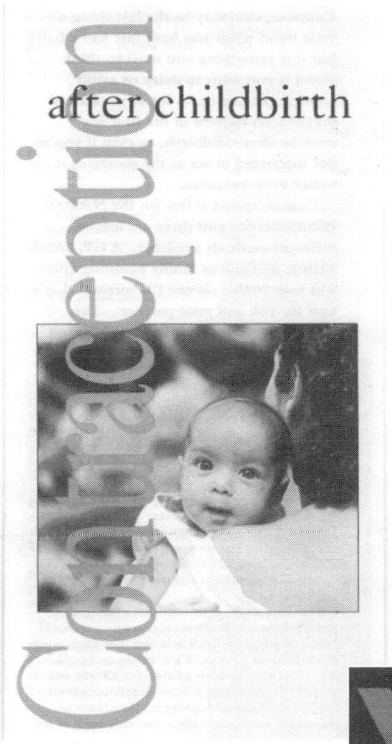

the development of an embryo in case the egg is fertilised. If it is, a pregnancy has begun. If not, the womb lining breaks down and the blood is lost as a period.

The male testes produce sperm. When sexually excited, the penis fills with blood and becomes erect. The sperm mixes with seminal fluid to become semen and is ejaculated. (It is thought that each ejaculation contains at least 300 million sperm.)

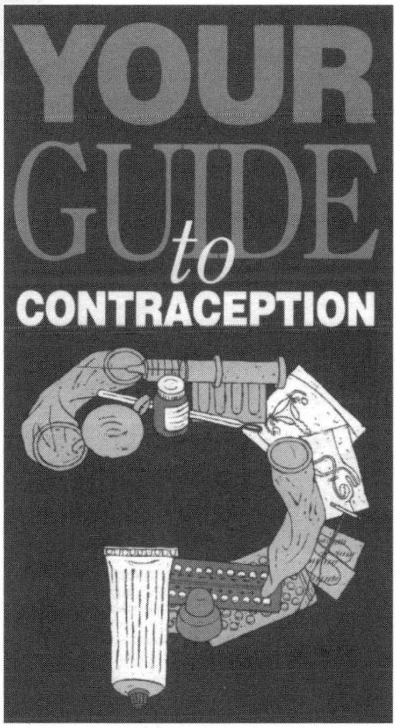

Nature has designed the male and female reproductive systems to complement each other for the purposes of reproduction. During sexual intercourse, the penis enters the vagina and sperm can then be ejaculated closer to the area where fertilisation takes place. The sperm is able to 'swim' its way from where it is ejaculated, through the cervix and into the Fallopian tubes to fertilise the egg. The fertilised egg will then move down from the tube to embed itself in the wall of the uterus where its development will begin. Each method of contraception aims to interfere with this process in one or more ways. Figure 19.12 shows the different methods of contraception and explains how they work.

Each of the different methods of contraception has its own disadvantages and advantages (Figure 19.13), and individuals need to decide what is best for them according to their circumstances. For example, a couple in a long-standing relationship may not be so concerned about the risk of contracting a sexually transmitted disease and therefore do not want a barrier method; whereas an adolescent, in a relatively new relationship, may feel that a barrier method of contraception, such as a condom, is best to reduce the additional risk of contracting HIV.

Sexually transmitted diseases

Sexually transmitted diseases (STDs) can be passed from one individual to another whether they are having sexual intercourse as part of a casual or long-term steady relationship. STDs are termed *genito-urinary diseases,* or GUs, by doctors as they tend to affect the urinary system as well as the genital area. It should be appreciated that anyone can contact an infection – men and women, heterosexuals and homosexuals. Getting an infection is not dependent on having lots of sexual partners; although the more partners an individual has, the greater the risk of contracting or passing on an STD. Sometimes, an infection can lie dormant in one of the partners and then reactivate itself to infect the carrier and his or her partner.

It is therefore important to know how to minimise the risks of infection. Barrier methods of contraception particularly the condom, are effective ways of minimising the risk of contracting STDs.

There are many different types of sexually transmitted diseases. They are often caused by bacteria or viruses. Figure 19.14 gives a summary of different STDs – their causes, symptoms and treatment.

HIV and AIDS

One of the most publicised sexually transmitted diseases in recent years has been HIV/AIDS. This is a relatively new fatal condition which has spread very rapidly. It has therefore been essential to increase awareness of lifestyle choices which can reduce the risk of contracting the virus.

HIV (Human Immuno Deficiency Virus) attacks and damages the body's defence mechanisms, preventing it from effectively fighting certain infections or illnesses. It lives in body fluids – blood, semen and vaginal secretions particularly.

Method	How it works
Combined pill (Progesterone and oestrogen)	Works in three ways: 1 Increases mucus in the cervix – prevents sperm entering womb 2 Prevents womb lining building up so it is unreceptive to the fertilised egg 3 Prevents ovulation Highly reliable
Mini pill	Thickens mucus in neck of womb which acts as a barrier to sperm
Male condom	Covers the penis and collects the semen in the tip, so preventing it from entering the vagina
Female condom	Lines the vagina to prevent the sperm reaching the egg
IUD (Intrauterine device)	A copper wire inserted into the uterus which makes the environment unsuitable for embryo development
Cap/diaphragm	Soft rubber cap with metal ring which fits over the cervix and prevents the sperm reaching the uterus. Must always be used with a spermicide and left for six hours after intercourse
Spermicide	Foam, cream, jelly or foaming tablet inserted high into the vagina before intercourse. They destroy sperm but also act as a barrier. Should always be used with a condom/cap
Sterilisation Male	Should be seen as irreversible Cuts and ties are made in the tubes which carry the sperm from the scrotum to prevent sperm being mixed with semen
Female	Cuts or ties are made in the Fallopian tubes to prevent the egg reaching the uterus or sperm passing up the tubes to the egg
Injection (Depo-Provera)	Similar to combined pill (injectable every three months)
Withdrawal (coitus interruptus)	Man removes penis before ejaculation occurs. Very unreliable as sperm can be released during love-making before full ejaculation
Rhythm method	Relies on estimating the time during the woman's monthly cycle when she is likely to conceive and avoiding intercourse then. Very unreliable as the time of ovulation is not easily predictable.

Figure 19.12 Methods of contraception

Method	Advantages	Disadvantages
Combined pill	Most reliable form of contraception. Reduces blood loss during menstruation. Relieves period pain. Easy to take. Does not interrupt the act of sexual intercourse.	Carries risks such as thrombosis and high blood pressure. Not suitable for women who smoke heavily because of this
Mini pill	Does not interrupt the act of sexual intercourse. Can be used while breast feeding	Must be taken at very regular intervals to be reliable. Periods can be irregular
Condom	Suitable for anyone, including those having unplanned or irregular sex. Helps protect individual from contracting sexually transmitted diseases Protects from the HIV virus	Interrupts the sexual act as it must be put on. Relies on an individual carrying one. Can dull the sensation for the male. Some people find them embarrassing to buy. Can be expensive
IUD	Does not interfere with the sexual act	Can cause heavy irregular and painful periods. Can cause fertilisation of the egg in the Fallopian tubes
Cap		Correct size needed for greatest reliability
Injectable methods	Very reliable. Do not have to think about regular medication	Menstrual cycle may be disturbed
Spermicide		Not very reliable if used alone
Withdrawal method	Does not require any preparation or resources	Not very reliable. Can be frustrating for the couple
Rhythm method	May suit those who, for religious reasons, do not believe in contraceptives, e.g. some Catholic Christians	Not very reliable
Sterilisation	Very reliable. Suitable for couples who know they do not want any more children	Considered irreversible; little opportunity to change your mind, although reversal operations are possible

Figure 19.13 Advantages and disadvantages of different methods of contraception

STD	Cause	Symptoms	Treatment
Gonorrhoea	Bacteria which live in warm moist internal linings of the body	– Discharge from vagina or penis – Irritation or discharge from anus – Pain in lower abdomen in women – Pain on passing urine	Antibiotics
Thrush	Yeast called 'Candida albicans'	– Thick white discharge from vagina – Itching around genitals – Soreness and pain on passing urine	Pessaries and/or cream
Genital warts	Virus	– Warts of varying sizes around genitals	Ointment
Genital herpes	Herpes simplex virus	– Small painful blisters in genital region – Tingling or itching in genital area – Flu-like symptoms (headache, backache) – Pain or tingling on passing urine	Ointment
Pubic lice	Small lice living in pubic hair	Itching and small eggs on pubic hair	Special lotion
Hepatitis B	Virus in blood and bodily fluids, resulting in liver inflammation	Two stages **1** Two to six months after contact with infection: flu-like symptoms including sore throat and cough. Feeling of fatigue, loss of appetite and joint pain. **2** Jaundice stage: skin and eyes take on yellowish tinge. Stools become grey and urine brown. Abdomen is sore	Bed rest and healthy food. Vaccinations are available for people in certain risk situations

Figure 19.14 The causes, symptoms and treatment of STDs

AIDS (Acquired Immune Deficiency Syndrome) is the end stage of a chronic infection by HIV. (A syndrome is a collection of illnesses.) An individual cannot 'catch' AIDS, only HIV. AIDS is said to be present if an HIV positive individual (i.e. after laboratory tests, an individual found to have HIV antibodies in the bloodstream) develops a particular infection or specific cancer with no apparent cause. AIDS first appeared in the 1970s but was not recognised until 1981. There is no cure for HIV or AIDS yet. The virus attacks and destroys certain types of white blood cells known as *lymphocytes*. It enters an uninfected individual through a break in the skin or pink lining tissue (mucosa).

Mode of transmission

Although the virus is known to occur in saliva, tears, breast milk and urine, the 'normal' routes by which it spreads are via blood, genital tract secretions or from mother to baby via the placenta. Main ways of spreading are therefore:

- Sexual transmission, because semen and vaginal fluid carry the virus. The greatest risks are male homosexual and heterosexual anal and vaginal intercourse, especially if there are ulcerations or erosions present. According to the World Health Organisation, nearly half of all newly infected adults are women. Anyone can contract HIV from unsafe sex (intercourse without protection against sexual fluids of a partner).
- From mother to foetus before birth, at delivery or soon after through breast feeding. At present 20 per cent of babies born to infected mothers will have the virus. As more women become infected so will the number of babies born with HIV rise.
- By sharing of equipment between injecting drug users, particularly syringes and needles. This is because they might receive contaminated blood or blood products from the equipment. The government, through the *Health of the Nation* document (1992) has set targets for reducing the numbers of drug users who report sharing injecting equipment within the previous few weeks by at least 50 per cent by 1997 and by at least a further 50 per cent by the year 2000. This would give a maximum of 5 per cent of drug users who practise the habit.

In the UK blood and blood products have been screened for HIV since October 1985, so both receiving and donating blood on this country are safe. All equipment for this purpose is sterilised. Most developed countries in the world share these safe practices but this may not apply to all countries. (Advice can be obtained from the Medical Advisory Service for Travellers Abroad 0171-631-4408.)

In the early years of the disease, many haemophiliacs contracted HIV and AIDS because their blood transfusions were not screened for the virus as they are now.

The virus is fragile and cannot live outside the body for long. It is also inactivated by disinfectants such as alcohol, bleach, peroxide, etc. This means that the virus cannot be passed on by:

- eating food prepared by an HIV infected individual
- being in the same room as, or by coughs and sneezes from, an infected person
- swimming in the same water
- mosquito or other insect bites
- casual contact such as touching, kissing, hugging
- using the same cutlery or crockery as an infected individual
- giving first aid treatment provided that safe hygienic practices are used, for example disposable gloves, disinfecting body fluids, etc.

How do HIV and AIDS affect the body?

Many people infected with HIV are not aware they have the virus and carry on a normal working life, feeling healthy and well.

There is no evidence that rest, exercise or sensible nutrition stops transmission or progression of the infection (Figure 19.15).

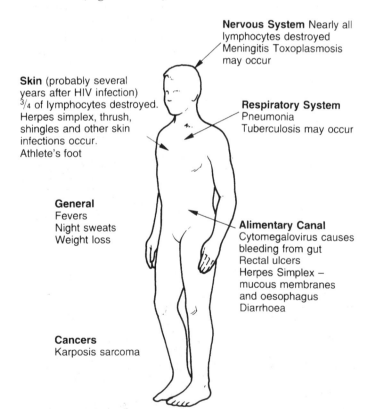

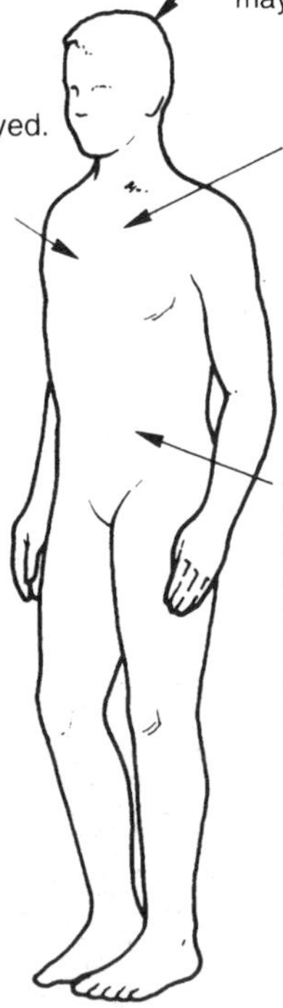

Figure 19.15 AIDS-related illnesses

One of the longest studies so far carried out suggests that about half the number of HIV positive individuals will develop AIDS within 10 years, and eventually 99 per cent will contract it. How long it takes to develop depends on the individual. When AIDS develops, some people die, but others can stay well for a long time if they have good care. Even if an individual becomes seriously ill he or she can often be nursed back to better health for a while. After several years during which the virus gradually destroys the lymphocytes, the body's defence system is unable to cope with certain infections and these are responsible for 90 per cent of the deaths from AIDS. It is believed that everyone who develops full-blown AIDS will die from one of the associated illnesses.

Strategies for control

At present there is no treatment or vaccination to prevent HIV infection, but the disease could be controlled by behavioural changes.

- Screening of blood – already implemented:
  - high-risk individuals excluded from blood donations
  - blood donors screened for antibodies against HIV
  - manufacturing processes for blood products incorporate heat treatment to inactivate HIV.
- Education programmes in schools, colleges and for the general public have raised awareness about the need for changing behaviour in homosexual and heterosexual males and females and intravenous drug users.
- Safe sex recommendations include:
  - limiting the number of sexual partners
  - use of (kitemarked/British Standard) condoms to create barrier between body fluids
  - encouraging non-penetrative sexual acts between partners such as kissing, touching, etc.
- Providing su pport and counselling to intravenous drug abusers to end practice but to take advantage of syringe exchange schemes if they persist.
- Treatment of other sexually retransmitted diseases.
- Safe hygienic practices associated with any procedures involving body fluids.

The government has set up a programme of anonymous surveys to seek up-to-date information on HIV and AIDS.

Everyone is at risk from the virus. In the year June 1992 to June 1993, the Communicable Diseases Surveillance Centre stated, the number of reported cases of HIV rose by 13 per cent. Although the largest increase was in the category of transmission by sex between men (15 per cent), reports of heterosexual transmissions were also up by 12 per cent on the previous year (*Health of the Nation: One Year On*, 1993).

	AIDS (up to Sept. 1994)	HIV (up to June 1993)
Number of reported cases, UK	9900	–
Number of deaths, UK	6700	–
Incidence rate of HIV infection (from surveys of ante-natal clinics in London)	–	1 in 380

Figure 19.16 Some statistics relating to HIV and AIDS

Important points to note about Figure 19.16:

1 Many people are unaware that they are infected with HIV virus.
2 Experts agree that new HIV infection and AIDS cases among gay men will probably have peaked in 1993 or 1994. This is providing safe sex behaviour continues to be practised. There is some concern that this may not be the case with the younger generation of gay men.
3 Each year until 1997, nearly a hundred HIV positive haemophiliac cases will develop AIDS.
4 Heterosexual cases of HIV are steadily increasing – this is the fastest growing section of the community. Around 25 per cent of current HIV infections arise from heterosexual contact:
   a 73 per cent from exposure overseas
   b 13 per cent from high-risk partners.
   Now the virus is in the heterosexual community the infection will accelerate. About 7000 men and women in Britain have become infected by HIV through heterosexual intercourse (excluding drug users). It is thought by some researchers that as many as 80 per cent of the infected heterosexuals have no idea that they may carry the virus.

If you think you may have contracted the virus, it can take at least three months or longer to be sure because the blood has to be checked for HIV-antibodies. The body can take a few months to produce these.

People who contract HIV and AIDS and their families need a lot of support. Carers need to understand fully the nature of AIDS to be able to do this effectively.

To protect yourself from the risk of HIV and AIDS you should:

- always practise safe sex
- limit the number of sexual partners you have
- always use disposable gloves when dealing with other people's wounds, no matter how small
- wipe surfaces with a disinfectant immediately after dealing with any body fluids or blood.

The strategy set out in *The Health of the Nation: One Year On* (1993) to achieve a reduction in the transmission of HIV and consequently the incidence of AIDS has four elements:

- *prevention* through maintaining public awareness and encouraging behaviour change
- *treatment and care,* increasing awareness of testing facilities and developing care service to meet changing needs
- *monitoring* incidence and funding research into the condition
- *international action* to minimise the global impact of the disease.

It calls for concerted action involving all agencies from the voluntary and statutory sectors on both a local and national level. Also the 1993 Education Act makes sex education compulsory (although parents have the right to remove their children) and this will include information on HIV/AIDS and sexually transmitted diseases, thus drawing HIV under the wider umbrella of sexual health.

Examples of health promotion materials in this area clearly show how the information is targeted at different groups. Although the message is likely to be similar, it is particularly important that all vulnerable groups are reached and therefore that materials are specifically targeted.

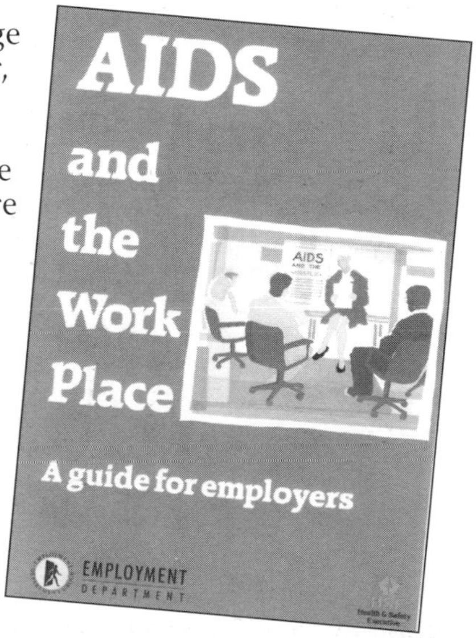

Because of the life-threatening potential of the HIV virus once contracted, a great deal of money has been spent on health education campaigns to inform and give protective advice. It is estimated that around £32 million was spent in 1993. This was divided between the National Helpline and local health authority initiatives. There are disparities between geographical areas as funds are allocated on the basis of adult population. In 1993, the South West spent £7 million on prevention schemes but had only 461 reported cases of AIDS, while London received £14 million but has many times more reported AIDS cases.

Substance abuse

Substance abuse is a broad term used to cover **alcohol**, **drugs** (including smoking) and **solvent abuse.** All three have socially acceptable uses. *Abuse* involves using substances in a way which is not socially acceptable and which can present a risk to health. Sometimes individuals make a conscious choice to take risks; sometimes people put themselves at risk because they are not fully aware of the consequences for their health. In this section, the risks related to alcohol, smoking, drugs and solvent abuse are explored.

Alcohol

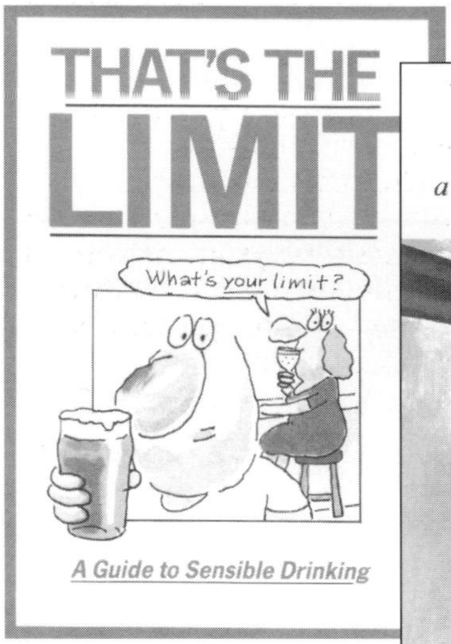

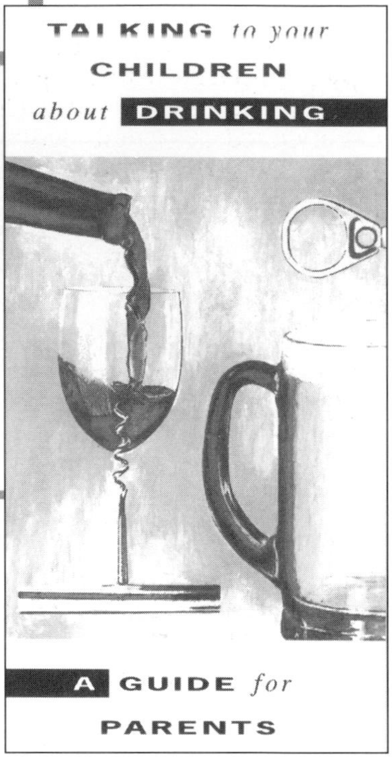

Alcohol is very much a socially accepted drug in the UK. It is an important part of many celebrations and festivities, such as weddings, Christmas, times of success. Alcohol is, however, a chemical substance and a drug – although it is not often seen in this way.

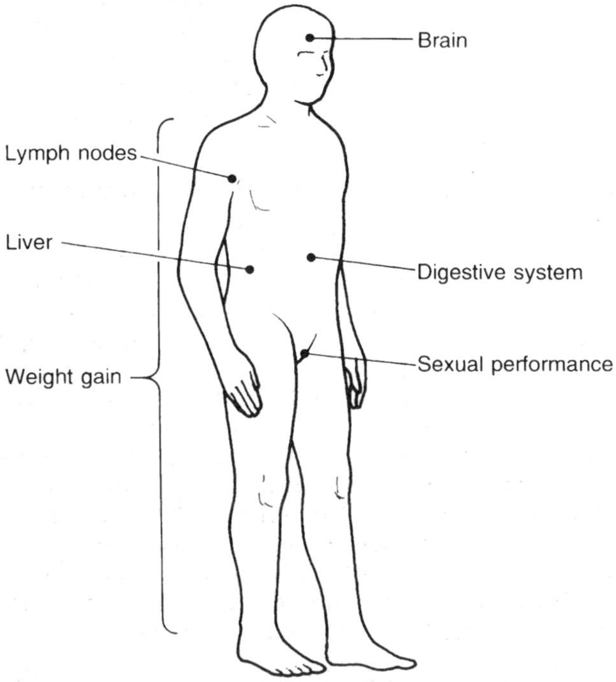

Figure 19.17 Where alcohol may attack the body

Some medical evidence seems to suggest that drinking alcohol in moderation may have a beneficial effect on health. It is suggested that red wine can help to reduce cholesterol in the blood, and cholesterol may be associated with heart attacks.

It is suggested that individuals do not exceed the recommended weekly intakes of alcohol, which are a maximum of 14 units for women and 21 units for men. A unit is roughly equivalent to one glass of wine, one measure of spirit or half a pint of lager or beer. A person who frequently exceeds these recommendations is thought to be placing his or her physical and mental health at risk.

The initial effect of drinking alcohol can be to make you feel happy. However, alcohol affects the speed with which the brain can make judgements. This might cause individuals to misjudge situations and distance when driving, which could lead to accidents. This is why even a moderate intake of alcohol is connected with so many road accidents. If excess alcohol is consumed by women in early pregnancy it can damage the development of the foetus, causing permanent harm to the baby. Excess alcohol is responsible for many lost working days due to sickness following a 'heavy session'.

Why do people drink?

Drinking often starts during socialisation. Drinking may be linked with eating and celebrations, and having an enjoyable time. Children have often experienced their first alcoholic drink long before the age of 16. Sometimes *peer pressure* plays an important role in the amount of alcohol consumed – whatever age you are. In some social contexts people can be ridiculed if they refuse a drink and feel uncomfortable doing so.

Some people also drink as a way to reduce stress or anxiety, or to forget any worries they may have. However, alcohol, in this context, works as a tranquilliser: it does not do anything to help the situation which has caused the drinking (and which may become worse because of it).

Try it

Choose a client group and design a questionnaire or survey to find out their perception of alcohol and its place in society. Assess their understanding of the health risks associated with drinking. Collate your findings. What conclusions can you draw? Compare your results with those of another client group. How are they similar or where do they differ?

Smoking

Smoking is another habit which has been part of western society for many years. It is the only retail product which when used as the manufacturer recommends – even in moderation – kills the consumer. It is the most significant cause of preventable disease and early death in Britain today. Approximately 111 000 people die each year because of smoking-related causes: 26 000 from lung cancer and the rest from other diseases caused by tobacco. Figures suggest that around 28 per cent of women and 29 per cent of men smoke; and that approximately 25 per cent of children smoke at the age of 15, despite the widely publicised relationship between smoking and health risks. It is believed that some smokers, while aware of the risks, take the attitude 'It won't happen to me'.

The acceptability of smoking has, it could be suggested, declined in recent years. There has been an increase in the number of smoke-free areas, especially in public places, as a response to raised awareness of the dangers of passive smoking. Increasingly, non-smokers are refusing to accept a cigarette-polluted atmosphere.

The adverse effects of smoking

Cigarettes contain harmful substances such as tar, nicotine and carbon monoxide – as can be seen in Figure 19.18.

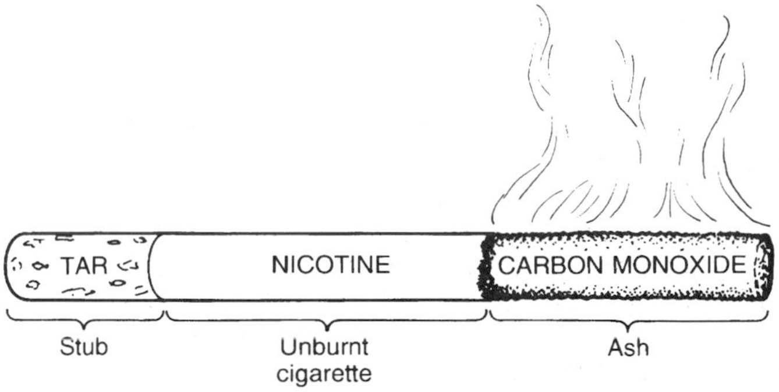

Figure 19.18 What a cigarette contains

Nicotine is the part of the cigarette that creates dependence on smoking. It is absorbed into the bloodstream and has numerous effects on the body including increasing the heart-rate, blood-pressure and hormone production. This explains why smokers are more at risk from heart attacks. Nicotine is also thought to thicken the blood and is therefore connected to an increased possibility of blood clots forming in the arteries, ultimately this could result in amputation of limbs.

Carbon monoxide is the poisonous gas found in cigarette smoke. It readily combines with *haemoglobin,* the part of the blood which carries oxygen, thus reducing the blood's oxygen-carrying capacity. As oxygen is essential for the functioning of tissues and organs in the body a reduction in supply can affect growth, repair and nutrient absorption. The body tries to compensate for this by producing more haemoglobin, in order to increase oxygen-carrying capacity, but this increases the risk of blood clots or *thombosis* – which ultimately could lead to limb amputation. It is also believed that carbon monoxide is connected to *atherosclerosis,* the depositing of fatty substances on artery walls. This contributes to a narrowing of the arteries, which in turn is connected with coronary diseases.

About 70 per cent of **tar** from cigarettes is deposited in the lungs. It is this tar which is particularly related to cancer: 81 per cent of people who died from lung cancer were smokers in 1991. Tar is also known to cause a narrowing of the bronchioles (small tubes in the lungs), along with increased coughing and bronchiole mucus. Tar damage affects the small hairs which line the lungs and help protect the lungs against dirt and infection. In this way the smoker can become more susceptible to chest infections, including *bronchitis* (an inflammation of the mucus membranes) and *emphysema* (emphysema involves the destruction of the walls of the air sacs in the lungs, reducing the surface area for gaseous exchange and consequently the ability to breathe).

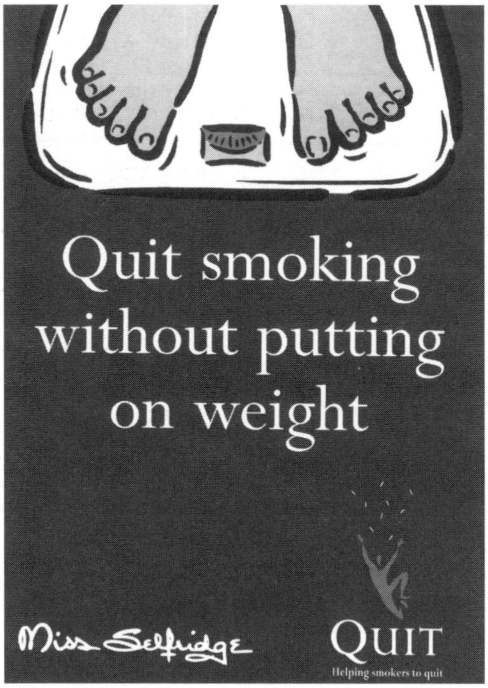

Smoking in pregnancy causes additional adverse effects. The reduction in the ability of the blood to carry oxygen has an effect on the amount of oxygen which can cross the placenta to the foetus. Therefore, smokers often give birth to smaller, lighter babies, who are weaker and more prone to infections. There is also an increased risk of miscarriage or spontaneous abortion as well as perinatal mortality (death around time of birth). The risk of illness is increased if parents or carers continue to smoke around the baby after birth. The child is effectively a passive smoker who, unlike many adults, has no choice over the matter.

Passive smoking occurs where a non-smoker breathes in the cigarette smoke of others: either in the form of the smoke the smoker has already exhaled (*mainstream smoke*) or the smoke from the

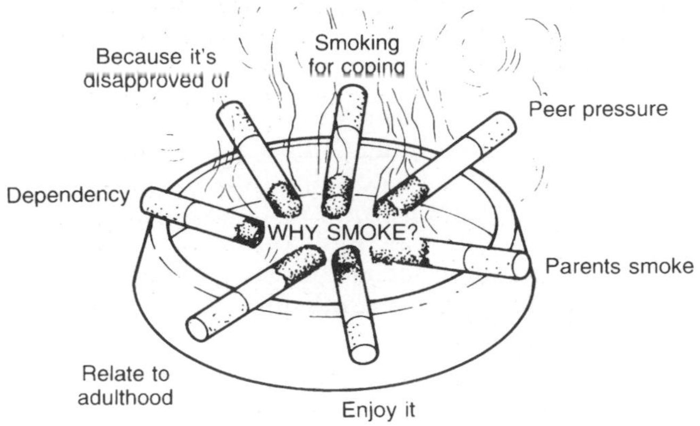

Figure 19.19 Why smoke?

tip of the cigarette (*sidestream smoke*). Passively smoking smoke from the tip of the cigarette is often worse than smoking itself as the smoke is not being filtered in any way. Recent research has shown that there is a 10 to 30 per cent risk of lung cancer in non-smokers as a result of passive smoking. However, despite these figures, the government appears reluctant to legislate to prevent passive smoking and prefers that smoking is reduced through a voluntary approach. The view taken is that legislation may only be considered if voluntary pressure does not work.

If employers fail to provide a safe working environment, they can be prosecuted by employees who believe that their health has suffered as a result. With compensation cases successfully being brought against employers by employees who have become ill due to passive smoking in the workplace, many employers will now be under strong pressure to ban smoking.

Think it over

Should smokers be allowed to smoke in public places and work situations? Whose responsibility is it to provide us all with a healthy environment?

Reducing the risks of smoking

Risk reduction should be considered for both the smoker and the non-smoker.

- Give up smoking completely. After giving up smoking, an ex-smoker's risk of getting lung cancer falls to being only slightly greater than that of a non-smoker after 15 years.

- Smoke lower tar cigarettes. But is should be remembered that just because a cigarette is low in tar, it does not automatically follow that it is low in other substances such as carbon monoxide or nicotine.
- Try using nicotine substitutes, such as the nicotine patch, to help lose the dependency on nicotine. (These substitutes can be expensive as they are not currently available on the NHS.)
- Try smoking only in certain places, as this will cut down the opportunity to smoke and, therefore, the amount smoked.
- Cut down the amount smoked generally.
- Increase your intake of vitamin C through fresh fruit and vegetables, and fruit juices, as this is believed to help the body get rid of nicotine.

Think it over

How could society in general help to cut down risks from smoking? Should there be policies on smoking in public places?

Try it

Choose a client group and develop a plan to help them stop smoking. Include in the package a way to promote the message that smoking is not healthy. Ensure that your plan promotes accurate evidence on the effects of smoking while acknowledging individual rights and choice.

Health education campaigns on smoking usually aim to prevent people from starting smoking or to encourage and support smokers to give up permanently or at particular stages of life, such as pregnancy. Approximately £5.5 million was spent on this by the Health Education Authority in 1993. The UK government has banned cigarette advertising on television, but it is still allowed on billboards and in magazines.

Other drugs

As we have seen, both alcohol and nicotine are drugs – but socially acceptable drugs if used within limits. Other drugs, such as those included under the heading of substance abuse, are less acceptable. These may be found in cases of *drug abuse,* i.e. *drug misuse,* where a drug is socially acceptable (for example, used for medicine like tranquillisers), but is used in a socially unacceptable way.

The prolonged use of any drug is dangerous to health. But the level of risk varies according to the way the drug is taken; for example, injecting a drug into the bloodstream is more dangerous than smoking a drug. It should be understood that different people vary in their reactions to the same drug, depending on factors such as their body size, state of health, tolerance of the body to the drug and so on. This is why the same 'dose' of one drug can kill one person and not another. For analysis of some common drugs see Figure 19.20.

Why take drugs?

There are many reasons why people might take drugs:

- *dependence* – both mind and body can become dependent on drugs
- *escapism* – some people see drugs as a temporary way to escape difficulties in life, such as personal problems, financial worries or work-related dilemmas
- *boredom* – drugs can be seen as a way to escape boredom
- *lack of confidence* – some people who are shy and lack self-confidence may find that drugs can help them overcome their inhibitions
- *image* – drugs are seen by some people as being daring and exciting, partly due to the associated risks
- *peer pressure* – there may be pressure from friends to try drugs
- *opportunity* – some people just take drugs because they are available.

Reducing the risk from drugs

The only way to reduce the risk from drugs is not to take them at all. However, the way this message is put across is crucial: straight education, merely providing the facts, does not always work.

Think it over

Why do you think that simply informing people about the dangers of drugs does not always succeed in preventing them from trying drugs?

When talking to people about drugs, the following points are recommended (Boice and Gamble)

Type of drug	Form	Use	Effects	Health risks
Cannabis (pot/hash)	Resin in form of solid brown mass	Smoked usually crumbled and mixed with tobacco	■ Relaxation and talkativeness ■ Appear 'high' or drunk ■ Possible hallucinations ■ Unable to function logically. Heavy doses – distorted judgements of space, slow reactions, drowsiness and poor concentration	■ Psychological dependency for enjoyment/coping with life ■ Bronchitis, lung cancer ■ Heart disorders ■ Might lead to use of stronger drugs within some social contexts
Ecstasy ('E')	Tablet or capsule – white, brown, pink of yellow	Swallowed – effects begin in 20 minutes	■ Calmness with raised awareness of colour and sound ■ Loss of co-ordination ■ High doses result in anxiety and confusion	■ Prolonged use can reduce sleep ■ Those with high blood pressure, heart conditions, epilepsy or mental illness at risk due to stimulant effects ■ Possible death
Amphetamines and cocaine (coke) (stimulants)	White powder	Usually sniffed, but can be injected	■ Stimulates nervous system which can result in over-excitedness and sleeplessness. Also linked to aggressiveness ■ Breathing and heart rate increase, pupils dilate ■ Feel alert, energetic, cheerful and confident ■ Reduces tiredness for a time ■ Reduces appetite	■ Poor sleep, loss of appetite, bodily itching leading to scratching and anxiety ■ Lower resistance to disease ■ Damaged blood vessels and heart failure ■ Damage to nose membranes ■ Depression and suicidal tendencies
LSD ('acid') (hallucinogens)	Impregnated into small sheets, like blotting paper	Dissolved on tongue	■ Affects perception – can be visions of joy and beauty or nightmares ■ Confusion and disorientation. Distorts colour, space and time ■ Gives users unrealistic perceptions of ability (e.g. think they can fly)	■ Accidents due to confusion and distorted perceptions of reality ■ Can be a damaging experience to those with mental illness
Heroin	White or brown powder	Sniffed, smoked or injected	■ First alertness, then drowsiness ■ Detached feeling of relaxation ■ Overdose results in unconsciousness and death	■ Dependency on heroin ■ Poor health due to inadequate diet ■ Risk of AIDS if needles are shared
Magic mushrooms	A range of fungi	Tablets	Toxic effects, hallucinations, sleep disturbances and nervousness	Injury/death due to accidents whilst confused

Figure 19.20 Analysis of some common drugs

- It is important to keep an open mind.
- Be sure you are clear about the facts concerning drugs and their use.
- Develop good communication with the group or individual concerned. They need to value your opinion in order to take it on board.
- Try not to act hastily but consider how to approach the problem. Acting on the spur of the moment without fully thinking through the consequences of an action may well have an adverse affect.
- Develop positive values in other things. Encourage a strong self-image in the group or individual so they do not feel they have to use drugs to prove themselves and they are able to resist peer pressure.

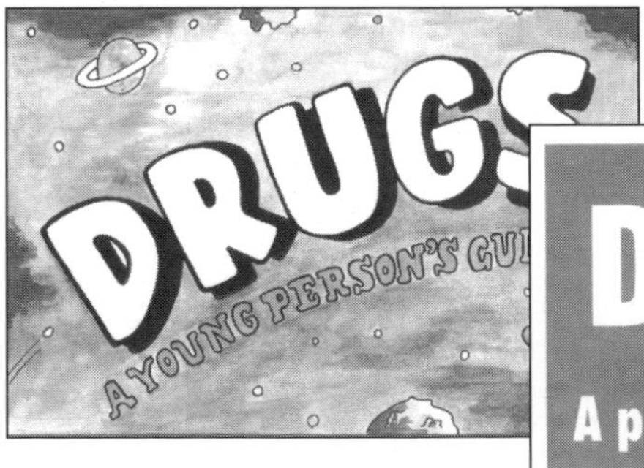

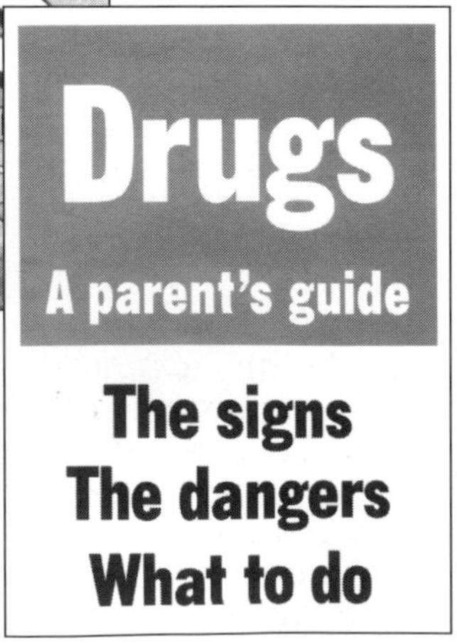

The focus of current health education programmes is on informing young children about the dangers of drugs from as early as 4 years of age. The White Paper 'Handling Drugs

Today' (1995), accepts that many young people will have contact with drugs, and published figures support this.

The White Paper focuses not only on reducing the acceptability and availability of drugs, but also on the importance of harm reduction by ensuring youngsters are aware of how to minimise risk. An £8.8 million drugs education scheme for UK schools draws together health, education and law enforcement to present a co-ordinated approach through vigorous law enforcement, accessible treatment for users and a comprehensive education package.

Solvents

Solvents are often classified in the same grouping as drugs. The term 'solvent' covers a range of products, including household products which give off gases or fumes, such as glue, lighter fluid, aerosol sprays, petrol and correction fluid.

Solvents are either sniffed through the nose and mouth, usually from bags (huffing), or sprayed directly into the mouth. Some solvents, such as thinners, may be sniffed from a cloth or coat sleeve in a similar way to nasal decongestants used for a cold. Because solvents are portable, sniffing can occur anywhere, but often people go to remote or isolated places to abuse solvents.

What are the effects of abusing solvents?

The effects of glue sniffing are very similar to the effects of alcohol but the 'drunkenness' occurs more quickly. This is because the vapour is inhaled into the bloodstream through the lungs and not through the stomach, which delays the effect (depending on what else is present). As the vapour is inhaled through the lungs, the effects also wear off quickly and so a sniffer has to keep sniffing to maintain the effects. People who sniff may experience hallucinations; unconsciousness is also possible.

The risks from abusing solvents

Possibly the greatest risk from solvent abuse is from what happens when the person who sniffs is 'intoxicated'. Substance abusers may not be realistic or 'aware' and may take risks they would not take under normal circumstances. In the same way abusers may be unable to react to danger. Accidents may result from this.

Sniffing solvents also has an effect on the heart and any physical exertion or fright following sniffing can result in death. If the solvent is sprayed directly into the mouth, this has been shown to cause a swelling of the throat tissues which can result in suffocation. It has also been shown that people who sniff can die from choking on their own vomit. As they often go to isolated places to sniff solvents, there is not always someone around who can help them in this situation.

Most of these risks are immediate and are directly connected to the sniffing of the solvent or the short-term intoxicating effect.

Why do people sniff solvents?

Solvent abuse is portrayed as a young person's habit. However, only about one in ten secondary pupils try sniffing and many do not keep up the habit for very long (Ives, 1992). As with the other 'drugs', people partake for various reasons, including:

- as an alternative to other drugs
- because solvents are cheap and easily available. Although the law makes it an offence (under the Substance Supply Act 1985) to sell a young person under 18 a substance if it is believed it will be used 'to achieve intoxication', this is very difficult to prove, and consequently there have been few prosecutions under this Act
- it can be exciting; and some people like the hallucinations that go with it
- because it might shock those seen as authority figures, such as parents and teachers
- because they enjoy it
- to avoid or blot out problems.

Promote personal safety and security

Electrical safety

Electricity is a utility used by everyone and so is not, perhaps, considered as a risk to personal safety. However, it is often overlooked as a significant cause of fire in the home. Figures from the Home Office (1991) state that approximately 28 000 domestic fires each year are caused by electrical faults, accidents or misuse of electrical equipment, and over 2500 people are killed in these fires.

The electric source comes into a building through the meter. The home has a wiring circuit which then takes the electricity to various points in the building.

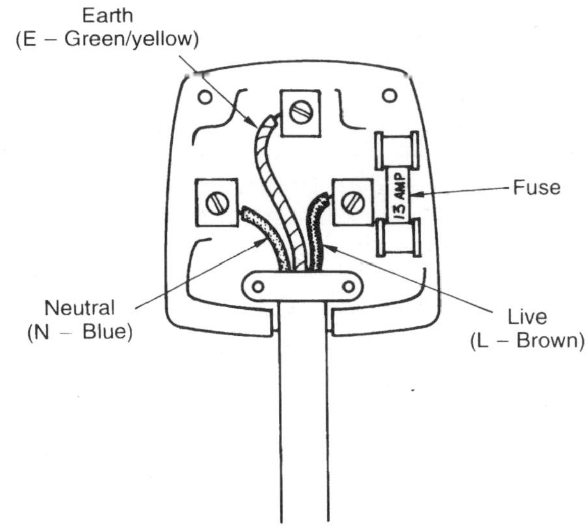

Figure 19.21 A plug and fuse

The wiring should be checked regularly to ensure it is safe. Signs of dangerous wiring include:

- hot plugs, sockets and switches
- fuses blowing for no reason
- lights flickering
- scorch marks on sockets and plugs.

The contact between the electrical current and the appliance is made by the plug. It is essential that a plug is wired correctly; all flexes are colour-coded to help (Figure 19.21).

It is also essential that the correct fuse is fitted as this could prevent a fire; if there is a surge of electricity, the fuse melts and breaks the circuit. An RCD (Residual Current Device) can also be used with electrical equipment. This will detect incorrect functioning in electrical cables or other faults in the system and will cut off the current in a millisecond, thus giving added protection against electrocution and electrical fires.

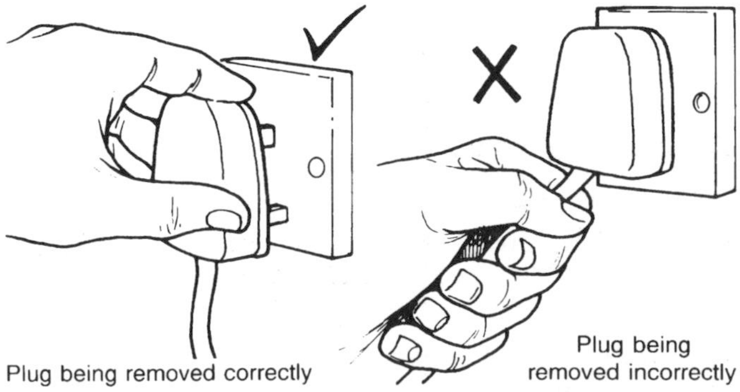

Figure 19.22 Removing a plug from the wall

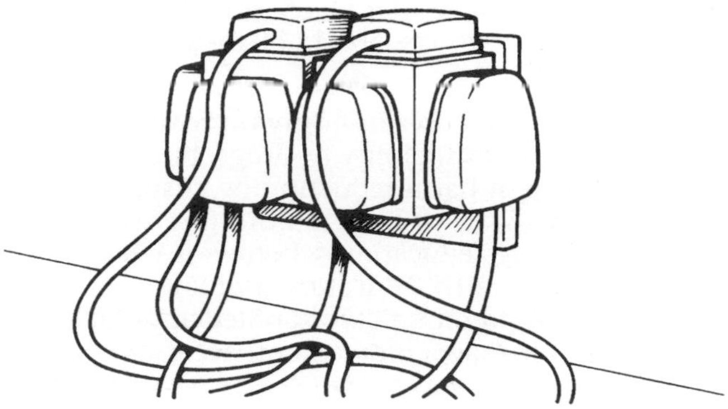

Figure 19.23 Overloaded plug socket.

When purchasing a plug, you should always use the three-pinned plug which conforms to British Standards. This carries the BS kitemark – the sign that it has been checked for safety.

When buying electrical equipment, always look for the BEAB Mark of Safety. This means the appliance has been checked by the British Electrotechnical Approvals Board. Most electrical equipment is now being sold with moulded plugs already attached and, unless absolutely necessary, these should not be removed.

Some types of electrical equipment are designed to be left on all of the time; others should be switched off at the mains and unplugged after use. Always check the manufacturer's instructions if you are unsure. Plugs should always be removed carefully and not by pulling the flex (Figure 19.22).

Sockets should not be overloaded with plugs/adaptors. If using the adaptor, ensure the correct fuse is used (Figure 19.23).

Electric shock

Electric shocks can occur on different levels. A minor electric shock may make you jump but not do any real damage. More severe electric shocks may cause burns, where the current enters and leaves the body; shocks can also cause muscle spasms. The electric current may affect the rhythm of the heart and possibly make it stop. It can also affect the brain and the way it controls the body's breathing.

If you suspect someone has had an electric shock, do not touch them unless you are sure that the current has been switched off as the current can pass to you and you then become a victim of the accident. If the

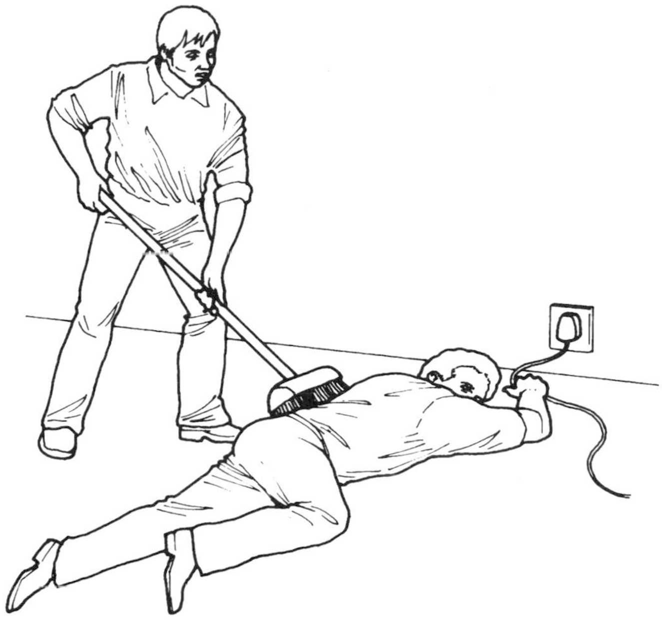

Figure 19.24 Moving an electric shock victim

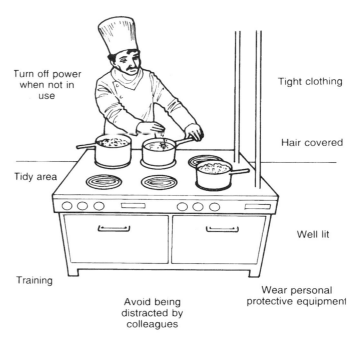

Figure 19.26 Ways to improve safety when using equipment

electricity cannot be turned off, you could use a non-metal item such as a wooden broom handle or walking stick to push or pull the person away from the electrical source (Figure 19.24).

Once the casualty is free of the electrical source, treat as for severe bleeding or shock as necessary. Call an ambulance if the accident appears serious.

Safe equipment

Besides ensuring that the electricity supply is safe and that the plug is wired correctly you should also check equipment regularly to ensure it is safe for use and not a safety hazard. Many tasks in the home and workplace involve the use of equipment which can make jobs both easier and quicker.

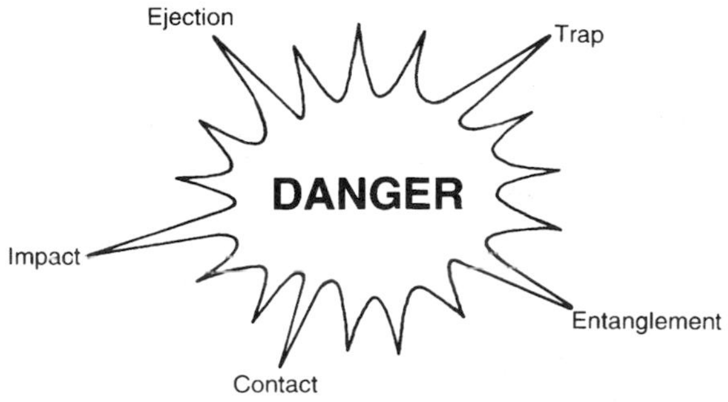

Figure 19.25 Danger from machinery

The Provision and Use of Work Equipment Regulations were introduced in 1992 to ensure that working equipment is safe and used properly to minimise risks (Institute of Environmental Health Officers, 1993). Employers have a duty to

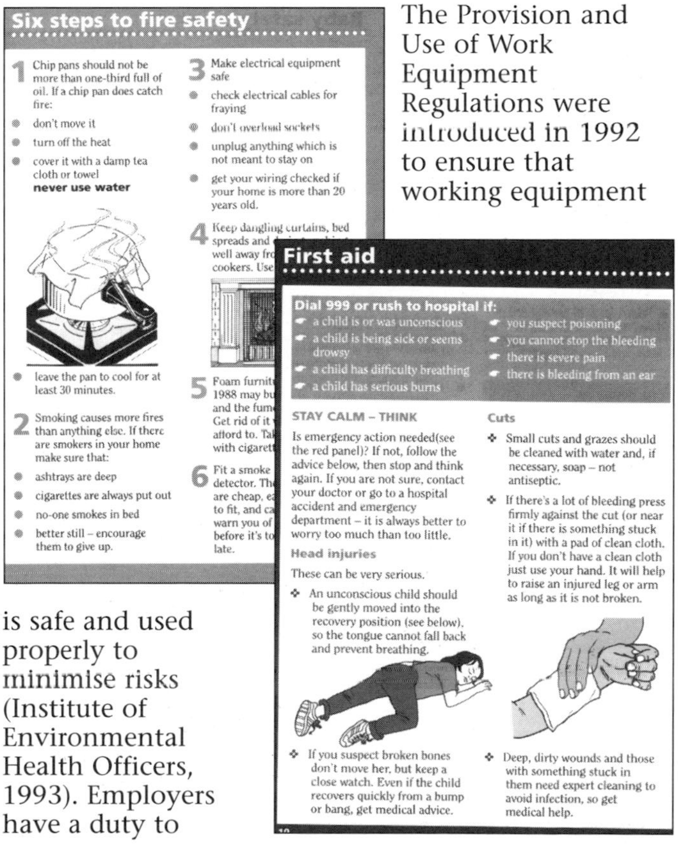

Six steps to fire safety

1 Chip pans should not be more than one-third full of oil. If a chip pan does catch fire:
- don't move it
- turn off the heat
- cover it with a damp tea cloth or towel **never use water**
- leave the pan to cool for at least 30 minutes.

2 Smoking causes more fires than anything else. If there are smokers in your home make sure that:
- ashtrays are deep
- cigarettes are always put out
- no-one smokes in bed
- better still – encourage them to give up.

3 Make electrical equipment safe
- check electrical cables for fraying
- don't overload sockets
- unplug anything which is not meant to stay on
- get your wiring checked if your home is more than 20 years old.

4 Keep dangling curtains, bed spreads and … well away fr… cookers. Use…

5 Foam furnit… 1988 may bu… and the fum… Get rid of it … afford to. Ta… with cigarett…

6 Fit a smoke detector. Th… are cheap, e… to fit, and ca… warn you of … before it's to… late.

First aid

Dial 999 or rush to hospital if:
- a child is or was unconscious
- a child is being sick or seems drowsy
- a child has difficulty breathing
- a child has serious burns
- you suspect poisoning
- you cannot stop the bleeding
- there is severe pain
- there is bleeding from an ear

STAY CALM – THINK

Is emergency action needed(see the red panel)? If not, follow the advice below, then stop and think again. If you are not sure, contact your doctor or go to a hospital accident and emergency department – it is always better to worry too much than too little.

Head injuries

These can be very serious.
- An unconscious child should be gently moved into the recovery position (see below), so the tongue cannot fall back and prevent breathing.
- If you suspect broken bones don't move her, but keep a close watch. Even if the child recovers quickly from a bump or bang, get medical advice.

Cuts
- Small cuts and grazes should be cleaned with water and, if necessary, soap – not antiseptic.
- If there's a lot of bleeding press firmly against the cut (or near it if there is something stuck in it) with a pad of clean cloth. If you don't have a clean cloth just use your hand. It will help to raise an injured leg or arm as long as it is not broken.
- Deep, dirty wounds and those with something stuck in them need expert cleaning to avoid infection, so get medical help.

provide and maintain suitable and safe equipment. Employers also have to ensure that anyone using the equipment has been appropriately trained. There are five main types of danger from machines, as can be seen from Figure 19.25.

Safer use of equipment can be ensured through:

- safe design to remove any potential dangers
- safe positioning in the workplace
- appropriate guards to cover dangerous parts.

Many workplaces have their equipment checked regularly, usually once per year. However, a piece of equipment is only as safe as the person using it.

Health education material in this area focuses on a range of topics.

Gas safety

Gas is an excellent source of energy. It provides fuel for cooking and is a versatile form of space heating. The main type of gas used today is non-toxic, like that extracted from below the North Sea. However, gas still has the potential to cause explosions if not treated with care. A few simple guidelines should be followed.

- Don't buy second-hand gas appliances unless you are sure of their safety. British Gas suggest that second-hand appliances cause most accidents that involve faulty equipment.
- Make sure you know where the main gas tap is (usually close to the meter). Ensure that it is not stiff and can be turned off (Figure 19.27).

If the tap is stiff, contact the local gas board and they will fix it. *Never* try to force the handle or fix it yourself.

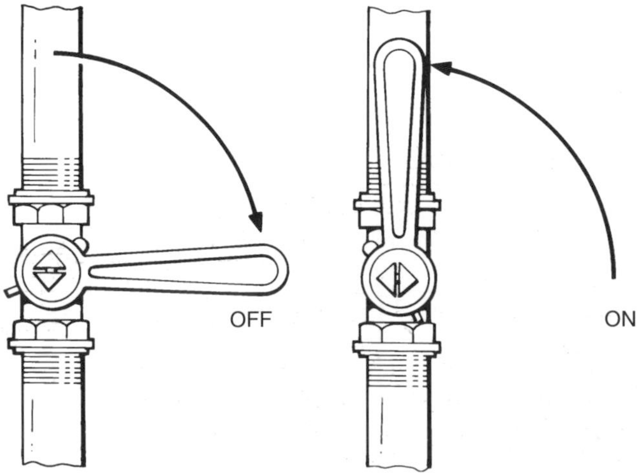

Figure 19.27 Switching off the mains gas tap

- Sweep a chimney before fitting an appliance into a fireplace – an air flow is essential for the removal of fumes. A blocked chimney will not allow the fumes to escape, and may become a source of carbon monoxide poisoning.
- Do not block ventilators as these are required to supply a constant stream of fresh air.
- Have appliances serviced regularly. Central heating and gas fires should be serviced every 1–2 years. A maintenance contract which includes regular servicing and a call-out service in case of breakdown is a good idea.
- Consider switching off the supply if you are going away, to reduce risk. In winter it would not be wise to turn off gas central heating as this could lead to water pipes freezing and later bursting, but the thermostat could be turned down.

> If you smell gas, you should
>
> - act immediately
> - put out all naked flames – do not smoke or light a match
> - open all doors and windows to allow the gas to escape
> - if possible, turn off the gas supply
> - call British Gas using the 24-hour service listed in the *Phone Book.*

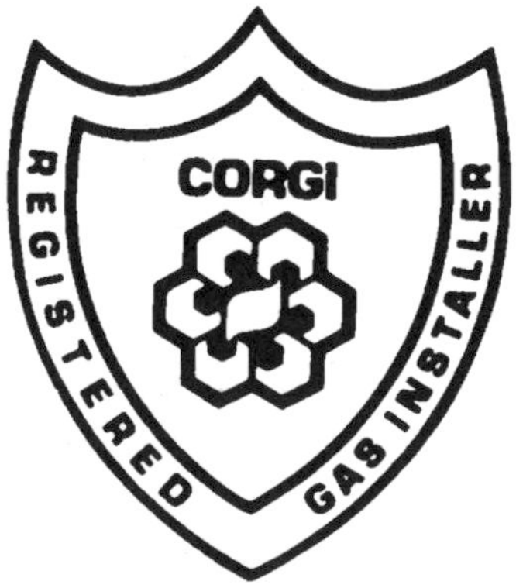

Figure 19.28 The CORGI symbol is awarded to registered installers of gas products.

The Council for Registered Gas Installers (CORGI) is the body given the responsibility by the Health and Safety Executive to maintain a register of approved gas installers in mainland Britain. Under no circumstances should you have a non-registered installer service, fit or mend a gas appliance.

Household security

With rising crime, household security has been the subject of a range of campaigns. A number of safety measures are recommended to increase household security.

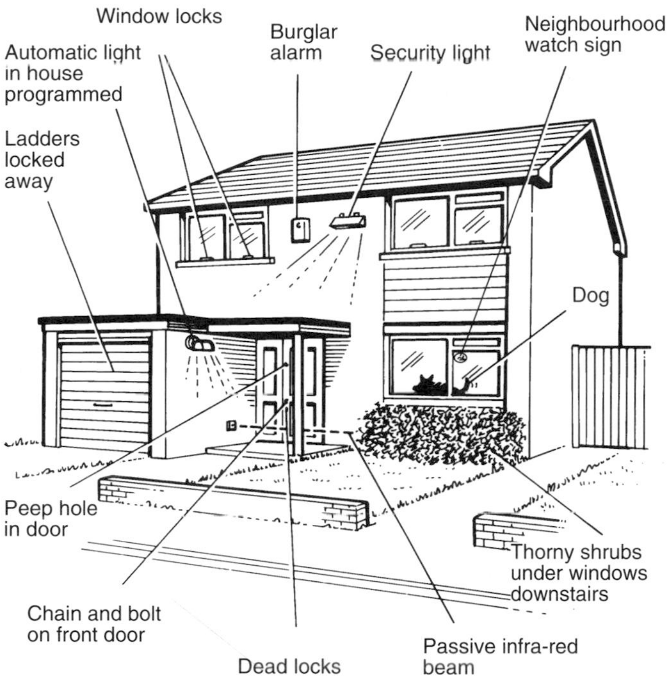

Figure 19.29 Household security

Campaigns on TV as well as in magazines, have attempted to raise awareness, using slogans such as 'Watch out, there's a thief about' as well as promoting concepts such as Neighbourhood Watch.

Road safety

It is estimated that about 16 people are killed on UK roads every day and that over 900 are injured. Young people are most vulnerable and have the highest accident levels. It is also interesting to note that most accidents occur in the early stages of learning to use a mode of transport, for example pedestrians of 5–9 years old, motor cyclists in the 16–19 age group and car drivers in their late teens and early twenties. Only with pedestrian accidents is there a fluctuation in this pattern with an increase in accidents occurring with old age, as individuals lose some of their faculties, and ability to judge distances and speed.

Figure 19.30 shows the number of accidents in one year.

Road safety has been the focus of a number of campaigns aimed at different aspects of this broad area. They have included campaigns aimed at the pedestrian, such as the Green Cross Code, and the

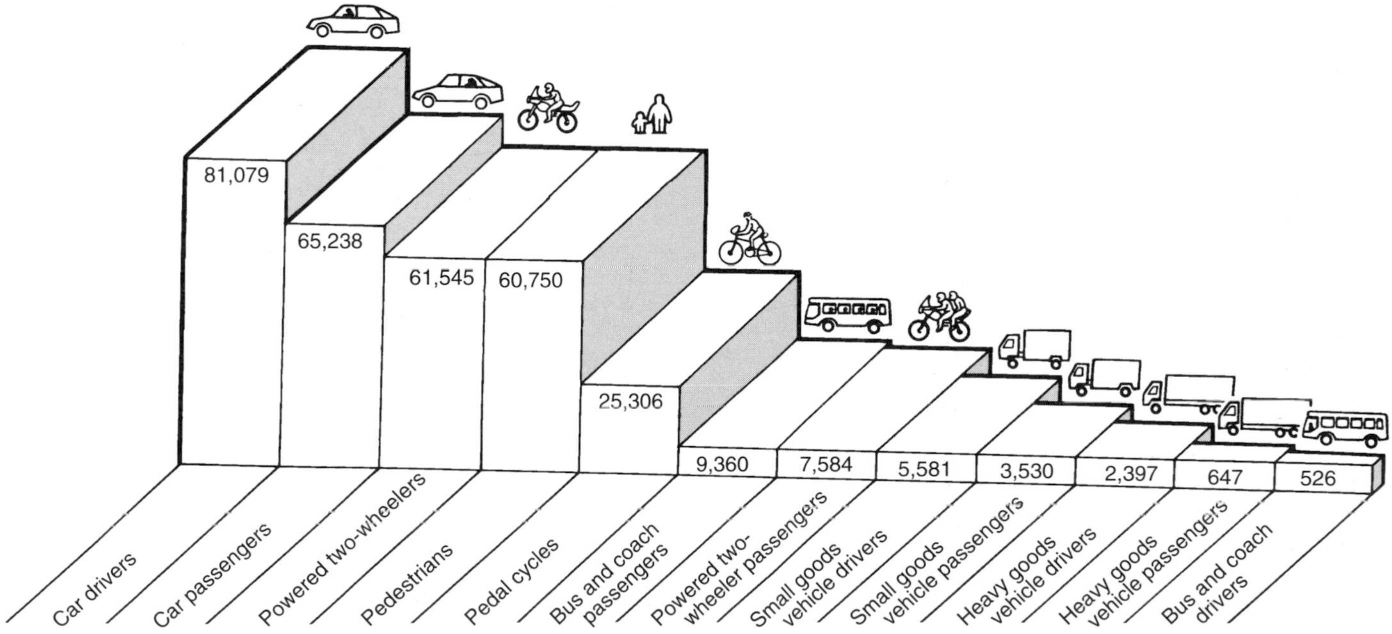

Figure 19.30 Number of road-user casualties

car driver, such as 'Clunk Click Every Trip' which promoted the use of seat belts before it became compulsory under the law to wear them. There are also campaigns aimed at other modes of transport besides the car, for example promoting the use of reflective gear for bicycle riders.

Also included in this area are the Drink Driving campaigns. It is suggested that a high proportion of people are killed on the roads as a result of driving after consuming alcohol. It has become increasingly unacceptable to drink alcohol and drive as the awareness of the potential results of driving after having a small amount of alcohol has risen. These campaigns are often more visible at certain times of the year. For several years there has been a successful campaign before Christmas on TV, supported by posters, aimed at preventing drinking and driving.

Think it over

Recent drink driving campaigns have used strong images and made their point very clearly. Why do you think this tactic is used? How effective do you think it is?

Evidence collection point

This chapter has provided an overview of the range of topics on which health education campaigns often focus. Choose three different areas of heath education, and produce a report for each which:

a identifies the objectives for the campaign and whether they relate to local and/or national targets
b sets out the main aspects for promotion in each campaign
c discusses how the emphasis for each area differs for different target groups
d evaluates the effectiveness of the material identified.

Chapter 20

The reasons for, sources of and methods used in health education campaigns

This chapter explores the sources of health campaigns and the methods used to put health messages across. This includes an investigation of:

- **the different sources and advantages and disadvantages of different outlets for campaigns**
- **the equipment and resources available for health education campaigns to help assess how well the message is put across**
- **the ways in which the messages are adapted to suit the needs of different groups.**

Sources of health education campaigns

Health education campaigns originate from a number of sources:

- public services
- private companies
- the voluntary sector.

Public services

The main public services in the UK involved in health education campaigns are the Health Education Authority (HEA) and the Department of Health.

National health targets

The government determines national health targets which are communicated to appropriate professionals and interested members of the public in documents such as *The Health of the Nation*. Targets are set for the improvement of health covering the five key areas of:

- coronary heart disease
- cancers
- mental illness
- accidents
- HIV/AIDS and sexual health.

Health education campaigns sponsored by public services operate on a national level to raise awareness in the hope of achieving these targets.

Local health targets

Public services can also operate health education campaigns on a local level in the form of local *health promotion units,* which have a role to play in achieving national targets.

Funding for services such as the health promotion unit and GPs can be based on achieving targets in health education, such as reducing the number of teenage pregnancies in an area. This gives them the incentive to run campaigns and access the appropriate client group, otherwise funding could be cut and they would have less money for their service.

Local health promotion units also provide health education to promote preventative action, such as immunisation programmes.

Services such as police and probation officers can also be considered health educators. Their aim is to protect the public from crime and help ensure road safety. They also have a role to play in preventing misuse of substances such as drugs and alcohol.

Private companies

Many private companies link a health message to a product or service that they offer. An example is the marketing of Flora margarine through adverts which link the product to the need to increase polyunsaturated fat in the diet in order to reduce the risk of heart disease.

The manufacturers of Flora were also quick to exploit media coverage on the antioxidant qualities of vitamin E by incorporating that too into their advertising campaign.

Since private companies need to make a profit to survive in business, it might be suggested that the main reason for private companies to promote a health message is to increase their profit margin.

The voluntary sector

Health education from the voluntary sector is likely to aim to promote the interests of a particular group.

Campaigns may simply seek to raise awareness of the work groups such as Cancer Research Campaign, carry out, in the hope of encouraging the public to donate money to them for their work.

Some organisations are pressure groups – they aim to lobby parliament on issues that they feel are important. Health education in this case may be to strengthen support for their campaigns. An example of this is ASH (Action on Smoking and Health) who provide education on the effects of smoking and passive smoking in support of the lobby for stricter laws against smoking in public spaces.

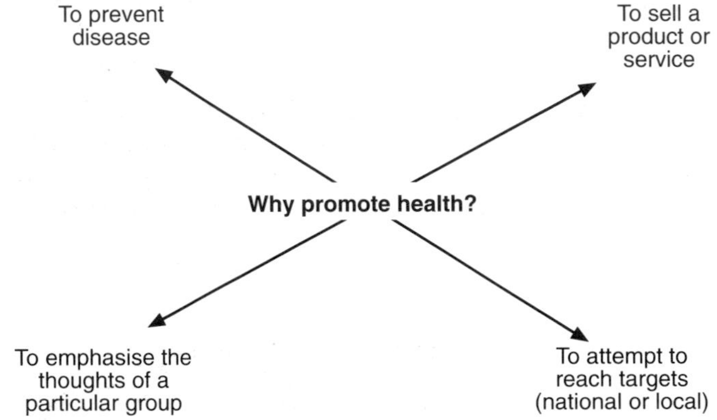

Figure 20.1 Why promote health?

Methods used in health education

Use of the mass media

One of the most common ways to promote health education is through the mass media. The term 'mass media' covers any channel of communication which reaches large numbers of people, for example television, radio, newspapers, magazines, exhibitions, displays and books. Leaflets and posters can also be classified as part of the mass media if used widely. (When they are simply part of a talk or presentation they would be described as a teaching aid.)

The mass media are used in a number of different ways to put over health education messages (Figure 20.2).

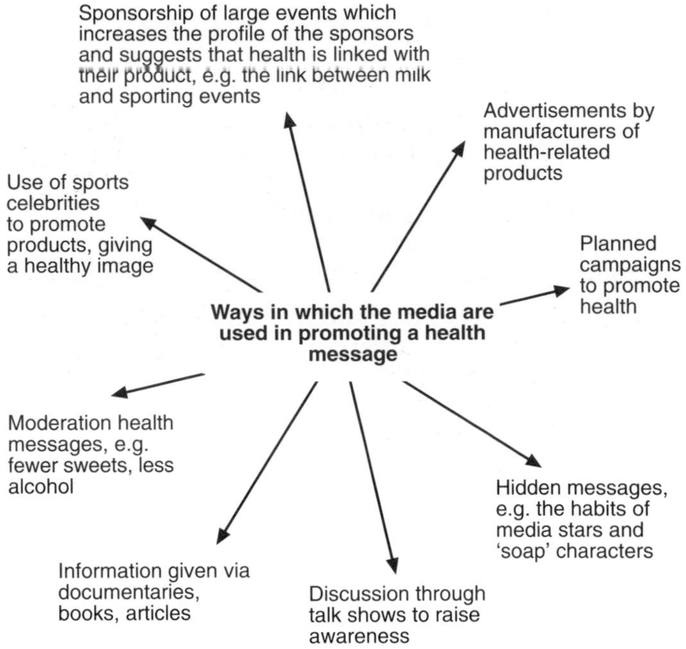

Figure 20.2 How the mass media are used to promote health education

Disadvantages of the mass media

One of the main disadvantages of using the mass media as the only outlet for a health education campaign is that it is difficult to obtain any immediate feedback from the target audience, and consequently it is difficult to assess whether the message is pitched at the right level or covers the right material. In situations where interaction is possible, the presenter can adjust the content and the level of the message as he or she goes through a presentation. The presenters can gauge the audience's needs and understanding from both verbal and non-verbal communication, i.e. body language and questions. Using the mass media makes it difficult to repeat, amplify or clarify a message. It may be, therefore, that the mass media are best used for simple messages. It is unlikely that mass media presentations alone will result in long-term changes in behaviour (Tones, Tilford and Robinson, 1990).

To ensure the mass media are used most effectively, the area must be well-researched by the promoter. This may be costly, but may be essential to avoid pitfalls, such as putting out an advertisement at the wrong time and therefore missing the target audience. In many ways, the mass media are not an effective tool for health messages, especially if the message involves unpleasant information. People can switch off or turn the page – they are not a captive audience. It may be easier for people to think 'this doesn't affect me' and one-way communication cannot argue a point as a discussion process can.

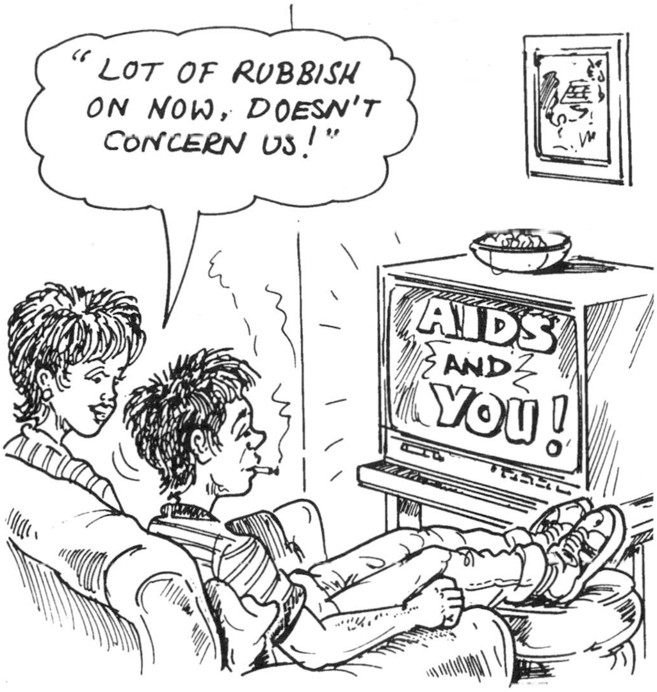
"LOT OF RUBBISH ON NOW, DOESN'T CONCERN US!"
AIDS AND YOU!

Advantages of the mass media

The mass media can be used effectively in the following way.

- *They can raise awareness* on a health issue, which can then be discussed by smaller groups.
- *They can increase knowledge* through information - giving.
- *They can influence behaviour change* by creating an emotional response which causes short-term changes. For example, a documentary on limb amputation due to arteriosclerosis associated with smoking may cause a smoker to think about cutting down or stopping smoking immediately after the programme. However, once the immediate effect has worn off, the smoker may think that the illness is a remote possibility and lose motivation to stop smoking.
- *They can influence changes in public attitudes* by producing a climate of public opinion which will then favour change, for example a discussion of the effects of smoking on non-smokers may promote gradual acceptance of non-smoking rules for public places including transport systems.

Creative designers can use colour and graphics to enhance the aesthetic appeal of advertisements, TV programmes, etc. to ensure they catch and hold the target audience's attention.

Using other methods

Besides the mass media, a health promotion campaign may choose to use methods which access smaller groups of people where individual interaction is possible. Here a range of methods and materials may be used, but there is the added advantage of the possibility of audience participation.

Characteristics of a good presentation

A presentation is a common method of health education and may incorporate any of the methods listed in Figure 20.4 on page 458. It is useful to be aware of the characteristics of a good presentation.

The *structure* of a presentation is important as it aids learning. A presentation should have clear sections rather like a sandwich with the introduction and the evaluation being the bread, and the middle sections being the filling.

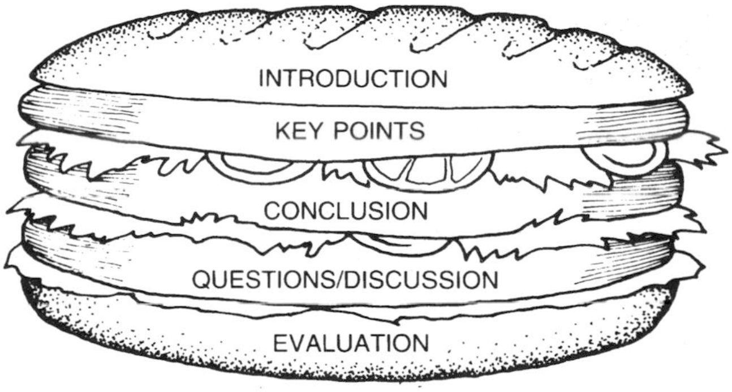

Figure 20.3 The presentation sandwich

- *Introduction* – setting out what you intend to cover. It is often suggested that the introduction should contain a startling fact or a joke, to gain the attention of the audience.
- *Key points* – areas which you discuss and expand upon. These key points could be given on an overhead projector (OHP) slide as a guide for the audience. Unless you are particularly confident, you will need to make notes on cards to remind yourself of the issues to be raised. It is easy for your mind to go blank when in front of an audience.
- *Conclusion* – an opportunity to sum up the main points you have covered.

Resource	Advantages	Disadvantages
Leaflets	■ Audience can use at own pace ■ Self-teaching ■ Reduce need to take notes ■ Often easy to produce and obtain ■ Can be free	■ Not always read ■ Cannot check if leaflets are understood ■ May be biased/used mainly as a means of advertising, (especially in support of a product)
Handouts	■ Easy to produce ■ Reduce need to take notes ■ Can allow audience to recap at own pace later ■ Can be used for self-teaching ■ Could expand on points raised in session	■ Not always read and could be regarded as producing waste material ■ Not everyone will fully understand content and there is no opportunity to clarify ■ Need to be trialled to ensure handouts are appropriate before fuller use
Posters	■ Useful to raise awareness on topic ■ Can attract attention if in a prominent place	■ Aimed at small audience ■ Not always read attentively
Videos	■ Most suitable for small to medium audiences ■ Can show real-life situations ■ Can be useful as trigger for discussion ■ Can have a lot of movement which keeps attention ■ Can be useful for self-teaching	■ Must be checked for relevance ■ Need to be sure of keeping attention ■ Length must be checked
Display	■ Can attract attention and raise awareness	■ Must be eye-catching to be successful
Games	■ Good way to check and confirm knowledge ■ Probably best used with groups which know each other reasonably well	■ Some people do not like a game as they may feel it shows their ignorance ■ Games can threaten individual self-esteem
Role play	■ Encourages audience to put themselves in the situation	■ Some people feel self-conscious ■ Audience may spend more time thinking about their 'performance' than the topic ■ Some people feel threatened by roleplay
Slides	■ Easy to use ■ Can help explain or clarify points	■ Lacks movement, so may fail to keep attention ■ Blackout conditions needed
Overhead projector and transparencies	■ Cheap and easy to produce ■ Illustrate point of talk ■ Can be used to show main point for audience and as reminder for speaker	■ Presentation is important ■ Too many can be confusing ■ Too much information displayed can lead audience to look at transparencies rather than concentrate on the talk

Figure 20.4 Advantages and disadvantages of other methods of promoting health education

- *Questions/discussion time* – this is extremely important and allows the audience to seek clarification if they need to. It is useful to tell the audience that there will be an opportunity to ask questions and discuss any points raised, so that they can note down anything they want to say as it is raised during the session. This will help avoid silence when question time arrives.

Discussion does not always happen naturally and sometimes you may have to initiate it. People are often more prepared to talk and offer ideas in smaller groups; and group work can be used to instigate discussion.

Other ways to get a discussion started include brainstorming and trigger materials such as photographs, statements or just a question for the group to work with.

- *Evaluation* – a very important section which allows you to analyse the programme and its value to the target audience.

With any programme, you may present ideas to an audience which could be in conflict with their current beliefs. Some individuals may choose to challenge what you say. For example, in a session on the effects of smoking on health, someone may quote the case of his or her grandmother who smoked 30 a day and lived until she was 90. Any feedback you give on comments made should always be constructive and non-judgemental. Avoid bringing your personal values and feelings into the discussion or it may become personal rather than general.

Present the facts, and allow individuals to make their own choices. You can only empower them to make an informed choice by offering clear and balanced information.

Content of message

Whatever method a campaign uses to put over a message, the content of the message may vary according to the approach the promoters wish to take. Many campaigns aim to offer *factual information* to enable the target audience to make its own choices based on full information, However, this approach can be presented in different ways. One method which is believed to be effective is to use an individual who has experienced the effects of the health message you are trying to put over, for example, by asking someone who has tobacco-related lung cancer to talk to a group of young smokers. The presenter might talk about his or her thoughts and beliefs when young, and the benefits of giving up smoking.

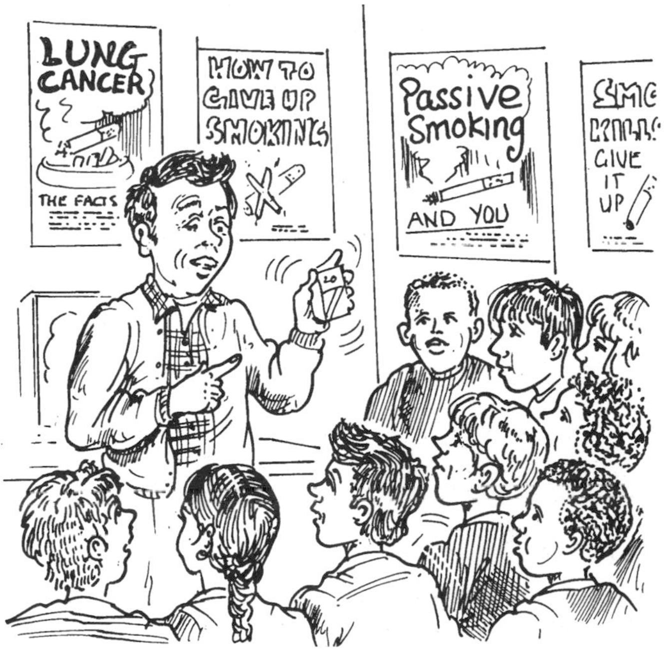

Scare or shock stories are sometimes used to try to make individuals change their habits, but this may not prove very successful as an individual may decide 'it won't happen to me'. Some individuals may respond to scare stories by believing that taking risks is a sign of courage.

Another method is to *promote the idea* and to suggest behaviour changes which could help the individual achieve this ideal, for example by using pictures of slim women to promote a particular breakfast cereal.

Whichever method is used and whatever the topic, as a health educator you will need to consider a number of factors before finally deciding on the method to be used.

In each target group, there will be wide variations on the types and levels of information required, but there are several points to be considered before planning a health education programme.

- What is the level of understanding of the target audience?
- What does the target audience already know? What is the starting point?
- What does the target audience need to know about the topic?
- How much is it reasonable to expect an audience to remember in the time allocated? The average person might only remember about four or five points from any one session.
- How do you involve the audience in the session? It is believed that people remember more if they are actively involved. However, you need to be quite confident and well-organised to develop audience participation to its fullest.
- How do you keep the concentration of the audience? This has a direct effect on maximising learning – a lot of talking can turn an audience off, so you need to include different methods within the presentation.
- Ensure the information being given is relevant to the topic.
- A presentation should take account of cultural issues where appropriate, as these can affect choices. This will also ensure you do not offend

Aims	Possible methods
■ To raise awareness of health issues ■ To increase knowledge	Lectures or talks in schools or colleges, use of mass media, displays, posters in work settings and public places, documentaries, articles, chat shows, debates (the audience is generally passive)
■ Self-empowerment ■ To change attitudes ■ To change behaviour	Group work, role play, case studies, assertiveness training, games in schools or colleges, counselling, indivudial or group therapy in self-help groups (interactive work with involvement is important)
■ To change a society's attitudes	Mass media, pressure groups, lobbying, community work, enforcing laws and regulations, local planning and policy-making

Figure 20.5 How selected methods can be used to achieve aims

anyone. For example, it would be inappropriate to suggest that Asian women should spend more time in the sun to increase vitamin D levels if their culture does not allow them to reveal their skin. Therefore another recommendation should be offered.

- Communication skills are paramount. Speak slowly and clearly. Try not to pack so much information into the presentation that the audience is lost.

Which method is most appropriate?

In most cases, the choice of the method used depends on the aim of the campaign. Some examples are given in Figure 20.5.

Evidence collection point

Investigate two different health education campaigns. For each, produce a report which:

a identifies the source of the campaign (give examples of other campaigns this source has produced)
b explains why the source is promoting the message
c identifies the promotional methods used, suggests why they were chosen and identifies the advantages and the disadvantages of the methods chosen
d discusses any shortfalls in the campaign and suggests how they could be overcome.

Chapter 21

Evaluating the effectiveness of a health education campaign

Chapters 19 and 20 explored the areas of health education campaigns and the methods used to promote the message. This chapter looks at one campaign in detail to illustrate how campaigns might be evaluated for effectiveness.

Whether you are going to evaluate a short-term campaign (for example, an hour-long presentation) or a long-term campaign, the evaluation process is the same. The only difference is that a long-term campaign may also be *monitored* as it progresses to allow changes to be made if and when necessary. This helps to ensure that time, money and effort are not wasted. Figure 21.1 sets out the stages of the evaluation process.

Case study: The materials

The stages of the evaluation process will be illustrated using the health education material aimed at promoting safe eating and avoiding infection from food in pregnancy.

The following materials have been used:

- Department of Health leaflet, *While you are pregnant: Safe Eating and How to Avoid Infection from Food and Animals.* This leaflet is produced to help prevent ill-heath during pregnancy which might result from poor food choice or infection.
- Milk Marketing Board leaflet, '*A Guide to Your Diet in Pregnancy*', obtained from The Nutrition and Education Dept., Milk Marketing Board, Thames Ditton, Surrey KT7 0EL. This is produced to promote health food choice in pregnancy.
- Ministry of Agriculture, Fisheries and Food leaflet, *Food Sense.* This was chosen as it has a section on healthy food choices in pregnancy, but unlike the other two, it was distributed through women's magazines and therefore should have reached the general public more readily.

Evidence collection point

Choose one health education campaign that you are familiar with to evaluate in depth. This could be a message which stands alone and uses discrete health education material, or it could be a message which is promoted through a range of methods. For example, campaigns against smoking focus solely on that topic, but non-smoking is also part of messages aimed at reducing heart disease. You could choose a campaign featured on the TV, in newspapers and magazines, in leaflet form only, or a presentation you have attended.

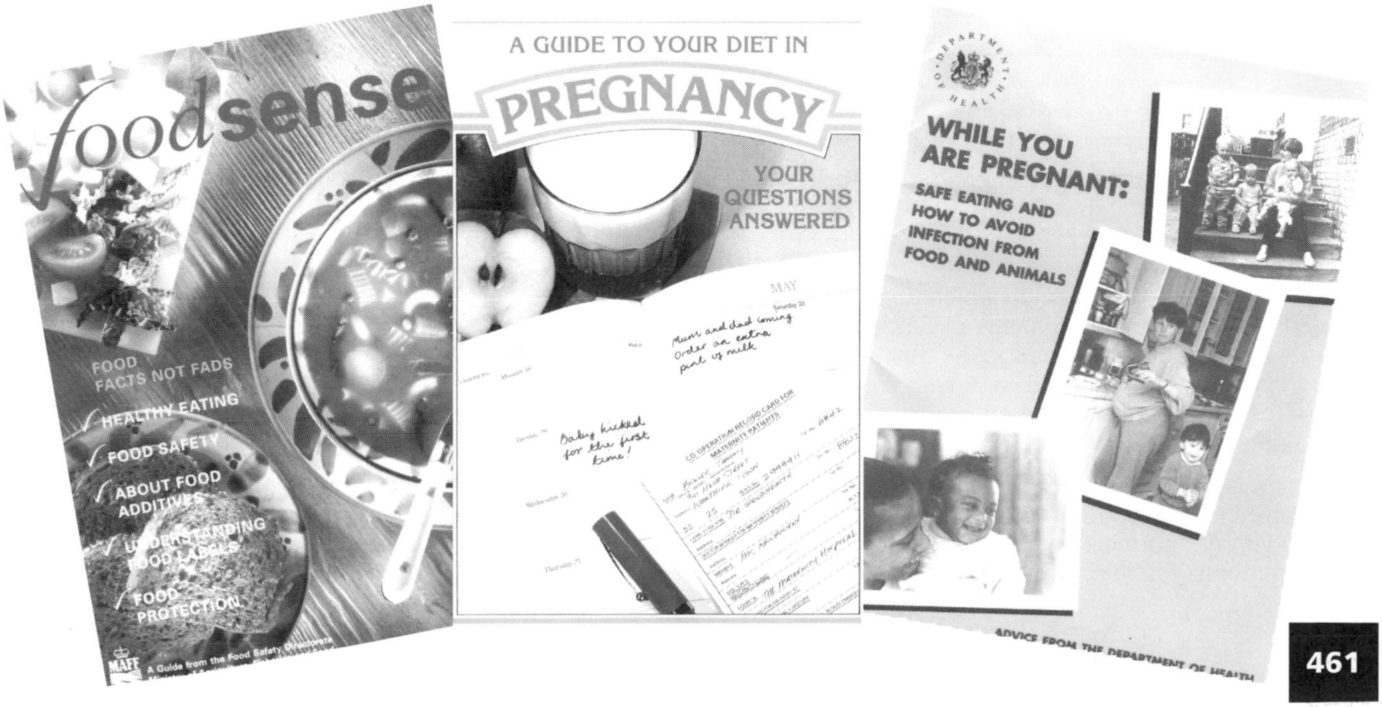

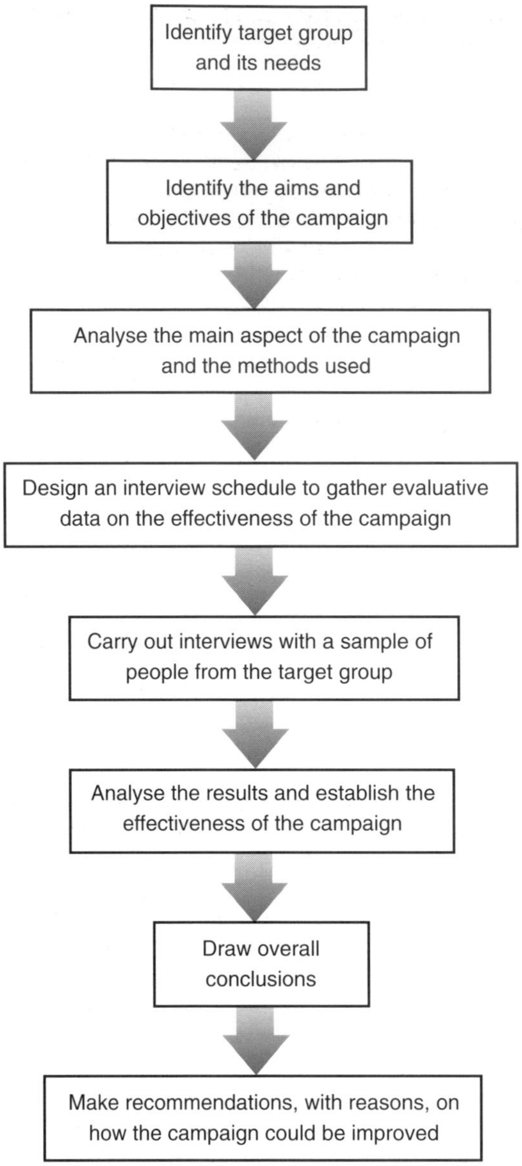

Figure 21.1 The stages in evaluating the effectiveness of a health education campaign

If possible, choose a campaign which uses a range of methods to promote the message or has a number of different sources of the message, as this will give you more material to analyse and work with. You will also need to be able to assess the effectiveness of the campaign.

Collect as much evidence of the campaign as you can. This might include tapes or videos of presentations (ensure you get permission first), copies of articles, advertisements, leaflets, videos of television material.

Use this material to work through the stages of the evaluation.

Identifying the target group and its needs

The target group

Material may be aimed at a very small specific group or at a wider audience.

Case study: The target group

Two of the materials we have selected are aimed at pregnant women or those who are intending to become pregnant. In these cases, the material is focused on a very specific group. There are a number of health education issues regarding pregnancy and food choice. Others include the importance of folic acid before conception and during the first three months to help prevent foetal abnormalities, and the need for increased iron in the diet during pregnancy. Health education focusing on a healthy pregnancy and consequent foetal development is very important as there are strong links between the two.

The third leaflet is aimed at a more general audience, but has a specific section on pregnancy. The message is one that the UK government is keen to put across and it is therefore highlighting it at any opportunity and aiming to get it read by as wide a target group as possible.

Needs

Needs must be identified for every campaign. The person to do this might be:

- the health educator, who will decide what the target group or individual might need to know on a subject
- the target group or individual who might themselves perceive a need to be informed about a topic and therefore identify what they want or need to be told.

These needs might be broad, for example 'more on smoking and health', or be more specific, such as 'the effect smoking has on the lungs'.

The needs may be so many that it is impossible to cover them all in the time allocated and so it may be necessary to *prioritise* according to decided criteria.

Case study: The needs of the target group

The needs of the pregnant women in this campaign have been identified by the professionals or health educators. They have identified what they feel the individuals need to know. The form of presentation suggests that they have assumed very little about the subject matter.

The Department of Health leaflet has a high percentage of writing, whereas the Milk Marketing Board has used a lot of diagrams and colourful pictures to support the text. This may prove more attractive and accessible to the reader.

The third leaflet is also full of factual information, but covers a wide range of topics. The section aimed at pregnant women is quite small and therefore its objective could be one of awareness-raising in the hope that anyone who reads it, who might be affected, will seek further advice.

These needs and priorities will naturally flow into aims.

Identifying the aims and objectives of the campaign

Think it over

Reread the section on page 431 to remind yourself of the difference between aims and objectives. You will need to establish the aims and objectives of your chosen campaign.

Case study: Aims and objectives

The *aims* of the campaign could be connected to achieving general government targets of improving the health of the nation and are:

- to increase knowledge on safe eating habits and food choice during pregnancy
- to raise awareness of the risk factors associated with infection from pets and other animals during pregnancy
- to promote and empower healthy choices which could reduce risk
- to support information which is given out in ante-natal classes
- to ensure the information reaches as wide an audience as possible.

The *objectives* of the campaign are

- to produce leaflet(s) for professionals to use with clients to increase knowledge on safe eating and the risk from animals during pregnancy
- to clarify facts on the dangers to the unborn child if the mother suffers food poisoning or contracts an infection from animals
- to give clear, simple advice on how to reduce risks through a checklist
- to identify where further advice may be obtained on the issues
- to distribute awareness-raising material to the general public on issues concerning safe food choice in pregnancy.

Analysing the main aspect of the campaign and the methods used

Often there is a range of ways to achieve the same aim or objective, but the way chosen may depend on a number of factors, such as:

- *cost* – if money is a problem, an educator is unlikely to buy expensive leaflets to cover a point, but may use an OHP
- *time available* – if a session lasts an hour, a 45-minute video is not likely to be used as there will be little time left for anything else
- *appropriateness for the target audience* – many health promotion topics are appropriate for many different audiences, but the way the message is put over varies
- *ease of use*
- *familiarity to the health educator* – it is very unwise to choose to use unfamiliar material when presenting a programme to a group
- *facilities available*
- *size of group* – for a group of 50, group work may not be appropriate, but it may work very well for smaller numbers.

Equally, health education campaigns may focus on just one aspect of a broad issue or aim to cover all very briefly.

Case study: Methods

The campaign uses leaflets and information prepared by professionals. It covers many of the risk factors associated with food choice and contact with animals. It includes information on listeria, salmonella, toxoplasmosis and chlamydiosis. It also has advice sections on safe food preparation and dealing with family pets.

It aims to provide advice without scare or shock tactics, and also to show that with simple precautions, the risk is minimal.

Once produced, the leaflets are a relatively cheap form of health promotion material as they are readily available through the health promotion unit. They are also given to every pregnant woman when she first registers with the hospital. However, this can be at four months pregnant or more, by which time she could already have been at risk from food poisoning and/or infection from animals.

Designing a structured interview schedule

Advice on how to construct an interview schedule is outlined in Chapters 22–24. A structured interview can be used when meeting individuals from the target group to obtain information from them regarding the effectiveness of the health education campaign.

If you are studying a new campaign, you may need to collect data on the target group's knowledge before exposure to the campaign and then, again, sometime after, to assess the long-term effects of the campaign.

Case study: The structured interview

A structured interview for evaluating this campaign might look like that shown below. This schedule could be used with each leaflet for comparative purposes.

In this interview, questions 4, 5, 8 and 9 allow the interviewer to assess the effectiveness of the message by testing awareness before and after seeing the leaflet. The interview also allows the respondent to comment on important aspects of the campaign such as source, target audience and presentation. This will allow you to assess whether it is perceived as relevant by the target audience, as this is one of the main reasons why campaigns fail – the message does not reach the target audience if they do not perceive it to be aimed at them. Additionally, you can comment on the aesthetics and language as this can be one of the major factors which makes someone read a leaflet or watch an advertisement.

Carrying out the interview

You are required to carry out the structured interview with at least six people. Before doing so, ensure you

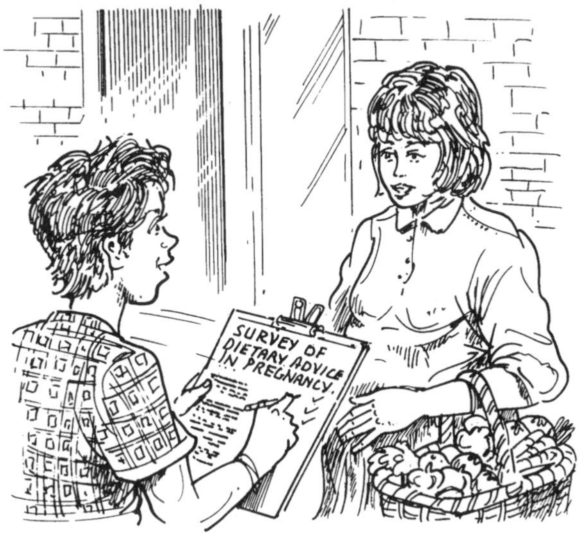

Structured interview schedule

1. Have you ever received any health promotion advice on safe eating in pregnancy?
   a. If yes, from where and in what context?
2. Have you ever received any adivce on risk of infections from animals in pregnancy?
   a. If yes, from where and in what context?
3. Have you ever seen this leaflet?
   a. If yes, where and in what context?
      If no, where might you expect to see it?
4. What foods should be avoided in pregnancy and why?
5. What are the potential risks from animals?
   Allow the respondent to study the leaflet.
6. Who do you think the leaflet is aimed at? Why do you think this?
7. Who do you think is responsible for producing this leaflet? Why do you think they have produced it?
8. What is the main message you think it is giving?
9. Is the message clear?
10. Do you think it is successful in putting over its message? Please explain your answer.
11. Is the presentation (e.g. language), use of pictures and diagrams appropriate for the target audience?
12. How might you adapt your lifestyle if you wanted to reduce the risk of food poisoning and infection from animals when pregnant?

are familiar with all the suggested techniques of carrying out a structured interview (Chapters 22–24). These techniques may help you to avoid bias and prevent distorted results

Analysing the results and establishing the effectiveness of the campaign

Once the interviews have been conducted, the results need to be collated so that you can draw conclusions on the effectiveness of the campaign. Chapters 22–24 deal with using and presenting the data.

Case study: The results

Results on the pregnancy campaign might show the following for selected questions regarding the Department of Health leaflet, *While you are pregnant.*

Q3 4 out of 6 had not seen the leaflet before

Q4 5 out of 6 could list one food to avoid in pregnancy – raw eggs due to salmonella. 1 in 6 couldn't list any.

Q8 The main message, perceived by all, is informing the reader of what foods and animals are potentially a danger to pregnant women and their unborn babies. The respondents also identified that the leaflet gave suggestions for reducing risks.

Q10 6 out of 6 feel it is successful in putting over the message, but 4 out of 6 feel it is likely to be available too late in the pregnancy to prevent all risks and should therefore be more generally available.

Q12 5 out of 6 could list a range of foods which should be avoided to reduce risk from both listeria and salmonella. 3 out of 6 were able to discuss practical tips to reduce the risk of Toxoplasmosis.

Presentation of results

You might present this information in a pictorial format using, for example, graphs, pie charts and pictograms, which would provide evidence for the core skill Application of Number.

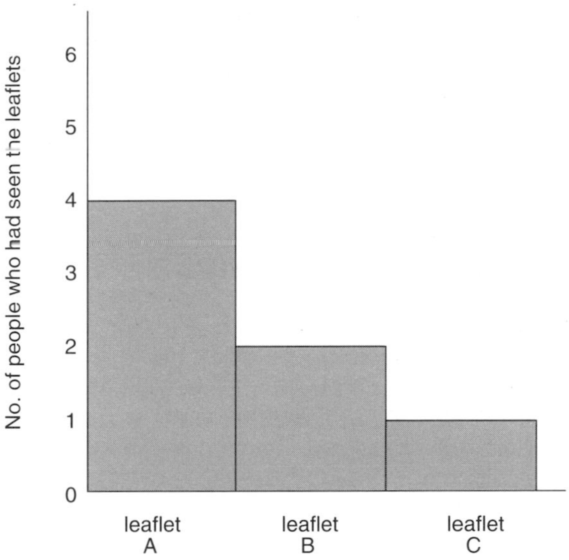

Histogram showing number of respondents who had not seen the leaflets

Figure 21.2 An example of a graph used to present results

If you can use a computer to produce the graphs, you would be able to claim some IT core skills too.

Analysis of results

From your results you could draw some conclusions, such as the following.

- Perhaps the leaflets are not completely successful in reaching the target audience because (say) few people have seen them.
- The message seems clear as all respondents could identify it.
- The leaflet would be successful in increasing knowledge and awareness levels of factors that contribute to risks from food and animals in pregnancy. Awareness of possible lifestyle changes rose following study of the leaflet.

You may also be able to conclude which was the most effective leaflet in meeting the needs of the target group.

Drawing overall conclusions

At this stage you may want to reflect back over all the information you have gained to draw some broad conclusions. You may compare your initial ideas about the target audience and the main message of the campaign with those expressed by respondents of the interview. This may highlight whether or not the campaign is correctly pitched and meets the needs of the target audience. This final analysis will help to formulate recommendations for the last section.

Case study: Conclusions

One overall conclusion of the pregnancy campaign might be that it could meet the needs of the target audience if only it were more readily available at an earlier stage in pregnancy – ideally when individuals are planning pregnancy. The aim of the campaign was to increase awareness and reduce incidence of infection, which the leaflets have the potential to achieve if used properly.

Making recommendations for improvement

The overall conclusions will form the basis of this section. Any recommendations must be valid, achievable and based on evidence gained through study of the effectiveness of the programme.

Case study: Recommendations

Recommendations for the safety in pregnancy campaign would include:

1 to ensure wider distribution of the leaflets in easily accessible places for the target audience, for example in doctors' surgeries, chemists' shops, supermarkets, health clubs
2 to adapt the message to aim it at all people in the childbearing age range, in order to reduce risk at earlier stages in pregnancy.

A sample size of six people may provide you with ideas about the effectiveness of a campaign. But it is important to recognise that such a small sample may not provide firm or final conclusions about a campaign. See Chapters 22–24 for a further discussion of using samples to research data.

Think it over

You may like to evaluate your research in order to contribute to the grading criteria. Evaluation is a vital skill which allows you to review and assess your methods and approach. It allows you to assess the strengths and weaknesses of your work and adjust future work in the light of your findings.

Evidence collection point

At this stage you should have chosen a health education campaign to evaluate. You are requested to:

1 Identify the aims and objectives of the campaign.
2 Analyse the main aspects of the campaign and the methods used.
3 Design and carry out a structured interview with at least six members of the target group to assess the effectiveness of the campaign.
4 Analyse the results and draw conclusions.
5 Make recommendations for changing the campaign.

Self-assessment test

1 A rise in the risk of blood clotting in the arteries can be a result of:
   - a Drinking a brandy last thing at night, every night.
   - b Inhaling lighter fuel.
   - c Smoking and inhaling nicotine from 20 cigarettes every day.
   - d Taking amphetamines.

2 Many of the lifestyle choices that people make can lead to risks to health. Which is associated with smoking?
   - a Cirrhosis of the liver.
   - b Emphysema.
   - c HIV.
   - d Influenza.

3 It is important that an individual is aware of electrical safety. Which of the following might cause an electric shock?
   - a Frayed insulation on flexes.
   - b Not earthing an appliance correctly.
   - c Double layer of insulation.
   - d A blown fuse.

4 Glue, lighter fluid and petrol all belong to the group of substances known as:
   - a Drugs.

- **b** Solvents.
- **c** Tranquillisers.
- **d** Amphetamines.

5 Unprotected sex can put an individual at risk from a number of sexually transmitted diseases. Which of the following is a symptom of gonorrhoea?
- **a** Severe pain on passing urine.
- **b** Thick vaginal discharge.
- **c** Menstruation stops.
- **d** Blisters on the genitals.

6 Drug misuse is the term used to describe the:
- **a** Use of socially acceptable drugs in an unacceptable way.
- **b** Use of socially unacceptable drugs.
- **c** Use of many different drugs at the same time by one person.
- **d** Injection of drugs into the blood stream.

7 You are asked by a client about the best way to reduce his alcohol intake. Which is the best advice to offer?
- **a** Drink with a straw as the alcohol will have less effect.
- **b** Choose half pints rather than shorts as they contain fewer measures of alcohol.
- **c** Use mixers to dilute and lengthen drinks and drink more slowly.
- **d** Avoid alcohol-free drinks.

8 An example of a drug classified as a stimulant is:
- **a** LSD.
- **b** Ecstasy.
- **c** Valium.
- **d** Cocaine.

9 One of the members of a local youth group has just been diagnosed as having HIV. What would be your first main objective with the rest of the group?
- **a** Tell the whole group how to practise safe sex.
- **b** Reassure the group by telling them not to worry; the risk of contracting the disease is small and it is unlikely to happen to them.
- **c** Ensure they all go for medical check-ups.
- **d** Give the opportunity to clarify facts about the virus and AIDS, and discuss any concerns.

10 At the start of a health education session, a speaker makes the following statements. Which one tells the audience about the objective of the talk?
- **a** Some people believe that those who smoke should not get free hospital treatment.
- **b** Can you all hear at the back?
- **c** I am going to talk about smoking and its effects on the body.
- **d** How many of you smoke?

11 For health reasons, doctors recommend a maximum unit intake of alcohol for males and females each week. These are:
- **a** 10 females; 14 males.
- **b** 14 males; 21 females.
- **c** 21 males; 14 females
- **d** 10 females; 20 males

12 When pregnant, you should not drink alcohol because:
- **a** It increases the chance of high blood pressure.
- **b** It crosses the placenta in the blood to the foetus.
- **c** It causes the foetus to put on body fat.
- **d** It always leads to miscarriage.

13 A health educator is presenting information to a group of adolescents on health food choices. The objective of the session would be:
- **a** To provide knowledge to enable the audience to make an informed food choice on diet.
- **b** To advertise low-calorie products.
- **c** To scare people into the right food choices.
- **d** To sell services which could promote health.

14 One way that the HIV is passed from an infected person to a non-infected person is through:
- **a** Kissing.
- **b** Drinking from the same cup when it has not been washed.
- **c** Sharing hypodermic needles.
- **d** Swimming in the same water.

15 There are many different contraceptives available on the market. Each suits differing needs. Which offers the highest protection rate against pregnancy?
- **a** Condom.
- **b** Combined pill.
- **c** IUD.
- **d** Spermicide gel.

16 Smoking is a worldwide habit. Smokers should know that:
- **a** Pipe smokers do not get cancer.
- **b** Smokers do not get lung infections because the smoke kills bacteria and viruses.
- **c** They are at a higher risk of contracting lung cancer.
- **d** Nicotine is not a poison.

17 If a faulty electrical connection is found on an electrical appliance you are using, you should:
- **a** Continue the task then call an electrician once finished.
- **b** Fix it yourself.
- **c** Buy new equipment.
- **d** Stop using the equipment immediately and report it to the appropriate person or call an electrician.

18 Coronary heart disease is caused by a range of contributing factors. Which of the following is *not* one of those factors?
- **a** Smoking.
- **b** Diet high in saturated fat.
- **c** Diet high in salt.
- **d** Varicose veins.

19 Aims and objectives are used to:
- **a** Focus a health education programme.
- **b** Tell the presenter what to say.
- **c** Evaluate the session.
- **d** Pick the topic of a session.

20 Which of the following actions is *not* likely to lead to the increased risk of contracting HIV?
- **a** Injecting heroin.
- **b** Sniffing glue.
- **c** Having unprotected sex.
- **d** Having unscreened blood in a transfusion.

21 Excess alcohol intake is linked with:
- **a** Cirrhosis of the liver.
- **b** Varicose veins.
- **c** Glaucoma.
- **d** Contracting HIV.

22 When talking to a 6-year-old about the importance of effective hand washing after using the toilet, the most effective way to present the message would be:
- **a** An animated cartoon.
- **b** A leaflet.
- **c** A lecture.
- **d** A discussion.

23 The most appropriate way to present health promotion advice on safe sexual practices to a group of school leavers would be:
- **a** A cartoon.
- **b** A two-hour lecture.
- **c** A 'reveal your sexual habits' game.
- **d** An informal discussion.

24 Health education advice on risks to personal safety covers a range of issues. Which would you present to young drivers?
- **a** Road safety.
- **b** Operating electrical machines.
- **c** Lifting techniques.
- **d** Electrical hazards in the home.

25 A health visitor is giving advice to a group of expectant parents. She is discussing smoking. The main emphasis of the talk will most likely be on:
- **a** The best choice of cigarettes.
- **b** The effects of smoking on the unborn child.
- **c** Where to smoke to prevent passive smoking risks to a partner.
- **d** Long-term effects of smoking on the mother's health.

26 In a health education session on drug addiction, where the audience is mainly drug users, you are most likely to focus the talk on:
- **a** Different types of drugs on the market.
- **b** How to spot a drug user.
- **c** How to reduce risk from drug-taking.
- **d** Why people become users.

27 A good health promotion plan has a number of elements. Which offers the target audience the opportunity to assess the success of the programme in meeting their needs?
- **a** Introduction.
- **b** Key points.
- **c** Conclusion.
- **d** Evaluation.

28 An example of a private company as a source of health education campaigns on fat in the diet is:
- **a** Health Education Authority.
- **b** Department of Health.
- **c** The Flora project.
- **d** *Health of the Nation* document.

29 The Campaign for Cancer Research would be classed as health education from the:
- **a** Voluntary sector.
- **b** Private sector.
- **c** National public sector.
- **d** Local public sector.

30 A private company is most likely to use a health message in connection with a product because:
- **a** It believes it will increase sales.
- **b** Its mission is to promote health.
- **c** Its role is education.
- **d** It is promoting the interests of a particular group.

31 An example of a education programme where the aim was preventative action is:
- **a** Immunisation programme.
- **b** Weight Watchers.
- **c** Anti-abortion campaigns.
- **d** HIV testing.

32 A GP's surgery is promoting a contraceptive advice clinic for teenagers. This is an example of a health education campaign started to:
- **a** Meet the national targets.
- **b** Promote the interests of the contraceptive companies.
- **c** Promote the work of charities.
- **d** Provide a screening programme.

33 A newspaper uses the headline 'Smoking causes limb amputation'. This is an example of using:
- **a** Shock/scare tactics.
- **b** An analogy.
- **c** An ideal model.
- **d** Factual information.

34 When referring to the aesthetic appeal of a health education leaflet, you are referring to:
- **a** The style of writing.
- **b** The use of graphics.
- **c** The attractiveness to the target group.
- **d** The level of language used.

35 Health education using the TV is considered to be less successful that a presentation by an individual because:
- **a** There is not opportunity to clarify points made.
- **b** Illustrations are not possible.
- **c** It lacks meaningful representation.
- **d** It does not appear realistic.

36 A health education campaign on TV is likely to bring about short-term change in behaviour because:
- **a** It promotes an emotional response.
- **b** It promotes a reasoned response.
- **c** Everything on TV is always believed.
- **d** The message is not always clear.

37 The term 'rationale' in relation to a health education campaign refers to:
- **a** Choosing a topic.
- **b** Identifying a method of presentation.
- **c** Justifying why you are approaching something in a certain way.
- **d** Reflecting on the campaign.

38 A health education message on immunisation which needs to reach a wide audience of parents is likely to use:
- **a** Magazine advertisements in *Farmers' Weekly.*
- **b** A television campaign.
- **c** Leaflets in a doctor's surgery.
- **d** Posters at a health clinic.

39 The term 'shortfall' used in a health education campaign means:
- **a** Not reaching the target group.
- **b** Not completing a session.
- **c** Having too few leaflets for a session.
- **d** Not having a full session.

40 Which of the following is *not* an example of a shortfall:
- **a** Misinterpretation by the target group.
- **b** Not identified by the target group.
- **c** Not accessed by the target group.
- **d** Being identified by more than the target group.

41 One of the disadvantages of using TV for promoting a health message is that often there is no feedback from the audience to clarify or discuss points made. This can lead to misinterpretation. One way to reduce this would be to:
- **a** Have subtitles on the text.
- **b** Repeat the programme later in the week.
- **c** Have a phone-in session as part of the programme.
- **d** Offer a transcription of the dialogue.

42 Mass media are often used for 'agenda setting'. This means they are used to:
- **a** Discuss a health issue in depth.
- **b** Devise a list of priorities of health issues for the public.
- **c** Raise general awareness on a topic and so encourage public debate.
- **d** Clarify complex messages on health issues.

43 An example of a health education campaign which is aimed at preventative action would be:
- **a** Animal rights campaign.
- **b** Immunisation campaign.
- **c** Anti-abortion campaign.
- **d** Uptake of benefits campaign.

44 If a health message is misinterpreted by a target group, it means it:
- **a** Is not fully understood.
- **b** Is aimed at the appropriate level.
- **c** Contains factually incorrect information.
- **d** Is broadcast at the wrong viewing time.

45 A cartoon programme on smoking and the dangers to health aimed at 7–8-year-olds is shown at 8.00 pm. This is likely to produce a shortfall in the number of the target audience it reaches because:
- **a** The message will be open to misinterpretation.
- **b** The target group will not identify with it.
- **c** It is unlikely to be seen by the target group due to screening time.
- **d** It is an inappropriate way to present this health message for the age group.

46 A government document stresses the need to reduce the number of teenage pregnancies. Consequently, GP practices set up adolescent advice groups on sex education and contraception. This is a response to:
- **a** Local targets.
- **b** Interests of a particular group.
- **c** Organisational targets.
- **d** National targets.

47 When evaluating the success of a health education campaign, you will evaluate the appropriateness of any published material used. The best use of published material would be:
a To leave it on the table at the front of the room.
b To devise a group exercise around it, requiring feedback.
c Hand it out on leaving a session.
d Pin it up on a board as a display.

48 An effective health education programme is well planned to maximise learning. It might include several aspects. If you were evaluating a campaign to reduce the incidence of smoking in young people, which aspect of a programme would you expect to be most useful?
a Providing facts.
b Exploring attitudes and values.
c Helping them make life choices.
d Helping them to change lifestyles.

49 Leaflets can provide a useful addition to a health education campaign. Their main advantage is that they:
a Are easy to obtain.
b Are easy to distribute.
c Promote local products.
d Give clear information which can be referred to later.

50 When evaluating the effectiveness of a leaflet on healthy diet aimed at primary school children, it is important to ensure that:
a It contains detailed written facts.
b It includes brightly-coloured pictures and diagrams.
c It is scientifically accurate.
d It uses a lot of jargon.

51 If you were evaluating the effectiveness of a campaign which conveyed real-life scenarios, which visual aid would you feel was most appropriate?
a A poster.
b A video and screen.
c Textbooks.
d A flip chart.

52 When evaluating a video for use in a primary school, which of the following would the *most* suitable video include?
a Warnings about what will happen if the advice is not followed.
b Scare tactics.
c A lecture by a children's personality.
d Simple messages in a pictorial form.

53 When evaluating a long presentation, you may focus on the methods used to keep the audience's attention. This may be achieved by using different aids. If evaluating a session on safe sexual practices, which method/aim would be most appropriate for giving information on new contraceptive methods?
a Brainstorming session using flipchart paper on the new methods of contraception.
b Video tape including a demonstration of use.
c Leaflets and discussion.
d Audio tape of a doctor describing use.

54 A health education campaign you are evaluating is aimed at encouraging the sale of nutritious foods from a school tuck shop, working with both parents and teachers. This strategy is trying to:
a Improve self-esteem.
b Change the physical environment.
c Increase knowledge.
d Increase awareness of health issues.

55 You are evaluating the success of a publican attempting to reduce smoking in his pub. Which of the following would be among his objectives?
a Setting up a smoke-free bar.
b Putting out more ash trays.
c Encouraging pipe smoking rather cigarettes.
d Increasing the number of cigarette vending machines in the establishment.

56 Structured interviews can be used to gain information for an evaluation of a health education campaign. Which of the following is a characteristic of a structured interview?
a All questions have yes or no answers.
b It always uses closed questions.
c It is only carried out with less than 10 people.
d It has a schedule of set question to follow.

57 When carrying out a structured interview to assess a campaign, you should talk to members of the target group for that campaign. This means:
a You can ask anyone.
b You can ask those the campaign was aimed at.
c You identify any one group to question.
d You target every fourth person who walks past you in the street.

58 When evaluating a health education programme, you need to establish if it has met the needs of the target group. You are evaluating a session where the need has been identified as offering advice to people affected by chronic health conditions – on how to adjust and improve their lifestyles. Which target group would it be aiming at?
a Adults in a busy shopping centre.

b Inactive people in wheelchairs.
c 5–6-year-olds.
d Pregnant women.

59 When evaluating the appropriateness of the level of a session for a target group, which of the following might *not* be an essential part of the evaluation?
a Seating arrangements.
b Audience's concentration span.
c Extent of vocabulary used.
d Audience's literacy skills.

60 A good health education session gives the audience the opportunity to seek clarification. This can most effectively be achieved by:
a The audience completing an evaluation.
b Having a question and answer session.
c Ensuring the speaker sums up the main points.
d Having a display available on the topic.

Fast Facts

AIDS Acquired Immunodeficiency Syndrome – the illness that HIV creates.

Aims Broad statements which outline goals people are hoping to achieve.

Alcohol A drug; a colourless, flammable liquid which forms the intoxicating part of drinks. It is produced by fermenting sugars.

Aspects of health education Topics or areas which health education focuses on, such as smoking, alcohol, drugs, road safety, accident prevention, etc.

Bronchitis Inflammation of the bronchial tubes caused by bacteria, a virus or irritation of the respiratory tract, for example by smoking.

Carbon monoxide A poisonous gas found in cigarette smoke which combines with haemoglobin and reduces the amount of oxygen the blood can carry.

Conclusion A summing up of the main facts.

Contraception Ways to reduce the risk of fertilisation of the female egg by the male sperm as a result of sexual intercourse.

Coronary heart disease A condition where the functioning of the heart is impaired by a build-up of fatty plaques in the arteries. It has a number of risk factors such as smoking, a diet high in saturated fat and lack of exercise.

COSHH Control of Substances Hazardous to Health: regulations that require that all employers carry out a risk assessment of any substance which might be considered hazardous to their employees' health and minimise that risk.

Dependency Relying on something for physical or mental functioning.

Disease Any reduction in the normal physiological functioning affecting all or part of the body.

Drug abuse The use of socially unacceptable drugs in a socially unacceptable way.

Drug misuse The use of socially acceptable drugs, such as tranquillisers, in a socially unacceptable way.

Emphysema A condition where the air sacs of the lungs are enlarged causing breathlessness and wheezing.

Equipment and resources Necessary materials or items of support which might be used in a health promotion programme, for example OHPs, leaflets.

Evaluation A way to review the success of something such as a health promotion programme or materials used. It is used to assess successful aspects as well as less successful aspects and is therefore used as a tool to improve future performance.

Feedback Information which is give back in response to an enquiry, perhaps a question or statement.

Free response A question which allows the respondent to answer however he or she wishes.

Fuse A protective device which safeguards electrical circuits and will break the circuit if it becomes overloaded and therefore a fire risk.

Genital urinary infections (GUs) Infections which affect both the sexual organs/reproductive system and the urinary system.

Hazard Anything that has the potential to cause harm to someone in some way.

Health The state of being physically and mentally free from disease; the general condition of the body and mind.

Health education Advice to encourage informed individual health choices.

Health promotion Advice to further or encourage healthy choices on a larger scale, for example the environment.

Human Immunodeficiency Virus (HIV) The virus which causes AIDS.

Introduction The start of something, such as a talk or book. It should set out briefly what is going to happen; a way of setting the scene.

Key points The main areas that a health promotion presentation is covering; the main issues the presenter is hoping to focus on.

Mass media Channels of communication to large numbers of people, such as TV, newpapers.

Mental health The health of the mind; the ability to think clearly and carry out intellectual processes.

Objectives Linked to aims, but are more specific and measurable. Statements saying what an individual is hoping to achieve and possibly how he or she intends to do it.

Passive smoking A non-smoker breathing in cigarette as it burns or the smoke the smoker has exhaled.

Physical health The health of the body and its organs.

Planning A detailed scheme or method for achieving an objective; may have a timescale.

Primary health education The process of informing different groups about aspects of health care before they risk their health.

Prioritise A way of ranking a number of issues or tasks according to importance to allow some but not all to be covered if time is limited.

Recommendations Suggestions made for development or change.

Residual current device (RCD) A device used with electrical equipment. It can detect damage to electrical cables or other faults and will cut off the electric current extremely quickly, thus protecting against electrical accidents.

Risk A measurement of how likely a potential hazard is to cause harm.

Secondary health education Health advice which aims to encourage people to change existing habits, which have the potential of being health risks, to healthier habits.

Sexually transmitted diseases (STDs) Diseases which are passed from one individual to another through sexual contact.

Shortfalls Where a health education programme does not meet its aims or target audience.

Social health Being able to form and keep relationships going with other people both on a personal and professional level.

Tar A substance in cigarettes which causes narrowing of the bronchioles and damages the small hairs which line the lungs. It makes the lungs less efficient and more prone to infections.

Target audience/group The potential audience at whom health promotion material is aimed. The type of audience will determine the material and approach used.

Tertiary health education The re-education of an individual to get the most from life when he or she has an irreversible or chronic illness.

Unit The way alcohol is measured and individual consumption assessed.

References and further reading

BMA, 1993 *Complete Family Medical Health Encyclopedia,* Dorling Kindersley

Department of Health, 1992, *The Health of the Nation,* HMSO

Department of Health, 1993, *Health of the Nation: One Year On,* HMSO

Department of Health, 1995, *Tackling Drugs Together,* HMSO

Ewles and Simnet, 1992, *Promoting Health: A Practical Guide 4,* Scutari Press

Institute of Environmental Health Officers, 1993, *Basic Health and Safety at Work,* Environmental Health Training

Tones, Tilford and Robinson, 1990, *Health Education Effectiveness and Efficiency,* Chapman & Hall

World Health Organisation, 1984, *Health Provision*

Leaflets

Boice & Gamble, 'You don't need to be an expert', Health Education Authority

Department of Health, 1991, 'While you are pregnant', HMSO

Flora Project for Heart Disease Prevention, 'Smoking'

HEA, 1991 'Smoking – The facts', Health Education Authority

HEA, 1992, 'That's the limit', A guide to sensible drinking, Health Education Authority

HEA and the Department of Health, 'A guide to childhood immunisations', Health Education Authority

Home Office, 1991, 'Electrical Safety leads to fire safety', HMSO

Ives, 1992, 'Solvents: A Parent's Guide', Department of Health

Milk Marketing Board, 'A guide to diet in your pregnancy'

Ministry of Agriculture, Fisheries and Food, 1991, 'Food Sense', HMSO

Pharmacy Health Care, 'It's time to stop smoking'

Portman Group, 'Talking to your children about drinking. A guide for parents'

QUIT, 'Smoking – your pregnancy, your baby: The facts'

QUIT, 'Quit smoking without putting on weight'

Chapter 22

The research process

Whatever field of work people are involved in, they need to be able to find things out. Information and knowledge are needed by scientists, economists, and practitioners in all fields, including health and social care. *Research* is the process of finding things out in an organised, systematic and thoughtful way. It can take a variety of forms, and use different methods, depending on the field and the question that you are interested in. As carers, our field of study is people, and this chapter deals with the methods of research used in health and social care.

This chapter focuses on:

- **the role of research**
- **research questions and research structure – quantitative and qualitative data, secondary and primary data**
- **research methods – including the uses and limitations of experiments, questionnaires, interviews, observation, and the reliability and validity of these methods**
- **ethical issues in social research**
- **the research process.**

The role of research

In our everyday lives we are frequently confronted with assumptions about social issues. They are often stated in the media, and crop up in conversations as 'common knowledge'. You may have heard statements like 'women don't really want a career' or 'people on state benefits are actually well-off', and have given your views on the subject in response. However, without research this is just argument and opinion. Several centuries ago it was 'common knowledge' that the earth was the centre of the universe, and that it was flat. European people were afraid to sail too far to the west for fear of falling off! This dramatically illustrates how incorrect assumptions about the world can affect people's behaviour, as well as their views. Eventually research showed that the earth was round and progress was made possible. Social research can address the social assumptions that we live with today, and allow progress to take place here too.

Social research involves collecting information about people's opinions and circumstances. It is a fairly widespread activity carried out by governments, businesses, organisations and individuals. Research of any type involves time and effort, so we could begin by asking why people make this investment in social research, and why they consider it to be so important. What is the role of research in the work of such a wide variety of users?

Research is often used to assess the effectiveness of policies and practices. Organisations, including governments and health and care organisations, develop policies for dealing with the issues that they face. Practitioners put these policies into practice. In health and social care organisations there are likely

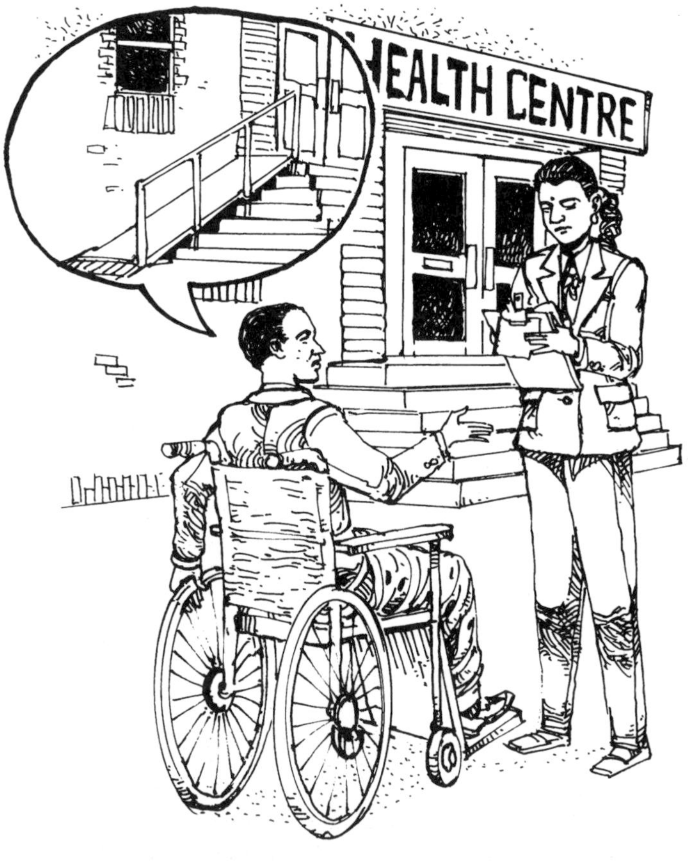

Figure 22.1 Research can help suggest improvements

to be policies covering dealings with clients, equal opportunities, and other aspects of their work. Organisations and individuals involved in social care need to know that they are achieving what they set out to do. They need to check that the policies they have adopted are working as they intended, and that the practices they are carrying out are supporting these policies. One of the roles of research is to discover how effective a policy is, and how well the working practices of staff support the policy.

For example, a local health centre may have developed an equal opportunities policy, aimed at preventing discrimination in its dealings with clients, in staff recruitment, and other areas of its work. Policy and practice need to go hand-in-hand. So putting the policy into practice means developing ways of working that support the equal opportunities policy. This may include changes to the environment to ensure that physical access is available to all, and changes to administrative procedures and publicity materials so that all potential users are fully informed and made welcome. A research investigation into the effects of these policies and practices can help to show whether the aims are being met. The results may indicate that changes to the policy are necessary and suggest more effective approaches. They may indicate that working practices need to be altered to allow the policy to work.

Research is also conducted by social scientists to disprove *propositions* about people and society. Propositions are statements which describe a situation or a relationship. They are framed as though they are a fact, and give an accurate description of the true state of affairs. The statements 'elders prefer being at home to attending a day centre' and 'students who spend the most time studying always get the best results' are examples of propositions. A proposition may be a statement of a commonly-held belief. The statements of 'common knowledge' mentioned earlier could also be described as propositions. Propositions that are carefully framed and worded so that research methods can be used to test them are known as hypotheses.

The notion that a proposition can never be proved, but can be disproved, comes from ideas about scientific method which are used in both the natural and social sciences. Physicists, chemists and other natural scientists work on the principle that a theory, or proposition, is never accepted as absolutely true, however many examples may seem to agree with it. If research reveals just one exception it shows that the proposition doesn't always hold. A counter example forces scientists to revise the proposition so that all cases are accounted for. The same method can be applied to propositions about social issues. For example, the proposition 'elders prefer being at home to attending a day centre' would be disproved if research showed that there were elders who preferred being at a day centre to being at home.

Research results may give indications of how propositions, and theories, should be revised and improved. In our fictitious example it may have been noticed that those elders who did prefer being at home often had family members living with them. This might suggest other lines of enquiry and the framing of new propositions. In this way the disproving of propositions can help to improve our understanding of how the world works, and help us to develop better theories to explain it. This relationship between theory and research is an important aspect of scientific methods of enquiry.

Research has a crucial role to play in extending our collective knowledge and understanding. For example, research results linking smoking to ill-health can help everyone to understand the risks that smokers face. The results of professional researchers help to develop knowledge in the field that they are involved in, and so develop understanding of the world for all people.

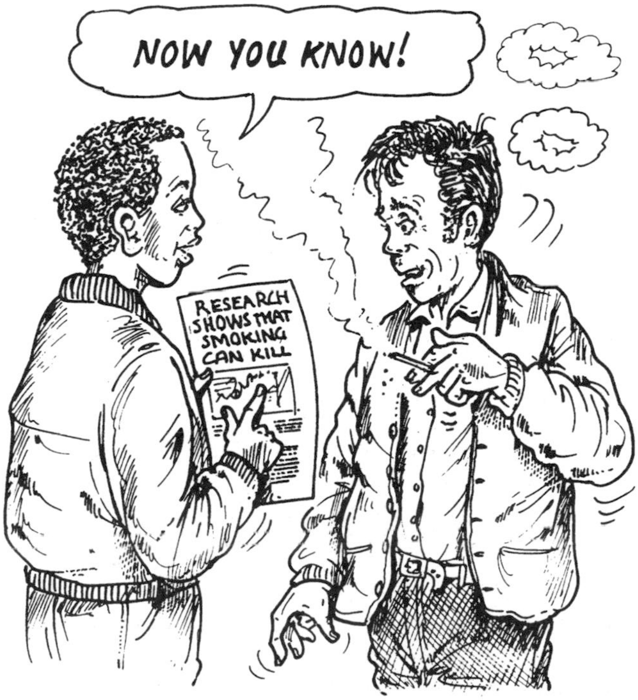

Individuals too can develop their knowledge, and improve their own professional practice, by finding things out. As a GNVQ Health and Social Care student you will be carrying out research of one sort or another throughout your studies. Research does not have to be carried out by large organisations and professional scientists to be useful. Small-scale research projects are not automatically less valuable than well-resourced professional studies. The thing that distinguishes good research from bad is how well other people can be convinced that the results are accurate and useful, and this means thinking carefully about what you are doing every step of the way.

The many organisations and individuals who investigate and carry out research may have different ideas about the role it plays in their work. They may be looking for definite conclusions and recommendations for practical action, or they may be content to allow their results to lead to further enquiry as part of the development of scientific understanding. Whatever reasons people may have for carrying out research, they are all involved in the process of seeking answers to research questions that they are interested in.

Research questions and research structure

All research begins with an area of interest. This may be discrimination, health and lifestyle, clients' feelings about the care they receive, or any other area relevant to health and social care. From this area of interest, specific questions emerge. Questions may be about situations people are in, such as 'What percentage of households live on low incomes?' or 'What is the ratio of male to female students on the GNVQ Health and Social Care course you are following?' They may be about their behaviour, such as 'How many people watch football on television?' or 'What percentage of students on your course smoke cigarettes?' They may be about their beliefs and options, such as 'Do people think that the National Health Service is improving?' or 'Do young people believe that sex before marriage is morally wrong?' The type of question you are interested in, and the people it applies to, will have a large influence on the planning and conduct of your research.

The research question will set the boundaries, or parameters, within which the work will take place. This means that you are able to define and clarify the area of study you are involved with. When you are clear about what you are looking at, it becomes possible to seek out work by other people that is relevant to your question. You can relate your research to existing findings and theories. This is important if you are to show that your research is serious and well prepared.

Research questions also set the *parameters* of hypotheses that researchers develop for testing. Most research questions can potentially yield many different hypotheses, and there are methods to help you uncover them. But however it is arrived at, the hypothesis must address the research question at hand.

For example, suppose that you are interested in clients' experiences of health and social care provision, and particularly in the question of how elders feel about the care they receive. Within this question there are many possible areas of enquiry and further focusing is needed before practical research can begin. You may come up with a number of possible hypotheses during this process. For instance, the hypothesis 'most elders attending the local day-care centre are satisfied with the care they receive there' might be one possibility. However, the hypothesis 'most elders using public transport are satisfied with the service they receive' would be rejected. It is not about health and social care services, and falls outside the parameters of the research question.

Try it

Think about the general question of how elders using the health and social care services feel about the care that they receive. Try to narrow the question down to a more specific focus. You may have some experience of local health and care facilities and their users which will help you to do this.

Now try to write down *three* statements which could be hypotheses to be tested for accuracy by research.

The research question may also suggest how you go about doing the research, and the type of information you need to collect. A range of research methods is available and the question you are addressing is likely to indicate which is suitable and which is not. For example, long drawn-out interviews are not usually appropriate when studying young children.

Whatever the methods used, your research will involve finding things out, and the information that is collected is called *data*. Your research question may suggest likely sources of data to you. If you are interested in the number of disabled students attending a local college then the college's own records could be a good data source. If you are interested in disabled people's opinions about the college, then you need to get data directly from them. Most good research draws data from different sources so that background and context is provided for the results.

The research question itself is thus responsible for much of the structure of the research that addresses it. It defines the area of study, indicates relationships with existing theories and findings, sets the parameters of hypotheses, and suggests research methods and data sources. It is important to remember that research is not about collecting as much data as possible without considering why it is needed or what use it will be put to. Above all, research is a planned process which always keeps the research question in view.

Types of data

Data can take different forms. Some data is numerical, for example the number of people attending a day centre for elders. Other data may be more descriptive and personal, for example people's feelings about attending the day centre.

Data which is numerical and can be analysed using statistical methods is known as *quantitative data*. The number of single-parent families in an area, or the number of people giving the same answer to a particular question are examples of quantitative data. Quantitative results can be displayed using graphs, charts and tables.

Data which concerns attitudes, opinions and values is often unable to be expressed in numerical form. It may include comments people have made about a subject, or accounts of their feelings about it, or reactions to it. This information is known as *qualitative data*. Qualitative data is expressed in words, not numbers, and cannot be analysed and reported using statistical methods.

It is important to understand that both quantitative and qualitative data can provide important and useful results. One is not better or more scientific than the other. The main issue is to choose the right type of data, and collection technique, for the questions you are interested in. Most really good research includes both types of data. This is the best way to provide background and balance in social investigations.

Think it over

Suppose that you are planning to collect data from fellow students to find out how effective a recent anti-smoking poster campaign has been. Divide a sheet of paper into two columns, one headed 'Quantitative data' and the other headed 'Qualitative data'.

Try to think of examples of data that you might collect and write each one under the appropriate heading. An example of qualitative data might be people's feelings about smokers. An example of quantitative data might be whether a person smokes or not.

Sources of data

Whether you are looking for quantitative numerical data or descriptive data, there are basically two ways of getting information. You can find out yourself by carrying out an original research project, or you can look at work that has been done already by other people. Carrying out your own research project is called *primary research,* and data you gather in this way is known as *primary data*. Looking at the work of others is called *secondary research,* and data taken from the work of others is called *secondary data*.

Secondary data

Collecting secondary data means looking at existing sources that contain information useful to your research. All researchers use secondary research methods to some extent. In fact some research is stimulated by interesting results that others have published. Doing secondary research, or 'reading around' the research question, is important for any investigation and there are good reasons for looking at secondary sources at an early stage.

- You may pick up useful ideas and concepts about the subject you are interested in. You can relate your research question to existing theories and findings.
- You may get ideas for methods you could use for your own primary research. You may discover that others have already carried out basically the same research project that you are interested in! This last point shouldn't put you off. It can be very

interesting to compare the results of your own carefully conducted research with other published results. It is often through repeating the work of others that new insights arise, and differences may point to interesting new areas of investigation.

- Secondary sources can provide data that it would be impossible to collect for yourself. For example, the government collects and publishes official statistics on a wide variety of topics. These include information on income, birth and death rates, and other features of the population at national and local level. Governments need these statistics, and have the resources to collect them. No research organisations can easily duplicate the endeavour needed to collect this data, and none would bother as the government's statistical department has an international reputation for the quality of its work.

The places you look for secondary data will depend upon the subject you are interested in. Information of all sorts is published in books, government publications, newspapers, journals and in a variety of other places. Whatever you are researching, it is likely that useful information exists somewhere. Your research reports should always list secondary sources that have been consulted. If statistics and other material have been quoted or used to help the research work, it is particularly important that the source is stated clearly in the report. Readers should be suspicious of anonymous or poorly attributed data since there is no way to gauge its accuracy.

Primary data

Collecting primary data means carrying out research work for yourself. The study of people is a wide and difficult area, and the range of research methods that have been developed reflect this. There isn't one best way to carry out social research. The methods used need to be suited to the research question and the people being studied.

Who could the data be collected from? The term *population* is used to describe the total number of people that the research is interested in. For example, if you are researching the attitudes of students towards smoking then your population would include all students. Unless the population is particularly small, only vast projects like the government's census can survey all or most of the student population. This means that a smaller group, a *sample,* must be selected for questioning. Sampling methods have been developed to help make the sample as representative of the whole population as possible.

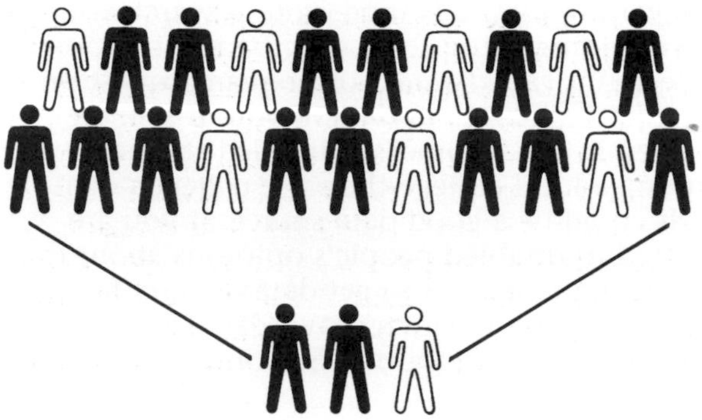

Figure 22.2 The sample should be as representative of the whole population as possible

Research methods

Primary research methods include experiments, questionnaires, interviews and observation. Researchers may use more than one of these methods if their work suggests that it would be useful to do so. Each method has advantages and limitations. and some are often associated with particular disciplines or theoretical approaches.

Experiments

Experiments are often used by psychologists as a way of discovering how individuals behave. Scientists such as chemists and physicists use experiments as their main method of testing theories and hypotheses, and psychologists attempt to apply experimental techniques to the study of people. The principle of the experimental method is that the scientist has control of all the variables in the situation that he or she is studying. For example, a chemist can control variables like temperature, the amounts of each chemical, and the length of time allowed for them to react. By altering one variable and measuring the effect on another, the chemist can establish the experimental relationship between them and make predictions about the future behaviour of the same chemicals in similar circumstances.

However, applying the experimental method to the study of people is not so straightforward. The behaviour of a person is vastly more complex than that of a chemical substance. The range of variables that may influence a subject's behaviour is so large that it is difficult to list them, let alone control them. This becomes even more problematic when the behaviour of groups of people is being studied. One result of this difficulty is that experiments usually deal with a very narrow range of behaviour in very specific circumstances. Predictions about future behaviour need to take account of the complexity of real life where people's actions and behaviour are affected by ideas and influences that the experimenter cannot measure, and may not even be aware of.

Most social experimenters are sensibly cautious about the claims that they make for their research. Provided this scientific honesty is kept in mind, experiments can be a useful way of testing hypotheses about human characteristics and behaviour.

Pros	Cons
Can be designed to test very specific theories and hypotheses	Range of enquiry limited to the specific aims of the experiment
The experimenter can control the circumstances in which the experiment takes place	Difficult for the experimenter to control all factors affecting the bahaviour of subjects
Data collected is nearly always quantitative allowing statistical interpretation of the results	Artificial circumstances of the experimental situation may distort subjects' behaviour
It is possible to duplicate the experiment and test the replicability of the results	'Scientific' conduct of the experiment and statistical presentation of results may lend more credibility to the work than it deserves

Figure 22.3 Some pros and cons of experiments

Social surveys

Other research methods study people in their normal environment, without imposing artificial conditions upon them. *Surveys* are the most common method used to collect data about people's circumstances, behaviour and opinions. There are different types of survey but all involve asking people questions. It is the circumstances under which the questions are answered, and the degree of flexibility allowed for answers, that distinguish one type of survey from another. There are advantages and disadvantages to each survey method. The research question, and the population it concerns, usually suggest which is the most appropriate.

Questionnaires

Self-completion questionnaires, as the name implies, are given to members of the sample group for them to complete themselves. It is up to the sample member, or *respondent,* to read and interpret the questions for him or herself. If it is a postal questionnaire, the respondent is entirely alone; if not, then the researcher may be present to help interpret the questions.

Questionnaires are used extensively in social research, and they can have several advantages.

- They give you the chance to collect information from a large sample of your population. It is fairly cheap to reproduce and distribute large numbers of questionnaires.
- There is no danger that the behaviour or appearance of an interviewer could affect the results. This problem occurs in all research which involves interaction between the researcher and the subjects. Distributing questionnaires is one way to avoid it.
- Respondents have time to consider their answers, and consult others if necessary. For example, if

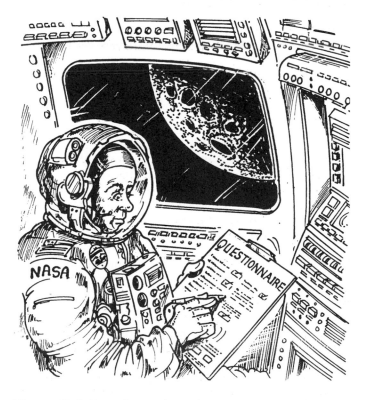

Figure 22.4 Postal questionnaires can reach people too far away to interview

you stop someone in the street and ask them how much their household spends on food per week, they are likely to respond with 'don't know', or make a guess. To get an accurate answer, it is probably better to give respondents time to think, and to ask other family members.

- Postal questionnaires may be the only practical way of contacting members of some populations. Postal questionnaires can be sent to people that physical distance makes it impossible to interview.

Some people, such as doctors or other professionals, may be more willing to fill in a brief questionnaire than give up time for an interview.

Most questionnaires are designed to collect quantitative information. This means that results can be compared between respondents and analysed statistically. This can be seen as another advantage. Remember though that good-looking statistics may mask sloppy research work. Well-presented results are not necessarily good results.

When the information required is comparatively straightforward, a questionnaire can be a very effective research instrument. However, there are problems associated with questionnaires that must be set against the advantages.

- A major problem is that questionnaires often attract a very low response rate. Those who do respond cannot be taken as representative of the whole population, however carefully you selected your original sample group. Statistical analysis of the data collected has little value in this situation. A poor response rate may be due to bad questionnaire design. Long or confusing questionnaires usually end up in the bin. Another possibility is that questions are asked which people are reluctant to answer, perhaps because the subjects are too personal or sensitive. The only answer to a low response rate is to make the subject and content of your questionnaire sufficiently interesting to members of your sample that they are motivated to complete and return them.
- A related problem is that the responses that you do receive are likely to be from those with a view on the subject. This can mean that you get many extreme answers indicating strong, but divided opinions. In fact, opinion may be much more evenly spread within the population, but non-response by those who aren't particularly interested will hide this.
- Questionnaires assume a certain level of literacy amongst respondents. This makes them inappropriate for surveying certain groups, such as small children. Even when this is not expected to be a problem, misunderstandings can and do occur. Without an interviewer present, there is no check that the questions have been understood. Respondents cannot ask for clarification and may guess an answer, or throw the questionnaire away. Either way the quality of the results will be reduced.
- The researcher has no control over who actually completes a questionnaire. It may be passed on to other members of the family. It may be filled in as a joke by a group of friends in the pub! Uncertainty over whose answers you actually receive can completely invalidate careful sampling work.

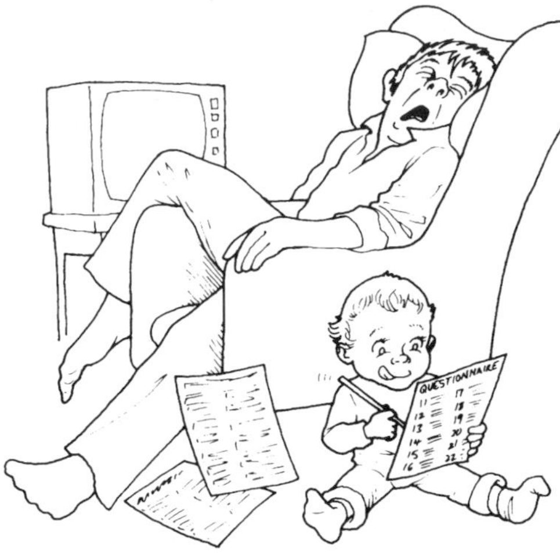

Figure 22.5 You have no control over who completes a postal questionnaire

- Sometimes researchers want to get people's spontaneous response to a question. Respondents may give accurate answers to personal questions if they reply spontaneously, but if allowed time to think they can pick answers that support the image they wish to project. You cannot expect to receive spontaneous responses from questionnaires.
- Respondents can see all the questions at once. An interviewer can control the order in which questions are delivered, so that answers are not prejudiced by knowledge of questions still to come. For instance, in a postal questionnaire it is no use asking 'Can you name the body set up by the government to promote good race relations?' If a later question asks 'Do you think that the Commission for Racial Equality is effective in promoting good race relations?' Another thing

that interviewers can do is to observe people's reactions to the questions as they are asked. This potentially useful information is not available with questionnaires.

Pros	Cons
Data can be cheaply collected from a large number of respondents	Postal questionnaires often suffer from a poor response rate
No problem with the behaviour and appearance of the interviewer influencing results	Responses may be largely from people who have strong opinions on the subject
Respondents have time to consider answers and consult others if necessary	No check on whether respondents have really understood the questions
Postal methods may be the only way to contact some respondents	No control over who actually completes the questionnaire
	No opportunity to observe respondents' reactions to the questions
	Cannot expect to collect respondent's spontaneous answers
	No control over order in which questions are answered
	Respondents are limited to the question and answer options presented and their authentic views may not be revealed

Figure 22.6 Some pros and cons of self-completion questionnaires

Try it

Self-completion questionnaires are a cheap and fairly easy way to collect data from a large number of people. Think about some of the areas you are interested in researching. For each area, assess whether a self-completion questionnaire would be appropriate. List the pros and cons of using this approach in these specific areas of research.

Questionnaires have their advantages, and their limitations, but the researcher has so little control that the quality of the information obtained may be poor. A survey method which allows the researcher more control is the *interview*.

Interviews

Interviews involve the researcher meeting individual subjects and collecting data directly from them. It is up to the researcher to decide whether to make the interview a more or less formal meeting. An interview can follow an inflexible schedule, or it can be conducted in more relaxed, less structured way. Interviews which follow a well-defined and fairly rigid plan are known as *structured interviews*. Interviews which allow the researcher more freedom to explore interesting answers further are known as *semi-structured interviews*. Interviews where the researcher allows the respondent to explore a question in their own way are called *unstructured* or *in-depth interviews*.

Structured interviews

A main aim of structured interviews is to ensure that each interview is carried out in exactly the same way. Any factors that could bias a response are thus minimised, or at least theoretically the same for all respondents. Uniformity in interviews is important if valid statistical comparisons are to be made between responses of different subjects. Interviews follow an *interview schedule* which dictates their input into the interview meeting. Interview schedules contain a list of questions, similar to a questionnaire. They also contain instructions for the interviewer to follow. Questions are read out to respondents and their answers recorded by the interviewer. To help maximise uniformity the schedule contains set comments to prompt a reply or probe an area more deeply. Interviewers are not allowed to deviate from the questions, prompts and probes provided in the interview schedule.

In practice, the degree of uniformity described above is often very difficult to achieve. Nevertheless, the structured interview is a useful and widely-used research technique which has several advantages.

- The response rate obtained by structured interviewing is likely to be good. Provided that the sample chosen is small enough to handle and is easily accessible, the only difficulty is in pinning respondents down for an interview.
- Misunderstandings over the meaning of questions can easily be dealt with. Interviewers can repeat the question and add prompts allowed by the schedule.
- Interviews can be designed to follow up interesting lines of enquiry that a respondent's answers might suggest. The schedule can be

structured so that certain responses result in an extra range of questions being asked.

- The pace of questioning is up to the interviewer, which allows him or her to draw subjects into giving quick answers. The result can be spontaneous responses which the subject hasn't had time to consider.
- Interviewers may pick up useful background data from observing respondent's reactions to the questions. These observations can be recorded on the interview schedule if space is reserved for them. Of course, the responses can be guaranteed to come from the respondents themselves. There is no danger of collusion with others if the subject is 'trapped' in an interview.
- A main advantage of the structured interview technique is that quantitative data collected can be analysed statistically, and conclusions made about the population as a whole.

Many of the pitfalls of postal questionnaires are avoided because of the control an interviewer has over data collection. Uniformity of method attempts to offset any distortion that the presence of the interviewer creates. Structured interviewing attempts to be as 'scientific' as possible so that the results can be convincingly applied to the whole population.

However, structured interviews also have disadvantages. Well-presented results can look convincing, particularly if charts and graphs are used to demonstrate a point. But structured interviewing can produce distorted data, and thus distorted results.

- Sample size is often small. Interviewing is very time-consuming. Contacting a representative sample may mean travelling, or waiting for respondents to turn up. Interviews that are really useful are likely to last for several minutes, and you need to add time to complete your notes. The lone researcher cannot hope to complete a large number of structured interviews and must select a sample small enough to be interviewed in the time available. But a very small sample is unlikely to be representative of the population as a whole.

One way to overcome this problem is to set less ambitious aims for your investigation, and select a research topic which has a smaller population. For instance, if you are interested in attitudes to smoking, choose to research attitudes among local students, rather than attitudes among all young adults. This makes it much easier to select and interview a representative sample. The results may not be as far-reaching, but they are far more likely to be accurate.

- The interaction between respondent and interviewer is a source of distortion that can never be completely eliminated. An interview is a type of conversation. Even when verbal messages are standardised by an interview schedule, the interviewer's appearance, accent and personal characteristics can affect what takes place. Non-verbal signals pass between the participants, and the respondent may be looking for cues that indicate what sort of answers the researcher wants. If they have negative perceptions of the interviewer, respondents may give deliberately provocative answers. If they wish to impress, they may give answers that project a positive image of themselves.

Distortions caused by interviewer–respondent interaction are difficult, if not impossible to assess. There is no doubt though that they do occur. Studies have repeatedly shown that different interviewers often get different answers to the same questions. Awareness of this issue has led to attempts by researchers to reduce its effect. The formal nature of the structured interview is itself an attempt to minimise interviewer influence.

Pros	Cons
Very good response rates are possible	Time-consuming interviews can mean that only small unrepresentative sample is chosen
Interviewer is available to clarify questions and prevent misunderstandings	Interaction between respondent and interviewer can lead to distorted answers being given
Probes allow extra lines of enquiry to be foillowed up	Respondents are limited to the question-and-answer options presented, and their authentic views may not be revealed
Pace of questioning can induce spontaneous responses	Respondents need to be easily contactable
No uncertainty over who actually answers the questions	
Interviewers can observe and collect useful background data	
Uniformity of interview technique and content makes quanitiative analysis of the data possible	

Figure 22.7 Some pros and cons of structured interviews

- Interviews rely on the honesty and good intentions of interviewing staff. Honesty can be checked, particularly if the data collected by one interviewer differs widely from everyone else's. Deliberate influence by gesture, tone of voice or deviations from the schedule, is much more difficult to detect.
- A structured interview is only as good as the questionnaire design and content allow. A poorly considered set of questions will not give useful data, however scrupulously the interviews are conducted and the results calculated.

Structured interviews and questionnaires are both very useful for collecting quantitative data. Questions on circumstances, behaviour and attitudes can be answered using some type of scale so that number values can be applied and results analysed statistically. However, both data collection techniques have similar limitations. Many aspects of opinion are difficult to explore through a fixed set of questions. People's attitudes, beliefs and opinions are a personal matter and formal quantitative techniques may not be the best way to bring out authentic views. Respondents often find it easier to make a safe, respectable response rather than think deeply about a sensitive issue on which their real views are not so clear cut. Authentic opinion is more likely to emerge in a relaxed, less formal meeting.

Because questions are fixed, the respondents have no room for manoeuvre. They may be forced into making choices, possibly between a set of equally inappropriate alternatives. Respondents may have other, strongly held, views that the questions fail to bring out and the interviewer never becomes aware of. The questionnaire and interview schedule define the territory to be explored, and define it in the researcher's terms. Answers may be obtained, but are they important or relevant to the lives and outlook of the respondents themselves?

In-depth interviews

In-depth interviews are less fixed and formal than structured interviews. At the extreme, an in-depth interview can be more like a chat, with the interviewer supplying only the topic for conversation. The interviewer can provide guidance as things progress, to keep the topic in view. The aim of in-depth interviews is to encourage respondents to open up, and provide as much detail as possible.

In-depth interviews have big advantages when it comes to finding out what people really think.

- Subjects don't have to choose between alternative answers.
- They can introduce areas for discussion that are important to them, and they can give any information that they feel to be relevant. This means that the data is given according to the respondents' frame of reference and view of the world. Connections may be made that would never have occurred to the interviewer.
- A good deal of information is likely to be collected since in-depth interviews can last for a fairly long time, sometimes for several hours.

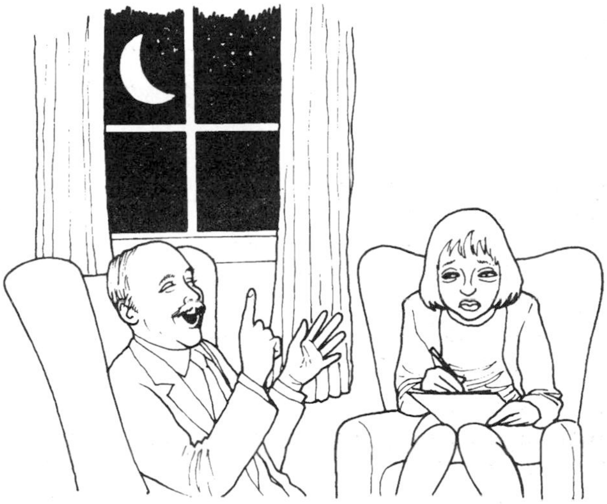

Figure 22.8 In-depth interviews can last for a long time

This open and flexible approach may be the best if not the only way to get information about people's real attitudes, values and opinions. In the informal atmosphere of the in-depth interview the respondents' inhibitions are reduced. They can be encouraged to talk about sensitive subjects and give views that they would not usually reveal to others. If interesting points arise that merit further investigation the interviewer has the freedom to steer the discussion towards them.

In-depth interviews provide rich information which is likely to represent accurately respondents' views. Of course, almost all the data collected is qualitative and the results cannot be analysed statistically. Comparing results between respondents is usually impossible, since each will have given information in their own terms. Respondents may approach the same topic from a completely different viewpoint. Different people will provide different items of data. Apart from this the sample size is likely to be very small because of the length of time needed to carry out and report on interviews. Even if comparisons between respondents can be made it is meaningless to try projecting the results onto the wider population. This is a characteristic of in-depth interviews, not a weakness of them. Researchers using the technique are aiming for depth and authenticity in difficult areas of enquiry, not for quantitative results.

The main issue that arises in in-depth interviewing is the level of skill required of the interviewer. Respondents must be put at ease and feel happy about talking openly to a stranger. Interviewers need to encourage their subject to speak, while subtly keeping the conversation focused on the topic they are interested in. As well as this, interviewers must try to avoid imposing their own bias on the discussion. Egging on respondents to make out of character comments will not produce accurate results.

All the problems of interviewer influence that can occur in structured interviews apply also to in-depth interviews. In fact, the freedom and depth of interaction that occurs in in-depth situations make the problem even more serious. To some extent the length of the interview can help, since subjects have time to get used to the interviewer and begin to behave naturally. Apart from this, it is the skill and integrity of the interviewer that is relied upon to make the interview useful.

In-depth interviews also pose practical problems. It is important that a suitable place is chosen for the interview. Time and privacy are needed and this may be difficult to arrange for some subjects. Recording the information is another problem. Taking notes is slow, and may inhibit the subject, reminding them that they are in an interview situation. Quickly jotted notes are likely to be at best a brief précis of the conversation, and later interpretation may lead to distortions. You cannot hope to remember all the information you receive, and things you have been too slow to write down are gone forever. One way to solve this is to record the interview on tape. Nothing verbal will be missed, but visual data about the subject's behaviour during the interview is not recorded. Some people are put off by the presence of a tape recorder and will not speak freely if you use one. Planting a hidden recorder is unethical practice, and you should resort to note-taking if a tape recorder puts subjects off.

Pros	Cons
Subjects have the freedom to give an answer in their own terms	Interviewers must have very well-developed communication skills
A large amount of information can be collected from each respondent	Each interview is time-consuming so it is only possible to carry out a few
Answers can be very accurate representations of the subjects' real opinions and feelings	Personal characteristics of the interviewer can affect answers given
Respondents have time to 'open up' on sensitive issues	Time and privacy are needed to carry out the interviews
Interviewers are free to explore any interesting areas that arise	Qualitative nature of data collected and small sample size limit the broader applicability of the results
Rich qualitative data can be gathered	

Figure 22.9 Some pros and cons of in-depth interviews

Semi-structured interviews

Semi-structured interviews have some of the characteristics of structured interviews, and some of in-depth interviews. They allow the researcher to get both quantitative and qualitative data from the interview. The semi-structured questionnaire is similar to the structured questionnaire in that questions are precisely worded and asked in a specified order. However, most questions are *open-ended* and respondents are encouraged to give as full an answer as they wish. Interviewers are usually free to probe for full answers, and all the respondents' comments are recorded. Because all respondents are asked the same list of questions, their answers are

Pros	Cons
More opportunity for respondents to answer in their own terms than structured interviews	Meaningful analysis of answers requires expertise
More control over subjects covered than in-depth interviews	Interviewer's personal characteristics can influence results
Less interviewer skill needed than for in-depth interviews	Researcher's frame of reference may be imposed by the set of questions asked
Relationships between different respondents' answers may be assessed	Time and privacy are needed for the interviews

Figure 22.10 Some pros and cons of semi-structured interviews

quantifiable to some extent. The relationships between different respondents' answers can be assessed, and content analysis can be used to give a fuller picture.

Semi-structured interviews have the advantage of being quicker to carry out than in-depth interviews. This means that more of them can be carried out in the research time available. They also require less skill on the part of the interviewer. There is a better likelihood that respondents' answers can be compared than with in-depth interviews, though meaningful quantitative analysis of answers requires considerable expertise. It is possible to explore issues in more depth than structured interviews allow. However, there is a limit to their flexibility. Because a fixed set of questions is being asked, it is still possible for the researcher's frame of reference to impinge on answers.

Think it over

Think about subjects you are interested in researching. Write down any that could be researched using in-depth interviewing. Write down the pros and cons of using in-depth interviews for each of the specific areas.

Choose the area that seems most suited to using in-depth interview techniques. How could you justify your use of this method to research that particular subject?

Reliability and validity

There is a marked contrast between the uniformity of the structured interview and the flexible openness of an in-depth interview. The differences between the two methods go further than interview style.

Structured interviews stress *reliability*. This means that repeats of the research using different samples should reliably produce the same results. Every aspect, from question design to interviewer style, is planned to maximise reliability. If the results of structured research seem not to be reliable, then the research has failed on its own terms. Reliability can be assessed only if results are expressed statistically.

In-depth interviews stress *validity*. This means that information collected comes very close to the subjects' real views. It gives a valid picture of what they truly believe. In-depth interview data is not expected to have reliability. Subjects' responses are individual, and are not intended to be compared directly. Certainly they cannot be compared statistically since the data is qualitative.

Research which emphasises reliability may lose validity in the process. Questions that reliably receive a similar range of responses have to be carefully designed in order to achieve this. Questions which produce conflicting or erratic responses are pruned out so that reliability is ensured. This can result in questions that ask only about trite, safe subjects. More seriously it can result in real variations of opinion and attitude being ignored because they don't fit the researcher's notion of what he or she is trying to find out. Questions may reliably receive invalid responses.

Research which emphasises validity makes no attempt to be reliable. It is not expected that different respondents will give comparable data. Comparisons may be suggested, but there is no list of allowed responses against which reliability can be assessed. The results don't help us to gauge the views of the wider population, and without wider applicability the research may be regarded as merely interesting.

In this discussion we have looked at two extreme positions in research methodology. In practice, many researchers pitch their work somewhere between them, or try to use both methods. In-depth interviews may give you information that suggests a pattern of opinion worth exploring further. Structured interviews may be used to check how far that pattern of opinion extends into the wider population. Different research aims and methodologies should be seen as complementary, not in opposition to one another.

Observation

Observation is another popular and useful research technique. There are two variants: *direct observation,* where the researcher remains detached from the subjects, and *participant observation* where the researcher joins in with the people being studied. Observation means studying by looking. To be classed as research, rather than merely looking on, observations need to be structured. As with other research techniques, data collection has to be organised so that relevant and useful information is sought and recorded. Well-organised observation has several advantages as a research technique.

- You can observe what people actually do, not what they tell researchers that they do. People are studied in their own environment and should be expected to behave as they do naturally.

Observation can detect 'taken for granted' behaviour that subjects are not aware of, and would thus not report if asked in an interview.

- Groups, and the interaction between their members, can be studied. Other research methods look at individuals, making group behaviour difficult to investigate.
- Observations can be done over time, allowing changes in groups or situations to be revealed.

Direct observation

Direct observation is rather like bird-watching. Subjects are watched as they go about their normal lives and observations recorded by the researcher. Naturally, observations can usually only take place where permission has been granted – otherwise observation could be unethical.

Both qualitative and quantitative data can be collected through direct observation. For example, quantitative data about playground usage is probably best collected by this method. Observers can count arrivals and can group them in terms of sex, age and other observable characteristics. Observers can also record qualitative data, such as how the children behave towards each other in the playground, and who seem to be friends.

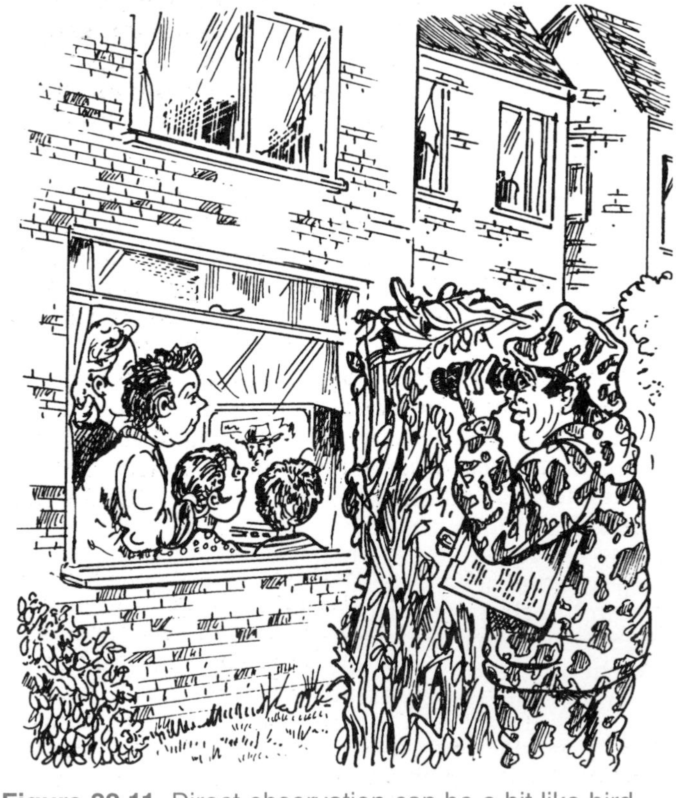

Figure 22.11 Direct observation can be a bit like bird-watching

Direct observation may be the only way to observe some groups, such as small children. It can be useful in any situation where your presence would be unobtrusive. Remember, permission to undertake observation will often be necessary. However, direct observation also has problems associated with it.

- One simple problem is that of *recording* the data. Making notes distracts the researcher from observation. It may be easy to miss something important, particularly when a fairly large group is being studied.
- Some methods of observation can raise ethical problems. Should researchers use secret techniques for collecting and recording data? This could be something fairly innocent, like fixing an electronic counter to a door to check how many people use it. However it could include bugging phones, or using two-way mirrors to observe private behaviour.
- A more serious difficulty is *interpreting* what is observed. Direct observers are not 'inside', and they cannot see behaviour from the subjects' point of view. For example, children may believe that they are playing a boisterous game, while the observer perceives a violent confrontation. Observers may project their own theories on to what they see, and fail to understand what is happening so far as the subjects are concerned.

It is because of the difficulties with interpretation that direct observation is a poor way to research

Pros	Cons
Observers see what people actually do, not say that they do	Observers may miss important behaviour while note-taking
Subjects studied in their natural environment	Secretive observation leads to significant ethical problems
Can detect behaviour that subjects are unaware of	Inferences drawn from observed behaviour can lead to serious misinterpretation, so a poor way to look at values and beliefs
Can look at group behaviour and interactions between members	Lack of control over the sample limits broader applicability of results
May be the only suitable method with non-literate subjects, such as small children	

Figure 22.12 Some pros and cons of direct observation

opinions and values. Inferring beliefs from observed behaviour is likely to produce highly distorted results. Of course, observed behaviour may suggest lines of enquiry that can be followed up with other methods. For example, you may observe that staff at a day centre seem to spend less time talking to black clients. Further research using interview techniques could probe staff attitudes to race and discrimination.

Participant observation

Participant observation means that the researcher becomes part of the group being studied. There is probably no better way of really getting to understand the way groups work than to join them. Several classic social research projects have involved this method. Researchers have sometimes spent years living and working with their subjects, while at the same time recording data about them. This clearly requires dedicated professionalism, and a good deal of time. The commitment required puts participant observation beyond the scope of most researchers. Nevertheless, there are several strengths to the technique.

- The data provided by participant research is likely to be very valid. Researchers are living alongside their respondents and can see things from their point of view. There is little danger that serious misinterpretations will occur. Researchers can get to know their subjects so well that a valid picture of their values and opinions can be built up. Participant observation can produce excellent qualitative data.

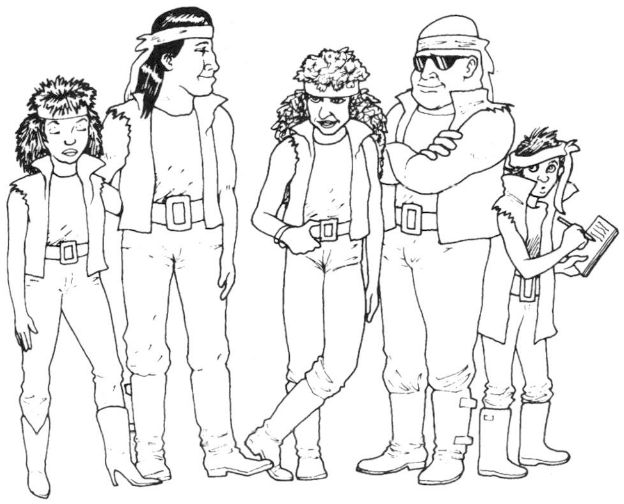

Figure 22.13 Participant observation may not suit everyone

Pros	Cons
Can produce very valid and accurate qualitative data	Researcher needs time, commitment and high order social skills
May be the only method possible with closed or hostile groups	Researcher needs skills of objectivity and detachment
Little likelihood of serious misinterpretation of data	Researcher's influence on group behaviour almost inevitable
	Observer may be unknowingly ignorant of important aspects of group behaviour
	Secretive participant observation leads to serious ethical difficulties

Figure 22.14 Some pros and cons of participant observation

- Participant observation may be the only way to study some groups. For example, people who are homeless and sleeping rough may only open up to someone who has become a familiar part of their world. Other groups, like delinquent gangs, may be so hostile to outsiders that participant observation is the only way to get close to them. This sort of social science is not for the faint-hearted.

The main limitation of participant research is the time and commitment it demands. Apart from this, participant researchers need special skills if the study is to remain objective. It is all too easy to get sucked into the world you are now a part of. This can mean that things are only seen from the subjects' viewpoint. Researchers have to remain detached while being fully involved. Involvement can mean that only unusual events are noticed and recorded. Valuable background data may be unnoticed because it is now such a familiar part of everyday life for the researcher.

Where the researcher is so fully bound up in the life of his subjects, it is certain that they are influenced by him to some degree. The effects of this depend very much on the skills of the researcher, and how the research is being conducted. Some researchers reveal themselves to the group and seek acceptance as a harmless observer. This makes it much easier to take notes, and gives an excuse for the occasional probing interview. Others may try to pass themselves off as ordinary group members, and must thus scribble their notes in secret whenever they get a chance. This sort of secretive observation has ethical difficulties. Is it right to record people's private lives in detail without their knowledge, particularly if you intend to publish the results?

Participant observation can lose quality if the researcher is not fully accepted by the group. He may be kept on the fringes of the group's activities and never really find out what is going on. The observer may not be aware that this is happening and report what is observed as the whole picture.

Ethical issues in social research

As we have seen ethical concerns are important and obvious in the application of observational methods. The use of two-way mirrors or hidden tape recorders by researchers is hard to justify. We would all wish to protect ourselves from becoming the victims of investigators using these sorts of methods. However, ethical issues run through all social research and need to be considered seriously by researchers whatever method of data collection they employ.

Social research deals with people, and there is considerable evidence to show that being the subject of research has an effect on individuals who are aware that this is happening. Some of these effects may be perceived as desirable by the subject. People may be flattered to be chosen as a sample member and feel that helping social researchers makes them special or important. If the research method involves a self-completion questionnaire or an interview, it is possible to refuse to participate. Researchers are aware that non-participation by sample members will affect how representative the sample becomes. They will seek to persuade people to take part so that the scientific qualities of their research are maintained. The question is how far should researchers go with this persuasion to remain within the bounds of good ethical practice?

With self-completion questionnaires, it is only possible to add a statement to the questionnaire form explaining the importance and relevance of the research in the hope that respondents will agree and go on to complete it. Adding statements which are threatening or intimidating is completely unethical, and could be regarded as unlawful!

Similar considerations apply to experiments and interview methods. Now the researcher is present to do the persuading, and this is one reason why interviews tend to get much better response rates than self-completion questionnaires. In fact, the ability of an interviewer to encourage participation is an important part of the selection process in professional research organisations. Again, the ethical issue is how far researchers should go to generate involvement. Lies or threats are unethical here too, and could be seen as threatening behaviour. People have a right to choose whether or not to become involved in a social research project and this right must be respected. Researchers can explain the importance of their work, and in fact should always explain truthfully what the research is about. This may be enough to convince the slightly reluctant subject. Also reassurances about anonymity are always necessary and this may help a subject to agree.

If people still refuse, researchers need to be able to judge whether further discussion might be seen as unreasonable pressure. There is no simple guide to follow here, but perhaps putting yourself in the position of the reluctant respondent will help. Would you be happy to be on the receiving end of the persuasive techniques that you, as a researcher, intend to use? If the answer is no, then you should thank the person for their time and leave. A friendly, open and honest approach is the best way to find willing subjects, and data collected will be more accurate than that obtained through coercion.

Think it over

Suppose you intend to use interview methods to collect data for a research project. Think about the range of reactions that you might encounter when you introduce yourself and your purpose. In particular try to imagine how you would deal with people who said 'no' to an interview. Think about the things you might say to encourage co-operation. List all the things you can think of at this stage.

Now review your list and consider the ethics of using each one. Try to decide where you think it is reasonable to draw the line and strike out those you think go too far. Look at those that are left. You may be able to use these approaches when carrying out your own research.

Because observation can take place without subjects being aware of it, there is an even greater need to consider the ethics of your research. Much depends on the type of things being observed, and on the use that the data will be put to. If a researcher wants to collect data on the usage of a facility, counting heads may be the best way. Collecting this data may raise few ethical issues. But if the data being collected is more personal, then subjects have a right to choose whether to participate or not. In practice, it may be difficult or impossible to inform all subjects of your activities fully. In this case you may have to consider whether the research should carry on. If it seems that secretive observation will be the only way to deal with the research question, data and population that you are interested in then the research should be abandoned.

Another ethical issue is the subjects' right to confidentiality. Research reports should never identify the subjects personally, and should be written so that respondents cannot be identified. For example, if you are looking at a small group with easily identified members you must avoid giving clues about who gave what response to particular questions. If the group has only one male member, then pointing to the differences between the sexes clearly identifies the responses of an individual and is unethical.

Researchers using participant observation have many ethical problems to face. It is likely to be a small group being studied, and the quantity of data gathered makes it hard to disguise who is being reported on. It is possible to be completely open about your intentions and seek the willing co-operation of your subjects. Though this may deal with the issue of participant's rights to refuse to participate, it still leaves open the question of confidentiality. The research should be abandoned if it seems that confidentiality is impossible to preserve.

Subjects also have a right to view the results of the research and to comment on its outcomes. Self-completion questionnaires usually have a box to be ticked if respondents wish to see the results. The same consideration should be given to people agreeing to be interviewed. This can lead to difficulties if the research is carried out by street interview methods. Here the subjects are met in public and cannot be easily contacted to view the results. One simple solution is to offer subjects the opportunity to supply their address so that the results can be sent to them. Research reports should include comments that respondents have made on the results, and researchers need to allow time for these comments to arrive before completing their report. This is not only good ethical practice, but could generate interesting and relevant observations on the quality of the results.

A more subtle ethical problem concerns the way in which a researcher's own background can lead to presumptions and distortions in the analysis and reporting of data. All researchers carry with them their own cultural backgrounds and world view. They have attitudes and opinions just like everyone else. Social researchers need to be aware that this can lead to ethical difficulties. The danger is that researchers impose their own norms and values on the data they collect, and interpret the results in their own terms. This can distort the objectivity of the research and misrepresent the real meanings that lie behind their subjects' responses. Where there are significant differences between the culture of researcher and subject, this may become an insurmountable difficulty. It is unethical to proceed with research in these circumstances. Imposing your own cultural values on the views of your subjects is arrogant, and leads to the production of irrelevant and unscientific results.

A final consideration in the ethics of research practice is the potential benefits of the research. This is sometimes set against the ethical issues outlined above, and used to justify continuation of the work when it may seem unethical to do so. There is a difficult moral problem here. Is it right to ignore the rights of the minority (the sample being looked at) if the majority will clearly benefit from the results? Sometimes it is decided that society's need for information outweighs the rights of individuals. This is the case with the government's national census. This massive research project takes place every ten years and legislation has been passed to compel people to respond. However, other rights, such as confidentiality, are carefully preserved in the census reports.

Arguments about the benefits of research can be used to justify other, more contentious research. For instance, secretive studies of deviant groups may claim that society's need to understand criminal behaviour allows researchers to disregard the rights of their subjects. Again this is a difficult moral area and judgements are not easily made. The general principle to be followed is that subjects' rights come first. Research which breaks this rule needs to have very exceptional reasons for doing so.

Research organisations and professional bodies have published codes of conduct to guide their members in considering ethical issues. The British Psychological Society has produced 'Ethical Principles for Conducting Research with Human Participants'. These principles are intended to apply to all psychological researchers, from GCSE to postgraduate level. They cover areas such as participants' consent, researcher deception, confidentiality, and the protection of participants from physical and psychological danger. Another example is the 'Code of Conduct' produced by the Market Research Society. This code is intended to cover all market and social research. It is based on the principles of willing co-operation of respondents, and their right to full confidentiality. It also covers the rights of children as research subjects.

These published ethical guidelines are easy to obtain (see page 535) and should be examined before any research project goes ahead.

The research process

All research projects, large or small, should follow the same basic process. When examining the work of other researchers you need to be able to identify the aspects of this process within it.

Research begins with a question. This should be explicitly stated early in the report. The overall aims of the research should be made clear at this stage, and the relationship of the research to existing findings and theories. The identification of the population concerned and the type of data to be obtained from them should follow from an examination of the research question. The research methods decided upon will be linked to this and should be justified with reference to the question, population and data required. The next stage is the data gathering itself, and research reports should explain how this was carried out and comment on how it went.

The data analysis stage comes next. You should expect to find details of how the data was dealt with and any problems that may have occurred, such as the response rate, or unforeseen difficulties with applying the chosen research method. The last stage is the report itself. This should contain the conclusions that the researcher has drawn from the data collected. The style of the conclusions will depend on the purpose of the research project. They may include recommendations for action, or an assessment of whether a hypothesis has been disapproved or not.

Finally you may find that examples of the research instruments used are included as appendices. Good researchers are as open as possible about their work, and the questionnaire, interview schedule, or

Planning	1	Identify the research area and narrow it to a research question to be studied. Identify links with existing findings and theories
	2	Identify the population, the research concerns, and the type of data needed from them
	3	Decide upon appropriate research methods to gather the data
	4	Design suitable research instruments to gather the data, and plan how to implement them
	5	Select a representative sample from the population to collect data from
Collecting data	1	Contact the sample and gather the data
	2	Summarise and organise the data in preparation for analysis
Analysis and interpretation of data	1	Relate the data to the research question and the research aims
	2	Draw conclusions from the data analysis
	3	Evaluate the research, assessing problems in execution and the limitations of the results
	4	Offer suggestions for further study in the light of the results

Figure 22.15 Stages in the research process

observation checklist will allow readers to judge the quality of the methods used for themselves.

Reviewing the work of professional researchers is a very good way of developing your understanding of the research process. An even better way may be to carry out a structured piece of research for yourself.

Evidence collection point

To pass Element 8.1 you need to examine and report on two research studies into health and well-being. One of these is to use qualitative research methods and the other quantitative.

Your report needs to cover:

a the nature of the research process
b the different stages in the process
c how the stages are interlinked

Try to pick studies that have been clearly written, and which consider questions that you know something about. Well-written reports should make it easy for you to identify the process that underlies them. Avoid complex work, or studies that deal with unfamiliar areas.

Chapter 23

Planning research and gathering data

This chapter is about planning your own research project. It covers:

- **developing a research question**
- **the rationale for the research**
- **doing secondary research – secondary sources, using secondary sources**
- **doing primary research – the research population, sampling methods**
- **collecting data – choosing and using a research method, designing questionnaires, designing structured interview schedules.**

Developing a research question

The *research question* is the starting point of the research process. At first the question may cover a broad area which is too big to be dealt with. The question 'What perceptions do disabled people have about the social care services that they receive?' is interesting and important, but it is also extremely wide. To be able to answer with confidence you would need to check on all the possible options, or sub-questions, that the question contains. There are many sorts of disability, and many types of service that people need to use. Perceptions about one service may be different from perceptions about others. After a few moments thought, the range of permutations and combinations can be seen to be vast. The question needs to be narrowed down to something workable for research purposes.

Exploring the range of possibilities in a question is easier if you structure your approach to it. You can begin to 'unpack' the question by thinking about the range covered by each part of it. In our example your could begin by considering the range of disabilities that could be included, listing them on paper. Next, you could think about the range of services that are available and list these also. Now the two lists could be related to each other. Looking at each entry in the list of disabilities in turn you could try to imagine which services may be particularly likely to link with it. For instance, you may have listed wheelchair-users on the one hand and homecare services on the other. It is possible that some wheelchair-users get help around the home from homecare services and you could indicate a link there. You should end up with many links between the two lists.

Now you need to make some decisions about which links to develop. It is probably best to choose links that are clear cut, or that you already know something about. You should also think about the ease with which you will be able to get data. The subject you pick will imply a particular population for your work, and the accessibility of the population is important whatever research method you eventually use. Bearing this in mind, it should now be possible to make a list of the possible questions that could be written around the links you have made.

Each potential research question in the list can now be checked in detail by repeating the methods we have discussed. Further unpacking may show that the subject is still too broad, or that the population is still too large to be easily sampled from. Eventually, a list of workable questions should emerge from which you can pick a specific research question to work on.

How far you take the unpacking process will depend on how wide you want your research projects to be. In principle you could carry on unpacking until you have questions which cover a minute area of interest. Stop when common sense indicates that you have a question that is within your scope. Further unpacking will now lead to lists of areas that you need to gather data about when carrying out your research.

Often the research question will be stated as an *hypothesis,* a statement which can be disproved or supported by the research results. There should be clear indications of the population concerned, and, of course, they need to be people that you can easily contact.

Try it

You can use the methods we have looked at to develop workable research questions in several areas of your GNVQ Health and Social Care studies. First, decide upon a research area that you are currently interested in developing. You could choose a client's experience of health and care provision (Element 6.3) or an evaluation of the effectiveness of a health campaign (Element 7.3). Or you could pick a research area from another part of the course.

Try to unpack the research area and develop a workable research question. Write your chosen question as an hypothesis that could be tested by research. Check that you have not still got too broad a question by trying to unpack it further.

The rationale for the research

The final chosen research question can now be considered in detail. All research needs to have a rationale – a purpose and a set of reasons for taking place. Researchers must check that they have a clear rationale for their research question before spending time and effort on it. Although you may not compose a detailed rationale until you come to write the research report, you should be sufficiently aware of the issues to confirm to yourself that it is worth proceeding.

One thing to consider is the original purpose of the research. Has the unpacking process drifted away from the reason why research was decided upon in the first place? You need be able to state what it is that the research is now going to try to find out. Associated with this is the importance of the research to your own goals. Why is it useful for you to research this particular question? You should think about these points seriously before embarking on the considerable effort that research can involve. If you are not certain that the research question will serve the purpose, then this is a good time to abandon it.

You should also think about who the *audience* for your research will be. Part of the rationale for the research should be an awareness of who is likely to be interested in the results. If you are not sure who the target audience is, then the purpose of the research is not yet sufficiently clear. Another aspect of your rationale is the links that may exist between your research and other existing findings. The research question may have arisen through looking at other people's research, or you may have discovered them later through secondary research. If you know that the question has links with other work, this too establishes the purpose and context of your research.

Finally, you should think about how widely your results are likely to apply. How far do you think the results of your research will be able to be generalised to other situations and contexts? This may be a difficult question to answer precisely, but you should be able to suggest some possibilities. For example, you might think that the results of your local enquiries could be relevant to the experiences of people in similar circumstances living in other parts of the country.

A clear statement of the rationale for the research covering all these points should show precisely why the work is taking place, and demonstrate the value of carrying it out. You can then proceed without doubts that you might be wasting your efforts on pointless work.

Evidence collection point

You need to be able to describe the rationale for any research you undertake during your GNVQ Health and Social Care studies. This is required as evidence for Element 8.2, and research without a rationale is usually wasted effort.

Choose an area of your studies where you intend to do research and have a research question in mind. Think about the factors involved in the research rationale and check your ideas about each one. You need to think about:

- what the research question is trying to find out
- the relevance of the work to you, and your learning goals
- the intended target audience
- links with previous research
- the extent to which the results could be generalised.

Try to write a rationale for the research question which covers these points. If you are not sure that you have answers to each issue yet, think how you might work towards them.

You must have clear ideas about the rationale before you begin your research planning. All your research reports need to contain a description of the rationale covering each of the above points.

Doing secondary research

Doing secondary research around the question at issue is a good way to begin your research development. There are many sources of secondary data and you need to begin by thinking about what sorts of information might be helpful and relevant to your research question. You may want statistical information about your population, and you may want to look at other studies that are related to your own. When you have some idea what you are looking for, you then have the problem of finding it!

Actually this need not be so difficult as it may sound. Your thoughts about the research question might suggest where appropriate secondary data could be found. Tutors, library staff and other advisers should make it easier to identify and obtain useful secondary source materials. Other problems crop up when you have found the material. All secondary sources need to be treated with some caution, and there are several points to bear in mind when using them.

- It is important that you understand the information you have found. Sometimes data appears in forms which are difficult to follow unless you are familiar with the field.
- You must assess how relevant the information is to your work. The people who collected and published the data will have had their own purposes in mind, and they are likely to differ from yours.
- There is the crucial question of the quality of other people's research work. Published data is by no means guaranteed to be accurate. Errors and distortions can result from careless or misguided research work. They can also occur because of deliberate bias. Unfortunately, the quality of the research in secondary sources is often hard to judge.

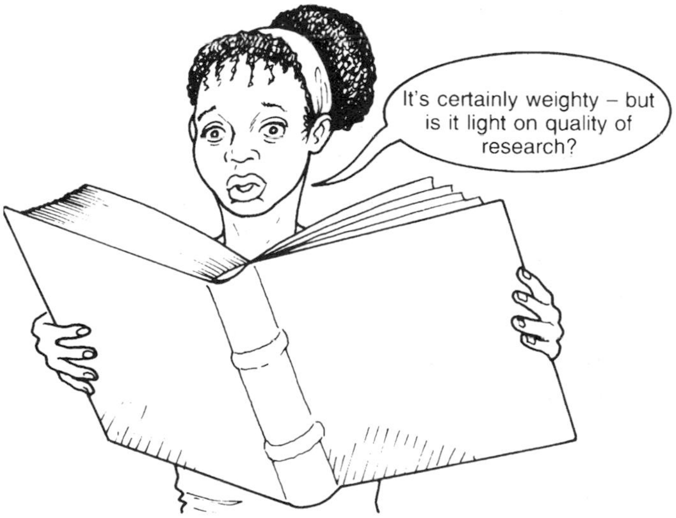
It's certainly weighty – but is it light on quality of research?

Secondary sources

Official statistics

National and local government organisations produce a wide variety of official statistics. These bodies need facts and figures of all sorts to assist in planning and decision-making.

The government carries out a census of the UK population every ten years. The last one was in 1991. Every household in the UK is required to fill in a questionnaire which asks about such topics as families, housing, education and work. Also many other surveys and research projects are carried out by, or on behalf of, government departments. These are not as comprehensive as the census, and usually concern specific topics such as transport or health.

There is a variety of books available which contain official statistics, all of which should be in local reference libraries. The census results are published in book form. They contain both national and regional information on a variety of topics. Remember though that some census results take several years to be published. The *Annual Abstract of Statistics* contains important government statistics. *Social Trends* is similar to the *Annual Abstract of Statistics* but may be more useful as it includes some discussion. It also looks at changes over time, and is also published annually. *Regional Trends* is similar to *Social Trends*, but contains information for particular regions. *Key Data* is an annual publication and covers important social and economic statistics. If you talk to the librarian you should easily be able to find these and other books containing official statistics in your local reference library.

Official statistics are usually straightforward and understandable. Most appear in the form of tables. You must make sure that you have read and understood the headings, and what the figures represent.

There is such a wide range of statistics available that you are likely to come across some data that is relevant to your work. One danger may be that you find a lot of interesting data and try to include too much of it in your final research report. Remember to use secondary sources as a guide to carrying out your own research project. Quote secondary data only when it adds useful background to your work, or when it provides interesting comparisons with your own results.

Very large-scale official surveys, like the census, are carried out extremely carefully. Methods of data collection and analysis used by the UK government's statistical staff have helped to define good practice. The results which emerge are likely to give a pretty accurate picture of things like housing, income or family composition in UK households.

Unfortunately, however, the quality of all official statistics cannot be taken for granted. Though scrupulous care may be used in data collection and analysis, some official figures may not represent the true picture. For example, statistics on crime may seem straightforward to collect. Crimes known to the police are recorded, and totals for different types of crime can be presented as results. But figures can shift if the police decide to 'crack down' on particular offences. A sudden apparent increase in cases of fraud, for example, may be the result of increased police activity in fraud detection. Also campaigns in the media can result in increased reporting of certain crimes by the public.

Think it over

Other official data may suffer from problems of distortion. Statistics on unemployment are also apparently easy to collect, but may not reflect the situation accurately.

Think about ways in which unemployment statistics may be affected by official policy and public behaviour.

Books

Whatever you are interested in, there are probably books that can help you in libraries you have access to. Books could include textbooks, reference books, or the published work of social researchers. Any of these may provide useful background, and introduce you to concepts and definitions relevant to your research. You may also find published results that you can compare with your own. If you make good use of library filing systems, and the advice of staff, you should find plenty of material.

Using books also has its pitfalls.

- The published research of social scientists is sometimes difficult to understand, and lengthy to read. It is often better to look at textbooks containing brief, condensed accounts of their work.
- Another problem is that data in textbooks and reference books may be out-of-date. Even recent works will have taken time to write and publish. Always check the age of any statistics quoted.
- The accuracy of data from books is usually extremely difficult to gauge. Research methods may not be fully explained, or they may be hard to understand and evaluate.
- Also it is possible that the researchers' own bias has influenced the results. Without detailed knowledge of the field, this may be difficult to gauge.

You can certainly refer to the data produced by others, but don't assume that it is correct.

Newspapers, magazines and journals

Newspapers and magazines print information of all types. Apart from quoting data produced by official sources they sometimes print the results of their own 'polls'. Articles are likely to be easy to understand, but the big problem is with quality. Newspapers tailor their content to suit the politics and expectations of their owners and readers. Stories can easily be slanted in the direction the editor wishes. Statistics quoted may have been carefully chosen to project a particular point of view. The problem of bias makes it difficult to rely on information found in newspapers and magazines.

Journals and professional publications usually print much more reliable information than newspapers. Because they are aimed at people who are specialists in a particular field, they report seriously on professional research results. The problem is that, because they are aimed at specialists, some articles may be written in technical language. Also, as with books, there is still no guarantee that the research reported has produced results that are free from bias.

Publications by other groups

Many groups and organisations produce information. Some are funded by government, like the Commission for Racial Equality. Some, such as Amnesty International or the RSPCA, are funded by donations from the public. Others, like the Trades Union Congress or the Confederation of British Industry, are paid for by members whose interests they represent. Political parties also sponsor and publish research.

These organisations are usually happy to send you any data they have, if you write and ask for it. The major drawback is that information from pressure groups may be heavily subject to bias, since the group is keen to get their message across. This is not likely to be a problem with officially-sponsored organisations, but data produced by privately-funded pressure groups should be treated with considerable caution.

Using secondary sources

Secondary sources have an important role to play in helping you to prepare your research project, and in providing material for background and comparison. Despite the reservations expressed above, it is always a good idea to consult the work of others when planning your own investigation. When referring to secondary sources it helps to follow some basic guidelines.

- Remember to be critical in your approach to secondary data. Taking other people's results as proven fact is not good practice.
- Only quote material that is really relevant to your research topic, or that adds useful background information. Don't pack your work with lengthy sections of irrelevant, second-hand data.
- Remember to keep a list of sources you have looked at, even if you don't use them in your final report. Showing that you have read around a topic helps to establish the credibility of your own research work.

Evidence collection point

Secondary research will be a part of any research project that you conduct during your GNVQ Health and Social Care studies. You are expected to show that you have found and consulted secondary data sources as part of the evidence needed for Element 8.2.

Take a research question that you are working on and look for secondary sources of information relevant to it. Try to find data that you can use or quote in your report. Any secondary source you intend to use should be considered in the light of the following points:

- Have you understood the data, and will your research audience?
- What is the purpose of using the data? Is it really relevant to your work?
- How old is the data?
- What is the quality of the data? Is it likely to be free from distortions or bias?

Check this list against the data you have found and use only that which meets the above requirements. Keep a record of all the works you look at. These can be included in your bibliography as evidence of wider reading.

Doing primary research

Your secondary research should help to broaden your knowledge of the issues surrounding the research question, and may provide usable secondary data. Now you need to plan the collection of your own *primary data*. You could begin by considering the people you are going to collect it from, your population.

The research population

Defining your population clearly is very important. It is a statement about who your results can be applied to, and who your sample must be selected from. Remember that it is likely to be easier to select a representative sample if the population is not too large. The hypothesis 'Most students believe that smoking is harmful to health' implies that the population includes all students. Does this mean all students in the UK, or is the research world-wide? Suppose we alter the hypothesis to 'Most local students ...'. How do we decide what 'local' means? Does 'students' include people studying at school, or older people attending evening classes? To define the population even more closely we could say 'Most full-time students at this college (or school) believe that smoking is harmful to health'. Now it is much clearer who we are talking about, and we know exactly who to take a sample of.

When the population has been defined, you can start to note down things you already know about them. Be particularly careful not to note assumptions which are unproved, however widely held or taken-for-granted they may be. Characteristics of the population will affect the research method that you can use. If they are geographically spread and likely to be interested in the subject, a postal questionnaire may work well. If they are easy to get hold of and likely to need encouragement to give the data you need, then interviews would probably be better.

You will need to select a sample of your population which is small enough to be handled, but large enough to be representative of the population as a whole. *Random selection* of the sample is important if the results are expected to be analysed quantitatively and generalised to the whole population. Methods for selecting a random sample are discussed on the next page, and all truly random sampling methods require you to have a list of the members of your population. A list containing the names of people from which a sample is to be drawn is known as a *sampling frame.* How easy will it be to get hold of a sampling frame listing the members of your population? Difficulties here often lead researchers to resort to less random sampling techniques, but this isn't always necessary. If you are studying your fellow students, then the college or school will have a list. Whether you can get access to it though is another matter. If the group is small enough, you can make up your own sampling frame. Another approach is to tailor your research to a sampling frame you can obtain. For instance, you could use a street directory to select a sample and treat people living in the area covered as the population. The danger with this is that you may end up researching a different group than you intended, and one that is not very interested in the subject.

Evidence collection point

You will need to consider the population of interest in each research project you undertake during your studies. Your notes and ideas are evidence towards Element 8.2.

Think about the population concerned in a research question you are working on.

- **a** Write a definition of the population so that it is absolutely clear who is included and who is not.
- **b** List things that you already know about the population.
- **c** Consider how you might get a list of members to use as a sampling frame.

It is essential to do this exercise so that you can choose the right sampling and research methods for the population of interest.

Sampling methods

Whatever research technique is used, researchers must decide who to collect information from. Without vast resources, or a particularly small population, it is impossible to cover everyone. This means that a sample must be selected. Many researchers seek quantitative results, and want to apply their findings convincingly to the whole population. To be able to do this, they need a sample which is as representative of the population as possible. This means that the proportions of people with different characteristics in the sample should reflect the proportions in the population as a whole. The sample should be a *representative cross-section* of the population being studied.

Careful sampling is crucial if quantitative results are to claim broader applicability. Even if research is qualitative, subjects must be chosen. This is sampling of a sort, though being representative is seldom such an issue. All researchers should be able to explain how their sample was selected, and how representative it is likely to be.

How big should a sample be? To be representative, it needs to contain a similar range of people to the population being studied. Very small samples run the risk of missing important groups. Social researchers want their sample to reflect the spread of things like age, gender, ethnic group and class background. The spread of such characteristics within a population is called *variance.* Some populations have much more variability than others. For example, children in the same class at a primary school serving a local estate will have a lot in common. But variance among the passengers travelling on a bus is likely to be far greater. In practice, the size of samples usually depends on the researchers' resources. If you select as big a sample as you can manage, then you have helped to make it representative and cover variance in the population.

Think it over

Think about the population concerned in a research project you are working on. What do you know about the variability in the population? You may know some things, such as age range within the population. Are there ways you can find out more?

Variability in some areas may not affect your research, whereas in other areas it may be important. Are there personal characteristics that you know will probably affect the answers given by different members of the population? Can you list these characteristics? You need a sample big enough to cover important areas of variability in the population. How big a sample do you estimate that you would need to cover variability in your population?

Random sampling

Even if samples are of a reasonable size, it is possible for distortions to occur. If sample selection is left entirely to the choices of researchers, then their own personal bias will be a problem. Random sampling methods are designed to eliminate the chance of personal bias influencing sample selection. Rules of sample selection are strictly applied by professional researchers so that sampling errors can be calculated and stated mathematically. Of course other factors such as interview bias, or poorly-designed questionnaires, can influence and distort results in ways which are difficult to estimate. But if random sampling methods are used then at least errors due to sample selection can be precisely estimated.

Basically, random sampling means that a group is selected randomly from the whole population. All members of the population must have a measurable chance of being selected. Where all members of the population have the same chance of selection the method is known as *simple random sampling*.

To begin random sampling the researcher needs to have a sampling frame. It is important that the sampling frame provides complete coverage of the population. If the sampling frame is incomplete then some members of the population can never be selected, and the principle of randomness begins to break down.

A sample can be selected from the sampling frame in different ways. One method is known as *systematic sampling*. Names are picked at regular intervals from the sampling frame until the required size of sample is obtained. All members of the population must have a chance of selection and it is important that the size of the interval allows this to happen. For example, if the sampling frame has 1000 names, and you want to select a sample of 100 then you need to select every tenth name. This will give you a sample of the required size. The number of the first name picked also needs to be randomised.

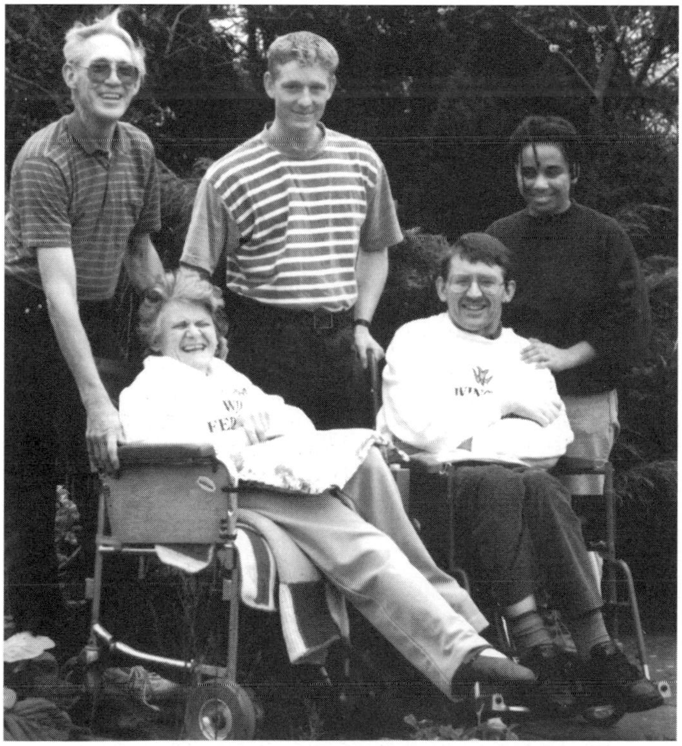

Figure 23.1 Your sample should be a representative cross-section of the population
(Photo courtesy of Winged Fellowship Trust)

There can be problems with the systematic sampling method. Sampling frames are usually acquired by researchers, seldom created by them from scratch. Most lists are not at all random in order. Many will be alphabetical, and some are grouped in other ways. In our example above, a list which is grouped in sets of ten would give a very biased sample. You could try to randomise the sampling frame before systematic sampling. However, this is a long process, and introduces the problem of how to make the list truly random.

A solution to the problem of systematic selection is to use *random number tables*. These consist of lists of randomly chosen numbers which are used to select a sample from the sampling frame. This is a better method than systematic sampling though it takes a bit longer.

One problem with simple random sampling is that a biased sample may be chosen by chance. For example, suppose the population consists of 500 males and 500 females. It is quite possible, though extremely unlikely, for a random sample of 100 to be entirely composed of one sex, giving seriously biased results. A larger sample size does not guarantee balance, unless the whole population is selected. To overcome this *stratified random sampling* may be used.

Stratified random sampling

Stratified random sampling is a way of making sure that important groups are represented in a sample. The sampling frame is split up into groups that need to be represented. Random methods are used to select a proportion of the sample from each group. In our example, the sampling frame is split into two lists – one containing 500 males, and one containing 500 females. To get a sample of 100 subjects we randomly select 50 males and 50 females. Our sample is sure to reflect the gender balance in the population and has still been chosen randomly.

The method described above is an example of *proportionate stratified sampling*. The proportions of each group chosen for the sample were the same as their proportions in the population. If the population had consisted of 600 males and 400 females we would have chosen 60 males and 40 females to get our sample of 100.

Sometimes though groups within the population may be small, but still important to the research. For example, a day centre may cater mainly for able-bodied people, but have a few disabled clients. Proportionate stratified sampling may allow only one or two disabled clients to be selected. The sample will thus fail to represent fully the views and needs of an important group. *Disproportionate stratified sampling* can be used to get over this problem. The researcher deliberately weights the proportions of different groups in the sample to include greater numbers of small but important groups.

Stratified random sampling is an improvement on simple random sampling, but it has some drawbacks. To stratify a sampling frame you need some prior knowledge of the groups within it. Unless the list contains extra information you may have to guess which groups people belong to. If you only have a list of names to go on, even guessing who is male or female can lead to mistakes. Apart from this, going through a sampling frame and identifying groups and proportions is a long process.

Another problem is that you could choose to stratify by characteristics which are not useful to your study. For example, you may stratify according to gender but not according to age. Later you could find that important differences of opinion occur between age groups. It is difficult to know how to stratify a population, even if it is possible to do so.

Pros	Cons
Aim to ensure that results can be generalised to whole population	Researcher must be able to obtain a sampling frame
Sampling errors can be assessed and quantified mathematically	Simple random sampling may still give a biased sample
Stratification can ensure the inclusion of small but important groups	Implementing random sampling methods can be time-consuming
Stratification can minimise the chance of selecting biased samples	Stratification requires you to have prior knowledge about the proportions of different types of people in the population

Figure 23.2 Some pros and cons of random sampling methods

Both simple and stratified random sampling need a sampling frame. The problem is getting hold of a suitable list. Records kept for many purposes may be useful as sampling frames, but most are also confidential. Even if you do obtain a suitable list there is no guarantee that it is accurate and complete. Also it may be ordered in ways you are unaware of, making systematic sampling liable to bias. There are populations for which it is impossible to find or create a sampling frame. Then other sampling methods have to be used.

Quota sampling

Suppose you are interested in people's opinions about a new health education exhibition at a local hall. In this case, it is impossible to draw up a suitable sampling frame for your population. The best way to find a sample is to hang around the exhibition exit. You simply stop and question some of the people who come out. This sort of sampling has the advantage that the sample can always be ensured to be of the desired size. If there is a problem with non-response from one person, you simply ask another. The major problem is that the selection of the sample members is entirely at the interviewers' discretion. Interviewers may pick people who they like the look of. They are likely to avoid those who they perceive as looking demanding or threatening. One way of dealing with this is to introduce some controls on who the interviewer can choose.

Quota sampling is a type of stratified sampling, though it is not a random sampling method since the final selection of the sample is left to the interviewer. In quota sampling, interviews must pick a specified number of people from certain defined groups. For example, an interviewer might have to pick 50 men and 50 women for their sample. Quota sampling is much used for market research and opinion polls. Street interviews are the usual method, and interviewers have a quota of people in different categories to stop and question.

Quota sampling has several advantages.

- It is cheap and quick to do.
- There is no need to find a sampling frame and select a sample randomly from it.
- There is no problem with non-response. If you need a particular quota of women with children you simply carry on until you have interviewed enough of them.

Quota sampling gets quick results from a varied sample.

One problem with quota sampling is that it is not a random method. The final decision on who to talk to is left to the interviewer, and this introduces the problem of bias in selection. Even if interviewers must speak to a quota of people in a group their selection may still be biased. It may be easier to stop a parent with one child than one with four children to handle. Quotas of 'over 65s' are likely to under-represent older members of the age group, particularly if interviewing is done in the street.

Most quota samples use gender, age and social class as the basis for setting quotas. Interviewers generally have no trouble identifying gender, and only a little more estimating age. However, the identification of class by appearance is a risky business, likely to be heavily influenced by the interviewers' perceptions and ideas.

Another problem is in drawing up the quotas for interview. Decisions can only be made if researchers have some prior knowledge of the population they are researching. This does not mean that a sampling frame is needed, but statistics indicating proportions of different groups in the population must be found.

Another important issue is where and when the sampling and interviewing takes place. If you interview in an upmarket shopping street, it is likely that you would get a different type of sample than you would in a less prosperous area. If you interview on a midweek afternoon you are likely to miss working people. Unless you interview door-to-door you will miss people who are house-bound. In short, quota sampling misses people who are difficult to 'bump into'. Quota sampling is fine if you need simple, approximate data from a section of the general public. It is less helpful if your population is more precisely defined.

Pros	Cons
No need to obtain a sampling frame	Not a truly random sampling method
Refusals do not prevent the required sample size being achieved	Interviewers' choice will influence sample selection
Can be a quick method to implement	Quota setting requires prior knowledge of the proportions of groups in the population
May be the only way to sample views on an exhibition or event	Misses people who are difficult to bump into, e.g. people who are house-bound or in hospital

Figure 23.3 Some pros and cons of quota sampling

Sampling and observational research

The sampling methods we have looked at can be used to select subjects for self-completion questionnaires, for interviews, or for experiments. If you decide to use observation as a research method you also have to make choices which result in sampling of a sort. Observation often deals with particular groups over time. Both group activities and group membership may vary at different times of the day or week. There may be regular patterns to these changes that the observer is unaware of. An observer who visits a day nursery every day just after lunch will get a biased view of the children's activity levels.

The timings of observations could be randomised to minimise distortions of this sort. Other types of observational study may be randomised in similar ways. The main point is that you should try to imagine what factors could introduce sampling bias into your observations, and attempt to deal with them.

The sampling method you choose will depend on who you are studying, and the resources available to you. Whatever method you pick, try to think out your decision. Will your method give a biased result? Can you do anything to improve how representative and random your sample selection has been?

As a warning, consider the case of the disastrous poll carried out in 1936 by the American periodical *The Literary Digest*. They intended to predict the result of the forthcoming presidential election between Landon and Roosevelt. A sample was chosen randomly from telephone directories and car registrations, and the result predicted an easy win for Landon. Roosevelt won. The problem was that the sample was not representative of voters. Only the well-off had telephones and cars at that time. Poorer people were not asked and Roosevelt's popularity was seriously under-estimated. *The Literary Digest* claimed too much for their research. If you are aware of the problems that may have occurred due to your sampling method, you can be more realistic about the accuracy of your own results.

Evidence collection point

Every research project you carry out during your studies will involve choosing a sample to gather data from. Details of the methods you have used, and problems that you are aware of, can act as evidence towards Element 8.2, and they should always be included in your research reports.

Think about the characteristics of a population that you are intending to sample from. Will you be able to use random sampling methods? You must obtain a sampling frame to be able to use this method. Can you find out enough about your population to stratify it and use proportionate random sampling?

If you think that you need to use quota sampling, how will you determine the size of your quotas? Can you get access to demographic data that will help you to do this?

Explain the reasoning behind your decisions on sampling methods clearly in the research report. Outline the factors that led to your final decisions, and discuss any unforeseen difficulties that cropped up during the sampling process.

Collecting data

When you have decided who your population is, and how you might choose a sample, it is time to think about the sort of data you want to collect from them. Will it be quantitative or qualitative, or a mixture of both? All research collects some quantitative data from subjects. Information like age and gender are recorded, even if in-depth interview methods are being used. Personal data like this is sometimes called *demographic data*, as it is factual information concerning the personal characteristics and circumstances of the subject.

Your research may need much more demographic data than age and gender. Some projects, such as the government's census, aim to collect little other than demographic data. There is a wide range of possible information that you could seek. Facts can be collected about health, income, family composition, lifestyle, work, and all other areas of people's lives. The range of demographic data you need will depend on your research question and the research methods you use.

An issue here is that subjects may be unwilling to give accurate data on personal or sensitive issues. Demographic data can be very personal. For example, questions on income or disability can make respondents ill at ease and lead to inaccurate responses, or even rapidly terminated interviews! Some people find it difficult to give their correct age. In fact careful questionnaire design and skilful interviewing can usually minimise this problem. You just need to remember that there are limits to the range of demographic data you will be able to collect.

Other data may be about the subject's behaviour. This is also often quantitative data and could concern things like the sorts of food usually eaten, or how often a daily paper is read. Answers to behaviour questions may require the subject to think and make estimates. This can mean that inaccurate guesses are made which lead to distorted results. Sensitive areas of enquiry are also an issue, and it may well not be obvious to the researcher that an area is sensitive until data collection begins. You need to imagine the point of view of your respondents. Will they feel happy to give accurate data about the aspects of behaviour you are asking about? If the answer seems to be 'no' then you should look for other ways to approach the research question.

Your research may call for data concerning people's attitudes, beliefs and values. This is probably the most difficult data to collect and deal with. Questions about circumstances or behaviour are likely to be understood in exactly the same way by both researcher and subject. Misunderstandings can usually be dealt with since both parties share a common frame of reference towards the subject of the question. This is not necessarily the case with attitudes and values. For example, take the question 'Do you think that sex before marriage is morally wrong?' There may be many ways of interpreting what 'morally wrong' means. Two people may both answer 'yes' while having completely different views about sin. They may also have differing concepts about sex and marriage which are crucial to a full understanding of their answer.

There are basically two ways of dealing with this problem and each tends to lead towards a different research method and style of data. Both are aiming to ensure that the data gathered gives as accurate a representation of people's real views as possible.

One way is to 'unpack' the question to reveal the possible interpretations that different parts may suggest. This produces a set of extra areas to be explored so that the subject's personal interpretation is made more clear. In our example, you could ask a number of questions around the concept of morals to discover more about the meanings placed upon it by the respondent. This method is usually associated with the collection of quantitative data. Several questions with restricted answer options are asked and a numerical coding system is applied to the answers. Researchers can analyse these responses later and categorise respondents according to the pattern of answers they gave.

This approach to collecting attitude data is extremely widely used. Professional researchers have developed sophisticated question sets to explore attitudes, and statistical techniques to aid accurate analysis of the results. Though this level of technical expertise is beyond the scope of this book, there are more simple methods that you can use to get quantitative data about attitudes and values in your own research.

Some researchers reject the idea that things like attitude can be scaled numerically. They see the designing of question sets and attitude scales as an imposition of the researchers' frame of reference onto the views of the subjects. Thus, they believe, the research is introducing distortions even before data has been collected.

These researchers believe that attitudes must be revealed by subjects in their own terms, and that direct comparison between subjects is usually impossible. They often gather quantitative data using in-depth interviewing methods. The research reports sometimes contain rich passages, quoting the comments made by the respondent, which seem to get to the heart of the feelings they have about a particular issue. The logic of an individual's view, and the connections he or she makes, can surprise and illuminate in a way that quantitative methods would not. Unless the quantitative researcher has predicted all the issues surrounding a question, these are not going to be brought up by the research. However, qualitative data may be so personalised that it cannot be easily compared with that given by other respondents or generalised to a wider population.

Suppose you are working on Element 4.2 and are interested in people's beliefs about the role of a wife and mother. You could take a quantitative approach and try to design a questionnaire that asks a number of questions about the concepts involved. You would be attempting to pin down exactly what subjects think a 'wife and mother' means, and what sorts of things they think are included in the role. At the data analysis stage, these different views can be quantified and compared statistically. Interesting links, or *correlations*, between different data items can be detected. For instance, expectations of the role of a wife and mother may be found to differ between people of different age groups, or different genders.

You could approach the same research topic using qualitative methods. Now you would use in-depth or semi-structured interview methods and encourage respondents to give details of their feelings about the role of a wife and mother. It is far less likely that you will misrepresent or misunderstand the views of your subjects, or that you will miss important aspects of the question that hadn't occurred to you in advance. However, you will be unable to apply the results to a wider population or make statistical comparisons between the responses of different types of people.

In practice it is common for researchers to use a combination of methods to collect data on attitudes and values. *Closed questions*, with a limited range of allowed responses available, can be included alongside *open questions*, where the subject can answer in his or her own words. The results obtained through one question style can help clarify and confirm the results obtained with the other.

Your choices about the type and range of data you intend to collect will be influenced by the issues we have discussed. As you list the things you want to find out, think about what difficulties each one presents. Will the subjects think the information too personal to reveal? Will they actually know the answer? Will they have complex views and opinions which are hard to categorise and assess?

There is also the question of the ethics of collecting the data you are interested in. You need to be certain that you are collecting data that you actually need, and that you could be reasonably expected to ask for. Skilled interviewers may be able to draw all sorts of revelations from their subjects but, unless the research question demands this information, it is bad practice, and ethically questionable, to collect it.

Evidence collection point

You will need to make decisions about data in all the research that you carry out. Evidence of your thinking and decision-making can be used towards Element 8.2.

Make sure that you have good reasons for needing the data that you intend to collect. Your research report should list the data areas you decided on. It should also include an explanation of your need for the data with reference to the research question.

At this point in the research process you should have thought about who the population is, how easily a sample can be chosen, and what range and type of data you need to collect. The next stage is to choose a research method which suits the population and the data required.

Choosing and using a research method

This section is about using different research methods for yourself. It covers:

- experiments
- self-completion questionnaires
- structured interviews
- in-depth interviews
- direct observation
- participant observation.

Experiments

Carrying out experiments in health and social care research can be difficult. Experiments are usually employed by scientists like biologists, or by psychologists who are interested in very specific aspects of people's abilities or behaviour. Chapter 22 outlines some of the problems of applying the experimental method to the study of people. Controlling, or even estimating, all the variables affecting human behaviour may be impossible. Researchers need to set up highly structured experimental situations so that outside influences are, as far as possible, identical for all the subjects tested.

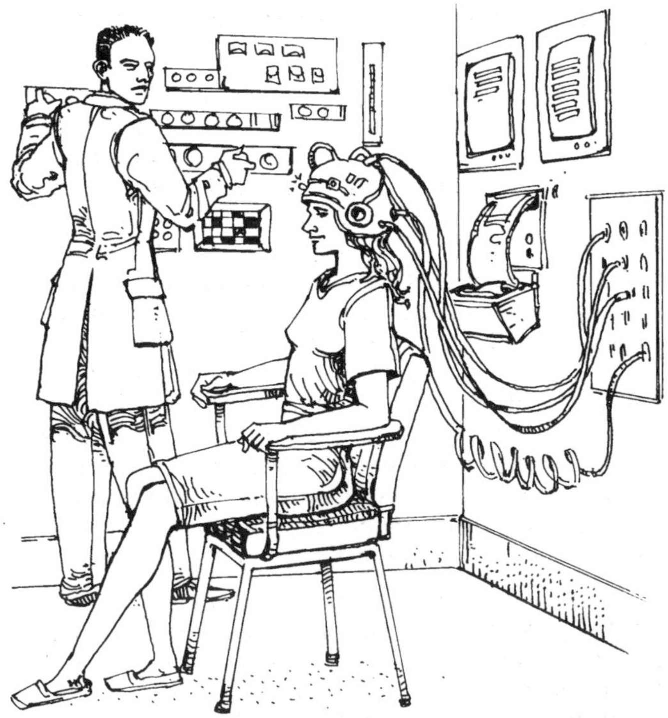

Figure 23.4 Specialised experimental equipment may not be available

Another difficulty is that experiments set out to measure things. This could be something like how far a person can jump, or how quickly they can press a button when ordered to do so. Taking measurements will mean having equipment available. Psychological and medical experiments often employ sophisticated equipment that has been specifically designed and constructed for the research in question. This sort of specialised equipment is usually not available to the student researcher.

Even where everyday equipment is used, experimenters must be sure that they are able to carry out measurements accurately. For instance, you may decide to set up an experiment to find out how quickly and effectively the students on your course are able to apply a particular style of wound dressing. It is easy to time each subject's efforts, but it is much more difficult to judge the quality of his or her work. It would need someone with skill and experience to make accurate judgements.

Another thing to consider is safety. You are setting up a situation and are responsible for the outcomes. Apparently simple experiments can be hazardous to some subjects, and you may not be aware of personal circumstances that could make the experiment dangerous to a particular individual.

You also need to think about the ethics of the experiment you are planning. Researchers often need to keep subjects ignorant of the true purpose of the experiment because knowledge of this will affect how they behave. Psychologists may tell subjects that they are researching one thing when they are really looking at another. Many classic psychological studies have relied on subjects being duped in this way, and a variety of tactics have been used to achieve it. The ethical considerations may have been ignored, or taken to be less important than the advancement of human understanding. While professional researchers working in important areas may have some justification for their methods, it is generally not ethical to keep subjects in the dark about the true nature and aims of an experiment. If you feel that your experimental research will demand that subjects are fooled about your real intentions then you should abandon the method and carry on your research using other means.

If you do decide to carry out an experiment you must try to make the experience similar for all subjects. Carry out the method in a uniform way so that each subject has, as far as possible, a similar set of influences to all the others. Try to make sure that each subject has the same prior knowledge of what they will be asked to do. If some have been told what to expect well in advance their results may differ from those of subjects given less warning.

Finally, remember that there can be difficulties generalising the experimental results to other populations or situations. You have set up an artificial situation and the results may not apply outside that context. For example, our wound dressing skill experiment may have shown that one particular student excelled over all the rest, both in quality of the dressing and speed of execution. However, unknown to you, the person may have a serious aversion to the sight of blood which prevents him or her using their skills effectively in a real emergency. What experiments show is how people have behaved on a particular occasion and under a particular set of circumstances. Going beyond this requires care and scientific honesty.

Evidence collection point

Think about which areas of your studies may suggest an experimental approach to data collection. For example, Element 2.2 asks you to gather data to evaluate interactions. You are expected to exert some control over the circumstances of the interaction so that participants are supported. Also you are expected to behave in such a way as to optimise effective interaction between participants. You could keep records of the things you decide to do to achieve these aims, and assess how effective each measure seemed to be. You could try varying aspects of the situation or your behaviour and repeating the interaction. This could help you assess the influence and effect of the measures you have been taking.

Your use of experimental techniques could count as evidence towards Element 8.2.

Self-completion questionnaires

If you want to get information from a number of people quickly then a self-completion questionnaire may be a good way to go about it. Unfortunately, self-completion questionnaires have a reputation for achieving poor response rates when postal methods are used. One answer to this is to make your questionnaire as interesting and relevant as possible to your subjects. And, of course, it needs to be clear and simple enough not to put people off. Information technology resources can help you to produce a professional looking and easy to follow questionnaire. Subjects are much more likely to respond if your questionnaire has these qualities.

Postal questionnaires are simple to administer. You just send a copy of your questionnaire, together with a suitable covering letter, to each member of your sample and wait for the replies to come rolling in. In practice, it may be necessary to include a stamped, addressed envelope to encourage people to return their questionnaires. This could be costly, but that is the price you pay for more accurate results!

If you are able to hand the questionnaires to your subjects, and collect them personally, your response rate should be much better. You may have thought of leaving a stack of questionnaires in a suitable place and providing a box for completed questionnaires to be placed in. This can be tempting if you want quick returns from people who use a particular facility. Beware though, because this method may give very distorted results. You are asking for a sample to select itself. Those who reply may do so because they have time or motivation. You will miss people in a hurry, and those who have moderate opinions on your research subject. People with strong opinions might fill in several forms so as to make their point. It is much better to take the trouble to use a simple sampling method and improve the quality of your results.

Element 6.3 asks you to evaluate clients' experience of, and influence over, the health and social care services they receive. Self-completion questionnaires could be used to gather data on clients' views. You need to follow the research process and begin by developing a research question that is workable. From this a definition of your population should emerge, and you can begin to think about drawing a sample from it. If you have decided to use postal methods you will need the addresses of all members of your population. This sounds impossible, but may not be for all populations. For instance, if you intend to research the experiences of local people using their GP service then a street directory will provide you with a sampling frame and allow you to randomise your sample selection easily.

However, if you are interested in the experiences of disabled people you are likely to have more difficulty conducting a postal survey. You may have to resort to distributing your questionnaires to people attending a day centre, and accept that you will miss those who don't attend it. Be honest about sampling difficulties in your report as it will help to establish your credibility as a researcher.

Next decide the types of data you intend to collect. Element 6.3 identifies the areas that you need to enquire about. They centre on clients' perceptions of the health and care services, and of their perceptions of a continuum of care. You can design a questionnaire which seeks data concerning these areas. It would probably be best to finish reading this chapter before beginning your research. It will help you with questionnaire design, data analysis and reporting.

Remember that this research deals with sensitive areas of people's lives. You need to take care that your questions are relevant and necessary, and that they are not liable to offend your respondents. Also remember that clients, and respondents, have a right to confidentiality. Respect this right in your research and assure your respondents that you are doing so.

Evidence collection point

Think about areas of your studies where you might use self-completion questionnaires to gather data. We have already mentioned Element 6.3. What other opportunities exist for you to use this method of data collection?

Research work that you carry out using self-completion questionnaires can count as evidence towards Element 8.2.

Structured interviews

Structured interviews are one of the most commonly used research methods and the features of them that we have looked at help explain why this is so. The method can be useful in several areas of your GNVQ studies. In particular Element 7.3 requires you to use structured interview methods to evaluate the effectiveness of a health education campaign.

This will mean going through the stages of the research process that we have looked at. To some extent the research question has been set for you, but you still need to choose which health campaign to focus on, and define the population it is aimed at. Secondary research will include finding out more about how the campaign was designed and conducted, and should help you to define the aims of the campaign in detail. The campaign organisers may be prepared to help you. Failing this, you could draw your own conclusions based on the material that the campaign produced. If the campaign is any good you should have little trouble identifying its message.

You may be able to find useful secondary data which you can use in your work. For instance, if the campaign aims to alert young people to the dangers of smoking, then statistics on the numbers of young people who smoke would be useful and relevant. Knowledge of the proportions of young smokers in the general population could help you to assess how typical your chosen sample is.

The campaign you choose will have its own target audience and they will form the population for your study. You will have to select a sample from this population for interview. If you are looking at a promotional event, then quota sampling methods will be best. You could use official statistics to get some idea of the proportions of different types of people in the general population. Next carry out a brief pilot of your questionnaire so that you know how long it will take to complete an interview, and in the light of this decide on the total number of interviews you intend to conduct. Now fix quotas of people you intend interviewing so that the proportions of different types of people in your sample are similar to those in the general population. All you need to do is stop people who seem to fit your quota categories as they leave the event. Remember that your questionnaire needs to begin with demographic data so that you can check whether a person fits a category you need.

Other types of campaign may aim at specific populations, or the public. It will help your work if you try to randomise sample selection as far as you can, but don't try to be too ambitious. It may be impossible to get hold of a sampling frame, and you may be dealing with a sample that is too small in size to be representative, however randomly chosen. The main thing is to be honest about what you have done, and about compromises you have been forced to make. This will demonstrate that you are aware of the issues and have considered solutions.

Next, you need to decide what data to collect so that you can begin to design the questions you will ask in order to obtain it. The details of this will again depend on the campaign concerned, and the section on questionnaire design should help (see page 509). You will need some demographic data so that comparisons between the responses of different types of people can be made. This means collecting data on age, gender and other relevant characteristics.

Think it over

You may have begun to think about which campaign you intend to focus on for

Element 7.3. Try to imagine what demographic data you will need, given the population that the campaign is aimed at and its message.

Finding out about the campaign's effectiveness can be approached in several different ways. You could ask the questions about behaviour to assess whether the campaign may have had an effect. Other questions could ask subjects to give their own views on the effects of the campaign on their behaviour or attitude. If the campaign sets out to inform, then you could test subjects' knowledge in the areas the campaign deals with. A combination of these and other question types can be included to give a range on data for analysis. When you have decided what data to collect, you can go on to design your questionnaire, or interview schedule.

When doing your interviews you should try to stick to the principles that underlie the use of this research method. Structured interviewing stresses *uniformity*. It is essential that the effect of the interviewer on a respondent's answers is as small as possible. Even the stress interviewers put on words when reading out a question can exert an influence. Try reading aloud the question 'Do you believe the government is doing a good job?' a few times, putting the stress on different parts of the question. Stress the word 'good' implies that there may be some doubt. Stressing the word 'government' implies that it is being compared with something else. Interviewers should read out questions in as neutral a way as possible to reduce the possibility of biasing an answer.

Of course, the questions asked must not be varied by the interviewer. If this is allowed, it is even more likely that bias will occur. This is fine provided an interview goes smoothly, but in practice interviewers don't always have such an easy time. Problems with responses can take a variety of forms, but fortunately there are ways of dealing with them. You may get only a partial response, where the respondent does not give enough information for the response to be recorded. Or the response may be irrelevant to the question. Respondents could side-track the questioning process, perhaps by commenting on a previous question instead of answering the one just asked. Some responses are inaccurate, and obviously so. This may be an indication that the question has been misunderstood. Also you may get no response at all. Your question could be met with silence, perhaps because respondents are thinking it over, or because they don't know what to say.

Interviewers have the problem of dealing with response problems without biasing the results. The solution is to have a prepared list of statements which can be used to tackle response problems. They can be printed on the interview schedule to ensure they are used similarly for each respondent (see Figure 23.5). If interviewers vary the content and wording of these comments it defeats the object of using them.

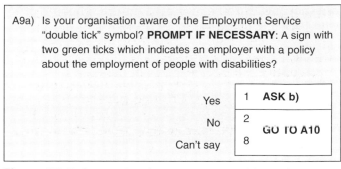

A9a) Is your organisation aware of the Employment Service "double tick" symbol? **PROMPT IF NECESSARY**: A sign with two green ticks which indicates an employer with a policy about the employment of people with disabilities?

Yes	1	**ASK b)**
No	2	**GO TO A10**
Can't say	8	

Figure 23.5 A question from a structured interview questionnaire, aimed at employers and used in the evaluation of the Access to Work Scheme in 1995. The question includes a precisely worded prompt to be used in the event of a response difficulty

Sometimes a non-verbal cue will help. If the problem is non-response, it may be best to stay silent and allow a noticeable pause to develop. Respondents may pick up that it is their turn to speak and provide you with an answer. Another method is to use a nod, raised eyebrows or a similar non-verbal signal to indicate that you are waiting for a reply. Remember to standardise the non-verbal cues you intend to use as haphazard use can introduce bias. If these tactics don't work, you could ask if they would like you to repeat the question.

Partial responses may be solved by using silence or non-verbal cues. If there is no improvement verbal follow-ups could begin with 'I see' accompanied by a nod to indicate you want more, or, more directly, 'Can you tell me more?'

Responses which are irrelevant or inaccurate may be the result of a misunderstood question. This can be tricky since you need to avoid insulting or belittling respondents by highlighting their mistake. You could try saying 'I'm sorry, I may not have asked that question very clearly,' and then repeat the question. Respondents may take care to listen closely as you have indicated that a problem of some kind has occurred, and the error has been transferred onto you. You could try stating the subject clearly before repeating the question. A statement like 'This question is about ...' can cover questions on many subjects. To minimise bias, the subject of each question needs to be indicated on the schedule in case this statement has to be used.

Think it over

Think about how you might deal with response problems during your interview. Try to imagine the sort of problem that could occur and what you could do or say to help.

Make a list of your ideas. You can decide which approaches to allow when you come to design your interview questionnaire.

When carrying out the interviews try to be friendly but professional. A standardised welcome and explanation of the purpose of the survey is needed, as are introductions to new parts of the interview. Remember that all the input of the interviewer needs to be scripted. Keep introductions brief and friendly, and be sure to stick to them with each respondent. Things go much more smoothly if the interviewer's input is clearly highlighted on the interview schedule, so use IT resources to make yours clear and well-organised.

The analysis of the data and reporting of the results and conclusions is the final step. These areas are dealt with in Chapter 24. It is probably best to complete your reading of this chapter before you begin your research.

Evidence collection point

You will be carrying out a research project using structured interview methods in Element 7.3. This work will be able to be used as evidence towards Elements 8.2 and 8.3.

There are other opportunities to use this research method, such as in Element 6.3. This could again generate evidence towards Unit 8.

In-depth interviews

Carrying out in-depth research may seem to need less planning and preparation than methods which use questionnaires. However, there are other demands placed on the researcher which require care and skill. In-depth interviews are about allowing people to 'open up'. This is how you expect to be able to collect accurate data from them. However, encouraging people to think and speak about deep personal feelings or events can lead to an interaction that you will need to handle with great care. Some respondents may find the interview a traumatic or even damaging experience. You need to prepare and carry out your research so as to avoid this happening, and to ensure that you are doing useful work towards your research question.

You can use in-depth, or unstructured, interview methods in your work towards several elements of the GNVQ Health and Social Care course. Element 6.3 asks you to evaluate clients' perceptions of health and social care provision. We have already mentioned one of the ways you could collect quantitative data towards this question. You could also use in-depth interviews to collect qualitative data from a small sample.

There may be advantages to using qualitative methods, perhaps before going on to design and use quantitative research approaches. You are likely to hear comments that you would never have expected, and you will have a much better understanding of the issues when your unstructured interviews are completed. You can use this knowledge and data to help you create a questionnaire that is interesting to your respondents and covers the things that concern them. Qualitative research helps you to design better quantitative research instruments.

The principles of the research process apply equally to in-depth research methods. You still need to begin by defining your research problem and the population it concerns. Secondary research is important for helping you to put your work in context. Quantitative data can be included in your research report to give background and to help readers to assess how typical your subjects might be.

Next you need to decide who to interview, and how many interviews to carry out. You will probably want to allow at least an hour for each interview, perhaps much longer. How many will you be able to conduct in the time you have available? Each interview must be carried out somewhere private and quiet, where the respondent feels at ease and where interruptions will not occur. One suitable place could be the respondent's own home, if you know them well enough to suggest it. Otherwise you may need to use a room in a suitable place. This may be a facility such as a day centre. Now you will have to consider whether you can get uninterrupted use of the room at times convenient to you and your subjects. All these issues will affect the number of interviews you can handle, and who you can use as subjects. If you intend to use in-depth techniques you should consider these implications at an early stage. You may need to re-format your research question so that it concerns a population that you can easily contact and meet in private.

Another thing to plan is how you are going to record the data. A tape recorder is probably the best way, if your subjects are happy about it. Of course it is unethical to record secretly. You must always warn respondents of your intentions, and most people will be happy if you use this method. You might want to keep notes as well to record background data such as the respondent's appearance and body language. Also, you can note the time and content of important parts of the interview. This may speed things up later when you need to find them on the tape. Note-taking can act as a barrier between you and your subject. This may not be a bad thing since it reminds you both that you are having an interview, and may make it easier for you to keep the point in view.

The content of the interview will depend on your skills, the person you are interviewing, and the subject being discussed. An important issue that you need to think about in advance is the sensitivity of the research question for your respondents. For Element 4.1 you need to look at how individuals have coped with expected and unexpected transition and change in their lives. In-depth interviews could be used to gather data about this issue. Such potentially traumatic events need handling with great care. You must pick respondents, and areas of change, that minimise the likelihood of your interview causing someone serious upset. Areas like bereavement or the break-up of a relationship may become so upsetting that the interview becomes harmful to the respondent's psychological well-being. If you think that this is possible, it is unethical to continue your research along those lines.

Another ethical issue is the subject's right to confidentiality. In-depth methods collect a lot of data, and you will be reporting results from a very small sample of people. This might mean that respondents can be identified from your report if they are known to members of your target audience. Simply avoid using subjects who may fall victim to this, and write your report carefully to prevent such identification.

In-depth research reports can help to remind us that social research really is about people. When writing your report try to include some quotes from your respondents that seem to sum up their views in their own words. It is rich original data of this sort that in-depth researchers are looking for.

Evidence collection point

You could use in-depth interview methods in several areas of your GNVQ Health and Social Care studies and two of these have been mentioned above. Another possible application is in Element 2.3 – you could use in-depth research methods to develop case studies concerning the effects of care settings and care relationships on clients.

Your in-depth research work can be used as evidence towards Elements 8.2 and 8.3.

Direct observation

Direct observation is a research method that is often used in combination with others. As we saw in Chapter 22, observers can detect behaviour that participants are unaware of, but they are also capable of misinterpreting what they have seen. On its own observation has major weaknesses if used for anything more complex than counting heads. But if other methods are also used to confirm or illuminate the observations, it can be a useful research tool.

Observation is one of the data sources suggested for use in Element 2.2. Here you are asked to gather data to evaluate the effectiveness of small and large group interactions. Used in conjunction with the other data sources suggested, observation will provide helpful data.

You need to organise your observations to make them useful. As usual this begins with the research question and the population it concerns. Thinking about these things should help you to decide what behaviour you are going to be looking for. Observers are not trying to record everything that they see. They begin with a research plan that demands certain data and set out to collect only what they need. This means that you should think about what you are going to look for and devise ways of noting it easily. An observation checklist can be drawn up so that you can easily record incidents that fit your data needs. For Element 2.2 there is a list of evaluation criteria in the Range which will help you. It includes items like participation and quality of contribution on which you could gather data by observation.

You may decide to look at other things, like body language or how relaxed participants appear to be, if you think this data is relevant to the participants and the contact of the interaction you are observing. The observation checklist can include anything that you feel in necessary. However, using a checklist in a live interaction might be very difficult if it is too complex. If you expect to be participating in most of the interaction, it may be impractical to try to keep notes, even if they are merely ticks in a column when a particular behaviour is observed.

You could use a video recorder to tape the interaction, and play it back with your checklist in front of you. Now you will have plenty of time to note interesting observations in detail, and better still you can replay them if you are not sure what you saw. Remember that ethical standards demand that you must get your subjects' permission before using video equipment. If anyone objects then you can't use it. Also don't expect a video to pick up everything. You may not be able to film the whole group wherever you place the recorder, and you will have to rely on your own notes to record anything it misses.

When writing up your research report try to be honest about the quality of observational data. Don't assume that, because you didn't record seeing something, it didn't happen. Try to relate your observational results to data gathered by other means. For example, do your observations on levels of participation agree with the views expressed by the participants themselves? You may be able to draw interesting conclusions by comparing data in this way.

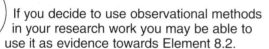

Evidence collection point

If you decide to use observational methods in your research work you may be able to use it as evidence towards Element 8.2. Include full details of your planning and methods in your report, and remember to evaluate the results.

If you are using observation in combination with other research methods, you should explain how the data gathered by each is related. Report any apparent inconsistencies in the results honestly. You may have uncovered interesting issues that deserve further investigation.

Participant observation

The discussion of participant observation in Chapter 22 stressed the time and commitment needed to join a new group and develop an understanding of the members. This is certainly true if you have no connections at all with the subjects of your enquiry. However, you are already a member of many groups. You could include your family, your close friends, or your fellow GNVQ students in a list of groups that you belong to.

For Element 4.2 you need to look at social constructs such as gender roles, and ideas about deviance. All your fellow members in the groups you belong to will have their own ideas of what these social constructs mean for them. You may already have a pretty good idea what they think.

It is possible to look at the behaviour or opinions of people you know and the data could be useful to you. There are dangers though in using family and friends as a data source. One problem is that of your own objectivity. Your existing relationships with the group members, as well as your role and status in the group, will affect your views of what you see and hear. This is a major problem even for experienced social scientists working amongst complete strangers.

Another problem is that you could easily run into ethical difficulties. If you intend to try to shift from group member to observer you must tell the other members that you are doing so and ask their permission. If anyone objects, you must abandon this method. Failure to do so is not only ethically wrong, but could jeopardise your personal relationships. Confidentiality is another problem, and you must be careful to report your observations in such a way that it is preserved.

You may find that members of a group you belong to have no objections to your recording their understanding of certain social constructs for a student research project. Your research must be organised and you need to be certain about what you are setting out to observe. You may want to instigate discussion on the ideas people have about a particular social construct so that you can collect the data you need. This also has the advantage of making it clear to the group when you are observing and when you are an ordinary member. It might make your relationships difficult if people are not sure whether you are 'on duty' or not. To record the data you could make notes and you could, with permission, tape the session. The data you are gathering will be qualitative. Good data may take the form of quotable passages which sum up in their own words a person's views on a particular social construct.

Where you are working with subjects who are so close to you, it is particularly important to make sure that they are happy with the way you have reported your findings. Show your report to all the people concerned before you finalise it. If any object then be prepared to make changes, or even abandon it altogether.

Evidence collection point

If you do decide to use data gathered through participant observation in a research project you may generate evidence towards Element 8.2. Bear in mind the problems mentioned above and use such data only when you are convinced that it is safe and ethical to do so.

Your report will need to explain why the method was used and how you went about it. Don't try to generalise your results to a wider population. You must accept the limits of this research method.

Designing questionnaires

This section is about how to write better questions and how to construct a questionnaire. It covers:

- open and closed questions
- measuring opinion
- writing questions
- question order
- layout and presentation of self-completion questionnaires
- designing structured interview schedules.

Open and closed questions

Whether you intend using self-completion questionnaires or structured interviews, you will need to create a questionnaire. The quality of your questionnaire largely depends on the questions it contains and you need to spend time and care getting them right.

Question style is an important aspect of questionnaire design. There are two basic types of question – *open* and *closed*. Open (or *open response*) questions allow respondents to answer in their own words. Closed (or *fixed response*) questions ask respondents to choose from a set of alternative answers provided. Most surveys use both types of question.

Open questions can give very useful background data. Respondents don't have to choose between alternatives and can answer in their own terms. Open questions can be especially useful in a *pilot survey*. This is a small-scale trial of the survey proper which is intended to test the method and research tools to be used. Here, open questions can indicate the sorts of things people regard as important to an issue, and help in the design of more relevant fixed response questions.

One problem with open questions can be that respondents' answers become rather lengthy. In self-completion questionnaires answers can be limited by providing a restricted amount of space for them. The main limitation of open questions is that replies can't be analysed statistically. Nevertheless they can be useful at the beginning of questionnaires as icebreakers, and they can be used to break up long strings of fixed response questions. Also they can be used to get people thinking about a topic, and establish a frame of reference before fixed response questions probe more specifically.

Fixed response questions restrict respondents to a choice between fixed alternatives. They can be used to collect data which is demographic or factual, such as gender, age group or religion. This data allows you to classify your respondents during the analysis stage and link, or correlate, their characteristics to their opinions. If quota sampling is used, demographic facts are vital to check that the respondent falls into a group you need to question. Responses to demographic questions can lead to a particular set of follow-up questions being asked. For instance 'yes' answers to the factual question 'Do you smoke cigarettes?' can lead to a set of questions specifically directed at smokers. This is usually known as *routing* (see Figure 23.6).

Other fixed response questions seek data on opinions. There are different ways to design these questions, and the style of response required varies between them.

7b) What are you doing <u>now</u>?

Please tick <u>one</u> box

In a full-time job (30 or more hours a week)	1	**Now please go to Question 8**
On a training scheme (YT or other scheme)	2	
Out of work	3	**Now please go to Question 14 on page 5**
Full-time at school	4	
Full-time at college or university	5	
Doing something else (please say what) ____	6	

Figure 23.6 An example of routing from a self-completion questionnaire used in the Scottish School-leavers Survey in 1994. The first two options lead to questions about the subject's job or training place. The other options lead to questions about educational courses and job-seeking

Measuring opinion

The most basic opinion question asks 'Do you agree with ...?' and allows respondents to choose between 'yes' and 'no'. Usually, however, it is better to allow more options so that *strength of opinion* can be indicated. Most opinion questions use some form of scaling or ranking method to allow differences between respondents to be measured more closely.

Rating scales are a way of measuring the strength of a person's opinion on an issue. A number of options, often five or seven, are offered for selection in answer to an opinion question. Options can be presented in a number of ways. They may be expressed verbally, say from 'strongly in favour' to 'strongly against', with tick boxes. Or you could use a graphical scale with fixed points for respondents to indicate how strongly they are for or against. (See Figure 23.7.)

The number of scale points offered can be odd or even. If an odd number is used respondents can select a safe, middle of the road position. Respondents may cluster round this 'safe' option if it is available. An even number of options prevents respondents remaining neutral.

This form of rating scale is the most basic. Professional social researchers often use more sophisticated scaling methods (see Figure 23.8), where responses from a group of questions are linked to give an overall view of opinion. Respondents are very sensitive to things like the order or wording of questions, and there are a vast number of different ways of asking questions about a subject. Scaling methods involve selecting a sample of these questions so that the overall result will be as representative as possible of the respondent's true opinion. The technical details of these sophisticated scaling methods are beyond the scope of this book. For more information see the recommended reading on page 535.

C2.26 Would you say that job opportunities for women are, in general, better or worse than job opportunities for men with similar education and experience?

Please tick **one** box only	(✓)
Much better for women	1
Better for women	2
No difference	3
Worse for women	4
Much worse for women	5
Can't choose	8

Figure 23.7 An example of a rating scale from a self-completion questionnaire used in the British Social Attitudes Survey of 1994. It is one of a number of questions used by the researchers to explore the beliefs about women's roles and circumstances

C2.01 To begin, we have some questions about women.
Do you agree or disagree ...?
Please tick **one** box on each line

	Strongly agree	**Agree**	**Neither agree nor disagree**	**Disagree**	**Strongly disagree**	**Can't choose**
a. A working mother can establish just as warm and secure a relationship with her children as a mother who does not work	1	2	3	4	5	8
b A pre-school child is likely to suffer if his or her mother works	1	2	3	4	5	8
c All in all, family life suffers when the woman has a full-time job	1	2	3	4	5	8
d A job is all right, but what most women really want is a home and children	1	2	3	4	5	8
e Being a housewife is just as fulfilling as working for pay	1	2	3	4	5	8
f Having a job is the best way for a woman to be an independent person	1	2	3	4	5	8
g Most women have to work these days to support their families	1	2	3	4	5	8

Figure 23.8 An example of a sophisticated approach to scaling, from a self-completion questionnaire used in the British Social Attitudes Survey of 1994. The questions have been carefully developed and tested so that combining a respondent's answers gives a reliable measure of attitude

You could use sets of questions to seek opinion on a topic from different angles. This prevents a small aspect of opinion from giving a distorted impression, which could happen if only one question was asked. For example, a respondent may say that he believes doctors to be very well qualified. He may, nevertheless, not believe their ability to cure him. A grouped set of questions using a scaling method would reveal more accurately his lack of faith in doctors. You could try to design your questions so that different approaches are taken to the same subject. This allows a check on consistency of response, and helps to minimise the effects of badly constructed questions.

Ranking alternatives is another method of recording responses. Respondents are asked to rank a list in order of preference, quality or some other factor. This method has the advantage of making direct comparisons between alternatives. Items must be familiar to respondents, and seen by them to be related. Things that don't seem to fit will lead to confusion.

Items can take a variety of forms. They could be associated with nurses. Here respondents could be asked to rank which qualities they thought most important. Or items could be posts within the caring services, such as doctor or care assistant. Respondents could be asked to rank these in terms of the level of help they offer, or how hard working they seem to be. Ranking allows opinion on a linked group of items to be scaled, and is very useful when comparisons need to be made. (See Figure 23.9.)

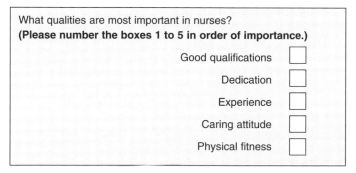

What qualities are most important in nurses?
(Please number the boxes 1 to 5 in order of importance.)

Good qualifications	☐
Dedication	☐
Experience	☐
Caring attitude	☐
Physical fitness	☐

Figure 23.9 An example of a ranking order question

In this discussion we have looked at the styles of question that questionnaires can contain. Another important aspect of question design to be considered is the wording and content.

Try it

Think about an area of attitude or opinion that you need to collect data about. It could relate to any of the research projects you will carry out during your studies where you intend using a self-completion questionnaire or structured interviews.

Try to think of a range of questions which you could ask that approach the attitude from different angles. Examine the list and make sure that there are no repetitions or questions that stray from the point. All the questions in the set need to complement each other. Your question set can use a scale to allow respondents to indicate the strength of their opinion on each question in the set. Pre-coded number values in the scale give numerical scores for strength of opinion on each question. Combining a respondent's scores for the whole question set gives a value for strength of opinion on the issue which can be compared with that of other respondents.

Writing questions

The quality of the questions is one of the most important aspects of survey design. All your careful planning is invalidated if the questions fail to collect the data intended. Sadly, there are no strict rules to follow which will always give good questions. However, there are points to guide you which, together with your judgement, should make the job easier. Knowledge of your population, common sense, and a pilot survey will all help you to write better questions.

One thing to decide is how many questions to include. Too many will exhaust the respondent and the interviewer. Postal questionnaires are likely to suffer from a particularly poor response if they are too long or complicated. On the other hand, too few questions will give very sketchy results. Try to strike a balance by thinking about your respondents. How long would they be prepared to spend on your questionnaire? How long will it take to carry out an interview? Guesswork can give you an idea of the answers, and a pilot survey will help refine them.

Question length is also important. Long questions should be avoided as they are likely to bore and confuse respondents. If you seem to be producing long questions, try to split them into a number of shorter ones. Long questions may occur because you want to set the scene for respondents. You could get around the problem by using a general introduction and then asking several shorter questions around this theme.

Question content is crucial to the survey process. Respondents must be able to give answers to the questions they are asked. Questions about things that respondents have no knowledge of, or no opinion on, will produce worthless results. It is also important that questions are about subjects that respondents are willing to discuss. Even answers to factual questions can be biased by choice of subject. For example, responses to 'How often do you clean your teeth?' are likely to be biased in the direction of respectability. Opinion questions are even more likely to be affected by a respondent's willingness to answer on a particular subject.

Questions need to offer options which cover the full range of possible answers. Fact questions must have an option for every possible member of the population. For instance, if you ask 'How do you travel to college?' your options need to cover all possible modes of transport. You should always add an 'Other…' option though, for those whose response you failed to predict.

Another aspect of option choices is exclusivity. This means that respondents belong exclusively in one category, and are not left confused about which box to tick. The question above may have a problem with exclusivity. What about people who use both bus and train to travel? The need to cover all possible options may lead to a long list being created. In interviews this can lead to respondents forgetting earlier items, and inaccurately picking one they can remember in order to save face. A solution to this is to have a card containing the options which is given to the respondent as the question is read out. This is known as a *prompt card.*

The wording of opinion questions needs to be looked at carefully if bias is to be minimised. Questions must be specific. If you ask 'How would you rate the service in this canteen?' some respondents may have difficulty in answering. They may think that some staff give good service whereas others do not. They may think service is good at lunch times, but poor during morning breaks. A more specific set of questions would get a more accurate, and fuller, response. Wording needs to avoid being vague. Questions like 'Do you use this canteen often?' leave the respondent to decide what often means. The frame of reference of the question must be spelled out in specific terms.

Your questions must not make presumptions about the respondent. For example, if you ask elders 'Do you find it easy to live on a state pension?' you are presuming that they have no other source of income. Answers could often be a guess about how easy

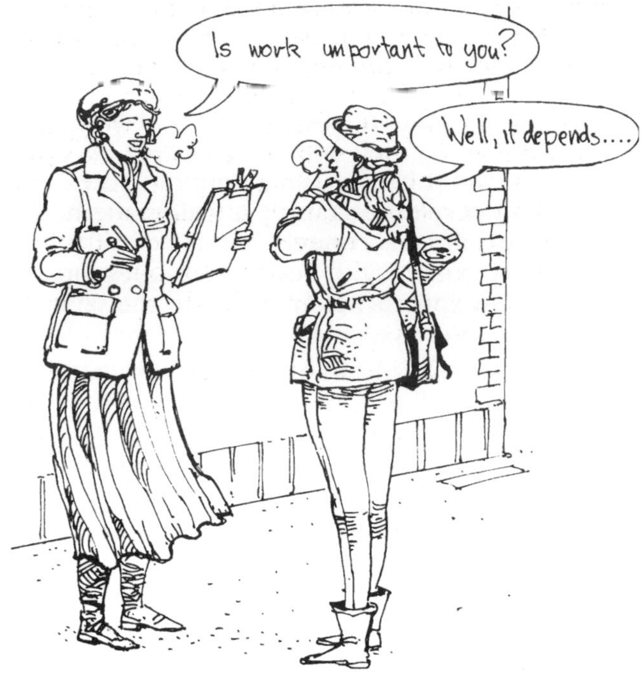

Figure 23.10 Make your questions specific so that subjects can choose an option easily

others may find it. Some respondents may be offended. You can insert factual questions to identify people who fit a certain category, if you need to ask particular questions of them.

Wording needs to be easy for respondents to understand. This means that language should be kept simple and non-technical. Try to avoid using an uncommon word when one or two simple ones would do. For example, use 'end' instead of 'terminate', 'worker' instead of 'practitioner', 'say' instead of 'state', 'need' instead of 'require'. There is nearly always a simpler way of expressing something. Clarity can also be obscured by a confusing use of double negatives. The question 'Do you think that not having enough money never affects people's quality of life?' is fairly difficult to understand. It is easy to reword it so that the double negative doesn't appear.

Wording also needs to be unambiguous. All respondents must understand the question in the same way. For example, the question 'Is work important to you?' is very ambiguous. Does it mean important in financial terms, or is it asking about personal attachment to a job? Is it about paid work, or about work in a more general sense? The same word can mean different things to different people.

Questions must not lead respondents into giving a particular answer. If you ask 'You don't think that the health service is improving, do you?', you are obviously leading the reply. Questions can also lead in more subtle ways. If you ask 'Do you think that social workers should get involved in people's private lives?', you are suggesting that they are being nosey rather than developing caring and supportive involvement. Leading questions can be difficult to spot. Try to examine the wording for signs that a loading, or value, is implied. Ask others how neutral the question sounds.

An important issue in question wording is that respondents don't find questions embarrassing or threatening. This can apply to factual questions, as well as opinion questions. For instance, questions on income may seem threatening, and some respondents may find information on age or disability hard to give.

Opinion questions may be perceived as threatening if they touch on sensitive subjects. One problem is predicting which areas respondents are likely to find sensitive. Once again, a pilot survey with open questions will help. Sometimes threat can be reduced by careful wording, or by projecting the opinion onto someone else. For example, asking retired people 'Do you feel less fulfilled now than when you were working?' is fairly threatening. You could change the question to 'Some people find that they feel less fulfilled during retirement than when they were working. What do you think could cause this feeling?' A follow-up question can ask whether respondents feel themselves to be a part of that group, and the question is now less likely to offend.

An important influence on how people respond to sensitive subjects is the way they are presented in the questionnaire or interview schedule. This brings us on to the issue of *question order, layout* and *presentation.*

Try it

Look at the questions that you have written for a questionnaire you are designing. Use the following checklist to assess the quality of your questions.

- Are there too many, putting respondents off, or too few to get the data you want?
- Will your subjects know the answer?
- Will they be willing to give the answer?
- Are any of the questions long and confusing?
- Do any questions make presumptions about respondents?
- Is each question specific enough to avoid ambiguity?
- Have you used wording that all respondents will understand?
- Are there any leading questions?
- Are any questions threatening or embarrassing?
- Do the options available cover all possible answers?
- Are the options offered mutually exclusive? (i.e. could someone need to choose more than one option?)
- Do some questions need a prompt card?

Use this checklist before finalising your questions, and revise any that fall below standards. *Remember that your research will only be as good as the questions you ask allow it to be.*

Question order

The way you order and present your questions can influence the responses you receive. There are no strict rules on question order, but there are guidelines to help improve the quality of responses in different situations.

Respondents in interview situations must be put at ease early on. This means that opening with a sensitive opinion question is usually a bad idea. Opening with a battery of demographic factual questions can also put respondents in a less co-operative frame of mind. It is generally better to put these items lower down in the schedule. You could start with an open question which introduces the survey topic in a broad, non-threatening way. This should stimulate respondents' interest in the questions that follow, and prepare them for the sorts of answers that may be expected of them.

If quota sampling is being used, it is important to collect some demographic data fairly early on. Interviewers and respondents' time will be wasted if interviews are conducted with people who don't fit the quotas. Usually only a few details are needed to establish whether a person fits a category needed for interview. These can often be found by a combination of observation and a couple of brief introductory questions. It is always a good idea to explain to respondents why you need to ask demographic questions, whenever they appear. This will make your enquiry seem less intrusive, and may help to get more accurate answers.

The order of the bulk of the questions is very much up to the researcher. One common device is to begin with general questions on a topic, then gradually narrow down the field of enquiry. This is intended to focus respondents down onto a topic by taking them

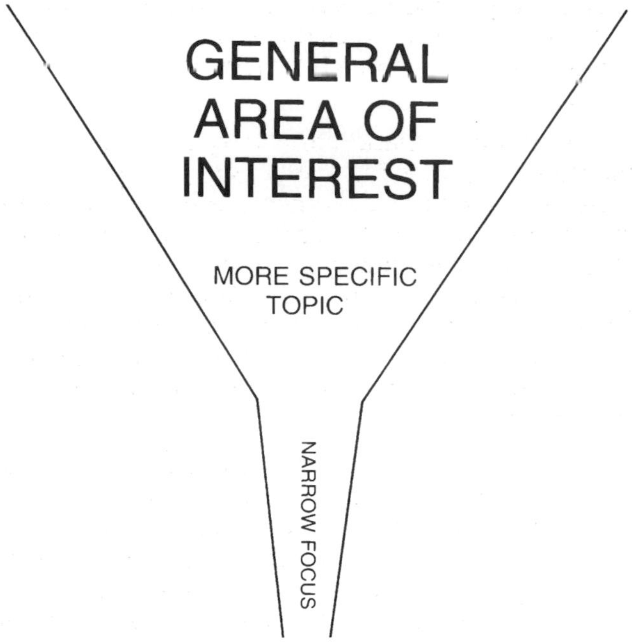

Figure 23.11 The funnel method can bring your questioning to a focus

from the general to the specific. It is sometimes known as the *funnel method* (Figure 23.11). The idea is that respondents are prepared for the specific questions when they arrive because they have been gradually oriented towards them. They may thus be more prepared to divulge sensitive information, or consider threatening topics. Also respondents' answers to later questions may be more accurate because they have had time to think out their opinions.

There is another reason for putting general questions before more specific ones. Answers given to specific questions can bias answers to general questions which follow. People may have strong views on a narrow aspect of a subject. If reminded of these by a specific question they may distort or exaggerate their response to questions about the subject as a whole.

Another point concerning question order is that perfectly good questions can become leading questions if they are badly placed. For instance, suppose you asked a string of questions designed to measure people's views on violence against children. If you followed these with the question 'Do you think that police and social workers should be given more power to deal with violence against children?', it is likely that some respondents will bias their answer because of feelings aroused by the preceding questions. The way to eliminate sources of bias caused by question order is by careful reading through of your questionnaire or interview schedule. A solution tried by some researchers is to randomise the question order for different respondents. However, this is time-consuming and complicated to do. Also, it doesn't attempt to eliminate bias. A randomised question order ensures that bias occurs with some, unidentified, members of the sample.

Try it

When designing your own questionnaire, try to put questions in an order which minimises the problems mentioned above. Look at the questions you intend to ask and order them with the following points in mind.

- Begin with easy questions that help set the context of the research.
- Don't begin with a battery of demographic questions. Sprinkle them around the questionnaire.
- Avoid a question order which may lead respondents' answers.
- Use the funnel method to focus on specific issues.

When you are satisfied with the order of your questions, show the whole questionnaire to other people and get their opinions on the content and order of your questions. Be prepared to make changes if this brings problems to light.

Layout and presentation of self-completion questionnaires

Layout and presentation are particularly important with postal questionnaires. If they are cluttered or confused they will probably end up in the bin. Respondents must find questionnaires clear and easy to follow. They should also find them friendly. Introductions and directions that sound too scientific and formal can put people off.

You should always introduce your survey with an explanation of what the research is about and why you are asking them to respond by questionnaire. Failure to 'sell' your questionnaire at this stage may mean that a respondent never completes it. Keep the introduction short and simple, but try to convince respondents that the questionnaire is worth filling in and returning.

Questions should be clearly separated so that respondents have no difficulty making their way through them. Keep the layout neat and uncluttered to prevent confusion. Respondents must decide where their response to a particular question should be recorded. A clear layout should make it obvious which responses link with which questions.

Make sure that it is also clear how responses to particular questions are to be recorded on the questionnaire. If you use rating scales or ranking techniques you will have to explain how you want respondents to indicate their answers. Keep these explanations simple and brief, but make sure that they give clear and adequate instructions.

When planning the layout of questions and answers in your questionnaire, you should remember that the respondent is not the only person you need to consider. If everything goes according to plan you will be receiving a large number of completed questionnaires, and will need to collate the data from them. If you lay the answers out clearly, it can make this task much easier. *Collating* involves putting answers from different respondents together to build a picture of the overall response. This task is made very much easier by the use of a computer, and Chapter 27 on Information Technology shows you how this can be done. However you collate responses, it is far easier and quicker is you *pre-code* the answers.

Pre-coding means assigning a number or letter to the possible responses for each question. For example you may code gender as simply M or F. Responses to a rating scale question could be coded 1 to 5, or however many are needed to cover all available

C2.32a Thinking about a single mother with a child under school age. Which one of these statements comes closest to your own view?

Please tick **one** box only (✓)

She has a special duty to go out to work to support her child	1
She has a special duty to stay at home to look after her child	2
She should do as she chooses, like everyone else	3
Can't choose	8

Figure 23.12 This example of a pre-coded question is taken from a self-completion questionnaire used in the British Social Attitudes Survey of 1994. Pre-coded responses are easily entered into a computer for data analysis

answers. If pre-coding is not done the reply must be coded when the completed questionnaires are gone through, which is a much longer process. (See Figure 23.12.)

The overall presentation of your questionnaire should be as professional as possible. People perceive professional-looking documents as more important then those which look amateurish. They are more likely to take your survey seriously if the questionnaire looks impressive. Your response rate is likely to be higher which makes the research far more useful. The best way to produce a professional-looking questionnaire is by using Information Technology.

One final point on postal questionnaire design is to remember to add a thank you at the end. Respondents need to feel motivated to return the completed form and a final word may help. You can use the opportunity to remind them why the research is important and increase the likelihood of getting a return. For example, if the survey is about services for the disabled you could end with, 'Thank you for taking the time to fill out this questionnaire. Your answers will greatly help our research into services for disabled people.'

Try it

You will have several opportunities to use self-completion questionnaires for carrying out research during your studies. The quality of your layout can be checked against the following list of recommendations.

- Include a brief, friendly introduction explaining the purpose of the research.
- Use a neat, uncluttered layout.
- Give clear instructions on how questions are to be answered.
- Make routing instructions easy to understand.
- Control the length of answers to open questions by limiting the space provided.
- Pre-code answer options to aid data analysis.
- Use IT resources to produce a professional-looking survey document.
- Always add a thank you at the end, and perhaps a statement encouraging return of the questionnaire.

Check that any self-completion questionnaire you create follows these guidelines. Poor questionnaires may well not be returned.

Designing structured interview schedules

Structured interview schedules don't need such care in presentation as questionnaires, but layout is important if things are to go smoothly. A professional approach can again improve the quality of responses. Professionalism is likely to be judged on how smoothly the interview is conducted, and a well-organised schedule can help with this. Interviewers must be able to keep track of the interview process.

This may be straightforward when questions simply follow one after the other. But often interviews branch into different areas, depending on the responses given to certain questions. If you ask 'Do you smoke cigarettes?', you may have prepared separate sets of supplementary questions to ask smokers and non-smokers. Interview schedules can turn into complicated documents. It may be best to put questions belonging to a particular branch together on a separate sheet of paper. This way you can quickly flip to them, and return to the main run of questions when you have finished. Remember to include guidance notes, even if they are to yourself! It is all too easy to forget where to return to when a branch of questions has been completed.

As with self-completion questionnaires, make sure that answers are clearly linked to questions and are pre-coded. Try to make the schedule as easy to use as possible. Don't forget to allow sufficient space for recording answers to open questions. You could also leave space for your own comments to collect qualitative background data. It is best to use Information Technology resources to design and create your interview schedule. A printed schedule is much easier to follow. You can use effects like *italic* and **bold** to separate clearly interview instructions from things to be read to respondents. The document will be much clearer, and easier to use. (See Figure 23.13.)

B13a) Suppose you had an applicant for a job who you knew was disabled, who showed you an Access To Work card, would this

... **READ OUT** ...

... encourage you,	1	**ASK b)**
or discourage you from employing this person,	2	
or, would it make no difference?	3	**GO TO B14**
(Can't say)	8	

IF ENCOURAGE OR DISCOURAGE

b) Why do you say that?
PROBE FULLY, RECORD VERBATIM

Figure 23.13 A question from a structured interview questionnaire, aimed at employers and used in the evaluation of the Access to Work Scheme in 1995. The interviewer's instructions are in bold capital letters and are easy to follow. The coding and routing instructions are also clear. Note that the follow-up question allows the interviewer freedom to seek full details if people have expressed a definite opinion

Prompts may be used to make respondents aware of the possible answers to a question. The interviewer can read out the options, prompting a respondent to choose one. Sometimes, however, it is useful to write prompts on a card which is handed to the respondent for them to pick an option.

Prompt cards have been discussed in connection with questions with many options, where respondents may have difficulty remembering the list if it was read out. They are also useful where information is sensitive or threatening. For example, questions on income may seem threatening, particularly if asked in a street interview. Respondents can be given a prompt card with income groups listed on it and coded. They only have to answer with a code number which the interviewer notes down. This can seem far less intimidating than saying an income level aloud. Prompt cards are also useful for ranking-type questions. Here respondents need to consider comparisons, and putting all the options in front of them will help you get more accurate results.

Evidence collection point

You will be creating a structured interview schedule to collect data during your GNVQ Health and Social Care studies. When designing the document you should keep the following recommendations in mind:

- Make routing easy to follow so that interviews go smoothly and you don't get lost.
- Leave sufficient space to record answers to open questions.
- Pre-code answer options in fixed response questions.
- Allow space for your own observations and comments.
- Provide yourself with any prompts that you may need.
- Create prompt cards where necessary.

- Use bold or italic highlights to separate clearly questions from interviewer instructions.
- Use IT resources to create a smart, easy-to-use questionnaire.

Try to design a structured interview schedule that meets all these points. Remember that you are going to have to use it in the field. A well-designed document will make the interviews and data analysis far easier to do.

Chapter 24

Producing and presenting research findings

This section is about dealing with research data to produce conclusions, and presenting research to others. It covers:

- **analysing data – qualitative data, quantitative data, statistical analysis, making comparisons, sources of errors**
- **drawing valid conclusions**
- **producing a research report**
- **presenting a research report.**

When you have finished all your interviews, or collected in all your questionnaires, it is time to begin dealing with the data you have collected. You may have gathered data that is quantitative or qualitative using any of the research methods we have discussed. Whatever form your data takes, it needs to be processed before you can analyse what it might mean. You may have gained impressions about your research results as you collected the data, particularly if you used in-depth research methods. To find out whether your impressions are supported by the data, you need to organise it.

Analysing data

Analysing qualitative data

Data that you intend to use towards your research needs to be relevant to the research question. With quantitative data collection methods, you can make sure that this is the only data collected. Your questionnaire should aim to collect no more information than you need. With qualitative data collection methods, however, the researcher has less control over the data coming in. This is particularly true of in-depth interview methods where respondents may have ranged into areas which are of great interest, but have nothing to do with your research question.

Interviews are frequently taped, and professional researchers may have them transcribed into print so that they are easier to examine and analyse. You will probably have to compromise and listen carefully through the tape yourself, pausing it and noting down passages that seem most useful to you. Your interview notes should help you with this, especially if you noted the time or tape counter number when interesting things came up.

Although you don't need to make a verbatim (word-for-word) transcript, you will need to make sufficient notes so that you can analyse them further. You will also need to record verbatim any responses that could be quoted in your research report. It is a good idea to take down several quotes for each respondent, possibly covering different aspects of the issue. This will give you some choice later when you are more sure of what you need to use to illustrate your conclusions.

Further analysis of qualitative data from in-depth interviews requires imagination and sensitivity to the meanings your respondents were expressing. You should sum up respondents' comments and opinions in a way that conveys accurately what they really think. Quotes used should clarify and establish your description of a respondent's views. At the same time, you must relate these views to the research question, and to comments made by other respondents. You can use quotes to illustrate points of agreement, or otherwise.

Your analysis may seem to be more like reporting, but if you keep referring back to the relevance of the data to the research question a meaningful picture should emerge. You may find patterns which suggest further study. For instance, your subjects might have expressed similar views on a health and social care service that they all use. The conclusions that you draw will inevitably be difficult to generalise, but you should be able to claim that you have given a very accurate picture of your respondents' views.

Evidence collection point

You will collect qualitative information of this type during some of the research work that you do during your GNVQ Health and Social Care studies. Your analysis of this data will provide evidence towards Element 8.3.

Use the methods described, and do your best to express respondents' views clearly and accurately. Remember to limit your expectations of the data in terms of generalising the results.

Qualitative data may also have come from semi-structured interviews, or open questions in a structured interview or self-completion questionnaire. Here, responses are more controlled since the space for a response is limited and context is set by the surrounding questions. Subjects may still drift away from the point though, and you need to assess all qualitative data in terms of its relevance to the research questions.

Short pieces of qualitative data gathered using these more controlled methods should be easy to deal with. Semi-structured questionnaires may allow about one side of a sheet of paper for each answer. Respondents may be aware of this and keep to the point. Also the interviewer controls what is noted down. It is usually good practice to try to record comments verbatim, since judgements about data should not be made in the heat of an interview. In practice you may find it hard to keep up with your subject and end up making decisions about what to jot down. This means that some, hopefully unneeded, data will be pruned out.

With fairly brief answers you can read through them and strike out any information that is irrelevant to the question. This leaves you short pieces of useful qualitative data. You can use a similar approach to editing open questions in questionnaires, and here again short answers should minimise irrelevant data. Often open questions are seeking reasons for opinion expressed in a previous fixed response question so answers should be fairly specific and relevant.

Try it

Look at data you have gathered by using short-answer open-question methods. Think about the question at issue and try to decide on the relevance of the data you have collected. Delete any items that go off the point and are irrelevant to the research question.

With data from semi-structured interviews and open questions you can take a structured approach to data analysis. Here, you may expect respondents' answers to cover broadly similar points. If the questions asked were direct enough you should find that a range of possible answers emerges for a particular question. You can code the answers to get a much clearer view of the patterns in your subjects' responses.

Coding the results of open questions means drawing up a **coding frame** for the question. This is simply a list of all possible answers, with each one given a code. The difficulty is that each respondent's answer has to be read and judged to decide which code to apply. This process can introduce errors. Respondents will have expressed themselves in different ways, and you must use your judgement as to whether one answer means the same as another. The range of answers in your coding frame may not cover all the responses you get. You need either to extend the range of the coding frame, i.e. add extra answers, or try to fit an answer into an existing slot.

In practice, it is unlikely that all answers can be neatly pigeon-holed, and there is a practical limit to the length a coding frame can be allowed. A certain amount of approximation is likely to occur. The important thing is not to claim scientific accuracy for data that has been coded in this way. So long as you are honest about potential errors, the procedure is perfectly valid. The results of your analysis can be examined statistically, and displayed on graphs or charts, using the methods outlined later in this chapter.

Evidence collection point

You will need to draw up and use a coding frame to analyse the responses to open questions that you have received. Your application of this method may be used as evidence of data analysis and contribute to Element 8.3.

Draw up a coding frame for each open question. You could begin by listing the answers that you can predict, or remember respondents giving. Now go through each subject's responses and attempt to allocate them to appropriate answer options. Be prepared to add extra options if necessary. Take care to code answers as accurately as possible.

Analysing quantitative data

The analysis of quantitative data may initially seem to be more an arithmetic process than a creative one. You will be expecting this sort of data to demonstrate patterns or relationships numerically, and this means beginning to count and total the answers you have received. It is possible to do this using pen and paper, and until quite recently this was the only way. Nowadays, however, most researchers will use a computer to help with data analysis, You are expected to use information technology in your

GNVQ studies and research is a good opportunity to do so. Chapter 27 will describe how you can use a computer to deal with your results.

Whether you use IT or paper, the process of analysis begins with looking at each questionnaire form and listing the answers given for each question. You can summarise each respondent's answers into a list of codes. Hopefully, you will have been wise enough to pre-code each answer as you go. Any open questions will need a coding frame so that you can assess and code respondents' answers.

As an example of summarising responses, let us look at a fictitious questionnaire containing ten fixed-response questions. Two demographic questions asked for gender, coded 1 or 2; and age, recorded in age bands coded 1, 2 and 3. The other eight questions had five coded fixed-responses each, with an extra code for 'don't know'. Thus answers to these will be recorded as a code number from 1 to 6. Figure 24.1 shows how the answers from three respondents have been summed up as rows of codes. The same principles are used in computer-based analysis, and this method makes it much easier to quantify totals and relationships.

	Question number									
	1	2	3	4	5	6	7	8	9	10
Respondent 1	1	2	1	4	3	4	5	6	1	2
Respondent 2	2	3	3	5	6	3	1	2	1	4
Respondent 3	1	2	4	2	4	1	6	5	2	4

Figure 24.1 An example of a table of coded results

When all the data has been taken from the questionnaires, you can start to examine it. A good starting point is to look at the total responses for questions which are demographic or factual. How many men and women responded? What are the proportions of respondents in different age groups? These figures give a profile of the people who responded. They allow you to check whether your respondents were a representative sample of the population. Remember that even if your original sample was representative, the group who actually responded from that sample may not be. Or course, if quota sampling was used you should already know the proportions of different people amongst your respondents.

The other set of totals you need are those for opinion questions. These will reveal how many people gave particular answers for each question. You can record numbers of people giving each answer and build up a picture of the way opinions differ within your sample. These totals, along with demographic totals, can be presented as tables. They can also be presented in graphical form as graphs or charts. Chapter 26 deals with presenting data in these ways. You may also be able to use IT methods to create graphs and charts (see Chapter 27).

Evidence collection point

You will need to deal with quantitative data collected by your research work during your GNVQ Health and Social Care studies. This aspect of your data analysis can contribute to the evidence needed for Element 8.3.

You are strongly advised to use IT methods to help you process quantitative data. Enter the data from each respondent into suitable software and obtain totals for demographic data items.

Although these totals are useful, the point of social research is usually to identify links between items of data. Your research question may indicate a need to do this. For example, suppose your hypothesis is 'Female students are more aware than male students of the risks of smoking'. To test the hypothesis, you will need to link answers indicating awareness of the risks of smoking with the gender of respondents. The term used for linking responses in this way is **correlation**. In this example, we are looking for a possible correlation between gender and smoking awareness. There are sophisticated statistical methods that can be used to give precise mathematical measures of correlation and significance. These methods are beyond the scope of this book, but you can perform simple **statistical analysis** on your data to help you understand it better.

Statistical analysis

Frequency distribution

When you have totalled the responses received, you can begin a more detailed examination of your results. A good starting point for a closer examination of data is to draw up a *frequency distribution diagram* for the answers to each question. This is a graph which shows how often each answer has been reported. As an example, suppose we had asked the question 'Do you think that the caring

Response		Number of answers
1	Strongly agree	2
2		4
3		6
4		9
5	Neutral	10
6		8
7		6
8		4
9	Strongly disagree	1
Total responses		50

Figure 24.2 A table showing responses to the question 'Do you think that the caring services do a good job?'

services do a good job?' We have allowed respondents to select an answer from a nine-point scale ranging from 'Strongly agree' to 'Strongly disagree'. Our scale is coded from 1 (Strongly agree), to 9 (Strongly disagree). We have received 50 answers from our sample and the results as shown in Figure 24.2.

A frequency distribution diagram for these responses is shown in Figure 24.3.

The data gives a roughly curved shape with a peak near the middle value, which indicated a neutral opinion on the question. The number of answers tapers off towards each end of the diagram,

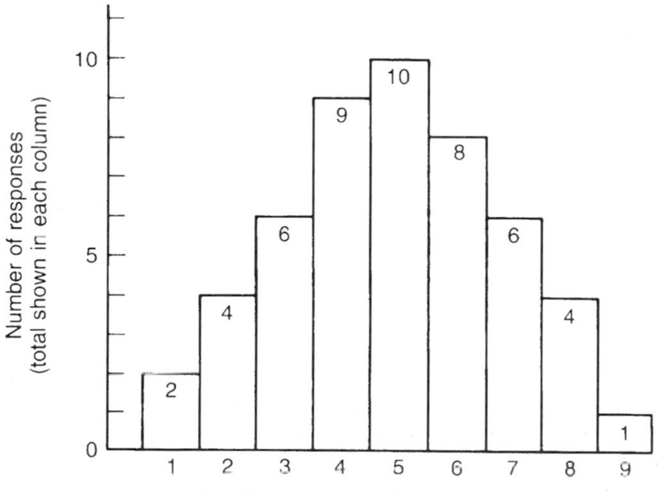

Figure 24.3 A frequency distribution diagram for responses to the question 'Do you think that the caring services do a good job?'

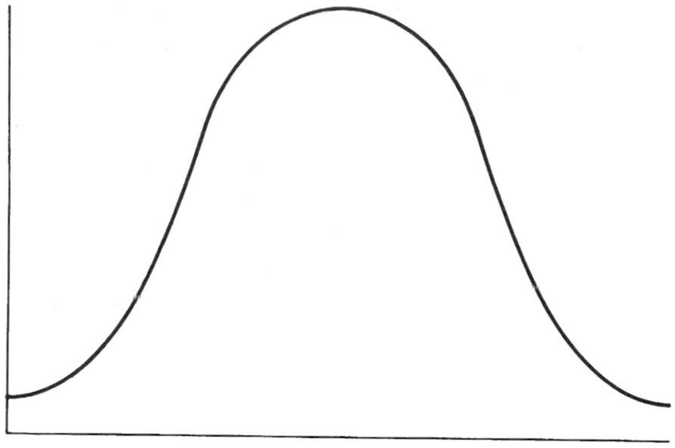

Figure 24.4 A normal distribution curve

indicating that extreme views are far less widely held. The shape of the diagram in our example is a familiar one in statistics. For many types of data a frequency distribution diagram will resemble a bell-shaped curve, referred to as a **normal distribution curve** (see Figure 24.4).

All kinds of data give approximations to a normal distribution when plotted on a frequency distribution diagram. Things like shoe sizes, income or opinion, tend to follow the basic pattern. Most cases fall near the middle, and the numbers tail off towards the extremes. It is so common that researchers are alerted when a distribution fails to approximate to the normal curve.

The normal distribution curve has some very useful mathematical characteristics which can make data analysis easy and precise. These mathematical techniques are really a way of expressing

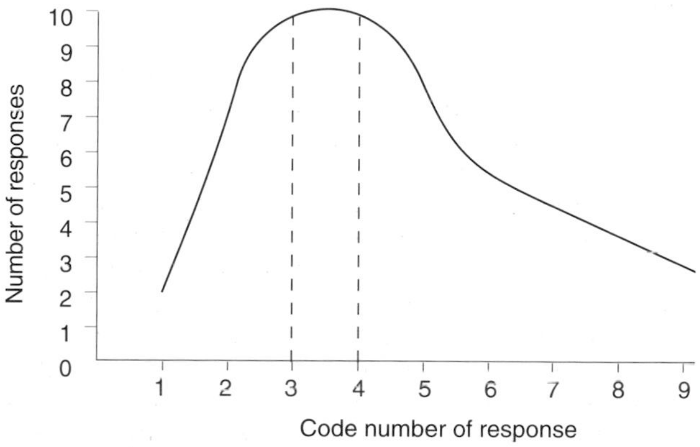

Figure 24.5 A possible alternative frequency distribution curve for responses to the question 'Do you think that the caring services do a good job?'

quantitatively the messages that lie within the shape of the distribution curve for a particular set of data. For instance, look again at the fictitious distribution of opinions on the caring services. The data could have been very different and we might have found that the distribution curve looked more like that in Figure 24.5.

In Figure 24.5 the peak is over to the left of the neutral position. This indicates that opinion is clustered towards the 'satisfied' end of our response scale, which may be seen as an important finding. Other statistical measures can help us clarify these implications.

Mean values

One commonly used statistic is the **mean value** – the average of a set of data. Methods for calculating the mean value are described in Chapter 26. The mean gives the point around which the data is clustered and can be marked on your frequency distribution diagram. In our example, the numbers 1 to 9 indicate the strength of respondents' opinions. Our first distribution curve (Figure 24.4) showed responses seeming to cluster around the neutral central position. The mean of this data is 4.94, which is very close to the neutral value of 5, and confirms our interpretation of the distribution curve.

In our second example (Figure 24.5), however, the curve was skewed over to the left-hand side. Calculation of the mean here would confirm our understanding of this distortion. Now the mean is likely to be somewhere between 3 and 4, indicating that people are inclined to agree that the caring services are indeed doing a good job. You have statistically identified the levels of satisfaction within your population.

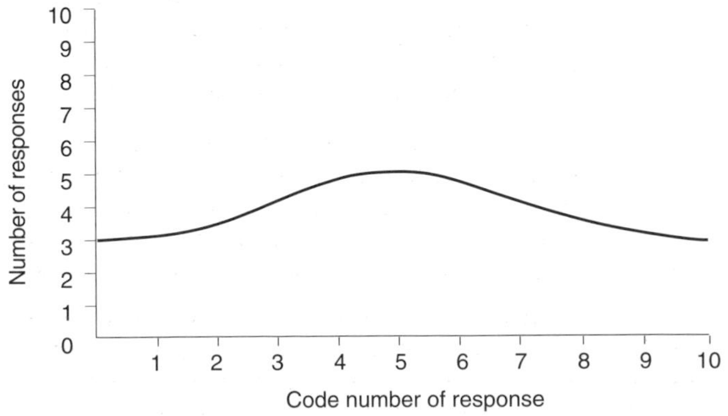

Figure 24.6 A distribution curve showing a spread of opinion

However, the mean value is not always so useful. Look at the distribution curve in Figure 24.6. Here the curve is much flatter which indicates that opinion is much more evenly spread across the range of possible views. It is easy to see that there is much less agreement in the sample on the question at issue. However, the mean value of the data could still be around 5, indicating neutral feelings. *The mean shows only part of the picture.* The shape of the distribution curve shows how people have deviated from the mean value. It gives a graphic view of the **variability**, or spread, of the results. You can see how much people's responses seem to have deviated from the mean. To get even more precision into your analysis you can use statistical methods to measure and quantify this deviation.

Standard deviation

If data is normally distributed, or at least approximately so, variability can be shown by calculating the **standard deviation** of the data. This is a way of showing how much the data varies from the mean. The size of the standard deviation indicates how spread out opinion on an issue really is.

To calculate standard deviation you need to measure the distance between each response and the mean value. Some data is higher than the mean and so gives a positive number. Other data is below the mean and so has a negative one. If you add all the deviations together, the result should be zero, since this is how the mean is defined. To get positive numbers to work on, the deviations from the mean are squared, and these squares are then added together. This total is known, logically, as the sum of the squares. You are trying to find the average deviation from the mean, so now you need to divide the sum of the squares by the number of data items. This gives the mean of the squares, also known as the **variance**. The standard deviation is the square root of the variance.

The calculations are not particularly difficult and can be made even easier if a computer is used. The point of finding the standard deviation is that you can now exploit some of the useful properties of the normal distribution curve. Fixed proportions of the curve fall within standard deviations from the mean. For example 68.27 per cent of all responses fall within one standard deviation either side of the mean. Figure 24.7 shows the proportions of the curve that lie within standard deviations from the mean.

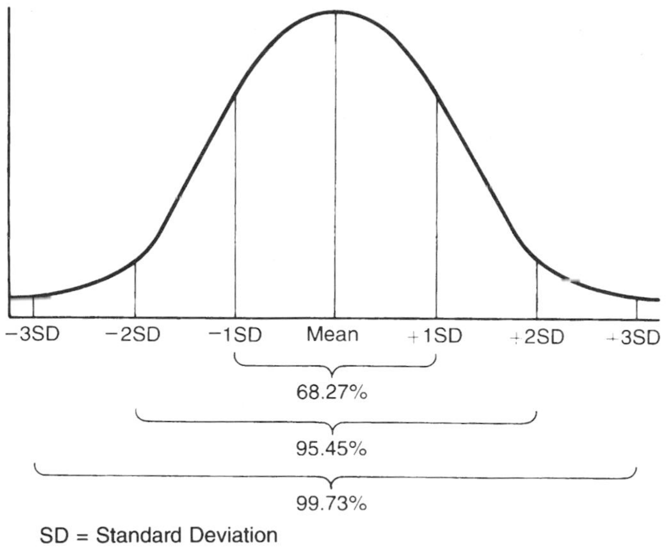

Figure 24.7 Percentage proportions of a normal curve between standard deviations

Standard deviation is often used to express probabilities associated with the data. You could say that there is a 68.27 per cent chance that an answer will lie within one standard deviation of the mean. There is a better than 99 per cent chance that an answer will lie within three standard deviations of the mean. To put it another way, you can say that there is a 68 per cent probability that an answer lies within one standard deviation from the mean, and a 99 per cent probability that it lies within three. Expressing your results in this way gives a statistical probability that future results will have a particular value. You have quantified your predictions based on statistical analysis of your data.

Mode and median

Calculations of mean and standard deviation may not be necessary, or possible, for all your data. If you have asked people to state their religion then the responses are not a measure of quantity or degree. Here it is more useful to take the **mode** – the most frequently occurring response.

Another statistic which is sometimes used is the **median**. This is the value which divides respondents so that an equal number lie above and below it. The median takes no account of the strengths of individual responses.

Evidence collection point

You should use statistical techniques to analyse the quantitative data that you have collected during your research. Your work can be used as evidence towards Element 8.3.

Try drawing up frequency distribution tables for questions with a scaled range of responses. Calculate the mean value of the data. What conclusions can you draw from this analysis? How do they relate to the research question? If possible, find the standard deviation for the responses to important questions. This is easy to do if you are using a computer to process the data, but don't go out of your depth mathematically if you are unsure about the method.

If necessary, find the median or mode of the data. The statistical measures you use must be appropriate for the data being analysed.

Making comparisons

The point of statistical analysis is usually to compare results from different questions and draw conclusions based on this. Comparison of means and standard deviations can show up differences in opinion between different sections of the population. For example, results of a question on income may indicate that females have lower values for mean and standard deviation than males. This shows that on average women's pay was found to be lower than men's. It also implies that variability is higher amongst men, i.e. that women's income is more tightly clustered around the mean, whereas men's is more spread out across different income levels.

Another way of analysing data is to look for relationships between two variables. Suppose you are interested in the relationship between age and opinions on the quality of the health and caring services. If you plot a graph of age against opinion you could get results like those in Figure 24.8.

Each dot in Figure 24.8 represents the age and opinion of an individual respondent. The graph is known as a **scattergram**, and more details can be found in Chapter 26. Here, there seems to be a clear trend for opinions to become lower as age increases.

A **line of best fit** would make the relationship more specific. The relationship between the two variables is called **correlation**. If correlation was perfect all the points would lie on a straight line. There are mathematical techniques for finding the line of best fit exactly, and for expressing the degree of

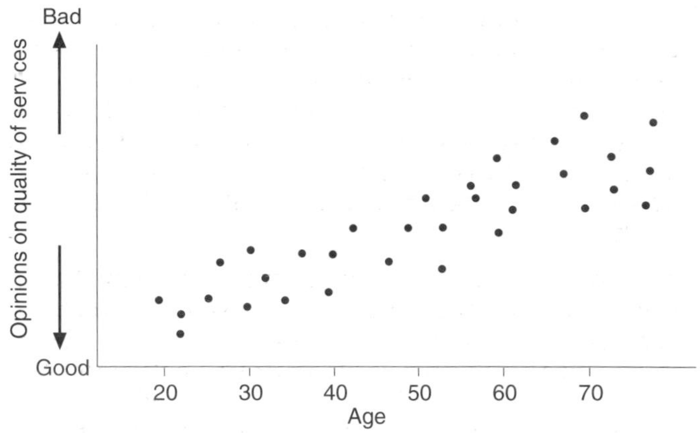

Figure 24.8 A scattergram of age against opinion of the quality of health and social care services

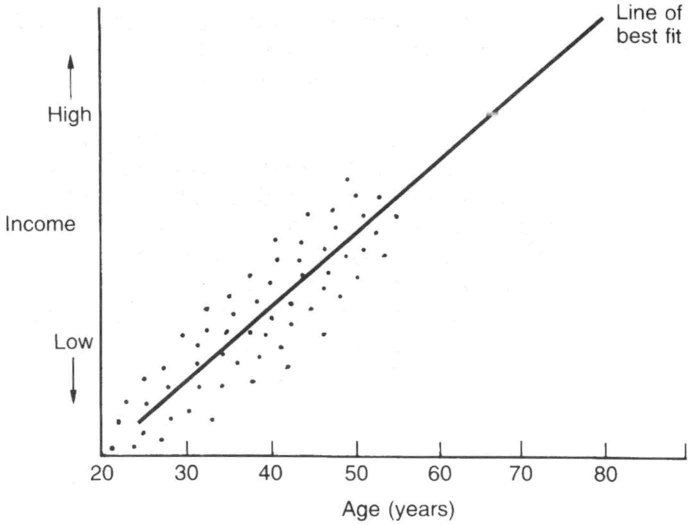

Figure 24.9 A scattergram of age against income showing the dangers of extrapolation

correlation shown by the data. These lie outside the scope of this book, but more information can be found in the recommended reading on page 535. Often a correlation is fairly easy to spot. If your scattergram shows a random pattern of dots, however, it implies that there is no relationship between the variables you have chosen to plot.

You may wish to compare different combinations of statistics in this way to check how groups in the population differ. Ideally you should have predicted which comparisons are relevant to the subject of your research. If you are researching with an hypothesis in mind then comparisons need to be related to it.

Sources of error

Beware – statistical analysis of your results can lead to errors and distortions. It is always possible that you have carried out the calculations incorrectly, though if you use a computer this risk is reduced. A more likely source of error is the way the statistics have been used.

One problem is misreading correlations between items of data. Correlations are often easy to identify, but difficult to explain or account for. You may find that a correlation seems to exist between two variables and wrongly assume that one is the cause of the other. There could be a third factor which is the cause of both effects. For example, there is a correlation between the number of leaves on oak trees and the amount of clothing people wear. This is not because oak leaves themselves bring about the wearing of light clothing, but because oaks bear their leaves during summer when the weather is warmer.

Another source of error when using statistics is **extrapolation.** This means extending your results beyond the range of your data, and attempting to predict what values a variable would have in extreme circumstances. The dangers of this can be shown by the scattergram in Figure 24.9.

In Figure 24.9 the relationship between age and income has been plotted for people between the ages of 25 and 60. If the line of best fit is extended beyond the range of the data it seems that most people are on a very high income indeed by the time they reach 80 years of age. In fact, we know that this is not the case, and income usually drops off sharply after retirement. Extrapolation is a very hazardous process. You should check your ideas carefully against other data, and in the light of common sense.

Errors can occur in the collection method. Was the method right for the population you are concerned with? Was it able to collect the data that you wanted? If you used a postal questionnaire, the number of responses you received is a good measure of the suitability of the method. A low response is a major source of error and should be indicated in your report. If structured interviews were used, a likely source of error is interviewer–respondent interaction. These are very hard to estimate, but you should be able to remember how the interviews went. If respondents proved uncooperative, or you needed to use probes not written into the schedule, then it is likely that significant bias has occurred.

The collection tools themselves may have introduced errors. This may be shown by returned questionnaires that have obviously been misunderstood. Or your interviewing experiences may have revealed that certain questions simply didn't work, needing many probes to get the desired answer. Non-returned questionnaires can leave you guessing at the source of the problem. Was a questionnaire using the wrong approach, or were some of the questions too intrusive or confusing? Whatever the reason, non-returns represent a source of error in the results. Problems with interview schedules will be only too familiar to you by the time you have finished the fieldwork.

Errors can also occur through the sampling process. There are ways of estimating errors when random sampling methods are used, though it is probably not worth calculating them for your research. For small samples such estimates are meaningless – as small samples are always prone to errors because they are not fully representative of the population. Representativeness can be checked by looking at the demographic balance among your respondents. Proportions of people within your sample should be available from your results, and can be compared with the profile a representative sample should have. Sometimes a sampling method is thrust upon you because no other is available. You need to consider how errors might have occurred through the method you ended up using.

Evidence collection point

You need to look for relevant connections and correlations in quantitative data that you are analysing. Your analysis could contribute to the evidence needed for Element 8.3.

You could draw up scattergrams, if appropriate, or compare response patterns from different groups in the population using frequency diagrams and statistics drawn from them.

Be careful not to make inappropriate correlations, or extrapolate your results beyond their capabilities. Also make sure that all the analysis you do is aimed at the research question.

Drawing valid conclusions

Analysis of your quantitative and qualitative data will help you to interpret what you have found out. The point of collecting and analysing data is to draw conclusions about the research question you began with. Now you need to consider the implications of your results for that question. It may be that all the results seem to agree and you feel fairly confident about declaring what your research has shown. More often, however, you will find that some results indicate one thing while other results indicate another.

Perhaps one section of your population seems to have different opinions from the rest, or people's feelings about different aspects of an issue are varied so that clear conclusions are hard to state. Don't feel that your results should always lead to definite conclusions. You must be prepared to conclude that the results don't allow you to give a clear answer to your research question, if this is what your data analysis indicates. The point is to make sure that *the conclusions you do draw are supported by the data you have collected.* The conclusion that further research is needed is a perfectly valid outcome.

The conclusions must also be clearly directed at the research question, and the purpose of the research. You may feel that your results allow you to draw conclusions about other things that lie outside the scope of your question. These findings can appear in your report, with suggestions that further research should be done. But remember that the main point of the report is to outline the relationship of your results to the research question, and the conclusions you are able to draw about it.

Another point to consider is how confident you can be that your conclusions are accurate. Being honest about sources of error has been stressed in relation to all the aspects of the research process that we have looked at. Making valid claims for your data means being realistic about sources of error that may have occurred.

However, you don't need to write your report as a catalogue of disaster! All you need to do is briefly state the error factors that you are aware of, and estimate the possible effects of these factors on the conclusions you are able to draw. You need to state the confidence limits that surround your conclusions. In fact, few social researchers ever suggest that they are completely confident about the conclusions they have come to. They are aware of the many factors that can influence their results.

Evidence collection point

You need to draw up conclusions from your analysis and relate them to the research question. These conclusions form part of the evidence needed for Element 8.3.

Make sure that your conclusions are based on the data that you have collected, and that they relate to the research question. Try to gauge the effects of errors that may have occurred, and be honest about them. Decide how the errors you have identified limit the quality of the results. Can you set confidence limits for your findings?

Producing a research report

The research report is the culmination of all your hard work. It is worth spending time to make the report as thorough and professional as possible or the care you took during planning, data collection and analysis will have been wasted. It is on the research report that the quality of your work will be judged by others.

The report is to some extent a catalogue of the research process.

- Begin with a statement of the research question and the rationale for conducting research upon it. This will be easy to state as you should have been aware of it from the start.
- Deal briefly with your choice of research method. This means referring to the factors that influenced your decision, such as population characteristics and the nature of the research question.
- Describe the sampling method you used in the same way.
- Outline how you implemented your data collection. This doesn't have to be a very full account of your experiences, but should explain the procedures you followed, and the research tools you created and employed. Always attach a copy of your questionnaire to the report as an appendix. It will help readers to understand what you have done, and it is good scientific practice to be as open as possible about the tools used in research work. Also include any comments you may have about possible sources of error that occurred in the data collection stage. This could form a brief 'how it went' section after your account of the procedures used.
- Explain how you analysed the data. This is also part of the research method and important in establishing the credibility of your conclusions.
- Present your data, and the conclusions you draw from it. The way you do this depends on the research question and the data you wish to present. Qualitative data from in-depth interviews may be presented entirely in written form. You need to explain the threads that ran through the interview and relate them to the research question. Attempt to sum up your respondents' views, and include quotes from them which illustrate the points that you are making. Provided that you keep to the point of the research question, you have a lot of freedom in how you report this sort of data.
  Quantitative data is usually easier to understand when presented in the form of charts and graphs. Using IT methods you can quickly produce good-looking graphics to display your results. Of course, displaying your data is only part of the story. Your report must explain what the data shows, and what conclusions you have come to in your examination of it. Here you are summarising the thinking that led you to your research conclusions, so it is important to be convincing. If you really believe that the data analysis has implied a particular conclusion then you must explain why this is so. Use charts and graphs to help you to make this point, but they are not an end in themselves.
- Write a summary of your conclusions in relation to the research question. You should also outline the **recommendations** that your conclusions lead you to make. These may concern a need for further research work that is indicated by your findings. They may be recommendations for practical action to deal with problems in the situation you have been looking at. Whatever form they take, your recommendations must be clearly linked to the conclusions your research has come to. Finally consider how far your findings may be able to be generalised and applied to other people and situations. Remember to be honest about the limitations of the methods you have used, and the errors that might limit the broader applicability of your results.
- Include a list of the references that you have consulted. This can appear as an appendix, along with a copy of your survey instrument, your covering letter if you used one, and any other research tools that you employed. The appendix can contain any documents that give background information about your research, but are not directly relevant to the main thrust of your report.

Your report should also include an account of the **ethical issues** that arose during your research. How you structure this is up to you. You could identify each issue in the part of your report which covers the stage where it occurred. Alternatively, you could have a section of the report devoted to ethical issues which discusses them in relation to the research project as a whole. However you deal with it, you must identify the issues and explain how you dealt with them.

Use IT resources to produce your research report. Chapter 27 will help you to do this. Make sure that the language you use and the style of the report are at an appropriate level for your target audience.

Evidence collection point

All the research work you do during your studies will need to be reported on. These reports are important evidence towards Element 8.3.

Write reports following the guidelines above. Use IT resources to make each report easy to read and as professional-looking as possible. Make sure that you include all the necessary content, and that it covers each part of the research process. Remember to keep the research question in mind and don't report on things that fall outside its scope.

Presenting a research report

Presenting a research report is rather different from writing one. It is not just a matter of reading your written report aloud. You need to tailor your message to the medium and present the information in a way that is appropriate to your audience and the research itself.

You need, above all, to *plan* what you are going to do. Find out where the presentation will take place and what resources you will have access to. Will you be able to use equipment such as an overhead projector? Find out who the audience will be. This will influence the style and content of your delivery. Now plan how you will outline your research.

The structure can follow the same basic pattern as that used in the written report. You need to cover planning, data collection, data analysis, conclusions and recommendations, and ethical issues. It is best to work from notes rather than trying to write out what you intend to say word for word. Reading extensive passages in a presentation is often difficult, and is inclined to bore the audience. If you glance at your notes and then put it into your own words you will find that you put much more life into the subject. An exception to this rule is the quotation of comments from respondents which are included as useful qualitative data. As with written reports, these will help to make your point, but should be used only when they really do so.

Use an overhead projector (OHP), if available, to display results as tables, charts or graphs. Try to get some practice if you've never used an OHP before, and make sure that your transparencies are readable from where your audience will sit. Tiny, blurred images will not improve the quality of your presentation. You can also use OHP transparencies to list important points during your delivery. Some people like to cover up the transparency on the OHP machine and reveal each point in their presentation as they come to it. This lets the audience see memorably how your argument has progressed, and it has the added advantage of acting as notes for the speaker.

Don't go to the extreme of putting all you intend to say on transparencies and reading them off. This is as unimpressive as simply reading out the written report. If no OHP is available, you will have to find some other way of showing graphical evidence to your audience. You could make large copies of the charts and graphs for display on a suitable surface. Alternatively, you could make smaller copies and hand them to each member of the audience. One final point on OHPs is that they can be very noisy. Try to remember to switch it off when a display is no longer needed.

An important part of the presentation is the question-and-answer session that follows your delivery. Don't be too frightened by this, By the time you come to present your findings, you will be pretty familiar with the research question and the issues it raises. You will find that you are able to deal with questions on the methods used, and your findings, if you have carried out your research in a thorough, scientific way. In fact, you may have become quite passionate about your research findings and will welcome the opportunity to explain them in detail.

Evidence collection point

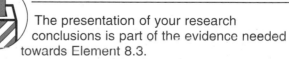

The presentation of your research conclusions is part of the evidence needed towards Element 8.3.

Follow the guidelines above for preparing and delivering your presentation. You might like to make a video recording of the presentation to submit as evidence towards this element.

Self-assessment test

1 Which of the following is the best description of research?
  a Collecting data by carrying out interviews.
  b Looking at books written by other people.
  c Any process which aims to find things out in an organised, systematic and scientific way.
  d Sending out questionnaires by post.

2 Research is sometimes used to attempt to disprove propositions. A proposition is:
  a A statement that is obviously untrue.
  b A theory.
  c A statement that is obviously true.
  d A statement that is framed as though it describes a situation accurately.

3 A local health centre carries out a small research project to find out clients' views on a new appointments system. Which of the following statements best describes the role of the research?
  a To assess the effectiveness of policies and practices.
  b To disprove a proposition.
  c To advance human knowledge and understanding.
  d To save the health centre money.

4 The information that is collected during the research process is known as:
  a Knowledge.
  b Opinions.
  c Data.
  d Statistics.

5 In-depth interviews collect mainly qualitative data. Which of the following statements best describes qualitative data?
  a Information about people's views and circumstances which is expressed verbally.
  b Statistical data.
  c Information about people's views and circumstances which is expressed numerically.
  d Information which can be displayed easily using charts or graphs.

6 Quantitative data is often collected using questionnaire methods. Though it is widely used there are drawbacks to relying on quantitative data in social research. Which of the following is a limitation of quantitative date?
  a Results cannot be displayed graphically.
  b Does not allow comparisons between respondents' answers to be made readily.
  c Answers given may not reflect the thinking behind a respondent's views.
  d Data cannot be analysed statistically.

7 Researchers often collect primary data. Primary data is:
  a Data that is found in official publications.
  b Data that you collect for yourself.
  c Data that is published in newspapers and journals.
  d Data that is found in libraries.

8 Carrying out secondary research is a useful starting point for any project. Which of the following statements offers accurate advice for secondary researchers?
  a Official statistics can always be relied on to clearly represent the true picture.
  b The original works of social researchers are usually quick to read and easy to understand.
  c Newspapers always publish accurate and unbiased statistics.
  d Secondary sources should always be assessed in terms of the quality of the research behind them.

9 In research the word population is used to describe:
  a The whole group of people that a research project applies to.
  b The people who respond to a questionnaire.
  c The group of people who researchers choose to interview.
  d The people who live in Great Britain.

10 Experiments are sometimes used as a research method. Which of the following is an advantage of using the experimental method in social research?
  a People can be studied in their natural environment.
  b There is little chance of the experimental situation influencing people's behaviour.
  c The experiment can be set up to test a particular hypothesis.
  d People's views and outlooks can be probed deeply.

11 Postal self-completion questions are often used as part of a research project. Which of the following is an advantage of this method?
  a Can allow data to be collected from people who are too far away to be interviewed.
  b Always tends to get a good response rate.
  c Allows the collection of valuable background data.

d Avoids the danger that respondents may misunderstand the questions.

12 Structured interviews are intended to be carried out in a similar way with each individual respondent. Which of the following is a reason for this?
- **a** It saves interviewers spending too much time with one person.
- **b** It helps to minimise the influence of the interviewer over the answers given.
- **c** It makes it easier for the results to be analysed.
- **d** It helps to make respondents believe that they are part of a scientific research project.

13 In-depth interviews are sometimes used to collect data. Which of the following is an advantage of using this method?
- **a** Gives a large amount of data which can be analysed statistically.
- **b** Data can be quickly collected from a large sample of people.
- **c** It is easy to make comparisons between the views of different subjects.
- **d** May give an extremely authentic representation of people's views.

14 Semi-structured interviews use a series of open questions to collect information from respondents. Which of the following is an advantage of this method?
- **a** Mainly quantitative data is collected.
- **b** People have a chance to explain their answers in detail.
- **c** It is easy to analyse answers statistically.
- **d** Respondents are free to bring any areas that they wish into the discussion.

15 Some research methods, such as structured interviewing, are designed to achieve reliability. Which of the following describes what is meant by reliability?
- **a** Repeat runs of the research produce similar results.
- **b** Results accurately describe people's real views.
- **c** Results are reported honestly by researchers.
- **d** Findings relate directly to social theories.

16 Direct observation is often used as a research method. Which of the following is an advantage of this method?
- **a** Accurate data on people's opinions can be collected.
- **b** Researchers have a lot of control over the research situation.
- **c** People's authentic behaviour can be detected.
- **d** Ethical issues seldom present problems.

17 Participant observation has been used as a method in some classic social research studies. Which of the following is an advantage of this method?
- **a** Requires little skill on the part of the researcher.
- **b** A quick method to carry out.
- **c** Allows the collection of accurate and deep data about group behaviour.
- **d** Results have a direct relevance for social policy development.

18 An interviewer tries to persuade a reluctant person to respond by claiming that the research is much more important than it actually is. Which of the following is the main problem with the interviewer's behaviour?
- **a** It could bias the answers given by the respondent.
- **b** It is unethical to lie about the research to respondents.
- **c** It could make the respondent nervous.
- **d** It might not work.

19 There are many factors that can cause problems for researchers. Which of the following statements describes a potential ethical problem?
- **a** The cultural background of the researcher is different from that of the subjects.
- **b** It is hard to choose a random sample of the population.
- **c** Only quantitative data has been collected.
- **d** Many respondents have refused to be interviewed.

20 All research projects should follow the research process. This is because:
- **a** It makes the final report much easier to follow.
- **b** The process is based on good scientific practice.
- **c** It helps researchers to do their work more quickly.
- **d** It is guaranteed to make the results more accurate.

21 All research needs to have a purpose, and reasons for being worth carrying out. This is known as:
- **a** The justification for the research.
- **b** The value of the research.
- **c** The rationale of the research.
- **d** The accuracy of the research.

22 All sources of secondary data should be assessed for possible bias. Which of the following sources is most likely to suffer from bias?
- **a** A pamphlet produced by a small political pressure group.
- **b** A government report.
- **c** The published report of a professional social research project.
- **d** An article in a professional journal.

23 A group of GNVQ Health and Social Care students are researching the question 'What do disabled people think about the local community transport service?' Which of the following best describes their research population?
- **a** Everybody living in Britain.
- **b** Disabled people living locally.
- **c** Disabled people living in Britain.
- **d** People living locally.

24 A sampling frame can be described as:
- **a** A definition of the people in the sample.
- **b** The proportion of people in the research population who are selected for the sample.
- **c** A list of all members of the research population.
- **d** A method of selecting a sample from the research population.

25 Many researchers try to use random sampling methods. Which of the following statements best describes the reason for this?
- **a** It helps to minimise the researchers' influence on the results.
- **b** It is seen as unfair if some people have no chance of being sampled.
- **c** It is much quicker than non-random methods of picking a sample.
- **d** It is traditional for researchers to use random sampling methods.

26 Research projects can collect different types of data. Which of the following statements is true about research data?
- **a** Quantitative data can only be collected by using structured interviews or questionnaires.
- **b** Quantitative data is more accurate than qualitative data.
- **c** Researchers using in-depth interviewing methods never need to collect quantitative data.
- **d** All research collects some demographic data.

27 Some researchers use experimental methods. Which of the following is important to getting good results?
- **a** Equipment used must be as sophisticated as possible.
- **b** Researchers should be qualified to use experimental methods.
- **c** Subjects should not be told the true purpose of the experiment.
- **d** The experimental circumstances should be, as far as possible, the same for all subjects.

28 Sometimes researches carry out a short preliminary investigation to test and refine their research tools before commencing the research proper. This is known as:
- **a** A questionnaire.
- **b** A pilot survey.
- **c** Secondary research.
- **d** Primary research.

29 Structured interviews may suffer response problems. Which of the following is good advice for interviewers to follow?
- **a** Try to stick to standard prompts with each respondent.
- **b** Use only body language to help people to understand the questions.
- **c** Ignore obvious misunderstandings to avoid embarrassing people.
- **d** Use any means you can think of to help people to give an answer.

30 In-depth interviews are sometimes used to collect data. Which of the following should you remember when using this method?
- **a** Each subject should have, as far as possible, a similar experience to all the others.
- **b** You will need a detailed questionnaire to use during the interviews.
- **c** Interviewers require good interpersonal skills.
- **d** You should secretly use a tape machine to record the interview.

31 Direct observation is sometime used as research methods. Which of the following is good practice when using this method?
- **a** Make sure that you observe in secret.
- **b** Don't try to infer the reasoning behind observed behaviour.
- **c** Try to record all that you see.
- **d** Try to observe at the same times each day.

32 Which of the following is true of participant observation?
- **a** Observers should never let subjects know their true intentions.
- **b** It helps if the researcher begins to think like a

typical member of the group.
- **c** It should only be used to collect quantitative data.
- **d** It is often difficult, or impossible, to analyse the results quantitatively.

33 A researcher wants to investigate the play activities of children under five years old. Which of the following research methods is likely to be suitable?
- **a** Direct observation.
- **b** In-depth interviews.
- **c** Participant observation.
- **d** Postal questionnaires.

34 A researcher wants to find out how a small group of disabled people feel about the respect that they are shown by carers. Which of the following research methods may get results which most accurately reflect the subjects' true feelings?
- **a** Postal questionnaires.
- **b** In-depth interviews.
- **c** Direct observation.
- **d** Experiments.

35 Questionnaires often use a combination of open and closed questions. Which of the following is an open question?
- **a** What is your date of birth?
- **b** Do you think that the health and social care services are doing a good job?
- **c** Are carers generally well qualified, in your opinion?
- **d** What improvements would you like to see in the services that you receive?

36 A researcher want to assess the strength of people's opinion on a range of issues, and display the results using graphs and charts. Which of the following approaches to questionnaire design will help?
- **a** Using mainly fixed-response questions, with a scale of option choices available.
- **b** Using mainly open questions.
- **c** Using fixed-response questions with 'yes/no' answers.
- **d** Asking a single fixed-response question for each issue.

37 Sometimes questions ask respondents to order a list of items according to their preferences of views. This is known as:
- **a** Routing.
- **b** Fixed response
- **c** Prompting
- **d** Ranking.

38 Sometimes questions can lead respondents to give a particular response. Which of the following questions is most likely to lead respondents?
- **a** Do you think that the care services do a good job?
- **b** Don't you agree that the care services do a good job?
- **c** In your opinion do the care services do a good job?
- **d** Thinking about the care services, do they do a good job in your opinion?

39 Questions need to be clearly written so that respondents understand what is being asked. Which of the following versions of a question is most clearly put?
- **a** Approximately how many informational exchanges have you had with the health campaign's materials?
- **b** Can you quantify, within reasonable limits, the number of times you have seen materials produced by the health campaign?
- **c** Can you state the approximate number of occasions on which you have perceived stimuli generated by the health campaign?
- **d** Please state roughly how many times you have seen materials produced by the health campaign.

40 The options available in fixed-response questions are usually pre-coded. Which of the following is the main reason for this?
- **a** It helps respondents to choose the right answer.
- **b** It makes the questionnaire look more professional and scientific.
- **c** It makes it easier for the researcher to collate responses.
- **d** It makes it clear to respondents which answers belong with which questions.

41 Qualitative data is often collected during research projects. Which of the following is true about the analysis of qualitative data?
- **a** Comparisons between the answers of different respondents can be made easily.
- **b** Charts and graphs can be used to display qualitative results.
- **c** Quotes which sum up a person's feelings should be looked for.
- **d** Unexpected comments or views should not be included as useful data.

42 A researcher has collected a large amount of qualitative data, but much of it is off the point of the

research questions. Which of the following is the researcher's best course of action?
- a Report honestly on what happened and use only relevant data.
- b Try to rewrite the research question to fit the data that has been collected.
- c Use quantitative methods in future.
- d Try to alter the data so that it fits the research question more closely.

43 A coding frame may be described as:
- a A list of people in a population used to draw a random sample.
- b A coded list of the possible answers to an open question.
- c The pre-coded options available as answers to a fixed-response question.
- d A method used to gauge the strength of people's feelings on an issue.

44 A researcher finds that a response collected by using an open question does not fit the answer categories available in the coding frame. Which of the following should the researcher do?
- a Fit the answer into the response slot with least entries in it.
- b Discard the responses from that particular respondent.
- c Fit the answer in the responses lot with the average number of responses in it.
- d Create an extra response option in the coding frame.

45 Some data concerns facts about people, like their gender, or age. This is known as:
- a Qualitative data.
- b Quota setting.
- d Information.
- d Demographic data

46 Researchers sometimes look for direct relationships between different items of data. This is known as:
- a Seeking correlations.
- b Data analysis.
- c Data processing.
- d Quantitative analysis.

47 Researchers sometimes draw up frequency distribution charts for answers that they have received. A frequency distribution is:
- a The average value of the responses.
- b A chart showing the number of people who responded to the survey.
- c A graph showing how many times each possible answer to a question was given.
- d A measure of the spread of opinion within a population.

48 A normal distribution curve is:
- a A mathematical concept based on the idea of a typical pattern of data distribution.
- b A curve based on the responses of normal people.
- c A graph based on the results of your research.
- d A graph used by researchers to assess the average response they have received.

49 A researcher has drawn up a distribution curve for the data obtained from a question and found that it is quite flat, with hardly any peak in the middle. What does this shape imply?
- a The researcher had a poor response rate for the survey.
- b Opinion on the issue is fairly evenly spread through the population.
- c People can't make up their mind on the issue.
- d Most people seem to feel the same way about the issue.

50 A frequency distribution curve of answers to a fixed-response question about opinion has a peak skewed well over to one side of the neutral response value. What does this indicate?
- a Most people have similar views on the issue.
- b Opinion is fairly well spread out on the issue.
- c The researcher has made mistakes when analysing the data.
- d The standard deviation of the data is likely to be small.

51 Researchers sometimes find the mean of a set of data. Which of the following defines what is meant by the mean?
- a The number of times a particular answer has been given.
- b The answer which is given most often.
- c The item which lies in the middle of a set of data, so that an equal number of items lie above and below it.
- d The average value of a set of data.

52 Researchers sometimes calculate the standard deviation of a set of data. Standard deviation helps researchers to:
- a Decide how accurate their results are likely to be.
- b Find the mean of a set of data.
- c Assess the variability of the data.
- d Assess the validity of the data.

53 One way to look for correlation is to use graphical methods and draw a line of best fit. What is the name for the type of graph used for this purpose?

- **a** Pie chart.
- **b** Scattergram.
- **c** Frequency distribution curve.
- **d** Bar chart.

54 Researchers may try to extrapolate from correlations that they have identified in their data. Which of the following describes extrapolation?

- **a** Making predictions about circumstances which lie outside the range of the data collected.
- **b** Making recommendations for policy based on the data.
- **c** Deciding to carry out further research to gather more information.
- **d** Drawing up graphs and charts to display the results.

55 The point of research is to draw conclusions. Which of the following is good advice to follow when drawing conclusions?

- **a** Conclusions should always be definite.
- **b** Conclusions should always suggest practical improvements.
- **c** Conclusions should always be related to the research question.
- **d** Conclusions may sometimes not be related to the research data.

56 There are potential sources of error in all research. Which of the following is good practice when dealing with research errors?

- **a** Trying to be honest about errors that may have occurred.
- **b** Mentioning only those errors that are your own fault.
- **c** Trying to play down sources of error to improve the reputation of the research.
- **d** Quantifying all errors mathematically.

57 The research report is how others will see your research efforts. Which of the following is important when writing research reports?

- **a** Always include full details of your experiences when collecting the data.
- **b** Include only as much detail as is needed to show how you planned and carried out the research.
- **c** Include as many graphs and charts as possible to help keep readers' interest.
- **d** Don't clutter up your report by including letters and questionnaires that you have used.

58 Which of the following is good practice when reporting on qualitative results?

- **a** Always try to include a chart or graph to display your findings.
- **b** Try to draw conclusions that can be applied to the wider population.
- **c** Include data on all areas that respondents have commented on.
- **d** Try to include quotes which seem to sum up respondents' views.

59 When compiling a research report you should remember to:

- **a** Include an account of any ethical issues that may have arisen during the research.
- **b** Mention ethical issues that may have affected the final results.
- **c** Try to play down the ethical issues that may have arisen.
- **d** Try to show that your research was designed to avoid all ethical problems, and that it was thus not an issue for you.

60 You will have to present research findings to a small group of people. Which of the following is good practice when presenting to others?

- **a** Read out your report as it was written.
- **b** Try to work without notes so as to avoid looking unprofessional.
- **c** Avoid using equipment such as overhead projectors.
- **d** Create transparencies or handouts of relevant charts and graphs.

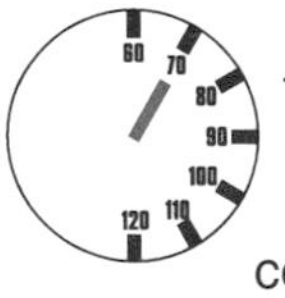

Fast Facts

Census A vast social survey, carried out by the government every ten years. The census attempts to collect information from every household in the UK.

Closed question A question which has a fixed set of possible answers pre-determined by the researcher. Closed questions produce quantitative data.

Coding frame A list of the possible answers to open questions used by researchers to code responses.

Correlation Making links between separate groups of data. Correlation shows how changes in one area relate to changes in another.

Data Information collected in the course of a research project.

Demographic data Data about respondents which is basically factual. Age, gender and income group are examples of demographic data.

Direct observation A method of social research in which the behaviour of people and groups is watched by a researcher. Direct observers do not become involved with the subjects.

Extrapolation Extending results beyond the range of data to make predictions about other members of the population.

Frequency distribution A graphical method showing how often different answers to a question have been given. Frequency distributions often approximate to the normal distribution curve.

Funnel method A way of ordering questions in which general areas are covered first and more specific topics gradually introduced.

Hypothesis A statement which is able to be tested by research.

In-depth interviewing An interviewing method which has a fairly loose structure. Respondents are encouraged to open up and provide detail on their views.

Interview A meeting between a researcher and a respondent where data is collected.

Interview schedule A document used in structured interviewing to direct and control the process. A schedule contains the questions, and strict instructions for the interviewer to follow.

Mean The average value of a set of data.

Median The value that occurs in the middle of a ranked list of responses. The median is chosen so that half the responses lie above, and half below it.

Mode The mode is the most frequently recorded response in a set of data.

Normal distribution curve A bell-shaped curve which often results when frequency distributions are plotted. The mathematical properties of the normal distribution allow percentage probability statements to be made.

Official statistics Data collected by national and local government. Official statistics cover a vast range of topics.

Open question A question which respondents answer in their own words. Open questions are often used to collect qualitative data.

Opinion poll A survey method intended to collect information on public opinion. Opinion polls often use street interviews and quota sampling techniques.

Participant observation A method of social investigation in which the researcher joins in with subjects and observes them from inside the group.

Pilot survey A test run of a survey which is carried out on a small sample. Pilot work is intended to help evaluate and refine the research method.

Population The whole group that a survey or research project is concerned with. A population usually consists of people, although it can be other things such as households.

Postal questionnaire A research method where questionnaires are sent to respondents by post.

Pre-coding Giving a code to each available answer for a question. Pre-coding makes it easier to deal with the data during compilation of results.

Primary data Data that you have collected yourself. Primary research involves carrying out your own investigation to collect primary data.

Probes Comments designed to get further information from a respondent. Probes can help deal with response problems, and follow up lines of enquiry.

Prompts Statements which are read out to respondents to make them aware of possible answers to a question.

Qualitative data Data which cannot be expressed in numerical form. Qualitative data is descriptive, and is often about attitudes, opinions and values. Qualitative research methods seek to collect this type of data.

Quantitative data Data which is expressed in numerical form. Quantitative research methods seek to collect this type of data.

Questionnaire A list of questions designed to collect primary data. Questionnaires are often filled in by the respondents themselves, without an interviewer being present.

Quota sampling A method of sample selection where a population is stratified into types of people. Interviewers are given quotas of people to interview from each category.

Random sampling A method of choosing a sample which uses random methods to eliminate bias in selection.

Ranking A method of obtaining respondents' opinions of the differences between items in a group. Respondents rank the group in terms of the criteria set by the researcher.

Rating scale A method recording answers to closed questions. Respondents indicate the strength of their opinion by choosing a scale point.

Reliability The quality of research results. A result is reliable if it can be obtained again by repeating the research on another sample.

Research The process of finding things out in an organised and thoughtful way.

Respondent A person who provides data for a social investigation.

Response rate The proportion of sample members who return information. Postal questionnaires often have a poor response rate.

Routing Instructions included in self-completion questionnaires and interview schedules which indicate which question is to be answered next.

Sample A group chosen from the population on which research is conducted directly. Samples are intended to be representative of the population as a whole.

Sampling frame A list containing all members of a population from which a sample can be chosen.

Scattergram A graphical method of showing correlations between different sets of data.

Secondary data Data that has been collected by other people. Secondary research involves looking at existing sources of information.

Semi-structured interview A method of data collection which uses a series of open questions. Semi-structured methods are less flexible than in-depth interviewing, but not as rigid as structured interviews.

Standard deviation A way of indicating the variability in a set of data. Fixed proportions of the normal curve lie within standard deviations of the mean.

Stratified sampling A method of making a sample more representative. The population is grouped and a proportion of the sample picked from each group.

Structured interviewing A method of social research which uses tightly controlled interviews to collect data. Structured interviewing aims to minimise differences between each interview to help eliminate bias.

Survey An enquiry designed to collect primary data. Social surveys usually involve asking people questions.

Systematic sampling A method of choosing a random sample from a sampling frame. Names are picked at regular intervals from the list, for example every fifth name.

Validity A quality of research results. A result is valid if it accurately represents the view of respondents.

Variability The degree of spread of a feature within a population.

References and further reading

Dixon, B., Bouma, G., and Atkinson, G., 1987, *A Handbook of Social Science Research,* Oxford University Press

Dooley, D., 1990, *Social Research Methods,* Prentice-Hall

Hemmersley, M., 1993, *Social Research: Philosophy, Politics and Practice,* Sage

Hoinville, G., Jowell, R., *et al.*, 1978, *Survey Research Practice,* Heinemann Educational

Jowell, R., *et al.*, 1994, *British Social Attitudes: the 11th report,* Dartmouth Publishing

Kidder, L., 1981, *Research Methods in Social Relations,* Holt, Rinehart and Winston

Langley, P., 1987, *Doing Social Research: A Guide to Coursework,* Causeway Press

Moser, C. A., and Kalton, G., 1971, *Survey Methods in Social Investigation,* Heinemann

North, P. J., 1980, *People in Society,* Longman

Shipman, M., 1988, *The Limitations of Social Research,* Longman

Walker, R., 1985, *Applied Qualitative Research,* Gower

Research ethics and codes of practice

British Psychological Society, 'Ethical Principles for Conducting Research with Human Participants', in Robson, C., 1994, *Real World Research,* Blackwell

'Code of Conduct' (for social and market research), 1994, from: The Market Research Society, 15 Northburgh Street, London EC1V 0AH

Chapter 25

Communication

This chapter will help you to develop your communication skills. It begins with some advice on GNVQ grading themes - planning, information-seeking and handling, evaluation and quality of outcomes. It then goes on to deal with each element of this core skill unit:

- **taking part in discussions**
- **producing written material**
- **using images**
- **reading and responding to written materials.**

Introduction

Everyone communicates throughout their lives, but to work in a caring situation requires you to develop these skills so that you will be able to communicate *effectively*. Many of the clients you will work with will depend on you to evaluate their needs and help to resolve their problems. You will only be able to help them with this if you have developed appropriate skills. Clients will only be able to relate to you if you show that you value them as individuals and you will be best able to show this by how you communicate with them.

Communication is a two-way process with both parties giving and obtaining information, and you will need to develop skills in both of these areas. Carers in health and social care require high levels of communication as this is integral to all aspects of caring, when working as part of a team as well as working directly with clients.

Communication is also an essential part of the GNVQ Advanced Health and Social Care units, most specifically Unit 2: Interpersonal Interaction. To communicate effectively, you need to place yourself in other people's positions to try to understand the person you are communicating with.

Grading

There are two grading themes common to all GNVQ courses:

- the *process grading theme*, which consists of planning, information-seeking and handling, and evaluation
- the *content grading theme*, which is based on quality of the work you produce (quality of outcomes).

These relate specifically to the elements of the core skills in Communication.

Planning

The following points are important in relation to communication:

- *Why are you communicating?*
  Are you trying to give, obtain or exchange information? Good communication usually involves an exchange of information, with everyone involved contributing.
- *Who are you communicating with?*

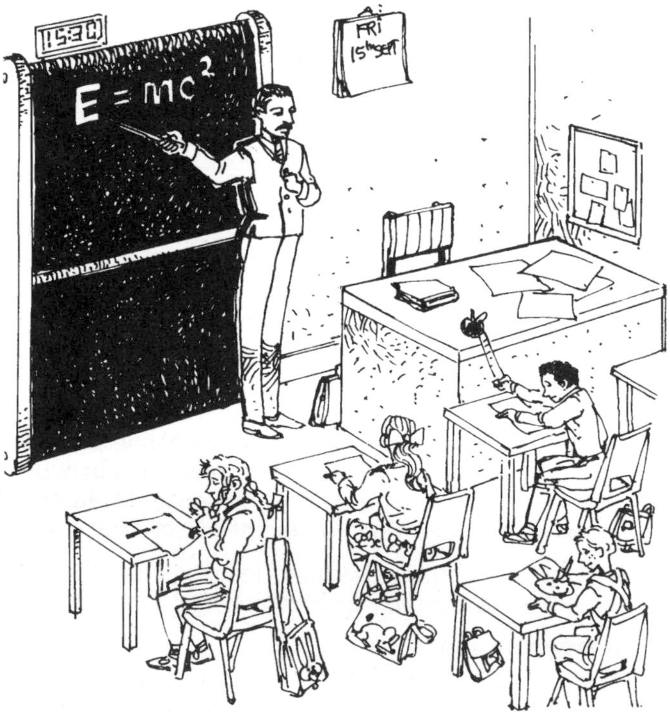

Figure 25.1 It is important to consider the age and abilities of your audience

What level of knowledge and skill do they already have? Do they have any specific difficulties in communicating?

- *How are you going to communicate?*
  Is it verbally, in writing, using images, or a combination of these?
- *Where are you communicating?*
  Is the setting appropriate? Can everyone hear, see and contribute easily?
- *When are you going to communicate?*
  Is it an appropriate time? What is the attention span of the participants? How long have you got, and how should you divide up this time?

Information-seeking and handling

Sources of information

Your first source of information is yourself. Make a list of things you know about the topic you are researching and note alongside each one where you think you got that information. For example, you probably obtained the information from one of the following.

- A lesson on this or a previous course. Have you still got notes or handouts from it? Look them up.
- A previous piece of coursework. Consider whether the work was of sufficient quality and of an appropriate level for you to use.
- A visit, or a talk for a visiting speaker. What organisation did the speaker represent? Can you contact anyone for further information?
- A book, magazine or newspaper. Where did you read it? Have you still got it, or do you know where it can be obtained?
- Personal experience, or from the experience of someone you know. Most people have had experience of the provision of health, education and social services. Personal experience, although it is often limited in scope, is a justifiable source of information and can give fresh insight when compared with more orthodox sources. Remember that confidentiality should be maintained when using other people's experience in a piece of work, and you should check with your tutor before including it in a piece of work (see the Introduction).
- A video, radio or television programme or even on a computer. Unless you can review the material then your memory might be faulty and it is difficult to use this material as a source. Some radio and TV stations sell transcripts of their material, and some transcripts are published in *The Listener* magazine. It is possible to print out most material on computers, and you should gain experience of this as evidence of your IT skills.

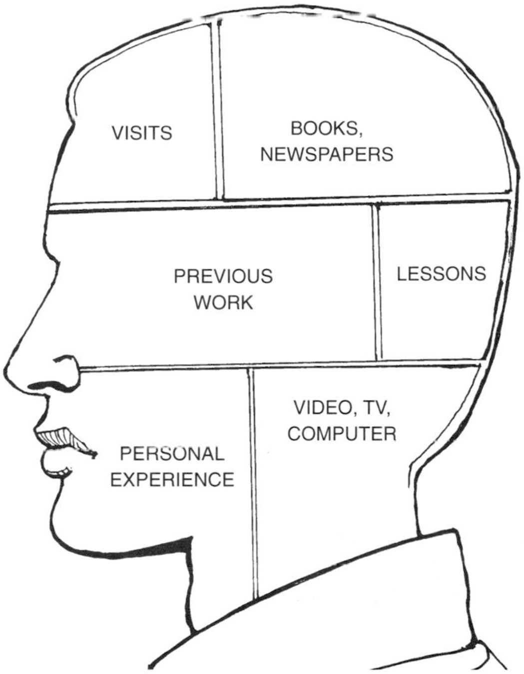

Human sources

After yourself, the most obvious people to ask for information are your teachers, supervisors and fellow students. There are many other people, working for a range of statutory and voluntary bodies, who can also provide information such as people who work for:

- local councils
- schools
- charities
- campaigning groups
- government departments
- politicians and political parties
- businesses.

You will usually need to contact them by phone or letter, but some leaflets are freely available in shops, libraries, doctors' surgeries and community centres.

It is possible to obtain information more quickly from people than from written sources, but you have to know which questions to ask and how to ask them in order to get positive responses. However, the information obtained from people is more likely to be wrong, biased or misinterpreted than that from written sources and, unless you use a tape recorder or video camera, it is more difficult to record. Remember that any recording should be with the full agreement of those people involved, and in some cases the permission of the relevant authority.

Try it

Chinese whispers is a good demonstration of how messages can become changed in transmission. Try if for yourself with a group of friends. Someone makes up a short complex message and whispers it to the person next to him or her. That person then whispers it to the next person, and so on through at least six people. Compare the original and final message. Has the meaning changed much?

Who to ask?

If you are stuck, ask your tutor or supervisor for advice. He or she should be able to give you a list of organisations who might have information. You can find their names and addresses in *The Phone Book, Yellow Pages* or *Thomson's Directory*.

Try it

Find out the following information from telephone directories.

1 How many local hospitals are there? Do any have specialist units listed?
2 How many primary schools are funded by your local council? How many are run by the Roman Catholic or Church of England religions? Are there any private schools in your local area?
3 What number should a person who is hearing-impaired use to contact the police if he or she is using Text Telephones?
4 Find the name and address of a charity or voluntary organisation dealing with each of the following:
   a special needs
   b medicine
   c children
   d elderly people.

Hints if you need them:

1 Look under 'Hospitals' in the Business and Services section of *The Phone Book.* They should be listed alphabetically with their addresses, which can be used to check whether they are in your local area or not. There is a map of the postal districts in the front of the directory. You can also look up individual hospitals under their names and some of these have more details about departments. Do not telephone the hospitals to find out how many departments they have, since this just wastes their time.
2 Look under the name of your local authority in the Business and Services section of *The Phone Book*, and the schools should be listed in alphabetical order under 'Education Department'. They usually state whether they are religious or direct-grant schools. Private schools are listed in *Yellow Pages* and *Thomson's Directory* under 'Schools, Private'.
3 Look at the 'Useful Numbers' section of the information section in the front of any directory and the number is given under 'Police'.
4 Look up the 'Charities' section of *Yellow Pages* or *Thomson's Directory,* or alternatively the Business and Services directory under 'National' and 'Royal' since many charities' names begin with these words.

Written sources

These are often the most useful sources, since they potentially contain far more information and are more easily accessible than other sources. First, consult any notes, handouts and any textbooks you have which are relevant to the topic. Note relevant sections, taking care also to note any references they contain to specific publications and authors. These can then be used for further research. To make your search easier, practise using the following items:

- *contents lists* this is towards the front of the book, magazine or journal and gives the titles of chapters in the publication together with the page number. There is sometimes further detail about the sections within each chapter, and in some books a brief summary of what is covered in it. In some books the chapters are organised into larger sections.
- *index* this is at the back of the book and gives an alphabetical list of the subjects covered in the book. This is often in a very incomplete form, so you must consider what other titles the subject might be found under. Some examples are given below:

Subject	*Related titles*
Down's syndrome	chromosomal changes, polysomy, genetic disability, special needs
Life expectancy	population, demographics, infant mortality – morbidity, health statistics
Condoms	contraception, birth control, sex, reproduction, disease, AIDS, prophylactics

Sampling	statistics, surveys, random sampling, experimental, questionnaires, data

Magazines and journals often publish an index every few months or once a year which makes it easier to find relevant articles.

- *glossary* this is a short dictionary defining specialist terms found in the article or book. The Fast Facts at the end of each section of this book are a form of glossary.
- *references* references give specific detail about where information, ideas or quotes referred to in the text were researched. They are usually numbered, and the section of text relating to the material is indicated by a small number raised above the line. The references are listed at the bottom of the pages, at the end of chapters or before the index at the end of a book. The convention for references is author's surname and initials, year of publication, title of journal or book, volume or edition, page number. For example: Smith A. and Jones P. (1994) Brit.Med.J., 36, 254.
- *bibliography* this is a list of books and articles used in the research for a piece of work. It is constructed either in order of importance or in alphabetical order, and is structured in the same way as the references.

Libraries

You should make sure that you have access to as many libraries as possible. There will be a range of libraries available to you.

Local libraries

You may be a member of your local library already. You will then have access not only to the material in that library, but also in all the other libraries in your local area. The indexes should list all the books found in any of the libraries run by the local authority, and you should be able to get books transferred from these to your local library. Main libraries often have a reference section where you can consult books, newspapers and journals, but you are not usually allowed to take these materials home.

Some local councils have agreements with neighbouring councils whereby users can use each other's services. It is worthwhile checking this with the librarian, especially if there are few appropriate sources available in your local service or if you live close to the border of your local council area.

University libraries

It may be possible to use these facilities, but it usually requires special permission which you can obtain by contacting the chief librarian. It might be helpful to gain the support of your tutor or college librarian when applying to show that you will use the services responsibly. There are often restrictions as to when you can use the facilities as there is often a high level of demand on them already, and it is unlikely that you will be allowed to take books home.

Specialist collections

These are libraries which specialise in a restricted range of subjects, and can be part of a council or university library, or attached to another organisation such as a museum or institute. You will need special permission to use some of these, and they often have restricted access. Many councils run a special library section, called an *archive,* which contains documents and maps relating to the local history of the area, and it is fairly easy to gain access to these.

Using a library

Librarians are skilled in finding sources of information, and can usually help you if you get stuck. However, you should not rely upon them to do your work for you and you should practise using the authors and subject index to find appropriate texts.

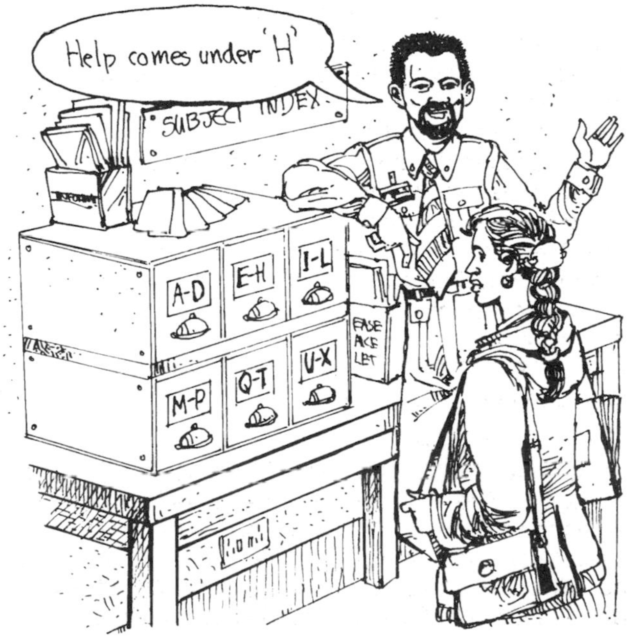

Dewey Decimal System

This is the system of reference numbers on the spines of books in libraries. The numbers are also found on the bookshelves around the library. The numbers relate to subject areas.

You should find out and list what the reference numbers are for the subjects you will be interested in, and find out where they are in the library. For example, for Unit 3 you would need books on biology and possibly health and medicine. Find out the Dewey decimal numbers for these sections. Within these sections there will be more restricted numbers for more specialised topics. List the numbers associated with the following topics: the heart and circulatory system; reproduction; contraception; the brain.

Indexes

The two most common indexes are the Author Index and Subject Index. The advantages of using these rather than looking on the shelves is that they will tell you if the library has the book even if it is out on loan, and whether there are spare copies on the reference shelf or obtainable from the librarian. In many cases, the indexes also contain information about books stocked in other libraries but available on request.

Many libraries have their indexes on computer, which means that you can use a search facility rather than flicking through a filing system. Other libraries have indexes on microfiche. These are sheets of photographic film with the index on them in a much reduced form. They can be studied using a viewer which magnifies them. The advantage of these over card files is that they take up a great deal less storage space.

An author index lists the names of authors in alphabetical order with surname first followed by initials. Remember that there are many thousands of authors, and so there is likely to be more than one with a common name such as Smith, J. or Patel, R. Look at the titles of the books which they have written, are they appropriate to the information you are seeking?

You can obtain the names of authors who specialise in particular topics by making reference to your notes or by looking up the references and bibliography in textbooks and other relevant texts.

Subject indexes list books according to the subject area. If you look up a very general title such as Sociology then there will probably be a lot of books listed under it. However, if you look up a more specific area, such as 'deviancy', the list will be more restricted.

Newspapers

Most libraries have copies of a wide range of national and local newspapers, and often have back (old) copies. The broadsheet papers usually have special sections on topics such as health, society and education on specific days of the week, and these are usually worth looking at quickly if you have the time.

Journals and magazines

Journals tend to be more specialised and have a more restricted subject matter compared with magazines, and the information in them is usually checked for accuracy by experts.

Find out which journals and magazines are available from the libraries you use. You might find some of the following useful on the course: *The Nursing Times, Social Work Today, Community Care, New Statesman and Society, Trends in British Society, Scientific American, New Internationalist.*

Constructing your own indexes

It is a good idea to make a note of those texts which you have found useful. You can consider different ways of constructing an index, including information on the author's name, which topic or GNVQ unit it covers, and where you obtained it.

Abstracts

These are compilations of summaries of articles and papers found in different magazines and journals. They are more commonly found in university libraries.

Evaluation

Evaluating your successes and failures is very difficult since it requires you to look at your own strengths and weaknesses. Nobody is perfect, but none of us likes admitting to failure, and some people find it hard not to over-exaggerate their success. To evaluate your work fully, you should use both **objective** and **subjective assessment.**

Objective evaluation

This means considering the facts uncoloured by feelings or opinions. An example of objective evaluation would be to compare your performance with set standards and criteria. The basic standards you have to attain are set in the GNVQ criteria – did you meet them? These standards are often interpreted by your tutors – did you meet their criteria? You might have personal standards which you wish to attain – did you meet your own standards?

Subjective evaluation

This means giving prominence to personal feelings and opinions.

Do you feel that you performed as well as you could in a given situation? What do you feel helped you work well, or caused you to under-perform?

If something worked well, can you transfer what you have achieved to other situations? Can you use this as a basis for further improvement?

If you under-performed, what factors were involved? Was it your responsibility or did external factors play a large part? Write out a plan of how you aim to improve, and list future activities where you can demonstrate this improvement.

Think it over

Nafisha was demonstrating the recovery position as part of a first aid exam, but had great difficulty in placing her casualty into it. Her evaluation was:

'I failed the exam because I could not get Tony into the recovery position since he is a lot bigger than me. I have only previously practised on people of my own size and I found I could not move a larger person. I found that I was getting better as I worked with Tony, and feel that with some practice I will improve my skills at it.

I feel it was slightly unfair to place me in the position of dealing with Tony in the exam. Although Tony did not actively hinder me, I feel he could have been more supportive, and I was annoyed when he made a silly remark about my being "feeble".'

Evaluating others

You might well be asked to evaluate other students in the group. Try to be fair, balanced and sympathetic. Remember they could soon be evaluating you

Try to start with an objective point of view. Have they attained the stated criteria? Which parts were the most successful? Was there anything new or innovative in what they did? Do you think they put in a lot of effort? Were there improvements when compared with previous attempts? Can you make any positive suggestions as to how they could improve?

Responding to criticism

You are entitled to respond to critical evaluations of your performance, but you must try to be as objective as possible. Try to relate your response to the set criteria, especially those set for GNVQ. You will need to provide evidence to show that you have met these criteria so that you can get people to reconsider their evaluation. There are appeal mechanisms as part of the course – find out about them and use them.

Quality of outcomes

Quality may be affected by the structure, language used and presentation of the piece of work, so these should be considered when completing an assignment. For further details, see the Introduction.

Taking part in discussions

In all GNVQ courses discussions form an important component of the learning and assessment processes, and this is particularly true for the Health and Social Care programme.

Think it over

Many people find it difficult to take part in discussions because they feel shy, particularly when they have to speak to large groups of people they do not know. You might have had to do this at the start of the course, when you first met your fellow students, even if it was only to tell them your name.

How do you feel in this type of situation?

Does your body feel as if it is reacting in a particular way? Does your heart seem to beat faster, your throat go dry, your mind stop working?

Try feeling your pulse and regulating your breathing so that it slows. If you breathe too quickly, you hyperventilate and feel faint. If you have a talk for a longer period, have a watch or clock handy – it can help you to pace yourself.

If possible have something written down, even if it is only the name of the person you are talking to – at least you won't forget his or her name.

Taking part in discussions (one-to-one, in a group or on the telephone) is a part of everyday life, but you should improve your skills and learn to adapt them to a new range of situations.

Types of discussion

Three general purposes of discussion are:

- to give information
- to obtain information
- to exchange ideas.

Try it

1 Make a table of all the activities you do as part of the course and beside each one make a note of the purpose it serves.
2 Consider which of the activities you find the most difficult.

Do they have any similarities? Do you find it easier to talk or to listen? Do you tend to contribute too much or too little in different situations? Do you have the patience to concentrate on activities for extended periods of time, or do you need to work on your concentration span?

Your list of activities should have included most of the following: lessons, discussions, seminars, role plays, brainstorms, simulations, talks, visits, meetings, interviews, tutorials, practicals, telephone calls, opinion surveys, debates and discussions with clients, supervisors and other workers during work experience placements.

Evidence collection point

You need to demonstrate that you have contributed to different types of discussion.

Keep a log of each time you take part in one of the activities listed above. Once you have logged a type of discussion more than twice, only log those times that you made a major contribution to an activity or for which there is evidence of your contribution in the forms of a recording, minutes, or if it was evaluated by someone else, especially a qualified assessor.

Preparing for a discussion

Many of the discussions you take part in are straightforward, and do not require you to prepare specially for them. Sometimes, however, a discussion will be complicated by particular factors, and you need to prepare yourself carefully for it.

New situations

If you are taking part in an activity which you have not experienced before, you should consider how you can best prepare yourself for it. Examples of this would be starting at a new work experience placement, working with an individual who has a special need of which you have no previous experience, or preparing for an interview at a college or university.

Think it over

How did you prepare for your interview for this course when you applied? Was your behaviour different from normal on the first day of the course? Were you quieter or more talkative than usual? Do you handle new situations well, or do you need to prepare yourself thoroughly?

Reasoning

Some activities need logical reasoning, and so you should think before you talk. Examples of this are the interpretation of scientific or sociological data, defining causes and effects, or discussing the validity of results and limitations to conclusions. These activities are often complicated because you have to consider many factors or large amounts of data.

Another reason that it might be complicated is if it is necessary to balance opposing points of view, or if it challenges you to consider objectively something on which you have a strong subjective opinion.

Think it over

Are there any topics, such as abortion, child abuse, religion, evolution or drugs, which you would find it difficult to talk about and to see justification for the opposing point of view?

Sensitivity

Any discussion with or about clients automatically involves **confidentiality** and must be handled with sensitivity. You should be careful not to make value judgements about clients, and you should reflect upon how your views are affected by the biases and prejudices you have.

Naturally you should be sensitive to the needs of your fellow students, supporting any who might have problems explaining themselves, and being aware when someone is feeling tense due to personal problems.

Think it over

You may have come across the theory of constructive criticism before. It means to balance negative aspects with positive ones. Don't just make negative comments, but suggest how the work could have been improved and mention aspects which you can praise.

Technical terms and concepts

In some cases it is necessary to understand technical terms to contribute effectively to a discussion. In other cases using the same terms might exclude people from contributing since they might not understand you. You must vary the language you use according to your audience.

Think it over

You are working in a hospital when a patient collapses, and you have to communicate with the medical staff, relatives and the patient when he or she recovers. With whom do you use the following explanations: myocardial infarction: heart attack: a blockage in an artery in the heart leading to damage to the muscle?

Evidence collection point

Keep copies of the following: notes you have made for a presentation, minutes of meetings when you are preparing a group presentation, evidence that you have adapted materials or ways of presenting information to suit a specific audience.

Giving information

Practical aspects of speaking

Some people talk too quickly, without leaving the gaps and pauses which add meaning to what we say. Others talk too slowly and have too many pauses, which also makes it hard to understand them. People often make these mistakes when they are unsure of what they are talking about.

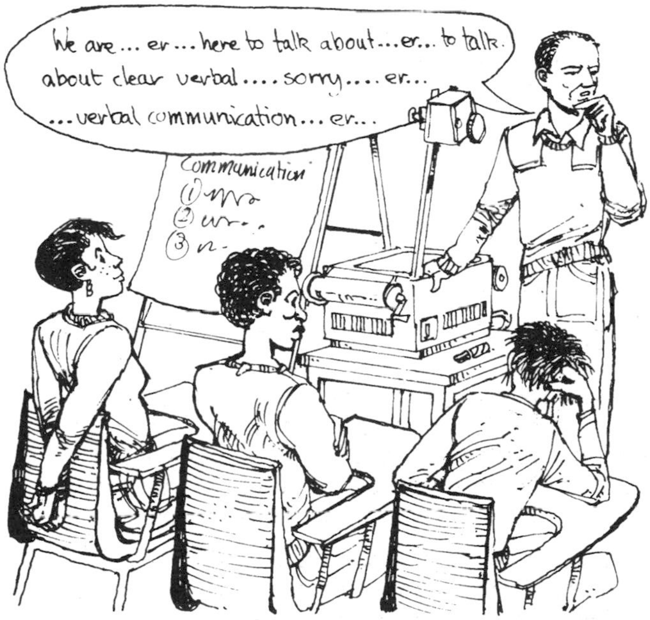
We are ... er ... here to talk about ... er ... to talk about clear verbal .... sorry .... er ... ... verbal communication ... er ...
Communication

Try it

If you talk too quickly or slowly then you will need to improve your verbal skills. Try timing how quickly you speak. Is it too fast or too slow? Ask other people to assess your performance.

When you read out a piece of work, you should usually leave short pauses at commas, longer ones at the end of sentences and larger gaps at the end of paragraphs. You can also use a pause to stress a word or phrase you consider important.

If you are talking from notes then your notes should contain markers to show which words and phrases to stress, and where you should leave longer gaps in your speech.

Read or talk?

Talking while referring to notes is a far more effective way of communicating then reading material word-for-word. The major reason that people read is because they lack self-confidence and are scared of forgetting what they want to say. This can be improved by having headed and highlighted notes and something to read if you suddenly get stage fright.

Think it over

Why is talking directly to people more effective? You should consider eye contact, body language, gaps and stresses in speech, ease of responding to questions, adaptability and ability to respond to the audience. Why is it easier if you are reading from a book to children?

Formal situations

Whether it is a first meeting with a supervisor, a visit, or a presentation to a group of external professionals, you should consider the overall impression you are giving.

Is your dress and overall image suitable for the occasion? Try to keep a good posture – use positive body language. Make eye contact appropriately. You should also use formal titles and surnames, only using forenames if asked to do so. A group of people is usually referred to as 'ladies and gentlemen'.

You should start by introducing yourself and your group and organisation, and making the other people welcome.

Try it

Below are notes from the case study of an individual. Have different members of the group present the same information and discuss whose was the best presentation and why.

Application for sheltered housing

Name: Olive Smith

Date of birth: 18 April 1914

Address: 32 Bingham Road, Midtown

Marital Status: Widow

Social history: Two daughters both married and living out of the country. Husband died ten years ago. Lives in a damp second-floor flat. Has two small pensions, one from her late husband, but still has to claim income support.

Medical history: Recently broke hip in a fall. Will be released from hospital in three weeks but will find flights of stairs difficult to handle. Some signs of arthritis in wrists and ankles, and has a cataract in her right eye.

Current provision: Home help twice a week. Uses local luncheon club three times a week.

Plan to provide temporary place in sheltered accommodation until her mobility improves then reassess situation.

Aids to discussions

Images

A picture is worth a thousand words, but only if it is appropriate. The use of images should complement the points you make and not distract from them.

Handouts

The use of handouts means that your audience needs to make fewer notes and can therefore pay more attention to what you are saying, but they can also be distracting.

If you distribute them before you start talking, then people can use them to back up what is being said, but it can also mean that they read them instead of listening. If they are distributed during a discussion, they can cause interruptions, although this can be useful as a break during a long presentation. If they are distributed at the end of a session, then the information within them should be referred to during the talk.

Evidence collection point

Keep copies of recordings of discussions, evaluations by others, detailed notes from preparations for discussions.

Recording information

Taking notes is an important skill which you will need to develop, since at this level you will be expected to take notes as people are speaking and not just copy them from a board or OHP. It will be impossible to note everything that a person says, so you must use abbreviated forms.

Shorthand

This is quicker than ordinary writing, but takes a lot of time and practice to use well. You can use standard abbreviations instead, such as 'Soc.' for society or social and 'psy' for psychology.

Try it

Work out what the following abbreviations could stand for. They all relate to the field of health and social care.

Standard abbreviations: CQSW, EOC, RNIB, NCH, OPCS, DSS, UBO, AIDS, RHE, PC, SD

Non-standard abbreviations: bio, pop, med, stat, Q&A, disab, gen, est, pro

These might appear difficult to work out, but are easier when put within a context. Hence 'gen' could stand for general, gender or genetic.

Headings, sub-headings and lists

These allow you to organise your notes and quickly take down the general topics covered in a discussion. You should use upper and lower case letters, and decimal and Roman numbers to help you organise them.

Try it

Below is a short section of notes from Element 3.2 about the structure of the heart. See if you can decode part of it and translate it into sentences.

Heart & circ.sys.

A) Heart – coronary/cardiac

a) structure – left (bigger) and right

– 4 chambers; 2 atria (top) 2 ventricles (bottom)

– valves. mitral (between atria & vents) and semi-lunar (in blood vessels). Connective tissue. Regulate blood flow.

– mostly specialised muscle

– encased in membrane (thin skin) Pericardium

– size, lightly clenched fist

b) location – slightly left of centre below rib cage.

c) function – pumps blood round double circ. sys.

I) Pulmonary – r.vent – pulm artery – lungs – pulm vein – l atrium

II) Systemic – l. vent – aorta (biggest blood vessel) – arteries – body organs (except lungs) – veins – inf & sup vena cava – r.atrium

d) control – more details next week

I) Internal – pacemaker function of Sino-atrial note – beat starts, spreads across heart along fibres.

II) External – vagal nerve from brain, regulates speed and power of beat.

Underline and highlight any points or words which are of particular importance.

Graphical representations

These can contain more information in a more easily accessible form than notes. Consider how much more easily you could record the information in the example above on the structure of the heart by using a diagram or a flow chart.

Try it

Draw a quick diagram showing what you know of the structure of your school or college, showing the position of yourself within it. Estimate how much writing it would have taken to convey the same information.

Evidence collection point

Keep copies of notes written in a variety of formats from different situations. Most of this will be primarily assessed in Communication Element 3.2.

Questions

Questioning can be negative or positive. You can put people under a great deal of stress by asking them challenging questions in an inappropriate setting, or you can make them feel valued and supported by questions showing that you have been listening and understand what they are saying.

First of all you must work out what you are going to ask, and how to ask it.

Make notes on what you want to ask, it can be indicated as simply as a question mark added to your notes or to a handout.

When to ask questions

The best time to ask questions is usually after the person who is speaking has finished talking. If the question is of immediate importance then you can interrupt the speaker, but make sure that it is not something which could be asked later, since you will be disrupting what they are trying to say.

Clarification

Seeking clarification involves asking questions to check that you have understood something correctly. You should relate your questions directly to what the person you are questioning has said.

You might state that you have understood one part of what has been communicated, but are uncertain about a related area. You could check the meaning of terminology used by checking if the person agrees with your definition.

You could check facts which you think might have been wrong or which have been presented confusingly.

Remember, if you are confused about something which has been said, it is likely that other people are as well.

Evidence collection point

Keep copies of videos of a range of discussions, evaluations of discussions by others, results of surveys and interviews described in assignments.

Confirmation

Providing confirmation is in many ways similar to giving clarification by answering questions, but also includes the provision of further information and the reiteration of points.

Providing further information

The additional information you supply should be appropriate to the point being made, and can come from any source – books, personal experience or research you have completed. You should state its source if you can.

It is also a good idea if you can apply concepts and data which you have covered in one unit or element to other units and elements.

You should indicate how certain you are of your information, and be open to challenges as to whether it is applicable to what is being discussed.

Reiterating points

This means repeating a point that has been made, but using a different context, new information or different terminology to make it.

It is important to reiterate points if they are of particular importance and need stressing, if people seem confused and unsure, or if the audience includes people who find things hard to understand due to their special needs or learning difficulties.

Evidence collection point

Evidence of confirmation may come from recordings of discussions, minutes of meetings, evaluations, aids to discussions (such as OHPs), models, flip charts.

Taking discussions forward

This is the use of information and ideas which have been presented to generate new ideas. You can use information you have previously learnt and new information given in the activity to generate new concepts. You might also have practical examples from your own experience which can add insight to a topic.

A useful technique for thinking up new ideas or solving problems is **brainstorming.**

Try it

In a small group, discuss 'What I would do if I won £1 million'. Make a chart of questions and decisions that your group can come up with in a brainstorming session. It could include sections on how much should be invested, and where it should be invested. You should end up with a chart with lots of interlinked sections.

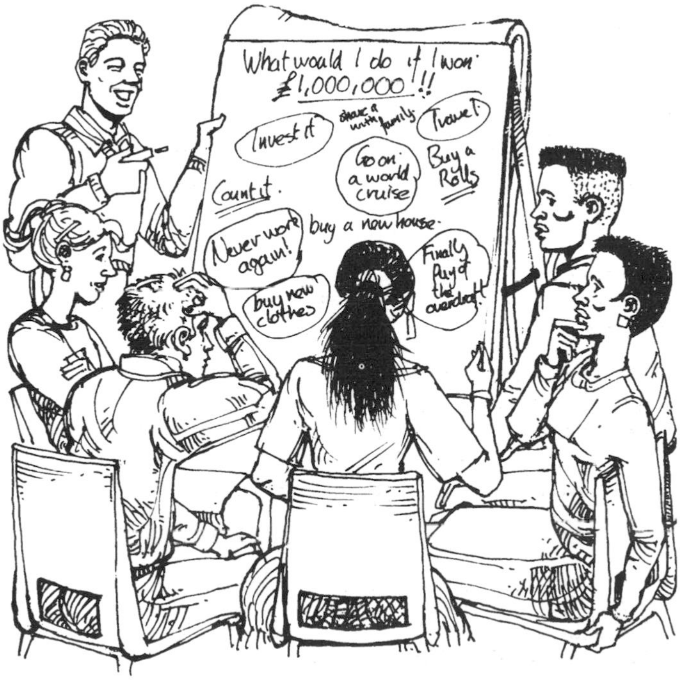
What would I do if I won £1,000,000 !!
Invest it
Travel
Go on a world cruise
Buy a Rolls
Count it.
Never work again!
buy a new house
Finally Pay of the overdraft!
buy new clothes

Evidence collection point

Evidence may be found in recordings of discussions, evaluations, notes made at the time, minutes, flip charts and brainstorming sessions.

Creating opportunities for others

Many people do not have the confidence to contribute to discussions, but by asking the right question they can be encouraged to contribute without being patronised.

In any group there are often people who crave attention, and they can gain it by monopolising discussion time. Their points might not be valid, but they have a lot of them to make. Most of the time they do not realise what they are doing, and do not deliberately exclude other people, but if others in the discussion are more shy they can be inhibited from making their contribution.

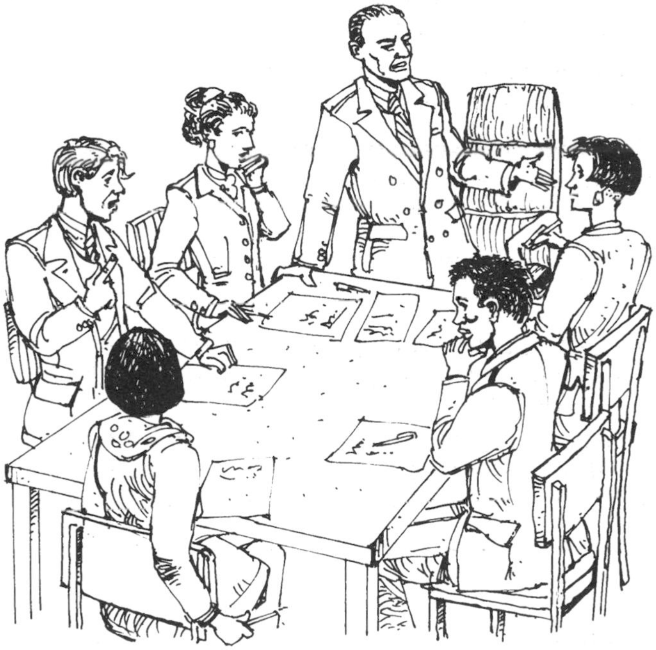

Formal discussions need a chairperson to control the situation, and in the classroom this is usually the tutor. At some point in the course you may be expected to act as the chairperson for a discussion, and will have to consider the best ways of controlling the situation.

Think it over

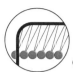

Which of the following attributes does an effective chairperson need to have?

a sensitivity to individuals' needs and abilities
b a loud voice
c fairness
d knowledge about the topic being discussed
e tolerance
f good eye contact
g a clear voice
h a sense of humour
i an upright and alert posture
j the respect of the rest of the group

How did you get on?

a Yes. It helps a lot to know the participants, since you will be more aware of any difficulties that might arise.
b No. If you have to shout, it means that you have already lost control of the group. If the chairperson is loud it encourages others to be.
c You should treat everyone equally, with no preferences. Although you are participating in the discussion, you should not take sides or show who you agree with. If in doubt, favour 'the underdog' since he or she needs more help.
d You do not need to know the subject and, if you do, you are more likely to act partially. You do need to be clear about the rules you are setting. How long will you allow people to speak for? Will you allow questioners to interrupt the speaker? What level of personal abuse will you stand?
e Chairpersons can be too tolerant. Remember, you are the person who has to control the discussion.
f Good eye contact is necessary to show that you are alert and listening. If you lack concentration, the rest of the group will as well. Remember that you will often be facing the other people in the group for the whole of the discussion, so they will see a lot of your face.
g A clear voice is an advantage when communicating, so try to open your mouth more when you talk than in normal conversation.
h This is not necessary but it helps defuse some situations.
i Yes, see (f).
j The participants should respect the status of the chairperson, but you will have to earn it by acting firmly but fairly.

Special needs

When you are working with people with special needs, you will need to make sure that they are included in as many activities as possible. You will have to adapt your behaviour to make sure that they are not excluded, possibly disregard some activities which they cannot contribute to and concentrate on those which they can take an active part in.

Evidence collection point

Evidence may include minutes of meetings you have chaired, recordings, evaluations, plans of how you have worked with people with special needs and how you tried to adapt the conditions.

Using the telephone

Using the telephone puts us in contact with more people far more quickly than any other form of communication. Most people use the telephone to contact friends and family and are often less confident when using it to contact strangers.

The telephone has a narrow range of sound and so people's voices change and they sound less clear. Also you cannot see people's body language which would help you interpret their meaning. Both of these factors inhibit total communication. In addition, the fact that you do not know the person on the other end of the telephone is inhibiting.

Using telephone directories

See the section on researching sources on page 538.

Sending a message

You should always prepare yourself before contacting someone new on the telephone. Make notes or even write out a script of what you wish to say. If necessary, rehearse it aloud. Have an abbreviated form of it handy in case you have to leave a message.

If you do not know the name of the person you wish to contact, you may know his or her title or the name of the department or section in which he or she works. If you are unsure, ask the receptionist or secretary, who will usually have a list of the people in an organisation, together with their job titles and where they can usually be found. If the person is not available, ask for the correct extension number for when you phone again.

Taking a message

Keep a pen and paper handy beside the telephone so you can take messages. On answering the telephone, state your name and your locations clearly and ask if you can help the caller. The messages you take should be written in memo form as shown on page 557.

If you need to go and find the person the caller is trying to contact, always ask for the caller's name and details of what he or she wants. This is useful if the caller becomes disconnected or rings off. Details of aids for people with impaired hearing are available from the telephone companies and in some directories.

Think it over

How could you help someone with partial hearing contribute to a discussion?

Evidence collection point

Evidence that you can collect may include records of information collected using the telephone, recordings or evaluations of simulated telephone calls, copies of messages taken by telephone.

Crossing the language barrier

How do you communicate with people who have verbal communication difficulties?

Think it over

Below is a list of groups of people who you might find it difficult to talk to. How do you think you could make communication possible or easier?

- **a** People whose first language is not English, or people who have no common language with you.
- **b** People with sensory disabilities: people who are blind or partially sighted and people who are deaf or those with partial hearing.
- **c** People with moderate or severe learning disability, including autism.
- **d** People with speech impediments, including stammering and stuttering.
- **e** Young children.
- **f** Older people.

Hints

- **a** *People with no common language*. Speak slowly and clearly. Use a restricted language and grammar, and use the same words and phrases repeatedly. Use images and body language to check that both you and they understand what has been said. Try to learn some words in their language – communication is a two-way process. Check whether a translator might be available from the local council or from a community organisation.
- **b** *Sight-impaired people* may wish to use recorders so that they have records of discussions. They should have access to RNIB services. Help them by staying in one place when you speak. It helps prevent disorientation.
  People with impaired hearing. Lip-reading requires the speaker to speak slowly and clearly facing the reader, giving them an unobstructed view. Although many deaf people have partial hearing, this is unlikely to be improved by talking loudly. Use a normal tone unless asked to speak up. You can use writing, but it is slow and limited. Use body language and gestures to add more meaning to words. Alternatively, you can learn sign language, but you need to know which system would be best.
- **c** For *people with learning disabilities,* body language is important since they can often use it to decode how you feel. They often have difficulty in receiving or giving information, and can find this frustrating. Be patient, people with learning disabilities have very individual disabilities and often you need to get used to the way in which they communicate.
- **d** *People with speech problems* should not be interrupted. Do not finish what they are saying (this is very patronising). Putting pressure on them often makes their condition worse.
- **e** *Young children* have a more restricted vocabulary and syntax (the way they structure sentences), and may react better to higher voice pitches.
- **f** *Older people's* abilities will often vary a lot from day to day. Individuals may become confused as to who you are and what you have been talking about. Remember their preferred name and some details of their life history which you can use as a basis for conversation.

Produce written material

During your GNVQ course you will produce a wide variety of written material. This will include notes, action plans, forms, CVs and letters of application, memos and reports. You will have to produce at least six pieces of material for assessment of

Communication Element 3.2., at least four of which must be written about complex subjects. The pieces of work should relate directly to the course, and be appropriate to the purpose and audience they are aimed at.

Try it

The best way to improve the way you write is to read widely, not just textbooks, and to analyse how other people communicate in writing.

Imitate those writers whose style you consider to be effective and appropriate for its purpose, and learn from the mistakes of those writers whose work is less readable.

Grammar

Below is a quick revision of basic grammar points.

Nouns

These are the names of things, whether they are people, objects, places or concepts. To show that a noun is plural (i.e. there is more than one 'thing'), most nouns have -s or -es added at the end, for example 'students', 'tomatoes'. There are some exceptions to the rule such as 'fish' and 'sheep' which do not change, and 'person/people' and 'baby/babies' which change in different ways.

Subject

This is the topic of a sentence (the 'thing' the sentence is about). It may be a noun or a pronoun (see below).

Proper nouns

These are the names of specific people, places (roads, towns, regions, countries) or objects, and begin with capital letters. For example, John Smith, North Road, Oxford, England.

Adjectives

These are words which describe nouns, for example in terms of colour, size, age or behaviour.

Think it over

We can often link adjectives with nouns without thinking, and show the way we *stereotype* groups of people in society. An example of this would be the noun 'delinquent', which means an offender or someone who neglects his or her duty. Not all delinquents are juvenile (an adjective), but adults are very seldom described in this way, and it is a term which was often used to stereotype young people (juvenile delinquent).

Think of all the different groups of people in our society and consider which adjectives are most often used to describe them. How many of them might show prejudices against that group?

Pronouns

A pronoun is a word used in place of a noun to designate a person or thing. The noun must already have been used, or be known from the context of what is written. Examples of pronouns are: 'this', 'that', 'each', 'some', 'who', 'which', 'I', 'you', 'they', 'my', 'your,' 'their', 'myself' and 'yourself'. The pronoun can either be singular or plural.

Verbs

These are action words describing what the subject of the sentence is doing.

They have *tenses* which indicate when the action occurs: in the past ('The old lady's neighbour *telephoned* the doctor'), in the present ('The old lady's neighbour *telephones* the doctor regularly'), in the future ('The old lady's neighbour *will telephone* the doctor in the morning') and the future in the past ('The old lady's neighbour *will have telephoned* the doctor by the morning').

Try it

Construct sentences using the following phrases and state what the tense of the verb is:

- **a** I am ...
- **b** she was ...
- **c** they were not ...
- **d** it will have ...
- **e** we will ...

You should check that you have a reasonable understanding of tenses and can use them appropriately since they are important in conveying the meaning to sentences.

Verbs may either be

- *active* – where the subject of the verb is doing the action, as in the examples above, or
- *passive* – where the subject of the verb is 'suffering' the action, for example, 'The doctor was telephoned by the old lady'.

The passive form is usually used, with the past tense, for reports (see the example in Figure 25.2, page 535).

Adverbs

These are words which add descriptions of verbs and come either before or after the verb. For example, 'The ambulance arrived *very quickly.'*

Sentences

A sentence may express a statement, a questions, an exclamation or a command. It is a group of words starting with a capital letter and ending with a full stop and which has a subject (a noun or pronoun) and a verb. It may also have an object (a noun or pronoun). For example, 'The old lady (*subject*) went out (*verb*)' and 'The old lady (*subject*) telephoned (*verb*) the doctor (*object*)'. These are examples of simple sentences – the basic structure of language.

Compound sentences

A sentence can become more complex by using *co-ordinating conjunctions* (such as 'and', 'but', 'or', 'not only ... but also') to join two sentences to become a compound sentence.

Clauses

A clause is a group of words making a single statement and containing a verb. A simple sentence can be described as having one *main clause,* while a compound sentence may have two (or more) main clauses.

Subordinate clauses supply additional information and cannot stand alone.

Complex sentences

In a complex sentence, there is a main clause and one or more subordinate clauses, joined by *subordinating conjunctions* (such as 'because', 'when', 'as', 'if', 'although', 'until'), relative pronouns (such as 'which', 'that') and adjectives, with commas separating the clauses.

For example, the following sentence is both a compound and a complex sentence: 'I went to meet my supervisor, having previously phoned her to make an appointment, but there was an emergency, which meant that she would be unavailable that afternoon, so I went home and completed my course work'.

Write in clear, simple sentences until you are confident in your ability to construct longer, more complex sentences.

Punctuation

Punctuation is the system of marking and dividing up your writing to aid understanding. It indicates where pauses and intonation would be used in speech.

Full stop

As already mentioned, every complete sentence should have a full stop at the end.

Comma

This indicates a slight pause in speech, and is used to separate clauses in sentences, lists of adjectives and items in lists of nouns. For example, 'The nursery was in a large, well-ventilated, brightly painted room, and was full of noisy, happy, active children taking part in painting, reading and modelling activities'. Note that there is no comma after the last adjective before a noun.

Colons and semi-colons

These are not used very frequently today. The *colon* (:) is most useful for introducing lists and before speech (although a comma is often used instead). For example:

> 'We cleared a space and assembled the equipment: buckets, spades, sieves, modelling shapes, paints, brushes, and rags for cleaning.'
>
> 'I heard him shout: "Goodbye".'

The *semi-colon* (;) is most useful for dividing items in long, complex lists and for joining two sentences which are closely linked in meaning. For example:

'We cleared a space and assembled the equipment: yellow, plastic buckets; red, plastic spades; a variety of sieves; all sorts of modelling shapes; washable, watercolour paints; brushes of different thicknesses; and, most importantly, rags for cleaning.'

'We cleared a space and assembled the equipment; this consisted of most of the items in the cupboard.'

Apostrophe

The apostrophe is used in two different ways:

- to indicate where a letter or letters have been *omitted*
- to show that something *belongs* to something or someone.

To show that a letter has been missed out, we put it where the missing letters would have been. For example, we sometimes shorten 'is not' to 'isn't'. In this case, the apostrophe in 'isn't' goes where the 'o' would have been in 'is not' if the full words had been written. In the same way the apostrophe in 'I'm' goes where the 'a' in 'am' would be. Sometimes people put the apostrophe in the wrong place because they have not learned the rule. Have you ever seen 'is'nt' or 'Im'?

If the owner of something is *one* person or thing, i.e. a mum or the car, the apostrophe would be before the 's'. For example, 'It was mum's outing' or 'The car's doors were damaged.' However, if the reference was to more than one mum or one car the apostrophe would be after the 's' to indicate this. For example, 'It was a mums' outing' or 'The cars' doors were damaged'.

The only exception to this possessive use of the apostrophe is with the word 'it'. When you see 'it's' it always means 'it is' and the belonging use is written just as 'its' *without* the apostrophe. For example, 'It's a lovely tree but some of its branches are rotten.' Mistakes are commonly made, so watch out for this!

Paragraph

This is the separating of distinct sections of writing. When you structure your work, you divide it up into sections, and these often naturally form paragraphs. At the beginning of a new paragraph you start a new line, and you can either leave an indentation at the start of the line to emphasise this or leave a space between each paragraph.

Question mark

A question mark (?) should appear at the end of every sentence which asks a question such as who, where, why, what or when.

Exclamation mark

An exclamation mark (!) should be used mainly in reporting speech when someone says something loudly, with anger, pain or surprise. In other cases, it should be used rarely, and only to stress a point.

Inverted commas

Inverted commas ('...', or "...") are the same as quotation marks or speech marks. They have several uses:

- for reporting direct speech
- for quotes from books and articles
- for titles of books, films, etc.
- for specific uses of words or phrases
- for nicknames.

For example:

> The speaker, John 'Chalky' White, said, 'There are good examples of "cognitive differences" between psychiatric carers and clients in the film "One Flew Over the Cuckoo's Nest".'

Inverted commas are often over-used or used incorrectly.

Brackets

These are generally used for inserting clauses which are separate from the main subject of a sentence, or example lists, examples, definitions, or comments about material in the text.

Conventions

Grammar and punctuation are conventions of how we should write, but there are also conventions relating to how different forms of writing should be structured and how they should be presented. In many ways, writing is similar to speaking – people automatically adjust what they say and how they say it according to their audience.

Formal language

This is used for reports, minutes, applications, official forms and business letters. The communication should be properly structured according to convention and any abbreviations and technical terms should be defined. The use of slang should be avoided, and the grammar, punctuation and spelling should be checked. Any graphs, tables or images used should be properly labelled, supplied separately from the text, and be referred to in the text.

> <u>Testing foods for sugar</u>
>
> The food material was weighed into one-gram samples and these were mixed with 10 cc of distilled water and heated to boiling point. The samples were then filtered and the filtrate poured into labelled test tubes.
>
> 2 cc of Benedict's solution were then added to each of the labelled test tubes. The solutions were then carefully heated to boiling point and were allowed to cool.
>
> The solutions were then examined for any colour change, and the results recorded in tabular form.

Fig 25.2 An example of a scientific report

Think it over

The extract from the scientific report in Figure 25.2 is written in the past tense describing what was done. It is in the passive form (see page 551). Note also that it doesn't say who did it (i.e. not 'I' or 'we'). This is an appropriate form of writing for science and medicine, but it is very austere and not necessarily applicable to social care situations.

In most cases it is an advantage for formal work to be word-processed, although some companies ask for handwritten covering letters to accompany application forms or CVs.

Informal language

This is used in notes, memos, personal communications and thank-you letters. In informal language abbreviations and slang may be used provided the recipients will know their meaning. The structure of the communications can also be more flexible, and images can be incorporated freely into the text. The work should still be checked for grammar, punctuation and spelling, but it need not be as rigorous as when using formal language.

Pamphlets, leaflets, handouts and advertisement may be either formal or informal depending upon their purpose and audience. The use of images is important when considering these forms of writing since their purpose is often to inform or persuade their target audience.

Conventions vary between countries, although most are broadly similar. One point of confusion occurs when material from the USA is used, since some words, such as colour (color), and oestrogen (estrogen), are spelt differently. Americans also use different words from those used in the UK such as elevator for lift.

Some European countries use a different convention for numbers, with 2,550.7 for example, being written as 2 550,70.

Try it

1 Read the passage below, which is without punctuation. See if you can put in the capital letters, commas and full stops to make it understandable. Suggest where new paragraphs might start.

> centres vary enormously in how much guidance and support they offer students to make realistic and considered progression plans it was found important that the regular planning and review sessions throughout the programme do not concentrate solely upon performance on the current programme some review of longer term goals should also take place checking that the process of narrowing down options is happening without support at this time hasty decisions may be made at the start of the second year on the basis of limited and inadequate information students need to be encouraged to make use of open days and other he taster opportunities taking place throughout the year ideally he visits should take place towards the end of the first year but if this does not occur early in the second year work experience outside speakers and feedback

from former students could all be used to clarify students thinking about particular courses

Here is a corrected version, which should be easier to understand!

Centres vary enormously in how much guidance and support they offer students to make realistic and considered progression plans.

It was found important that the regular planning and review sessions throughout the programme do not concentrate solely upon performance on the current programme. Some review of longer-term goals should also take place checking that the process of narrowing down options is happening. Without support at this time, hasty decisions may be made at the start of the second year on the basis of limited and inadequate information.

Students need to be encouraged to make use of open days and other HE taster opportunities taking place throughout the year. Ideally, HE visits should take place towards the end of the first year, but if this does not occur, early in the second year. Work experience, outside speakers and feedback from former students could all be used to clarify students' thinking about particular courses.

2 Correct the following passage for spelling, punctuation and grammar.

the family with its strengths and its weeknesses and it possibilities for the future is today at the center of a lively and concerned debate Legislators consider the roll of the family in shaping social policy and social workers academics and churchmen organise conferences nad symposia around such themes as 'the future of the family' or The Family Today . some sea in an apparent decline of the families and the erosian of familial values a threat to the future of Civilisation itself while others sees the institution of the family was the main barrier to the liberation of woman – indeed of humanity – in our society. some see in the apparent weakness of the contempory family and parentals authority the sauce of many contemporary evils such as juveniles crime vandalism and drug abuse.

This passage comes from *Introducing Sociology* by Peter Worsley, published by Penguin. It is the first paragraph of Chapter 4, 'The Family' on page 165, if you want to check your work.

Evidence collection point

Pieces of written work from any part of the course, which demonstrate the correct use of grammar, punctuation and spelling, will be useful evidence indicators.

Research

We have already discussed how to research information, the use of written and verbal sources, and how to use libraries (see pages 537–540). How do you ensure that the information you present is accurate and relevant to the subject?

In simple written pieces of work this is relatively easy and can be accomplished by referring to one or two sources. When dealing with more complex subjects, however, you should refer to a number of sources and check that notes you have taken are consistent with those sources. Detailed statistics and complex arguments found in reference books can be photocopied so that you can refer back to them.

Relevance

It may be tempting to plan your work according to the sources you have at hand. This may mean that you include a mass of irrelevant material. So always start with a general plan of your work, which you can then update to accommodate changes.

Beware of your own preferences. Although personal experience is a valid source of information, it can tend to be one-sided. Don't use it unless it's relevant and balanced (see below).

Balance

If you find yourself strongly agreeing with one side of an argument, you should always present the counter-arguments dispassionately, and compare the two sides.

Balance also means that you should read all the specifications of an assignment and try to complete

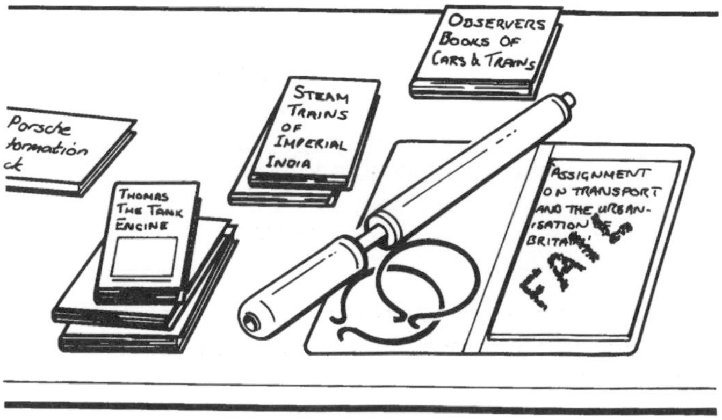

all tasks equally. Concentrating your effort on one or two parts of an assignment will mean neglecting other parts and possibly not meeting the assessment criteria.

Plagiarism

This is the copying of work, either from a fellow student or from a book, without acknowledging its source. Your best proof against this accusation is to keep your original notes, plans and rough drafts, to show how you produced the work. While phrases can usually be used without having to attribute them, if you copy whole sentences from a source, you should indicate which parts are not original, and where you obtained them.

Checking text

One advantage of using IT is that it allows you to run a spell-check and grammar check on your work to eliminate some of the silliest mistakes. This will not help, however, if you have mixed up similar-sounding words, misused a term or used it in the wrong context.

Try it

Below are 12 pairs of words which are often confused. See if you can distinguish between the pairs of words.

accept	except
emend	amend
there	their
embryo	foetus
diagnosis	prognosis
depress	repress
inter-	intra-
physician	physicist
necessary	necessity
mean	average
affect	effect
practice	practise

If you have a lot of trouble with this you might consider constructing your own glossary of terms which often get confused.

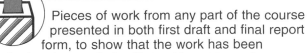

Evidence collection point

Pieces of work from any part of the course presented in both first draft and final report form, to show that the work has been checked and corrected, will provide evidence for Element 3.2.

Legibility

Even if you do not have attractive handwriting, you can usually improve its legibility. Producing a well-presented piece of work does not take much longer than an untidy one. Follow these simple rules.

- Always produce a plan – it saves time in the end.
- Write your first draft without worrying about presentation.
- For your draft(s), use paper with wide rules and wide margins, so it is easy to make changes.
- Think carefully about your first draft and make any changes necessary before you start on your final report.
- For your final report, use good quality paper.
- Use a pen with which you can write comfortably, with the best type of nib for your writing and with plenty of ink in it so you don't have to change pens.
- Use correcting fluid over mistakes, but make sure that is diluted with thinner so it doesn't make a mess.
- If you are copying work out from notes, be careful not to work when you are too tired. It's easy to make silly mistakes when you are over-tired and lose concentration.

Evidence collection point

A piece of neatly presented, handwritten work, will provide evidence of legibility.

Formats

Types of format include pre-set, outline and freely structured. You should have examples of all three types as evidence of your written communication skills.

Pre-set formats

These are usually forms where the information required has to be entered in prescribed places with restricted space. Forms vary in length and complexity from simple order forms to complicated application forms, such as an UCAS form applying to university.

Order forms

The information required on order forms is usually very limited, with little use of grammar and punctuation. (See Figure 25.3.)

GREENGATE COLLEGE

AUDIO-VISUAL AIDS EQUIPMENT LOANS

Name: Joseph Kikuyu

Group: GNVQ H&SC   Year: 2

Tutor: Helen Smith   Department: Social Studies

Equipment	Ordered for	Due for return
Video pack	10/2/95 14.00 p.m.	11/2/95 16.00 p.m.
Video player		
SLR camera	9.00 a.m. 10/2/95	11/2/95 16.00 p.m.
Kodak camera		
Tape recorder	9.00 a.m. 10/2/95	11/2/95 16.00 p.m.
OHP		
Others (please specify)		

Tutor's signature: ....

You are reminded that all materials such as tapes, films, acetates and markers are to be provided by the student or the department, and will not be provided by the AVA staff

Figure 25.3 An example of an order form

Memos and telephone message forms

These usually have an informal structure and language, but should include information on who the memo or message is for, who it is from, the date sent, and who took the message. There should also be a short heading referring to the subject matter in the memo or message.

Answering the telephone

When you answer the telephone at work you are acting as a representative of your organisation. It is important, therefore, that you give the impression of being business-like and efficient. You should give the telephone number or the name of the establishment first and then say, 'x speaking' (giving your own name). The caller will then usually say who he or she is. But if not, ask who is speaking so you can make accurate notes. It is very annoying to receive a message about a phone call only to be told that the person who took it doesn't know who it was from!

Below is a conversation between a clerk in the Special Services Division of an Education Department and a teacher from a local school.

Teacher 'Hello, could I speak with Ian Lovell, please?'

Clerk 'I'm sorry he's not in the office at the moment, could I take a message?'

Teacher 'Yes, it's Mr Holt from The Mount School, I'm ringing about Sudeb Kumar Mandal. He got all his 9 GCSEs and 'A' grades – but he's partially-sighted and he started his 'A'-level Design and Technology course in September and he still has not had his equipment upgraded. It is February now and he can't produce his assignments until he has a computer and the necessary software to work with. The IT Support Service came to school to make an assessment in October and we are still waiting. Sudeb's parents are getting very irate and threatening to write to the Director of Education to say his statemented needs are not being met. I know it's difficult with the funding but this lad's work is brilliant but it's full of mistakes he can't see when he's working on the PC. Will you ask Mr Lovell to ring me back on 01977 324750 tomorrow between 11 and 12. Thanks, goodbye.'

The message might look like Figure 25.4.

Try it

1 You have organised a group visit to a specialist play association which works with children with special needs, but the appointment has had to be rearranged for the following week when no children will be present, or until the week after when you will be able to meet the

MESSAGE

For: Ian Lovell   Date: 6/2/96

From: Mr Holt   Time: 11.35 a.m.

The Mount School

Tel. no: 01977 324750   Taken by: Karen Jones

MESSAGE:

Sudeb Kumar Mandal (a partially sighted pupil) has still not had his IT equipment upgraded and he can't proceed with his A-level coursework.

Mr and Mrs Mandal are threatening to contact the Director of Education if the equipment does not arrive soon.

Please telephone Mr Holt tomorrow (Wednesday) between 11 and 12.

Figure 25.4 A nessage form

children as well. Write a memo to your tutor stating the changed circumstances and asking for a rapid decision on when the group will make the visit. You can include your own opinion as to which date is preferable.

2 You are contacting a college by telephone to find out information about the social care courses they offer, and what qualifications they require. Construct a brief plan of what you want to say.

Accident and incident report forms

Whenever there is an accident or incident at college on placement, it should be reported on the appropriate form or book. The structure of these forms varies but a typical example is given in Figure 25.5.

Try it

Create a scenario in which you have been injured in an accident in your school or classroom. Fill in an accident report form giving as many details as you think necessary.

GREENGATE COLLEGE
ACCIDENT REPORT FORM

Please be as precise as possible and give complete details.

Date and time of accident: 3/3/96 12.30 p.m.

Site of accident: Corridor outside of room A32

People affected: Rahima Patel and George Drake both from Health and Social Care Advanced.

Injuries caused and treatment given: Rahima had a small cut on her leg which was cleaned and covered with a plaster. George had a sprained ankle which was bandaged by the first aider, and an ambulance was called in case it was broken. The hospital confirmed it as a sprain.

Details of how the accident occurred: George was pushing Rahima in a wheelchair as part of an exercise, but was going too fast and slipped on a wet patch on the floor caused by a leak in the ceiling when it rains. The wheelchair went out of control, and Rahima fell out colliding with a radiator and George collided with the wheelchair.

Signature of member of staff: Isobel Haigh

Figure 25.5 An example of an accident report form

Evidence collection point

Examples of order forms, accident reports, memos and copies of phone messages taken as part of the course or on work placement will provide evidence for this element.

Application forms

The structure of application forms varies slightly from one organisation to another. However, the basic design is usually fairly similar. Application forms are usually divided into sections for personal details, education details, employment details, other relevant details and a personal statement. The overall

College Application Form for Higher Education

Application No.

Personal details

Surname/Family Name (BLOCK CAPITALS) HADJI CHARITOU

First names[s] ELIAS

Previous surname, if changed

Correspondence address 31 THE GROVE,
MANCHESTER

Post Code M40 2HJ

Telephone No [including STD code] Daytime 0161 243267 Evening [if different]

Fax No.

Home address if different
SAME

Post Code

Telephone No. [including STD code] Daytime Evening [if different]

Fax No.

Sex: Male ☑ Female ☐

Date of Birth

Day	Month	Year
04	09	75

Year age on 31 December in year of entry

Years 19 Months 03

Special needs or medical condition
Please tick this box if you have a physical, sensory and/or other learning disability which might in some way affect your studies at the college or may require special facilities or treatment. ☐

Country of birth GREECE

Nationality GREEK

Country of domicile or area of permanent residence
ENGLAND

Applicants not born in the European Community please state:

Date of first entry to the EC

Day	Month	Year

Payment of fees
Who is expected to pay your fees? [eg Research Council, LEA, yourself, family member, employer, other]

If an LEA, which one?
MANCHESTER

Details of course[s] to which you wish to apply

Month and year in which you wish to start

Course Title	Preliminary choice of main subjects/options [if appropriate]	Mode of study: full-time/sandwich/ part-time/other. Please specify
HIGHER NATIONAL CERTIFICATE IN		
CARING SERVICES (CARE MANAGEMENT)		P. T.
Please indicate how you heard of these courses		

Last two educational establishments attached Name and address of the two most recent educational establishment attended	From		To		FT or PT
	Month	Year	Month	Year	
ROUNDWOOD HIGH SCHOOL, UPPER LANE, MANCH.	9	1985	7	1992	FT
CITY COLLEGE, PARK STREET, MANCHESTER M40 8QT	9	1992	7	1994	FT

Record of Achievement
Do you have an up-to-date (post 16) Record of Achievement?

Yes ☑ No ☐

Academic Qualifications
Applicants should, if applicable, list all subjects taken, whatever the result, in chronological order. If you are awaiting the result of any examination recently taken, write PENDING in the result column.

Level eg GCSE, A Level, RSA, Access, Degree, Professional	Subject	Date: Month	Date: Year	Place of Study	Result [grades or bands]	CATS points
GCSE	ENGLISH LANGUAGE	7	1992	ROUNDWOOD HIGH SCH.	B	
	ENGLISH LITERATURE	"	"		B	
	MATHMATICS	"	"		C	
	HISTORY	"	"		C	
	CHEMISTRY	"	"		D	
	BIOLOGY	"	"		C	
	DRAMA	"	"		A	

Qualifications awarded by
BTEC, SCOTVEC, NCVQ.

Title of award held

Title of current qualification
GNVQ HEALTH & SOCIAL CARE (ADVANCED)

BTEC registration number for current qualification

Name and brief address of college
CITY COLLEGE, PARK ST. MANCHESTER M40 8QT

Unit, module or component title				
ACCESS, EQUAL OPPS. & CLIENT RIGHTS	94	ADVANCED	1 UNIT	PASS
INTERPERSONAL INTERACTION	"	"	"	"
PHYSICAL ASPECTS OF HEALTH	"	"	"	"
PSYCHOLOGICAL & SOCIAL ASPECTS OF HEALTH & SOCIAL CARE	"	"	"	"
HEALTH PROMOTION	"	"	"	"
STRUCTURE & PRACTICES IN HEALTH & SOCIAL CARE	"	"	"	"
CARE PLANS	"	"	"	"
RESEARCH IN HEALTH & SOCIAL CARE	"	"	"	"
WELFARE SERVICES & SOCIAL CHANGE	"	"	"	"
HUMAN BEHAVIOUR IN THE CONTEXT OF HEALTH & SOCIAL CARE	"	"	"	"
SPECIAL NEEDS	"	"	"	"

Unit, module or component title				
ENVIRONMENTAL HEALTH & SAFETY	94	[illegible]	1 UNIT	PASS
DEVELOPMENT OF SOCIAL POLICY	94	"	"	"
COMMUNICATION LEVEL 3 (ADVANCED)	"	3	"	"
I.T	"	3	"	"
APPLICATION OF NUMBER	"	3	"	"
IMPROVING OWN LEARNING & PERFORMANCE	"	3	"	"
WORKING WITH OTHERS	"	3	"	"
PROBLEM SOLVING	"	3	"	"
AWARD OF GNVQ EXPECTED				
AT MERIT LEVEL.				

Work Experience
Beginning with most recent.

[Give details of work experience, training and employment]

Job Title Nature of work/training	Name of organisation	Full time or Part-time	From		From	
			Month	Year	Month	Year
CLASS ROOM ASSISTANT	ST. PETERS SCHOOL	P.T.	03	1993	04	1993
CARE ASSISTANT	THE GROVE	P.T.	05	1993	06	1993
CARE ASSISTANT	PENNINE HOUSE	P.T.	01	1994	02	1994
SUPERMARKET ASSISTANT	SUPERDRUG	P.T.	09	1992	TO DATE	

Further information
Please use this section to provide any additional information in support of your application. For example skills; relevant work experience [including voluntary work or time spent at home with your family]; reasons for choice of course; career aspirations etc.

DURING MY GNVQ PROGRAMME I HAVE WORKED WITH CHILDREN, ELDERS AND PEOPLE WITH PHYSICAL AND LEARNING DISABILITIES. MY EXPERIENCE OF WORKING WITH PEOPLE WITH PROFOUND LEARNING DISABILITY HAS PARTICULARLY HELPED ME TO UNDERSTAND AND INTERPRET NON-VERBAL COMMUNICATION. PLACEMENT WORK HAS HELPED ME TO DEVELOP SUPPORTIVE SKILLS AND TO FEEL CONFIDENT WHEN WORKING WITH INDIVIDUALS AND GROUPS.

THE COLLEGE PART OF MY GNVQ PROGRAMME HAS ENABLED ME TO DEVELOP SKILLS IN PLANNING, INFORMATION HANDLING AND EVALUATION. I HAVE CLAIMED A MERIT GRADE FOR THE PORTFOLIO OF EVIDENCE THAT I HAVE COMPLETED FOR GNVQ. I AM FAIRLY CONFIDENT THAT I WILL BE AWARDED A MERIT GRADE AT THE FINAL ASSESSMENT BOARD.

DURING MY TIME AT COLLEGE I HAVE HELPED WITH STUDENT UNION EVENTS AND WITH FUND RAISING FOR CHARITY. IN MY OWN TIME I TAKE PART IN THE LOCAL DUKE OF EDINBURGH SCHEME. THIS INVOLVES PHYSICAL AND SPORTING ACTIVITIES SUCH AS WALKING AND SAILING. I HAVE ALSO TAKEN PART IN A RANGE OF COMMUNITY PROJECTS SUCH AS WORKING WITH THE LOCAL HOSPITAL RADIO TEAM. I HAVE GAINED PART-TIME EXPERIENCE IN CARE WORK AND BY WORKING AS A SUPERMARKET ASSISTANT. THESE ACTIVITIES AND EXPERIENCES HAVE ENABLED ME TO FEEL CONFIDENT IN MY ABILITIES TO WORK WITH OTHERS AND ENABLED ME TO DECIDE ON A CAREER IN CARING.

I AM APPLYING FOR A PLACE ON THE PART-TIME HNC COURSE SO THAT I CAN GAIN PRACTICAL EXPERIENCE IN CARING BY WORKING AS A CARE ASSISTANT, WHILST ACHIEVING FURTHER ACADEMIC QUALIFICATIONS. MY LONG TERM AMBITION IS TO WORK IN CARE MANAGEMENT AFTER GAINING PRACTICAL EXPERIENCE.

Special Needs
Please give details of any physical, other disability, or medical condition, including any which might necessitate special arrangements or facilities.

Creche
Do you wish to request a place in the college creche.

Yes ☐ No ☒

References
Please give the names and addresses of two referees

1 Name J. MARLEY	2 Name M. McMANUS
Address BEDE HOUSE, COLLEGE GROVE	Address 17 THE GROVE
MANCHESTER M12 4E2	ALWOODLEY, LEEDS LS17 8QT
Telephone No. 061 247 839	Telephone No. 0532 610 543
Post/Occupation/Relationship TUTOR	Post/Occupation/Relationship FAMILY FRIEND

Declaration
I confirm that, to the best of my knowledge, the information given in this form is current and complete.

Applicants Signature Elias Hadjicharitou

Date 17 MAY 1994

Please return this form to the Enrolments Officer.

Tip: Whenever you have an application form to fill in, always take a photocopy first. Then *practise* on the photocopy so you know exactly what is going in each box and how much you can write in any 'further information' spaces. It is much better to make mistakes on a photocopy than on an original that you are sending to a prospective employer or admissions tutor!

Figure 25.6 An example of a completed application form for a course at a college presentation of the form is important since the recipients are often sorting through hundreds of applications.

Higher National Certificate in Caring Services (Care Management)

Attendance
1 day per week over 2 years

Course aims
To meet the needs of students working in a range of care settings, for example, social services, private and voluntary care, social security, police, housing welfare. These staff will acquire and demonstrate skills to allow them to develop the new management roles required by the changes taking place in the care sector.

Course content
The first year provides a broad based education in social policy, applied social sciences, methods of social research, developing human resources, the legal environment. Students will also gain experience in the use of information systems and technology. In the second year, students concentrate on care management and work, or a consultancy project as a group.

Entry requirements
The minimum age of entry is eighteen. Students should hold either an appropriate BTEC National qualification or GNVQ Advanced or A-level equivalent. Entry will also depend on the student's relevant experience. Applicants with other entry qualifications will be considered if they can provide evidence of relevant experience and ability to study at an advanced level.

Assessment
Assessment is continuous throughout the course. Academic study and practical experience in the workplace are linked to produce an integrated programme of learning. Students will work on assignments individually and in groups. Links with the line manager and tutor will develop a work based assessment of the student.

Additional information
This is a new course running for the first time in September 19–. The college is currently negotiating with a number of universities to develop links with their Diploma in Social Work programmes.

Figure 25.7 The details of the college course

Curriculum vitae

A curriculum vitae (CV) is very similar to a standard application form, but is not specific since it contains the appropriate information for most applications. Many job advertisements ask applicants to send a CV and a personal statement rather than fill in an application form. By the end of the course you should have a CV which you can update as your career progresses.

Outline formats

Personal statements

These are commonly used to support applications. They should refer to the information to be found on the form or CV. They should specify how the information relates to the requirements of the application and should answer the question of how your experience makes you suitably qualified.

A personal statement should also state how the position relates to your interests and desired career progression. For the people reading the statement this tells them about your motivation and desire to succeed.

Finally you should relate how your personal qualities, possibly shown by specific experience, make you a person able to work in a team, deal appropriately with the public, and work to deadlines (or whatever the requirements are).

You should finish by summarising why you consider yourself to be a suitable candidate. (See Figure 25.8.)

Try it

Find a copy of a local paper or a journal such as *Nursing Times* or *Social Work Today*. Pick out one or two suitable jobs advertised in it, and write some notes which you could use to write a personal statement in support of your application.

Evidence collection point

Evidence may include photocopies of UCAS and other application forms for courses, your formal CV and a personal statement relating to an application for a specified job.

Personal statement

During my present course I have worked with children, elders and people with physical and learning difficulties. I have particularly enjoyed my present placement with children with profound learning difficulties. This has developed my ability to communicate with people in different ways, according to their needs. Through my placements I have gained confidence to approach new people and situations with a positive attitude. (Please see enclosed open reference.)

The course has developed my skills in information seeking, planning activities and evaluating the results. I have had experience in assessing people's needs, listening to and then carrying out instructions. I have gained additional core skills in the GNVQ units 'Working with others' and 'Improving own learning'.

Throughout my recent studies I have been actively involved in fund-raising activities. This has helped me work as part of a team, take responsibility and to be innovative. I help with organising student union events and this has developed my organisational skills and required commitment. During my spare time I take part in the Duke of Edinburgh scheme which involves me in outdoor activities, such as walking and sailing, and working in the community. One of my projects has been working with the local hospital radio team to broadcast programmes to the wards. This has been a creative challenge and helped me develop confidence. I also have a part-time job in a supermarket which has given me experience of relating to a range of customers and responsibilities for personal time management and presentation.

I would like to take the Higher National Certificate course to enhance my academic qualifications and give me further experience of the work opportunities in the field of social care.

Figure 25.8 An example of a personal statement

Business letters

These have a standard format and should use formal conventions (see Figure 25.9).

- *Addresses.* Your address should be in the top right corner, and the recipient's in the top left (slightly lower than your own). The date should be a few lines below your address.
- *Salutation.* You should start your letter with 'Dear Mr/Mrs/Ms/Miss' together with their surname if you know the name of the person you are sending it to. If you don't, then you should use the form 'Dear Sir or Madam'.
- *Reference line.* You should then state the subject of your letter in a brief heading. It may be about an invoice, a bank account, or a general enquiry, for example.
- The *main body* of the letter should give the details of your enquiry.
- *Complimentary close.* You should finish with 'Yours sincerely' if you have used the addressee's name, or 'Yours faithfully' if you have not.

The Oaks Registered Home for the Elderly
329 High St
Midtown
MN6 8SG

Branch Manager
National Bank
Midtown Branch
27 Green St
Midtown
MN9 0FT

23 November 1995

Dear Sir or Madam

Account no. 0776539, Mrs Sophie Tucker

I am sorry to inform you that Mrs Tucker died in her sleep yesterday after a long illness. Her financial affairs are now in the hands of her solicitors, Sinclair & Howards of Longbridge. They have been informed and should contact you shortly.

In the meantime, if there is any information you require please do not hesitate to contact me at The Oaks.

Yours faithfully

R. E. Jones

Matron

Figure 25.9 An example of a business letter

Try it

Write a business letter to a bank querying details of a statement you have received.

Evidence collection point

Evidence of business letters may include writing to an organisation requesting information, or arranging a visit, or letters to businesses asking whether they are prepared to make donations for a community-based activity, such as arranging a Christmas party for children or for elderly people.

Agendas and minutes

An agenda is a list of items to be discussed at a meeting. It should include the following information: the name of the organisation or committee calling the meeting; where and when it is taking place; who the agenda has been distributed to; a list of items to be discussed.

The agenda should be distributed several days before the meeting to allow people time to consider the items on it, to add items of their own, and to make sure they can attend or send their apologies.

The items on the agenda are usually:

1 Apologies – sent by people who cannot attend
2 Minutes of the previous meeting – a reading of the minutes of the previous meeting
3 Matters arising – a discussion of any matters arising from the minutes of the previous meeting
4 Reports of activities and other meetings
5 The main items on the agenda, sometimes with details of what they will cover
6 Any other business – this allows people to bring up any other relevant matters
7 A decision about the date and time of the next meeting.

The **minutes** are notes of decisions arrived at by the meeting, whether they come about by a formal vote or are decided informally, and any actions to be taken by individuals attending the meeting. They do not require details of any of the discussion, but members may specifically ask for any points about which they feel strongly to be noted in the minutes.

The agenda and minutes are usually sent out either by the chairperson or secretary, if there is one. In many cases, members of the committee or organisation take it in turns to take notes and write up the minutes.

Structured reports

Some of the reports you will be asked to write will have defined structures. You will be told what should be included in each section and the number of words for each section, or an overall length.

Reports require careful planning before you start writing. Read through the structure you have been set and note the information that you should include. Decide how many words should be used on each section, and how many should be used on each of the pieces of information you have noted down.

Try it

Decide how many words you think should be used in each section of the following report:

Write a report comparing the advantages and limitations of the use of different imaging techniques on different anatomical features. You should use the three techniques of X-rays (plain, contrast media and body scanning), ultrasound, and magnetic resonance imaging. You should consider the chest, soft tissue and the foetus as features. You should use 3000 to 3500 words.

Hints. There are five techniques, each of which requires an explanation of how it works, what its advantages and its limitations are, and then how they apply to the three features. This means that there will be sections for each technique, which together with an introduction and a conclusion make a total of 32 sections. The average section should therefor be about 100 words in length. You will need to decide which sections require extending and which can be shortened. Remember that the use of illustrations will reduce the number of words you need to write.

Evidence collection point

Work experience placement reports are good examples of structured reports, although their length is not usually specified. Other examples that could be used as evidence include scientific reports from Unit 3, and survey reports from Unit 8.

Freely structured formats

Student-structured report

Many of the reports you will be assigned to do will be given only as a title, with some basic guidelines.

In most cases you should use a formal structure and standard conventions for writing a report. It may be a good idea to start with a table of contents if the report is of any great length. Use an introduction to state your interpretation of what the report covers and how you have structured it. It can also include some general information about which you will give more detail later in the text.

The report should be divided into sections, using appropriate headings and sub-headings. You can indicate the structure in the table of contents, or signify it in the text by applying alphabetical or numerical lists to the headings.

For example, an assignment for Element 5.3 might be to write a report on a local family planning clinic. You might structure it like this:

A Introduction
- a Where is it?
- b What does it do?

B Who runs it?
- a A brief history of the Family Planning Association
- b Present funding
- c Management

C Who works there and what do they do?
- a Advisers
- b Doctors
- c Administrative staff
- d Other staff

D Services provided
- a Opening hours
- b Services provided on-site
- c Off-site services
- d Liaison with other providers

E Clients' needs
- a Number of clients
- b Types of clients
- c Limits on range of clients
  - i By age
  - ii By gender
  - iii By ethnicity

F Physical structure of building, equipment and resources

G Possible future developments

H Conclusion

Remember to keep all your notes from the planning and information-gathering phases as these can be used to provide evidence for the grading themes.

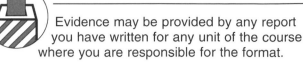

Evidence collection point

Evidence may be provided by any report you have written for any unit of the course where you are responsible for the format.

Leaflets, pamphlets and brochures

The structure of leaflets, pamphlets and brochures varies depending on the target audience they are aimed at. Care needs to be taken with layout and illustrations since many people will not bother to read them if they seem to consist of lots of words. Many pamphlets are aimed at a wide range of different groups and therefore the language in them may be relatively simple, with as many relevant illustrations as possible to make the text clear.

There is a delicate line between making leaflets as accessible as possible, and patronising the people you are trying to communicate with. If possible, translate parts of a leaflet into a another language used in your community . Note how difficult it is to translate exact meanings from one language to another.

Think it over

A drug information leaflet for teenagers would be different from one for their parents. Consider what the content of each should be.

Both leaflets might contain information on the range of drugs commonly available, their effects and the dangers associated with them. Both might contain the contact details of organisations involved in drug counselling. Both leaflets might contain information on the legal status of drugs and the penalties for their possession.

The major differences are in the aims of the leaflets and how they are illustrated. How are these achieved?

Leaflets are usually just a piece of A4-size paper, often folded in half to make four A5-size pages. Pamphlets are usually the same size but longer. Brochures are usually A4-size, and advertise a particular product or service.

Examine examples of leaflets, pamphlets and brochures in local health and community centres, libraries, post offices, banks and building societies and supermarkets. Which do you think are effective in their use of language and layout, and which are not?

Evidence collection point

Evidence may be provided by any information leaflet you have produced for an assignment. For example, an information booklet for a nursery or primary school where you have done work experience, a leaflet giving instructions for a first aid technique, or a publicity leaflet for a charity or voluntary organisation.

Using images

Presenting a large amount of material, whether in a written or verbal form, usually only holds people's attention for a maximum of about 20 minutes. There are limits to what you can present effectively in these forms since descriptions of objects or people require a great deal of detail.

Think it over

Attempt to describe the physical appearance of another member of your group, remembering to show sensitivity and tact. How long do you think it would take you to complete this so that a stranger could identify the person in a crowd? Compare your description with the effectiveness of a photograph.

Images are very powerful means of expression, which is why they are often used in advertising with very little text attached.

However, images can also be very misleading. They can reinforce negative stereotypes, and may be considered objectionable by groups being represented in them.

Think it over

Images of women have been central to the debate over women's rights. Consider the range of representation of women in advertisements. How many of them are stereotypes? Is it easy to distinguish those aimed at women and those aimed at men? Is it only the image which is objectionable, or the context in which the image is used?

Take care when deciding which images to use in discussions and as part of your written course work. Try to understand the views of others who might find the images objectionable.

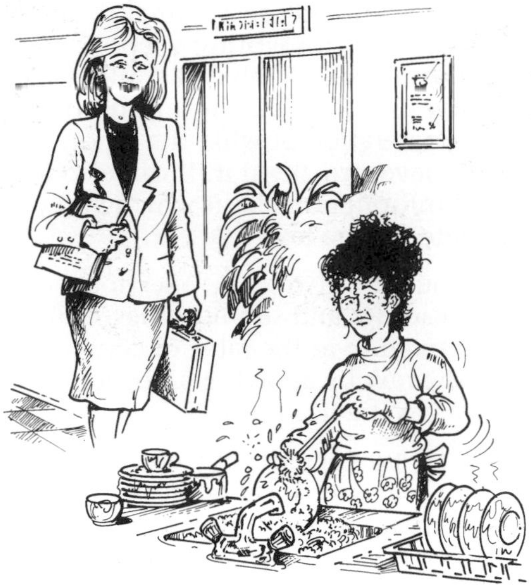

Types of image

Any graphical representation can be considered an image, and you will be expected to demonstrate the use of a range of images in at least four discussions of which two should be group discussions, and in at least four pieces of written work.

You will be expected to demonstrate skills in selecting images from a variety of sources and to construct or manufacture your own images. Where you have used images from external sources you will need to state where they were taken from.

Remember to label images clearly when it is necessary, otherwise the meaning of the images within the text may be unclear. Images used should also be referred to directly within the text, otherwise they become mere design features and lose their importance.

Symbols

Symbols are important in transmitting essential information very quickly and clearly. They are usually simple in structure and may be brightly coloured to gain attention. Good examples are traffic signs and health and safety signs, both of which follow similar conventions.

Negative instruction signs

These are contained within a red circle. If they convey the message not to do something, then they

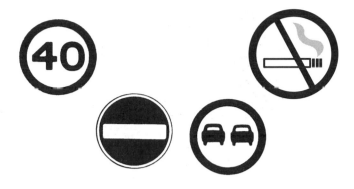

Figure 25.10 Some negative instruction signs

often have a red diagonal bar across them. Look at the examples in Figure 25.10. Do you know what they mean?

Positive instruction signs

These are shown by blue squares. Examples of this are instructions to use safety equipment such as goggles and hard hats. Can you interpret the meaning of the signs in Figure 25.11?

Figure 25.11 Some positive instruction signs

Hazard warning signs

These are usually in a red triangle for traffic signs, and in a yellow or orange triangle or lozenge (diamond) for safety signs. Can you interpret the signs in Figure 25.12?

Evidence collection point

Evidence may be collected if, for example, you do any laboratory work as part of Unit 3 or you may be given a health and safety assignment for Unit 7, including the use of safety symbols. You might be asked to do a health and safety review as part of a work experience placement.

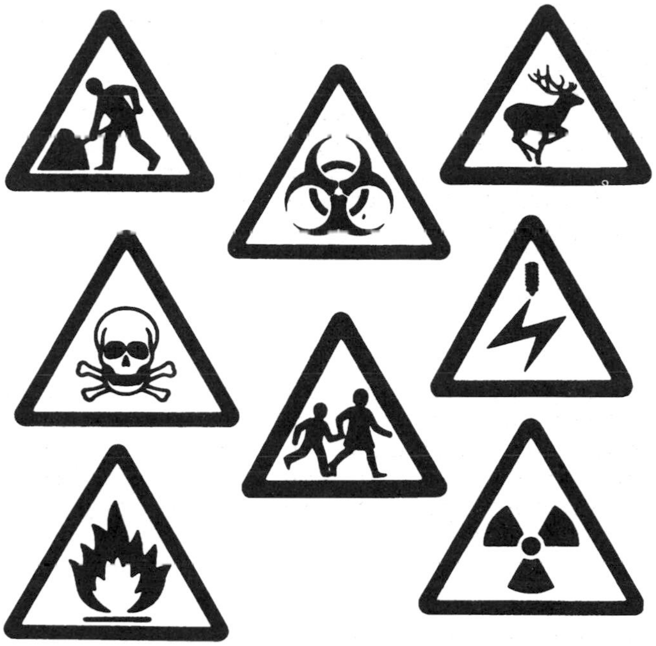

Figure 25.12 Some hazard warning signs

Maps

It is difficult to present geographical information without the use of maps, and they are used

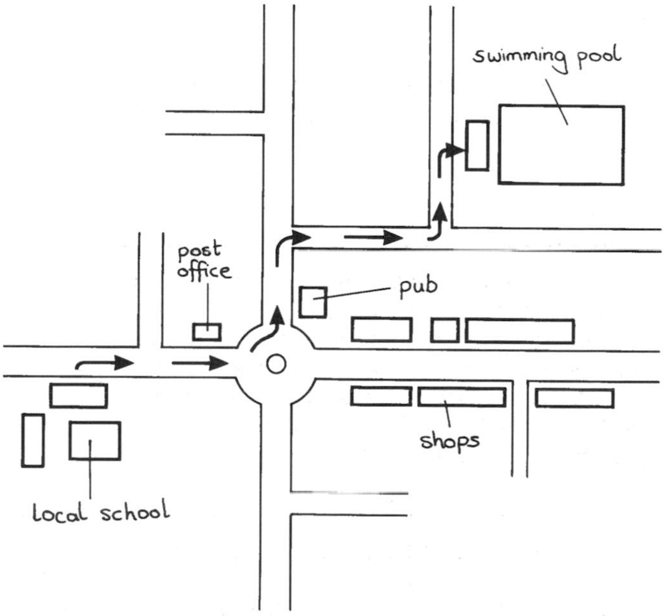

Figure 25.13 A simple map

extensively in topics where, for example, it is necessary to show the distribution of specific diseases and death rates. You might also use them to show the distribution of local health, social service, educational and leisure facilities.

Maps convey a lot of information using symbols. The interpretation of maps is dealt with in greater detail in Communication Element 3.4 but the construction and use of simple maps also comes under Element 3.3. Figure 25.13 shows a simple map showing details of how to get from a primary school to a local swimming pool.

Try it

Look at the example in Figure 25.13 and try to construct a similar map from your school or college to a local facility such as a sports centre, library, etc. Compare using the map with following verbal instructions on how to get to the facility.

Evidence collection point

Evidence may be provided by using maps to show statistical information, using appropriate symbols, and by using simple maps to back up instructions on how to get from one site to another as part of arranging a visit, for example.

Charts and tables

Charts are used to track information over a specified period of time, for example music charts or medical charts (see Figure 25.14).

Medical chart Mrs Yin-Poon 22/7/96			
Time	Blood pressure	Pulse	Respiration
00.00	145/70	133 bpm	22 pm
03.00	145/70	130 bpm	22 pm
06.00	140/70	120 bpm	18 pm
09.00	130/70	108 bpm	16 pm
12.00	120/80	95 bpm	15 pm

Figure 25.14 An example of a medical chart

Charts are also used to show lines or organisation and responsibility, such as those for the different types of care services within a local health authority. They are usually *hierarchical,* with the people (or bodies) with overall responsibility at the top, with those with the least responsibility at the bottom (see Figure 12.15).

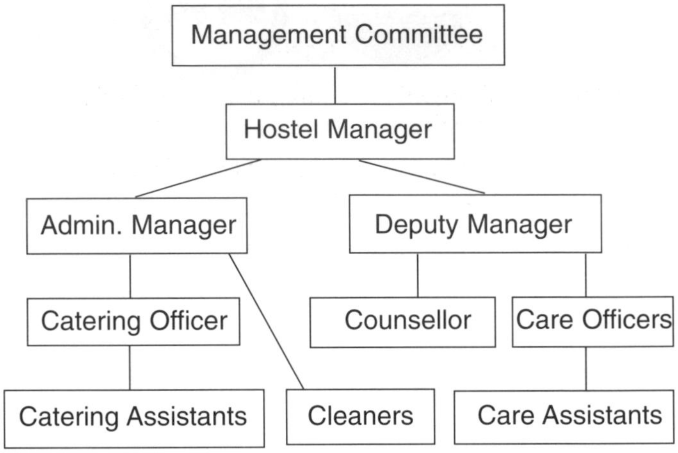

Figure 25.15 An example of an organisation chart for a hostel for young homeless people

Charts may also be used for other purposes, for example to show how systems within the body interact.

Evidence collection point

You will be expected to chart your own progress in meeting performance criteria and attaining elements and units of the GNVQ course. These will be used in tutorials to assess your achievement. On work experience in hospitals and primary schools you will also come across charts used in connection with the national curriculum and standard assessment tests, and also medical charts showing how patients progress.

Tables are similar to charts, but they do not necessarily correlate and record information hierarchically or with specific variables such as time. They are an effective way to display information in a condensed and accessible format. The columns and rows should be clearly labelled (see Figure 25.16).

Day	Time 9 a.m.–12 noon	1 p.m.–4 p.m.	5 p.m.–8 p.m.
Mon.	Toy library	Help the Aged	Youth club
Tues.	Playgroup	Women's Institute	MP's surgery
Wed.	Health visitors	Help the Aged	Youth club
Thurs.	Women's health	Playgroup	Weight Watchers
Fri.	Literacy class	Claimants' Union	Council surgery
Sat.	Tai chi & yoga	Tenants' Assoc.	Youth club

Figure 25.16 Table of weekly activities held at Northton Community Centre

Evidence collection point

You should use tables to present information and data in most units of the course.

Plans and diagrams

Plans are representations of buildings or objects drawn to scale. You should measure or carefully estimate the dimensions of the object, decide upon an appropriate scale, and produce its outline. You can then fill in the details within the outline also to scale, and decide how you are going to represent them, using symbols if necessary (see Figure 25.17).

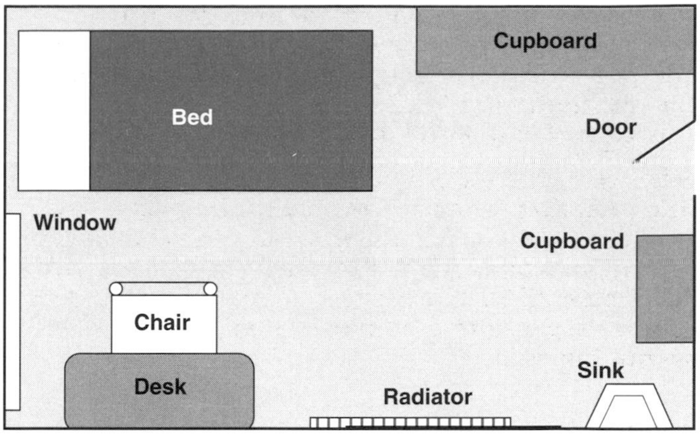

Figure 25.17 A plan of a clients' room in Midshire Hostel, scale 1:100

Evidence collection point

When on work experience or on visits you could draft plans of the rooms or of the equipment used. You do not have to be exact in the measurements, but the overall dimensions should be approximately correct and in proportion.

Diagrams are graphical or symbolic representations of objects or processes, and have a wider use than plans. They are often used to illustrate processes and concepts as well as structures and objects, and therefore their construction is less predetermined than plans. Their effectiveness depends more upon good design and imagination.

Plans and diagrams must be clear, and as simple as possible. Unnecessary detail can be confusing and may distract attention from the points you want to illustrate. They are not meant to be pictures or drawings and so it is not necessary for them to be works of art. You should refer to these illustrations in the text and explain their meaning and purpose.

Sketches and drawings

It is said that 'a picture is worth a thousand words'. Sketches and drawings not only contain a lot of information, but also help to illustrate feelings and emotions. Your choice is very important, and as a rule it is a good idea to attempt to make them as simple as possible.

Try it

Autism as a disability in its own right has only been recognised for the past 40 years, and its causes are still not fully understood. The syndrome has a range of symptoms which vary in severity and form from individual to individual. All the symptoms disrupt the development of social and communication skills, leading to difficulty with social relationships and communication problems.

It is fairly rare, with about 5 people in every 10 000 having the classical (or typical) form, but over 100 000 people in the UK suffer from autistic-like symptoms. The

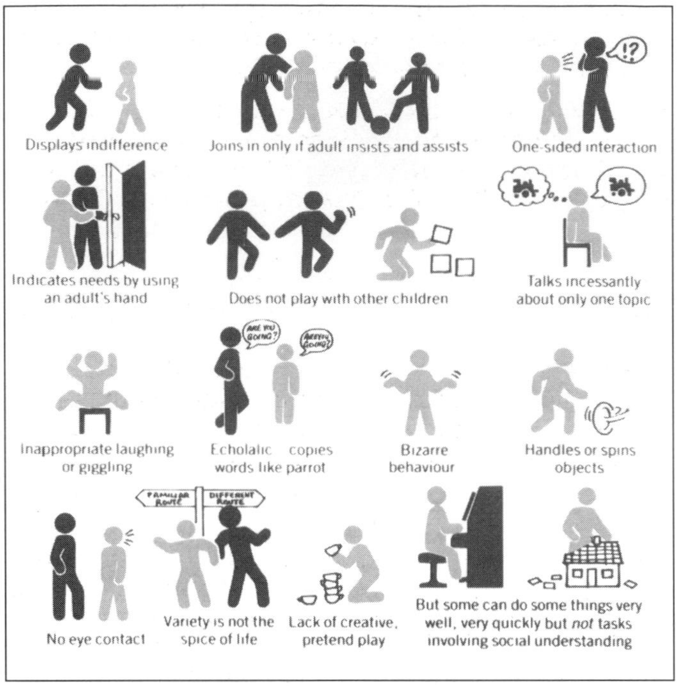
Displays indifference
Joins in only if adult insists and assists
One-sided interaction
Indicates needs by using an adult's hand
Does not play with other children
Talks incessantly about only one topic
Inappropriate laughing or giggling
Echolalic – copies words like parrot
Bizarre behaviour
Handles or spins objects
No eye contact
Variety is not the spice of life
Lack of creative, pretend play
But some can do some things very well, very quickly but *not* tasks involving social understanding

Figure 25.18 The symptoms of autism, from a leaflet produced by the National Autism Society

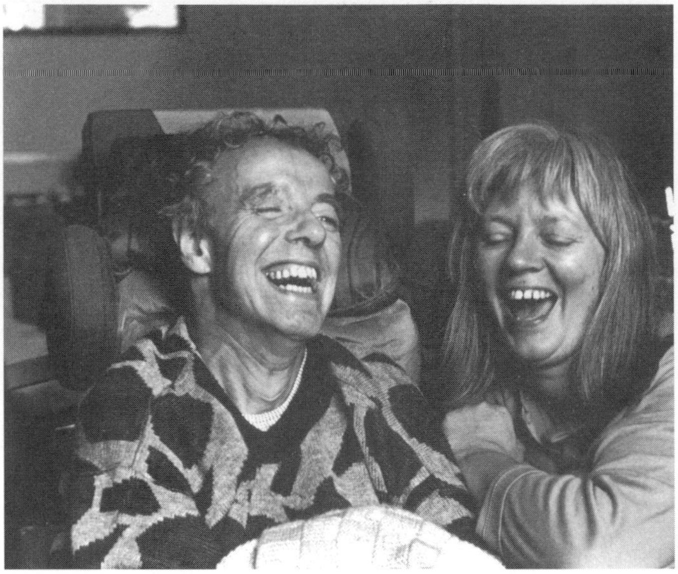

Figure 25.19 Photographs should be of good quality as well as showing appropriate subject matter
(Photo courtesy of Winged Fellowship Trust)

National Autistic Society publishes leaflets describing the main symptoms, and using the series of pictures shown in Figure 25.18 to illustrate them.

Look at the illustrations and consider how effective they are at conveying information. Choose another disability and attempt to illustrate its symptoms and effects using similar pictures.

Photographs

Photographs are valuable images since they are less open to individual interpretation and are therefore more reliable as a form of record. However, you must remember that they are selective – the photographer decides which images to capture, and the editor decides which parts of an image to use.

If you use photographs from personal sources, either your own or from someone you know, you should gain permission from the people represented in the photographs to use them. If you plan to take photographs on placement or on visits, you should always get the permission of the supervisor before using a camera.

Although colour photographs contain more detail, they are sometimes less effective than black-and-white photographs, which are also easier to photocopy.

If you are using photographs extensively for a presentation, it is worth considering using slide film, since slides can be projected onto a screen or suitable white surface. Slides usually have a fine grain and so when enlarged they show more detail. If you want to use the same photographs for inclusion in a written report, it is easy to have prints made.

The alternative to slides is to photocopy pictures onto a special form of OHP acetate sheet, but these are normally only black-and-white images, and the level of detail and the overall contrast produced is not as good.

Use and purpose of images

Use of images

You might make use of images to support both your written and spoken communications. They should illustrate points you are making, and help others to understand them. You can use the same images for both written work and for discussions, and an evaluation of the different ways the same image can be used within different contexts can help you use images more effectively.

You should adapt the images you use to the audience they are aimed at, and integrate their use fully into the overall design of your communication.

Images should be used to punctuate your communication, so that they occur at appropriate points to break up a presentation or report, rather than appearing in extensive blocks without comment or interpretation.

Producing images

Images can be obtained from a variety of sources, be personally produced by you or be copied.

If you are producing the images yourself, it is a good idea to use a separate sheet of paper, and then to cut them out and paste them into your text. The advantage of this is that if you wish to enlarge or reduce the image then you can use most types of photocopier to produce them at exactly the size you require to fit your text.

Using images from other sources requires the selection of appropriate material. Cutting out images from books and journals is destructive, and you may only do this when *you* own the book or magazine. Newspapers and magazines are a good source of images, but their quality is not always very good, and the ink can smear if you use a lot of glue to affix them to your work.

Copying images is usually easier, and can involve: tracing them onto tracing papers, greaseproof paper, or thin white paper; photocopying the original source; or scanning them into a computer and then transferring the image to the appropriate space in your text. Photocopying and scanning have the advantage that you can enlarge and reduce the size of the image to fit the space you have available.

Remember that copyright applies to images. Although this will usually not be a problem, you should be aware of it if you are copying a lot of material or are making multiple copies for distribution in pamphlets and leaflets.

The use of appendices

Appendices (singular 'appendix') come at the end of a piece of communication, usually in reports.

Some images are best placed in an appendix, for example if you want to use images which do not directly relate to the major points of your communication and hence are not directly referred to, if they expand at length on points you have made, if they relate to many different sections of communication, of if they contain a large amount or data.

In spoken communications, image can be held in reserve to deal with questions which might arise, of if a different approach is needed to get your points over if your initial plans do not prove to be effective.

Read and respond to written material

Some basic research skills were discussed at the start of the chapter, but finding appropriate sources is only part of the problem. Interpreting and extracting information can be very time-consuming, especially if you have a lot of research to do and have located a large number of relevant sources.

You will have to select your sources of information carefully, since you will sometimes find that they will contain inaccurate, outdated or conflicting information. This is why it is important to use a variety of sources and to find a number of reference books to consult.

Set texts and reference lists

Some courses have an extensive recommended reading list, while on others students consult as wide a variety of sources as possible and so very few books are recommend. It is a good idea to borrow books from libraries and to read them before deciding to buy a copy if you can. It might be possible to buy second-hand books from the previous year's students. But, *beware.* Courses frequently change and last year's book may not cover the material you need for this year's programme.

Evidence collection point

Keep lists of the books and other sources of information you use to complete assignments. These are also evidence for the grading themes of planning, and information seeking and handling.

Fact or opinion?

It is important to try to distinguish between opinion and fact when researching a subject. Even when information is presented as fact, it can still be biased by the opinion of the person who selected it, and by the way in which it is presented. This is discussed in greater depth in Unit 8.

Think it over

Can you distinguish between fact and opinion? Which of the following are facts and which are opinions?

1 AIDS started in America.
2 The average woman's brain is smaller than the average man's.
3 Margarine is healthier than butter.
4 Smoking causes lung cancer.
5 It is better for women to have children before the age of 25.
6 More children have been murdered in recent years compared with the past.

Hints

1 Opinion. There is some evidence that HIV infection has been present in America for some time, but there is no proof about where AIDS started.
2 Fact. But the ratio of brain size to body size is the same for both sexes – men just tend to have bigger bodies.
3 Opinion. Both are fats which make up too high a proportion of most people's diets. Margarine tends to contain less cholesterol and saturated fat, but it has more trans-fatty acids and can contain fewer nutrients.
4 Opinion. Smoking is a major cause of lung cancer, but there are often many other factors involved, such as diet, genetic inheritance and environmental pollution.
5 Fact. There tend to be fewer medical problems for women having children in their early twenties rather than later, but there is some evidence that there are fewer social problems for women having children later in life.
6 Opinion. The number of children murdered each year by people other than their family has remained constantly very low for the past 30 years, and has not increased at all.

Reference books

Dictionary

A dictionary defines the meaning of words. Dictionaries range in size from pocket versions, containing several thousand words, to the *Oxford English Dictionary*, which contains millions of words. There are also subject dictionaries available which contain more detailed explanations of words and terms associated with a particular area, such as sociology or medicine.

Thesaurus

This is a type of dictionary which lists words according to their meaning. It can help you find words with a similar meaning (*synonyms*), so you don't use the same word throughout an assignment.

(a) **Care 1.** *noun.* Trouble, anxiety; occasion for these; matter of concern, task; serious attention, caution. **2.** *verb.* Feel concern, interest, regard or liking (about, for, whether).
(b) **Care**
Meaning: responsibility (noun).
Synonyms: responsibility, custody, burden, supervision, guardianship, keeping, charge.

Figure 25.20 Examples of entries for 'care' in (a) a dictionary and (b) a thesaurus.

Encyclopaedia

These are books giving information on every branch of a subject and are usually arranged alphabetically. They are good for finding basic information but usually do not go into enough detail for most assignments at this level.

Extracting information from sources

Scanning

This process allows you to assess sources of information rapidly to get an overview of their structure. The first way of doing this is to look at any table or list of contents, and to see whether there is any index. The contents can give you some idea what is in the book, while the index can give you specific pages to consult.

If there is no contents or index, it is sometimes possible to flick through the pages looking at headings and sub-headings and the titles of illustrations.

Skimming

Once you have located the information by scanning, you will need to identify the key points it contains. When reading through material you will find a lot of information that is irrelevant to your research, which you do not need to read. Sometimes the opening paragraphs of an introduction, or the start of a chapter, contain a brief summary of the main points covered and this is an indication of whether it will be of any use.

It is useful if you can develop the ability to skim read. Sometimes it helps if you have a list of key words which are important, and as you look down the pages you search for these words. Once you find a section you might find useful you should consider whether the information is relevant, how recent it is, and whether you have already found the same or similar information in another source.

Key points

These are the main ideas contained in a piece of material, and can usually be summarised briefly under headings and sub-headings. Any tables, charts, graphs or diagrams can also be noted under they key points, especially if they are of direct relevance.

Evidence collection point

Any references included as part of an assignment will be useful evidence. They should include the author, title, publisher, date of publication, and volume and page number. Keep copies of notes you have made as part of researching an assignment, including key points from a number of sources.

Interpreting information

The material you read will not only be in written form, there will also be maps, charts, diagrams, tables, graphs and photographs to consider.

Maps

Maps of the world often show inherent cultural bias and suffer from inaccuracy. For example, most world maps you will come across show Greenwich meridian in the middle, so Europe is in the centre of the globe with Eastern Asia and the Pacific on the outside. This is a product of the colonial past, when European empires dominated world trade.

The inaccuracies present in world maps come from the attempts to represent a three-dimensional globe on a two-dimensional piece of paper. It is possible for the shapes *or* the size of the countries to be accurate, but it is impossible to do both at the same time.

Evidence collection point

On your course maps will mainly be used to show national data relating to the UK, or more local information, such as distribution of health, educational or leisure facilities in your local area. You may also use maps to find the locations of places you are to visit, and to work out directions on how to get there.

National data is available from sources such as the Office of Population Censuses and Surveys (OPCS), and the journal *Trends in British Society* (TIBS). These publish maps relating to population, birth and death rates, employment and unemployment statistics, income distribution and the prevalence of particular diseases.

Local maps of your area are available from a number of sources and contain varying levels of detail. Road maps showing street names can often be obtained from libraries, town halls, local estate agents or shops. Larger urban areas are often covered by the A-to-Z and Streetfinder range of books, which have indexes with all the street names at the back. Another source of maps is the Ordnance Survey, although these do not show street names and contain more geographical information, such as contour lines. Thomson Directories usually have

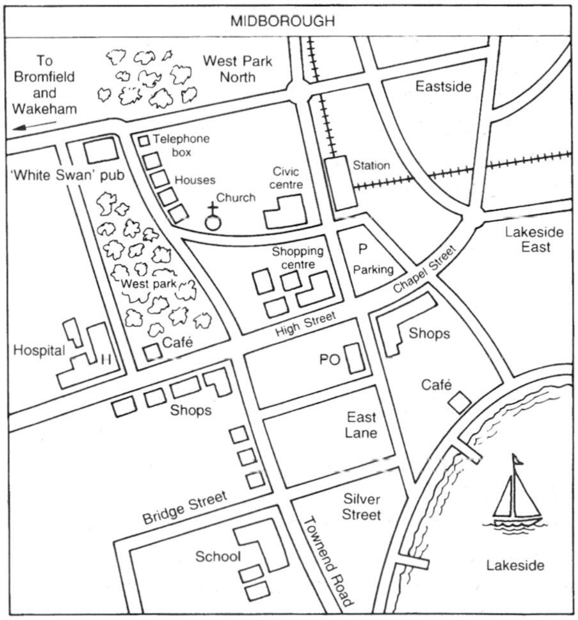

maps of local centres as well as telephone numbers, but these show very limited areas.

Try it

Your group has travelled by minibus from Bromfield to Midborough to visit a hostel for homeless people. The driver knows the way as far as West Park North. Using the map, produce written instructions on how to get from West Park North to Chapel Street where the hostel is.

Tables

Tables are sets of facts or figures systematically arranged, usually in columns. The columns and rows should be labelled. Where figures are presented, the units used should be specified.

Tables should include notes on where the information was obtained, the sizes of any samples used, and any other details of importance. Notes are often in small lettering at the bottom of the table.

Evidence collection point

1 While Sharon Lee was on placement at the community centre she often had to help people read tables and charts. Below is part of a table on the back of a packet of dried baby milk.

FEEDING TABLE

Approx. age		1–3 weeks	6 weeks	3 months	4 months
Approx. weight	kg	3.5	4.5	5.5	6.5
	lb	8	10	12	14
Number of feeds per 24 hours		5	5	5	5
Number of scoops per feed		4	5	6	7
Water per feed	oz	4	5	6	7
	ml	115	140	170	200

a How much milk should Sharon advise a mother to give a baby who weighed 4.5kg or 10lb?
b How many feeds a day would the baby need?

2 Another client, Mr Nicholaus, has been referred to the clinic by his doctor who has told him he is overweight. He is 1.75 metres tall and 40 years old.

WEIGHT CHART FOR MEN
(in stones and pounds)

Height without shoes (m)	25 yrs+	23–24 yrs	21–22 yrs	19–20 yrs
1.52	9.12–8.3	9.11–8.2	9.9–8.0	9.7–7.12
1.55	10.1–8.6	10.0–8.5	9.12–8.3	9.10–8.1
1.57	10.4–8.9	10.2–8.8	10.0–8.6	9.13–8.4
1.60	10.8–8.12	10.7–8.11	10.5–8.9	10.3–8.7
1.63	10.12–9.1	10.11–9.0	10.9–8.12	10.7–8.10
1.65	11.2–9.4	11.1–9.3	10.13–9.1	10.11–8.13
1.68	11.7–9.8	11.6–9.7	11.4–9.5	11.2–9.3
1.70	11.12–9.12	11.11–9.10	11.9–9.8	11.7–9.7
1.73	12.2–10.2	12.1–10.0	11.13–9.12	11.11–9.10
1.75	12.6–10.6	12.5–10.4	12.3–10.2	12.1–10.1
1.78	12.11–10.10	12.10–10.8	12.7–10.6	12.5–10.4
1.80	13.2–11.0	13.1–10.12	12.13–10.10	12.11–10.8
1.83	13.7–11.4	13.6–11.2	13.4–11.0·	13.2–10.12

How much would Mr Nicholaus be advised he should weigh according to the table shown here?

3 Convert a sample of these measures to kilograms as part of your Application of Number evidence.

4 In order to lose weight, Mr Nicholaus will need to be aware of how many calories he is eating in different foods. He has been told to cut down on fat but is not clear about what energy value different foods have. He likes cakes and biscuits. He needs to know how much he can eat of different foods to keep him at the correct calorie intake.

Below is a list of different foods and their calorie values. Make a simple chart of different food types and their calories for Mr Nicholaus, so he will know when he is being naughty. You can use this as evidence of 'Responding to written material' .

Caramel wafer, 54 each
Baked beans per oz, 26
Tomato soup per oz, 10.8
Toast and butter, 119
Mars bar, 284
Mayonnaise per oz, 105
Sausage roll, 112
Frozen peas per oz, 18.5
Medium pork sausages, 72 each
Choc ice, 145 each
White bread per oz, 69
Apple, 46 each
Packet of peanuts (small) 160
Crumpet per oz, 54
Weetabix per oz, 100
Prawns per oz, 29.5
Orange, 10
Cheddar cheese per oz, 120
Melon per oz, 6
Cola per oz, 12
Brown ale per 10 oz, 80
Steak and kidney pie per oz, 87
Ovaltine per oz, 109
Pork chop (grilled) per oz, 129
Butter per oz, 226
Clear mints per oz, 100
Corn flakes per oz, 102
Whisky per pub measure, 60

Banana, 119
Cod in batter, 210 per portion
Raspberries per oz, 22
Fish fingers per oz, 54
Chips per oz, 68

5 Convert ounces to grams as evidence for gathering and processing (Application of Number core skill).

Timetables

You may need to use timetables when you are planning visits. For example, you may need to compare modes of transport (bus, train or car) to decide the quickest or least complicated way to travel.

Try it

Your group has decided to travel by train on the next visit to the hostel in Midborough. You have to arrive there by 2 p.m. and you will need to allow at least an hour to get from the rail station to the hostel.

Bromfield and Wakeham → Midborough

Mondays to Fridays

	Bromfield depart	Wakeham Westgate depart	Midborough Central arrive
✕	—	**0512**	**0726**
✕	0541f	**0827**	**0833**
	0636f	**0712**	**0906**
	—	0732	0919
⊠	—	**0752**	**0945**
✕	0705c	**0807**	**1025**
✕	0834f	**0917**	**1125**
	—	0935e	1219
✕	0926c	**1017**	**1230**
✕	1041f	**1117**	**1333**
	1126c	**1217**	**1430**
✕	1241f	**1317**	**1532**
✕	1326c	**1417**	**1630**
✕	1441f	**1517**	**1704**
	—	1535e	1808
	1526c	**1617**	**1825**
	1541b	1635e	1918
	1641f	**1717**	**1930**
	—	1734e	2015
✕	1723c	**1817**	**2040**
	1841b	1932e	2159
	1918c	**2017**	**2248**
	1941b	2035e	0023

Saturdays

Bromfield depart	Wakeham Westgate depart	Midborough Central arrive
—	**0517**	**0731**
—	**0622**	**0836**
—	0634e	0916
0636f	**0717**	**0921**
—	0739e	0951
0735f	**0816**	**1031**
—	0842e	1115
0834f	**0916**	**1129**
—	0935e	1202
0941f	**1017**	**1231**
—	1035e	1312
1041f	**1117**	**1331**
—	1135e	1414
1141f	**1217**	**1432**
1241f	**1317**	**1530**
1341f	**1417**	**1631**
—	1435e	1716
1441f	**1517**	**1730**
—	1535e	1828
1549c	**1647**	**1901**
1650c	**1747**	2001
1801c	**1852**	**2106**
1849g	1941e	2234
1941f	**2033**	**2251**

Sundays

Bromfield depart	Wakeham Westgate depart	Midborough Central arrive
—	0802e	1150
—	**0832**	**1210**
0806g	1014e	1350
—	**1032**	**1410**
1054g	1214e	1550
—	**1232**	**1610**
1254g	1414e	1725
—	**1432**	**1735**
1406c	**1532**	**1800**
1454c	**1632**	**1910**
1621c	**1732**	**2004**
1722c	**1832**	**2110**
1851g	2005e	2323
2021c	**2112**	**2350**

Notes
b Change trains at Wakeham Westgate
c Change trains at Newton
e Change trains at Southford
f Change trains at Wakeham Westgate
g Change trains at Newton and Southford
⊠ Restaurant (First Class only).
✕ Restaurant.
• No catering available.
Times in **bold** type indicate a direct service.
Times in light type indicate a connecting service.
All services shown in this timetable offer
– First Class and Standard accommodation.
– Light food, hot and cold drinks for most of the journey.
– Reservable seats available.

Using the timetable below, answer the following questions.

1 Which train will you have to catch from Bromfield to get the group there in time?
2 What services/restrictions will be available on this train?
3 Will you have to change trains?

Graphs and charts

Graphs and charts can display information in tables in a more accessible way. There are several types with pie charts, bar charts, histograms and line graphs being the most common. It is easier to distinguish trends and anomalies in graphs that it is in tables, and it is possible to extrapolate these further. Read Chapter 26 for more information about graphs.

Graphs and charts may be misleading, and you should evaluate how they are presented before using them. Graphs should be properly labelled and titled, with the scales and units shown on each axis. They should also contain information about where the data used to construct them originally came from.

Think it over

Look at Graph A and consider its shape. How would it change if the vertical (y) axis started at 200 instead of 0? What effect would there be if the horizontal (x) axis was made a lot narrower or a lot wider?

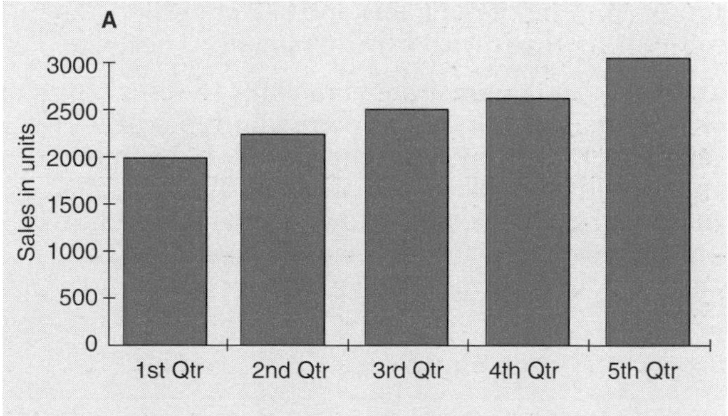

Graph B uses the same data, but shows the percentage rate of increase each quarter instead of the actual figures. Notice that it has a completely different shape to Graph A.

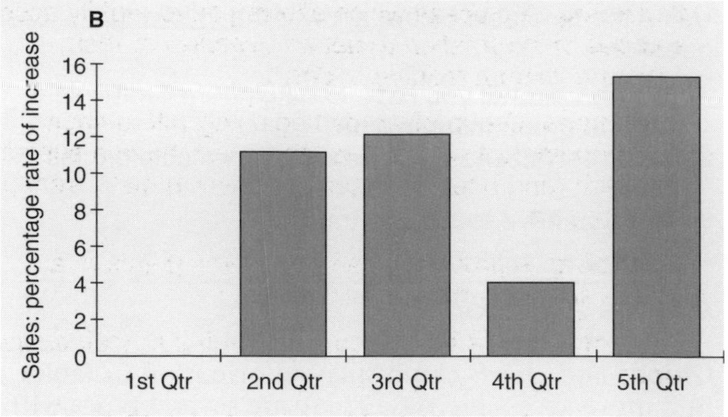

You will need to analyse and interpret any graphs you find in your research, and to select your sources of data carefully.

Diagrams and sketches

These can contain a lot of information, but need to be carefully analysed to extract the relevant information. These are especially important when they are part of the instructions for using a piece of apparatus or as part of a technical manual. You can demonstrate your use of diagrams by following a set of illustrated instructions to construct or utilise a piece of equipment in a practical setting.

A second important use of diagrams is in describing the biology of the human body. These range from micrographic representations of cells and organelles, to whole body diagrams showing entire systems such as the circulatory, skeletal or digestive systems. It is important to read a diagram's title carefully, and also to consider the scale used. You can demonstrate you understanding of diagrams and sketches by annotating them with brief explanatory notes.

You can also demonstrate your skills in responding to written materials by using particular types of diagrams but adding extra information. Examples of this would be drawing the physical structure of a building or explaining the management structure of an organisation using standard conventions, but adding your own information.

Fast Facts

Abstracts Compilations of summaries of articles and papers found in different magazines and journals.

Adjectives Words which describe nouns, such as giving their colour, size, age or behaviour.

Adverbs Words which describe verbs.

Agenda A list of topics to be discussed at a meeting.

Appendices Supplementary sections found at the end of a piece of writing which give additional information on specific points. (Singular 'appendix'.)

Author index A list of names of authors in alphabetical order with surname first followed by initials.

Bibliography A list of books and articles used in the research for a piece of work.

Charts Tabulated or diagrammatic information.

Clarification Asking questions to check that you have understood something correctly.

Clauses A main clause is a group of words making a single statement (such as a simple sentence). A subordinate clause within a complex sentence gives additional information but cannot stand alone.

Commas Used in writing to indicate a pause in speech, and to separate clauses, adjectives and items in lists.

Confirmation Similar to clarification through questions, confirmation also includes the provision of further information and the reiteration of points.

Contents A list of chapter titles in a book together with the page number, and sometimes the main subsections of each chapter. It appears at the beginning of a book.

Curriculum vitae A summary of your career so far.

Dewey Decimal System A system of categorising non-fiction books and pamphlets in which they are numbered according to their subject area. The numbers on the spine of books and the numbers on the book racks around a library are Dewey decimal numbers.

Encyclopaedias Books giving information on every branch of a subject, usually arranged alphabetically.

Format The style or manner of arrangement of a written or verbal presentation. Pre-set formats have a specific style.

Glossary A short dictionary defining specialist terms found in an article or book.

Index An alphabetical list of the subjects covered in a book. It appears at the end of a book.

Intonation and modulation The adjustment and variation in your tone of voice. It adds interest to your speech, and should change according to your audience.

Inverted commas Used to indicate direct speech or words quoted from another source.

Memorandum A note or record kept for future use, or a

fairly informal message. (Plural 'memoranda'.) Usually known as a 'memo'.

Minutes Notes of decisions made at a meeting, whether they come about by a formal vote or are decided informally, and of any actions to be taken by individuals attending the meeting.

Nouns The names of things, whether they are people, objects, places or concepts.

Objective evaluation A consideration of facts uncoloured by feelings or opinions, for example when you compare your performance with set standards and criteria.

Paragraphs Groups of sentences which have the same basic subject or topic.

Plagiarism The copying of work, either from a fellow student or from a book, without acknowledgement of the source.

Pronouns Words used instead of a noun to designate a person (or persons) or thing already mentioned (he, she, they, it).

Proper nouns The names of specific people, places or objects. They begin with capital letters.

References Found either at the bottoms of pages, at the ends of chapters or before the index at the end of a book, they give specific details about where information, ideas or quotes were researched.

Reiteration Repeating a point that has been made, but using a different context, new information or different terminology to make it.

Scanning A process which allows you to rapidly assess sources of information to get an overview of their structure without reading in detail.

Sentences Group of words beginning with a capital letter, ending with a full stop, and which have a subject and verb (and often an object) and which make sense on their own.

Skimming A process whereby the key points of a written source can be identified.

Subject index A list of books according to their subject area.

Subjective evaluation An evaluation which gives prominence to personal feelings and opinions.

Symbols Marks or characters taken as a conventional sign of an object, process or idea.

Tables Similar to charts but do not necessarily correlate and record information hierarchically or with specific variables, such as time.

Thesaurus A type of dictionary which lists words according to their meaning, and gives words of similar meaning (synonyms).

UCAS University Central Admissions System. The system for applying for a place on a course at a college or university for higher education.

Verbs Action words describing what a subject of a sentence is doing.

Chapter 26

Application of number

This chapter is designed to be an aide-mémoire, to remind you of the various techniques you will need to use achieve your core skills in the application of number.

If you have completed an Intermediate GNVQ you will already have mastered many of these skills. The chapter covers:

- **collecting and recording data**
- **tackling problems using calculations**
- **interpreting and presenting data.**

Collecting and recording data

When you need to carry out a task involving numbers (quantities, amounts, volumes, angles, etc.) ask yourself the following questions:

1 What am I trying to find out?
2 Is there more than one thing that I am trying to find out?
3 If so, what is the order of the things I am trying to find out? Take particular care to note whether the solution to one problem is necessary before you can complete another. If the problems are not dependent on one another, tackle easier ones first to give yourself practice and gain confidence. Take one problem at a time.
4 What do I already know about the problem?
5 What data have I got?
6 What data do I need?
7 How will I collect the extra data?
8 Do I need measuring instruments?
9 Once collected, how will I record the data?
10 What will I do with the recorded data to find out the answer to my problem?
11 What is the next problem to solve?

Carry on until you have found out everything you need to know.

Example

Sandcastles, a privately owned day nursery, has found that the number of its vacant places is increasing by

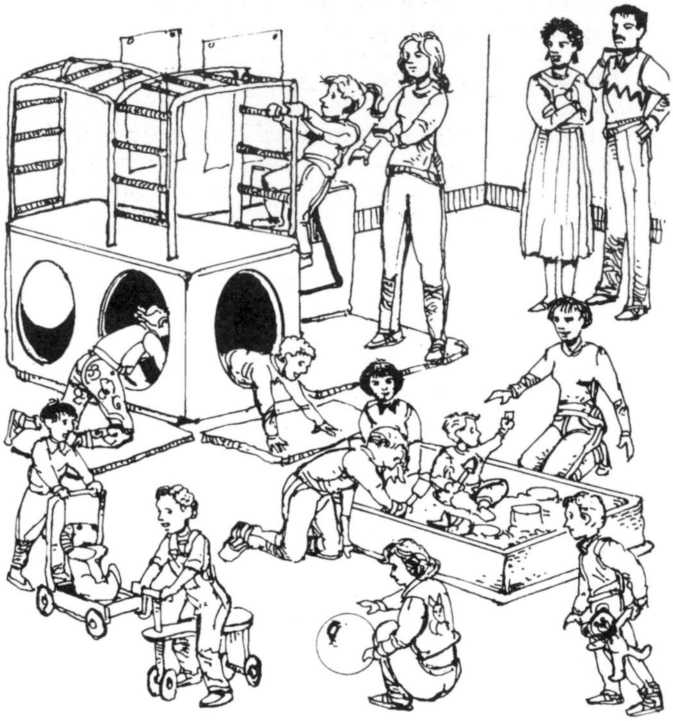

three each year, as a result of competition from a local authority nursery that has opened nearby.

Sandcastles can take 25 children on a full-time basis and charges £70 for a 5-day week, including meals. This year, the nursery has 19 children and has already reduced the number of its staff to five full-time nursery nurses. The salary bill is £31 200 per year, catering is £12 350 per year, and rental and maintenance of the premises is £250 per month. The owner, Anne Gregory, says that she has to make a 15 per cent profit to cover her living expenses; otherwise Sandcastles will have to close. Total profit which includes Anne's share, is taxed at 25 per cent. Anne knows she can only increase fees by the rate of inflation or the parents will go elsewhere. Find out the following.

1 How long can Anne continue to run the nursery if, overall, she loses three children a year to school or the rival nursery? (She will lose more than this, but some new children will enrol so the net loss will only amount to three.) You should assume a ratio of one

member of staff to four children. Catering costs £12.50 per week per child. Staff supply their own meals.

2 The staff agree to a 10 per cent cut in salary. Will this enable the nursery to stay open for a further year?

3 If fees were increased by 3 per cent (the current rate of inflation), will this enable the nursery to remain open for a further year?

4 Construct a line graph showing Anne's profit share for four years if the nursery stays open.

Anne wishes to give her staff sufficient time to find other jobs, so she has to work out these figures in advance and have them checked by the nursery supervisor. If you were the supervisor, could you work this out?

Answers

1 **Income**

This year = 19 × £70 × 52 = £69 160
Year 2 = 16 × £70 × 52 = £58 240
Year 3 = 13 × £70 × 52 = £47 320
Year 4 = 10 × £70 × 52 = £36 400

Outgoings (£)

	This year	Year 2	Year 3	Year 4
No. of children	19	16	13	10
Premises	3 000	3 000	3 000	3 000
Staffing	31 200	24 960	24 960	18 720
Catering	12 350	10 400	8 450	6 500
Owner's 15%	10 374	8 736	7 098	5 460
Total	56 924	47 096	43 508	33 680

Profit = income – expenditure

Therefore profit:

This year = £1316
Year 2 = £224
Year 3 = – £7108 (a loss!)

Tax to be paid on profit and owner's share:

This year = £1316 + £10 374 = £2922.50

Anne needs to consider closing down immediately as she will not be able to pay her tax bill and take her 15 per cent profit.

2 If staff take a 10 per cent cut in salary this year, the nursery could be run as the saving of £3120 would cover the tax bill. Next year's tax bill would be:

£224 + £8960 × 25 per cent = £2240

Profit after Anne's share is £224 plus a saving of £2496, equal to £2720 which would cover the tax bill, so the nursery would survive next year (Year 2) with the cuts in salaries.

3 Year 3 looks impossible because of the huge loss, but let's see what happens if fees are raised to help as well. An increase of fees at 3 per cent will increase the income to £48 739.60, an increase of £1419.60 but not enough to pay the tax bill on Anne's share, 25 per cent of £7098 equals £1774.50.

4

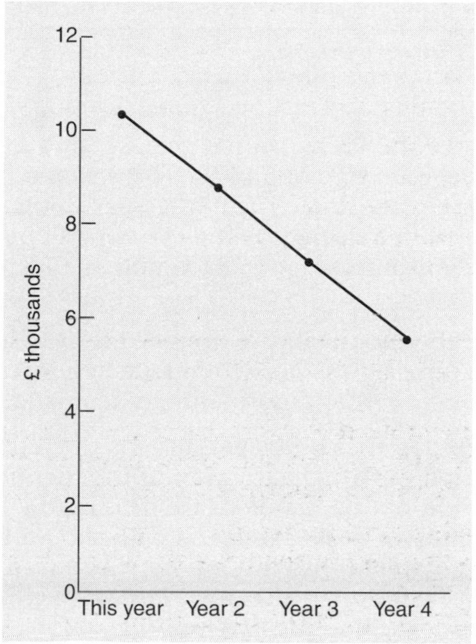

Figure 26.1 Value of the owner's profit share

Conclusion

If the staff are prepared to accept a salary cut of 10 per cent the nursery can survive for the remainder of this year and one further year. The nursery will definitely have to close after that: Anne's share is decreasing significantly each year and she cannot afford to take less than 15 per cent profit.

Measuring instruments

Thermometer

There are many different types of thermometer, but the most common are those containing mercury (silver) or alcohol (coloured; frequently red). Both types either have a scale running alongside the column of liquid or a scale engraved on the glass or plastic wall of the container.

Temperature is usually measured in degrees Celsius (°C), but some older thermometers, particularly in people's homes, may measure in degrees Fahrenheit (°F), a measurement no longer in common use. Thermometers normally read from 0°C (the freezing point of water) or a few degrees below, to 100°C (the boiling point of water). Thermometer scales are usually divided into intervals of 10°C by long marks and 1°C intervals by much shorter marks.

Clinical thermometers

They have scales in one-degree intervals, with tenths of a degree shown by shorter marks. You can read off a body temperature of 36.9°C. There would be no point in having smaller markings, say of one-hundredth of a degree, as the eye would not be able to distinguish between 36.91°C and 36.92°C with any accuracy.

Clinical thermometers are designed to read body temperature, so it is only necessary to measure a few degrees either side of normal body temperature.

The bulb of a thermometer contains the reservoir of liquid used in the construction of the thermometer, and should not be handled. To measure the temperature of a substance the bulb should be carefully lowered into it. Care must be taken that the substance has an even temperature throughout or inaccuracies will result. For example, taking the temperature of water being heated in a beaker with the thermometer resting on the base of the beaker will result in a higher temperature being recorded than if the thermometer was held or clamped off the base.

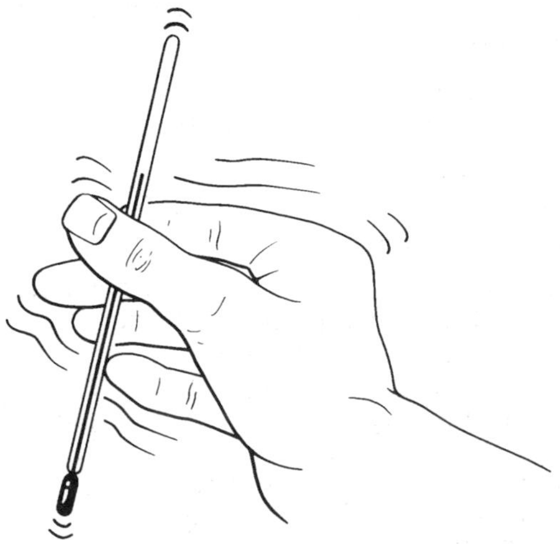

Figure 26.2 Always shake the thermometer before and after use

With a clinical thermometer, you must make sure that it is shaken before and after use. This is necessary to ensure that the mercury thread links directly with the mercury in the ball and that the thread is well below the expected reading. The thermometer is usually placed in the client's armpit, or less commonly these days, under the tongue. Allow sufficient time for the thermometer to register the highest temperature – 2 minutes. Shake and clean the thermometer after use.

Weighing scales

Just as there are many types of thermometer, there are even more types of weighing scale. Digital reading scales are simple to use as long as the scales are given sufficient time to come to a steady state. You can then read off the quantity direct. Other types may involve moving weights along a balance arm until the arm is balanced neither up nor down or reading off a scale at a point reached by the marker when the item is on the scale pan.

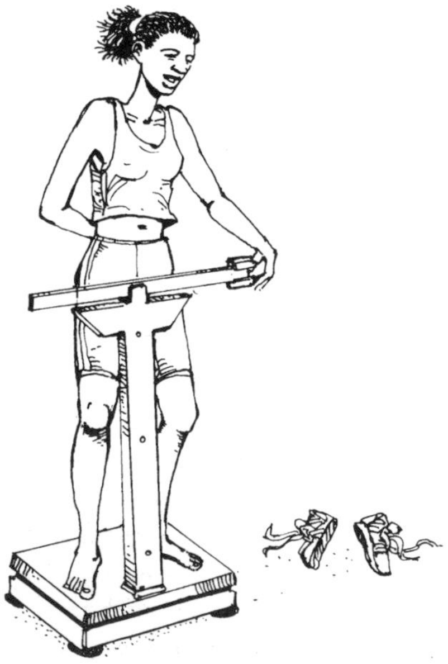

Weight is measured using either the metric or the imperial system, although the metric system is becoming the more common. As many people in the UK still use the imperial system, you will need to be familiar with it. The two systems are:

Metric system

1000 micrograms (µg)	=	1 milligram (mg)
1000 milligrams	=	1 gram (g)
1000 grams	=	1 kilogram (kg)
1000 kilograms	=	1 tonne (t)

Imperial system

16 ounces (oz)	=	1 pound (lb)
14 pounds	=	1 stone (st)
112 pounds/8 stone	=	1 hundredweight (cwt)
160 stone/20 cwt	=	1 ton

The choice of which weighing scales to use depends very much on what you are weighing. For example, it is no good weighing 4 oz of jelly babies on a weighing machine meant for commercial lorries full of gravel – the machine would not register as the quantity is too small. Similarly, in a school laboratory you would need a scale which measure to 0.1 g, but not to µg, as you would be unlikely to deal with anything quite so small.

Scale rule

Measurement of length is today most often carried out using the metric system. However, you will also need to understand the imperial system. The two systems are:

Metric system

10 millimetres (mm)	=	1 centimetre (cm)
1000 mm/100 cm	=	1 metre (m)
1000 metres	=	1 kilometre

Imperial system

12 inches	=	1 foot
3 feet	=	1 yard
1760 yards	=	1 mile

Some engineering industries do not use the centimetre, while in other contexts it is a very useful measure indeed.

School rulers tend to display both the metric and the imperial systems, so as to be as useful as possible. A ruler is a very useful instrument and you should not be without one when studying.

In a laboratory, wooden metre and half-metre rules are available for measuring. Unlike school rulers, there is no unmarked end section, so if the end of a metre rule is damaged or worn, the measurement might be inaccurate. To avoid this, it is often better to start measuring a length at the 10 cm mark and then take 10 cm off the final measurement.

Protractor

This is a semi-circle of plastic, marked with graduations around the edge and lines coming to the midpoint of the straight base. It is used for measuring angles. Do not use a scratched or faded protractor; it will lead to inaccurate results.

An angle is formed where two lines meet. To measure an angle already drawn or to draw one, you must begin by placing the line running parallel to the straight base of the protractor over a drawn line on the paper. Then read off where the other line meets the scale around the edge of the protractor. The answer will be in degrees. There are 360 degrees in one full circle, 180 in a semi-circle and 90 in a quarter circle.

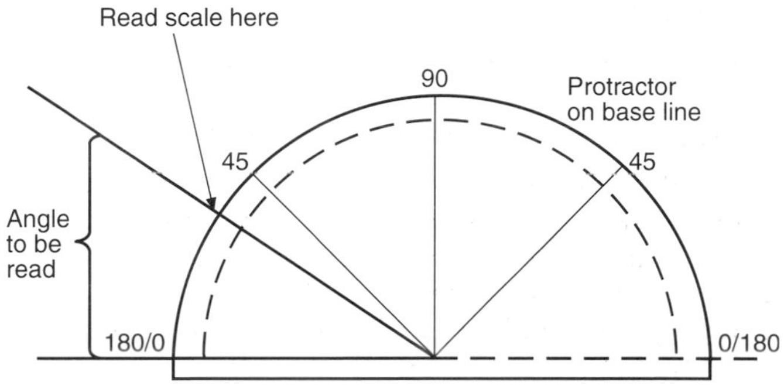

Measuring jug

Volume or capacity is measured by the metric system or the imperial system.

Metric system
1000 millilitres (ml) = 1 litre (l)

Imperial system
20 fluid ounces (fl oz) = 1 pint (pt)
8 pints = 1 gallon

A measuring jug has a scale printed or etched into the glass with either imperial or metric units. The interval between marks will depend on the size of the jug. For example, a small jug might measure individual millilitres, but a large one might only record in 100, 250 or 500 millilitre intervals.

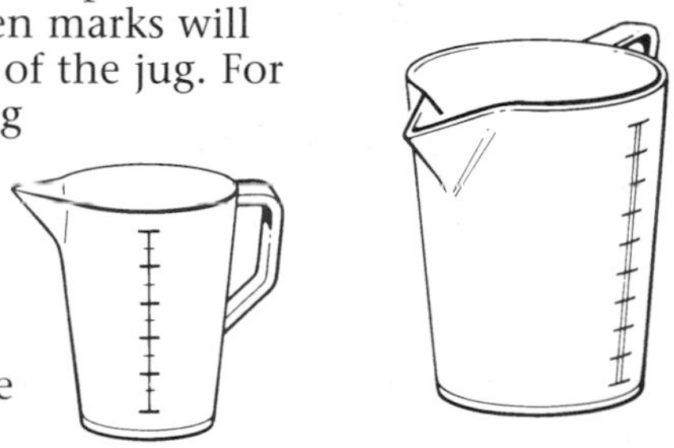

Money

In 1971, decimal currency was introduced in the UK (decimalisation), but you will still come across people who think of money in pre-decimal terms.

Pre-decimalisation money
12 pennies (d) = 1 shilling (s)
240 d/20 s = 1 pound (£)

Post-decimalisation money
100 pence (p) = 1 pound (£)

Time

Time is measured in seconds, minutes, hours, days, weeks, months and years:

60 seconds	=	1 minute
60 minutes	=	1 hour
24 hours	=	1 day
7 days	=	1 week
28–31 days/4–5 weeks	=	1 month
365 (or 366) days/52 weeks/ 12 months	=	1 year

There are two systems for measuring clock time:

12-hour clock	*24-hour clock*
12.00 a.m. (midnight)	24.00 hours
1.00 a.m.	01.00 hours
2.00 a.m.	02.00 hours
↓	↓
12.00 p.m. (12 noon)	12.00 hours
1.00 p.m.	13.00 hours
2.00 p.m.	14.00 hours
↓	↓
11.00 p.m.	23.00 hours
12.00 a.m. (midnight)	24.00 hours

e.g.
7.45 p.m. → 19.45 hours

Timetables, public services, the armed services and other organisations use the 24-hour clock.

Units of rates of change

These describe the rate (speed) at which a task or action is completed and includes:

- speed of travel – for example, miles per hour (mph)/kilometres per hour (kph)/metres per second (m/sec)
- movement of materials – for example, litres per minute (l/min) if calculating how long it might take to fill a bath with water
- inflation – expressed as a percentage
- consumption – for example, miles/kilometres per litre/gallon of petrol.

Using units of measurement

It is very important that, whether you are measuring length, weight, volume, speed or any other quantity, you use the same units consistently. It would be of no use to weigh a baby in kilograms one week and in pounds and ounces the following week; similarly, it would make life very difficult if you were carrying out a survey on drinking habits and you collected data from some people in terms of units of alcohol consumed, others in litres drunk, and yet others in pints. Always compare like with like, and measure using the same system. If you need to convert measurements between different units, use conversion tables – see page 590.

Estimation

This means an approximate judgement. It is very useful to have a rough idea of what your answer should be so that you know when you have made a mistake.

For instance, many people do not realise that when two fractions are multiplied together the answer is *smaller.* Take two simple fractions you are familiar with, $\frac{1}{2}$ and $\frac{1}{2}$. Multiply them together and you get $\frac{1}{4}$. This may seem puzzling because you are used to thinking that $\frac{1}{2} + \frac{1}{2} = 1$, and indeed it does. But when multiplying these fractions together you are in fact saying a half *of* a half and when you reflect on that, the answer *is* a quarter.

Another estimating tip, useful with both fractions and decimals, is to look at the whole-number parts. For example, if adding together 16.956 and 2.305 look at the whole numbers 16 and 2 (added together = 18). Next look at the decimals – the first shows 9 in the tenths position and the second shows 3, so when added together these are going to make at least another whole one. So your answer is going to be 19 point 'something not very big'.

Also try to get into the habit of 'rounding' in your estimates. Take for example 3.75×5.02. This sum is 'nearly 4' multiplied by 'just over 5', so your answer must be in the region of 4×5, which is 20.

Hints on estimation

Practise estimation in your work – it only takes a few seconds, but pays off in accuracy.

Another useful tip is to get used to the mental images of lengths, areas, volumes, weights, etc. so you have a better understanding of them. For instance:

- The average weight of an adult man is 70 kg, but it is not unknown for a care worker to write someone's weight as 7000 kg. Clearly, the unit has no real meaning for such a person.
- A litre is approximately $1\frac{3}{4}$ pints – we are all familiar with a pint milk bottle, so a pint is roughly $\frac{1}{2}$ a litre (just over in fact).
- Most people know the feel and size of a 2 lb bag of sugar, but many have not noticed that sugar comes now in 1 kg bags (= 2.2 lb). They did not notice that it had changed because the weight is so similar. (Since 1 October 1995, all pre-packaged food has had by law to be sold in metric measures.) So, try to remember that a pound is *roughly* half a kilogram, or 500 g (just under in fact).
- Fabric used to be measured by the yard, and a popular way of 'measuring' in the UK was to hold the length of fabric between your nose and fingers of an outstretched arm – this was approximately a yard. Now, a metre is only about 3 inches longer than a yard, and this is about the length of a nose – so if the head is turned away from the outstretched fingers, one can still use the old-fashioned way to measure a metre!

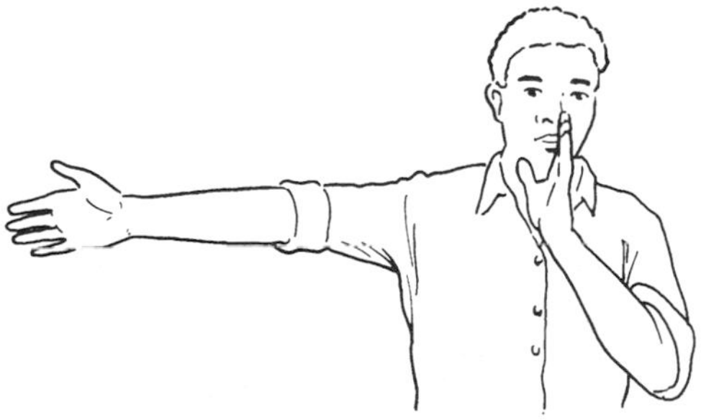

- An excellent way of estimating some lengths or heights is to use your own body. Get to know your own height in metres and in centimetres (or millimetres). The average height for a woman is 1.60 metres, and her fully stretched handspan (from little finger tip to thumb tip) is about 20 centimetres. Measure yours to check.
- Measure your biggest stride and you will always be able to pace out a distance.

When you get a feel for measurements, estimating will be that much easier for you.

Data handling

The core skill Application of Number requires you to be able to use a number of methods to collect, record, analyse and present data – from written sources (*secondary data*) and from people (*primary data* – your own research). Chapters 22, 23 and 24 cover Unit 8, Research Perspectives in Health and Social Care, in detail. The areas covered include:

- research methods – secondary research and primary research (questionnaires, interviews, observation and experiments)
- sampling methods
- designing questionnaires and interview schedules – types of question, trialling
- recording and analysing data – frequency distribution curves, scattergrams
- producing a report of your research
- presenting a report on your research.

You should read these chapters in conjunction with the information in this chapter on techniques for presenting data.

Types of data

Discrete data and continuous data

When data is collected as separated items, such as counting the number of different blood cells in a sample, these are known as *discrete data.*

Sometimes it is necessary to collect data such as a person's hourly body temperature and pulse rate over a continuous period of time. Data such as this is called *continuous data.*

Large data sets and frequency tables

As an Advanced-level GNVQ student you should be able to collect and handle large amounts of data. *Raw data* is information which has not been arranged in any order and it can be very difficult to handle.

Clearly there needs to be a plan for handling large sets of data and one way is to organise the information is the form of *frequency distribution.*

First, find the range of data – from the smallest figure to the largest. If you have a large set of numbers you may wish to group them into classes or categories.

Example

The number of clients visiting a day centre under threat of closure has been counted. The results are as follows:

6	5	10	2	12	13	11	8	15	20
18	6	12	12	4	21	10	8	13	19
13	15	11	22	6	18	23	19	11	19
14	15	7	17	19	7	22	9	14	20

This set of numbers is fairly meaningless. If you know that the set of data is likely to be a large one, a *tally chart* is a good way of collecting the information right from the start, rather than just jotting down numbers. (See Figure 26.3.)

Number of clients	Tally	Frequency
1		0
2	1	1
3		0
4	1	1
5	1	1
6	111	3
7	11	2
8	11	2
9	1	1
10	11	2
11	111	3
12	111	3
13	111	3
14	11	2
15	111	3
16		0
17	1	1
18	11	2
19	1111	4
20	11	2
21	1	1
22	11	2
23	1	1

Figure 26.3 A tally chart

As you can see, this would be giving a level of information too detailed for the task, and if you were counting for a long period of time, it would be quite laborious. A far better arrangement would be to group the data as in Figure 26.4.

Number of clients	Tally	Frequency
1–9	~~1111~~ ~~1111~~ 1	11
10–19	~~1111~~ ~~1111~~ ~~1111~~ ~~1111~~ 111	23
20–29	~~1111~~ 1	6

Figure 26.4 A grouped tally chart

Notice how the count of five in the tally is an oblique mark across the previous four. This is so that the surveyor can add up the marks quickly and does not get confused by too many marks. You can complete the tally by adding a total figure and checking this against your number of raw data to make sure none has been missed. The information gained from this chart is much more useful and quick to understand. If the day centre is expected to accommodate 30 clients each day then it is certainly under-used, if it is meant for 20 clients daily, then there is now a valid reason for keeping it open.

The figures of 1 and 9, 10 and 19, 20 and 29 are the *class limits;* 1–9, etc. are the *class intervals.* A word of warning – when you are dealing with grouped data, choose the number of groups carefully – too many destroy the pattern of distribution, while too few give too little detail. With large sets (larger than the example) between five and twenty will be sufficient. Also take care not to make the class intervals overlap, for example, 1–10, 10–20, etc. – where would you tally 10? This is a very common mistake.

If the example given dealt with, say, lengths of catheters rather than numbers of people (who are always whole numbers!) how would you mark 9.6 cm? It is over nine and under 10. By convention, the numerical limit is the mean of the highest limit for the lowest class and the lowest limit for the higher class. For example, 9 + 10 ÷ 2 = 9.5 cm. Therefore, 9.6 cm would be tallied in the 10–19 class, 9.4 cm would be tallied in the 10–19 class, 9.4 cm would be in the 1–9 class. A division like this, 9.5 cm, is the *class boundary.* The width of a class interval is the difference between the upper and lower class boundaries *not* the class limits – again a common mistake.

Extraction of data from secondary sources

It is often necessary to interpret and extract data from a mass of information at source.

Example 1

Figure 26.5 shows the blood sugar of a healthy person before and after lunch.

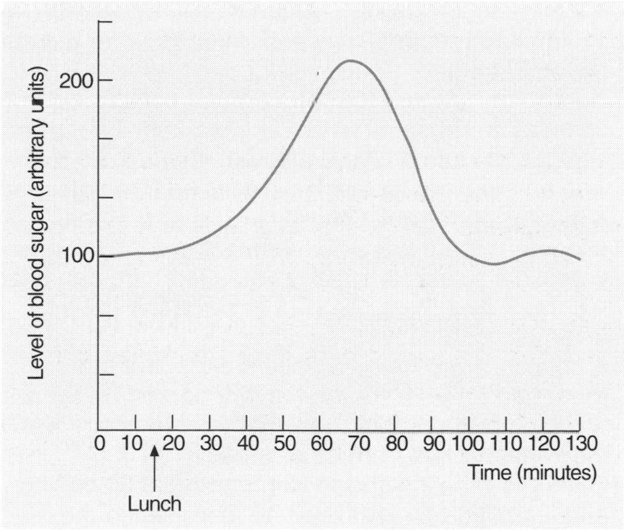

Figure 26.5 Blood sugar level of a healthy person, over a period of time, before and after a meal

a Find the blood sugar level 45 minutes after eating lunch.
b At what time did the blood sugar reach its highest level after the meal?

How to set about this:

a Lunch was eaten at 15 minutes on the graph, so 45 minutes after was 15 + 45 = 60 minutes on the graph. Find 60 minutes on the time axis and extend vertically until the graph line is crossed. At this point draw a horizontal line to meet the vertical axis and read off where it crosses the scale. This is the answer to **a**.
b Find the highest point on the graph and extend a vertical line from that point to meet the time axis. Where this line meets the axis read the scale figure. This is the answer to **b**.

Example 2

Examine the table for converting imperial volumes into metric volumes (Figure 26.6 on page 590). Find out how many millilitres is equal to 14 fluid ounces.

You will need to look up for 10 fl oz and then 4 fl oz and add them together to make 390 ml. You have extracted data from a table!

Levels of accuracy

Using a calculator

Calculators are important tools in today's society. They shorten the tedious business of long and complicated calculations and of repeating the same type of sum over and over again. Yes, of course, you should use a calculator in your GNVQ work, but a word of warning: *they cannot get the sum correct for you if you do not enter the correct data or use the right method.* It is therefore sensible to make sure you know what you are doing with the figures first.

People sometimes use a calculator to perform a long division sum and quote their answer to 6 or 7 decimal figures. They may be surprised or upset if tutors cross out all but the first decimal place or two. The fact is that those last figures are nonsense, because the data entered into the calculator may only have been gathered to an accuracy of one decimal place.

Using a ruler

If you take a ruler and measure the page width of this book, you will need good eyesight to be accurate in measuring to half a millimetre, and you certainly could not be accurate to 1000th of a millimetre. So it is usually nonsense to quote an answer to that degree of accuracy in health and care situations. A calculator will go on dividing as long as it has spaces to do so.

Decimals

A decimal number is one that includes a decimal point (for example, 0.681, 12.833, 143.99). The figures to the *left* of the decimal point count as a whole number. The place values of figures on the right of the decimal point are tenths, hundredths, thousandths, tens of thousandths, etc. For example, in the number 6.983 there are 6 whole numbers, 9 tenths, 8 hundredths and 3 thousandths.

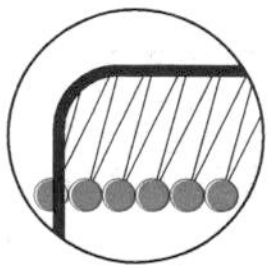

Think it over

If you get the places and decimal points in numbers muddled, for practice make a table like the one shown here and insert the following numbers into the table:

100.5	0.05	40.09
14.008	0.99	1.10
0.1	10.95	10.10

Hundreds	Tens	Units	•	Tenths	Hundredths	Thousandths
		6		9	8	3

The number 6.983 is said to have three decimal places. So has 0.003, but 142.89 only has two decimal places. The number of decimal places is simply the number of figures on the right of the decimal point.

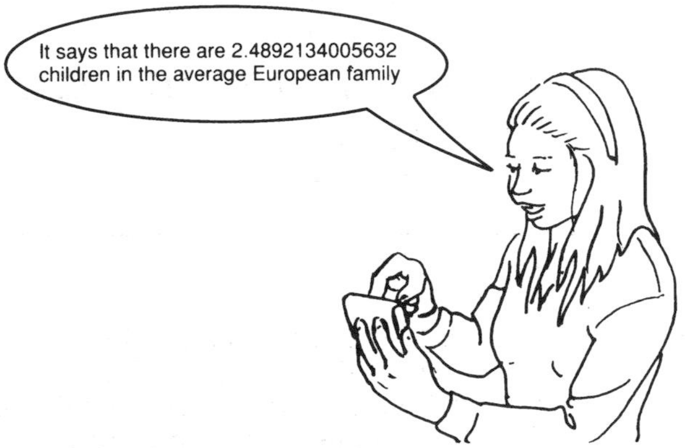
It says that there are 2.4892134005632 children in the average European family

When carrying out a calculation, you may be asked to present the answer to a particular number of decimal places. For example, to present the number 2.48821 to three decimal places, you should look at the number immediately following the third decimal place. If it is over 5 you will need to round up the third decimal figure, while if it is under 5 you leave the third figure as it is. In the example, 2.488 is the correct answer. However, if the original number was 2.48871, the correct answer would be 2.489.

Tackling problems using calculations

As a student on an Advanced GNVQ programme, you will have acquired many mathematical skills already. Check your arithmetic by working out the following problems. The answers are given on the next page. If you have any difficulties, check with your tutor.

Try it

1 The practice reception staff earned £100, £224, £226.91 and £437.28 last week. What was the salary bill for the week?

2 A locum doctor making six night calls travelled 6 km, 11 km, 4 km, 6 km, 8 km and 3 km. How far did she travel that night?

3 Nurse Troy wanted to represent her colleagues in the union at the hospital where she worked. Two other candidates' names were also put forward, so there was an election. Nurse Troy received 234 votes, and a theatre porter got 179 votes. She knows that altogether there were 534 workers in that union who voted. Calculate how many votes the third candidate received, and therefore who became the hospital union representative.

4 A hospital ward held 25 patient beds, but the day-room had only 18 chairs. If every person on the ward went to the day-room, how many more chairs would they have to find from other areas?

5 Gina, the practice supervisor, eartns £3.50 per hour, and is entitled to overtime pay at $1\frac{1}{2}$ times the standard rate if she worked more than 7 hours in any day. On Monday she worked 7 hours, Tuesday 7 hours, Wednesday 6 hours, Thursday $8\frac{1}{2}$ hours, Friday 9 hours, and Saturday $6\frac{1}{2}$ hours. What did she earn for the week?

6 The locum doctor in question 2 above is paid 20p per kilometre for travelling expenses. How much was she paid for her travel on the night in question?.

7 You have been asked to organise seating for a lecture on NVQ training at your workplace. The supervisor tells you that about 270 people are expected to attend. When you investigate the lecture hall you find it is already laid out in rows with 29 seats in a row. You do not want some people in the front rows nor others right at the back, so you decide to limit the number of rows to be used and mark the rest: 'Not to be occupied'. Work out how many rows you need. If there are 50 rows in total, how many need to be closed off? If the outside chairs of each row only will carry the closed notice, how many notices do you need to make? How many people could be seated in the hall if necessary?

8 A health visitor finds that she has almost no fuel left in her car's petrol tank. She is going on holiday by train tomorrow and she reckons on travelling by car to see four clients today. They are 16 km, 12 km, 8 km and 13 km apart. The health visitor is anxious not leave excess fuel in her car while she is away. She estimates that her car can travel 19 km on 1 litre of petrol. She certainly cannot risk running out of petrol because the area is mostly rural, there are

very few petrol stations around and her clients are expecting her to turn up. Work out how many litres of petrol will enable the health visitor to see all her clients.

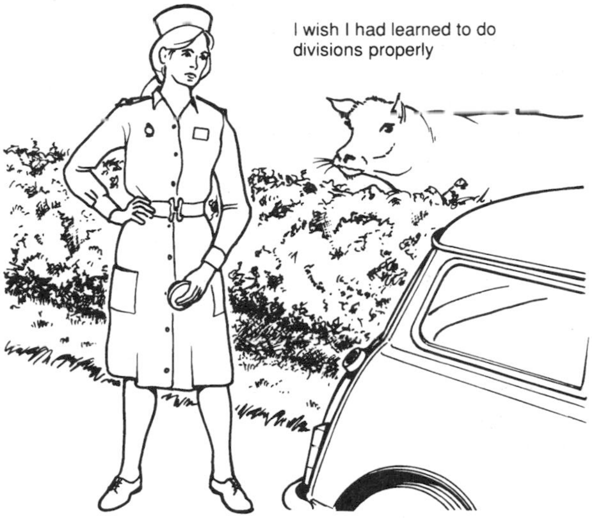
I wish I had learned to do divisions properly

Check your answers:

1 £988.19.
2 38 kilometres.
3 The third candidate received 121 votes, so Nurse Troy became the elected representative.
4 7 chairs.
5 £160.12.
6 £7.60.
7 10 rows were used, so 40 rows were blocked off, therefore 80 notices were needed. Total capacity of hall: 1450.
8 3 litres.

A word about brackets

Brackets are used with more than one number, when those numbers are to be treated as a single number. For example:

$$4 \times (6 - 2) = 4 \times 4 = 16.$$

The sums inside the brackets are always worked out first, as in the above. When more than one pair of brackets appears in a sum, the *innermost* ones are always worked out first, and then the next, and so on. For example:

$$20 - (4 \times (6 - 3))$$
$$= 20 - (4 \times 3)$$
$$= 20 - 12$$
$$= 8$$

Use of mathematical procedures in the correct order

It is important when carrying out calculations that a certain order is followed. The word BODMAS was coined by a mathematician to describe this order. It stands for the following items:

B Brackets
O Of
D Division
M Multiplication
A Addition
S Subtraction

BODMAS will help you to recall the correct order when tackling problems. For example, if you saw the sum $2 \times 3 + 4$, you would calculate the sum as:

$$2 \times 3 = 6$$
$$6 + 4 = 10$$

But if it was written as 2(3+4), you would calculate:

$$3 + 4 = 7$$
$$2 \times 7 = 14$$

Percentages

Percentage means exactly what the name tells us. 'Per' stands for 'for each' and 'cent' stands for 'one hundred'. So 'per cent' means 'for each hundred'. We can use the symbol % to represent a percentage. Percentages are really fractions which always have the denominator of 100%. Fractions and percentages are therefore easily interchanged.

To convert a fraction into a percentage, simply multiply the fraction by 100. For example:

$$\frac{6}{20} \times 100\% = 30\%$$

Example 1

Out of 396 people surveyed, 132 still smoked. Express this as a percentage.

$$\frac{132}{396} \times 100\% = 33\frac{1}{3}\%$$

To convert a percentage into a fraction, divide the percentage by 100 and simplify the fraction if possible. For example:

$$55\% = \frac{55}{100} = \frac{11}{20}$$

Example 2

In a nursing home with 40 residents, 15% of the patients had suffered a stroke in the last twelve months. How many patients did not have a stroke in that period?

Check your answer: Either (i) work out 15% of 40 and subtract the figure from 40, or (ii) work out (100 – 15)% of 40:

(i) $40 \times \frac{15}{100} = 6$, and $40 - 6 = 34$

(ii) $40 \times \frac{85}{100} = 34$

Ratios

A ratio is a comparison of two figures. We can either write the two figures like a fraction, or more commonly with the symbol : in between. For example, if one care worker earns £10 per hour and another earns £5, their earnings are in the ratio of 10:5, which is the same as 2:1. Note that in ratios the units for the quantities *must* be the same. You can multiply ratios up or down to simplify the figures as long *as you do the same to both sides* (as we did above). It is better to get one of the sides down to 1 as this gives you an idea of the relationship very quickly.

Example 1

Mr and Mrs Winston have discussed with the elder Mrs Winston whether it is the right time for her to stop living on her own and get expert care in a nursing home close by. They all decide to look further into the costs. There are two nursing homes nearby. The first costs £110 per week and the second costs £100 per 4-week month. Find out the ratio of the cost of the first home to that of the second.

First the costs must all be expressed in the same units, so it is important to bring the second home's costs to a weekly figure (or the first's to a 4-week month figure). So divide £500 by 4 to make £125 per week. Then:

$$\frac{\text{cost of first home}}{\text{cost of second home}} = \frac{110}{125} = \frac{22}{25}$$

The ratio is 22:25 in lowest terms.

Example 2

Nurse Osborne works 37 hours each week on ward 33. Find the ratio of his working hours to non-working hours.

Time working = 37 hours

Time in week = 24 × 7 = 168 hours

Time not working = 168 – 37 = 131 hours

$$\text{Ratio} = \frac{37}{131} \text{ or } 37{:}131$$

Try it

1 Mr Biggs received a very pretty card signed by all the residents of the nursing home to celebrate his 100th birthday. He is so attached to the card that everyone decides to pay a share so that the card can be framed. You decide it would be much better to enlarge the card at the colour copy centre in the next street and framed it so that Mr Biggs still has the original to look at and touch. The card measures 12 cm × 8 cm with a border 3 cm wide. It is increased so that the length becomes 27 cm.

- **a** What does its width become (it is increased in the same ratio)?
- **b** Find the ratio by which the area has increased.

2 The costs of three similar drugs for treating migraine are £3, £2.50 and £2 for 100 tablets, and the numbers of pharmacists who buy these drugs are in the ratios of 3:4:5.

- **a** Find the number of drugs bought in a locality if the total amount spent is £1914.
- **b** What fraction of pharmacists buy the cheapest drugs?

Check your answers: (1) (a) 18 cm. (b) Original area = $12 \times 8 = 96$ cm^2 and new area = $27 \times 18 = 486$ cm^2. So ratio of increase 96:486, which is the same as 1:6.

(2) (a) 79 200 tables. (b) $\frac{5}{12}$.

Proportion

If the ratio between two dimensions is always the same then the two dimensions are always in proportion. For example, if x is always in the same ratio to y, then if x halves so must y and if x doubles so must y.

Squares and square roots

When a number is multiplied once by *itself,* the result is known as the **square** of that number. It is represented by a small number 2 after and to the top of that number:

4^2 is the same as 4×4
25^2 is the same as 25×25

The square root is shown by a $\sqrt{}$. This symbol means that a number can be made from the multiplication of another number times itself (squared). For example, $4 \times 4 = 16$, so the square root of 16 is 4. The square root of 625 is 25, because 25×25 makes 625. These can be written:

$$\sqrt{16} = 4 \text{ and } \sqrt{625} = 25$$

Cubes and cube roots

Cubes are similar to squares, but this time the number is multiplied by itself *twice.* For example, the cube of two is

$$2 \times 2 \times 2 = 8$$

This can be written 2^3. Similarly, 2 is the *cube root* of 8.

Statistical averages

When you have collected a mass of data it will not be in a suitable form for analysis until it is arranged in a chart or graph format.

Another way of making data easier to understand is to try to find one value to represent several values in your data. This single value is called an *average.*

There are three kinds of average known as:

- The (arithmetic) *mean* which is equal to the total of all the values divided by the number of values.
- The *median* is the value which lies half-way along your values arranged in ascending or descending order of size. If there is an even number of values, take the mean of the two values.
- The *mode* of a set of values is the one which occurs most often. Should everything occur the same number of times there may be no mode, or conversely, more than one mode may occur.

See Chapter 24 for more about these.

Range

When considering data, you may wish to refer to the *range.* This is the spread of the values from the highest to the lowest.

For example, a hospital administrator was examining figures which counted the number of nights 14 patients stayed in a particular ward. They were as follows:

1, 4, 12, 3, 6, 11, 10, 7, 3, 5, 13, 12, 2, 4.

The report he prepared included the statement: 14 patients stayed in ward 32 overnight and the number of nights stayed ranged from 1 to 13.

Calculating rates of change

Speed is an example of rates of change. If a community nurse travels 3 miles by bicycle to visit a client and she takes 20 minutes to get here, her speed would be calculated as:

Speed (rate of change)
= distance travelled ÷ time taken

$$\text{Speed} = \frac{3}{20} \text{ miles per minute}$$

As it is usual to state speed in miles per hour (mph) or kilometres per hour (kph), it helps to convert the minutes to hours. As there are three lots of 20 minutes in one hour, she will travel three times the distance:

$$\text{Speed} = 9 \text{ miles} \div 1 \text{ hour} = 9 \text{ miles per hour}$$

Using graphs to calculate rates of change is described on page 597.

Converting between units of measurement

When you are carrying out numerical tasks such as comparing, multiplying, adding, dividing, etc. you must always make sure that your units are from the same numerical system and of the same size. If they are not, then you must convert them into the chosen size by multiplication, division, scales or tables. For example, if you are comparing the birth weights of babies born to smoking and non-smoking mothers, it would be pointless if some weights were in kilograms and others were in pounds and ounces.

Example

On a children's outing, you are trying to find out how many ice-creams you could buy for £3.00, assuming each ice-cream costs 45 pence, you would need either to convert your money to pence or the ice-cream costs to parts of a pound (this is a harder calculation and you would be very unlikely to do the sum this way).

£3.00 = 300 pence

Number of ice-creams = 300 ÷ 45 = 6 with 30 pence change.

Conversion tables

It is useful to have conversion tables (or scales) to help you convert measurements from one system to another. Figures 26.6–26.8 show some examples. You should note that these tables give *approximate* conversations for convenience.

To use the tables, find the figure on the reading you have taken and read directly across the adjacent figure. That is the equivalent in the other scale.

Using calculation

You can also convert by doing simple calculations. To convert *to* metric *multiply* by the figure shown. To convert *from* metric *divide* by the figure shown.

miles/kilometres	1.61
feet/metres	0.30
inches/centimetres	2.54

imperial (fl oz)	metric (ml)	imperial (fl oz)	metric (ml)
1	30	8	230
2	60	9	260
3	85	10 ($\frac{1}{2}$ pint)	280
4	110	15 ($\frac{3}{4}$ pint)	425
5 ($\frac{1}{4}$ pint)	140	20 (1 pint)	570
6	170	40 (1 quart)	1140
7	200	160 (1 gallon)	4500

Figure 26.6 Approximate imperial to metric conversion table for volumes

metric (g)	imperial (oz)	metric (g)	imperial (oz)
10	$\frac{1}{3}$	100	3
20	$\frac{2}{3}$	120	4
30	1	150	5
40	$1\frac{1}{2}$	200	7
50	$1\frac{3}{4}$	250	9
60	2	300	$10\frac{1}{2}$
70	$2\frac{1}{2}$	400	14
80	3	450	16
90	3	500	$17\frac{1}{2}$

Figure 26.7 Approximate imperial to metric conversion table of weight

Gas Regulo	Centigrade	Fahrenheit	Gas Regulo	Celsius	Fahrenheit
	°C	°F		°C	°F
	70	150	4	180	350 (normal hot frying)
	80	175	5	190	375 (upper limit for frying)
	100	212 (boiling point of water)	6	200	400
$\frac{1}{4}$	120	225	7	220	425 ('hot' oven)
$\frac{1}{2}$	130	250	8	230	450
1	140	275	9	240	475 ('very hot' oven)
2	150	300	10	250	500
	160	310 (normal gentle frying)		270	525
3	170	325		290	550

Figure 26.8 Cooking temperatures conversion table

pints/litres	0.56
pounds/kilograms	0.45
ounces/grams	28.34
stones/kilogram	6.35

For convenience, these figures are sometimes rounded to the nearest whole number – so 400 grams would be 14 ounces. You can use these conversion figures to make *estimates* of the approximate answer before you complete the calculation. This will help you to judge whether your final answer is likely to be correct.

For example, if you are converting 4 inches into centimetres, a rough estimate of the result would be $4 \times 2.5 = 10$ cm (2.5 is used because it is close to the actual figure and easy to multiply). (See Estimation on page 582.)

Remember

- You can check your result by converting the answer back to the original figure (for example, 10 cm ÷ 2.5 = 4 inches.)
- You can use estimates and checks like this for many kinds of calculations.

Two-dimensional shapes

A *plane shape* is one that is flat (i.e. not curved or round).

Rectangles and squares

Area

To calculate the *area* of a square or a rectangle, multiply together the lengths of two adjacent sides, (using the same units). The answer is expressed in 'square' units. For example, the area of a rectangle with sides of 6 cm and 4 cm is:

$$6 \times 4 = 24 \text{ cm}^2$$

and the area of a square with sides of 1 metre is:

$$1 \times 1 = 1 \text{ m}^2$$

We can construct a simple *formula* for calculating area:

$$\text{Area} = \text{length} \times \text{width}$$

Perimeter

The **perimeter** of a rectangle is the distance around the edge. It will therefore be twice the length and twice the width added together. For the rectangle mentioned above this is $6 + 4 + 6 + 4 = 20$ cm.

(Note that as we are simply adding up lengths there is no 'square-ing' involved.) The square mentioned above has a perimeter of 4 metres. We can construct a simple formula for working out perimeters:

$$\text{Perimeter} = 2 \times (\text{length} + \text{width})$$

The two formulae above are *word equations* to which you may wish to refer to produce core skills evidence.

Circles

Area

The formula for the area of a circle is πr^2, where:

π = the ratio between the circumference of the circle and its diameter – this is a fixed value for all circles and is 3.142 or $\frac{22}{7}$ (π is the Greek letter pronounced 'pie')

r = the radius of the circle (distance from its centre to its outside)

For example, the area of a circle with a radius of 2.5 cm is:

$$3.142 \times 2.5^2 = 3.142 \times 6.25 = 19.6 \text{ cm}^2$$

Triangles

To calculate the area of a **triangle** you need to multiply the base by the height and divide by 2.

$$\text{Area} = \frac{\text{base} \times \text{height}}{2}$$

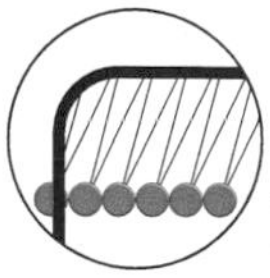

Think it over

Can you say why you have to divide by 2? Think of a rectangle cut in half diagonally.

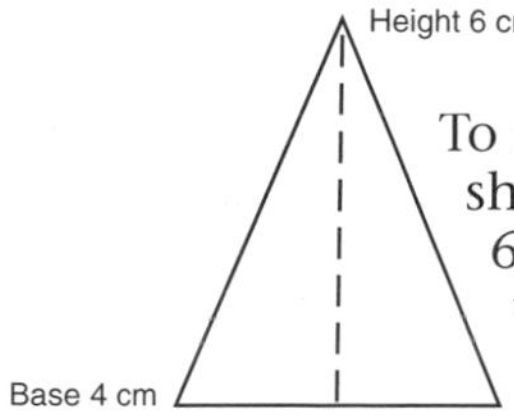

To find the area of the triangle shown here, multiply 4 cm by 6 cm and divide by 2. Note that we are 'square-ing' again, so the answer will be in 'square' units. It is:

$$\frac{(6 \times 4)}{2} = 12 \text{ cm}^2$$

Complex plane shapes

Many shapes are *combinations* of rectangles, squares and triangles, and appropriate dividing lines can be drawn if the areas or perimeter need to be calculated.

Try it

A group of students held a fund-raising activity to carpet a newly opened day-centre for older people in their neighbourhood. They chose a carpet priced at £25 per square metre and decided to make a plan of the area to find out how much money they needed. Their plan is given below. Work out how much money they needed to raise.

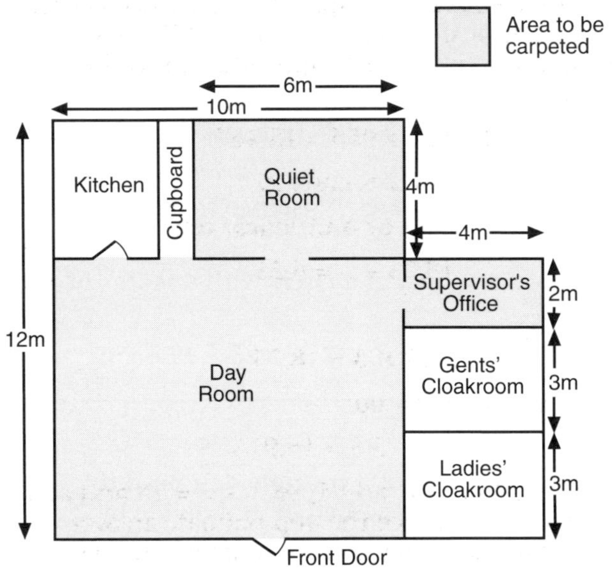

Check your answer: Area of day room = (12 – 4) × 10 = 80 m^2. Area of quiet room = 6 × 4 = 24 m^2. Area of supervisor's office = 4 × 2 = 8 m^2. Total area to be carpeted = 80 + 24 + 8 = 112 m^2. Cost of carpet = £25 × 112 = £2800.

Irregular shapes

Occasionally you may be required to measure the area of something which cannot be divided into rectangles and triangles and where you want more accuracy than rough estimation. An example might be a hand!

A reasonably accurate method is to draw around the shape on to a piece of squared paper such as graph paper. With larger objects you might need to make

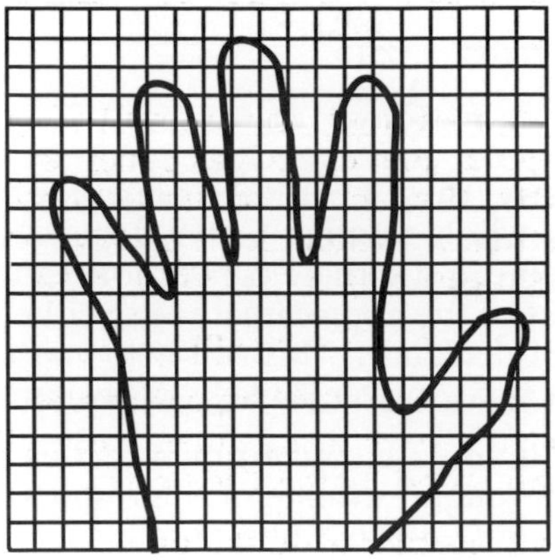

your own squared paper in bigger units. Having done that, count the *number of squares* the shape occupies.

Have a system for counting parts of squares. For example, if half or more than half a certain square is included in the shape outline then count it as a whole one, but if less than half ignore it. Finally, multiply the number of squares you have counted by the area of a single square. A surface calculation for the hand would be doubled as there are two surfaces, the palm and the back of the hand. Remember that your answer is in 'square' units (for area).

Three-dimensional shapes

One way of showing three-dimensional objects on paper is to show **elevations**. An elevation is a picture of what an object looks like if you see it from the front, side or above. These are known as the **front, side** and **plan** elevations. For example, the box in Figure 26.9 (a) can be represented as three elevations, as shown in Figure 26.9 (b).

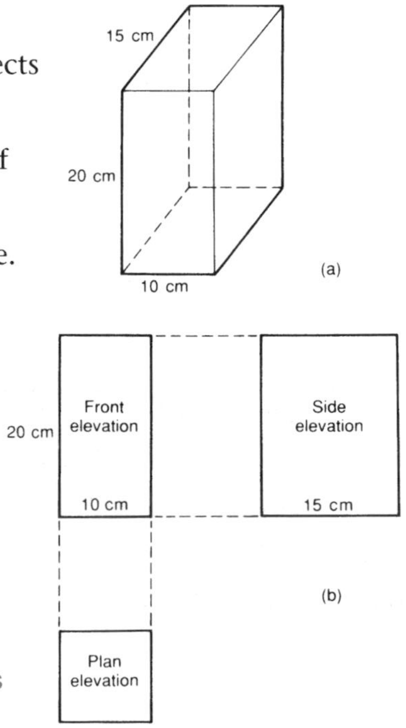

Figure 26.9 Elevations of a box

Volume of a simple solid

The **volume** of something is the amount of space it occupies. For regular shapes such as cubes or rectangular blocks, the lengths of the sides are multiplied together. For example, the volume of a block with sides measuring 5 cm, 3 cm and 4 cm is:

$$5 \times 3 \times 4 = 60 \text{ cm}^3$$

Note that this time we are dealing with three dimensions, so the answer is in 'cubed' units. This is shown by a small raised 3 after the units.

We can construct another formula for this:

$$\text{Volume of solid} = \text{length} \times \text{width} \times \text{height}$$

Always remember to make all the units the same before multiplying (for example, all in millimetres, or all in inches).

Volume of a cylinder

The volume of a cylinder is found by multiplying the area of its cross-section (a circle) by the length.

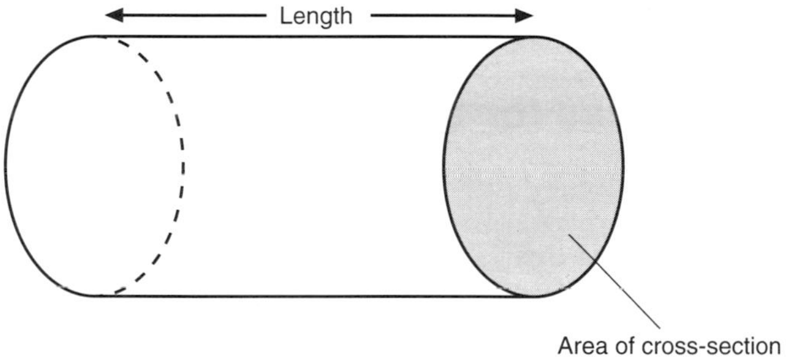

We have already seen (on page 591) that the area of a circle with a radius of 2.5 cm is:

$$3.142 \times 2.5^2 = 3.142 \times 6.25 = 19.6 \text{ cm}^2$$

Therefore, the *volume* of a cylinder with a radius of 2.5 cm and length of 10 cm is:

$$3.142 \times 2.5^2 = 10 = 196 \text{ cm}^3$$

or $19.6 \text{ cm}^2 \times 10 = 196 \text{ cm}^3$

The formula is:

$$\text{Volume of cylinder} = \text{area of cross-section} \times \text{length} = \pi r^2 \times \text{length}$$

Try it

A baby's feeding bottle has a diameter of 6 cm and it is 15 cm long. What is its capacity when full? Give your answer in cubic centimetres. Also try converting the capacity to fluid ounces (fl oz) and pints, making use of the table in Figure 26.6. One millilitre (ml) is the same as 1 cm^3.

Check your answer: Volume = 424 cm^3. Did you remember to take half the diameter to get the radius before doing your calculation?

Checking procedures

Many errors are made if simple checks are not carried out on calculations. For example, if 15 467 – 956 = 14 511, then to check this simply add 956 to the answer, i.e.

$$14\,511 + 956 = 15\,467$$

so you know the answer is correct.

Similarly, with division or multiplication:

$$18.75 \div 3 = 6.25$$

check:

$$6.25 \times 3 = 18.75$$

Also check by rounding up:

$$4.85 \times 3.5 = 16.975$$

We know that 4.85 is nearly 5, so 3 × 5 = 15 and add on half of 5 = 17.5. Since the approximate answer must be slightly less than 17.5, our actual answer is likely to be correct.

Rounding up to 10 or 100 is another way of checking whether your answer is likely to be accurate.

$$9.85 \times 19 = 187.15$$

This can be checked by approximation 10 × 19 =190, so the answer will be slightly less than this.

Predictions

This is a forecast of what is to come, usually based on a few results when many are expected. Predictions can turn out to be fairly accurate or wildly inaccurate. If you have ever watched television on general election day, you will see predictions: a multitude of different graphical displays show how

Parliament will be made up and which will be the party of government. As the night wears on and more and more results are announced, the predictions become more accurate. So with a few results, questionnaires, surveys, etc. a prediction can be made, but its accuracy is questionable. As more results become available, the accuracy of the prediction increases.

Margins of error

A measurement can never be exact, even if you are very careful. A good piece of work always includes an evaluation of the possible deviations of the results. Sometimes, particularly in scientific work, a calculation of error can be just as important as the numerical calculations involved in the work. For example, a body temperature reading of 38.3°C can point to hyperthermia (fever) if the thermometer used has an accuracy of + or – 0.2°C, but if the thermometer has an error of + or –5°C then the hyperthermia is questionable as the temperature reading could be anywhere between 37.8 and 38.8°C, the former being rather low to identify as a fever.

A method of recording margins of error is to follow the number with the range of uncertainty, for example 38.3 ± 0.2°C. It would be nonsense to record 38.328 ± 0.2°C because the extra two decimal points do not add to the accuracy of the information. (The information is also deceiving as it implies that the thermometer has an accuracy to thousandths of a degree, whereas when using a clinical thermometer the human eye is unable to distinguish to such an accuracy between each 0.1°C mark on the glass scale.)

If measurements of temperature in °C were likely to be: 36.3, 35.8, 36.1, 36.0, and the thermometer had only an accuracy range of + or – 0.5°C, it would make more sense to round up the figures to 36°C in each case.

Examples

A student is measuring a volume of urine in a measuring jug which is calibrated in 50 cm^3. He or she might feel able mentally to divide up the distances between two marks into five portions, i.e. 10 cm^3 intervals, but certainly not into 50 or even 25 parts by eye. The accuracy will be to + or –10 cm^3.

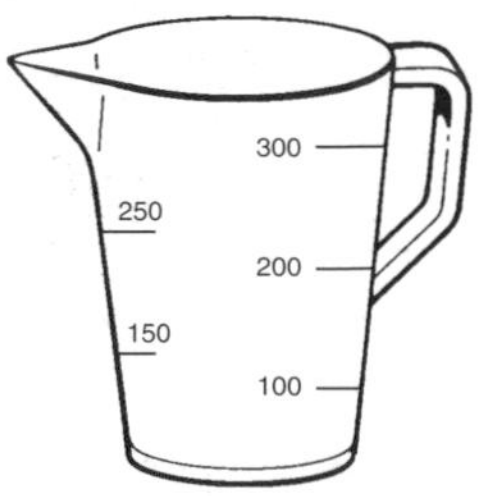

On the other hand if you are measuring the length, of say, a limb with a ruler which is divided into tenths of centimetres, and you estimate the accuracy to be 0.01 cm, you need to remember that you could make an error at both ends of the ruler so the error estimation is ± 0.02 cm.

A rough guide is that the final result should not contain more significant numbers than the measurement with the largest error calculation. For example, if you were calculating the area of a skin graft 4.2 ± 0.02 cm × 3.3 ± 0.1 cm, there would be no point in quoting the result at 13.86 cm^2 – 13.9 cm^2 or even 14 cm^2 would be accurate enough.

An alternative way of quoting error is by the use of percentages. In the example used above:

$$0.02 \times 100 \div 4.2 = 0.4\%$$
$$0.1 \times 100 \div 3.3 = 3.0\%$$

The final result would be 13.86 cm^3 ± 3.48%. Note that the final result has added the percentage errors. This has led to quite a large error estimation which some might feel is too great. A modification of this by some people would be to use the percentage error of the least accurate factor rather than by adding the two together, for example 13.86 cm^2 ± 3%.

Techniques for presenting data

There is a range of different ways to present data you have collected. Graphs are often used to show *changes* in data over a certain period of time. Graphs, bar charts, pie charts and tables can be used to illustrate text, and doing this will help you gain core skills in Communication.

Whatever method you choose to present your data, you should *always* label the presentation clearly. The work should be neat (and coloured if appropriate).

If you are using figures to work out an anwer, *always* show your workings. Core skills credit the methods used and the process followed, as well as getting the answer right.

Tables

A table can be used to present a range of information in a neat way. It is particularly useful if you want to compare data.

For example, Figure 26.10 shows the formal qualification of staff in a nursery at two different times since it opened.

Qualification changes of staff	1985	%	1991	%
NNEB	2	20	5	50
BTEC Nursery Nursing	0	0	2	20
Teaching	1	10	1	10
PPA	3	30	2	20
None	4	40	0	0
Total	10	100	10	100

Figure 26.10 Tabulated data

Pie charts

If a circle is divided into 1-degree segments, there will be 360 segments in total. Segments of varying size in a circle are often used as a clear way of showing shares of a whole.

Example

Using the example of Sandcastles Nursery (on page 578), we can immediately see the different amounts spent on keeping the nursery going (Figure 26.11).

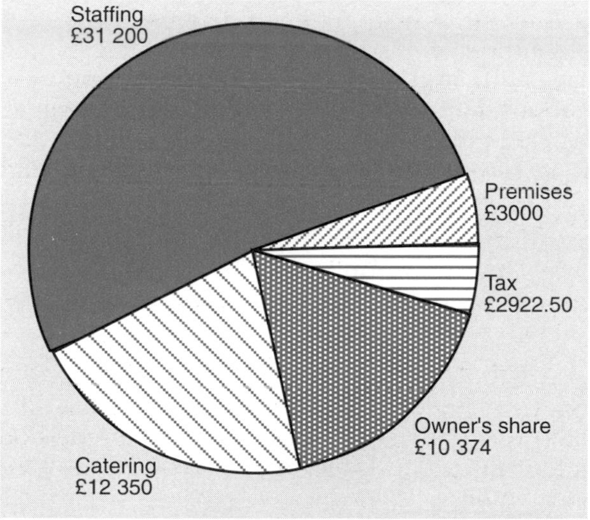

Figure 26.11 Sandcastles Nursery – expenditure for this year

As with almost all other care establishments, staffing Sandcastles accounts for most of the outgoings, – approximately half the outgoings. The owner's share and the catering are almost identical, as are the premises and the tax. The pie chart allows us to evaluate the data quickly and easily. Now you can see how useful pie charts are.

Try it

Seaview, a day centre for people with learning difficulties, found that it spent its money in the following way:

Salaries £60 000
Premises £15 000
Catering £9000
Maintenance £3000
Other items £3000

Construct a pie chart to illustrate this so that some clients and relatives might understand where the income goes.

First, find the total of the expenditure or outgoings, so add all the figures together

$$= £90\ 000$$

This must be equal to 360 degrees. Therefore, to find out how many pounds each degree is worth divide £90 000 by 360.

$$\frac{90\ 000}{360} = 250$$

So, each degree of the circle represents £250. We know the value of every item of expenditure, so if we divide each one by 250, we will find out how many degrees of the circle individual segments need to be. For example, premises cost £15 000 so:

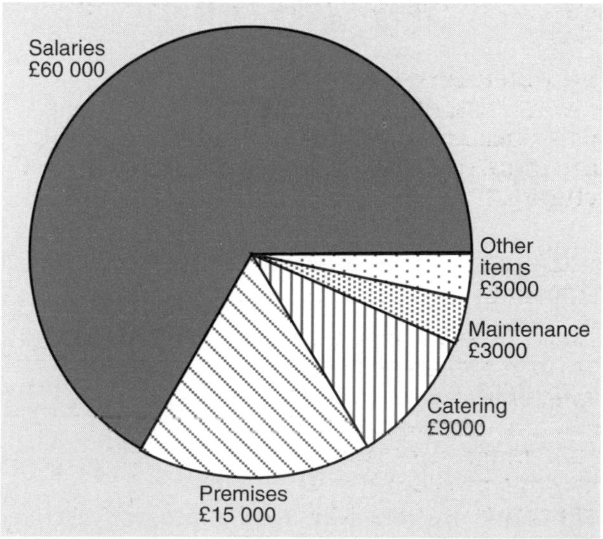

Figure 26.12 Expenditure of Seaview day centre, 1995

$$\frac{15\,000}{250} = 60 \text{ degrees}$$

Place your protractor on a faint pencil line through the centre of the circle to get a start and measure 60 degrees – label this segment, 'Premises'. (See page 581 for information on using a protractor if you are unsure.)

Work through the other costs in the same way and you should have a pie chart like the one in Figure 26.12.

If you are using a computer you may be able to construct graphs and pie charts quite easily. Discuss this with your IT tutor.

Pictograms

These are bar charts made up of pictures rather than bars.

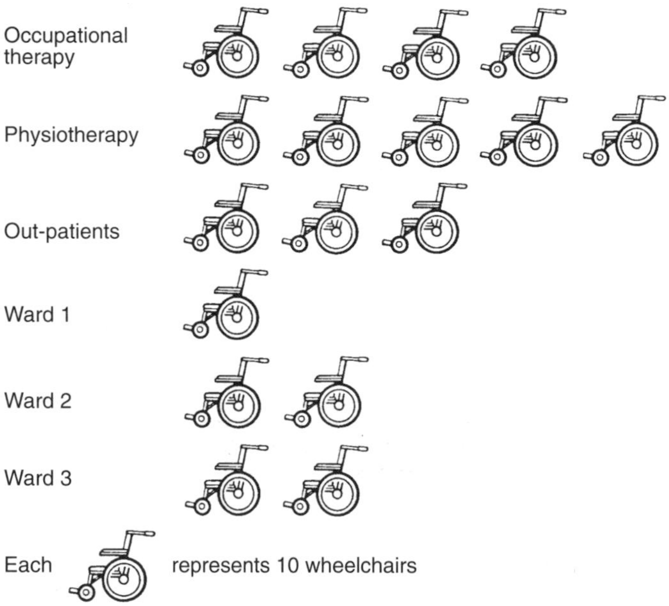

Figure 26.13 Number of wheelchairs in Turley Hospital departments

Bar charts

One common (and simple) type of graph is a bar chart. An example is shown in Figure 26.14.

- Bar charts are generally used to present discrete data, i.e. where it is collected as separate items. In Figure 26.14 the numbers of patients were collected separately on each day of the week.
- All the bars are the same width.
- The height of the bar indicates the frequancy.
- Only the vertical axis has a numerical scale.

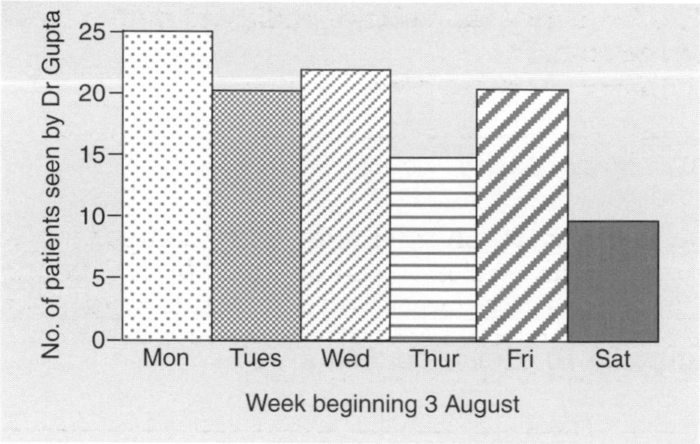

Figure 26.14 Number of patients seen by Dr Gupta in the week beginning 3 August

Histograms

Histograms look like bar charts, but there are in fact quite different. A histogram is a diagramatic representation of *frequency distribution* (see Chapter 24, page 520), and is therefore used to present continuous data (data collected over a continuous period). Figure 26.15 shows the number of clients visiting a day centre over a certain period of time. The most common number of daily visitors in 10–19.

- In a histogram, the width of the columns is always in proportion to the size of the class or group it represents. Therefore columns may have different widths.

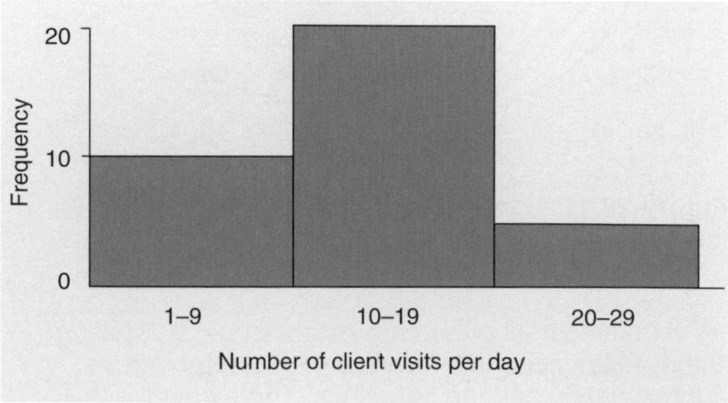

Figure 26.15 Number of clients visiting Hewland Day Centre

- The frequency for a class is indicated by the area of the column.
- Both axes have numerical scales.

Interpreting a histogram

If the columns are all the same width, comparison of the frequencies of classes can be made by comparing the height of the columns. If the column widths are different, comparison can only be made by calculating the area of each column.

Line graphs

A line graph can be used to show clearly how values have changed over a period. It can also show cumulative information. An example of each is shown in Figure 26.16.

Graphs have two axes at right angles to one another:

- *horizontal axis* (the *x* axis) – for data over which you have control, for example, months of the year, years, times, etc.
- *vertical axis* (the *y* axis) – for data over which you have no control, for example blood sugar levels recorded, incidence rates.

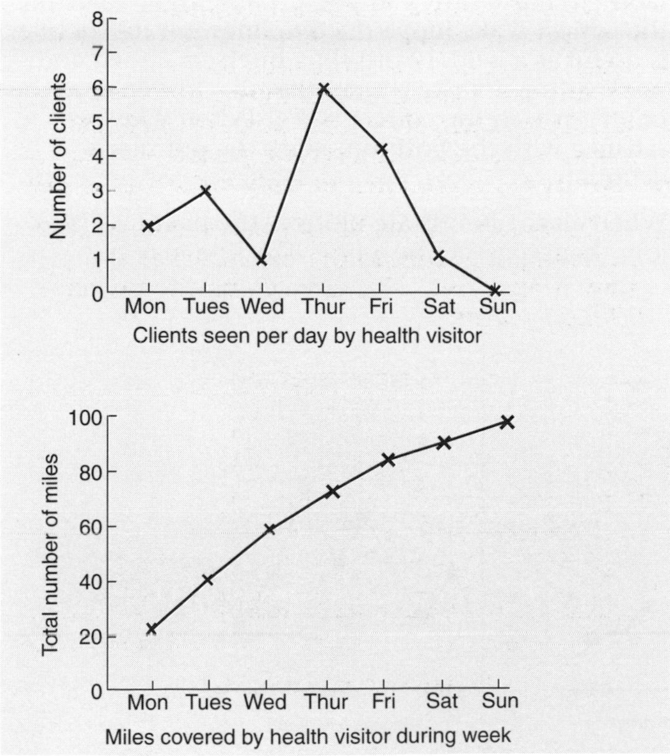

Figure 26.16 Examples of line graphs

Each axis should be neatly and clearly labelled with its units. Some may have arrowheads alongside or end in an arrow to indicate a continuing increase. The point where the axes meet usually represents zero on both scales, although this is not always so.

On graphs where the overall fluctuations are more important than the units measured, *arbitrary units* may be used on an axis.

Each graph graph should have a title to explain what it is showing. (See Figure 26.16.)

Always look carefully at the axes of graphs. Both graphs in Figure 26.17 show the weight gain of a newborn baby. You might think the baby in graph (b) is doing much better. But look carefully – the weight gain is the same, but because of the choice of scale for the vertical axis (which does not start at zero) the weight gain appears to be much more dramatic.

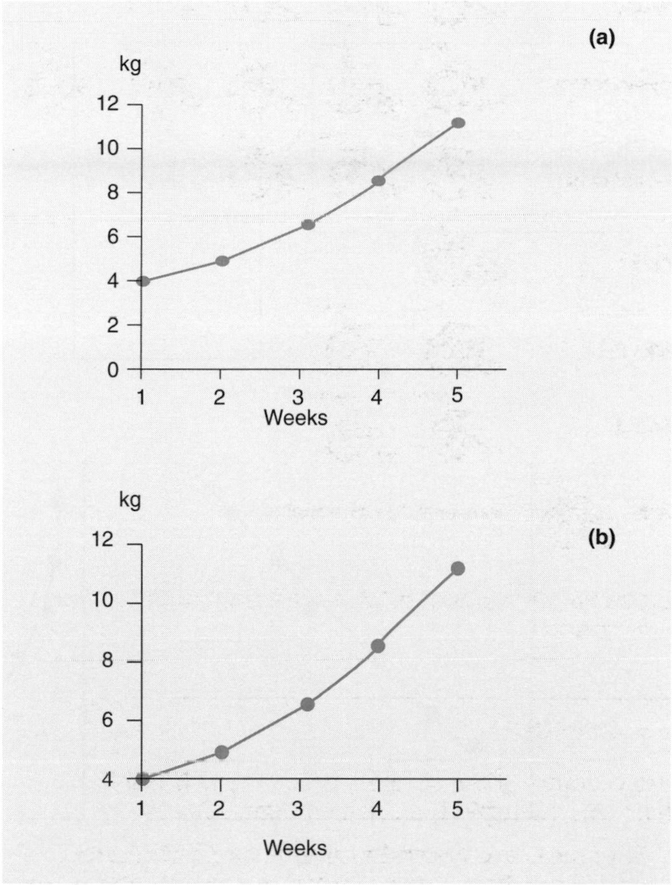

Figure 26.17 Two ways of presenting the same data

Example

Let us take a simple example, a temperature chart for a client with a fever.

Body temperature is going to be measured every 4 hours or every 2 hours or every hour – you set the interval. However, you do not know what the temperature is going to be (that is why you are measuring it); you only know the extremes between which it will be. Therefore, the chosen time interval will be on the *x* axis and the temperature on the *y* axis.

Choosing a scale

One of the most confusing things in drawing graphs seems to be choosing a suitable scale. You will have your lists or charts of data, so find the smallest and the largest values. For example, in a graph to show how rate of growth varies with age, age runs from 0 to 25 years. The graph paper to be used has 28 cm squares vertically and 19 horizontally. Would it matter if the graph was drawn in landscape format?

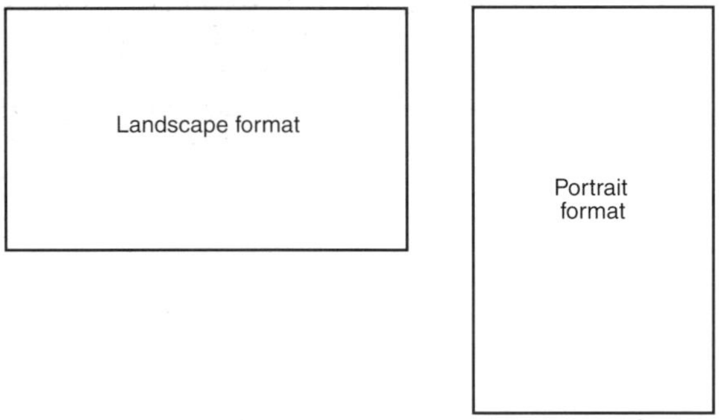

In this case, the answer is no, so the paper is turned around: 25 intervals will fit well into 28 spaces at 1 cm per year interval. What about the other scale? Rate of growth will range from 0 cm/month to about 10 cm/month, i.e. 10 intervals, and that will also fit well at the same scale on the vertical axis.

Sometimes, however, it is not possible to turn the paper to suit the graph, particularly if there is text before and following the graph. In portrait format, 25 intervals have to fit on to paper 19 cm wide; clearly, the same scale of 1 cm per year cannot be used. Could 1 cm represent 2 years? Yes, but that would leave nearly one-third of the paper blank, so try 0.75 cm per year for 25 years, which equals 18.75 cm, about the right size for the paper.

Now is the time for individual choice. If you are not very experienced at plotting points, you may choose the first easier scale, but the graph will not look quite so well on the paper. If you are experienced and can plot 0.75 cm accurately, then the second scale would be preferable. You should now be able to follow the same procedure to work out the scale for the *y* axis.

Plotting points

You will generally have two sets of data, usually in a table. To make sure that you find the right value on the correct scale, move the two lines inwards (a ruler is useful as a guide) until they intersect (cross) and mark with a dot. Take away the ruler and look at the point – is it in the correct place? When you are satisfied with the position, mark the dot more definitely.

When all the points are plotted, the next task is to join them together by a line. The line may be

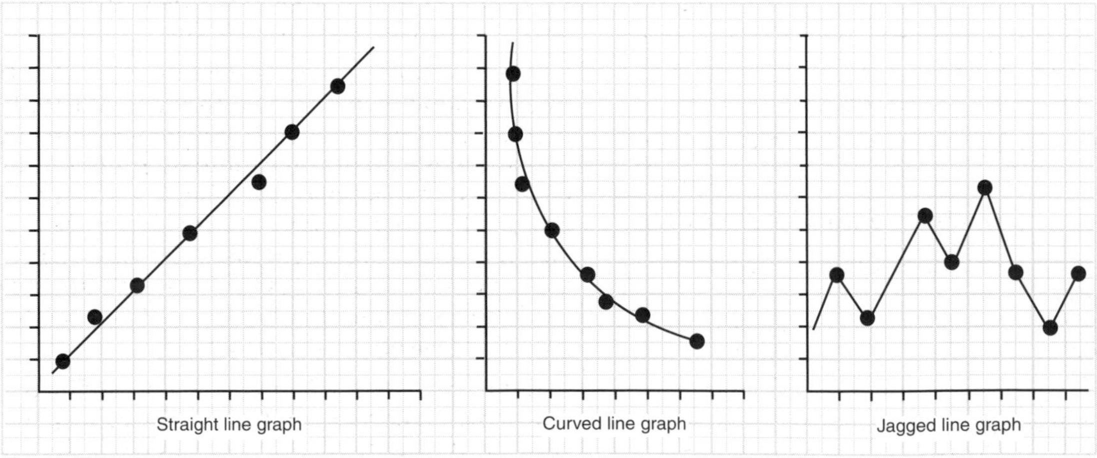

Figure 26.18 Types of line graph

straight, curved or jagged. If it is clearly straight or curved, but one or two points do not quite fit, then make a straight line or curve using the line which best fits most of the points – do not worry if one or two points lie outside the line. It would be quite unusual to have everything matching perfectly! (See Figure 26.18.)

To ensure that the graph shows data to the best advantage:

- Use graph paper whenever possible to present your information.
- Use the paper to the best advantage – do not squash the graph into a corner and leave the rest of the paper blank.
- Draw the graph axes in pencil, but with label lines and titles in ink.
- Plot the points carefully, using either a cross (the centre of which coincides with your desired point) or a dot surrounded by a circle. Use a sharp pencil so that errors can easily be corrected.
- If there is more than one line on the same graph, try to avoid using colour – use the different ways of plotting points as described above.
- Label each line neatly.
- Make sure that the interval between scale marks is the same along your axis – pay particular attention to decimal intervals, which are often confusing.

Cumulative frequency graphs

This is a variation of frequency which looks at running totals and gives rise to a smooth *cumulative frequency curve* (or *ogive*).

Example

Sixty nursing students in their last examination scored the following results on a 50-mark test paper:

Test marks	10–19	20–29	30–39	40–49
No. of candidates	3	17	37	3

The cumulative frequency (cf) table would look like this:

Marks	Cumulative frequency
Less than 20 marks	3 cf
Less than 30 marks	20 cf
Less than 40 marks	57 cf
Less than 50 marks	60 cf

The results are then plotted to give a cumulative frequency curve (Figure 26.19). See also Frequency distribution in Chapter 24.

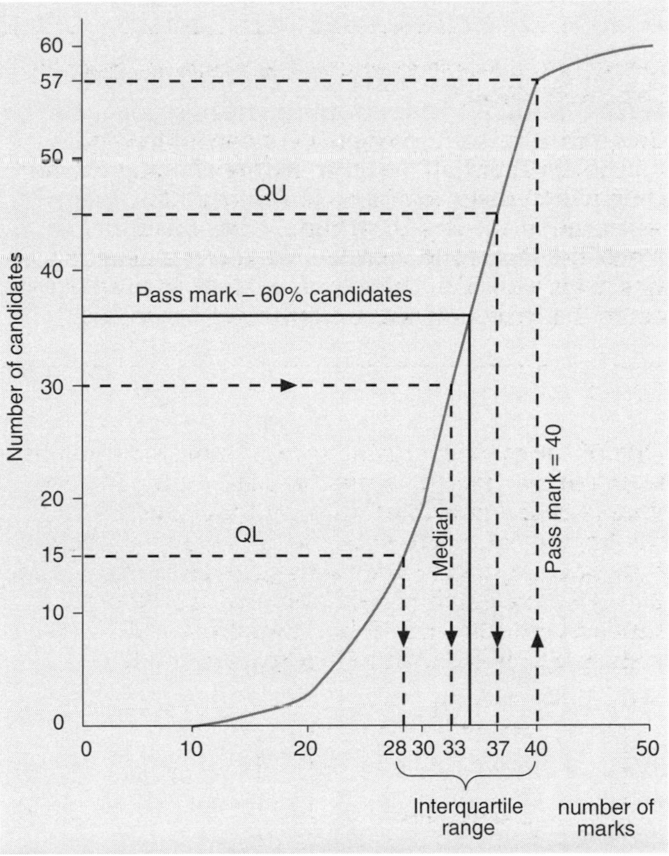

Figure 26.19 Cumulative frequency curve for nursing test

Interquartile range

The interquartile range is a more appropriate measure of *dispersion* (the spread of data) than the range, because it is unaffected by extreme (one or two very low or very high) values.

When a set of data is arranged in size order, the middle value is the *median*. In Figure 26.19, the median can be obtained from the value read off from 30 candidates (half the candidate number). In this case, it is 33 (rounded up). The lower quarter (Q_L) is the value below which a quarter of the data lies – 28, and the upper quartile (Q_U) is the value above which a quarter of the data lies – 37. The interquartile range lies between these two figures – 28 and 37. So this is a better measure of the range.

If the pass mark is 40, then only 3 candidates (60–57) will pass. If the nursing tutors wished to pass 60 per cent of the candidates, i.e. 60 × 60% = 36 candidates, then the pass mark should be 34 marks.

Graphs to calculate rates of change

A community nurse travels by car for 7 miles to reach a farm, 2.5 miles from the nearest road. She gets a lift from a farmer on a tractor for 1.5 miles, taking another half an hour, before walking the last mile which takes a further 30 minutes. She seems surprised at the length of time it has taken her to reach the farm, and wonders what her average speed has been. How can this be calculated? It can be done quite easily by drawing a graph (see Figure 26.20).

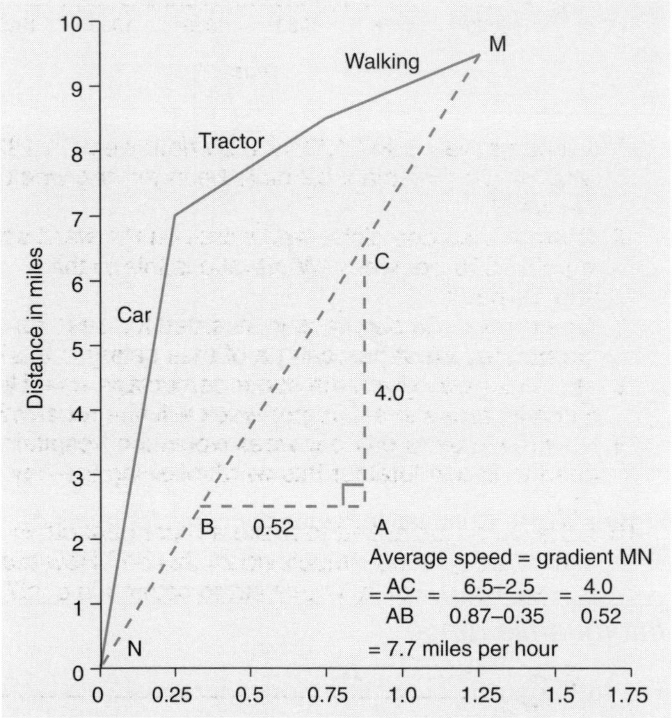

Figure 26.20 Distance–time graph to determine the average speed of community nurse

The average speed could be found by joining the points M and N, and calculating the gradient of the slope (B–C) of the right-angled triangle of the graph (of which the slope is the hypotenuse). The calculation is shown in Figure 26.20.

Other rates of change follow a similar pattern to speed.

Try it

A nurse has to provide a client with medication intravenously. She needs to give 500 cm^3 in four hours. When she checks the drip after the first hour, it has delivered 130 cm^3. She slows down the rate of delivery to 125 cm^3 per hour and checks again 1.25 hours later. The drip is running well and she slows it further to 120 cm^0 for the rest of the time.

When the doctor arrives to check the client, she wants to know the average speed at which the IV drip has been operating. Plot a volume–time graph and calculate the average rate of the drip.

Scatter diagrams

Scatter diagrams (or scattergrams) can often be useful if results appear to be widely variable. They may be influenced by more than one factor. With a scattered distribution of results, it may be important to know of any interdependence or *correlation*.

- Positive correlation occurs if the distribution appears from left to right across the graph.
- Negative correlation runs from right to left, and a cluster of no direction shows no interdependence (see Figure 26.21). See also Chapter 24.

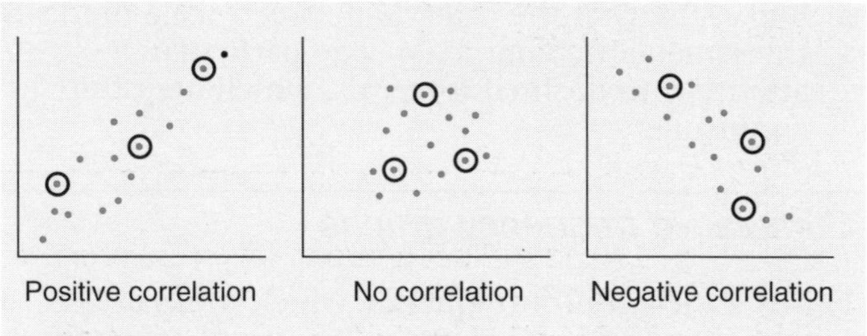

Figure 26.21 Scatter diagrams

Probability

If a coin is tossed it has an equal chance of coming down heads or tails. In this case we often say there is a 50/50 chance (or an even chance) that it will show heads (or tails). In number work we give a value to the likelihood of a particular outcome.

For instance, the likelihood of heads turning up with a tossed coin is 1 out of 2 (= $\frac{1}{2}$ or 0.5). The probability of a particular score on a die (singular of dice) is 1 out of 6 (= $\frac{1}{6}$), as there are 6 possible numbers. Similarly, the probability of producing the queen of hearts from a pack of cards is 1 out of 52.

Example

Suppose now we have two dice, one with numbers and one with colours. What is the probability of a red and a 6 turning up? What is the probability of blue and an odd number being thrown together?

The following table will help us to work this out.

Colours	Numbers					
	1	2	3	4	5	6
Yellow	×	×	×	×	×	×
Green	×	×	×	×	×	×
Blue	**✘**	×	**✘**	×	**✘**	×
Brown	×	×	×	×	×	×
Red	×	×	×	×	×	**✘**
Black	×	×	×	×	×	×

All the equally likely outcomes are shown with a cross, and we can see that there are 36 possibilities (= 6 × 6). The favourable ones we are seeking are shown in bolder type. From this we can see that 'red + 6' can only happen in one way, so that the probability of this happening is 1 out of 36, or $\frac{1}{36}$ (= 0.028). On the other hand, 'blue + any odd number' can happen in three ways, so the probability of this happening is 3 out of 36, or $\frac{3}{36}$ (=0.083).

Try it

1 Find a client group that you can access in a group setting.
2 Choose an aspect of their physical development which can be measured and recorded accurately (e.g. height, age, mass, shoe size).
3 Collect the appropriate data from the clients, and collate it in a pictorial form.
4 Calculate the mean from your sample (show your workings).
5 Draw conclusions from your findings and justify why you have drawn those conclusions.

Try it

Study the chart below and answer the questions, showing your workings.

1 What trend can you identify from the data?
2 What reasons can you give for this trend?
3 What was the increase in places between 1970 and 1990?
4 The ratio of nursing staff to clients is 1:4. How many nurses were needed in 1970, 1980 and 1990?

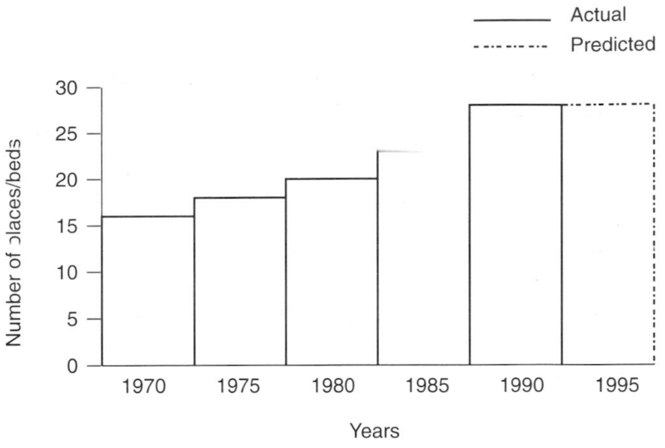

5 If a nurse was paid £120 for a 30-hour week in 1990, what would the salary bill have been for one week in the ward?
6 There is also one sister who works on the ward who is paid £200 per week. What ratio is this to the nurse's pay?
7 A pay rise of £6 per week is awarded for 1991 for the nurses. What percentage of their salary is this?
8 The sister was given the same percentage rise. How much increase in salary per week will she receive?
9 How much extra pay per week would the hospital need to find in total for this ward following the pay rise?
10 If the ward was asked to make a 5 per cent cut in its staffing budget, how much would this be? How many nurses' hours would it have cut to cover this cost?

Fast Facts

Area The space covered by a shape. It can be a regular shape (for example square) or irregular.

Area of a circle Pie (π) multiplied by the radius squared.

Area of a rectangle Length multiplied by the width.

Area of a triangle Half the base length times the height.

Axes The lines containing the scales which form the framework of a graph. They usually meet in the left-hand corner of the page. The horizontal line is called the *x* axis and the vertical line is the *y* axis.

Calculator A device for calculating quickly. Beware of quoting answers to large numbers of decimal places – rounding to two is usually enough (for example, 6.3486 would be 6.35).

Circumference of a circle Pie (π) times the diameter.

Closed questions Questions with closed types of answers (e.g. yes/no).

Conversion Changing one unit into another (for example pounds to ounces or ounces to grams). If you are using any of the **four rules of number,** *always* check that all figures are in the same unit.

Decimal number A number which includes a decimal point. Remember during calculation, moving the point to the left makes the figure smaller; moving the point to the right makes the figure larger.

Estimation Making a close guess or approximate judgement as to the value of your answer. This helps to check that no serious mistakes have been made.

Four rules of number Plus, minus, divide and multiply. (Remember always to line your units under one another if not using a calculator.)

Fractions Expressing a part in relation to the whole. The upper number is the *numerator,* the lower figure is the *denominator.* Remember when using the four rules of number with fractions, you must work out a *common denominator.*

Generalisation Picking out the pattern or trend shown by a set of figures or chart.

Justification Reasons or proof used to back up statements made.

Landscape format Paper turned so that the greatest length goes horizontally, like a landscape painting in an art gallery.

Mean The average of a set of values. The total amount of a set of values divided by the number of values.

e.g. 1, 3, 3, 3, 4, 6, 9, 15, 19 mean = 63 ÷ 9 = 7

Median The half-way value of a series of values.

e.g. 1, 3, 3, 3, 4, 6, 9, 15, 19 median = 4

Mode The most common value in a set of values.

e.g. 1, 3, 3, 3, 4, 6, 9, 15, 19 mode = 3

Percentage Rate or proportion per hundred (per cent). A fraction can be converted to a percentage by multiplying by 100. The symbol is %.

Perimeter The distance around the outside of any shape. The perimeter of a circle is the same as its circumference.

Pictogram An eye-catching method of presenting data which is quick and easy to understand.

Portrait format Paper turned so that the greatest length goes vertically, like a portrait painting.

Range The spread of values from the highest number to the lowest number.

Ratios Ratios are a way of comparing two or more quantities.

Recording The noting down of information.

Scale An item marked in such a way that the distance between two marks measures a quantity.

Sequence Doing a calculation in the correct order for example, BODMAS – this gives you the correct order for calculating – Brackets Of (usually means multiplying) Division Multiplication Addition Subtraction.

Three-dimensional object One with depth as well as area. Everything in the world is really 3-dimensional. A piece of paper is 3-dimensional because it does have some depth (its thickness).

Two-dimensional object A shape that is flat on the page and which is therefore reckoned to have an area but not a volume.

Volume The volume of a container is the same as its capacity. It is the amount of space inside the shape.

Volume of a cylinder Pie (π) times radius squared (i.e. πr^2) times length. The radius is half the diameter.

Volume of a rectangular block Length times width times height.

Chapter 27

Information technology

This chapter deals with introductory issues and general topics relevant to all information technology users. It covers:

- **hardware and software**
- **input devices**
- **saving your work**
- **computer networks**
- **files and directories**
- **errors and faults**
- **working safely with computers**

What is information technology?

Information technology (IT) is now very much a part of everyday life. It is essential to your studies, and it will be increasingly important at work, whatever career you follow. Wherever modern electronics technology is applied to handling, the term IT may be applied. It doesn't refer just to computers – developments in computing, video and communications are rapid, and they are increasingly becoming aspects of the IT field.

All GNVQ students are expected to have a certain level of skill and knowledge in the use of IT, whatever the area of their studies. The IT core skill unit sets standards that you have to meet, just as other units do. You will find that most of the evidence you need to pass the IT unit will be there amongst the work that you do during your Health and Social Care studies. This chapter will help you to use IT effectively by showing you how it can be applied to things you will be doing in Health and Social Care. It will also help you to identify work which may count as evidence towards the IT unit.

Hardware and software

Hardware simply means the physical **equipment** used in IT. This includes the **computer** itself (sometimes referred to as the base unit), the **monitor** (screen), the **keyboard** and the **mouse**. Hardware also refers to other physical equipment such as the **printer** and the cables that connect it all together.

There are other devices that are described as hardware, and you may have access to some of them. For example,

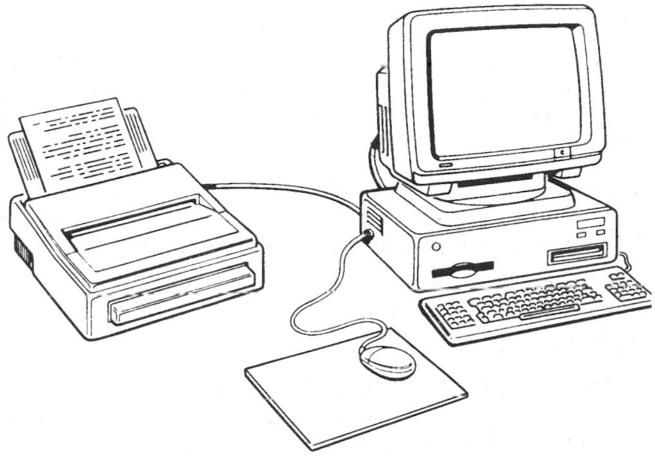

Figure 27.1 Hardware is the physical equipment used in IT

scanners can be used to enter a picture (or **graphic**) into the computer from a paper-based copy.

Software is the term used for the set of instructions which the computer follows when performing a task. You may have heard this referred to as a **program**, or as an **application**. This can be confusing, but remember that they are basically just different words for the same thing.

System software

One important type of software is known as system software (or the operating system). This is used to get the computer up and running, and controls the flow and processing of information when it is in use. The operating system runs automatically when you start up the computer.

Different types of computers use different operating systems, but fortunately you are only likely to encounter the two most common systems. These are IBM-compatible computers and Apple Mackintosh computers. Most IBM-compatible computers use Microsoft Windows (or simply Windows), which means they are similar in use to the Apple system. Both provide the 'WIMPS' user environment: this stands for **W**indows, **I**cons, **M**ouse, **P**ointer, and describes the way instructions are given to the computer using a mouse. This chapter describes the use of software offering a WIMPS environment to users.

Applications software

Applications software is required to make the computer perform different tasks. There are several types that you will come across.

Word processors are used to handle text (i.e. words and numbers) and produce letters, reports and other documents. Word processing is one of the most common uses of IT. **Database software** is used to work with information in the form of lists. Your address book and a book of recipes are forms of non-computerised database. **Spreadsheets** are designed to handle numerical information. With a spreadsheet you can enter numbers, perform calculations and present your results neatly as charts or graphs. **Graphics applications** are used to create and edit drawings, illustrations and other types of graphics.

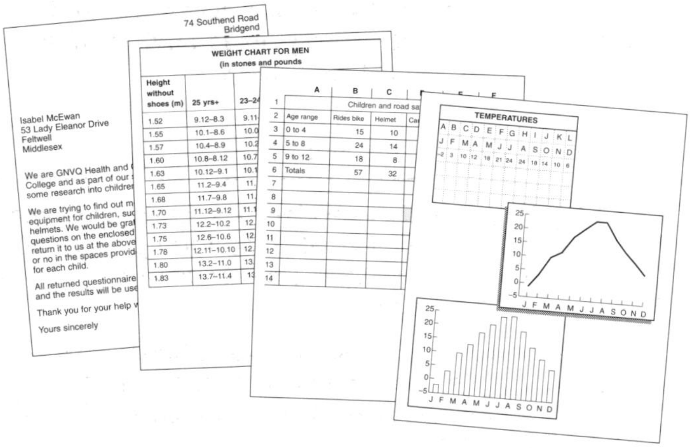

Figure 27.2 Software can handle a range of information

All of these applications are powerful tools, and each has a wide range of uses which fall beyond the scope of this chapter. They can be even more powerful when used together. For example, a graph of results from a spreadsheet, or a graphic from a drawing application, can be put into a word-processed report. A word-processed letter can be blended with a list of names and addresses in a database to send a mass 'mail shot'. This ability to share information between applications opens up many possibilities, and we will be looking at some of them later.

There are other types of software that may be available to you. For example, **desk-top publishing** (DTP) software is like a cross between a word processor and a graphics application and allows you to produce high quality printed material from leaflets to books. There are also specialised applications designed to help you do a particular job, such as creating survey questionnaires and processing the results, or keeping financial accounts. Your tutors and IT staff will advise you which software you have access to. The most important thing you need to do is to actually use the equipment and software that is available to you.

Input devices

Input devices are items of hardware that are used to give data and instructions to the computer. This includes the **keyboard** and the **mouse**. The keyboard is the main input device for most purposes, but the mouse is also important in modern computer systems. This mouse controls the movement of an on-screen pointer. You can use the pointer to perform tasks within software applications. You can also use the mouse and pointer to start up software. When you switch on the computer you will see a number of small graphic pictures, known as icons. Each icon represents a different piece of software. You simply position the pointer over the icon for the software you need and double click the mouse button. The software then starts up. The mouse makes it very easy to use some software features, though there are usually ways of using the keyboard to do the same job. One exception is with graphics software – the mouse is an essential tool when using a drawing or painting application.

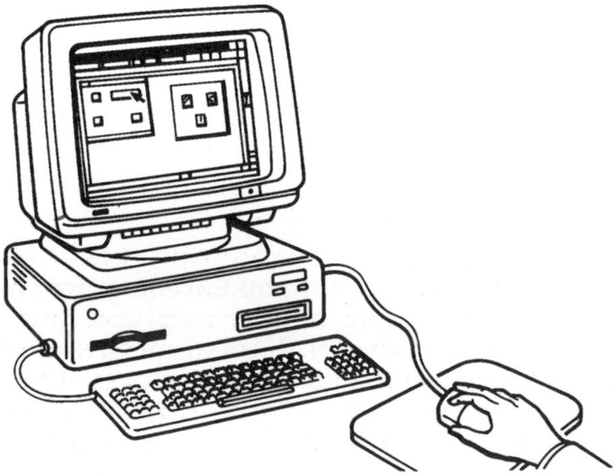

Figure 27.3 The mouse can be used to start software

Saving your work

The computer's memory is known as **RAM** which stands for Random Access Memory. The RAM holds the information and instructions that are being used by the computer during your work sessions. But RAM is not a permanent storage place for your work as everything is deleted from it when you turn off the computer. You need to save your work before closing the application and switching off the machine. Where do you save your work ? The answer partly depends on the equipment you are using, but it will be some form of electronic storage **disk**. There are two types of disk that you are likely to encounter, **hard disks** and **floppy disks**.

Hard disks

Most computers have a hard disk installed in them. It can be used to store large amounts of information (including the operating system and applications software) and it is also possible to save your own work there. However, it is unwise to rely on the hard disk for this purpose. This is because any work saved on the hard disk can be called up later by other people using that computer, which could result in tampering or even accidental, but complete, erasure of your work ! This can easily be avoided by saving your work on your own floppy disk too.

Floppy disks

Floppy disks are a compact, cheap and secure way to save your work. You can buy a disk for well under £1 and it will hold a large amount of data. Floppy disks are the best way of keeping your work secure. You can insert your own disk into the computer's disk drive and save your work onto it. When you then shut down the application, a copy of your work remains on your floppy disk. Wherever you save work always keep a copy on your floppy disk. This is called **backing-up** your work.

New floppy disks need to be formatted before work can be saved onto them. To format a disk simply insert it into the floppy disk drive slot and instruct the computer to format it. Beware when reformatting a used disk, however – formatting permanently removes any work that was previously stored on it and you could lose something you didn't mean to! You can avoid this by closing the **read/write 'gate'** on your floppy disk to prevent the contents being erased. When the tab is closed you can still read the

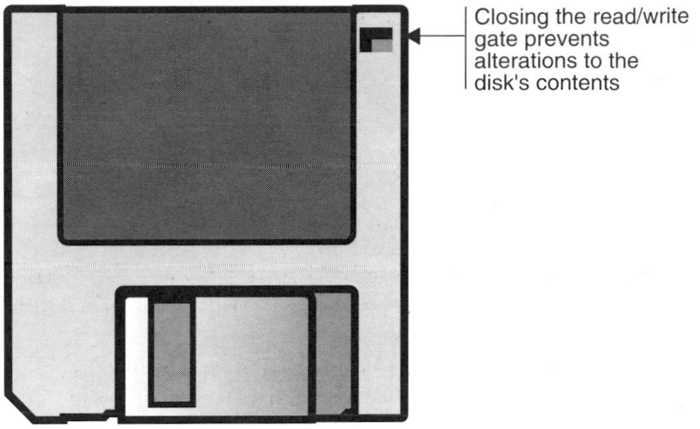
Closing the read/write gate prevents alterations to the disk's contents

Figure 27.4 A $3^1/_2$-inch floppy disk

information on the disk, but you cannot alter or delete it. This is very secure but, of course, prevents you saving any new files on the disk, and prevents you from reformatting it.

You will need to format your disk according to its storage capacity. Check with your IT advisers if you have any doubts about this process.

Evidence collection point

As part of the evidence required by Element 3.1 of the Information Technology unit you should keep back-up copies of work you have done using IT. You need to:

- have you own floppy disk with you when you work with a computer, and find out how to format it
- save your work regularly onto your floppy disk, and make back-up copies
- save examples of your work at different stages to show where improvements have been made .

Computer networks

The computers we have discussed so far are complete machines in themselves. They can keep applications software on their internal hard disk and save your work there. They need to be connected to a printer to get paper copies, but they are not connected to other computers. Machines like this are known as **stand-alone computers**.

Nowadays many organisations, including educational institutions, are linking computers together to form **computer networks**. It may well be that you will be using a machine on a network during your studies.

All the machines in a network are linked to a piece of hardware called a network server. This is effectively an extremely large hard-disk drive which can hold a vast amount of data. Each separate computer, or workstation, loads software from the server, and can usually save work on it. A workstation computer doesn't even need to have its own hard disk-drive inside it, because the network server can act as a hard disk for all the machines on the network.

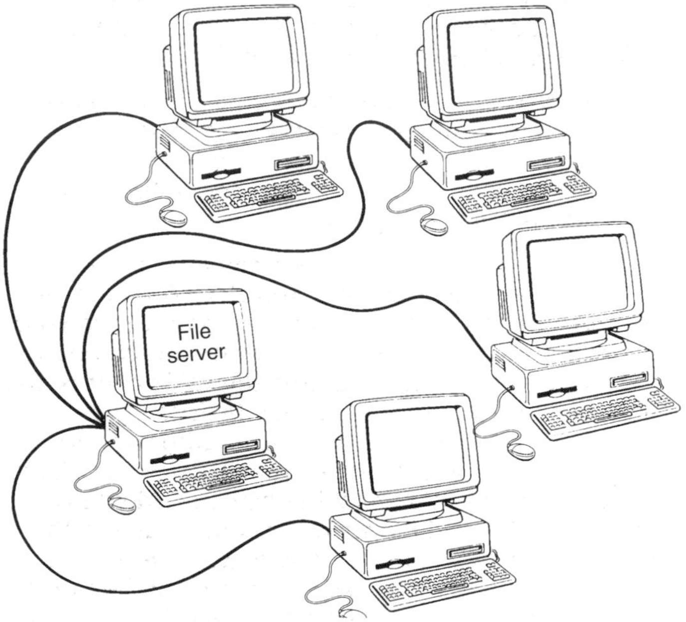

Figure 27.5 Networks allow information and software to be shared

Networks have big advantages over stand-alone computers.

- The file server can hold a much greater range of software than a stand-alone computer's hard disk, and this range is available to users at each workstation.
- Specialised hardware can be connected to the server and so made available to all users. For example, a *CD-ROM* (Compact Disk – Read Only Memory) device can allow encyclopedias and other reference work to be used at each workstation without the need to install expensive hardware in every machine.
- Another big advantage, in most situations, is that information can be shared between different computers in the network. Businesses use networks to help information flow between parts of the organisation. If you use a local hard disk or a network server, to save work you should always keep back-up copies on a floppy disk which you can keep securely.

Files and directories

Files

Each separate piece of work that you create and save on the computer is known as a *file*. Files are linked to the applications that they were created in, so that a word-processed letter is saved as a word-processor file and a database listing books you have read is saved as a database file. The computer will ask you to give your files names as you save them, and it will add its own bit of code at the end to remind you what application the file belongs to. The problem is that you are restricted to a maximum name length of only eight characters when you save. As you add files to your floppy disk it can soon contain a confusing list of meaningless initials, unless you organise it.

Directories

The computer can set up a storage system on a disk so that files that you want to keep together are stored in the same place, in a **directory**. Suppose you were doing a piece of work towards Element 7.3 and had used IT to help you to research people's views on the effectiveness of a health education campaign. You may have produced a word-processed questionnaire, and created a database file containing the names of the respondents you intend to interview. Later you may have used a spreadsheet to help you analyse the results, and word-processed a report on the research project. You can create a directory called RESEARCH to hold all the work that you do towards that research project. The directory can be used to save any type of file, so you can save a word-processed letter together with a spreadsheet in the same directory.

In our example, you are intending to split the work into two parts, and keep each part separate within the RESEARCH directory. You can create further divisions within your directory, known as **sub-directories**. You could create a sub-directory called PLANNING to hold your questionnaire form and respondents database, and another called RESULTS to hold your spreadsheet and final report.

You save each file in its appropriate sub-directory. Now there is a 'path' to each file. For example, you may have called the questionnaire file FORM, and saved it in the PLANNING sub-directory of the

RESEARCH directory. The path to your questionnaire file would be written as RESEARCH\PLANNING\FORM, showing the route to be taken to the location of your file on disk. This path provides a unique address for your file which you use to reload it for editing or printing (see Figure 27.6).

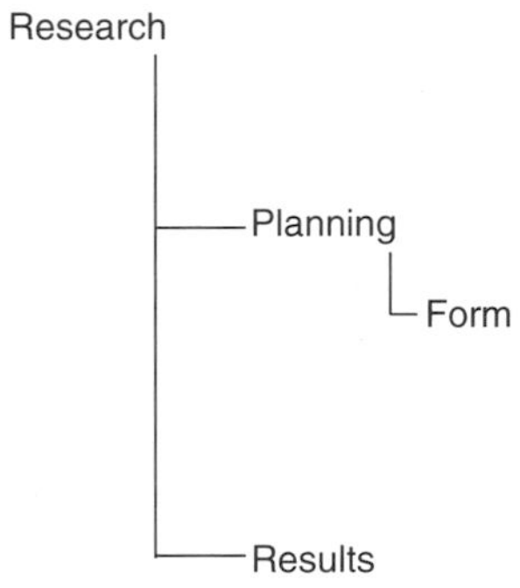

Figure 27.6 A simple directory structure

You can easily keep track of your work by thoughtful use of directories and sub-directories. The computer can quickly show you the layout and contents of directory structures that you have created so there is no need to remember the paths to all your files.

Try it

1. Talk to your IT tutor about the equipment you will be using during your studies.
2. Find out which software applications you have access to, and check that they are able to share data.
3. Find out what hardware may be available, such as a scanner or a CD-ROM.
4. Check where you will be able to store your work. You should always keep back-up copies on a floppy disk so find out how to format a disk on your equipment.
5. Find out when you can get access to a computer, and the days and times that there is someone there to help you.

This piece of initial research will help you to plan your use of IT facilities in your work, and to get the most from them.

Errors and faults

Generally speaking, using IT should make work easier and should be trouble-free. Occasionally, however, problems do occur. These could be due to errors made by the user (you!), or to faults with the equipment itself.

Some faults are caused by the user. Everyone makes the odd mistake, and experienced users expect to make occasional errors when learning to use new software. Most errors are easy to spot as you go. For example, pressing the wrong key generally shows instantly on the screen and can be corrected right away. Other user errors may be less easy to detect. Don't worry – as you become familiar with the software you are using the errors you are likely to make become familiar to you as well.

Sometimes you may find that the problems you are having are not caused by mistakes you have made but are the result of faults in the equipment. Generally, IT equipment is remarkably reliable, but occasionally things do go wrong.

One simple cause of problems is cables that are poorly, or even incorrectly, connected. For example, the reason that the printer is not responding to your request for a paper copy may be that your computer is not connected to it. Similarly, the cable connecting the base unit to the monitor may be loose, accounting for the fact that your monitor has no image on it. If the computer suddenly stops working, it could be due to the machine being accidentally being turned off. More rarely it could be due to the equipment breaking down. The biggest problem for you in this situation is that your work will be lost. If you have made regular back-ups, this will not be so serious. Remember that switching machines off when software is running can damage information stored on the hard disk. Always take care to close down properly, following the steps shown to you by your IT tutor.

You should be able to deal with simple equipment problems yourself, but always check with your IT tutor that you have diagnosed the problem correctly, and that you have chosen an appropriate solution.

Evidence collection point

Part of the evidence needed towards Element 3.4 of the IT core skill unit is a record of user errors and equipment faults that have occurred while using IT resources.

Whenever you use IT keep a log of the errors that you make, and record your evaluation of their effects on your work.

Also record equipment faults, and solutions that you have found. Again make comments on the effects of equipment faults on your work.

Keep a 'faults log book' so that the information is easily available for assessment.

Working safely with computers

It is important to follow safe working practices when using IT. This means avoiding risks to yourself and other users, and to the equipment. It also includes risks to the information that computers work with.

The equipment that you are using has been designed to be as safe as possible. The computer itself and peripheral equipment, such as printers, are powered from the mains electricity supply. You should observe the normal precautions as you would with any mains-powered electrical equipment. Cables must be arranged so that they don't endanger health and safety. They must not be damaged, or laid where they may form a hazard in themselves. If you connect items of equipment like printers be sure to arrange the cables tidily.

Never eat or drink around IT equipment ! Liquids are particularly dangerous, and a spilled drink can cause a serious electrical hazard, as well as causing considerable damage to equipment.

Another health and safety issue is the way your equipment is arranged physically. As part of the health and safety laws, the Display Screen Equipment Regulations lay down certain standards on equipment, seating and lighting. Monitors may be swivelled left and right, and tilted up and down. This allows you to turn the screen to a position where it is facing you directly, so that you are not forced to sit in an awkward or uncomfortable position to see it clearly. You should have a chair that can be adjusted to different heights, has an adjustable back rest for support and is on castors for mobility.

Screens are also adjustable for brightness and contrast and you need to set these so that you can see your work clearly. It is important not to work with the screen turned up too brightly. Prolonged use of a bright screen at close quarters can strain eyes and should be avoided. The lighting conditions in the room affect the visibility of monitor screens. It will need to be turned up much more brightly to be seen in a well-lit room, particularly if lights are reflected directly onto it. A screen facing a sunny window is very difficult to see. Adjust the lighting conditions so that you do not need to have your screen excessively bright to be able to work.

Apart from protecting yourself and the computer hardware from damage, it is also important to look after your stored data. Though floppy disks are durable when used and stored correctly, they must be protected from physical damage. Keep them in a dry secure place as you would a CD or cassette tape.

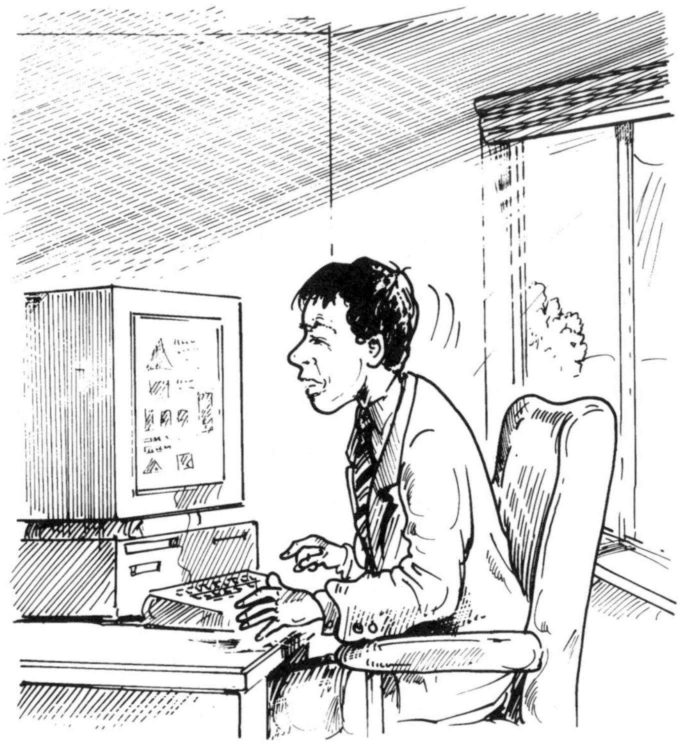

Figure 27.7 Control lighting to improve monitor visibility

Information is stored electrically on floppy disks and this can be damaged or erased if the disk is exposed to strong magnetic or electrical fields. Many domestic appliances produce electrical fields so the best rule is to keep disks away from electrical apparatus.

Data can also be damaged if the computer is switched off while you are working. You will lose any work that you haven't already saved. In addition to this, important data stored on the hard disk can be damaged if software is exited incorrectly. Always shut down the computer as directed by your tutor.

Evidence collection point

As part of the evidence needed for Element 3.4 of the Information Technology unit you need to explain the importance of working safely, and in line with good working practices.

Develop a checklist of 'Do's and Don'ts' to be observed when using IT equipment. Your checklist should include recommendations for the safety of users, for the protection of equipment and for the protection of information from loss, corruption or unauthorised use.

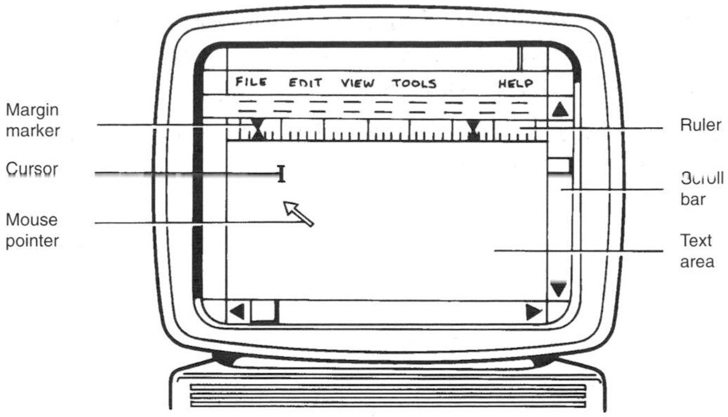

Figure 27.8 A word processor screen

Word processing

This section is about applying a word processor to the tasks you will be doing during your studies. It covers:

- planning a document
- templates and style sheets
- creating questionnaire forms
- copying text.

What is a word processor?

Word processors are used to work with text – words and numbers. They have many features designed to make it easy to produce high-quality written documents.

With a word processor you can:

- enter any text you wish
- make corrections, revisions, and even major changes
- create special styles for headings and important points
- alter the layout to suit your requirements
- create and save templates, or style sheets, for document styles you use often
- add headings and page numbers
- import information from other applications such as a spreadsheet or database, and incorporate it into your document
- print your work when you are satisfied with it
- save your file so that you can reload it later and make further changes and copies, if you wish.

You might have used word processors before and may recognise the typical screen layout shown in Figure 27.8. The flashing **cursor** (insertion point) shows where your typing will appear. It will be blinking towards the top left of the **text area.** Above it is the **ruler** with **margin markers** at either end indicating the left and right boundaries set for your text. There is a narrow strip running up the right hand side of the screen alongside the text area, with arrows at the top and bottom. This is a **scroll bar** which allows you to use the mouse to move through your document.

What appears above the ruler will depend on the word processor that you are using. There may well be one or two rows of graphic buttons which you use with the mouse pointer to select quickly some of the word-processing facilities available with the software. You can find out what each one means by asking your tutors, or by using the on-line help available within the word processor.

Near the top of the screen there is usually a row of words such as 'File', 'Edit' and 'Help'. These are **menu headings** and you can use the mouse or the keyboard to open the menus they represent. On-line help is found by opening the 'Help' menu and selecting the option you need. You use the 'File' menu to start a new document, open an existing one, or obtain a printout. It is a good idea to look at the contents of the menus in your word processor. You may not understand what all the options mean at this stage, though some may be easy to guess. Don't select an option until you are sure what it will do, and know how to reverse it if necessary. Use the on-line help to find out what the options refer to. This is an excellent way to explore the capabilities of any application.

Try it

Find out how to open the on-line help on your word processor, and how to use it. Explore the help system to find out what the software is capable of. If there is an automatic tutorial available, work through it.

Check whether there are any help shortcuts that you could use. For example, some software will display help information for the specific job you are engaged in if key F1 (F1) is pressed.

Planning a document

You will use a word processor to produce a range of written documents during your studies. This could include reports, letters, questionnaire forms, or any text-based work where presentation and flexibility are important. Whatever the final product, the first step is to *plan* your document before you begin to create it. This means deciding on content, layout and style. The content depends, of course, on the purpose of the document and you may prefer to work from notes, or alternatively write it out fully by hand first.

The purpose of the document will also indicate an appropriate layout and style. All documents have their own format affecting things like line spacing, margin settings, and the size and shape of letters and numbers (**characters**). These can be set before you begin a new document, or you can accept the normal (**default**) settings and make changes later. Even if you expect to edit it later, your planning needs to consider how you want your document to look.

Character formatting

You can control the look of characters in the document. Text that is displayed and printed out by the computer has a consistent shape and style, whether it includes letters or numbers, and the term for a full set of characters in a particular style is a character set or font. (Each font has a different name, such as Helvetica or Times.) You can use whatever fonts your word processor has available, and mix them in the same document.

Text size is measured in points. Normal text is usually formatted at 10 point or 12 point; 6 point is getting too small to read and 24 point is too large for general use.

You can vary the font and size of text and greatly alter its appearance. Careful selection of fonts and sizes can improve the look of the whole document, as any available fonts can be applied to any part of the text. Other effects can be applied to characters in the selected font. You can use **bold**, or *italic*, or

GNVQ Advanced Health and Social Care

Times 12pt

GNVQ Advanced Health and Social Care

Avant Garde 10pt italic

GNVQ Advanced Health and Social Care

Univers 8pt bold

Figure 27.9 Examples of different text styles

underline, or CAPITAL LETTERS, or even ***ALL FOUR***, to make parts of your text stand out.

Use of different fonts and effects can add emphasis to headings, create good-looking title pages, and make complicated documents, such as questionnaires, easier to follow. Beware, however, because it is easy to ruin a perfectly good-looking document by going wild with too many fonts and effects. The golden rule is to keep your character formatting simple and neat for the best presentation.

Page formatting

Formatting can also be applied to paragraph layout and the page margins. You can change the position of the margins for particular paragraphs or for the whole document. There are also margins at the top and bottom of the page and you can vary these too. Remember that your text needs some space around it on the page and set reasonable margins for printing. You are able to control the alignment (**justification**) of paragraphs and the line spacing within them. Printed text is aligned between the margins of the page in one of four ways, as shown in Figure 27.10.

Line spacing within a paragraph can also be adjusted if you wish. The standard spacing is one line, but you can increase this in half-space steps.

By using these formatting features you can put any type of text virtually wherever you want to on the page. You can set the format before you begin, and alter any aspect of it as you work. Also, you can select a part of your document using the keyboard or the mouse and apply any format to the selected text. This gives you the chance to experiment with different formats on-screen, as well as enabling you to edit the content. It is a good idea to explore the

Left-aligned text is arranged so that lines are even on the left-hand side, but the right-hand side is ragged

Right-aligned text is similar to the above, except that it is lined up on the right.

Justified text is adjusted by the computer so that the lines are of an even length, though it can lead to a lot of extra spaces being added. Newspapers are printed with justified text.

Centred text is centred.

Figure 27.10 Styles of text justification

range of effects that the word processor can create by producing sample documents using different fonts and styles. Your samples will show you what the format options actually look like when printed. This will help you to make choices when planning a new document.

Evidence collection point

The evidence required towards Element 3.1 of the IT unit includes the source information that you have used for IT work. Keep your planning notes covering layout, style and format, as well as the source information from which a document has been created.

Templates and style sheets

A template, or style sheet, is a special document that acts as a blueprint for the text style and formatting of documents created from it. When you accept the normal settings for a new document you are agreeing to use the **default** template with its particular format and text style. There may be a list of existing alternative templates that you can choose from which offer suggested formats for particular types of document, such as a letter or memorandum. You can also create and save your own templates for document styles that you expect to use again. Your templates can include text and graphics, as well as character and paragraph formatting instructions. This means that you just need to fill in the gaps when creating a new document based upon it.

As an example, suppose you want to create a template for a font sheet to use with the assignment work you do on your course. You would begin by planning the layout and content of a typical frontsheet. Details like your name, the date, the course title, and the title of the assignment need to be included. You may also want to include a numbered list of contents. Your original ideas may look something like the example from a fictitious student in Figure 27.11.

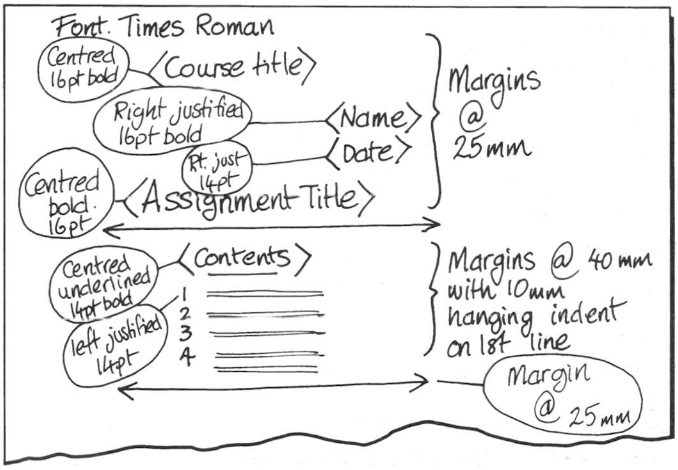

Figure 27.11 Formatting details are shown on a student's hand-written template plan

The notes in the example in Figure 27.11 are specific enough to show all details of font size and type, paragraph alignment, margin settings and added graphics. To create the template, start a new document on the word processor, accepting the default settings. Now you need to make the changes you have planned and save the result as a template.

In our example you would begin by choosing the margin settings for the first section. Both left and right margins are set to 2.5 cm. Now the font is selected, Times Roman at point size 16 and bold. You also need to centre the first line. The same course title will appear on each front sheet so this is typed in on the template. Now Return is pressed two or three times to make space and the paragraph alignment changed to right justified. The student's name can now be typed in. Following similar steps the date is added, and here point size has been reduced and bold removed. Size is increased again, and justification centred, for the words 'Assignment title:'.

The graphic line can be produced by holding down the shift and pressing the underscore key (–). Most word processors have a range of facilities for creating much more adventurous graphic borders than this example. The heading 'Contents' comes next with the addition here of underlining. For the list of contents, Return is pressed twice to position the cursor where the contents list will begin. Now the margins are set at 4 cm, with the first line 1 cm less than this. This produces a hanging indent and makes it easy to number lists. Some more Return presses and then the margins are returned to 2.5 cm for the bottom line.

The result is saved as a template and can now be used to produce front sheets for assignments. On screen, and as a paper copy, a template can look a rather empty document. Our example looks something like Figure 27.12.

GNVQ Health and Social Care Advanced

Asif Gupta

Date:

Assignment title:

Contents

Figure 27.12 A template

When the template is used the embedded formatting makes it easy to create a new document. You just need to move the cursor to the relevant place and type in the details. In the above example the contents list needs numbering. For each item the number is typed and then the Tab key is pressed. Now the item details are entered, and return is pressed to move on to the next item. Figure 27.13 shows a completed front sheet using the template we have looked at. It is for an assignment linked to Element 8.1.

You can create templates for any type of document that you intend to produce more than once. You should always save copies of your templates on a floppy disk, and get a printout of each blank template as it may be needed as evidence towards Element 3.1 of the IT unit. Don't forget that you are not committed to any of a template's settings when you edit a document. You can use a template that has settings close to what you need and make changes later to suit your current requirements.

GNVQ Health and Social Care Advanced

Asif Gupta

Date: 10 October 199–

Assignment title: An investigation into the research process

Contents

1 The nature of the research process

2 The different stages of the research process and how they interlink

3 An examination of a quantitative research study into health and social well-being

4 An examination of a qualitative research study into health and social well-being

5 Ethical issues in research

Figure 27.13 A completed front sheet using a template

Evidence collection point

As part of the evidence needed towards Element 3.1 of the IT unit you need to configure software to the needs of your task. Word-processor templates, or style sheets, are an example of **software configuration**.

You should keep copies of any templates that you produce, both on floppy disk and as paper copy. You will need at least one example of a word processor template in your evidence for Element 3.1.

Where can I use a template?

You can design and save templates for any documents you create during your studies. Whenever you set up the word processor with the format settings you require for a new document you have created a basic template. Why not save it ?

You can reload it later and make improvements if it seems to be useful. You could also set out to design and create templates for specific types of document, such as reports, letters and questionnaire forms, as the next section explains.

Creating questionnaire forms

One type of document that you will need on more than one occasion during your studies is a questionnaire form. Element 7.3 requires you to create and use a structured interview questionnaire, and there are other opportunities to use the questionnaire methods to collect information, for example in Element 2.2, Element 4.2 and Element 6.3. Chapters 22, 23 and 24 will help you to design the content of a questionnaire, and give advice on layout. This section offers advice on word processing questionnaire forms.

Questionnaire forms need to be clearly laid out and easy to read. Of course, this applies to all documents, but questionnaires are working research tools. Cluttered or confusing postal questionnaire forms end up in the bin, and poorly laid-out interview questionnaires can lead interviewers into making many mistakes. The first step, as usual, is to plan your questionnaire document before you begin.

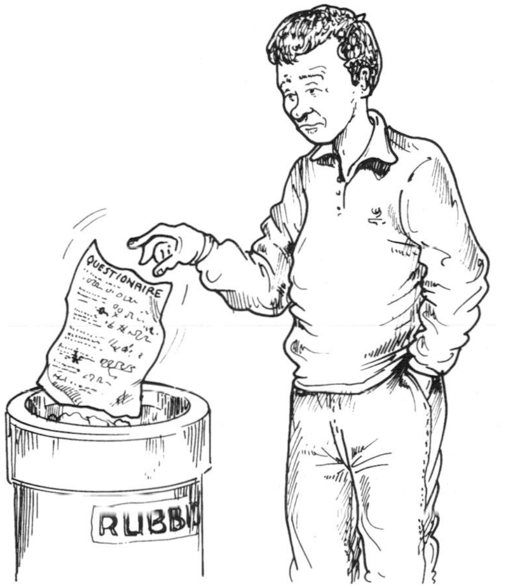

Figure 27.14 Cluttered and confusing questionnaire forms may not be returned

Basically, questionnaire forms consist of a numbered list of questions. They are easier to use if the format of all questions is similar, which is easy to arrange with the word processor. Choose a clear and simple font for the main text of the questions, not a fancy '*handwriting*' one that is difficult to read. Don't select any highlights or effects, you may need to use these later elsewhere in the form. Set up the left margin to give a hanging indent for question numbering. Set the right margin fairly wide, say roughly one quarter of the page width. Choose left justification and single spacing for the question paragraphs. You now have a basic questionnaire template and could save a copy at this stage. This template will produce a list of numbered questions, and you can provide answer space easily by pressing Return several times between each one.

Evidence collection point

Try producing the simple template described above. You can use it as the basis for the questionnaires that you will be creating during your studies. You can improve and adapt it as you become more experienced, and some suggestions are given below. Your template could be used as evidence towards Element 3.1 of the IT unit.

Questionnaires need more sophistication than this, however, and the basic template needs to be developed. Not all questions are of the same type. Some questions will be the fixed-response type with options to be selected; others may be open questions with space allowed for recording the answer. Your template is fine for open questions, but there are usually few of these, if any, in questionnaire forms. Fixed-response questions need a clear list of answer options, and a pre-coded space to mark the response next to each one. Often these appear as a right-justified column below the question, as shown in Figure 27.15.

There are different ways to produce a response column and the method you use will partly depend on the capabilities of the word processor you are using. More sophisticated word processors have facilities for creating and inserting tables in your document. A table is composed of rows and columns of **cells**, and may look a bit like a spreadsheet at first. You decide how many rows and columns the table needs and can control their size. Text and numbers can be entered into a cell, and formatted however you wish. In Figure 27.15 the option statements have been justified right and have the same font format as

6 Do you think that the publicity material produced for the health education campaign is likely to be seen by the people it is aimed at?

Please tick <u>one</u> box only

Very likely		1
Fairly likely		2
Even likelihood		3
Not very likely		4
Not at all likely		5
Depends/Can't say		6

Figure 27.15 An example of layout for a fixed-response question

the question text. The coding numbers are also right justified and are at a much smaller point size. One big advantage of tables is their ability to add **borders** to selected cells. The example shows borders added to the column of 'check-box' cells making them easy to use.

Try it

Find out whether the word-processing software that you are using is able to create and insert tables into documents. If it can, find out how to use them, and how to control their size, position and appearance in a document. Use the on-line help, consult a tutor, or look in the software manual to get this information.

If you can't create tables with your word-processor there are other methods available. Tab stops allow you to line up columns of text and can produce the effect we need. Change the paragraph to right justified and set up a tab on the ruler that gives you room for your longest option statement. In Figure 27.16, this is the 'Depends/Can't say' option. Now each option is typed in and the Tab key then pressed. Underscore is used to create a short line, and the font size then reduced for the coding number. After

Very likely	____1
Fairly likely	____2
Even likelihood	____3
Not very likely	____4
Not at all likely	____5
Depends/Can't say	____6

Figure 27.16 An alternative way of setting out a fixed-response question

typing the code number return the font size to normal. Finally, press Return twice to create space before typing in the next option. The effect produced will be something like that shown in Figure 27.16.

Tabs create a neat column effect for the response statements and the check-boxes, but bordering is more limited. Because of this you may want to leave more space between response options to avoid confusions over which check-box belongs to which option.

Copying text

Whatever method you use to create answer options, it will help if you try to use **copy and paste** methods to avoid having to start from scratch for each question. Begin by using the basic template to create a numbered list of questions that is the basis of your questionnaire. Leave an appropriate amount of space below open questions, and a couple of blank lines below questions needing response option columns.

You won't be using the same range of options for each question, but there may be some that you need more than once. For instance, you may use a five-option scale ranging from 'Agree strongly' to 'Disagree strongly' for several questions. This is a commonly used scale and an example is shown in Figure 27.17.

When you have created a response column for the first question requiring one, you can select it and choose the editing option to copy. Now move the cursor to where the next one is needed and paste in a copy of the response column using the editing option 'paste'. You may be using a sophisticated

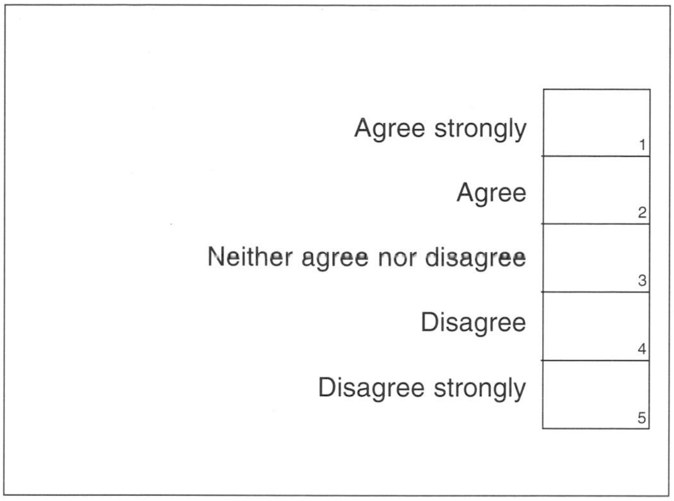

Figure 27.17 A five-option scale

word processor that allows you to save items of selected text as part of your template, thus creating a glossary of useful items that you can paste in whenever you need to. If so you could save your response column and recall it for pasting in this or later questionnaire documents.

You may wish to create a general response options column to speed up your questionnaire creation. This can be used in the current document, and saved in the template if possible. Use either the table or the tabs method to create a column of response options. Include all the formatting instructions we have mentioned, but don't type in any option statements at this stage. Make enough entries in the column to cover the question that has the greatest number of options. On screen you will only see the column of pre-coded check-boxes. Now you can select, copy and paste this column below every fixed-response question. It is easy to go through the document question by question filling in the necessary answer options and deleting the check-boxes you don't need.

Questions also require instructions to the respondent or interviewer on how they are to be answered. Fixed response questions may have 'Tick one box only' and open questions may instruct interviewers to 'Probe fully and record verbatim'.

These instructions need to be clearly separated from both question text and answer options. In the Figure 27.18, a different font has been used, with a bold highlight, to make the directions clear. Also it has been placed between the question and the answer options with space around it so that there is little chance of respondents being confused. Use these methods to add instructions to your questionnaire document.

There may be other instructions that you want to add to your questionnaire. These tell respondents, or interviewers, where to move on to if a particular answer is given. For example, you may ask 'Do you smoke?' and have separate follow-up questions for smokers and non-smokers. This is called **routing**. Routing instructions also need to be clearly separate from question-and-response options text, so you could use the same format as for other instructions. You could put your routing instructions below the response options column, and centre them so that they stand out clearly, as shown in Figure 27.18.

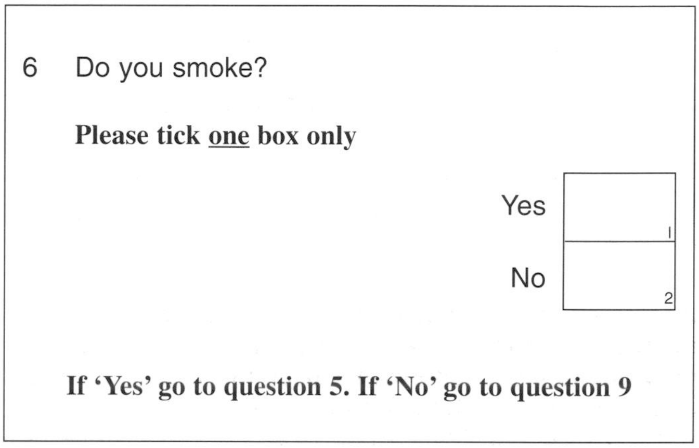

Figure 27.18 An example of a routing instruction

Using the methods we have looked at you will be able to produce good-looking and easy-to-use survey questionnaires. Remember to explore the potential of your word processor and make use of the facilities it offers. Keep copies of all your work as printouts and on a floppy disk so that you have evidence towards the IT unit.

Evidence collection point

The creation of a questionnaire form will allow you to collect evidence towards the IT unit. Keep records of your work at various stages, both as paper copy and as files on floppy disk. Particularly keep records of important editing changes – this is evidence towards Element 3.2.

Your completed document can be used as evidence towards Element 3.3. This element is concerned with the presentation of information. Other word-processed documents that are created for a particular purpose and audience may be useful evidence towards it.

Database software

This section looks at how you can use database software in your studies. It covers;

- setting up a database
- managing data
- creating and printing form letters
- using a database to handle research data.

What is a database?

Database software is used to handle lists. It could be lists of clients, of books read, or of respondents to a social survey. The software application that is used for this is properly called a **database manager**, though it is usually referred to simply as a database.

The sorts of things you can do with a computerised database include:

- locate particular information instantly
- add extra information
- update and alter information
- rearrange the order of the list
- make smaller sub-lists from your information
- share information with other software applications.

Setting up a database

Suppose that you want to create a database containing the details of people you are using as subjects in a research project. To begin setting up a database you first need to decide what information you want to record. You may intend to send postal questionnaires to the people on your list, and use the database to help with analysing the data. For each person you would want to store name and address, and possibly telephone number. Each of these categories of information is known as a **field**. The information held for a particular person is called a **record**, and in our example each record will contain fields for the title (i.e. Mr, Mrs or Miss), name, address and telephone number.

To set up a new database, you must tell the computer precisely what fields you need. It is a good idea to provide separate fields for first name and surname, and for each line in the address. This allows you much more control when managing the data. You also need to decide what type of fields you need. The information you are storing will be of different types, some will be numbers (**numeric data**) and some will be words or perhaps words and numbers together **(alphanumeric data).** Names, titles of books and telephone numbers are all alphanumeric data. Telephone numbers are not used to do calculations so it is easier to treat them as alphanumeric data. You need to decide the types of field necessary for your data and in our example we would need only alphanumeric fields as no numbers are being stored.

You also need to decide on the length of your fields which is specified by a number of characters. Let us allow four characters for the title field, 20 characters each for the surname and first name fields, 30 characters for the first three address fields, eight for the postcode, and 12 characters for the telephone number field. Now we give titles to the fields which indicate their contents.

When you have set up your fields you will have a blank record looking something like Figure 27.19. All you need to do now is enter the details of the first respondent into the fields. When you have finished you add another record and fill in the data for the next person. You carry on creating on creating new records until all your data is stored. When you have finished this process you have created a database.

Title:

Surname:

First_Name:

Address_1:

Address_2:

Address_3:

Postcode:

Telephone:

Figure 27.19 A blank record of fields

Evidence collection point

As part of the evidence required towards Element 3.1 of the IT unit, you need to create and use a database.

You need to:

- decide what information you want to include in each record, and thus what fields you would need in your database
- decide whether fields will be used for numeric or alphanumeric data, and how big each field needs to be
- enter the data for each record.

Keep copies of your work on floppy disk and on paper. Make a paper copy of a blank input screen where data for a new record is entered. This shows the field names, size and type and is evidence of the database structure that you have created.

Where can I use a database?

In Element 5.1 you will be investigating the provision of health and social care services and facilities. You could create a database of services and facilities that are available locally.

All the research that you carry out will generate lists. These may be lists of people, or of books and printed sources that you have consulted. A database is ideal for working on these lists. There will be many other opportunities during your studies to use database software for information that you need to store and work on.

Managing data

You are now able to look at the entries you have made in a variety of ways. Looking at records is known as **browsing** and you have a lot of control over how you arrange them. When you browse records, they are displayed in rows with the field names written as column titles at the top, as in Figure 27.20.

Title	Surname	First_name	Address_1
Mr	Adams	William	14 Park Drive
Mrs	Collins	Susan	8 Longfield Avenue
Mrs	Khan	Naeem	26 Weston Road
Mrs	Mann	Sarah	109 Cedar Drive
Mr	West	Steven	35 Station Road

Figure 27.20 An example of a list of records

You may find that not all the field columns are displayed on the screen at once. This is because they cannot be fitted onto the screen. You can think of the screens as a window that can show only part of the screen at once. You can move the window around to view other areas using the cursor keys or the scroll bar.

In our example the records have been displayed alphabetically using the surname field as the index. The records could be displayed sorted by the first names, or by using any of the fields.

You can ask the computer to search for and display a particular record in a database, and then edit the data it contains. You need to specify the text or numbers that you are looking for and the record that contains it will be displayed. You just need to move the cursor to the information needing alteration and make your changes. For example you could specify 'Collins' in the surname field to find and display the record for Mrs Susan Collins. You can now make any alterations you wish to the data contained in each field, and save them when you are satisfied.

Searching the database for a particular record is very useful, but what if you want to look at a group of records that have something in common? You can query the database to find out which records contain the data you are interested in. A query is made by specifying the fields to be queried, and the information to be searched for. The records which fit the requirements are displayed as a list and you can work on this list using the database management tools available.

Evidence collection point

Managing and editing the information in a database can form part of your evidence towards Element 3.2 of the IT unit. Keep records of your work before and after changes have been made.

Creating and printing form letters

A research project using postal questionnaires may involve sending letters to each respondent. If you have created a respondents database this is easy to do. You can automatically print personalised letters to all your respondents by using the word processor to create a letter and linking it with the database of names and addresses. This process is known as a **mail merge**.

The document that you create on the word processor for a mail merge is known as a **form letter**. Form letters are typed in like an ordinary letter except that you indicate the places where information from the database is to appear. We want to send the same letter to each person on the list, but will need to have a different name and address on each copy of the letter.

Create a form letter on the word processor in the same way that you would any other document. The difference is that form letters need to indicate where database information is to be included, so that the right things appear in the right places. This is done by typing the name of a database field into the letter, positioned where you want the data contained in that field to appear. It has to be made clear to the computer that you have typed a field name and not just another word, and the word processor you are using will have a way of indicating this. These specially marked field names are called **merge fields** and act as an instruction to the computer to bring information from a database file into a word processor file when it is printed.

It is important to realise that merging only takes place when the document is printed so that you do not see the details of particular records displayed on the screen in the letter, only the field names of the database which the records are stored in (see Figure 27.21).

The merge fields indicate where we want database information to appear. Also included is a special field for the current date to be inserted when the letters are printed. Field names have been typed exactly as they are written in the database file so that the computer can recognise them. Here they have been enclosed in angled brackets which some word processors use to define a merge field.

To print the letters you run the word processor and load the file containing the merge letter. You then tell the word processor to perform a print merge, which is one of the print options available. Take care to specify the path to the database file, and its name, so that the computer can find it. This produces a personalised letter for each record on the database. You can also print labels for the envelopes from the database. Run the database programme and load the mailing list file. The database should have address labels included in its printing options. You simply specify the fields to print and the position in which they are to appear on the label. When you instruct the computer to print it produces a label for each record in the database.

47 Princes Avenue
Myton
MY1 2BE
<DATE>

<First_Name><Surname>
<Address_1>
<Address_2>
<Address_3>
<Postcode>

Dear<Title><Surname>

I am a GNVQ Health and Social Care student at Myton College. As part of my studies I am carrying out some research into people's views on health and social care provision.

I would be grateful if you could answer the questions on the enclosed questionnaire form and return it to me at the above address. All returned questionnaires will be kept anonymous, and the results will be used only for my college work.

Thank you for your help with my research.

Yours sincerely

Figure 27.21 An example of a form letter

There may be occasions when it is only necessary to print a letter for a few records on the database and this can be done when printing the merge document with the word processor. As well as specifying the name of the database you can identify particular records that you want to use by using a method similar to querying the database. With the merge letter loaded into the word processor, you would need to select print merge and then specify not only the database name and path, but the particular field contents to look for.

Evidence collection point

You need to combine information from different sources as part of the evidence required towards Element 3.2 of the IT unit. Carrying out a mail merge is a good way of acquiring this evidence. Keep full records of your work at all stages. A printout of a record in a database together with a copy of a personalised form letter will show how data has been copied between applications and combined to form a document. A copy of a completed form letter can be used towards the evidence needed for Element 3.3 where printouts of presented combined information are required.

Using a database to handle research data

Database software can also be useful in the later stages of the research, when the data has been collected and needs to be compiled and analysed. Suppose that you have carried out structured interviews to collect data concerning the effectiveness of a health education campaign. You may have created a database to store the names and addresses of people you are interviewing, using fields similar to those in the example. Now you need to be able to enter the details of each person's responses into his or her record.

You would begin by creating extra fields in the database to hold the response data. If your questionnaire contained 20 questions then you need this number of new fields. The data will be entered in the form of numeric codes so you can choose to create numeric fields this time. This allows you to use the database to perform calculations on the field contents if you wish. You could use simple field titles such as Q1 through to Q20.

Now you need to call up the first record and enter the response codes for each question under the appropriate field heading. Repeat the process for each record until you have entered all the research data. You will need to code the responses to open questions before they can be entered. Chapters 22 and 24 give more detail on this. Code 'Don't know' options with a zero. This will prevent them influencing the results of any statistical analysis that you carry out later.

Think it over

You might have designed opinion scales which use numbers 1 to 5 to measure strength of opinion, with an extra 'don't know' option available. You may intend to average the opinion strength over several questions. What would be the effect on the averaging if you used a number code other than zero for 'don't know' answers?

When all the data has been entered you may want to consider whether you should make changes to the database for reasons of confidentiality. It is part of the ethics of the research process, and also of computer-based data storage, that only necessary data is collected and held. The names, addresses and telephone numbers of respondents clearly link them to the data in their record, and you are not likely to need these details when processing the survey data. You may want to keep part of the address data if you intend to make comparisons between responses from different neighbourhoods. Otherwise the information in the name, address and telephone number fields can be safely deleted. Personal details which are more useful, such as age and gender, should appear in coded form as responses to questions in the Q1 to Q20 fields.

There is no need to go through every record to delete the information. You can select the fields that you don't need and delete them from the database entirely. Removing complete fields means that they, and all the data they contain, are removed from every record simultaneously. Don't delete fields unless you are sure that no important data will be lost.

Now you can begin to analyse the data you have saved. You could begin with fairly simple queries to get a picture of who your respondents are. For instance, you may wish to discover how many women and how many men you have collected data from. You will have noted respondent's genders during the interviews, and coded the answer 1 for male and 2 for female. This data will have been entered into each respondent's record in the appropriate field, say Q1 in our example. You can query the database to find all records with the value 1 in the Q1 field. This will produce a list of all records concerning male respondents, and the total number of such records found will be displayed. Perform the same operation using the value 2 in the Q1 field to get the total number of female respondents.

You can use this method to find out the **frequency** with which particular responses in a question were given. For example, suppose that question 6 was similar to the one mentioned in the word-processing section of this chapter. This concerned the likelihood of publicity materials produced as part of a health education campaign being seen by members of the target audience. There were six possible codes for the answer, ranging from 1 ('Very likely') to 5, ('Not at all likely') with a 'don't know' option which you would have entered in the database as a zero (0). You can set up a database query that searches the Q6 field for records containing each of the codes. The first query is to find the number of '1' responses, and you can note the total given. Now make another query, changing the 1 to a 2 this time. Carry on the process for all the possible answer codes and you will have obtained the response frequency data for the question. (See Figure 27.22.)

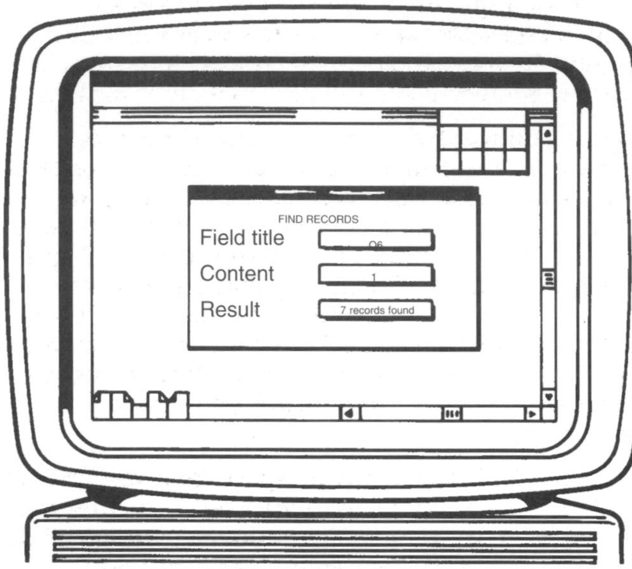

Figure 27.22 Query the database to get response frequency data

You may be interested in how response patterns vary between different types of respondent. For instance your research may have led you to suspect that there may be differences between men and women in the patterns of response to question 6. You can check this possibility by drawing up two sets of response frequency data for the question, one for men and one for women. Now your query carries two conditions. You specify a '1' in the Q1 field and a '1' in the Q6 field for the first query. For the next query you change the Q6 value to '2'. Work through the answer option codes as before, recording the totals given to get frequency totals for the male respondents. You now repeat the process specifying '2' in the Q1 field to get frequency data for female respondents.

You may also want to perform calculations on the data in some fields, and you can use the database to help. For example, you may want to find the mean response to question 6, and the standard deviation from the mean. The mean will indicate the average feeling on the question, represented as a number between one and five which can be compared with the option statements in the original question. The standard deviation will indicate the spread of opinion on the issue.

Database software can perform calculations on data in numeric fields and there are a range of mathematical and statistical symbols that you can use. These are known as operators. To find the mean value of the responses given to question 6 you need to specify the field containing the data, and indicate which calculation you wish to perform on it. Here you would indicate that you wanted the average value of the data in the Q6 field for all records in the database, and the mean response value is rapidly calculated and displayed. You can use similar methods to find the standard deviation of the data.

You may want to calculate separate values of the mean and standard deviation for male and female respondents in order to make comparisons between them. To do this you first need to query the database so as to draw out a list of the male respondents. Specify '1' in the Q1 field for your query to get this list. Now that you have only 'male' records displayed you can perform the calculations for mean and standard deviation on them using the methods discussed above. Do the same for female respondents to get the other statistics you need.

You can design queries that will help you to analyse your data from practically any angle. To avoid wasting time and becoming confused by the statistics that you are creating, always plan your data analysis in the light of your research needs.

Evidence collection point

The calculations that you make on database data can be evidence towards Element 3.2 of the IT unit. Your queries and searches are examples of processing data, and are also relevant evidence towards this element. Keep full records of your work at each stage.

Spreadsheets

This section looks at using spreadsheets to handle and present data. It covers;

- setting up a spreadsheet
- formulae
- copying formulae
- analysing research data with a spreadsheet
- creating a table.

What is a spreadsheet?

Spreadsheets are designed to work with numerical information. With a spreadsheet you can:

- enter numeric information in well-organised rows and columns

- give the rows and columns any titles you choose
- make changes to the number and titles in your spreadsheet whenever you wish
- perform calculations on the numbers in your spreadsheet
- make a graph or chart from numbers in your spreadsheet
- export results and other data from your spreadsheet to another application such as the word processor
- save and print your spreadsheet, and charts made from it.

Setting up a spreadsheet

The information in a spreadsheet is organised into columns and rows, and you can see this arrangement on the screen when running the spreadsheet software. (See Figure 27.23).

	A	B	C	D	E	F
1						
2						
3						
4						
5						
6						
7						
8						

Figure 27.23 Part of a typical spreadsheet screen

Each row and column is labelled. In Figure 27.23, letters are used to label the columns and numbers are used to label the rows, which is the system found on most spreadsheets. This labelling system means that each cell has a unique address, known as the **cell reference**, which is written using the column letter and the row number. The cell in the top left corner is highlighted and its cell reference is A1, as it is in the column labelled A and in the row labelled 1. You can move the highlight from cell to cell using the cursor arrow keys or the mouse, and highlight any cell in the spreadsheet. The highlighted cell is called the active cell. Information that you type in is entered into the **active cell**, and to enter information in a particular cell you need to highlight it as the active cell first.

The screen can only display a part of the spreadsheet at any one time, as happens with the other software applications that we have looked at. You actually have a large number of rows and columns available to you. As you move the active cell highlight across, or up and down your spreadsheet other parts will come into view. You can enter text or numbers into the cells of a spreadsheet. Text is used to label columns and rows, and to create spreadsheet titles. The job of a spreadsheet is to work with numbers, however, and there are a range of facilities for this.

Suppose you wanted to create a spreadsheet to calculate the costs involved in carrying out a research project using postal questionnaires, to help you decide how many subjects you can afford to include. Your first step, as always, is to plan the work. Begin by listing the areas of spending that are involved. You may include postage, reprographics, envelopes, and the cost of a good-quality printout of your word-processed form and covering letter. These spending categories can become row headings in your spreadsheet.

Leave Row 1 blank to provide space for a spreadsheet title. Now make cell 2A the active cell and enter the heading 'Postage' into it. Then move down to cell 3B and enter the word 'Reprographics'. Carry on entering spending categories as row titles into the cells in column A. The look of a spreadsheet can be improved by changing the size of rows and columns, and by formatting the text and number entries to suit your requirements. For instance, the word 'Reprographics' will not fit in the space provided, but this can be solved by increasing the width of the A column to allow enough room.

The spreadsheet recognises which cell entries are text and aligns them over to the left, whereas numbers are aligned to the right. You can control this arrangement, and change other formatting options for cell contents. Change the appearance of your row titles by selecting the cells in column A and choosing the formatting options you want for that column. Your spreadsheet will now look something like Figure 27.24.

	A	B	C	D	E	F
1						
2	Reprographics					
3	Envelopes					
4	Postage					
5	Printing					
6	Total					

Figure 27.24 A spreadsheet with row titles in place

The spreadsheet is intended to calculate the cost of producing and sending different numbers of questionnaires. Printing out your original document from the word processor is a one-off cost. The costs of the other items are found by multiplying the unit cost by the number of questionnaires being sent. These amounts are added together to give the total cost. This means that you need to enter the unit costs of reprographics, postage, and printing into vacant cells in the spreadsheet. Also you need somewhere to enter the number of questionnaires you intend to send out. The cost of printout and reprographics depends on how many sheets you intend to send to each respondent, so you will also need to find a cell for this information. The spreadsheet in Figure 27.25 has title, added to indicate where these items will appear.

	A	B	C	D	E	F
1						
2	Reprographics					
3	Envelopes					
4	Postage					
5	Printing					
6	Total				Unit	cost
7					Reprographics	
8					Envelopes	
9	Sheets/mailing				Postage	
10	No. to send					
11						

Figure 27.25 A spreadsheet with titles added

Headings have been added to cells A9 and A10 to indicate that cell B9 will contain the number of sheets per mailing, and that cell B10 will contain the number of questionnaires you intend to send out. A 'Unit cost' column has been created by entering the spending categories in cells E7 to E9.

The next space is to add numerical information and formulae into the spreadsheet so that it can begin to work. Suppose reprographics costs 5p per sheet, envelopes 2p each, and postage 20p per respondent. A high-quality laser printed copy of your word-processed questionnaire form and covering letter may cost 10p per sheet. Some items in the 'Unit cost' column can be filled in immediately. Envelope and postage unit costs can be entered directly into cells F8 and F9 as they will be the same regardless of how many sheets each mailing contains. However, for reprographic and printing costs you need to multiply the price per sheet by the number of sheets per mailing. This means entering a formula into the cell where you want the information to appear.

Formulae

Formulae (plural) use mathematical and other symbols to perform calculations on the contents of different cells in the spreadsheet. A formula (singular) is entered into the active cell and operates on the contents of the cells it refers to. The result is calculated and displayed in the active cell. The symbols used for basic arithmetic calculations are: + for add, – for subtract, *for multiply, / for divide, which are all available on the keyboard. Maths symbols like these which are used in formulae are called **mathematical operators**. Formulae can include a range of mathematical, statistical and scientific symbols, and your equipment will have a set of such symbols that it will recognise and use. You can also use parentheses (brackets) in formulae as you would in mathematical calculations.

To calculate the unit cost of reprographics in our example we need to enter a formula into cell F7 that multiplies the contents of cell B9 (number of sheets per mailing) by £0.05 (the cost of reproducing one sheet). Your spreadsheet will recognise a particular symbol as indicating a formula and it is essential that you enter it correctly, otherwise your formula will be treated as a text cell entry. In our example we have used the equals sign to signify a formula. Make F7 the active cell and enter the formula B9*0.05.
A similar formula can be entered into cell B5 to calculate the printing cost. Here the formula will be entered as B9*0.10.

Like other cell entries, the formula appears both in the active cell and outside the spreadsheet area until you press enter to confirm you entry. When you press enter, the formula is no longer displayed in the cell but the result of the calculation appears there instead. The formula remains visible in the other part of the screen so that you can recognise that the spreadsheet is displaying the result of a calculation. Our formulae will not be able to display a result until we specify the number of sheets being produced in cell B9, so let's say that we intend to send four sheets to each person. The formulae operate on this value in cell B9 and the spreadsheet now looks like Figure 27.26.

The result we want is the total cost of sending a certain number of mailings so now formulae can be entered into cells B2 and B6 to calculate this. The formula B10*F7 would display the total reprographics

= B9*0.05

	A	B	C	D	E	F
1						
2	Reprographics					
3	Envelopes					
4	Postage					
5	Printing	0.04				
6	Total				Unit	cost (£)
7					Reprographics	0.20
8					Envelopes	0.02
9	Sheets/mailing	4			Postage	0.20
10	No. to send					
11						

Figure 27.26 A spreadsheet with printing and reprographics calculated

cost cell B2. It will multiply the number of mailings, contained in cell B10, by the cost of reprographics for one mailing, which is contained in cell F7. We need similar formulae in cells B3 and B4 and can use the select and copy features of spreadsheets to help.

Copying formulae

You are able to copy cell contents to other cells in a spreadsheet, whether the cell contains text, numbers or a formula. If cells containing formulae are copied the cell references adjust to the new location so that the formula now refers to a different range of cells. Cell references in formulae which are able to adapt in this way are called relative cell references. All cell references in formulae are treated as **relative cell references** unless you indicate otherwise.

If we wanted to fix a cell in a formula, so that it doesn't change when the formula is copied to a different cell, we can indicate this using a symbol that the computer recognises. Cell references in formulae which have been fixed in this way are called **absolute cell references.** In our example, we need to copy the formula in cell B2 to cells B3 and B4. The reference to cell B10 in the formula must be fixed so that copies of the formulae still refer to it. However, we want the reference cell F7 to change when the formula is pasted to a new location. The formula in cell B2 needs to be written as $B$10*F7. The absolute cell reference is indicated by the use of dollar signs in this example. Next the formula is selected and pasted into cells B3 and B4. The relative cell references adapt to their new location, for instance the formula in cell B3 becomes $B$10*F8.

A formula is needed in cell B6 to total the costs in cells B2 to B5. You will be able to use a command like SUM to add together the contents of a number of cells along a row or down a column. First highlight cell B6 as the active cell then enter the formula SUM(B2:B5). The colon symbol (:) has been used here to indicate that the formula operates on a range of cells.

You can now use the spreadsheet to calculate costs. Enter a value for the number of questionnaires you intend to send into cell B10, and results appear in cells B2 to B6. Suppose we enter the number 50 into cell B10 as the number we want to send. The costs are calculated and displayed as shown in Figure 27.27.

50

	A	B	C	D	E	F
1						
2	Reprographics	10.00				
3	Envelopes	1.00				
4	Postage	10.00				
5	Printing	0.04				
6	Total	£21.40			Unit	cost (£)
7					Reprographics	0.20
8					Envelopes	0.02
9	Sheets/mailing	4			Postage	0.20
10	No. to send	50				
11						

Figure 27.27 A completed spreadsheet

What makes the spreadsheet so useful is that you can now experiment with different values for the number being sent, and the number of sheets per mailing, and instantly get a figure for the total cost of a postal research project. You can adjust the number of respondents, and possibly the number of sheets to be sent, until the total cost falls within your budget.

Evidence collection point

As part of the evidence required towards Element 3.2 of the IT unit, you need to set up and use a spreadsheet. You can create a spreadsheet to deal with any numerical information during your studies. Keep copies of your spreadsheets on paper and on floppy disk.

Analysing research data with a spreadsheet

Spreadsheets can also be applied to data analysis, and displaying the results. You can use a spreadsheet to examine in detail the responses to a question. Suppose that you have used a database to store the response data from the respondents and have examined the data by querying the database in various ways. You may have obtained response frequency information for the answers to some questions, and can now use the spreadsheet to analyse the data further.

Spreadsheets allow you to create graphs and charts from selected items of data. This can be used to give you a visual impression of the shape data makes when plotted as a graph. It is much easier to use visual methods for checking how well a distribution matches the normal distribution curve (see Chapter 24).

Suppose a question has five allowed responses scaled from 'Agree strongly' to 'Disagree strongly'. Examination of the response data using a database gives the response totals for each answer option in the scale. A spreadsheet is set up to store these total, and may look something like Figure 27.28.

	A	B	C	D	E	F	G	H
1	Question response frequency							
2								
3	Question 6							
4	Answer option:	1	2	3	4	5		
5								
6	Frequency (All):	7	10	14	11	6		
7								
8	Frequency (Male):	2	3	5	7	4		
9								
10	Frequency (Female):	5	7	8	4	2		
11								
12								

Figure 27.28 A spreadsheet showing the response totals for each answer option

Now you can select the data that you want to plot as a graph and choose how you would like it to be displayed. You could make bar charts which plot the answer options along the horizontal axis, and the number of responses up the vertical axis. Bar charts of the responses given by women and men can be compared visually to assess differences between them in the pattern of responses. Charts based on this data would look like Figure 27.29.

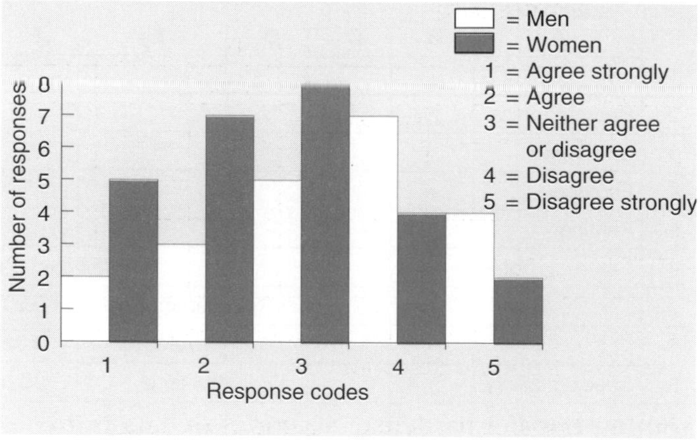

Figure 27.29 A chart showing research data

You can use a spreadsheet to calculate the mean and standard deviation of a set of data. You have seen how this may be done using a database, but many people refer to handle numbers in a spreadsheet since they have more flexibility in calculations than a database, and instant charting is available. To examine the data fully, it is useful to transfer items directly from the database records into a spreadsheet. You should find that you can share data easily with the software you are using. In our example, you have stored response codes for question 6 in the Q6 field of respondents database. You select the contents of this field for copying to the spreadsheet, and instruct the computer to carry this out.

In the example, there were a total of 47 respondents which means that a row of 47 cells in the spreadsheet now contains the data. Each cell displays a number from 1 to 5, indicating the responses given to question 6. To find the mean of the data you need to put a formula in the cell where the answer is to appear. The spreadsheet will have its own list of available functions, and the mean and standard deviation are standard ones that you will find on all spreadsheets. You move to the answer cell and enter your formula in the format your software recognises. Use the on-line help to check on the particular format you need to follow. Figure 27.30 shows how this may look.

There is data for 47 respondents occupying cells 1 to 47 in the A column, and Figure 27.30 only shows part of this. Formulae have been entered into cells D1 and D2 to calculate mean and standard deviation. As D2 is the active cell you can see its formula displayed above the main body of the spreadsheet.

= STD(A1:A47)

	A	B	C	D	E	F
1	3		Mean	2.28		
2	2		Std. deviation	1.26		
3	2					
4	3					
5	1					
6	5					

Figure 27.30 A spreadsheet showing the calculations of mean and standard deviation

You can transfer particular selections of data from the database to the spreadsheet if you want to make comparisons. For instance, you could query the database to obtain the records of male respondents. You can choose to transfer data from these records to a spreadsheet and thus perform separate statistical calculations on the responses from men and women.

Creating a table

Spreadsheets are often used to produce tables of results which can then be printed, or exported to other software applications such as word processor. You may wish to summarise some of your research findings as a table, and include percentages to help readers interpret the data. Suppose that you have been analysing the results from your structured interview research in Element 7.3. You may now have statistics on key issues that you want to display together, and may have noticed differences between the responses of men and women that you want to bring out.

To set up a spreadsheet you first need to enter column headings and row labels in appropriate cells, and format them appropriately. The column headings indicate where totals and percentages will be displayed for men, women and the respondents overall. Row labels include total responses, and four categories of data relating to the research question. The number of people who have seen publicity, understood the message, etc., have been found and can be entered straight into the appropriate cells (see Figure 27.31).

Now formulae can be added to calculate the percentages that are needed. The percentages of men and women who responded could be dealt with first. Cell C4 is intended to display the percentage of women amongst the respondents. The total number of respondents is displayed in cell F4, and the total number of women amongst them is in cell B4. The

	A	B	C	D	E	F	G	H
1		Research findings table						
2		Women	%	Men	%	Overall	%	
3								
4	Total responses	26		21		47		
5	Seen publicity	20		15		35		
6	Message understandable	18		13		31		
7	Message relevant	15		8		23		
8	Behaviour change	8		5		13		
9								

Figure 27.31 A spreadsheet table with information entered ready for calculation

formula needed to calculate this percentage is B4/F4(*100). This will divide the contents of B4 by the contents of F4, and multiply the results by 100. A similar formula is entered into cell E4 to find the percentage of male respondents. Here it will be D4/F4(*100).

The percentage of women who have seen the publicity is to appear in cell C5. It can be calculated by using the formula B5/B4(*100). Remember though that the formula will be similar for the percentages in cells C6, C7 and C8, and we can copy the one in cell C5 to these other locations. The reference to cell B4 will be unaltered in all the formulae, but the reference to cell B5 needs to be adapted to the other locations. Cell B5 needs a relative cell reference, and cell B4 needs an absolute cell reference. The formula can be written as B5/$B$4(*100) and entered into cell C4. Again dollar signs have been used to indicate an absolute cell reference. Now when it is copied to other cells in the C column the formula will adapt to give the result we want. For example, the formula becomes B8/$B$4(*100) when it is copied to cell C8.

Similar formulae are needed to calculate the percentages for male respondents, and the overall percentages. The cell references will be different, however, for example, the formula in cell E5 will be D5/$D$4(*100). Copying can be used to enter the formula in other cells, as before. The final result is shown in Figure 27.32.

You can use this spreadsheet as the basis of a table, and you could illustrate your conclusions by making charts or graphs. For instance, in this example the differences between responses from women and men could be shown by selecting the data in columns C and E and creating a bar chart which displays these percentages.

	A	B	C	D	E	F	G	H
1		Research findings table						
2		Women	%	Men	%	Overall	%	
3								
4	Total responses	26	55	21	45	47	100	
5	Seen publicity	20	77	15	71	35	74	
6	Message understandable	18	69	13	62	31	65	
7	Message relevant	15	58	8	38	23	49	
8	Behaviour change	8	31	5	24	13	28	
9								

Figure 27.32 The completed spreadsheet table

There are many other ways to use spreadsheets to analyse data. You can use your imagination, and refer to the needs of the research project to find the best approach in your own work.

Evidence collection point

Analysing and presenting data with a spreadsheet can produce evidence towards the IT unit. Your data analysis is evidence towards Element 3.2, as is the spreadsheet template you create to carry it out. Importing data from a database, and exporting charts and graphs to a word processor, are also evidence towards Element 3.2. The graphs, charts and tables you produce are evidence towards Element 3.3.

Graphics software

This section is about using graphics software. It covers:

- drawing software
- painting software.

What is graphics software?

If you want to produce a diagram, illustration or any other sort of graphic, computer-based methods could be used. There are two basic types of graphics software: drawing programmes and painting programmes. Each type produces work in its own style, but both share the advantages of using computer-based methods.

With graphics software you can:

- create diagrams and illustrations easily
- use powerful software features to develop and adapt your work
- save your work, and reload it later to make improvements and new versions
- export your graphic to another application, such as a desk-top publisher or word processor, and incorporate it in another document.

You may well have access to both types of graphics application, so we will look briefly at what each of them can do.

Drawing software

Drawing software is designed to create precise and clear illustrations and diagrams. Some specialised drawing software is intended to be used for technical drawing and computer-aided design (CAD). Other drawing packages are intended for more general use, though these are also capable of producing very accurate work. The drawing screen consists of a main working area in the middle, where your drawing is created, and a number of small graphic 'buttons' around the side. These buttons represent the different drawing facilities (**tools**) available within the software.

There are tools for creating standard geometric shapes, such as circles, ovals, squares and rectangles. Other tools allow you to draw smooth curved lines, do freehand drawing, and create polygons with as many sides as you wish. You can adjust the line thickness (**line weight**) and the colour of lines and fill effects. (Remember, though, that you will only get coloured printout with a colour printer. If you draw in colour and print in monochrome you will not be able to judge how the final result will look.) There will also be a text tool which lets you add text in whatever font shapes and sizes your machine has available.

The mouse is an essential tool with graphics software. You use the mouse to select a drawing tool, and to draw on the screen with it. It can be quite difficult to draw with the mouse at first, and practice is the best way to improve. Try experimenting with the tools available in the drawing package so that you are familiar with the shapes and effects that they produce. The on-line help will give guidance on what different tools can do, and how to select them. Figure 27.33 shows the effects produced by some drawing tools.

As you experiment with the drawing software you will notice that new shapes sit on top of existing ones, and cover up all or part of them. This creates

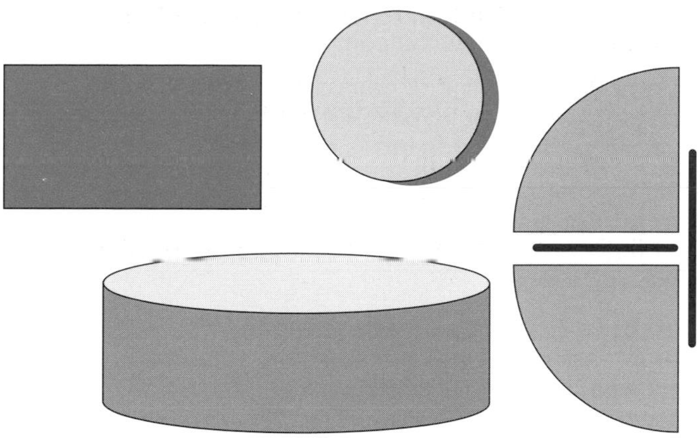

Figure 27.33 Using drawing tools

interesting effects, and you can control which object is displayed in front and which behind. All you need to do is select the object you are interested in and send it to the back or front. It will then be on top, or hidden, as required. You can use this feature with text to produce attractive bordered titles.

You can select any line or shape you create with a drawing application and edit it. Selected shapes are displayed with a group of small squares around them. There are many different editing facilities available. Selected objects can be copied, moved, reshaped, deleted, and even reversed (flipped). Each separate piece of a drawing can be individually selected and edited. In a way it exists in its own right, and so it is referred to as an object. You can make alterations to an object, leaving other parts of the drawing unaffected.

Sometimes, however, you want objects to stay together so that you can make editing changes without affecting the arrangement of the group. You can do this by **grouping** the objects. You just select the objects you want and define them as a group. Grouped objects behave as though they were a single object, and you can move and adjust them all together. When you have finished editing you can ungroup the objects again, and select individual parts for further editing if necessary. See Figure 27.34.

Painting software

Painting software is also used to create graphics and illustrations. Like drawing software, you will see the painting area in the middle of the screen and buttons to select the painting tools available. You can create circles, squares and other geometrical shapes. You can draw straight, curved or freehand lines, and you can add text. Using these facilities may not seem much different from using drawing software.

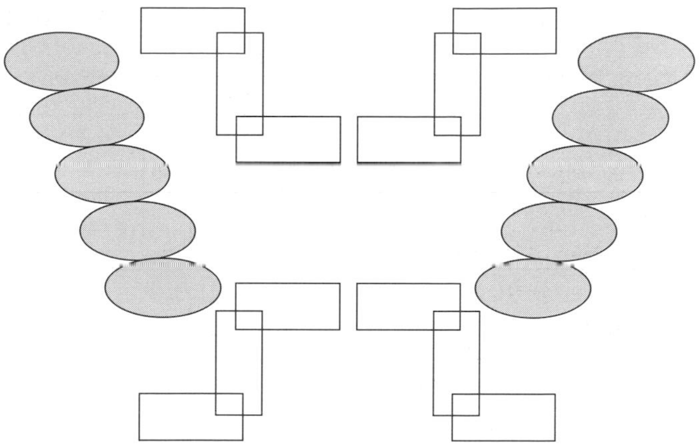

Figure 27.34 This illustration uses grouping, copying and flipping techniques

However, painting software has other characteristics which make it very different to use. You can apply colours, or grey tones, with a variety of effects. The shape and size of the brush can be altered, and you can use a spray effect to produce artistic looking shading. Another useful facility is the 'fill effect'. This fills a bounded area with any colour or tone you want. If you try to fill a shape that is not fully bounded, paint will spill out and fill your background too! Figure 27.35 shows the effect created by painting software.

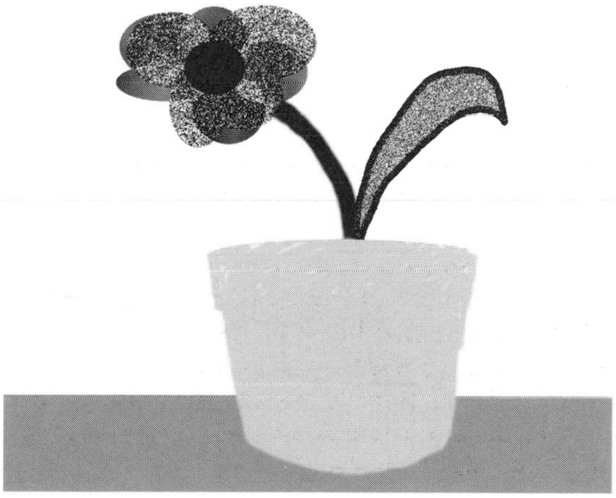

Figure 27.35 An illustration created using painting software

The big difference between painting and drawing software becomes obvious when you edit your work. Things that you draw with drawing software can be treated as separate objects, and individually selected for editing. Things you paint using painting software become part of the overall picture and cannot be separated from it later. You can go over bits of your painting with another colour to make changes, and do any touching up you wish, but you can't just pick up all the paint that is of a particular colour, or is in a particular shape. It is best to think of painting software as if it really does use paint.

Evidence collection point

You need to use graphics as part of the evidence needed for the IT unit. The creation and editing of graphics is evidence towards Elements 3.1 and 3.2. You can import a graphic into a word-processed document and produce evidence of combining information, which could be used towards Element 3.2. The presentation of your graphics, whether on their own or as part of another document, can be evidence towards Element 3.3. Remember, as always, to keep full records of your work on paper and on floppy disk.

Fast Facts

Absolute cell reference In a spreadsheet formula an absolute cell reference remains unaltered when the formula is copied to other cells. A special symbol is used to denote an absolute cell reference.

Application A word used for the set of instructions that the computer carries out. The word application refers to software that has been designed to be applied to a particular task such as word processing or spreadsheeting. See also **Software** and **Program.**

Byte A single piece of information – one keystroke is one byte. Bytes are used as a measure of computer memory size. See also **Kilobyte** and **Megabyte**.

Cell In a spreadsheet, a cell is the area where an item of data or a formula is stored. Spreadsheets are made up of a large grid of cells.

Cell reference The unique address of a cell in a spreadsheet. The cell reference is given by the row and column headings which apply to the cell.

Compatibility The ability of hardware and software to work together. Software packages that are compatible can share information. Hardware needs to be connected to other hardware that is compatible with it.

Cursor A blinking line or dash on the screen which indicates where your typing will appear, or your editing take place. Sometimes this is referred to as the insertion point.

Cut and paste A term used for the process of selecting and moving text. Text is cut from one place and pasted back in another.

Database A database manager (usually referred to simply as a database) is a software application used to deal with information in the form of lists. Strictly speaking, a database is any listed information and a telephone directory or your address book are databases.

Directories Electronically created compartments on a disk that are used to group files that you wish to keep together. Directories help you to keep track of your files.

Drawing application A graphics application that is used to edit and produce diagrams, plans and many other types of graphic. Drawing applications give a clean, designed look to graphic work.

Field A category of information contained in a database. Records contain data entered into fields.

File A piece of work that has been created and saved on the computer. Each file has a name. It also has a few characters indicating the type of file it is, and the software that it can be loaded into.

Floppy disk A portable piece of hardware used to store data. Floppy disks are small, lightweight and durable. You can store a large amount of data on a floppy disk.

Form letter A word-processed letter that contains merge fields linked to a database. Form letters are used to create mass mailshots.

Formatting documents This refers to alterations made to the way a document looks, either by changing character size and type, or by varying the arrangement of paragraphs.

Formatting floppy disks The process of electronically dividing a floppy disk into tracks and sectors. Disks must be formatted before files can be saved on them.

Graphics application A software application designed to deal with graphical information. There are two types of graphics application, drawing software and painting software. Graphics applications are used to produce plans and artwork of all types.

Grouping In drawing applications, separate objects can be joined together as a group. The objects can now be edited as a single unit.

Hard disk A piece of hardware used to store information. The hard disk is permanently fixed inside the computer's case and cannot be removed from it.

Hardware The physical equipment used in IT. This includes the computer, the monitor, the keyboard, the mouse, cables and other devices such as printers.

Information technology The term is used to refer to modern, scientific ways of handling information. It is applied to the fields of computing, video and telecommunications and the rapidly developing links between them.

Kilobyte A measure of amount of information. One kilobyte (K) = 1024 bytes. (See **Byte**).

Margins The boundaries within which your work is printed. There are margins at the top and bottom of the page, as well as on either side.

Megabyte A measure of amount of information. One megabyte (Mb) = 1024 kilobytes (or 1048546 bytes). (See **Byte.**)

Merge fields Specially marked parts of a form letter which contain the titles of fields in a database. Merge fields allow information in a database list to be merged with a word-processed document.

Mouse A piece of hardware used to communicate instructions and information to the computer. The mouse, and its on-screen pointer, are basic equipment these days, and are essential with graphics software.

Network When several computers are linked together so that information is shared they form a network. Networks allow a large range of software, and other facilities, to be used by many people at once.

Operator In a spreadsheet or database, an operator is a mathematical or statistical term that is used in formulae to perform calculations. Operators include terms like 'Average' and 'Sum', and make it easy to create formulae. Spreadsheets have a wide range of operators available.

Painting application A graphics application that is used to create and edit pictures and illustrations. Painting programmes produce a free, 'fine art' effect.

Program A word used for the set of instructions that the computer carries out. See also **Software** and **Application**.

RAM Random Access Memory. The RAM holds the information and instructions that are being used by the computer during your work sessions. It is completely cleared when you switch the computer off.

Record The information in a database on a particular item. Each record consists of data entered into fields.

Relative cell reference In a spreadsheet formula, a relative cell reference adjusts to its new location when the formula is copied to other cells.

Scroll bar Scroll bars are long bars with arrows at each end which are used in many applications. Scroll bars are used with the mouse to bring other parts of documents into view.

Scrolling Bringing other parts of a document into view on the screen. Scrolling is necessary because software usually has more information to display than can be fitted onto a single screen.

Selecting Identifying certain parts of a file with a highlight so that the selected section can be deleted, moved or copied. Usually both the mouse and the keyboard can be used to select text.

Software A word used for the set of instructions that the computer carries out. See also **Program** and **Application**.

Spreadsheet A software application designed to deal with numerical information. Spreadsheets store numerical data in a grid of cells, and can perform a wide range of calculations upon it.

Stand-alone computer A stand-alone is a computer that is a self-contained machine. It is not linked to other computers and works independently of them.

Style sheet A name used for a blueprint document which is created and used on a word processor. Style sheets contain formatting instructions so that each document based on it has a similar style. Style sheets are sometimes referred to as word processor templates.

Template A template is a file which has instructions embedded within it, and sets up the software for a task before you begin. Spreadsheet templates contain formulae, and labels and titles. Word-processor templates contain instructions on format and style. If you need to perform a task on more than one occasion a template prevents you having to start from scratch. Word-processor templates are sometimes known as style sheets.

Word processor A software application that is designed to deal with text-based information. Word processing is one of the most common uses of IT. Practically any kind of text-based document can be created with a word processor.

Self-assessment test answers

Answers to Unit 1

1 **False.** There are many differences between cultures, for example some value human life, whilst others value male aggression more highly. In some historical cultures, the more people a man killed the greater his social status and therefore his chance to marry and have children.

2 **True.** This is a central principle for Western democratic societies. Democracy encourages people to make decisions about how they wish their society to be organised. This is achieved through voting for a political party. In addition, competition for money and success is perceived as being essential. Ensuring that all groups of people are able to compete is seen to be an important issue.

3 **True.** The equality of opportunity legislation aims to ensure that issues like race, gender and disability do not artificially exclude groups of people from the chance to compete.

4 **False**. Legislation alone cannot ensure that all have the same chance in the competition. Legislation ensures the opportunity for different groups to compete.

5 **True**. They form an agreed way of reaching decisions within the health and social care professions. Ethical codes are based on essential values for health and care.

6 **a** Staff are in a powerful position to ensure all clients' rights are upheld in the care setting.

7 **c** By recognising cultural need, staff are working to sustain the individual client's self-esteem. Culture forms a major part of an individual's self-concept.

8 **b** Institutional racism includes any system within an organisation which places people at a disadvantage to others within an organisation, for example, male-only toilets when there are a few women working in an organisation.

9 **c** This Act applies to men and women to ensure neither are disadvantaged because of their gender.

10 **a** These codes set out the 'rules' of a given profession. They aim to ensure a consistently high-quality service. They are a guide for professionals regarding the expected behaviour within the profession.

11 **False**. As yet it is not illegal to discriminate against an individual on the grounds of sexuality.

12 **c** There is a growing movement to reduce the legal age to 16 years to come into line with heterosexual relations. As yet the law is unchanged at 21 years.

13 **False.** As yet there is no legislation in Britain regarding discrimination on the grounds of age. There is, however, some pressure from the EC to review this.

14 **d** The EOC offers advice and support to both men and women regarding rights under the Sex Discrimination Acts.

15 **d** The CRE offers advice and support regarding the rights of individuals under Race Relations legislation.

16 **c** There is legislation to support equality on grounds of race, gender and disability. Disability is the only one of the three not to have a government 'watch-dog' and therefore the legislation in this area lacks 'teeth'.

17 **True.** It is possible to appeal against the decision of an industrial tribunal. Certain cases may be taken to the House of Lords and finally to the European Court of Justice in Luxembourg. All decisions must comply with the EEC Equal Treatment Directive (76/207/EEC).

18 **c** The others raise funds and public awareness of the issues faced by their particular client groups. VOAL works to promote a change in public attitude to people with any disability. The aim is to tighten legislation for people with a disability to enable them to have a more equal opportunity to compete.

19 **b** Now that Britain is a full member of the EU it is influenced by the ruling of the European

Parliament, e.g. the EEC Equal Treatment Directive (76/207/EEC). The EEC Recommendations (OJL 86/225/43) were a factor in the introduction of the Disabled Persons (Services, Consultation and Representation) Act 1986 in Britain.

20 **d** None of the others directly affects employment opportunities for people with disability.

21 **d** Showing quite open disrespect for another through language or behaviour.

22 **b** This is less obvious and more subtle. In your view you are saving a possibly embarrassing situation at a party. By doing so you are discriminating against your friend because he or she is non-white.

23 **c** Knowingly telling jokes which devalue other people because they are different from you.

24 i **d:** implies only white-skinned people need apply.
ii **b:** implies only able-bodied people need apply.
iii **a:** implies only females need apply.

25 a **iv:** assuming the elder cannot decide for himself or herself.
b **i:** placing emphasis on the word 'only' implies that girls are inferior.
c **ii:** the facial expression and laughter are at the expense of someone in difficulty.

26 **b** This statement is discriminating against those who are retired.

27 **a** Both are true: words are very powerful ways of making others feel good or bad. The tone used can totally change the meaning of a word or sentence, for example, placing emphasis on the word 'silly' when used to describe a person can be shown as a joke if said with a smile in the voice or, said brusquely, can be used to put someone down.

28 **d** Institutional discrimination is the way an organisational culture promotes one group as superior to another. In this example the implication is that only men are thought to be suitable for senior positions in the company.

29 **c** The Race Relations Act is being contravened as Muslims are being discriminated against because of their culture, and this could be indirect discrimination.

30 **d** If an organisation considers it to be essential to have a balance of gender or ethnicity to meet the needs of the organisation, then positive action may legally be taken to redress the balance; for example advertising for staff fluent in Bengali to meet the needs of the Bengali community in a given area.

31 **d** The group leader is effectively blocking the person with disability out of the discussion by turning his or her back on the individual. In the other examples the body is used to reinforce the interaction between individuals.

32 **a** Both are true. (**i**) Women are openly being put down at work by the words or actions of others just because they are female. (**ii**) The person with the facial scars is being discriminated against in a more subtle way by some people avoiding him or her. If staff openly refuse to share tea breaks with this individual, then it would be direct as it would be open discrimination. In both instances there will be a negative effect on the individual concerned.

33 **c** By denying choice an assumptions is being made that the man is incapable of making his own decisions. Down's syndrome is a condition where there are varying degrees of cognitive ability.

34 **b** It is discrimination if the only reason this person was refused entry to the youth club is because he or she is black.

35 **a** As long as the women has the required qualifications, and meets the criteria for the job, there is no reasons to refuse her application.

36 **a** To treat people the same is to deny individuality. Each person has different needs which must be recognised and addressed to ensure equality of opportunity. All the other options acknowledge differences. (**d**) shows an awareness of inequalities in society. The carer must take steps to address the issues in the care setting to ensure equality of opportunity for the clients.

37 **a** Continuing with his usual social activities will encourage Jim to be more self-confident. He may fear rejection by his friends as he can no longer see. Being accepted as part of a circle of friends is an important step to rehabilitation.

38 **c** By learning new skills, Jim will gain in confidence. Work may have been a major factor in the way Jim saw himself as a father, husband and in society in general.

39 **b** By continuing an active role with his children, Jim will again build his self-confidence and self-image. Being able to contribute to the family in this way will maintain his social status as a parent. In turn this will boost his self-confidence as a 'worthwhile' individual.

40 **b** By avoiding stereotyping clients, the carer is recognising individuals rather than looking at an unrealistic mental image of what the client will be like.

41 **True.** Clear guidelines are set out in professional codes of practice. These aim to ensure that all staff work within the same value base with all clients whatever the situation.

42 **True.** Clients expect staff to be understanding of their needs and to respect issues like confidentiality of information. This enables clients to place trust in the carer as a professional. Without trust, it may be impossible to build a supportive relationship to meet client need effectively.

43 **b** Clients must be able to trust that any information they give to a carer will be held in strictest confidence. Clients know that records must be kept and that it is helpful to staff to know what they can tell others and what must be kept between themselves.

44 **d** It is important that the client understands why, in your professional opinion, you need to pass on the information in confidence to a senior member of staff. The aim is to gain his or her agreement. Should the client still refuse, you may need to make it clear that you have no choice in the matter.

45 **i** Both are true. All information held on file or on a database comes under the Data Protection Act to ensure confidentiality. Anyone may ask to see their file; however, where it is considered inappropriate for the mental well-being of a client to see his or her medical records, then this part of the file is kept for medical staff on a need-to-know basis only.

46 **ii** (**a**) is true – health and social care staff should continually work to raise their awareness of discrimination and the effects it has on individuals. (**b**) is false. Older people may find it harder to change long-held attitudes, but age is no excuse for causing harm to others by words or deeds. It is important to work with individuals to support them as they review the effect their attitude has on others.

47 **d** It is important to check that the client fully understands written or verbal statements of his or her rights. Time should be made available to answer any questions and to clarify any point.

48 **c** Helping her to gain a range of information so that she is able to make choices is essential. This is empowerment of the client – a key value in health and social care.

49 **d** Negotiating with her to continue to learn English will enable her to take a more active part in the care setting. It will also ensure that she has a better chance of employment when she is ready to take that step.

50 **a** By keeping in touch with members of her West African community, she will keep alive her own language and customs. These all form an essential part of her identity.

51 **d** Some people prefer a shower to bath. This stems from a preference to wash under running water rather than to sit in water considered 'dirty'.

52 **c** It is important to record any religion followed by a client. Religion often forms the guidelines for living for individuals and becomes an important part of their custom and practice. A contact name is useful and clients should be encouraged to continue their faith if they so wish.

53 **a** It is important to ensure that any establishment reflects the cultural diversity of the clients. This demonstrates value and respect for the richness of other cultures, rather than just a white Eurocentric culture.

54 **b** This is quite a dilemma for the night staff. They have to balance the rights of the man to do as he likes in the privacy of his own room, with the rights of the other residents to have a quiet night's sleep! As with most ethical dilemmas there is no one right answer. The key is to acknowledge the concerns of all parties and to negotiate a settlement which is seen as fair by all.

55 **i** **a** Kantians might consider that the principle of quality of life means that the child has a right to the best possible chance for recovery, so should be given the chance.

ii **b** A simple all-Unitarian view might consider that the greatest good must be made available to the greatest number of people. The child would receive the best possible treatment as long as this did not deny it to others.

56 **c** The Patient's Charter sets out waiting times for clinic appointments. The aim is to encourage each hospital to set targets to improve the service they offer the patients. Clear communication regarding patient expectations of the service is considered a way of improving quality.

57 **a** The Sex Discrimination Acts and the Race Relations Acts aim to ensure that applicants are not discriminated against on these grounds. Organisations have a duty to review all procedures for recruitment and selection to keep within the law.

58 **d** The aim of professional codes of conduct, e.g. of BASW or UKCC, is to give a framework to guide staff behaviour and decision-making as a professional.

59 **c** It is essential that clients are empowered to make their own decisions where at all possible. It would be unethical to make decisions on behalf of a client without discussing the issues and encouraging him or her to make an informed decision, if there is a possibility this can be done.

60 **b** The client has a right to independence; the carer has a responsibility for the safety of the client. The dilemma is that the client has the right to take risks in the same way that we all decide to take risks from time to time. By acknowledging the rights of the client, and by discussing the concerns from the carer's point of view, the rights and responsibilities of both client and carer are being addressed. A negotiated settlement should then be achieved. Remember that carers have rights too!

Answers to Unit 2

1	a	6	c	11	a	16	b
2	b	7	a	12	b	17	c
3	b	8	a	13	d	18	d
4	a	9	b	14	c	19	c
5	c	10	b	15	c	20	d

Answers to Unit 3

1	b	16	a	31	a	46	c
2	a	17	b	32	b	47	c
3	d	18	c	33	d	48	b
4	d	19	a	34	d	49	d
5	d	20	d	35	d	50	c
6	a	21	c	36	c	51	a
7	c	22	b	37	a	52	c
8	c	23	b	38	b	53	c
9	d	24	d	39	b	54	b
10	b	25	a	40	c	55	d
11	a	26	b	41	b	56	a
12	b	27	c	42	c	57	b
13	d	28	b	43	b	58	c
14	c	29	c	44	a	59	d
15	b	30	a	45	d	60	c

Answers to Unit 4

1	d	16	b	31	b	46	d
2	c	17	d	32	d	47	d
3	b	18	a	33	a	48	c
4	b	19	d	34	d	49	b
5	a	20	d	35	c	50	b
6	b	21	d	36	b	51	a
7	b	22	c	37	a	52	d
8	b	23	a	38	b	53	c
9	a	24	d	39	d	54	b
10	b	25	a	40	b	55	a
11	d	26	c	41	c	56	c
12	b	27	d	42	d	57	a
13	a	28	a	43	d	58	b
14	a	29	c	44	a	59	a
15	b	30	b	45	b	60	c

Answers to Unit 5

1	d	16	d	31	d	46	a
2	c	17	a	32	a	47	b
3	a	18	d	33	b	48	c
4	c	19	b	34	d	49	b
5	d	20	c	35	d	50	a
6	b	21	b	36	c	51	c
7	c	22	c	37	c	52	b
8	a	23	a	38	b	53	a
9	a	24	c	39	a	54	d
10	b	25	d	40	c	55	b
11	c	26	b	41	c	56	c
12	c	27	d	42	b	57	b
13	d	28	c	43	d	58	b
14	a	29	c	44	a	59	d
15	b	30	a	45	d	60	a

Answers to Unit 6

1	c	16	b	31	d	46	c
2	d	17	a	32	b	47	a
3	c	18	b	33	d	48	b
4	a	19	c	34	c	49	d
5	b	20	c	35	a	50	c
6	c	21	c	36	b	51	a
7	c	22	d	37	c	52	c
8	b	23	a	38	b	53	d
9	a	24	b	39	c	54	b
10	c	25	d	40	a	55	c
11	d	26	c	41	b	56	a
12	c	27	c	42	d	57	d
13	c	28	a	43	b	58	c
14	d	29	b	44	d	59	d
15	c	30	c	45	a	60	c

Answers to Unit 7

1	c	16	c	31	a	46	d
2	b	17	d	32	a	47	b
3	b	18	d	33	a	48	c
4	b	19	a	34	c	49	d
5	b	20	b	35	a	50	b
6	a	21	a	36	a	51	d
7	c	22	a	37	c	52	c
8	d	23	d	38	b	53	a
9	d	24	a	39	a	54	d
10	c	25	b	40	d	55	a
11	c	26	c	41	c	56	d
12	b	27	d	42	c	57	b
13	a	28	c	43	b	58	b
14	c	29	a	44	a	59	a
15	b	30	a	45	c	60	b

Answers to Unit 8

1	c	16	c	31	b	46	a
2	d	17	c	32	d	47	c
3	a	18	b	33	a	48	a
4	c	19	a	34	b	49	b
5	a	20	b	35	d	50	a
6	c	21	c	36	a	51	d
7	b	22	a	37	d	52	c
8	d	23	b	38	b	53	b
9	a	24	c	39	d	54	a
10	c	25	a	40	c	55	c
11	a	26	d	41	c	56	a
12	b	27	d	42	a	57	b
13	d	28	b	43	b	58	d
14	b	29	a	44	d	59	a
15	a	30	c	45	d	60	d

Icons for photocopying

Photocopy any of the range of icons below and paste on to your GNVQ assignments. This will enable you and your tutor to see at a glance those areas which have been covered in your evidence collection.

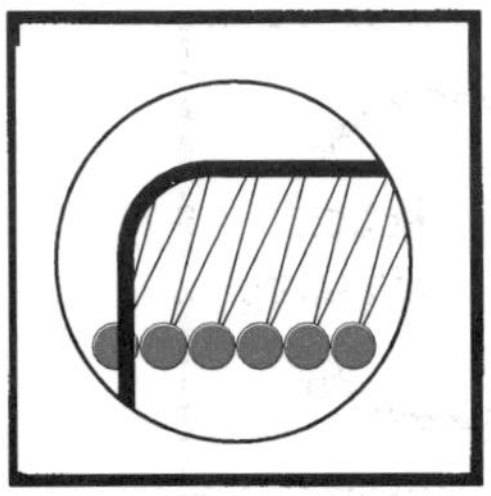

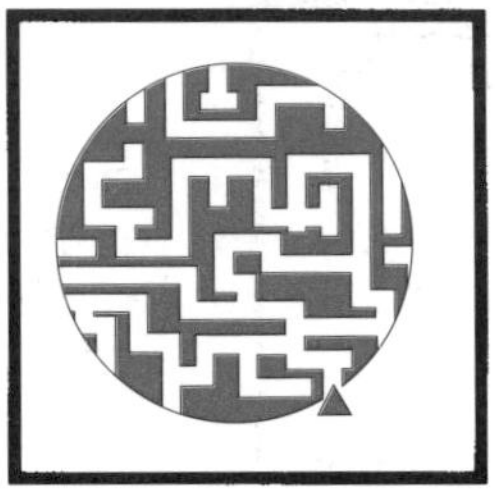

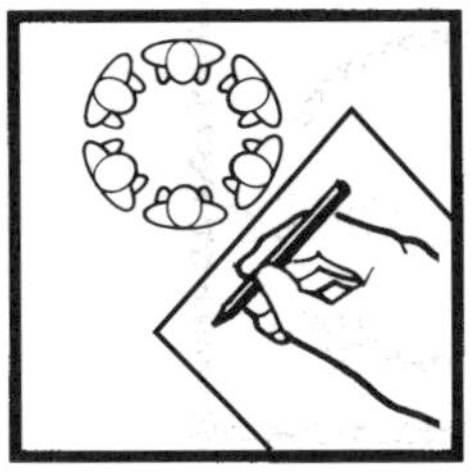

Communication

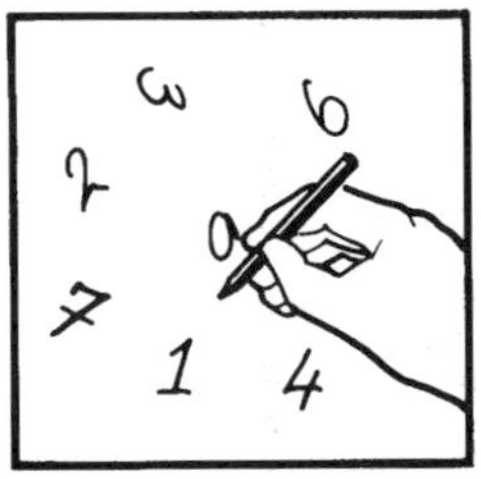

Application of number

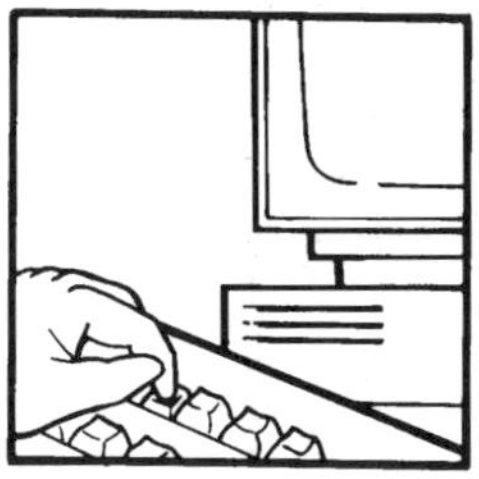

Information technology

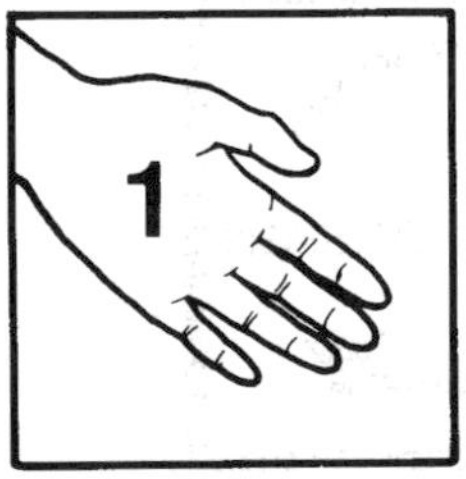

I did this independently without help

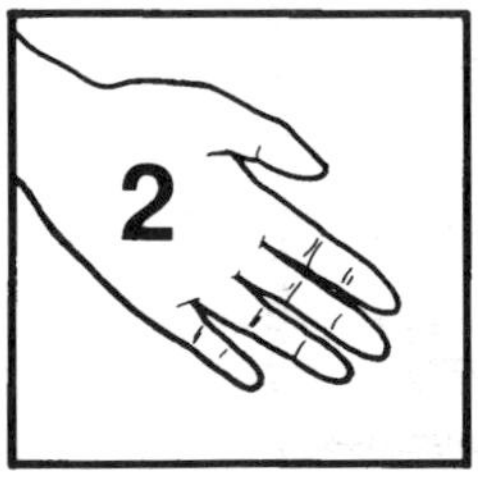

I did this with guidance

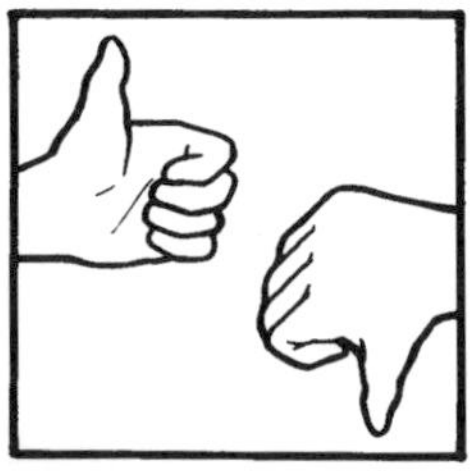

Equal opportunities and individuals' rights

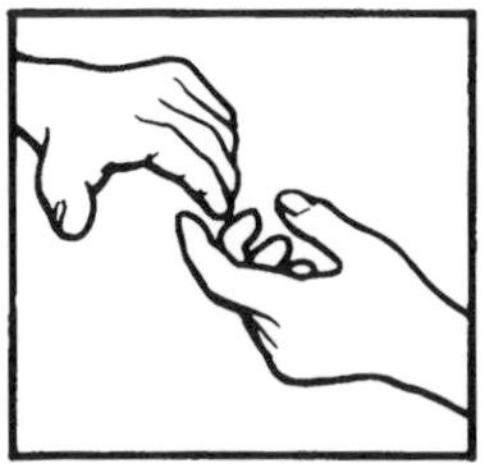

Interpersonal interaction

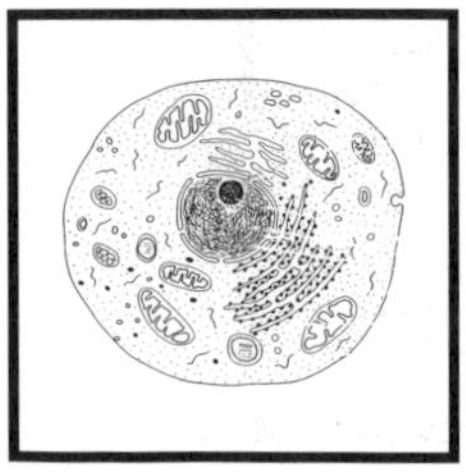

Physical aspects of health and social well-being

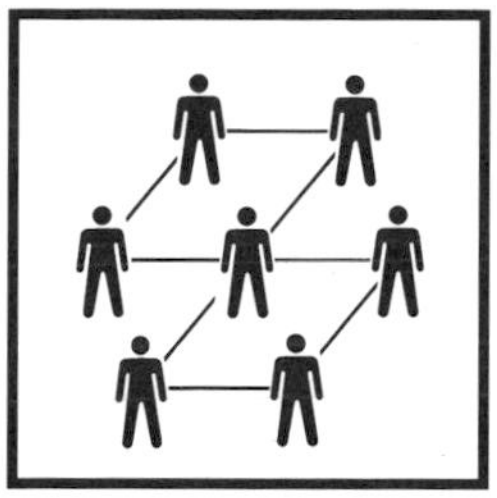

Psycho-social aspects of health and well-being

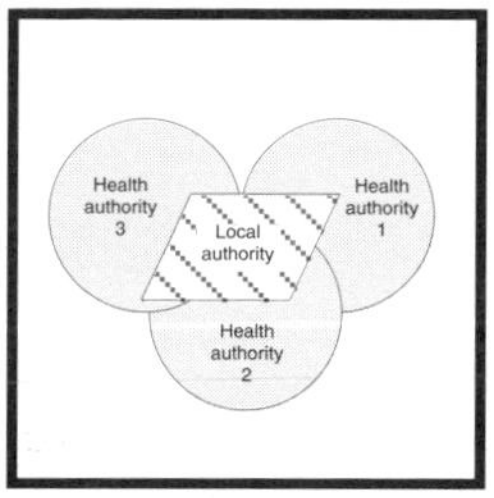

Structure and development of health and social care services

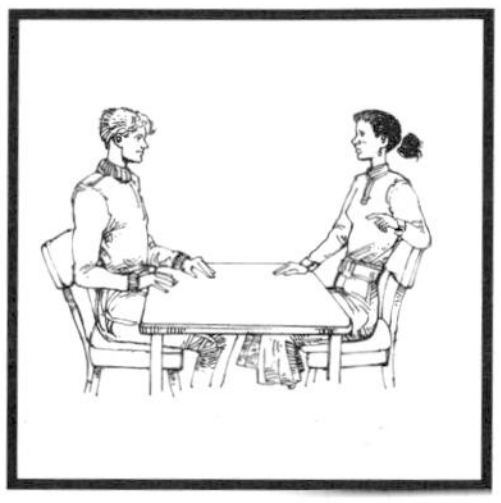

Health and social care practice

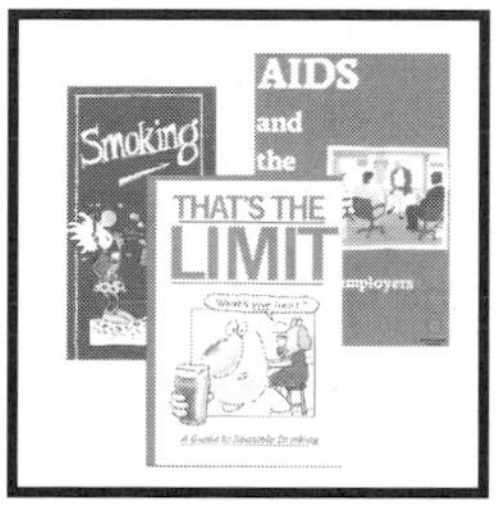

Educating for health and social well-being

Research perspectives in health and social care

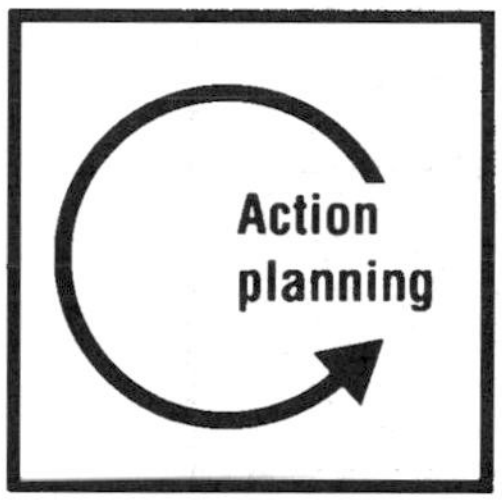

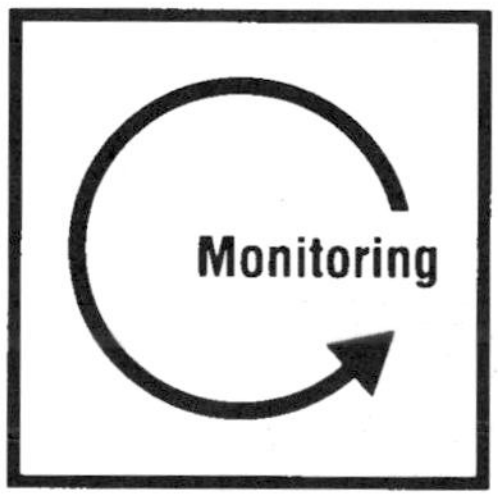

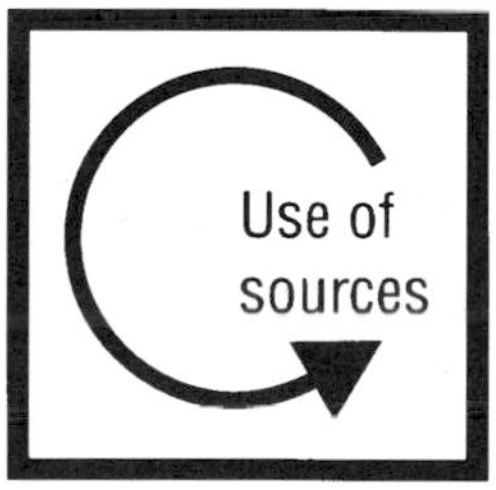

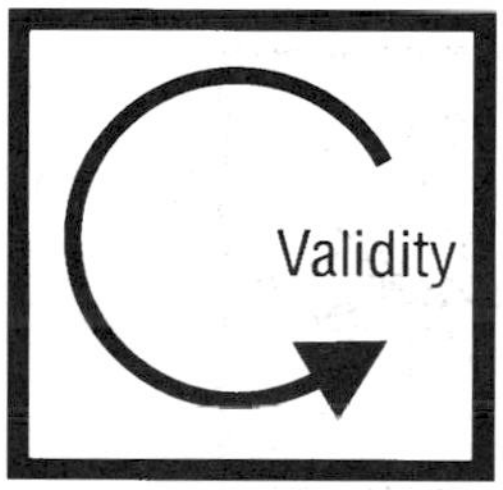

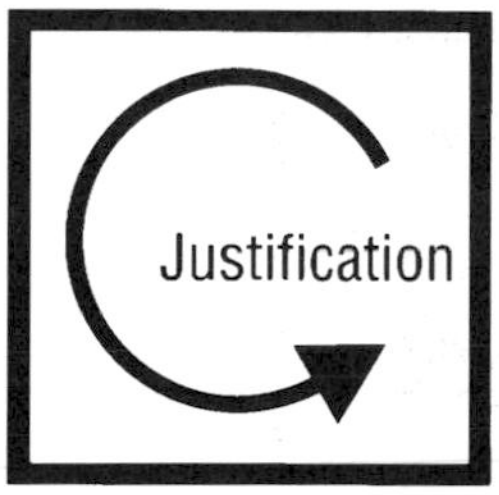

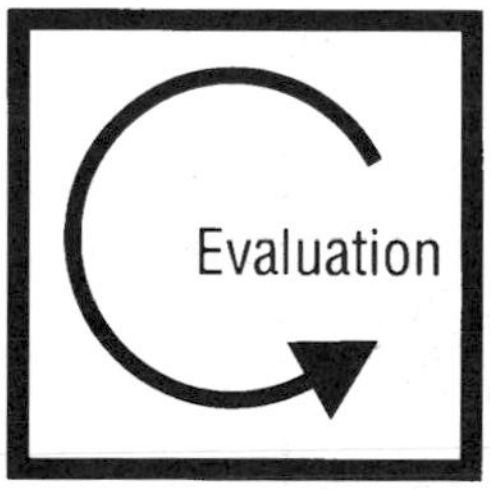

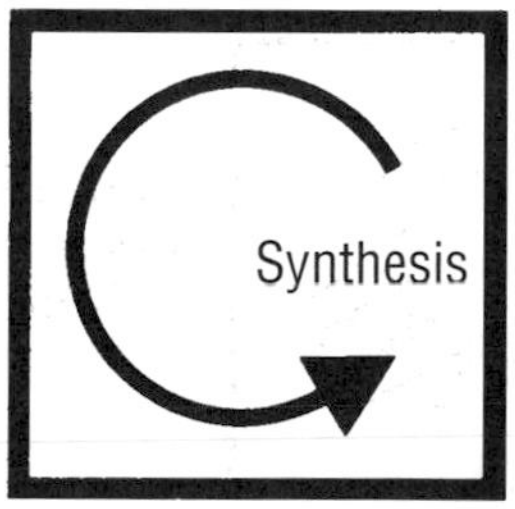

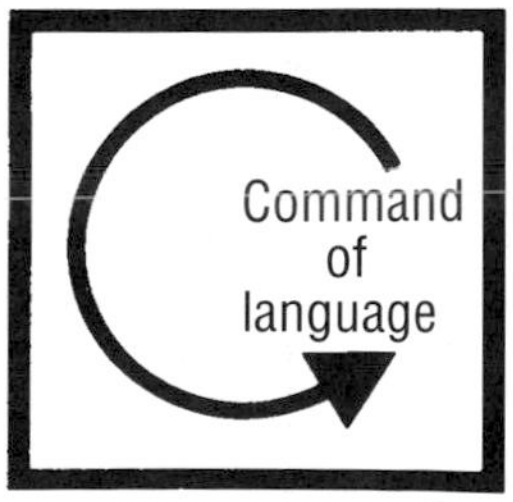

Index

The page numbers in brackets refer to Fast Facts

A

Absolute cell reference (628)
Abstracts (576)
Abuse 123, 124
Acceptability (425)
Accessibility (425)
Access to services 317,318
Accommodation (297) 219
Accuracy 585
Action planning (23) 11, 13
Action potential (197)
Adenosine diphosphate (197) 155
Adenosine triphosphate (197) 155, 171
Adjective (576)
Adolescence 206
Adrenaline 197
Adulthood 206
Adverb (576)
Advocacy (425) 126, 139
Aerobic respiration (197) 157
Ageing 181, 330
Agenda (576) 564
Age profile 266
Agranulocytes 176
AIDS (471) 439-444
Aims (471) 431, 432, 462, 463
Alcohol (471) 263, 444, 445
Amphetamines 448
Anaerobic respiration (197) 158, 159
Antibodies (197)
Anti-discrimination (141) 54, 55, 122
Antidiuretic hormone (197)
Antigens (197)
Appendices (576)
Aortic body (197)
Apostrophe 552
Appearance (141)
Application (628) 603, 604
Appropriateness (425)
Approved social worker (355)
Area (601)
Arteries 164, 165
Assessment (425)
Assessment (GNVQ) 6, 7
Assessment of client need 342, 358, 360, 361, 363, 364, 410
Assessor (425) (23)
Assimilation (297) 219
Assignments (23) 11, 12
Assumptions (141) 136, 474
Asthma (297) 270
Atheroma 435
Attachment 229
Attitude (73)
Auditory (141) 83
Author index (576)
Autism 569
Autonomic nervous system (197) 168
Awarding body (23)
Axes (601)

B

Babbling (297) 208
Baby talk (297) 209
Barriers to communication 77
Bases of discrimination 42
Belief (73)
Belonging (298)
Bereavement (298) 239, 240
Beveridge Report (355) 29, 321
Bibliography (576)
Bile (197)
Bilirubin (197)
Biological determinism 234-238
Bio-medical positivism (298) 281-283, 288
Black (73)
Bliss system 77
Blood 151, 161
Blood count (197) 189
Blood pressure (197) 185
Blood vessels 164
Body language (141) 46, 47, 78, 90
Body movements (141) 81
Bonding (298) 229
Boundaries (141)
Bourgeoisie 253
Brackets 587
Braille 77
Brain 167
Breathing rate 186
Bronchitis (471)
Buffering (141) (298) 88
Byte (628)

C

Calculators (601) 583, 586
Cancer (298) 233, 268, 437, 438
Candidates (24)
Cannabis 448
Cap 440
Capillaries 164
Carbon dioxide 174
Carbon monoxide (471) 445
Cardiac cycle 163
Cardiac muscle 162
Care in the community 323
Care management 358, 360
Care manager (425)
Care package (425)
Care planning cycle 358, 360
Care plans (425)
Care relationship 122
Care settings 119, 120
Caring for people (355)
Carotid body (197)
CD ROM 606
Cell organelles 147
Cell reference (628)
Cell (spreadsheets) (628) 613
Cell structure 146
Census (533)
Central nervous system (198) 167, 168
Change (298) 239-248
Charters 35, 36
Children Act (425) 34, 35, 308, 309, 395
Chiropodists 390
Choice (425) 55, 121, 122, 125, 126, 130
Chromatin network (198)
Chromosomes (198) 149
Chronically Sick and Disabled Persons Act 307
Cilia (198)
Circulatory disease (298) 267
Circulatory system 160-165
Circumference (602)
Classification (355)
Claudication 435
Clause (576)
Clients' rights (425) 374, 376, 377
Clients' view 410, 414
Closed question (533) (602) 96, 97, 509-514
Cocaine 448
Codes of practice (425) 39, 40, 61-63
Coding frame (533)
Cognition (298)
Cognitive development 212-220
Collagen (198)
Comma (576)
Command of language (24) 13, 16
Commission for Racial Equality (CRE) 33, 38
Communication 56
Community Health Councils (425)
Community psychiatric nurses 363
Compact bone 151
Compatibility (628)
Computer networks 605, 606
Concept map 230
Concepts (24) (298) 10, 100, 116, 216
Conclusion (471) 419
Concrete operations (298) 216
Condom 439, 440
Confidentiality (73) (141) (425) 55, 64, 125, 129
Connective tissues (198) 151
Conservation (298) 214, 215, 217-219
Constellatory 230, 231
Construction (298)
Constructs (298) 230
Contact tracing 394, 395
Contents list (576)
Continuum of care (426) 405, 415
Contraception (471) 438-440
Contracts 345, 348
Control of care 417
Conversational skills 97, 98
Conversion (602) 590
Core skills (24)
Coronary heart disease (471) 435-437
Corpus Luteum (198)
Correlation (533) 523
COSHH (471) 394
Counselling 247

Crime 273, 274
Criminal justice 400-402
Cristae (198)
Criteria (24)
CT scan (198)
Cultural needs 64, 65
Culture (73) (142) 90-93, 275-278
Curriculum vitae (576)
Cursor (628) 609
Cut and paste (628) 614
Cycle of deviance (298)
Cytoplasm (198)

D

Data (426) (533) 477, 500, 501, 578, 583
Database (628) 616-620
Data collection 500, 501
Death 266, 276
De-centring (298)
Decimal number (602) 585
Defence of the body 165
Degenerative disease 267
Dementia (298) 207, 208
Democracy 26, 27
Demographic data (534)
Demographic/Demography (298) (355) 265, 329-332
Dentists 389
Department of Health (355) (426)
Dependence/Dependency (142) (471)
Depression (298)
Determinism (298) 234-238, 253
Devaluing (142)
Deviance 257, 258, 261
Dewey system (576)
Diastolic (198)
Diet 432
Differential growth rates (298)
Dignity (426) 126, 131
Direct observation (534)
Directly managed units (355)
Directories (628) 606, 607
Disability (298) 36, 37, 43
Disabled Persons (Consultation and Representation) Act 305, 308
Disabled Persons Act 33, 308
Discrimination (73) (142) (426) 42-53, 125
Discrimination (direct) (74) 30, 43
Discrimination (indirect) (74) 30
Discussion 542-548
Disease (471) 434
Disempower (74)
Distance (142)
District Health Authorities (355) 337, 388
District nurses 362, 388
Divorce 272
DNA (198) 149
Downs syndrome 232
Drawing application (626)
Drug abuse (471) 447-449
Drug misuse (471)
Drug users 263
Dysfunction (298)

E

ECG (198) 188-189
Ecstasy 448
Edoplasmic reticulum 148
Education 41, 44, 45, 250
Effectiveness (426)
Efficiency (426)
Egocentricity (298) 215, 216, 218, 220-222
Ego identity 223
Ego integrity 240
Elder 260, 261
Electric shock 450, 451
Electrical safety 449
Electrocardiograph (198) 188, 189
Electrolyte (198) 190, 191
Elements (24) 5, 6, 7
Embryo (299) 201, 202
Emotion 222
Emotional development (299) 220-223
Emotional maturity (299) 223
Emotional support (142)
Empathy (74) 99
Emphysema (471)
Empiricism (74)
Empowerment (74) (142) 57, 61, 132-134, 406
Endocrine system 168, 169
Endoplasmic reticulum (198)
Energy supply 172
Environment (299) 93, 139, 277-280, 391-394
Environmental health officers (426) 390
Epithelium (198) 150
Equal opportunity (74)
Equal Opportunities Commission (EOC) 31
Equal Pay Acts 29, 30
Equity (426)
Erythrocytes 174
Estimation (602) 582
Ethics (74) 57-60, 402-404, 488-490, 526
Ethnic group (74)
Ethnic minority (74)
Eurocentric (74)
European union 41
Evaluation (24) (471) 15, 99, 118 458, 540, 541
Evidence (24) 8, 9
Evidence indicators (24) 6, 7
Excretion (198) 174
Exercise 434
Expectations (420)
Expected life events (299)
Experiments 478, 479, 502-504
Extrapolation (534) 524
Extroversion (299) 224, 225
Eye-contact (142)

F

Facial expression (142) 79
Family 250
Family Health Service Authorities (355) 337
Fat 432, 433
Feedback (142) (198) (471) 100
Female reproductive system 172, 438
Fertilisation (299) 201
Field (628)
File (628) 606
Flagella (198)
Floppy disk (628) 605
Foetus (299) 202
Form filling 556-562
Form letter (628) 617, 618
Formal operations (299) 216
Formatting documents (628) 610, 611
Formatting floppy disks (628)
Formulae (in spreadsheets) 622, 623
Four rules of number (602)
Fractions (602)
Free response (471)
Frequency distribution (534) 520-522
FSH (198)
Functionalism 253
Functionalist perspective (299) 253
Funding services 314-317, 326-329
Funnel method (534)
Fuse (471) 450

G

Gamete (198)
Gaseous exchange 173
Gaze (142) 79, 80
Gender 223
Generalisation (602)
General practitioners 388
Genetic code (299)
Genetics 232
Genital herpes 441
Genital warts 441
Genotype 232
Gestures (142) 80, 81
Glossary (576)
Glucagon (198) 179
Glycogen 171, 179
Glycolysis (198) 157
Goal 102
Gonads (198)
Gonorrhoea 441
GP-fundholders (355) 338
Grading 12, 16
Grading criteria (24) 12, 16
Granulocyte (198) 176
Graphics application (628) 604, 626
Grammar (299) 550
Graphs 575, 597-600
Griffiths Report (355) 347
Group (299) (142) 102-111
Group polarisation 107
Group values (142) 105, 110
Group work 111
Grouping (628)
Growth rates 204, 205
GUs-Genito-urinary infections (471)

H

Hallucinogens 448
Hand movement 204
Hard disk (629) 605
Hardware (629) 603
Haverian systems (198) 151
Hazards (471)
Health (299) (471) 428
Health and Safety at Work Act 393
Health care approaches 324, 325
Health education (471) 429, 430
Health Education Authority 388, 455
Health of the Nation (299) 267, 269, 270, 287, 343
Health promotion (426) (471) 385-391
Health promotion units 388
Health protection (426)
Health Services and Public Health Act 307
Health status 44
Health visitors 389
Healthy eating 432, 433
Heart 160-164
Heart attack 436
Heart disease 435-437
Hepatitis B 441
Heroin 448
Histogram 596

HIV (471) 439-444
Holmes-Rahe scale (299) 240, 241
Home care workers 363
Home life: A Code of Practice 39
Homoeostasis (198) 177
Homoeostatic mechanisms 177-181
Household security 453
Human body cells 146-157
Humanistic theory (299) 229
Hypothalamus (198)
Hypothesis (74) (299) (534) 478
Hypothetical constructs (299) 216, 217

I

Identity (74) (299) 56, 122, 223
Identity crisis 223
Images 566, 567, 569-571
Imaging techniques 191-193
Immunisation 269, 394, 434
Immunity (198)
Impairment (299)
Income (299)
Independence (142) (299) (426) 126, 130
Independent sector 332-335
In-depth interview (426) 483, 484, 506, 507
In-depth interviewing (534)
Individuality (142) 89
Industrial tribunals 39
Infancy (299)
Informal care 311
Injectable contraception 440
Inspection (426)
Insulin (198) 179
Interactionist perspectives (299) 281-284, 289
Interest (142)
Intervention 326, 363-367
Interview (534) 464, 481-485
Interview schedule (534) 464, 465
Intimacy 228
Introduction (471)
Introversion (299) 224, 225
Inverted commas (576)
Involuntary muscle (198)
Ion (198)
Islets of Langerhans 179
IUD 440

J

Joint consultative committees (355)
Joints 170
Justification (24) 15

K

Kantianism (74) 59-61
Key points (472)
Key worker (426)
Keyboard 604
Kilobyte (629)
Knowledge (24)
Kolb learning cycle 10, 115
Krebs cycle (198) 157, 158

L

Labelling (142)
Lactic acid (199)
Landscape layout (602)
Language 45, 46, 76, 430
Language acquisition device (299) 211
Language development 208-212
Leaflets (472) 458
Learning (143) 112, 113
Learning processes 111-115
Levels (24) 2
Library 539
Life chances (299) 280
Life crises (300) 228
Life expectancy 265
Life transition 120
Lifestyle choice (300) 280, 284
Listening skills (143) 84
Local Authority Social Services (426)
Local Authority Social Services Act 307
Log books 17
Loss 241-244
LSD 448
Lung cancer 268
Lung volumes 186, 187
Luteinising hormone (199) 172
Lymph (199) 177
Lymphatic system 177
Lymphocytes (199) 177

M

Macrophages (199)
Magic mushrooms 448
Magnetic resonance imaging 193
Male reproductive system 171, 172, 438
Mandatory unit (24)
Marginalise (74)
Margins (629)
Market economy (355) 340, 341
Mass media (472) 251, 456
Maternal deprivation (300)
Matrix (199)
Mean (534) (602) 522
Measuring instruments 579-582
Media (300)
Median (534) (602) 523
Medical ethics 67, 68
Megabyte (602)
Meiosis (199)
Memorandum (576)
Menopause (300)
Mental Health (472) 397-399, 428
Mental Health Act (426) 308, 397
Mental illness (300) 271
Merge fields (629) 618
Meshing (143)
Metacognition (300) 220
Methodology (24)
Midwives 389
Minutes (577)
Mirroring (143)
Mission statement (143) 105
Mitochrondria (199) 148
Mitosis (199)
Mixed economy of care (355)
Mode (534) (602) 523
Monitoring (24) (143) (426) 13, 377 378
Monitoring services 346
Monitoring worker (426)
Monocyte (199)
Motor development (300)
Mouse (629)
MRI (199)
Muscle (199)
Muscle co-ordination 204
Muscle tension (143) 82
Muscle tissues 152, 153

N

National Assistance Act 306
National Health and Community Care Act 34, 64, 309, 310, 314
National Health Service 306, 314, 320-322, 336-339
National Health Service Act 306
Nature-nurture debate (300)
NCVQ (24) 2
Needs (426) 64-66, 462
Nerves (199)
Nerve tissues 154
Nervous conduction (heart) 162, 163
Nervous system 165-168
Networks (629) 246
Neurones (199)
Neurotransmitter (199)
New public health care (300) 269
Nicotine 445
Noise 280
Non-judgemental 129
Non-verbal communication 76-85
Non-verbal signals (143)
Normal distribution curve (534)
Norms (74) (300) 223, 249, 261
Noun (577) 556
Nucleolus (199)
Nurses 388

O

Objective (577) 541
Objectives (472) 431, 432, 463
Object permanence (300) 214-217
Observation (143) 485, 486, 507-509
Occupational health nurses 389
Occupational therapists 362, 390
Oestrogen (300)
Official statistics (534)
Older people 206, 207
Olfactory (143) 82
Open question (534) 96, 97, 509 –514
Operator (629) 622
Opinion poll (534)
Opticians 390
Optimised interaction (143) 95, 123
Optional unit (24)
Organisational systems 138
Orientation (143) 82
Osmoreceptor (199)

P

Pace of communication (143)
Packages of care (356)
Pain 261
Painting application (629) 627
Pancreas (199)
Paragraph 577
Paraphrasing 85
Parasympathetic nervous system (199)
Participant observation (534) 487, 508
Passive smoking (472)
Patient's Charter (426)
Pattern notes
Peak flow (199)
Peer group (74) (300) 250
Percentages (602) 587
Perceptions of care 405
Performance criteria (24) 5
Perimeter (602)
Personal constructs 230
Personal space (143)
Personality 233-232
Personality traits 224-226

Phagocytosis (199)
Pheremones (143)
Phenylketonuria 233
Phenotype 232
Physical development 201-207
Physical health (472)
Physiotherapists 290
Pictogram (602) 596
Pie chart 595
Pilot survey (534)
Pitch (143)
Pituitary gland (199)
Plagiarism (577) 555
Planning (24) (472) 536
Planning services 343
Play 209
Plugs 540
Pollution 279, 280, 391, 392
Poor Law (356) 319, 320
Population (426) (534) 276
Portfolio (24) 16-18
Portrait layout (602)
Positive action (74)
Postal questionnaire (534)
Posture (143) 81
Poverty 275, 277, 278, 285-287, 289
Power (300) 105, 236, 237, 256
Practice nurses 388
Pre-coding (534)
Pre-conception (300)
Pre-emptive 230
Pre-operational (300) 214–216
Predictions 593, 594
Prejudice (74) 48, 49
Presentation methods 457, 458
Primary care 312
Primary data (534)
Primary health education (472)
Primary research 478, 495, 496
Primary socialisation (74) (300)
Primitive reflexes (300) 203
Priorities (472)
Privacy 130, 131
Private sector 311
Probability 600-601
Probes (534)
Problem solving 136
Program (629)
Programmes (24)
Proletariat 253
Prompts 253
Pronoun (577) 550
Proper nouns (577)
Proportion 588, 589
Propositional 231
Provider (356) (426) 346-348
Psychodynamic (300) 228, 229
Puberty (300)
Pubic lice 441
Pulse (199) 184
Punctuation 551
Purchaser (356) (426) 341, 342

Q

Qualification (25)
Qualitative data (426) (534) 518, 519
Quantitative data (534) 519, 520
Questioning (143) 96
Questions 458, 476, 491, 509-514, 546
Question mark 552
Questionnaire (426) (534) 479-481, 509, 514, 515, 613-615
Quota sampling (534) 498, 499

R

Race (74) 43
Race Relations Acts 31-33
Racial discrimination (74)
Racial prejudice (74)
Racism (74)
Radiation 280
RAM (629) 605
Random sampling (534) 496, 497
Range (25) (602) 5
Ranking (534)
Rating scales (535)
Ratios (602) 588
Residual current device (RCD) (472)
Recommendations (472)
Record (629)
References (577) 12, 14
Reflection (25) 9, 10, 100
Reflective listening (143) 84-86
Regional Health Authorities 337
Registrar-General's social classification (300) 275
Regulation (300) 219, 220
Relationships 239
Reliability (535) 485
Religion 38, 251
Reports 564, 565
Reproductive systems 171, 172, 438, 439
Research methods 412
Research reports (535) 411, 554
Residential staff 363
Resource allocation working party (356)
Resource constraints 138
Resource management initiative (356)
Respiration 155
Respiratory system 172, 173
Respondent (426) (535)
Responding skills (143)
Response rate (535)
Review 115
Reviewing (426) 379
Ribosomes (199) 148
Rights 55
Risk factors (301) (472)
RNA (199)
Road safety 453
Role (301) 249, 250
Role boundaries (143)
ROM 606
Routing 535
Rowntree Report 275, 278, 290
Royal Commission Report (356)

S

Safety 451-453, 608
Sample (427) (535) 412
Sampling frame 497
Sampling methods 496-499
Sanctions 252
Scale (602)
Scanning (577) 573
Scattergram (535) 523, 524
Schizophrenia 260
Scroll bar (629) 609
Scrolling (629)
Seamless service (427)
Secondary care 312
Secondary data (535) 477
Secondary health education (472)
Secondary research 492, 493
Secondary socialisation (74)
Secondary sources 493-495, 584
Seebohm Report (356)
Selecting (629)
Self-advocacy 126
Self-assessment (25)
Self-awareness 222
Self-concept (301) 223, 241, 242, 246
Self-confidence (301) (144) 88
Self-disclosure (144)
Self-efficacy (301) 227, 228
Self-esteem (144) (301) 88, 89
Self-fulfilling prophecy 252
Self-image (144)
Semi-structured interview 484, 485
Sensorimotor 212-214
Sensory contact (144)
Sentence (577)
Sequence (602)
Service delivery 137
Service provision 344
Service specifications (356) (427) 345
Sex Discrimination Act 30, 31
Sexism (74)
Sexual maturity (301)
Sexual practices 438, 439
Sexual orientation 66
Sexuality 37, 38, 66, 67
Sexually transmitted diseases (472) 439-441
Shortfalls 472
Sign language 77, 78, 208
Silence (144) 86
Sincerity (144) 99, 120
Skills (25)
Skin 175, 176
Skimming (577) 572, 573
Smog (301)
Smoking 445-447
Social class (301) 275–278
Social constructs (301) 255-259
Social context (75) (144) (310) 86, 87, 93, 94
Social development (301)
Social determinism 236, 237, 254
Social health (472) 428
Social interactionism 254
Social learning perspective (301) 226-228
Social networks (301) 246-248
Social positivism (301) 281-283, 288
Social relationships 87, 88, 239-248
Social role (75) (144) 52, 223, 249
Social Services 339, 340
Social status (75) 52
Social stratification (301) 275
Social support networks (301) 246, 247
Social surveys 479
Social workers 361, 362
Socialisation (301) 42, 249-252
Socio-economic conditions 392, 393
Software (629) 603
Solvents 449
Sources of data 477
Sources of error 524, 525
Spatial awareness (301) 212, 213
Special Health Authorities (356) 338
Speech therapists 390
Spermicide 440
Spirometer (199)
Spreadsheet (629) 604, 620, 621
Stand-alone computer (629)
Standard deviation (535) 522, 523
Standard spending assessment (356)
Standards (25) 4, 5

Statistical analysis 520-525
Statistical averages 589
Status (144) (301) 260
Statutory organisations (427)
Stereotype (75)
Stereotyping (144) 42
Sterilisation 440
Stratified sampling (535) 497, 498
Stress (144) 281
Stress-related illness (301)
Stress response (301)
Structural functionalism 253
Structuralism (301) 281-283, 288
Structured interviewing (427) (535) 464, 481-483, 504-506, 516
Style sheet (629) 611
Subjective (577) 541
Suicide 271, 272
Substance abuse 444
Supervision registers (427)
Supporting carers 409
Supportive skills (144) 127-129
Survey (535)
Symbols (577)
Symbolic interactionism 254
Sympathetic nervous system (199)
Synapse (199)
Synaptic knob (199)
Synovial fluid/membrane (199)
Synovial joint 170
Synthesis (25) 13, 16
Systematic sampling (535)
Systolic (199)

T

Tables (577) 568, 569, 573, 574
Tactile (144) 83
Tar (472) 445
Target audience (472) 462
Teeth 205
Telephone 548, 549, 556
Telegraphic speech (301) 210
Temperament (302) 224
Template (629) 610-612
Tertiary care 312
Tertiary health education (472)
Tests (25) 19-21
Theory (25) 10, 116
Therapeutic era (302) 269
Thesaurus (577) 573
Threat (302)
Three dimensional (602) 592, 593
Thrombosis 436
Thrush 441
Tidal volume (199)
Tissues (199)
Tone of voice (144)
Touch (144)
Trait (302) 244-226
Transitions (302) 239-246
Trusts (356) 338, 339
Tutorials (25)
Two dimensional (602) 591
Type A behaviour (302)

U

Ultrasound (199) 192
UN Convention of the Rights of the Child 35
Understanding (25) (144) 89-93, 128, 129
Unexpected life events (302)
Unit (alcohol) (472)
Units (GNVQ) (25) 3, 5
Urea (200)
Urine (200)
Use of sources (25) 14
Use of space 102, 103
Utilitarianism (75) 58-61

V

Validity (25) (535) 14, 485, 525
Value base (144) 27, 54-57, 122, 123, 132-134
Values (25) (75) (144) (302) 262
Valuing others (144)
Variability (535)
Veins 164, 165
Verb (577)
Verbal communication (144) 76
Verifier (25)
Visual communication 78, 79
Vital capacity (200)
Volume (602)
Voluntary muscle (200)
Voluntary organisations (427)
Voluntary sector 311, 455

W

Warmth (144) 97, 127, 128
Wealth (302) 274
Welfare state (356)
Wisdom 220, 228
Withdrawal method 440
Word processor (629) 609
Work 251
Working with patients (356)

X

X-ray image (200) 191, 192